DATE DUE

Complementary and Alternative Veterinary Medicine

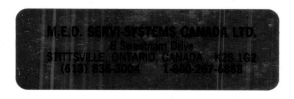

Complementary and Alternative Veterinary Medicine

Principles and Practice

Edited by

ALLEN M. SCHOEN, DVM, MS

Veterinary Institute for Therapeutic Alternatives
Sherman, Connecticut
Consultant, Department of Acupuncture, The Animal Medical Center
New York, New York

SUSAN G. WYNN, DVM

Department of Immunology
Emory University School of Medicine
Atlanta, Georgia
Wynn Clinic
Marietta, Georgia

with 100 illustrations

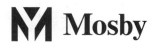 **Mosby**

St. Louis Baltimore Boston Carlsbad Chicago Naples New York Philadelphia Portland
London Madrid Mexico City Singapore Sydney Tokyo Toronto Wiesbaden

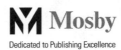

Mosby
Dedicated to Publishing Excellence

A Times Mirror
Company

Publisher: Don E. Ladig
Editor: Paul W. Pratt
Senior Developmental Editor: Teri Merchant
Project Manager: Linda McKinley
Production Editors: René Spencer, Jennifer Furey
Designer: Elizabeth Fett
Manufacturing Manager: Linda Ierardi

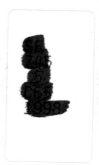

This book was written for use by licensed veterinarians in the practice of conventional and alternative medicine. Nonveterinarians are cautioned against practicing medicine on animals, unless permitted by law. Because the science of veterinary medicine is continually advancing, our knowledge base continues to expand. Although every effort has been made to ensure the accuracy of information contained herein, the publisher, editor, and authors are not legally responsible for errors or omissions.

Printed in the United States of America
Composition by Top Graphics
Lithography by Top Graphics
Printing/binding by R.R. Donnelley & Sons Co, Crawfordsville, IN

Mosby, Inc.
11830 Westline Industrial Drive
St. Louis, Missouri 63146

Library of Congress Cataloging in Publication Data

Complementary and alternative veterinary medicine : principles and
    practice / edited by Allen M. Schoen, Susan G. Wynn. — 1st ed.
        p.   cm.
    Includes bibliographical references (p.   ) and index.
    ISBN 0-8151-7994-4
    1. Alternative veterinary medicine.   I. Schoen, Allen M.
II. Wynn, Susan G.
SF745.5.C65   1997   97-10210
                                                            CIP

98 99 00 01 02 / 9 8 7 6 5 4 3 2 1

Contributors

SHELDON ALTMAN, BS, DVM
Small Animal Practitioner
Certified Veterinary Acupuncturist
VCA Animal Hospital
Burbank, California
savca@aol.com

STEPHEN M. BECKSTROM-STERNBERG, PhD
Faculty Research Associate
Department of Plant Biology
University of Maryland

WENDELL OLIVER BELFIELD, DVM
San Jose, California
www.belfield.com

STEPHEN R. BLAKE JR., DVM, CVA
Carmel Mountain Animal Hospital
San Diego, California

BRENDA N. BONNETT, DVM, PhD
Associate Professor, Epidemiology
Department of Population Medicine
Ontario Veterinary College
University of Guelph
Guelph, Ontario, Canada
bbonnett@ovcnet.uoguelph.ca

MARY W. BROMILEY, FCSP, RPT
Director
Downs House Equine Rehabilitation
Baydon, Marlborough, United Kingdom

CAROLYN L. BUTLER, MS
Director
Changes: The Support for People and Pets Program
College of Veterinary Medicine and Biomedical Sciences
Colorado State University
Fort Collins, Colorado
cbutler@vagus.vth.colostate.edu

ELAINE R. CAPLAN, DVM, DIPL ABVP
Acupuncture Consultant
The Animal Medical Center
New York, New York
Ercdvm@aol.com

CHRISTOPHER DAY, MRCVS
Alternative Veterinary Medicine Centre
Chinham House, Stanford in the Vale
Faringdon
Oxon, United Kingdom

ENRIQUETA DE GUZMAN, DVM, MS
Watkinsville, Georgia
deGuzman@Athens.Net

W. JEAN DODDS, DVM
Adjunct Professor of Medicine Clinical Sciences
University of Pennsylvania
School of Veterinary Medicine
President, HEMOPET
Santa Monica, California

JUDITH L. DUCELLIER
Plant Germplasm Program Assistant
National Germplasm Resources Laboratory,
Plant Exchange Office
U.S. Department of Agriculture, Agricultural Research Service
Beltsville, Maryland
peojd@ars-grin.gov

JAMES A. DUKE, PhD
Economic Botanist
USDA (Ret.)
Beltsville, Maryland
http://www.ars-grin.gov

DANIEL Q. ESTEP, PhD
Vice-President, Animal Behavior Associates, Inc.
Littleton, Colorado

PEGGY FLEMING, DVM
Owner, Florida Equine Acupuncture Center
Dade City, Florida

MICHAEL W. FOX, DSc, PhD, B.Vet.Med, MRCVS
Vice-President, The Humane Society of the United States
Washington, D.C.

JOYCE C. HARMAN, DVM, MRCVS
Harmany Equine Clinic, Ltd.
Washington, Virginia
DocHarmany@crosslink.com

SUZANNE HETTS, PhD
Certified Applied Animal Behaviorist and President,
Animal Behavior Associates, Inc.
Littleton, Colorado
shetts@aol.com

DONALD E. HUDSON, BSEE
President, Respond Systems, Inc.
Branford, Connecticut
respondsystemsinc@worldnet.att.net

DOREEN O. HUDSON, BS, CET
Vice President, Respond Systems, Inc.
Branford, Connecticut

ROGER V. KENDALL, PhD
Gladewater, Texas

MICHAEL D. KIRK-SMITH, PhD
Reader in Behavioral Sciences
Health Sciences
University of Ulster
Belfast, Northern Ireland
mks@ulst.ac-uk

LAUREL LAGONI, MS
Co-Founder and Former Co-Director
Changes: The Support for People and Pets Program
Veterinary Teaching Hospital
Colorado State University
Fort Collins, Colorado

ALAN E. LEWIS
Ann Arbor, Michigan
aelewis@aol.com

JOHN B. LIMEHOUSE, DVM, CVA
Limehouse Veterinary Clinic
Toluca Lake, California
jlime@aol.com

JEN-HSOU LIN, DVM, PhD
Professor
Department of Animal Science
National Taiwan University
Tapei, Taiwan, Republic of China

DAVID M. McCLUGGAGE, DVM, BS
Owner, Chaparrel Animal Health Center
Longmont, Colorado
BirdDocDav@aol.com

CONSTANCE M. McCORKLE, PhD
President, CMC Consulting
Falls Church, Virginia

GREGORY K. OGILVIE, DVM, Diplomate ACVIM
Professor of Oncology and Internal Medicine
College of Veterinary Medicine and Biomedical Sciences
Department of Clinical Sciences
Veterinary Teaching Hospital
Colorado State University
Fort Collins, Colorado

PEKKA J. PÖNTINEN, MD, PhD
Associate Professor of Anesthesiology
Institute of Extension Studies
Tampere University, Tampere,
Associate Professor, Chief
Acupuncture Research Project
Department of Physiology
Kuopio University
Kuopio, Finland
pontinen@sci.fi

MIMI PORTER, MS, AT, C
Equine Therapy, Inc.
Lexington, Kentucky
equinetherapy@uky.campus.mci.net

PHILIP A.M. ROGERS, MVB, MRCVS
Principal Research Officer
Department of Animal Nutrition
Grange Research Centre
Teagasc, Co. Meath, Ireland
progers@grange.teagasc.ie

SHERRY A. ROGERS, MD, FACAZ, ABFP, ABEM
Medical Director
Northeast Center for Environmental Medicine
Syracuse, New York

J.G.G. SAXTON, B.VET. MED., Vet M.G. Hom., MRCVS
Pool-in-Wharfedale, Otley
West Yorkshire, United Kingdom

C. EDGAR SHEAFFER, VMD
Clark Veterinary Clinic, Inc.
Palmyra, Pennsylvania

ALLEN M. SCHOEN, DVM, MS
Veterinary Institute for Therapeutic Alternatives
Sherman, Connecticut
Consultant, Department of Acupuncture
The Animal Medical Center
New York, New York

CHERYL SCHWARTZ, DVM
San Francisco Specialty Veterinarians
San Francisco, California

GREGG A. SCOGGINS, DVM, JD
McGuire, Woods, Battle & Boothe, L.L.P.
Richmond, Virginia

ROBERT J. SILVER, DVM, MS
Director, Holistic Wellness Center
Boulder, Colorado
rjsdvmms@aol.com

JOANNE STEFANATOS, BS, DVM
Director, Owner
Animal Kingdom Veterinary Hospital
Las Vegas, Nevada

PRISCILLA A. TAYLOR-LIMEHOUSE, DVM, CVA
Limehouse Veterinary Clinic
Toluca Lake, California
jlime@aol.com

DANA ULLMAN, MPH
President, Homeopathic Educational Services
Berkeley, California
mail@homeopathic.com

SHARON WILLOUGHBY, DVM, DC
Port Byron, Illinois

SUSAN G. WYNN, DVM
Department of Immunology
Emory University School of Medicine
Atlanta, Georgia
Wynn Clinic
Marietta, Georgia

HUISHENG XIE, DVM, MS
Department of Animal Science
University of Florida
Gainesville, Florida
xie@animal.ufl.edu

HARUKI YAMADA, PhD
Director of Research
Oriental Medicine Research Center
The Kitasato Institute
Tokyo, Japan
yamada-haruki@pa.aix.or.jp

JIANXIN ZHU, DVM, MS
Jiangxi Institute of Traditional Chinese Veterinary Medicine
Nanchang, Jiangxi Province, People's Republic of China

To all my teachers: two-legged, four-legged, and winged!

AMS

For Mom and Dad who taught me to wonder and to read; and to Duke, Eric, B.J., and all the other animals who taught me the need for a different approach

SGW

Preface

Complementary and alternative veterinary medicine (CAVM) is experiencing unprecedented attention in both popular and professional circles worldwide. A new understanding of these ancient and novel methods is slowly emerging as increased research funding has become available. Because CAVM is being integrated into all phases of veterinary practice, the American Veterinary Medical Association recently reviewed the guidelines pertaining to these therapies:

Holistic veterinary medicine is a comprehensive approach to healthcare employing alternative and conventional diagnostic and therapeutic modalities.

In practice, holistic veterinary medicine incorporates, but is not limited to, the principles of acupuncture and acutherapy, botanical medicine, chiropractic, homeopathy, massage therapy, nutraceuticals, and physical therapy, as well as conventional therapy, surgery, and dentistry. It is recommended that holistic veterinary medicine be practiced only by licensed veterinarians educated in the modalities employed. The modalities comprising holistic veterinary medicine should be practiced according to the licensure and referral requirements concerning each modality.

The nomenclature for this new field in human and veterinary medicine has been changing rapidly. No one name can describe this entire field appropriately for all the modalities involved. Names for this field have included terms such as *holistic medicine, integrative medicine, naturopathic medicine, complementary medicine,* and *alternative medicine.* Each name has its own limitations. *Holistic* has many negative connotations and misconceptions associated with it; therefore we decided this label might detract from the information provided here. *Holistic* does appropriately describe a field of medicine that assesses the entire animal and its environment and then attempts to treat the whole animal

rather than simply the disease at hand. *Naturopathic medicine* incorporates many of the different modalities but is also somewhat limiting. *Complementary medicine* suggests that this field is meant to complement conventional medical therapies such as pharmaceuticals and surgery but not replace them. However, many "holistic" practitioners feel that this term is condescending. It may imply that this modality is secondary to conventional treatment, whereas in some cases, the holistic approach is initially the most appropriate. *Alternative medicine* suggests that these additional options are alternatives to conventional medicine; the "either/or" mentality implied by this language may turn many practitioners away from open-minded education concerning the subject. Each name has its supporters and critics.

The National Institutes of Health recently changed the name of their Office of Alternative Medicine to the Office of Complementary and Alternative Medicine. The editors feel that, in keeping with the judgment of the leading research and political body in this field of medicine, CAVM was the most appropriate name for the first text addressing CAM in the veterinary field.

This text is intended not as a training program in CAVM but as an introduction to its philosophy, science, and clinical applications, presented as concisely as possible for such a huge and diverse group of modalities. It is designed to introduce the practitioner of veterinary medicine to applications of CAVM and to show how these methods may be integrated into a conventional veterinary practice. The current research and clinical applications are reviewed, and it is natural that some modalities have more documentation than others. Although some therapies discussed have limited documentation, the editors believe that they should be included in this text so that veterinarians are aware of them. Many clients may be using these therapies on their pets, and veterinarians should at least become familiar with the basic principles of these modalities. Future research will either document their efficacy or reveal that they produce nothing more than a placebo effect.

Although the functional mechanisms for many of the methods are not well understood, this particular obstacle has never stopped practitioners "in the trenches" from using drugs and procedures that they perceive as efficacious. Aspirin and vaccinations were used successfully for decades before their mechanisms were

understood; these procedures survived the scrutiny of science, once scientific methods were developed to examine them. Surgery for angina was used with great confidence before a brave researcher finally determined that it had no benefit beyond a placebo effect. Our hope is that in using this textbook, researchers and practitioners will develop ways to further examine these modalities, eventually separating the wheat from the chaff.

Although this is a rapidly expanding field, a 1000-mile hike must begin with one step. We hope this text provides the walking shoes for such a venture.

Acknowledgments

This book would not have been possible without the help of my teachers, colleagues, friends, and family. I am grateful to Susan Wynn, who shares a similar vision of the future of veterinary complementary and alternative medicine, its scientific basis, traditional medical theory, and clinical applications, for her wisdom, insights, and resolute attention to detail in coediting this text.

I am grateful to Paul Pratt, our editor, for his vision and support in creating this text. I would like to thank Teri Merchant, our developmental editor, for her invaluable assistance and her patience in helping us make this vision a reality. I also wish to thank René Spencer, our production editor, for her patience and wisdom in creating this text.

This text is a compilation of the knowledge, experience, and visionary efforts of all the contributing authors who have had the courage to explore new approaches to animal health care. I would like to acknowledge all of them for contributing their valuable time to write chapters for this text in order that the information can be made available for the first time in one text for veterinarians.

I would also like to thank my parents, who supported me in my desire to become a veterinarian and who honored my desire to march to the beat of a different drummer. I am also grateful to my wife, Barbara, for her patience, understanding, and support during the long hours of working on this text.

AMS

I had encouragement from so many sources that this book took on a life of its own. It would not be a reality without the consideration of Allen Schoen, for believing that this was a collaboration that would be fruitful. Thanks for the chance, Allen.

I could not physically have produced the manuscripts without the emergency data entry and computer specialist efforts of my parents, Jack and Linda Wynn. I also thank Linda Gooding, PhD, for her patience over the months of preparation of this work, and her efforts in teaching me that anything is possible, even in the field of medical science. I couldn't have gotten it done without the support of these people I love.

Phylis Austin, the consummate research librarian, kept me updated and made me aware of changes and news in the medical field. She has been extremely generous in sharing her discoveries and her time; this book would simply not have been possible without her.

I am honored to have been able to work with such a talented group of contributors. They exhibited patience and dedication when faced with my incessant questions, challenges, and demands. They have provided us with the cutting edge of knowledge in this field and an invaluable reference resource.

Teri Merchant went above and beyond the call of her editorial duties in helping this new writer understand the demands and oddities of publishing, and Paul Pratt was extremely understanding and gave us creative solutions and flexibility when we needed it.

My first and most durable mentor, W. Jean Dodds, has been an ongoing source of inspiration as a pioneer. I also thank Michelle Tilghman for her advice and patience when I first investigated this field of study.

I am indebted to my animal friends for their unearthly patience in teaching me why this collection of knowledge is vital. Sharon Harrison, who reappeared in my life with uncanny timing, made it possible for me to stay in medical practice while spending most of my time in the laboratory; this partnership made it possible for me to remember the important things.

Thanks to all of you for helping me through the production of my favorite accomplishment to date.

SGW

Contents

Complementary and Alternative Veterinary Medicine

Fundamentals

Chapter 1

Fundamentals of Complementary and Alternative Veterinary Medicine

SUSAN G. WYNN, ALLEN M. SCHOEN

The philosophies of one age have become the absurdities of the next, and the foolishness of yesterday has become the wisdom of tomorrow.

Sir William Osler
Aequanimitas and Other Addresses, 1942

Veterinary medicine, like all professions, is rapidly changing. As additional diagnostic and therapeutic modalities emerge, the veterinary profession must investigate and become acquainted with these new techniques to incorporate valid complementary and alternative medicine (CAM) into a new, integrated medical approach to health and disease. The purpose of this text is to introduce veterinarians to the scientific basis and clinical applications of many of these techniques. The authors who contributed these chapters have expertise in either the scientific or the clinical aspects of these areas. Although the latest research has been included whenever possible, the challenge in introducing some of these modalities into conventional medicine is that some are not yet well documented. This perceived lack of evidence is neither unique to complementary and alternative veterinary medicine (CAVM) nor an impediment to its use.

Definitions

Although the title of this textbook implies that the therapies described within are somewhat related, connected by the common thread of unusual methodology and questionable efficacy, the truth is not so simple. CAM is multidisciplinary in the broadest and most honest sense of the word. CAM modalities, if a seemingly diverse lot on the surface, are in fact strengthened by their association. The cross-pollination between the disciplines produces a synergy that has resulted in a unified assembly, one both attractive to medical consumers and fortifying to the practice of medicine as a whole. A quick perusal of the table of contents will suggest families of therapies, some of which are more familiar to the reader than others. In truth, the term *alternative medicine* is insufficient to describe the massive variety of therapeutic philosophies, treatment approaches, and tools used by the different systems.

What do they have in common then, and why address them in one textbook? The answer can best be supplied by attempting a few definitions. Most therapies have been called at one time or another alternative, unconventional, holistic, or complementary. Most fit all these descriptions, which makes them worth further definition.

Alternative medicine is the best recognized term for a group of treatments or therapeutic systems that lie outside mainstream or conventional medicine. Because they are unconventional, they have not been taught in U.S. medical or veterinary schools. In fact, Harvard University Medical School supplies this definition: "Alternative medicine refers to those practices explicitly used for the purpose of medical intervention, health promotion, or disease prevention which are not routinely taught at U.S. medical schools nor routinely underwritten by third-party payers within the existing U.S. health care system" (Micozzi, 1996). More recently, the terms *complementary* and *integrative* medicine have come into use to indicate that they are used with or in addition to conventional therapies. The NIH Office of Alternative Medicine now recommends the acronym CAM to describe complementary and alternative medicine.

Another term used to refer to CAM modalities is *holistic medicine*. The *New American Dictionary* defines *holism* as "the theory that reality is made up of organic or unified wholes that are greater than the simple sum of their parts." The simplest description of holistic medicine defines it as any system that diagnoses and treats a disease in the context of the "whole" patient; that is, in relation to the patient's general state of health, the presence of other diseases, and environmental influences, both physical and mental. Holistic systems do not address a disease entity alone, as, for example, surgery does. Therefore holistic therapies might not include such treatments as low-level photon or ultrasound therapies, even though these therapies may be considered unconventional.

One common misconception is that the terms *holistic* and *homeopathy* are synonymous and can be used interchangeably. Homeopathy is a complete and separate approach to health that is in itself considered a holistic modality. Homeopathy is the use of dynamized microdoses of herbs, minerals, and animal products to stimulate the body's innate healing mechanisms. This is an important distinction to remember during discussions of these modalities. Another large subset of CAM includes "traditional" or "natural" therapies. These modalities are often cultural or ethnic in origin. They may consist of nutritional, herbal, and manual therapies developed over time by a culture based on the materials locally available. Natural therapies are the mainstay of "naturopathic medicine." Traditional medical systems that developed from specific cultures include traditional Chinese medicine and Ayurvedic medicine. Because these ancient methods constitute traditional medicine in many cultures, some CAM practitioners object to the use of the word *traditional* to denote modern, scientific medicine.

Our current conventional medical system has been called Western medicine, modern medicine, scientific medicine, and biomedicine. Western medicine has pursued biomedical knowledge using the following criteria (Micozzi, 1996):

- Objectivism—the observer remains separate from the phenomenon being observed
- Reductionism—complex phenomena can be broken down into smaller and simpler parts to study and explain the original whole
- Positivism—information can be derived from physical observations and measurements
- Determinism—knowledge of the body of scientific data may allow prediction of phenomena.

Western medicine is subtractive and uses the reductionist philosophy in both scientific investigation and treatment of medical problems. In general, CAM promotes diversity and individualization and is synergistic in its use of various therapeutic tools. We prefer not to lend the name *scientific medicine* to the current modern system because as more research reveals mechanisms by which

CAM therapies work, our belief is that these new modalities will be embraced as "scientific" as well.

Philosophy

Conventional practitioners who do not use the techniques of CAVM often question the need for a different system of medicine, given the obvious successes of modern medicine. Practitioners of CAVM may point to glaring inadequacies in the practice of modern medicine. One difference in the interpretation of "cure" may explain these differences in philosophy. CAVM practitioners claim to address the root cause of a condition, and "cures" are aimed in this direction. For example, "allergy" does not really represent a diagnosis to many practitioners of homeopathy or Chinese medicine; it is simply a symptom of physiologic imbalance. Treating allergies with antihistamines or corticosteroids therefore does nothing useful for these patients in the long term. In modern medicine a cure has been accomplished when symptoms have been ameliorated and the patient is comfortable. As long as the patient gets better, conventional medicine is working, and continued medication for the inevitable flare-ups is not seen as a disadvantage of the system. The fact that differences in philosophy represent a major stumbling block in the integration of the two types of medical systems is hardly surprising.

Most systems of medicine use particular metaphors for the management of disease. Western medicine has used the battle metaphor: phrases such as "the war on cancer" and "vanquishing germs" exemplify this view. Doctors, their drugs, and surgery are perceived as warriors against the enemy disease. Other systems, especially Eastern medical philosophies, focus more on ways of strengthening physiologic defense systems and restoring homeostasis. This approach has been described as "teaching the body to heal itself." Acupuncture and homeopathy seek to utilize body "energy," already being affected by disease, to effect a cure. Disease is viewed as an imbalance in the body. The purpose of therapy is to bring the body back to a state of balance, or homeostasis.

David Hoffman, a well-known teacher in human herbal medicine, speculates that the recent trend in science toward the study of biologic response modifiers may reflect the ancient idea of "tonic" therapy. A *biologic response modifier* is defined as an agent "that modifies the host's response to pathogens with resultant beneficial prophylactic or therapeutic effects" (Campos and others, 1993). The therapy is used to manipulate the host's own physiologic defense systems. Conventional drugs in this category include cytokines such as the different interleukin (IL) agents IL-1, IL-2, IL-3, IL-4; tumor necrosis factor; and the colony-stimulating factors (Staren and others, 1989). Antibiotics may also work as potent immune modulators by initiating physiologic cascades that cause release of cytokines (Ritt, 1990). Biologic response modifiers (BRM) are usually native substances being used by the scientist or practitioner to bring about a desired therapeutic response. We would pose this question: How is this different from using nutritional supplements and phytochemicals? The answer may represent a bridge for two evolving philosophies of medicine.

One extremely important and controversial issue confronting the field of alternative medicine involves the evaluation of these therapies. Research design is challenging in this area, because of the emphasis on individualized interventions integral to the idea of holistic treatment. These difficulties are addressed in greater detail later, but the question for practitioners who subscribe to the philosophy of complementary, holistic treatment is an ethical one. Is using "unproven" therapies right? Is CAVM unethical to use because it is unproved, or would it be unethical to use only if disproved? Furthermore, is withholding therapies with thousands of years of effective use from patients who may benefit from them, patients for whom other treatments have not proved efficacious, a fair action? For example, this ethical problem was a major obstacle in the scientific evaluation of a Chinese herbal therapy for common warts. The Chinese herbalist involved would not handle a placebo group because it was unethical in the medical system in which she was trained to allow treatable patients to go untreated.

The future will surely prove that integrating the best elements of both these world views results in the best medical care. When neither conventional medicine nor CAM is effective alone, a combination may prove synergistic. For example, if a patient is fighting a bacterial infection, an antibiotic is probably appropriate. A chronic infection may indicate the presence of depressed immune function, and a reasonable adjunctive treatment would involve the use of nutritional supplements, phytochemicals, or acupuncture to support immune function and thereby help the animal fight the infection. An additional example of holistic assessment might be seen in the feline patient with a history of intermittent lower urinary tract disease, seborrhea sicca, obesity, and occasional herpetic keratitis. The CAVM practitioner goes much further than prescribing antiviral ophthalmic ointments and an acidifying diet. The holistic practitioner examines dietary and environmental factors that may predispose to a sedentary lifestyle (contributing to obesity and feline lower urinary tract disease [FLUTD]) and susceptibility to stress (contributing to FLUTD and herpetic ulcers).

These examples illustrate the ways in which different therapies can truly complement each other. If our true goal as veterinarians is to maintain animal health without doing harm, the integration of CAVM into conventional therapies surely represents the next logical step in the evolution of veterinary medicine.

Integration of the different medical systems may appear challenging because of the widely varying metaphors and paradigms by which practitioners view health and disease. Recently, a workable synthesis of the various systems has been proposed (Kemper, 1996). As the divisions between conventional and CAM practitioners erode, the current fragmentation in health care delivery must be corrected. Kemper (1996) has proposed a new system for categorizing the various holistic and conventional therapies:

- Biochemical therapies—drugs, herbs, nutritional supplements
- Lifestyle therapies—nutrition, exercise, environmental therapies, mind-body regulation, group support or counseling.
- Biomechanical therapies—massage, spinal manipulation, surgery
- Bioenergetic therapies—acupuncture, laying on of hands, homeopathy

At a time when veterinary medicine is becoming as specialized as human medicine, holistic practitioners may provide a therapeutic anchor. A more modern, holistic approach could minimize or prevent the number of dangerous drug interactions that result when specialists prescribe drugs without considering the patient's entire health situation.

History

The diverse group of therapeutic systems represents an equal diversity of historical traditions. Nutritional manipulation, herbal medicine, and manual therapies are thousands of years old, and these traditions continued to grow and develop until the rise of modern medicine in the nineteenth century. For the most part, modern medicine began in Western Europe. With the advent of bacteriology and antibiotics, science took its rightful place in the art of medicine, and doctors since then have never looked back.

In the mid 1800s, scientific medicine came to the fore. Two events shaped the new philosophy of medicine: the discoveries that (1) pathogenic organisms (bacteria) produced specific disease states and (2) antitoxins and vaccines could be produced and were effective in preventing these diseases. These findings led to the great quest—the belief that science would eventually reveal the cause of all diseases along with the appropriate treatment (Dossey, Swyers, 1991).

Medical schools of the 1800s and early 1900s were largely unregulated and variable in quality. The turning point occurred in 1910 with the publication of the Flexner Report, which recommended upgrading the medical curriculum with standardization and emphasis on scientific methodology. Funding for other types of institutions, such as homeopathic colleges, subsequently became less available, and most eventually closed.

Consumer confidence in conventional medicine began to wane slightly after a few decades. The American Holistic Medical Association was founded by Norman Shealy, MD, in 1978. By 1993, researchers estimated that 34% of the American public had used unconventional therapies (Eisenberg and others, 1993). In 1992 the Office of Alternative Medicine was formed by the National Institutes of Health to foster the study of CAM modalities.

Veterinary medicine has followed in the footsteps of human medicine. Traditional healers who specialized in the treatment of animals were described as early as 2200 BC as the *azu* depicted on the tomb of a Sumerian king and in 1900 BC on the Egyptian Kahun papyrus. Traditional Chinese medicine has a long history. Veterinary medicine was designated as a separate branch of traditional Chinese medicine during the Zhou dynasty (1122-770 BCE) (Jaggar, 1992). Veterinary medicine at this time consisted mainly of acupuncture and herbal medicine. One of the first texts in veterinary medicine is *Bai-le's Canon of Veterinary Medicine.* Veterinary folk remedies from Japan have recently been evaluated (Katsuyama, 1994). Traditional methods of animal disease prevention and treatment from Sri Lanka (Piyadasa, 1994), Croatia (Vucevqac-Bajt, Karlovic, 1994), and the Near East have been described (Haani, Shimshony, 1994).

In many areas of the world, traditional methods were developed and refined without the influence of scientific medicine until only recently. The first formal veterinary school was formed in Lyon, France, in 1761 to formalize the study of livestock disease. Even after a formal training curriculum was established in Europe, farriers were the practitioners most commonly called to treat animals. Treatments ranged from traditional herbal remedies to bleeding and toxic mercurial or arsenical compounds.

The U.S. Veterinary Medical Association (USVMA) was organized in 1863, and its membership consisted chiefly of self-educated veterinary practititioners. The USVMA was reorganized in 1898, becoming the American Veterinary Medical Association (AVMA); at that time, less than 40% of its members were graduates of North American veterinary colleges. As veterinary science evolved, veterinary practitioners published increasingly more sophisticated and comprehensive textbooks, and areas of specialization such as small animal practice emerged. In 1933, 13 years after the publication of the Flexner Report, the American Animal Hospital Association (AAHA) was formed. The goal was to standardize small animal hospital facilities and hold them to high standards of scientific medicine (Dunlop, 1996).

In response to consumer interest in alternative medicine and an apparent dissatisfaction with conventional medicine, more options became available. The National Association for Veterinary Acupuncture (NAVA) was instrumental in investigating and providing acupuncture for animals from 1973 to 1978, and the International Veterinary Acupuncture Society (IVAS) began training veterinarians to perform acupuncture in 1975 (see Chapter 10). IVAS has graduated over 400 veterinary acupuncturists worldwide.

The American Holistic Veterinary Medical Association was organized in 1982 to help establish a network for veterinarians interested in alternative medicine. The most eclectic of the veterinary CAM organizations, the AHVMA holds yearly conferences for continuing education in this area for veterinarians. Newer organizations include the American Veterinary Chiropractic Association (AVCA), which holds certifying courses for veterinarians and chiropractors, and the Academy of Veterinary Homeopathy, which holds certifying courses in the principles of classical homeopathy for veterinarians.

Current Status of CAM in Veterinary Medicine

As complementary medicine gains acceptance in the field of human medicine, veterinary organizations are beginning to take notice. In 1996, the AVMA revised its guidelines for alternative and complementary veterinary medicine (Box 1-1).

Controversies

Science and CAM

We walk a thin line, balancing open-minded investigation with the potential for loss of critical review. Maslow (1966) summarizes the dilemma as follows:

> If there is any primary rule of science, it is . . . acceptance of the obligation to acknowledge and describe all of reality, all that exists, everything that is the case. . . . it must accept within its jurisdiction even that which it cannot understand or explain, that for which no theory exists, that which cannot be measured, predicted, controlled, or ordered. . . . It includes all levels or stages of knowledge, including the inchoate . . . knowledge of low reliability . . . and subjective experience.

Practitioners of CAM modalities are often viewed as "true believers," gullible people unable to discriminate between the real and unreal, science and quackery. CAM practitioners often accuse conventional practitioners of narrow-mindedness. Few controversies in veterinary medicine engender such emotional intensity and heated debates. When any unproven medical treatment is examined, the key points to keep in mind are as follows:

- Is it safe?
- Is it efficacious?

Some points of arguments are discussed in the subsequent sections.

Poor quality of data

Some critics say that no data exist to support unconventional therapies; if data do exist, the therapies would

BOX 1-1

Avma Guidelines for Alternative and Complementary Medicine

PREAMBLE

Veterinary medicine, like all professions, is rapidly changing. Additional modalities of diagnosis and therapy are emerging in veterinary and human medicine. These guidelines reflect the current status of the role of these emerging modalities within the parameters of veterinary medicine for use in providing a comprehensive approach to the health care of nonhuman animals.

Use of these modalities is considered to constitute the practice of veterinary medicine. Any exceptions will be indicated in the following guidelines. Such modalities should be offered in the context of a valid veterinarian/client/patient relationship. It is recommended that appropriate client consent be obtained. Educational programs are available for many of the modalities. It is incumbent upon veterinarians to pursue education in their proper use.

It should be borne in mind that because the emergence and development of these modalities is a dynamic process, as time passes, the following information may need to be modified.

VETERINARY ACUPUNCTURE AND ACUTHERAPY

Veterinary acupuncture and acutherapy involve the examination and stimulation of specific points on the body of nonhuman animals by use of acupuncture needles, moxibustion, injections, low-level lasers, magnets, and a variety of other techniques for the diagnosis and treatment of numerous conditions in animals.

Veterinary acupuncture and acutherapy are now considered an integral part of veterinary medicine. These techniques should be regarded as surgical and/or medical procedures under state veterinary practice acts. It is recommended that educational programs be undertaken by veterinarians before they are considered competent to practice veterinary acupuncture.

VETERINARY CHIROPRACTIC

Veterinary chiropractic is the examination, diagnosis, and treatment of nonhuman animals through manipulation and adjustments of specific joints and cranial sutures. The term *veterinary chiropractic* should not be interpreted to include dispensing medication, performing surgery, injecting medications, recommending supplements, or replacing traditional veterinary care.

Although sufficient research exists documenting efficacy of chiropractic in humans, research in veterinary chiropractic is limited. Sufficient clinical and anecdotal evidence exists to indicate that veterinary chiropractic can be beneficial. It is recommended that further research be conducted in veterinary chiropractic to evaluate efficacy, indications, and limitations. The assurance of education in veterinary chiropractic is central to the ability of the veterinary profession to provide this service.

Veterinary chiropractic should be performed by licensed veterinarians; however, at this time, some areas of the country do not have an adequate supply of veterinarians educated in veterinary chiropractic. Therefore it is recommended that, where the state's practice acts permit, licensed chiropractors educated in veterinary chiropractic be allowed to practice this modality under the supervision of, or referral by, a licensed veterinarian who is providing concurrent care.

VETERINARY PHYSICAL THERAPY

Veterinary physical therapy is the use of noninvasive techniques, excluding veterinary chiropractic, for the rehabilitation of injuries in nonhuman animals. Veterinary physical therapy performed by nonveterinarians should be limited to the use of stretching; massage therapy; stimulation by use of (a) low-level lasers, (b) electrical sources, (c) magnetic fields, and (d) ultrasound; rehabilitative exercises; hydrotherapy; and applications of heat and cold.

Veterinary physical therapy should be performed by a licensed veterinarian or, where in accordance with state practice acts, by (1) a licensed, certified, or registered veterinary or animal health technician educated in veterinary physical therapy or (2) a licensed physical therapist educated in nonhuman animal anatomy and physiology. Veterinary physical therapy performed

From American Veterinary Medical Association: *Guidelines on alternative and complementary therapies,* Schaumburg, Il, 1996, The Association.

Continued.

BOX 1-1

AVMA GUIDELINES FOR ALTERNATIVE AND COMPLEMENTARY MEDICINE—cont'd

by a nonveterinarian should be performed under the supervision of, or referral by, a licensed veterinarian who is providing concurrent care.

MASSAGE THERAPY

Massage therapy is a technique in which the person uses only the hands and body to massage soft tissues. Massage therapy on nonhuman animals should be performed by a licensed veterinarian with education in massage therapy or, where in accordance with state veterinary practice acts, by a graduate of an accredited massage school who has been educated in nonhuman animal massage therapy. When performed by a nonveterinarian, massage therapy should be performed under the supervision of, or referral by, a licensed veterinarian who is providing concurrent care.

VETERINARY HOMEOPATHY

Veterinary homeopathy is a medical discipline in which conditions in nonhuman animals are treated by adminstration of substances that are capable of producing clinical signs in healthy animals similar to those of the animal to be treated. These substances are used therapeutically in minute doses.

Research in veterinary homeopathy is limited. Clinical and anecdotal evidence exists to indicate that veterinary homeopathy may be beneficial. It is recommended that further research be conducted in veterinary homeopathy to evaluate efficacy, indications, and limitations.

Because some of these substances may be toxic when used at inappropriate doses, it is imperative that veterinary homeopathy be practiced only by licensed veterinarians who have been educated in veterinary homeopathy.

VETERINARY BOTANICAL MEDICINE

Veterinary botanical medicine is the use of plants and plant derivatives as therapeutic agents. It is recommended that continued research and education be conducted. Since some of these botanicals may be toxic when used at inappropriate doses, it is imperative that veterinary botanical medicine be practiced only by licensed veterinarians who have been educated in veterinary botanical medicine. Communication on the use of these compounds within the context of a valid veterinarian/client/patient relationship is important.

NUTRACEUTICAL MEDICINE

Nutraceutical medicine is the use of micronutrients, macronutrients, and other nutritional supplements as therapeutic agents.

Communication on the potential risks and benefits from the use of these compounds within the context of a valid veterinarian/client/patient relationship is important. Continued research and education on the use of nutraceuticals in veterinary medicine is advised.

HOLISTIC VETERINARY MEDICINE

Holistic veterinary medicine is a comprehensive approach to health care employing alternative and conventional diagnostic and therapeutic modalities.

In practice, holistic veterinary medicine incorporates, but is not limited to, the principles of acupuncture and acutherapy, botanical medicine, chiropractic, homeopathy, massage therapy, nutraceuticals, and physical therapy, as well as conventional medicine, surgery, and dentistry. It is recommended that holistic veterinary medicine be practiced only by licensed veterinarians educated in the modalities employed.

The modalities comprising holistic veterinary medicine should be practiced according to the licensure and referral requirements concerning each modality.

not be unconventional. Others claim that data supporting unconventional methods are of poor quality. One question is whether unconventional studies are held to a higher standard than conventional medical science.

We are not aware of data comparing the quality of research in CAM with that of conventional medicine. However, recognition of deficiencies in the quality of conventional medicine is currently under discussion in many teaching institutions. The recent call for evidence-based medicine indicates the lack of research support for many popular techniques used worldwide by doctors in conventional practices. David Eddy of Duke University claims that only 15% of medical interventions are actually supported by strong science. He further states that only 1% of published medical articles are scientifically sound (Smith, 1991).

Further, McCance recently evaluated all articles with numerical data (133 total) published in the *Australian Veterinary Journal* between January 1992 and December 1993 for statistical flaws. He found that had a statistical referee been included in the review process, only 29% of the papers would have been acceptable without revision (McCance, 1995).

Without claiming that CAM research is in any way superior, we would suggest that true comparisons in data quality might soften the criticism that CAM research is usually without value.

Data are difficult to find

The truth is that data exist depending on the information the investigator seeks. For example, the difficulty in finding evidence of the efficacy of homeopathy and herbal medicine is illustrated in the following:

1. We want to know whether homeopathy is effective in the treatment of asthma. If we ask this very specific question, we find no veterinary trials but three high-quality human trials, two of which were published in the *Lancet* (Reilly, 1985, 1986, 1994). If we want to know about the efficacy of homeopathy in the treatment of meningitis, we will find no studies at all. We may find the same situation if we ask about the efficacy of any other drug for the treatment of a particular condition. Skeptics often dismiss an entire approach with the argument that a particular unconventional therapy has never been proved effective for a particular condition, but many untried treatments may be proved effective once studied. Clearly, investigating specific indications for specific clinical conditions is warranted, but because of the huge variety of treatments that fall under the umbrella term *alternative* or even all the treatments that fall within the system *homeopathy*, this information may not be available for a long time.
2. We want to know whether homeopathy is effective for a variety of diseases. In this case, we find a variety

of reports from both standard peer-reviewed journals and alternative, sometimes peer-reviewed journals. The quality and results of the trials are mixed, and because of the number of diseases and treatments, these results are rarely reported.

3. We want to know whether homeopathically prepared substances have any measurable characteristics apart from those of their solvent. These references are available in a variety of journals as well. A search, however, may prove confusing because the terminology for in vitro experiments in homeopathy may differ from that for clinical reports. In vitro papers studying homeopathy tend to refer to "serially agitated dilutions," rather than homeopathically prepared substances, so these studies may prove difficult to find.

Data may be useful but different than expected

The data may offer information that is useful but different from that which the investigator is seeking. If the investigator confines the search to "efficacy of a treatment" only, the approach overlooks other aspects of CAVM therapies. Much of the time, safety and efficacy are issues. For herbalists the potential toxicity of purified drugs is most important. If an herb is shown to work reasonably well for a particular disease condition compared with a drug that works very well but the herb proves to be much safer, the herbalist feels vindicated on the safety issue. The skeptic, however, may also feel vindicated for having proved that the drug was more effective than the herb, ignoring relative safety as a consideration in patient care.

The safety of CAM treatments is the major reason for their popularity. Some data suggest that up to 5% of all hospitalized patients are admitted because of an adverse drug reaction, and 30% may experience a reaction while hospitalized (Bukowski, Wartenberg, 1996). Another source claims that 40,000 to 60,000 annual average deaths resulted from approved drugs in 1991 (Classen and others, 1991). On the other hand, vitamins and uncontaminated amino acids caused no deaths (American Association of Poison Control Centers, 1990). The perceived safety of CAM is actually a double-edged sword because the public tends to believe that "natural" means "safe." Comfrey, hops, kava kava, lobelia, nutmeg, senna, and yohimbe have all been reported to cause toxicity (Ford, Olshaker, 1994). All are easily found on the shelves of health food stores.

A key difference between the herbal and chemical drugs is the history of their use. Herbs have been used for thousands of years, and poisonings from therapeutic (as opposed to recreational) use are quite rare statistically. Toxic ingestions rarely occur when the patient is under the care of a trained herbalist. On the other hand, chemical drugs, though subjected to a lengthy and expensive approval process, are still tested on only a small number of individuals initially. These trials are too small and too short to detect uncommon reactions (Bukowski, Wartenberg, 1996).

Inaccessible data

The data may be inaccessible. For example, very good data support the use of Chinese herbal medicine and acupuncture, but because the reports are published in Chinese, Western doctors may never be made aware of the findings. Second, "publication bias" may exist (Kleijnen and others, 1991). Authors of studies on alternative modalities tend to publish their studies in CAM journals for fear of rejection by conventional peer-reviewed journals. Widely published and well-respected conventional researchers may choose to publish their unconventional studies by other avenues (Doutremepuich, 1991). Other aspects of publication bias may include the potential for CAM journals to publish only positive studies and, conversely, for conventional journals to publish primarily negative reports (Richmond, 1992), or even reports that betray a clear misunderstanding of the tenets of the treatment involved (Barry, 1995).

Klein published the story of his efforts to report that the standard practice of performing episiotomies during childbirth is not well established except in the minds of practicing doctors. Klein's study was based on a large, rigorously conducted, randomized, controlled trial to determine the benefit of routine episiotomies. The results showed that episiotomy produces no additional benefit to the mother. Klein's story about the investigation, however, is much more interesting than the results. He encountered unusual resistance throughout the process, from acquiring funding through the publishing stages (Klein, 1995). Klein concludes the following:

> Those who struggle for paradigm change must be prepared for a long fight. It is well known and appropriate that editors scrutinize papers that contest existing realities more intensely. . . . Episiotomy is a marker for a range of other procedures, approaches, and attitudes.

An important factor in Klein's story is that he was not proposing an unconventional or unproven treatment; he was simply challenging a medical habit.

Unpublished data or data that do not conform to research design

The data used in CAM are not published by scientists in the accepted form and venues. Research in CAM is a relatively new area for those scientists trained by conventional methods to design and publish well-founded research. In this book, data that range from 2000 BCE to 1996 AD are presented. Still, compared with the mass of research funded by granting agencies, research in CAM is not well supported. The budget for the Office of Alternative Medicine was $7.4 million in 1996 and is $11.1 in 1997. CAM and CAVM have grown by popular mandate, and practitioners in the field are responsible for much of the material published. Because practitioners are not always well-versed in research design or even scientific jargon, the overall quality of publications suffers.

Research in CAM is made difficult by the individualized interventions

Individualized treatments are at the core of holistic evaluation and treatment. Controlled studies that propose to work within that framework may encounter methodologic difficulties. For instance, homeopathic and traditional Chinese herbal prescriptions for one recognized disease entity certainly vary, even with only one prescriber involved, because holistic evaluation requires that the prescriber consider the entirety of the patient's conditions in one prescription. Each patient is different; for 26 cats diagnosed with cholangiohepatitis, one prescriber will write many prescriptions. If more than one prescriber is involved, levels of competence or personal style may further complicate matters. Some researchers have developed creative approaches to this problem. One study admitted for trial only those patients who fit the prescription for one homeopathic remedy. Other approaches have also been tried with some success. For the manual therapies, controls may be difficult because the "operator" cannot be blinded. For example, acupuncturists in a clinical trial know placebo versus experimental acupuncture points. In addition, experts have argued that placebo acu-points do not exist and needling of real acu-points may produce very different sensations from the feeling that comes from needling a placebo point; therefore blinding the patient may not be possible. These difficulties are not, insurmountable, however, and as we learn more about the clinical indications and specific uses for various modalities, the development of creative approaches to their study will be more easily accomplished.

Other Controversies

The use of CAM therapies tends to give clients a false sense of security and delays the institution of vital conventional treatments until it is too late

The issue of whether CAM therapies dangerously delay treatment by conventional methods is a matter of public education that can be overcome only with the combined efforts of CAVM and conventional practitioners. If clients know that the veterinarian is open to a holistic approach, they will be more likely to see a veterinarian rather than a lay provider. In many cases the veterinary client approaches the holistic veterinarian at a very late date, claiming to have spent thousands of dollars and too many hours on lay providers of "alternative medicine" before finding or learning to trust a veterinarian who practices CAVM. Unfortunately, these people find a veterinarian trained in CAVM after the case has progressed too far or their money has been depleted.

Alternative therapies do not work

Practitioners may believe that alternative therapies are ineffective because clients are uneducated about the uses of CAVM and seek out complementary therapies only as a last resort or for confirmed terminal cases. Surgery is no more effective in curing metastatic cancer than is homeopathy or massage, and both types of practitioners would like to see these cases sooner rather than later. By working together from an early point in disease management, practitioners may be able to reduce morbidity and mortality.

CAVM modalities probably do not work, but they do not hurt

Because many CAM modalities have possible side effects or interact with certain drugs, practitioners should be thoroughly trained. Recently, the herb Ma Huang (Ephedra sinensis) has received a great deal of media attention as a "natural high" that has potentially lethal side effects. Consumers should remember that overdose problems are occurring among uneducated recreational users or those who self-medicate, not among patients seeing responsible trained herbalists.

In addition, CAM practitioners frequently discuss "healing crises," which are described as detoxification processes directly related to the treatment. In this medical model, healing crises cause the patient short-term discomfort in a variety of ways and are considered positive events because patients can be expected to improve rapidly afterward. To our knowledge, the physiology and epidemiology of this phenomenon has never been studied. No one can confirm its existence, yet most CAVM practitioners claim to have witnessed these healing crises. For our purposes the reality of the healing crisis is not as important as the idea that if it exists, it is a side effect of treatment. Because a healing crisis is usually not pleasant for the patient, CAM practitioners must assume responsibility for the fact that these modalities, although usually safe, do have side effects.

Human studies do not extrapolate well to animals

CAVM practitioners often rely on human studies and clinical findings, which may not extrapolate well to animals; therefore these therapies should not be used in animals until more studies are done. The reverse argument has been used for years by animal rights activists, who claim that studies on animals are meaningless when applied to humans. The truth is that findings from animal studies have been used in human clinical medicine for decades, and medical science has evolved at an impressive rate, in part because of these findings. Because the therapies that are used on humans are often based on laboratory animal studies, many interventions may be more valid for our patients. In an ideal research setting a controlled study exists for every condition in every species. Creating this situation would obviously be too time consuming and costly. However, how many double-blind studies were performed for open-heart bypass surgery in humans?

Where is the research funding?

Curiously, the companies who stand to profit from research in CAM do not seem to fund these badly needed studies. In many cases, treatments involve manual therapies, not products that can be sold for a profit. Consequently, organizations that exist for the advancement of these therapies are usually nonprofit and educational. Herbal remedies rely on plants, which are essentially unpatentable and therefore unlikely to be profitable. The total cost for new drug approval in the United States is estimated to be between $150 and $200 million. Unfortunately, herbal, nutritional, and homeopathic medications may never lead to a return on such an investment.

Can CAM systems be combined with each other or with traditional medicine?

Systems such as homeopathy, traditional Chinese medicine, and chiropractic often claim all-encompassing powers in the treatment of the sick—the practitioners may claim that the use of other therapies outside these systems is not indicated and may be harmful. However, no one form of medicine has all the answers to all disease conditions. If one did, other forms of medicine would not exist. If natural medicine had proved sufficient to manage the ills of humans and animals, modern medicine would never have surfaced and developed at such a rapid pace. If modern medicine were perceived as completely efficacious, CAM would not be gaining such rapid popular approval. Many CAM therapies overlap, which suggests that they may be designed to work cooperatively. For instance, homeopaths often counsel patients in ways to improve the diet to remove "obstacles to cure." Chiropractors and naturopaths counsel patients about diet as well as prescribe homeopathic remedies. The strength in the field of CAM is in the philosophy that an integrated approach to wellness and disease increases the odds that the patient will do well.

The disadvantage to this feature of CAVM is that learning these modalities for the first time can be a daunting and confusing project. A major stumbling block to acquiring knowledge in CAVM is the need to learn specific clinical indications for the different modalities. If clinical research and retrospective studies could accomplish one major goal, perhaps the most important accomplishment possible would be to determine the modality that works best for the particular problem.

The Future of CAM in Veterinary Medicine

Although CAM began as a popular movement, with the public opting for self-treatment with natural and easily available products, doctors are also beginning to recognize the value in acknowledging (if not using) these treatments. Positive papers continue to appear in medical journals (Alpert, 1995; Dyer, 1996; Kemper, 1996; Pavek, 1995). A recent metaanalysis suggests that physicians perceive complementary medicine to be moderately effective (Ernst and others, 1995); efficacy was rated at 46 ± 18 on a scale of 100. In response to the interest and need for more information in this area, the National Library of Medicine added many new MESH terms in alternative medicine for the 1996 year (NLM Technical Bulletin, 1995). A total of 32 medical schools now offer courses in CAM (Daly, 1996).

Veterinarians have not been far behind. Publications have appeared with increasing frequency as either advertisements for the booming natural-product industry (Langreth, 1996) or instructional papers in the journals (Mandelker, 1995; Wynn, 1996). A postdoctoral position in complementary methods became available at the University of Guelph's Ontario Veterinary College (DVM, 1996). At least one U.S. veterinary school will soon be offering a course in CAVM.

The continued growth of CAVM seems assured for the moment, despite the controversies and obstacles mentioned. The explosion in the popularity of products and publications assures us that this trend will continue. Another hint seems to come from the pharmaceutical industry itself.

Holistic evaluation and treatment stand in direct opposition to the modern trend in medical research. Research funding supports two goals: discovery of pathologic mechanisms and discovery of disease prevention and treatment. Funding agencies provide billions of dollars for the kind of study that defines mechanisms, with the apparent assumption that disease must be understood at the molecular level before a treatment can be devised.

However commendable their commitment to molecular research, medical practitioners must ultimately answer to the patient sitting in their waiting rooms. Research has established that the discovery of treatments for disease has slowed dramatically in the last 30 years (Wurtman, Bettiker, 1995). Although scientific discoveries have not slowed, effective treatments for some of the biggest killers in modern times have simply not been forthcoming. Important treatment advances have frequently been made when clinical investigators experimented with off-label drugs used for unrelated diseases. Examples include the use of antibiotics for peptic ulcers and aspirin for the prevention of coronary artery disease. This approach to clinical research has received little attention from funding agencies (Wurtman, Bettiker, 1995). We may predict a relative shortfall in research funding in CAM for exactly these reasons.

The complaint that little is known about mechanisms of alternative methods may certainly become less important as this biomedical research crisis is recognized. Many are becoming increasingly aware that drugs and treatments frequently arise from what is often called "folk medicine" (Wurtman, Bettiker, 1995). The major pharmaceutical companies have already recognized this fact; for instance, Ciba-Geigy tested 4000 samples of natural products in 1991, and Sphinx Pharmaceuticals receives 15,000 samples per year. These companies are screening plant and marine products, microbes, and even spider venoms (Balick and others, 1996). Although research into individual plant constituents (which are patentable) and pathogenic mechanisms will clearly remain foremost in these research laboratories, the sources of medical knowledge may be coming full circle.

This push for more knowledge about traditional medicine and interventions that are more acceptable to patients and pet owners is simply good for business. If the billion-dollar pharmaceutical industry is pursuing this line of reasoning, we believe that the veterinary industry cannot be far behind.

The definition of *medicine* is in itself interesting. The *New American Dictionary* defines *medicine* as follows: (1) the science of diagnosing, treating, or preventing disease and other damage to the body or mind; (2) the branch of this science encompassing treatment by drugs, diet, exercise, and other nonsurgical means; (3) the practice of medicine; (4) among North American Indians, something believed to control natural or supernatural powers and to serve as a preventive or remedy.

The definition of medicine certainly does not seek to exclude "unconventional" therapies, and it is holistic in scope. Carvel Tiekert, executive director of the AHVMA, defines holistic medicine as "everything that works"—a definition fairly reminiscent of the dictionary description of medicine itself.

Conclusion

Veterinary medicine is developing and expanding into new horizons. One horizon is complementary and alternative medicine. The integration of these therapies in mainstream medicine is inevitable; the only questions that remain are when, how, and by whom. The belief system that limits veterinary practice to medicine and surgery has become obsolete.

The timely and professional integration of the therapies that comprise CAVM is essential. If veterinarians do not train for and practice these therapies, individuals who have far less training will practice within this medical system on nonhuman patients. The public is searching for practitioners to trust, and it has no way of evaluating individual competence or training. Veterinarians are the most well-trained professionals to develop advanced training in these therapies and their practice. Ideally, rigorously controlled studies would exist to validate these practices, but if we wait for this ideal situation, many animals will die under our limited care. If we choose to integrate CAVM therapies in a professional and educated way, explaining their indications and limitations, clients and patients alike will benefit.

No one form of medicine has all the answers. If our primary concern is the welfare of animals, we must incorporate all reasonable forms of treatment into an approach that can offer as much as possible to help the animals under our care. The future requires us to take the best of the various diagnostic and therapeutic modalities and integrate them into a new paradigm of veterinary medicine. A world-renowned veterinarian and acupuncturist states (Lin, 19XX) the following:

> It matters not whether medicine is old or new, so long as it brings about a cure. It matters not whether theories are Eastern or Western, so long as they prove to be true.

Veterinarians would be prudent to respond to the call, study this new field in veterinary medicine, and integrate the appropriate therapies into their education, research, and practices. The future of CAVM is here; veterinarians have the opportunity to enhance animals' health care and benefit all life on Earth.

REFERENCES

Alpert JS: The relativity of modern medicine, *Arch Intern Med* 155:2385, 1995.

American Association of Poison Control Centers: Fact sheet 1983-1990, Washington, DC, 1990, The Association.

Balick MJ, Elisabetsky E, and Laird SA, editors: *Medicinal resources of the tropical forest*, New York, 1996, Columbia University Press.

Barry R and others: Feasibility study of homoeopathic remedy in rheumatoid arthritis, *Br J Rheumatol* 34(suppl 2):17, 1995.

Bukowski JA, Wartenberg D: Comparison of adverse drug reaction reporting in veterinary and human medicine, *JAVMA* 209(1):40, 1996.

Campos M and others: Symposium: immunomodulatory strategies for controlling infectious diseases of dairy cattle: the role of biological response modifiers in disease control, *J Dairy Sci* 76:2407, 1993.

Classen DC and others: Computerized surveillance of adverse drug events in hospital patients, *JAMA* 266(20):2878, 1991.

Daly D: Alternative medicine courses taught at U.S. medical schools: an ongoing listing, *J Altern Complement Med* 2(2):315, 1996.

Dossey L, Swyers JP: *Introduction in alternative medicine: expanding medical horizons*, Washington, DC, 1991, US Government Printing Office.

Doutremepuich C, editor: *Ultra low doses*, Washington, DC, 1991, Taylor and Francis.

Dunlop RH, Williams DJ: *Veterinary medicine: an illustrated history*, St Louis, 1996, Mosby.

Dyer K: Resident forum (letter), *JAMA* 275(8):1996.

Eisenberg DM and others: Unconventional medicine in the United States, *N Engl J Med* 328:246, 1993.

Ernst E, Risch K-L, White AR: Complementary medicine: what physicians think of it: a meta-analysis, *Arch Intern Med* 155:2405, 1995.

Ford MD, Olshaker JS: Concepts and controversies in toxicology, *Emerg Med Clin North Am* 12(2):483, 1994.

Hadani A, Shimshony A: Traditional veterinary medicine in the Near East: Jews, Arab Bedoins and Fellahs, *Rev Sci Tech Off Int Epiz* 13(2):581, 1994.

Kemper KJ: Separation or synthesis: a holistic approach to therapeutics, *Pediatr Rev* 17(8):279, 1996.

Kleijnen J, Knipschild P, ter Riet G: Clinical trials of homeopathy, *Br Med J* 302:316, 1991.

Klein MC: Studying episiotomy: when beliefs conflict with science, *J Fam Pract* 41(5):483, 1995.

Langreth R: "Heal Fido!" drug makers say, unleashing homeopathic pet care, *Wall Street Journal* Tuesday, June 4, 1996, p B1.

Mandelker L: Alternative medicine, *Vet Forum* June 1995, p 46, pp 46-47.

McCance I: Assessment of statistical procedures used in papers in the Australian Veterinary Journal, *Australian Vet J* 72(9):322-328, 1995.

Micozzi M, editor: *Fundamentals of complementary and alternative medicine*, New York, 1996, Churchill Livingstone.

Morris W, editor: *The American heritage dictionary of the English language*, Boston, 1976, Houghton Mifflin.

National Library of Medicine Technical Bulletin: News item, *DVM* 27(8):5s, 1996.

Pavek R: Current status of alternative health practices in the United States, *Contemp Internl Med* 7(8):61-71, 1995.

Piyasada HDW: Traditional systems for preventing and treating animal diseases in Sri Lanka, *Rev Sci Tech Off Int Epiz* 13(2):471, 1994.

Reilly DT and others: Is evidence for homeopathy reproducible? *Lancet* 344:1601-1606, 1994.

Reilly DT, Taylor MA: Potent placebo or potency? A proposed study model with initial findings using homeopathically prepared pollens in hay fever, *Br Homeopathic J* 74:65-75, 1985.

Reilly DT and others: Is homeopathy a placebo response? Controlled trial of homeopathic potency, with pollen in hayfever as model, *Lancet* ii:881, 1986.

Richmond C: A homeopathic fatality, *Can Med Assoc J* 147(1):97, 1992.

Ritt RE: Antibiotics as biological response modifiers, *J Antimicrob Chemother* 26(suppl C):31, 1990.

Smith R: Where is the wisdom? *Br Med J* 303:798, 1991.

Staren ED, Essner R, Economou JS: Overview of biological response modifiers, *Semin Surg Oncol* 5:379, 1989.

Vučevac-Bajt V, Karlović M: Traditional methods for the treatment of animal diseases in Croatia, *Rev Sci Tech Off Int Epiz* 13(2):499, 1994.

Wurtman RJ, Bettiker RL: The slowing of treatment discovery, 1965-1995, *Nature Med* 1(11):1122, 1995.

Wynn SG: Wherefore complementary medicine? *JAVMA* 209(7):1228, 1996.

Chapter 2

Evidence-Based Medicine: Critical Evaluation of New and Existing Therapies

BRENDA BONNETT

What is evidence-based medicine, and why is it one of the subjects in a book about veterinary alternative medicine? In this chapter we define this concept, which originated in human medicine, and discuss its application in the veterinary field. We talk about how we as a profession and as individuals should make decisions about what interventions we incorporate into practice. How should we proceed when evidence is lacking? What evidence is available relative to alternative modalities? As we discuss these topics, we will see that the debate surrounding alternative therapies is a spark that should set off a consideration of medical decision making in general.

Evidence-Based Medicine

Evidence-based medicine is an approach to the practice of health care that has recently been promoted by many human medical specialists and practitioners (Evidence-Based Medicine Working Group, 1992). These authors suggest that we must base our decisions about interventions, including diagnosis, therapy, and prevention, on quantitative evidence. They state that an understanding of basic pathophysiologic mechanisms of disease is necessary but is not sufficient grounds for decision making in clinical medicine. As important as clinical acumen, experience, and judgement are, we must move beyond a dependence on anecdote, personal experience, and expert opinion. We must have adequate evidence that our interventions do more good than harm.

What constitutes sufficient evidence? Ideally, interventions must be shown to be efficacious and effective (Box 2-1), and preferably of more benefit than harm, and cost-effective in randomized controlled trials (RCTs).

If this "scientific" evidence is unavailable, clinical experience may provide the only evidence. However, we know that memory is selective and not unbiased (even among experts). Therefore systematic, reliable, and reproducible recording of observations provides better information than unquantified experience and intuition. The formal rules of evidence that should be applied to any assessment of the association between an intervention and its outcome are also discussed later in this chapter.

In veterinary medicine, if we accepted as "proved to work" and therefore used only those interventions substantiated by a properly conducted RCT, few procedures would be performed. Quality formal clinical trials are rare in the field of veterinary medicine. Most studies of interventions have been descriptions of a series of cases, often done retrospectively and without an appropriate comparison group (Bonnett, Reid-Smith, 1996). As interesting as these studies may be, they are just descriptions of experience and provide only weak evidence for the usefulness of an intervention. For many other treatments, evidence from pathophysiologic or experimental studies may provide the answer to "might it work?" but not to "does it work in the clinical situation?" A lack of evidence is not proof of ineffectiveness. However, the search for better information must be ongoing.

The skills of information management, critical appraisal, and causal reasoning are necessary to apply the philosophy of evidence-based medicine. Blind acceptance of expert opinion and textbook platitudes is discouraged. Experts' opinions may be based mainly on personal experiences and knowledge of disease mechanisms. Textbook information is limited by delays in time to publication and may be nothing more than individual or combined expe-

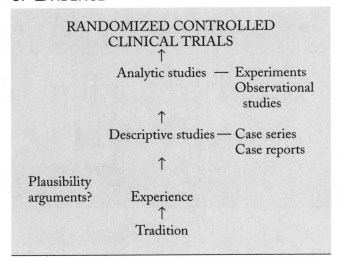
rience. Ideally, data on treatment should be sought in current literature on primary research studies. This literature must be critically appraised as to the validity and relevance of the design and analysis. However, veterinary practitioners may lack the skills necessary to do this.

Practitioners tend to review articles uncritically, perhaps hoping that the experts publishing the articles have done the critical appraisal for them. Unfortunately, many review articles are exhaustive summaries of the existing literature rather than critical assessments of what information can truly be gleaned from published articles. Two excellent articles that provide guidelines for reading overview articles are available (Oxman and others, 1988, 1994).

In the human field the suggestion is that evidence-based medicine can be practiced in the clinic by accessing computerized literature sources (Evidence-Based Care Resource Group, 1994 a, b, c). Additional resources are continually becoming available on the Internet, although in the veterinary field these are currently more limited. In human medicine, two initiatives are the American College of Physicians (ACP) Journal Club and the Cochrane Collaboration (Cochrane, 1979; Davidoff and others, 1995), both of which function with panels of experts in study design and appraisal who produce critical summaries of the clinical literature and RCT literature, respectively. Similar efforts are in the formative stages in veterinary medicine.

How Should We Assess "Evidence"?

A sufficient lesson in critical appraisal is beyond the scope of this chapter. Numerous resources are available. An extensive series of articles from the human field are excellent, but may be too detailed for the average practitioner (Guyatt, Drummond, 1993; Guyatt, Sacket, Cook, 1993; Jaeschke, Guyatt, Sackett, 1993; Laupacis and oth-

ers, 1994; Levine and others, 1994; Oxman, Cook, Guyatt, 1994; Oxman, Sackett, Guyatt, 1993). In the veterinary field, older and newer references are available (Bonnett, Reid-Smith, 1996; Dohoo, Waltner-Toews, 1985a,b,c; Reeves, Reeves, 1995). A brief outline of the relative strength of various study designs for providing evidence on the effectiveness of interventions is presented in Box 2-2.

The main failure of descriptive studies is that they lack an appropriate comparison group. Well-designed and correctly performed observational studies (e.g., case-control, cohort) can provide relatively strong evidence of an effect. Experimental studies may be appropriate for showing biophysiologic effects but may lack relevance to the clinical situation. In the "real world," disease development is usually a function of many factors (e.g., genetics, nutrition, environment) that affect the occurrence of health and disease and the success of therapies. The RCT therefore is the best design to evaluate the usefulness of most interventions. In any study, the selection of subjects has a major effect on the validity and relevance of the findings. An appropriate comparison group, generally receiving a placebo or standard treatment, must be in place. The method, preferably a formal randomized procedure, by which subjects are assigned to receive treatment, is also an important determinant of validity. Those responsible for assessing the outcome should not know which treatment the individual is receiving. This information may be withheld from both the owner and the clinician. The assessment of outcomes of interest (i.e., application of diagnostic procedures) should be equal in all patients (Martin, Meek, Willeberg, 1987).

BOX 2-3

*S*TEPS IN *B*ASIC *C*AUSAL *R*EASONING

- Does the proposed causal factor precede the outcome?
- Is there a statistical association between the factor and the outcome? If so, how strong is the effect?
- Are there other factors (intervening, preceding, or coexisting) that might have produced the outcome?
- Is there a dose response? (Does "more" of the factor result in "more" of the outcome?)
- Does the association make biologic sense (coherence)?
- Do the findings agree with previously published information (consistency)?

In veterinary medicine a major challenge for clinical trials is enrollment of a sufficient number of subjects to achieve adequate power (the ability to detect a difference or effect if one truly exists). One method to overcome this problem is the use of multisite trials (Bonnett, Kelton, 1995; Kelton, Bonnett, 1995). Assessment of alternative modalities may offer additional challenges (e.g., dealing with individualization of treatment to subject), but these should not be insurmountable. Even if a true RCT is impossible, clinical researchers should try to satisfy many of the basic criteria for validity. Otherwise the strength of evidence from the study is compromised.

Unfortunately, the control the investigator exerts to ensure validity in an RCT may make the results less relevant to the clinical situation. The acts performed in the study of disease may influence or change the nature of the clinical encounter, the attitudes and behaviors of participants, and the outcomes to be measured. Thus the results of any one trial, even if it is of high quality, may not offer all the answers about the effectiveness of an intervention under all circumstances. How available evidence is critically summarized to form health care policy or practice guidelines involves more layers of complexity. A series of articles addressing these issues has appeared in the *Journal of the American Medical Association* (Eddy, 1993).

In the assessment of evidence (causal reasoning) no ultimate test of proof exists. An inferential process should be performed with appropriate standards (Martin, Meek, Willeberg, 1987). (A basic outline of this reasoning is presented in Box 2-3.)

Unfortunately, the criteria of coherence and consistency are often relied on heavily. Many conventional interventions are accepted without rigorous assessment because they fit current pathophysiologic understanding or agree with experience or previous work (which itself may not have provided very strong evidence). However, if the criterion of coherence is relied on excessively, scientific breakthroughs will be rare or nonexistent. The current level of knowledge and prevailing theories are the limits in this approach. The consistency criterion is hampered by little research being performed in areas in which little research exists. New information has no standard of comparison. In addition, misinformation can be propagated. Axioms that have become accepted and are quoted repeatedly in articles and texts may have originated from anecdote or supposition (Bonnett, Reid-Smith, 1996).

How Do We Proceed in the Absence of Strong Evidence?

Without strong evidence from RCTs or correctly performed and relevant experimental or observational studies, individual, collective, or expert experience is the only information available. Coherence and consistency again come to the forefront. Medical practitioners are constantly faced with uncertainty. However, uncertainty can be quantified rather than ignored or couched in very subjective terms (Sackett and others, 1991). This can lead to improved comparison of experience among practitioners and across various health care settings. This can also provide a basis for improved communication with clients.

The discrepancies between what practitioners perceive that they do and what they actually do are well known. Memory is selective and often biased (Evidence Based Care Resource Group, 1994c). Computerization of medical records allows a great potential for improved quantification of experience and process and outcome assessment (Sackett and others, 1991).

How should a practitioner proceed in the face of uncertainty? A common way to proceed is to transfer the responsibility and go with prevailing theory, assuming the expert source can back up claims with "science." The most appropriate goal is to take personal responsibility for decisions and to be open and honest about the relative strength of available evidence.

Why Is a Discussion of Evidence-Based Medicine so Pertinent to Alternative Medicine?

Alternative interventions may deviate significantly from existing doctrines, thereby not satisfying the criteria of coherence and consistency. This should not be an overwhelming obstacle; coherence and consistency represent only two of many criteria that should be assessed. However, the emphasis on the necessity for new information to agree with existing concepts and information has resulted in a double standard. Most scientists and medical practitioners tend to view information that does not fit with existing theory with suspicion and (perhaps unconsciously) have a higher threshold of acceptance for something new. In other words, the strength of evidence about effectiveness required before a conventional intervention is accepted may be less than that demanded for an alternative intervention. The proponents of evidence-based medicine have suggested that a pathophysiologic understanding is a "necessary" criterion for "proof." However, throughout history, helpful treatments have been discovered and implemented long before the reasons and ways they worked were known (limes for scurvy are one classic example). Veterinary professionals should be able to agree on the guidelines of causal reasoning, the criteria for good and relevant study design, critical appraisal of the literature, and appropriately rigorous ways of assessing subjective findings and experience (in other words, the basis of evidence-based medicine). These principles can then be applied equally to assessment of all interventions.

Additional factors that must be considered when the literature is reviewed are the wish bias (Wynder and others, 1990) and publication bias (Rennie, Flanigan, 1992). Obviously, unless research is conceived of, supported (academically and financially), and accepted for publication, reports will not be available for appraisal. Demand from the public can have a major influence on direction of research. A diligent profession practicing evidence-based medicine places pressure on researchers to fill the void between published reports and the needs of daily practice (Bonnett, Reid-Smith, 1996).

In practical terms, how can veterinary professionals begin practicing evidence-based medicine? First, each time you state a "fact" or prescribe a treatment, consider and ideally verbalize the source and strength of evidence for that statement or decision. Although this is a time-consuming process, you will start to get a feel for those actions in which you have great confidence and understand the reasons for your approach. This process should be promoted in our veterinary schools and demanded of expert consultants in daily practice. A second approach is to critically appraise the evidence for certain conditions, diagnostic tests, or treatments for which you feel less confident. Organization of findings increases your database of critically appraised topics. Critical appraisal necessitates knowledge and continuous application of that knowledge. Many professional groups now include sessions on epidemiology and critical appraisal in their continuing education programs (Bonnett, Kelton, 1995; Kelton, Bonnett, 1995).

Researchers and academics can help practitioners by providing quality research that answers the right questions and critical though not exhaustive reviews. Regardless of the availability of data from researchers, practitioners must consider each case individually. Evaluation of medical practices in human medicine and critical assessments of the literature have shown an alarming lack of evidence, even for "established" procedures (Eddy, 1993; Smith, 1991). Eddy has suggested that only "15% of medical interventions are supported by solid scientific evidence" (Smith, 1991).

No doubt the situation in veterinary medicine is even worse. However, given that reappraisal of all current practices is an impossible task, application of stringent criteria to all new interventions is the minimal action needed. In conventional medicine, all alternative modalities are "new."

What Is the Current Evidence for Alternative Medicine?

At the time of writing, this author and others are working on a critical appraisal of the veterinary literature on alternative medicine. One major argument against holistic practices has been that scientific literature to support claims is nonexistent. A search was done of the computerized CAB Abstracts data base.* This resource includes academic and scientific publications (not lay press). A search of the years 1984 to 1996 has uncovered over 1000 articles relative to veterinary alternative medicine. Almost one third of these are in languages other than English. Many are case reports and review papers (as is true of much of the literature on conventional modalities). Work is underway on translation and critical appraisal. Many articles detail experimental studies conducted to examine the effects of herbal, homeopathic, and acupuncture treatments on biophysiologic functions (e.g., neutrophil migration). Some reports are observational studies and clinical trials. (A cross-reference by modality and species of a large portion of these articles is presented in Table 2-1.) The assessment of these articles will offer a more informative way to judge the evidence. Plans for Internet access of this information are continuing.

In the human field, similar assessments of the literature on alternative medicine have been and continue to be conducted. An interesting paper from 1991 in the *British Medical Journal* systematically reviewed trials involving homeopathic remedies (Kleijnen, Knipschild, terRiet, 1991). Using strict guidelines, the authors found at least 23 randomized controlled clinical trials that could not be faulted in study design and analysis. In 15 of these the homeopathic remedy was shown to have a significant beneficial effect. The authors concluded that the evidence presented suggests efficacy and that further studies should be performed.

Summary

The evidence-based medicine approach deemphasizes intuition, unsystematic experience, and pathophysiologic rationale as sufficient grounds for decision making. It suggests that appropriate guidelines for assessing the strength of evidence should be followed by the profession and individuals. Many practitioners may lack the skills or resources to currently practice this way for all patients and

---

*CAB International, Wallingford, Oxon OX10 8DE, UK.

TABLE 2-1

ARTICLES FROM A SEARCH OF THE VETERINARY LITERATURE 1984-96

SPECIES	MODALITY NO. OF ARTICLES/NO. IN ENGLISH		
	HOMEOPATHY	ACUPUNCTURE	HERBAL MEDICINE
Bovine	82/27	77/19	119/10
Canine	69/12	118/62	49/46
Equine	41/10	60/36	10/5
Feline	32/4	23/16	10/9
Porcine	30/3	16/8	20/10
Total	254/56	294/141	208/80

conditions. However, an honest appraisal of the way decisions about interventions are made is a good exercise for the veterinary profession. Discussion of acceptance of or resistance to alternative medicine cannot proceed without attention to critical appraisal.

Therapies should be rigorously assessed, regardless of whether they fit with existing doctrines. However, as a new modality (at least in North America) alternative approaches are under added scrutiny. Much quantitative evidence may already exist as to the efficacy of some complementary modalities. Continued assessment of the literature and expanded, quality research need to be conducted. With conventional medicine professionals should adopt a policy of "evidence not acceptance"; with alternative medicine, the policy of "evidence not avoidance" is needed. As the boundaries continue to blur between what is considered alternative or conventional and as new interventions continually come to light, evidence-based medicine will provide the most appropriate, substantive, and truly scientific approach to medical decision making.

ACKNOWLEDGMENTS

The assistance of Heather Reid in the literature search on alternative therapies is greatly appreciated. The interest and support of various private donors who have stimulated my work in this area also are greatly appreciated, as is financial support from the Pet Trust.

REFERENCES

Bonnett B, Kelton D: Clinical trials: what is needed to move from clinical impression to critical proof? Proceedings of the Fifth Annual Symposium, *Am Coll Vet Surg Vet Symp,* 1995, p 241.

Bonnett B, Reid-Smith R: Critical appraisal meets clinical reality: evaluating evidence in the literature using canine hemangiosarcoma as an example, *Vet Clin North Am: Small Animal Pract* 26:39, 1996.

Cochrane AL: 1931-1971: a critical review, with particular reference to the medical profession. In *Medicines for the year 2000,* London, 1979, Office of Health Economics.

Davidoff F and others: Evidence-based medicine, *Br Med J* 310:1085, 1995.

Dohoo IR, Waltner-Toews D:. Interpreting clinical research. I. General considerations, *Comp Cont Educ Pract Vet* 7:S473, 1985a.

Dohoo IR, Waltner-Toews D: Interpreting clinical research. II. Descriptive and experimental studies, *Comp Cont Educ Pract Vet* 7:S513, 1985b.

Dohoo IR, Waltner-Toews D: Interpreting clinical research. III. Observational studies and interpretation of results, *Comp Cont Educ Pract Vet* 7:S605, 1985c.

Eddy DM: Clinical decision making: from theory to practice. Three battles to watch in the 1990s, *JAMA* 270:520, 1993.

Evidence-Based Care Resource Group: Evidence-based care. I. Setting priorities: how important is this problem? *Can Med Assoc J* 150:1249, 1994a.

Evidence-Based Care Resource Group: Evidence-based care. II. Setting guidelines: how should we manage this problem? *Can Med Assoc J* 150:1417, 1994b.

Evidence-Based Care Resource Group: Evidence-based care. III. Measuring performance: how are we managing this problem? *Can Med Assoc J* 150:1575, 1994c.

Evidence-Based Medicine Working Group: Evidence-based medicine: a new approach to teaching the practice of medicine, *JAMA* 268:2420, 1992.

Guyatt GH, Drummond R: Users' guides to the medical literature, *JAMA* 270:2096, 1993.

Guyatt GH, Sackett DL, Cook DJ (for the Evidence-Based Medicine Working Group): Users' guides to the medical literature. II. How to use an article about therapy or prevention. A. Are the results of the study valid? *JAMA* 270:2598, 1993.

Jaeschke R, Guyatt GH, Sackett DL (for the Evidence-Based Medicine Working Group): Users' guides to the medical literature. III. How to use an article about a diagnostic test. B. What are the results and will they help me in caring for my patients? *JAMA* 270:2598, 1993.

Kelton D, Bonnett B: Multicenter clinical trials: can the community practice provide those needed numbers? Proceedings of the Fifth Annual Symposium, *Am Coll Vet Surg Vet Symp,* 1995, p 244.

Kleijnen J, Knipschild P, terRiet G: Clinical trials of homeopathy, *Br Med J* 302:316, 1991.

Laupacis A and others (for the Evidence-Based Medicine Working Group): Users' guides to the medical literature. V. How to use an article about prognosis., *JAMA* 272:234, 1994.

Levine M and others (for the Evidence-Based Medicine Working Group): Users' guides to the medical literature. IV. How to use an article about harm, *JAMA* 271:1615, 1994.

Martin SW, Meek AH, Willeberg P: *Veterinary epidemiology: principles and methods,* Ames, Iowa, 1987, Iowa State University.

Oxman AD, Sackett DL, Guyatt GH (for The Evidence-Based Medicine Working Group): Users' guides to the medical literature. I. How to get started, *JAMA* 270:2093, 1993.

Oxman AD, Guyatt GH: Guidelines for reading literature reviews, *Can Med Assoc J* 138:697, 1988.

Oxman AD, Cook DJ, Guyatt GH (for the Evidence-Based Medicine Working Group): Users' guides to the medical literature. VI. How to use an overview, *JAMA* 272:1367, 1994.

Reeves MJ, Reeves NP: Epidemiology and the veterinary oncologist—evaluation and critical appraisal of the scientific oncology literature: how to read the clinical literature, *Vet Clin North Am Small Anim Pract* 25:1, 1995.

Rennie D, Flanigan A: Publication bias: the triumph of hope over experience, *JAMA* 267:411, 1992.

Sackett DL and others: *Clinical epidemiology: a basic science for clinical medicine,* Toronto, 1991, Little, Brown.

Smith R: Where is the wisdom: the poverty of medical evidence, *Br Med J* 303:798, 1991.

Wynder EL, Higgins IT, Harris RE: The wish bias, *J Clin Epidemiol* 43:619, 1990.

Nutrition

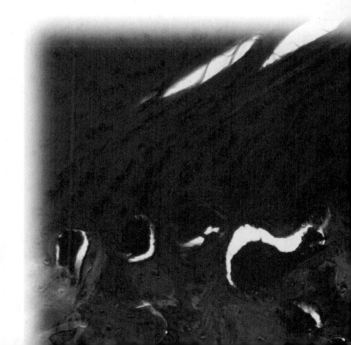

Chapter 3

Basic and Preventive Nutrition for the Cat, Dog, and Horse

ROGER V. KENDALL

Nutrition as actually practiced in the field of veterinary medicine may perhaps best be classified as (1) basic, (2) preventive, or (3) therapeutic. The term *basic nutrition* refers to the animal's daily food intake, which should meet the daily nutritional requirements based on the dietary guidelines of the National Research Council (NRC). Preventive nutrition involves adding nutritional and feed supplements to the basic diet to eliminate possible deficiencies caused by the diet and the animal's biochemical individuality. This approach seeks to prevent the onset of disease in animals that are still outwardly healthy. Therapeutic nutrition involves the use of nutritional supplements in animals who display specific health problems and disease conditions. Combining preventive and/or therapeutic nutrition with conventional veterinary drug treatment is one example of complementary therapy and is one of the fastest growing modalities in the field of modern veterinary medicine. (Therapeutic nutrition is detailed in Chapter 4.)

Basic Nutrition

Good nutrition and a sound, balanced diet are essential to the health, performance, and well-being of all animals. This simple statement is easy to dismiss as obvious and unworthy of further discussion. However, a holistic evaluation of diet and its effect on an animal is the cornerstone of good medicine. Slight dietary changes may produce dramatic alterations in most metabolic processes, influencing the development of disease and consequently an animal's susceptibility to disease. Many researchers have found, for example, that established animal models for disease absolutely depend on diet. In fact, changes in brand names of commercial diets have prevented investigators from producing valid disease models in more than one case (Bhatia and others, 1996; Pound and others, 1973).

An animal's *basic* diet must provide adequate water in addition to proper amounts of energy foodstuffs, protein, essential fatty acids, vitamins, minerals, and accessory food factors to maintain biologic and metabolic functions. If the basic diet fails to provide complete and adequate amounts of these macronutrients and micronutrients, a number of problems can result over time. Growth in juveniles can be impaired, performance reduced, and recovery from illness or injury delayed; greater susceptibility to infections may result as well as the early onset of degenerative conditions (Lewis and others, 1994; Simpson and others, 1993). The NRC has published dietary requirements for the dog, cat, and horse, among other species (National Research Council 1985, 1986, 1989). The NRC guidelines are based on average daily nutritional requirements for animal groups and designed to maintain health and prevent deficiencies. The NRC nutritional recommendations are not based on optimum levels but focus instead on the average needs of healthy animals. The NRC guidelines do not take into consideration actual food quality, nutrient bioavailability, breed differences (James, McKay, 1950; Kendall and others, 1983; Zentec, Meyer, 1995), and the all-important concept of *biochemical individuality* (Williams, 1963). Individual nutritional needs of animals vary widely. The quality of food varies depending on the commercial processing and storing methods used (Kronfeld, 1989; Lowry, Baker, 1989).

The term *basic nutrition* refers to the foundational dietary requirements of the animal that are best achieved using high-quality food ingredients (meats, concentrates, and roughages) and eliminating artificial preservatives, dyes, and flavors whenever possible.

The nutritional quality of commercial pet foods varies widely in sources of ingredients, biologic value, and digestibility. According to Morris and Rogers (1994), progress in understanding nutritional requirements for dogs and cats requires more precise information on the specific requirements for various life stages, including reproduction and maintenance, as well as values for the biochemical availability of nutrients in common dietary ingredients in pet foods. Sole dependency on the cheaper commercial products may cause dogs and cats to develop nutrient deficiencies and health problems (Sousa, 1987; Sousa and others, 1988). Premium commercial diets have been shown to provide higher-quality, more digestible protein elements (Case and others, 1995).

Many veterinarians who recommend home-prepared diets find that pets who eat the better-quality, human-grade ingredients therein exhibit even more dramatic health benefits. An additional advantage to feeding home-prepared foods may be to enhance dental health; several studies have shown that gristly foods such as tough beef remove and prevent subsequent accumulation of dental tartar (Brown, Park, 1968; Egelberg, 1965a, b). Pet-owning clients who prepare diets for their pets should follow published recipes to ensure proper balance.

Because nutritional biochemistry is constantly evolving, some have questioned whether a manufactured diet can ever contain "complete" nutrition. One example can be found in the fatal consequences of dietary taurine deficiency that occurred in cats being fed, interestingly, a high-quality premium diet (Pion and others, 1987). Because scientists cannot know everything necessary about animal nutritional requirements, many veterinarians choose to recommend various high-quality natural commercial diets or supplementation of fresh food in proper balance. The need for additives in commercial pet foods has also been questioned. (For a detailed examination of pet-food additives, refer to Chapter 5.)

In the horse, borderline deficiencies or marginal levels of certain nutrients in grains and hay may be common because of improper farming practices or deficiencies in local soils (Mortvedt and others, 1972).

Preventive Nutrition: The Role of Biochemical Individuality and Nutritional Supplementation

Nutritional needs vary greatly depending on type of species, age, size, physiologic state, and biochemical individuality. Biochemical individuality, a concept originally developed by Roger Williams, discoverer of pantothenic acid (vitamin B_5), refers to the idea that necessary levels of essential nutrients can vary widely for individual animals (Williams, 1956, 1963, 1971). Williams and Kalita (1977) proposed that the size, shape, and function of glands and organs in humans and animals can vary greatly among individuals, who may consequently have unique biochemical and nutritional needs. Based on the various nutrients evaluated in the literature, Williams (1977) has concluded that "the needs for all nutrients vary on the average over a fourfold range" (Rose, 1957).

Nutrient needs vary within a group of animals for several reasons. For example, animals under stress produce more epinephrine than normal. Epinephrine synthesis requires vitamin C (among other nutrients) for its production (Shils and others, 1994). The unstressed normal rat synthesizes ascorbic acid at the rate of 70 mg/kg of body weight per day, and the stressed rat increases production to 215 mg/kg per day (Conney and others, 1961). These findings suggest reasons that some stressed animals may benefit from vitamin C supplementation (Dabrowska and others, 1991; Gross, 1992; McKee, Harrison, 1995; Nakano, Suzuki, 1984). Williams (1963; 1977) found that some or all of the following factors can affect biochemical individuality and subsequent nutrient requirements: genetic makeup and heritability, environmental toxins, nutrient-deficient diets, illness and injury, stress, inadequate exercise, and long- and short-term drug therapy. One or more of these factors may cause potential deficiencies.

Nutritional supplementation should be used in conjunction with a high-quality basic diet. The use of nutritional products and daily supplements (such as a multiple vitamin/mineral formula) raises the nutritional availability of essential nutrients in the animal's overall diet. The purpose of incorporating supplements into the diet of work and companion animals is to provide a full spectrum of essential vitamins, minerals, amino acids, and other food factors that may be deficient in the animal because of biochemical individuality or low-quality food. Diets deficient in nutrients may lead to poor growth, frequent illness, poor appearance, and suboptimal performance. Left unnoticed and unattended, subclinical deficiencies and varying stress factors may contribute to the onset of more serious, costly health problems in the future.

Biochemical and nutritional research and clinical observations demonstrate the qualitative and quantitative benefits that result from combining high-potency, individualized nutritional supplementation with an animal's basic diet. Nutritional supplementation not only enhances recovery from stress, illness, and injury but also helps prevent the onset of many degenerative diseases, such as arthritis, cardiovascular disease, cancer, gastrointestinal problems, and skin disorders. This chapter reviews some current concepts of preventive nutrition and provides points of departure for their application in veterinary medicine.

Basic Dietary and Nutritional Management of the Cat, Dog and Horse: The NRC Guidelines

Kronfeld (1989) defines *nutrition* as "the whole flow of substances taken in as food and used in the body to build its structures and sustain its functions." A nutrient is any food component that aids and supports life. The basic daily nutrient requirements, which have been reported in the literature for the cat, dog, and horse and compiled by the NRC, represent average amounts of nutrients that a group of animals should consume over time to maintain growth and prevent deficiencies (National Research Council, 1985, 1986, 1989). The NRC guidelines provide useful reference points in managing the diet of the animal in various physiologic states (e.g., age, gestation, lactation, workload) but should not be considered the correct or optimum level for all animals in the group. Each nutrient has a normal range of variation in need, in which 5% to 10% of the population requires either much more or less than the calculated average (Williams, Kalita, 1977). Multiplying this variation by the 40 or more essential nutrients required for cellular function often reveals individual animals as deficient in at least three to five nutrients. Therefore the nutritional tables found in the NRC publications fail adequately to distinguish individual needs based on a wide range of physiologic, genetic, and metabolic conditions (biochemical individuality). *Biochemical individuality* may be defined as the animal's unique nutritional needs, which may differ quantitatively for each separate nutrient. In the case of certain nutrients, some individual animals may require from 2 to 10 times as much as others in the group (Williams, 1971). Statistical data that fail to account for an animal's unique nutrient requirements are of minimal value in discussing the relationship of nutritional intake to individual disease patterns.

In human medicine, researchers have already questioned the adequacy of published nutritional guidelines in maintaining health as opposed to preventing overt deficiencies (Willet, 1994). Calls for reexamination of the recommended daily allowances have also appeared in this context (Reynolds, 1994). The NRC guidelines are oversimplified; depending on the physiologic state of the animal, a range for each nutrient need is appropriate, not a fixed figure. Average nutritional requirements and optimal nutritional needs are not necessarily identical or even similar in an individual cat, dog, or horse. Nutrient needs are not static but vary widely depending on the state of the animal and the metabolic function to be met. Therefore the NRC tables may be satisfactory for some, but certainly not all, animals in the group.

Although commercial diets and feeding programs may adequately provide the foundational levels of nutrients needed for growth, reproduction, and maintenance, greater attention must be paid to the quantity, quality, and bioavailability of the nutrients in an animal's diet if a higher degree of health, fitness, and performance is to be realized (Morris, Rogers, 1994). The nutritional approach proposed by Roger Williams (1977) is useful in understanding the basics of an optimal dietary program. It provides a conceptual basis for nutritional supplementation and its role in preventive nutrition. Williams and Kalita (1977) also discuss the following topics: (1) food as part of the animal's environment, (2) suboptimal nutrition preva-

lent in nature, (3) biochemical individuality, and (4) the synergistic effect of nutrients.

Food as an Element of Environment

In addition to needing oxygen and water, an animal depends on approximately 40 essential nutrients plus additional factors that come from the diet to sustain life (Shils and others, 1994; Williams, Kalita, 1977). The diet must be based on high-quality food ingredients that are readily assimilated, as unprocessed as possible, and free of artificial preservatives, flavors, and coloring agents. Food processing lowers the nutritional quality of the diet (Schroeder, 1971), and excessive chemical additives may negatively affect an animal's health. BHT, BHA, and ethoxyquin, for example, are widely used in commercial animal foods because these additives can prevent oxidation and rancidity. (For additional reading on the potential deleterious effects of preservatives, see Chapter 5.) An animal's basic diet should provide a highly bioavailable, well-balanced program with adequate levels of all essential nutrients required for good health. A poor-quality diet, which may include additives to which an animal is sensitive, can have as dramatic an effect on the animal as the air and water it consumes. It can eventually lead to serious health problems.

Suboptimal Nutrition Generally Prevails in Nature

Williams and Kalita (1977) postulated that organisms in nature generally live under suboptimal conditions, which includes suboptimal nutritional intake. Cells and tissues of the body compete for available nutrients and may be unable to obtain consistently appropriate levels of individual nutrients for optimal growth, repair, and performance. The quality of the diet worsens when a large part of the diet is highly processed. Without attention to dietary management and individual nutritional needs, suboptimal nutrition can prevail.

Biochemical Individuality

Nutrient requirements can vary according to physiologic, environmental, metabolic, and genetic differences among individual animals (Williams, 1963). Variations can range from a factor of 2 to 4 times depending on the individual biochemical and nutritional needs within the group. Individual animals vary in their genetic makeup and can also differ in morphologic and physiologic aspects, including their endocrine activity, metabolic efficiency, and nutritional requirements. When environmental factors such as pollution, stress, age, and overall health condition are also considered, the reasons that some nutritional needs greatly exceed NRC guidelines are obvious.

Nutritional supplementation can be effective in overcoming nutritional deficiencies caused by unique biochemical needs. For instance, certain rats with a hereditary requirement for high levels of manganese develop severe inner-ear problems when fed ordinary rat chow. When they receive manganese supplements, the inner ear problems do not develop (Hurley, Everson, 1959). Assessing biochemical individuality is therefore essential when striving to optimize the health and well-being of an animal through nutrition.

Nutrient Synergy

No nutrient works alone in the body; each is linked by enzymatic reactions and metabolic pathways to other nutrients in the cell. For instance, the conversion of glucose into pyruvate involves 10 steps requiring multiple enzymes and cofactors (Lehninger and others, 1993). Adequate nutrition requires the presence of all nutrient factors at adequate levels for a particular pathway to function properly. If an animal's diet is severely deficient in one nutrient in a nutritional pathway using 10 nutrients, the same results may occur as would in the absence of all 10 nutrients (Williams, Kalita, 1977). In other words, the metabolic sequence cannot produce the desired product unless all 10 factors or nutrients are present. The nutritional chain is therefore only as strong as its weakest link or nutrient. When added as a supplement to the diet, a nutrient such as a mineral, an amino acid, or a vitamin can provide no favorable effect unless all other associated nutrients are present in adequate levels. Understanding how nutrients work synergistically is essential to knowing how foods and supplements can work together to build health and overcome disease. Providing animals with a broad-spectrum nutritional supplement raises their nutritional reserves and improves the availability of key essential nutrients.

Successful nutritional management of the cat, dog, and horse must go beyond the basic dietary needs outlined in the NRC publications. Such information is invaluable in establishing a general feeding program for animals in different physiologic states but may fall short of determining individual needs. Space constraints prevent a detailed discussion of the energy and basic nutritional requirements of the cat, dog, and horse, but the reader may refer to the NRC guidelines for this information.

Basic Classes of Nutrients

Although all nutrients are necessary to maintain health, absolute requirements vary widely depending on the animal under discussion. The six basic classes of nutrients are water, carbohydrates, fats, proteins, vitamins, and minerals.

Water

Water is the most essential nutrient because its absence causes death more rapidly than the absence of any other nutrient. Water is the most abundant substance in living systems, comprising between 60% and 70% of total body weight. This level cannot change appreciably without serious health consequences. Vital to the functioning of all living cells, water is the medium in which the transport of nutrients, the enzyme-catalyzed reactions of metabolism, and the transfer of energy occur. Structure and function of the cell are adapted to the properties of water. Most animals have a limited capacity to store water, and its deprivation can cause a loss of metabolic function and energy production and, if severe, eventually death. Water intake must balance water losses, which occur principally through exhaled air, perspiration, urine, and feces.

Because water quality may contribute to ill health in animals, veterinarians should consider water sources in diagnostic workups. Municipal water systems have been sources of epidemic parasite infestations (Communicable Disease Report, 1995; Kent, 1988). Chlorine, arsenic, and radioactive materials are additional toxic sources (Fuortes and others, 1990; Smith and others, 1992; Zierler, 1988).

Carbohydrates

Carbohydrates are the chief source of energy for the horse and also important to the cat and dog. All animals have a metabolic need for glucose to supply energy to vital organs and provide substrates for the synthesis of other compounds, including glycoproteins. Carbohydrates help regulate protein and fat metabolism. The principal carbohydrates in food include sugars, starches, and cellulose. All sugars, starches, and cellulose can be converted into glucose, which is the principal fuel used by the brain, nervous system, and muscles (Lewis and others, 1994). Dietary fiber is supplied chiefly by plant cellulose, pectin, hemicellulose, gum, and mucilage, which are primarily complex carbohydrate polymers. Supplemental soluble and insoluble fiber is useful in the treatment of constipation, hyperglycemia, gastrointestinal disorders, hyperlipidemia, and other veterinary disease entities.

Fats and Lipids

Fats and lipids are the most concentrated sources of energy in the diet, providing more than twice the number of calories per gram than do carbohydrates or protein. In the form of phospholipids and sphingolipids, lipids are the main constituent of cell membranes and make up a large number of metabolic regulators such as sterols and prostaglandins. Fats in the diet aid in the absorption of the fat-soluble vitamins from the digestive tract and help make calcium more available to the body.

Proteins

Made up of both essential and nonessential amino acids, proteins are essential for the growth and development of all body tissues. They are used for the production of enzymes, hormones, neurotransmitters, antibodies, and a variety of structural tissues such as muscle, skin, hair, nails, and internal organs (Lehninger and others, 1993). Essential amino acids found in protein are indispensable and must be supplied in the diet at appropriate levels. A protein deficiency can lead to abnormal growth and tissue development (Shils and others, 1994). Protein quality is directly related to digestibility and feed efficiency. For carnivorous animals such as the dog and cat, proteins with high biologic value such as meat should constitute the majority of protein supplied by the diet. Lower-quality sources increase the protein requirement (Case and others, 1995; Huber and others, 1986).

Vitamins

Vitamins, an essential part of an animal's diet, regulate a number of physiologic processes, including growth, maintenance, and energy production (Shils and others, 1994). (Table 3-1 reviews the main functions of the vitamins.) Vitamins aid in the reactions and synthesis of various cellular tissues and act as cofactors to many enzymes. Although dogs, cats, and horses (unlike humans) can synthesize their own vitamin C, during times of sickness, stress, or advanced age, supplemental vitamin C is beneficial because the animal may not be able to produce adequate levels to meet its needs (Hintz, 1988; Kronfeld, 1989). (Table 3-2 gives vitamin requirements for the dog and cat and clinical signs of deficiency and excess.)

TABLE 3-1

THE NAMES AND MAIN FUNCTIONS OF VITAMINS

VITAMIN	FUNCTION
Vitamin A (retinol)	Vision, a component of light-sensitive pigments in retina, rhodopsin and iodopsin
	Synthesis of mucopolysaccharides, hence integrity of mucous membranes (e.g., cornea)
	Immunity
	Reproduction
Vitamin D (cholecalciferol)	Precursor of active form, 1,25-dihydroxycholecalciferol, made in kidney
	Regulation of calcium and phosphorus, interacting with parathyroid hormone and calcitonin
	Mineralization of bone and teeth
Vitamin E (tocopherol)	Because of antioxidant activity, diminished production of lipid peroxides that damage cells, especially membranes; especially susceptible—erythrocytes, muscle, heart, liver, adipose tissues, brain
	Effect on synthesis of coenzyme A and adenosine triphosphate (ATP)
	Reproduction
Vitamin K (phylloquinone, menadione)	Necessary for activity of carboxylases in hepatic synthesis of blood-clotting factors II (prothrombin), VII, IX, and X
Vitamin B$_1$ (thiamin)	Precursor of thiamin pyrophosphate (TPP) or cocarboxylase, a coenzyme required by dehydrogenases in the citric acid cycle (Krebs' cycle) and by transketolase in the pentose phosphate shunt
	Effects on all tissue, most sensitive—nerves, stomach, heart
Vitamin B$_2$ (riboflavin)	Component of two coenzymes, flavin mononucleotide (FMN) and flavin adenine dinucleotide (FAD), involved in dehydrogenase reactions and serving as electron carriers in all tissues
	FMN and FAD linking metabolism of carbohydrates, proteins, and fats to the cytochrome system, the terminal oxidative pathway
	Desaturation of fatty acids
Niacin (nicotinic acid, nicotinamide)	Component of two coenzymes, nicotinamide adenine dinucleotide (NAD) and nicotinamide adenine dinucleotide phosphate (NADP), required by many dehydrogenases; reduced and acting as electron carriers
	Important in oxidative processes in all tissues
	Biosynthesis of long-chain fatty acids
Pantothenic acid	Component of coenzyme-A, which is involved in the metabolism of fatty acids
	Synthesis of steroids

Modified from Kronfeld D: *Vitamins and mineral supplementation for dogs and cats,* Santa Barbara, Calif, 1989, Veterinary Practice Publishing.

Continued.

TABLE 3-1

THE NAMES AND MAIN FUNCTIONS OF VITAMINS—cont'd

VITAMIN	FUNCTION
Vitamin B$_6$	Precursor of a coenzyme, pyridoxal phosphate (PDP), involved in metabolism of amino acids
	Synthesis of heme
Folacin (folic acid, pteroyl-glutamic acid)	Precursor of tetrahydrofolic acid (THF), a carrier of methyl groups in transmethylation reactions
	Synthesis of purines and pyrimidines
Vitamin B$_{12}$	Precursor of methylcobalamin, which is involved in certain transmethylations, interacting with THF
	Synthesis of deoxyribonucleic acid (DNA)
	Erythropoiesis, interacting with THF
	Myelin synthesis (specific for B$_{12}$, not interacting with THF and folacin)
	Synthesis of methionine and choline
	Conversion of methylmalonate to succinate
Biotin	Coenzyme in carboxylative reactions (e.g., those involving acetyl-CoA, crotonyl-CoA, propionyl-CoA, methylmalonyl-CoA, pyruvate)
	Integrity of skin and possibly claws
Choline	Synthesis of acetylcholine in nerves
	Synthesis of phosphatidylcholine, important in cell membranes and export of fat from liver (lipotrophic action)
	Synthesis of methionine and dimethylglycine
Vitamin C	Antioxidant cofactor in several hydroxylations, either proactive or protective
	Synthesis of collagen
	Synthesis of catecholamines
	Synthesis of steroids
	Synthesis of carnitine
	Iron absorption
	Cellular and humoral immunity

Minerals

Constituents of all body tissues and fluids, minerals are nutrients essential to many biologic functions. The macrominerals—calcium, phosphorus, potassium, sodium, and magnesium—are necessary for the regulation of pH balance, skeletal integrity, osmotic pressures, and nerve and muscle function. The microminerals, such as iron, zinc, copper, manganese, iodine, and selenium, help control and regulate a wide range of biochemical reactions as components of metalloenzymes (Shils and others, 1994). Mineral deficiencies are sometimes difficult to determine initially but can eventually cause major growth problems and metabolic imbalances. (Table 3-3 presents the main functions of the essential trace elements.)

Dietary management of minerals must consider the minerals as a group rather than in isolation because the intake of any mineral may affect the absorption and utilization of other minerals (Kronfeld, 1989; Lewis and others, 1994). The goal is to maintain the proper levels and ratios of minerals in the diet. An example of this relationship occurs with phosphorus, which can block calcium ab-

sorption when given in excess. Excessive zinc can disrupt copper, calcium, and phosphorus absorption. Therefore maintaining both the diet and mineral supplementation at the correct levels and ratios is important. (Table 3-4 presents the recommended amounts of minerals in the diet of the cat and dog and the major causes and symptoms of mineral deficiencies and excesses.)

Preventive Nutrition

Given the various risk factors to an animal's health, the role of preventive nutrition becomes apparent. For example, deficiencies of calcium or phosphorus result in improper bone development in growing animals; essential amino acid deficiencies can retard growth, impair performance and health, and reduce resistance to infectious diseases; a lack of essential fatty acids can lead to serious skin problems; and a deficiency of thiamine and riboflavin can cause inadequate energy production (Lewis and others, 1994). Nutritional deficiencies have also been linked to weakened immunity (Beisel, 1981)

TABLE 3-2

VITAMIN REQUIREMENTS FOR THE DOG AND CAT AND SIGNS OF DEFICIENCY AND TOXICITY

| | MG (OR FOR A & D IU)/KG | | | | |
| | DOGS[56] | CATS[55] | | MAJOR SIGNS | |
VITAMIN	BODY WT*/DAY	DIET†	DIET†	DEFICIENCY‡	TOXICITY
A (3.3 IU = 1 mg retinol)	110	5000	5000	Reproductive failure, retinal degeneration, tearing, papilledema, keratomalacia, night blindness, photophobia, conjunctivitis, poor coat, weakness of hind legs, increased susceptibility to infectious diseases; plasma vitamin A level less than 10 μg retinol or 45 IU/dl	Anorexia, weight loss, bone decalcification, hyperesthesia, plasma vitamin A level above 600 μg retinol or 1800 IU/dl (normal—40-100 μg/dl)
D (40 IU = 1 μg)	11	500	500	Rickets in young, osteomalacia in adults, lordosis, chest deformity, and poor eruption of permanent teeth	Anorexia, weight loss, nausea, fatigue, soft tissue calcification, hypercalcemia, diarrhea, dehydration, death
E (alphatocopherol)	1.1 Up to threefold increase with increased unsaturated fat intake	50	50	Reproductive failure with weak or dead fetus, muscular dystrophy, pansteatitis, progressive retinal atrophy, intestinal lipofuscinosis (brown gut disease), impaired immunity	Anorexia, none others recorded
K	Not required except during antibacterial therapy or chronic ileal or colonic disease			Increased clotting time and hemorrhage	None recorded but high levels probably dangerous
C	Not required for normal dogs and cats			Retarded healing, increased susceptibility to disease, hemorrhage, anemia, rickets	Generally considered nontoxic
Thiamin (B₁)	0.02	1	5	Anorexia, vomiting, weight loss, dehydration, paralysis, prostration, abnormal reflexes, ataxia, convulsions, cardiac disorders, ventral flexion of neck (called "Chastek paralysis"), mydriasis	Nontoxic
Riboflavin (B₂)	0.1	2.2	4	Dry and scaly skin, erythema, posterior muscular weakness, anemia, sudden death, cheilosis, glossitis, pannus, reduced fertility, fatty liver, testicular hypoplasia	Nontoxic

Modified from Lewis L, Morris M, Hand M: *Small animal nutrition III*, Topeka, 1994, Mark Morris Institute.

*Twice these amounts are recommended during growth and lactation.

†Based on a diet providing 4.0 kcal metabolizable energy/g. For diets with a different caloric density, multiply the amount given times the quotient of (kcal/g of that diet ÷ 4).

‡All result in retarded growth or weight loss and most in anorexia.

Continued.

TABLE 3-2

VITAMIN REQUIREMENTS FOR THE DOG AND CAT AND SIGNS OF DEFICIENCY AND TOXICITY—cont'd

| VITAMIN | MG (OR FOR A & D IU)/KG | | | MAJOR SIGNS | |
| | DOGS[56] | CATS[55] | | | |
	BODY WT*/DAY	DIET†	DIET†	DEFICIENCY‡	TOXICITY
Niacin	0.25	11	40	"Black tongue," hemorrhagic diarrhea, anemia, reddening and ulceration of mucous membranes of mouth and tongue, death; in cats only signs possibly diarrhea, emaciation, death	Dilation of blood vessels; itching, burning of skin
Pyridoxine (B₆)	0.02	1	4	Microcytic hypochromic anemia, high serum iron level, atherosclerosis, convulsions	None recorded
Pantothenic acid	0.22	10	5	Anorexia, hypoglycemia, hypochloremia, blood urea nitrogen level increase, gastritis, enteritis, convulsions, fatty liver, coma, death	None recorded
Folic acid (pteroylglutamic acid)	0.004	0.18	0.8	Due to blood loss, prolonged malabsorption, or sulfonamide administration; hypoplasia of bone marrow, macrocytic anemia, glossitis	Nontoxic
Biotin	0.002	0.1	0.07	Scaly dermatitis, alopecia, anorexia, dried saliva around mouth, secretions around eyes, weakness, diarrhea, progressive spasticity, posterior paralysis	Nontoxic
Cobalamin (B₁₂)	0.0005	0.02	0.02	No clinical occurrence, macrocytic anemia resulting in experiments	Nontoxic
Choline§	26	1200	2000	Fatty liver, hypoalbuminemia; increased alkaline phosphatase, prothrombin time, hemoglobin and hematocrit values	Persistent diarrhea caused by 10 g/day or greater

§Although routinely listed as a vitamin, it is not and is not needed for metabolism. It is needed as a structural component of fat and nervous tissue.

Preventive nutrition involves assessing the nutritional needs of the individual animal with consideration of the animal's physical condition and various physiologic and environmental risk factors that may exist. Preventive nutrition also involves adding nutritional supplements to the basic diet to correct deficiencies and provide an optimal nutritional environment and preventing cellular degeneration and suboptimal function. Obtaining information about the nutrient and its relationship to other nutrients in the diet is necessary. Effective use of supplements requires consideration of five factors: need, dosage, form, balance, and safety. To this end, using scientifically formulated, high-quality nutritional formulations from well-established, respected manufacturers can take much of the guesswork out of incorporating nutritional supplementation into clinical practice.

Need

A number of specific conditions exist that may require supplementation for proper nutritional management of the cat, dog, and horse. Nutritional supplementation is generally indicated during growth, gestation, lactation, breeding, old age, periods of high stress, times of excessive physical activity, and illness. Evaluation of an animal's physical state usually gives clues to suboptimal nutritional status. Practitioners should note that the mere presence of a nutrient in the animal's food does not ensure its delivery to the cells

TABLE 3-3

MAIN FUNCTIONS OF ESSENTIAL TRACE ELEMENTS

ELEMENT	FUNCTION
Iron	Component of oxygen carriers such as hemoglobin and myoglobin
	Cofactor of enzymes in heme synthesis
	Component of cytochromes in the terminal oxidative pathway
Iodine	Incorporation into thyroid hormones, therefore essential for regulation of energy metabolism
Zinc	Component of over 120 enzymes in plants and animals, including alcohol dehydrogenase, carbonic anhydrase, superoxide dismutase
	Polysome structure and function in protein synthesis
	Stabilization of cell membranes
	Insulin storage in pancreas
	Skin
	Reproduction
	Immunity
	Taste and appetite
Copper	Component of many enzymes that catalyze reactions involving oxygen or related radicals, including tyrosinase, cytochrome oxidase, and superoxide dismutase; limited factor often in metabolic pathway; hence, sensitivity of pathway to copper status
	Synthesis of melanin, affecting color of skin and hair
	Synthesis of heme
	Myelinization of nerves
	Mineralization of bone
Manganese	Component of pyruvate carboxylase and superoxide dismutase
	Activator of glycosyltransferases involved in synthesis of glycosaminoglycans and glycoproteins
	Organic matrix of cartilage and bone
Molybdenum	Component of xanthine oxidase, involved in purine metabolism and production of uric acid
	Oxidation of sulfite to sulfate
Selenium	Component of glutathione peroxidase
	Integrity of cell membranes
	Hepatic microsomal oxidation and detoxication
Fluorine	Incorporation into mineral crystals of bone and teeth
	Resistance to dental caries

Modified from Kronfeld D: *Vitamins and mineral supplementation for dogs and cats,* Santa Barbara, Calif, 1989, Veterinary Practice Publishing.

and tissues that need it. Assimilation, transportation, and utilization of nutrients in the body are adversely affected, especially during times of stress and illness. Without analysis the actual levels of nutrients delivered by the diet may be questionable, as well as the amounts being assimilated and utilized.

Drugs can impair absorption, increase excretion, decrease nutrient utilization, and cause a loss of appetite in general (Roe, 1978, 1992). Conditions such as high levels of stress, disease states, and parasitic infestation in the animal may also create a nutritional deficiency. Stress studies in chickens (Pardue, Thaxton, 1986), pigs, and rabbits (Verde, Piguer, 1986) demonstrated that certain conditions (e.g., heat, pathogens) may increase the requirement for vitamin C beyond the animal's ability to synthesize it.

Dosage

Once the need for supplementation has been established, proper dosage levels must be determined. Information from scientific literature and manufacturer's guidelines usually provide the best information regarding dosage. NRC guidelines are only minimal foundational levels and do not represent needs based on biochemical individuality or the actual amount of nutrients being utilized from the diet. The initial dosage of a particular supplement may vary from suggested published levels depending on the nutrient. This variation may be true for water-soluble vitamins such as C and the B-complex vitamins. The feeding program may also call for dosage adjustment once beneficial results are evident.

TABLE 3-4

MINERAL REQUIREMENTS FOR THE DOG AND CAT AND EFFECTS OF DEFICIENCY AND EXCESS

MINERAL	UNITS	REQUIREMENT (DOG AND CAT) IN DIET*	DEFICIENCY	EXCESS
Calcium	%	0.5†–0.9	Occurs when meat or organ tissue comprise majority of diet; **initially:** lameness, stiffness, reluctance to move, constipation, enlarged metaphyses, splayed toes, carpal and tarsal hyperextension; when **chronic:** spontaneous fractures, limb deviations, anorexia, dehydration, loose teeth; when **acute:** tetany	Most commonly caused by oversupplementation; may cause phosphorus, zinc, iron, and copper deficiencies; slows growth, decreases thyroid function, and may predispose to bloat
Phosphorus	%	0.2†–0.6	Generally caused by excessive calcium supplementation. Causes depraved appetite and same signs as a calcium deficiency	From oversupplementation or high P diets; causes Ca deficiency; Ca is increased enough to offset excess P, results in excess Ca; excess P promoting renal damage
Potassium	%	0.4	Caused by excess losses from diarrhea or diuretics, or inadequate intake because of anorexia; causes anorexia, weakness, lethargy, and decreased muscle tone, which may cause head drooping, ataxia, and ascending paralysis	Does not occur unless oliguria present; causes hyperkalemia, same signs as a deficiency, cardiotoxicity, and death
Sodium	%	0.1–0.5‡	Polyuria, salt hunger, pica, weight loss, fatigue, agalactia, and slow growth§	**Acute:** Occurs only with inadequate nonsaline, good quality water; causes thirst, pruritus, constipation, anorexia, seizures and death§; **Chronic:** high amounts in many pet foods may induce hypertension, resulting in increased heart and renal disease
Magnesium	%	0.05–0.10‡	Retarded growth, spreading of toes, hyperextension of carpus and tarsus, hyperirritability, convulsions, soft tissue calcification, enlargement of the metaphysis of long bones§	Acute excess intake causing diarrhea because of poor absorption§; chronic intake of high amounts present in many cat foods contributing to urolithiasis and cystitis
Iron	mg/kg	60	May occur if fed milk exclusively for an extended period or secondary to blood loss; causes microcytic-hypochromic anemia, anisocytosis, and poikilocytosis of erythrocytes	Anorexia, weight loss, hypoalbuminemia, hemochromatosis§; Death following excess administration to young, particularly if they are vitamin E or selenium deficient§

Modified from Lewis L, Morris M, Hand M: *Small animal nutrition III,* Topeka, 1994, Mark Morris Institute.
*Based on a diet providing 4.0 kcal metabolizable energy/g. For diets with a different caloric density, multiply the amount given times the quotient of (kcal/g of that diet ÷ 4).
†Ca should equal or exceed P, and twice these amounts are recommended during growth and lactation.
‡The greater amount is recommended during lactation.
§This mineral imbalance is rare in dogs and cats.

TABLE 3-4

MINERAL REQUIREMENTS FOR THE DOG AND CAT AND EFFECTS OF DEFICIENCY AND EXCESS—cont'd

MINERAL	REQUIREMENT (DOG AND CAT)		DEFICIENCY	EXCESS
	UNITS	IN DIET*		
Zinc	mg/kg	50	Anorexia, weight loss, slow growth, emesis, generalized thinning of hair coat, scaly dermatitis, parakeratosis, hair depigmentation, decreased testicular development and wound healing, depression, and peripheral lymphadenopathy	Causes a calcium and/or copper deficiency§
Copper	mg/kg	7	May be caused by excess zinc, iron, or molybdenum; slow growth, bone lesions similar to calcium deficiency, pica, and liver copper less than 20 μg/g wet weight. Reported that anemia, hair depigmentation, and diarrhea do not occur in cats as they do in other species	Occurs in Bedlington terriers because of their inability to mobilize hepatic copper, resulting in signs of liver disease
Manganese	mg/kg	5	Impaired reproduction, abortion, enlarged joints, stiffness, reluctance to move; short, thick, and brittle bones§	Partial albinism, impaired fertility§
Iodine	mg/kg	1.5	Hypothyroidism, goiter, alopecia, fetal resorption, cretinism, myxedema, lethargy, drowsiness, timidity; at necropsy, feline thyroid weight >12 mg/100 g body weight	Same as a deficiency§
Selenium	mg/kg	0.1	"White muscle disease," skeletal and cardiac myopathy	Based on data in other species: nervousness, anorexia, vomiting, weakness, ataxia, dyspnea, and death caused by pulmonary edema within hours to days§

Form

The form of a nutrient in a supplement may affect its assimilation and use by the animal. This is especially true of minerals in which inorganic salts are poorly absorbed (5% to 20%) compared with organic chelated minerals with significantly higher absorption levels (50% to 80%) (Ashmead, 1970). Although chelated minerals are generally more expensive, the improved assimilation and reduced interaction with other minerals make the product more cost effective because its dosage can be significantly lower than that of inorganic forms. Another advantage of chelated organic minerals is that the minerals are retained in the body longer than sulfates and chlorides (Jensen, 1979).

The form of a vitamin may also affect its bioavailability. Pyridoxal phosphate, the active form of vitamin B_6, is better absorbed and transported than pyridoxine hydrochloride (Henderson, 1984). When administered at high levels in the pure ascorbic acid form, vitamin C can cause some gastrointestinal tract disturbance because of increased acidity. A concomitant loss of minerals also occurs when excess ascorbic acid is excreted in the urine. Vitamin C given as calcium or magnesium ascorbate overcomes these limitations. Another improved form of vitamin C is the polyascorbate form, Ester-C, which has been shown to have improved absorption and retention properties compared with other forms of ascorbate (Bush, 1987; Verlangieri, 1987, 1991). It also contains other biologically active metabolites of ascorbic acid. Ester-C has been used effectively against osteoarthritis, rheumatoid arthritis, and canine hip dysplasia (Berge, 1990).

Balance

Balance refers to the relationship among nutrients in the diet relative to use and absorption. Higher levels of some nutrients can reduce absorption of other nutrients. Minerals with this relationship are calcium and magnesium, sodium and potassium, and zinc and copper. Minerals in these pairs affect each other; consequently the total intake of these minerals must be balanced to prevent problems (Lewis and others, 1994). Vitamins are less affected by these interactions, but a large dose of a single vitamin can also have implications for the absorption, use, and excretion of other vitamins. When a higher dose of a single nutrient is required, use of a broad-spectrum vitamin/mineral supplement is recommended because it helps maintain proper balance by raising the nutritional levels of other nutrients as well.

Rationale for Using Nutritional Supplements

The approach of preventive nutrition is to remove nutritional risk factors from an animal's diet to maintain optimal health and well-being and prevent the onset of disease. Providing an animal with the highest-quality diet is important but will not always accomplish the goal.

Studies of nutritional supplements have shown the effectiveness of using well-designed nutritional supplements to overcome subclinical deficiencies and health problems during times of growth, gestation, lactation, heavy stress, and work (Machlin, Sauberlich, 1994). Nutritional supplementation has also been shown to increase life span. In one study a group of mice received extra pantothenic acid in their drinking water with a commercial stock diet and were compared with a control group given only the commercial stock diet (supplying all nutrients, including pantothenic acid). The mice receiving the additional pantothenic acid had an increased longevity of nearly 20% (Williams, Kalita, 1977). Strengthening only one link in the nutritional chain produced this result. Essential nutrients in levels exceeding the basic requirements may significantly reduce degenerative conditions and increase the healthy life span of animals (Cutler, 1991). Nutritional supplements increase the efficiency of cellular regeneration, enhance the elimination of waste products and toxic substances, and decrease the damaging effect of free radicals (Halliwell, 1994; Sies, Stahl, 1995), all of which have been linked to the aging process. Better nutrition for the cell allows all organs and systems to recover faster from the stresses of pollution and deteriorative phenomena that occur over time. With further research and better assessment methods the benefits of short- and long-term use of nutritional supplements will be even more fully realized and understood.

The Role of Specific Nutrients in Preventive Nutrition

Vitamins

Vitamins are essential substances that cannot be produced in the body in levels adequate to maintain health. With some minor exceptions, vitamins must be supplied in the animal's diet. Vitamins function primarily as coenzymes to catalyze reactions in the body (Lehninger and others, 1993). When they are not present in adequate levels, metabolism slows and the deficiency disease associated with the vitamin eventually occurs. In addition to preventing deficiency diseases, most vitamins play other biologic roles. Deficiencies of certain vitamins and antioxidants have been linked to degenerative diseases such as cancer, heart disease, and cataracts (Machlin, 1995; Schalch, Weber, 1994). For instance, vitamins A, C, and E function as antioxidants and protect the cells from free-radical damage (Halliwell, 1994; Machlin, Bendich, 1987). (See Table 3-2 for a list of certain vitamins and their major clinical signs of deficiency in cats and dogs. Box 3-1 summarizes the major benefits of the vitamins.)

Minerals

Minerals perform many functions in the body. They are needed for the proper composition of body fluids, formation of blood and bone, and maintenance of healthy nerve function. Minerals also function as components of metalloenzymes in thousands of biologic reactions (Lewis and others, 1994) (Box 3-2).

Essential Fatty Acids

Dietary requirements for essential fatty acids (EFAs) vary among animals. EFAs are polyunsaturates and include members of the omega-6 series (linoleic acid, gamma-linolenic acid, and arachidonic acid) and members of the omega-3 series (alpha-linolenic acid, docosahexaenoic acid, and eicosapentaenoic acid). These fatty acids play a vital role in the structures of cell membranes. They are also involved in the synthesis of several series of prostaglandins and other eicosanoids that regulate various metabolic functions, such as platelet aggregation and inflammatory processes (Fig. 3-1). Essential fatty acids stimulate growth, benefit skin and hair, influence the inflammatory response, and affect the development of the nervous system, including the brain (Kendler, 1987; Thomsett, Lloyd, 1989; White, 1993) (Box 3-3).

Amino Acids and Derivatives

In addition to the essential and nonessential amino acids, which are the components of enzymes and other proteins, other amino acids and derivatives have important functions in cellular metabolism and structure (Blackburn, 1983). These include L-carnitine, taurine, L-glutathione, glutamine, and *N,N*-dimethylglycine (DMG).

L-Carnitine, produced in the cell from methionine and lysine, is needed to transfer fatty acids across the inner mitochondrial membrane of cells. Because L-carnitine is essential in the process of converting fatty acids into energy,

BOX 3-1

MAJOR BENEFITS OF VITAMINS IN PREVENTIVE NUTRITION

VITAMIN A
Prevents eye and skin disorders
Enhances immunity
Protects against air pollution
Helps maintain epithelial tissue
Acts as an antioxidant

VITAMIN B-COMPLEX
Maintains nerve function, skin, hair, liver, and muscle tone
Is needed for energy production
Is essential for red blood cell function
Acts to reduce the effects of stress

VITAMIN C
Enhances tissue growth and wound healing
Acts as an antioxidant
Enhances immune function
Acts as an antiinflammatory agent
Acts to reduce stress
Improves cardiovascular function
Helps lower cholesterol

VITAMIN E
Acts as an antioxidant
Improves circulation
Aids in preventing cataracts
Helps prevent cardiovascular disease
Improves the immune system

BOX 3-2

MAJOR BENEFITS OF MINERALS IN PREVENTIVE NUTRITION

CALCIUM
Is necessary for development of bones and teeth
Regulates nerve function
Is necessary for bone strength and integrity

MAGNESIUM
Is essential for energy production
Acts to reduce the effects of stress
Helps prevent muscle weakness
Helps maintain proper pH balance

PHOSPHORUS
Is necessary for bone and teeth formation

CHROMIUM
Is involved in glucose metabolism

COPPER
Aids in formation of bone, hemoglobin, and red blood cells
Enhances healing
Helps prevent osteoporosis

IODINE
Is incorporated into thyroid hormones
Is essential for regulation of energy

IRON
Is necessary for hemoglobin and myoglobin production

MANGANESE
Is necessary for protein and fat metabolism
Aids immune function
Is required for energy production
Aids bone growth and reproduction

POTASSIUM
Helps maintain heart function and the nervous system
Helps regulate blood pressure

SELENIUM
Acts as an antioxidant
Aids immune function
Aids in heart function

ZINC
Is necessary for protein and collagen formation
Aids the immune system
Enhances wound healing

a deficiency of L-carnitine may result in increased fat storage, decreased performance, and exacerbation of heart disease associated with mitochondrial defects (Shils and others, 1994). Some evidence indicates L-carnitine biosynthesis is reduced in the newborn offspring of several species, including the horse (Frankel, McGarry, 1980).

Taurine belongs to a separate group of amino acids not found in proteins that contain a sulfonic acid group. Synthesized from cysteine, it is found in high concentrations in the heart, skeletal muscle, and central nervous system. It is a key component of bile, which is essential for the digestion of fats, absorption of fat-soluble vitamins, and control of serum cholesterol levels (Blackburn and others, 1983). Taurine is an essential component of the cat's diet, in which a deficiency has been linked to retinal degeneration, reproductive problems, and dilated cardiomyopathy (Hayes, 1982; Pion and others, 1987).

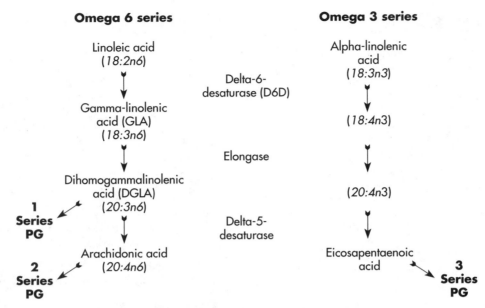

Omega 6 series

Linoleic acid
(*18:2n6*)

Gamma-linolenic
acid (GLA)
(*18:3n6*)

Dihomogammalinolenic
acid (DGLA)
(*20:3n6*)

**1
Series
PG**

Arachidonic acid
(*20:4n6*)

**2
Series
PG**

Delta-6-
desaturase (D6D)

Elongase

Delta-5-
desaturase

Omega 3 series

Alpha-linolenic
acid
(*18:3n3*)

(*18:4n3*)

(*20:4n3*)

Eicosapentaenoic
acid

**3
Series
PG**

Fig. 3-1 Outline of prostaglandin formation from essential fatty acids. (From Kendler B: Gamma-linoleic acid: physiological effects and potential medical applications, *J Applied Nutr* 39:79, 1987.)

BOX 3-3

BENEFITS OF OMEGA-3 AND OMEGA-6 FATTY ACIDS IN PREVENTIVE NUTRITION

LINOLEIC ACID
Maintains healthy skin and hair coats

GAMMA-LINOLENIC ACID
Is necessary for proper growth and development of the nervous system

ALPHA-LINOLENIC ACID
Is involved in prostaglandin synthesis

EICOSAPENTAENOIC ACID
Enhances reproduction processes
Prevents symptoms associated with allergic, inflammatory skin disease
Improves cardiovascular health

L-Glutathione is a tripeptide derived from glycine, glutamic acid, and cysteine. It is an important reducing agent in the cell and functions as a powerful antioxidant that inhibits the formation of free radicals (Levine, Kidd, 1985). It also helps detoxify heavy metals and drugs (Sies, Wendel, 1978).

Glutamine plays a major role in the health of the digestive system. Glutamine is the primary energy source of the intestinal mucosal cells during stress and illness, and during such times, demand for glutamine increases greatly (Souba and others, 1985). Glutamine is useful in treating conditions associated with the digestive tract and may be useful in inflammatory bowel disease (Burton, Anderson, 1983; Fox and others, 1987, 1988). Glutamine also strengthens the immune system, aids healing, and prevents muscle breakdown during times of injury or stress (Jepson, 1988; Newsholme, 1990; Welbourne, 1993). Glutamine is a precursor to glucosamines, which are used in the production of glycosaminoglycans in the body and the synthesis of purine nucleotides (Shils and others, 1994).

N,N-Dimethylglycine (DMG) is the dimethylated derivative of glycine. Produced naturally from choline and betaine in the body, DMG enhances immunologic processes by modulating the production of lymphocytes and antibodies, improves oxygen use, and decreases allergic responses (Graber and others, 1981; Reap, Lawson, 1990). DMG can enhance performance and reduce lactic-acid buildup in oxygen-deficient environments such as those experienced by equine and canine athletes (Gannon, 1983; Levine, 1982). (Box 3-4 summarizes the benefits of certain amino acids in preventive nutrition.)

Antioxidants

Antioxidants protect the cell from free-radical damage. Free radicals are highly reactive species containing an unpaired electron such as a superoxide, hydroxyl, or peroxide radical that, left unchecked, can cause extensive damage to cell membranes, enzymes, and genetic material (DNA and RNA) in the cell. Antioxidants help the body destroy these free radicals, which have been associated with a number of pathologic degenerative conditions such as cancer, arthritis, cardiovascular disease, and premature aging (Levine, 1985; Stocker, 1991). Free radicals may form from exposure to radiation, overexposure to solar rays, environmental toxins, heavy metals, pollution, and a

BOX 3-4

AMINO ACIDS' AND DERIVATIVES' BENEFITS IN PREVENTIVE NUTRITION

L-CARNITINE
Enhances lipid metabolism

GLUTATHIONE
Scavenges free radicals
Helps prevent cataracts

TAURINE
Prevents retinal degeneration
Reduces reproductive problems
Helps reduce elevated cholesterol levels

GLUTAMINE
Reduces muscle wasting
Helps reduce inflammatory bowel conditions

N,N-DIMETHYLGLYCINE
Enhances immune function
Improves endurance and performance
Protects cardiovascular system

BOX 3-5

ANTIOXIDANT NUTRIENTS THAT FUNCTION AS FREE RADICAL SCAVENGERS

Vitamin A
Beta-carotene
Vitamin C
Vitamin E
Glutathione
Selenium
Zinc
Cysteine
Methionine
Proanthocyanidins
Coenzyme Q_{10}

variety of natural processes such as cellular respiration and macrophage activity. Deficiencies of free-radical scavengers can lead to significant free-radical damage over time (Halliwell, 1994), causing inflammation and a weakened immune system. (Box 3-5 lists antioxidant nutrients that function as free-radical scavengers.)

Accessory Food Factors

Some dietary components may not be essential for the prevention of a specific degenerative disease but are useful in improving cellular efficiency and overall metabolic reactions. Important examples include coenzyme Q_{10}, bioflavonoids, and choline.

Coenzyme Q_{10} is found in the mitochondria of all cells and is essential for the production of adenosine triphosphate (ATP) in the cell. Research suggests that coenzyme Q_{10} may be useful in several disease states because of an increase in cellular energy. Coenzyme Q_{10} also improves cellular immunity and macrophage activity (Bliznakov, 1978, 1970). It has been used in the treatment of heart disease (Fujioka, 1983; Kamikawa, 1985; Kitamura, 1984; Langsjoien, 1990; Matsushima, 1992), periodontal disease (Wilkinson, 1976), and diabetes (Kishi, 1976). Coenzyme Q_{10} production declines with age, and supplementation in older animals may be especially helpful (Folkers, 1986).

Bioflavonoids, including the special class of polyphenols known as *proanthocyanindins*, work especially well with vitamin C to speed healing of wounds and bruises. Bioflavonoids help reduce inflammation (Amella, 1985;

Middleton, Drzewieki, 1985; Pearce and others, 1984), strengthen capillaries (Gabor, 1972), scavenge free radicals, have antiviral activity (Kaul and others, 1985), and enhance immune function (Facino, 1994).

Choline is a part of the phospholipid known as *phosphatidylcholine* and of sphingomyelin, essential components of all cell membranes. It is also found in acetylcholine, an important neurotransmitter, and choline supplementation may have some use in certain neurologic and behavioral problems (Harless, Turbes, 1982). Choline acts as a methyl donor in the oxidation process to form betaine and DMG. The demand for choline as a methyl donor is probably the major factor that determines the speed with which a diet deficient in choline induces pathologic changes. Choline can function as a lipotrophic agent to protect the liver. Rats fed a choline-deficient diet had reduced carnitine levels in liver, heart, and skeletal muscle, which was probably caused by methyl-group deficiency (Shils and others, 1994).

Preventive Nutrition for the Cat

Cats are carnivorous animals. Unlike canine carnivores, however, their ancestral predatory styles and eating habits directly relate to their unique metabolisms and different nutritional needs. Some special nutrients required by the cat include the essential fatty acids gamma-linolenic acid and arachidonic acid, taurine, and preformed vitamin A, which is needed because the cat cannot convert beta-carotene to vitamin A (National Research Council, 1986). Because of low activity of the enzyme pyrroline-5-carboxylate synthase, cats have higher requirements for the amino acid arginine. More details on the specific nutritional needs of cats for growth, maintenance, pregnancy, and lactation can be found in the NRC guidelines (National Research Council, 1986). (Table 3-5 lists the recommended minimum nutrient requirements for the adult cat.)

TABLE 3-5

RECOMMENDED MINIMUM NUTRIENT LEVELS IN DOG AND CAT DIETS

NUTRIENT	DOGS	CATS
Protein (g)*	22	28
Fat (g)†	5.5	9.0
Linoleic and arachidonic acids (g)†	1.1	1.0
Arachidonic acid alone (g)†	—	0.02
Calcium (g)	1.1	1.0
Phosphorus (g)	0.9	0.8
Ca/P ratio	0.8-1.5:1	0.8-1.5:1
Sodium (g)	0.08	0.2
Potassium (g)	0.5	0.5
Magnesium (g)	0.04	0.05
Iron (mg)‡	8.0	10
Copper (mg)‡	0.7	0.5
Manganese (mg)‡	0.5	1.0
Zinc (mg)‡	5.0	4.0
Iodine (mg)	0.15	0.1
Selenium (μg)	10	10
Vitamin A (IU)	500	550
Vitamin D (IU)	50	100
Vitamin E (mg)†	5.0	8.0
Vitamin K (μg)§	8.0	10
Thiamin (mg)	0.1	0.5
Riboflavin (mg)	0.25	0.5
Pantothenic acid (mg)	1.1	1.0
Niacin (mg)	1.2	4.5
Pyridoxine (mg)	0.12	0.4
Folic acid (μg)§	22	100
Vitamin B_{12} (μg)	2.7	2.0
Choline (mg)	125	200
Biotin (mg)§	0.05	0.007
Taurine (mg)‖	—	100 or 250

Values expressed per 400 kcal (1.7 MJ) metabolizable energy (ME), which approximates to 100 g dry matter (DM) in typical commercial pet foods.
Modified from Simpson J, Anderson R, Markwell P: *Clinical nutrition of the dog and cat*, London, 1993, Blackwell Scientific.
*Protein levels assume a balanced amino acid profile and satisfactory digestibility.
†Fat content stated only as a guide. Key nutrients are the essential fatty acids (EFA) linoleic and arachidonic acids. With high levels of EFA, vitamin E needs to be increased.
‡Figures assume high availability. It is particularly important to ensure that this is the case with these nutrients.
§A dietary requirement for these nutrients has not been demonstrated when natural ingredients were fed. Intestinal bacterial synthesis can meet the needs of the animal. Supplementation may be necessary if antibacterial or antivitamin compounds are being administered or present in the diet.
‖100 mg/400 kcal for dry foods, 250 mg/400 kcal for canned foods.

Cats have a limited ability to synthesize taurine and are susceptible to a dietary deficiency of this essential nutrient. A long-term deficiency of taurine can lead to retinal degeneration, dilated cardiomyopathy, and reproductive problems such as growth abnormalities and increased mortality in kittens (National Research Council, 1986; Simpson and others, 1993).

Calcium deficiency can lead to serious problems in growing kittens, including lameness, abnormal gait or stance, bone pain, and fractures. Such skeletal problems are generally caused by an incorrect relationship between calcium and phosphorus levels and ratios, which should

be approximately 1:1 (National Research Council, 1986). These mineral imbalances commonly lead to secondary hyperparathyroidism. A calcium deficiency usually occurs when cats are fed a diet consisting only of fresh meat or filter organs, a practice that is not uncommon among cat owners. Excess phosphorus, even in the presence of adequate calcium, can also lead to the same problem. (Table 3-6 lists the nutrient requirements of cats according to the NRC and CVMA Pet Food Certification Program.)

Cats cannot convert linoleic acid to gamma-linolenic acid (and therefore into arachidonic acid) because they lack the necessary Δ_5 and Δ_6 desaturase enzymes (National

TABLE 3-6

NUTRIENT REQUIREMENTS OF CATS* ACCORDING TO THE U.S. NRC AND THE CVMA PET FOOD CERTIFICATION PROGRAM

NUTRIENT	NRC† (1986)	NRC (1978)	CVMA‡ (1987)	CVMA§ (1987)
Protein (%)	24.00‖	33.30	28.00	55.00
Arginine (%)	1.00			
Histidine (%)	0.30			
Isoleucine (%)	0.50			
Leucine (%)	1.20			
Lysine (%)	0.80			
Met-cys¶ (%)	0.75			
Phe-tyr# (%)	0.85			
Threonine (%)	0.70			
Tryptophan (%)	0.15			
Valine (%)	0.60			
Taurine (%)	0.04		0.04	
Fat (%)			9.00**	50.00
Linoleic acid (%)	0.50		1.00	
Arachidonic acid (%)	0.02		0.01	
Minerals				
Calcium (%)	0.80		1.00	4.00
Phosphorus (%)	0.60		0.80	
Potassium (%)	0.44		0.30	
Sodium (%)	0.05		0.20	
Chloride (%)	0.19		0.30	
Magnesium (%)	0.04		0.05	
Iron (mg/kg)	80.00		100.00	1500.00
Copper (mg/kg)	5.00		5.00	
Manganese (mg/kg)	5.00		10.00	
Zinc (mg/kg)	50.00		30.00††	
Iodine (mg/kg)	0.35		1.00	
Selenium (mg/kg)	0.10		0.10	10.00
Vitamins				
A (IU/kg)	3333.00	27777.00	10000.00	87000.00
D (IU/kg)	500.00	1111.00	1000.00	10000.00
E (IU/kg)	30.00	151.00	80.00‡‡	1000.00
K (IU/kg)	—§§			2000.00
Thiamin (mg/kg)	5.00	4.40	5.00	5000.00
Riboflavin (mg/kg)	4.00	4.40	5.00	100.00
Panto ac§§ (mg/kg)	5.00	5.50	10.00	2000.00
Niacin (mg/kg)	40.00	44.00	45.00	
Pyridoxine (mg/kg)	4.00	2.20	4.00	50.00
Folic acid (mg/kg)	0.80§§		1.00	
Biotin (mg/kg)	0.07§§		0.05	1.00
B₁₂ (μg/kg)	0.02		0.02	6.00
Choline (g/kg)	2.40	3.30		

Modified from Kronfeld D: *Vitamins and mineral supplementation for dogs and cats,* Santa Barbara, Calif, 1989, Veterinary Practice Publishing Co.
*Expressed as a percentage or amount per kg DM.
†DM basis, 5 kcal ME/g.
‡DM basis, 4 kcal ME/g.
§Suggested upper limit.
‖Protein minimum if minimums are met for all essential amino acids.
¶Methionine-cystine.
#Phenylalanine-tyrosine.
**Fat needed for palatability and to reach 4 kcal/g DM.
††Zinc may need to exceed 40 mg/kg in vegetable-protein bsed diets.
‡‡Vitamin E may need to be higher, perhaps 90 to 120 IU/kg when large amounts of polyunsaturated oils such as tuna oil are used.
§§These vitamins may not be required in the diet except when antimicrobials or antivitamins are present.

Research Council, 1986). Cats must therefore consume preformed arachidonic acid, which is found only in animal sources. Deficiency of arachidonic acid can result in dry, scaly skin; a lusterless coat; and if the deficiency continues, skin infections, alopecia, edema, and lesion-forming moist dermatitis (MacDonald, 1984; Rivers, 1982). Cats also must have adequate amounts of antioxidants (e.g., vitamins C and E, selenium) to protect the unsaturated fatty acids from oxidation.

Zinc deficiencies in the cat usually appear as skin problems and allergic reactions. Cats may also show delayed growth, vomiting, and an overall poor appearance (Brown, 1990). In most cases, supplementation with a multiple vitamin and mineral product reverses these subclinical deficiencies without causing imbalances or excesses of any single nutrient. Other essential supplements are vitamins A, C, and E and other antioxidants, which prevent disease and are effective in keeping the cat healthy during times of stress. (Table 3-7 describes an effective multiple vitamin/mineral supplement for cats that focuses on form, balance, and appropriate potency.)

Preventive Nutrition for the Dog

Dogs have been with humans longer than any other domesticated animal. This relationship has been complex, with many breeds being removed from their natural environments. Breeding practices have attempted to control mutations, resulting in interbreed and intrabreed differences in physiology and nutritional requirements. A well-balanced diet accompanied by a high-quality nutritional supplement is therefore important in maintaining canine health. Manipulating the diet according to individual and breed requirements may be necessary.

The basic nutrient requirements for the adult dog are found in Tables 3-5 and 3-8. Because these values are based on averages, adjustments for specific nutrients based on each dog's biochemical needs is necessary. The key is to use a high-quality program from a variety of foods that provide nutrients according to individual need. The dog generally consumes sufficient food to deliver the metabolizable energy required, and therefore the overall quality of the diet is critical to ensure adequate intake of essential nutrients.

Dogs do not have as many unique nutritional needs as cats. Dogs do require certain polyunsaturated fatty acids, and a deficiency of dietary fat may result in slower growth and dermatitis. Studies have shown that members of the linoleic acid (n-6) series are the essential fatty acids required (National Research Council, 1985), although recent studies suggest a role for the n-3 fatty acids for skin health (Logas, Kunkle, 1994). Supplementation with a

TABLE 3-7

QUALITY FELINE VITAMIN AND MINERAL SUPPLEMENT: RECOMMENDED DAILY FEEDING PROGRAM

SUPPLEMENT	AMOUNT	SUPPLEMENT	AMOUNT
Vitamin A	900 IU	Gamma-linoleic acid	10 mg
Vitamin D_3	50 IU	Calcium (bonemeal)	50 mg
Vitamin E	5 IU	Phosphorus (bonemeal)	25 mg
Vitamin K	2 µg	Magnesium (citrate)	1.5 mg
Vitamin C (ascorbic acid)	20 mg	Potassium (citrate)	250 µg
Thiamine	2 mg	Taurine	200 mg
Riboflavin	2 mg	Iron (peptonate)	1.5 mg
Niacinamide	5 mg	Copper (gluconate)	30 µg
Pyridoxine	2 mg	Zinc (gluconate)	1 mg
Folic acid	2 µg	Iodine (kelp)	40 µg
Biotin	2 µg	Chromium (yeast)	3.5 µg
Vitamin B_{12}	2 µg	Selenium (yeast)	3.5 µg
Pantothenic acid	5 mg	Desiccated liver	600 mg
Paraaminobenzoic acid (PABA)	2 mg	Perna canaliculus	100 mg
Choline (Bitartrate)	5 mg	Digestive enzymes (enteric coated)	
Inositol	2 mg	Pepsin	1.5 mg
DL-Methionine	10 mg	Papain	1.5 mg
Cystine	5 mg	Bromelain	1.5 mg
Betaine HCl	10 mg	Protease enzymes	1.5 mg
Lecithin	5 mg	Ox bile	2.5 mg
Linoleic acid	25 mg	Lipase enzymes	2.5 mg

Courtesy VetriScience Laboratories, Essex Jct, Vt, 1996.

TABLE 3-8

NUTRIENT REQUIREMENTS OF DOGS* ACCORDING TO THE U.S. NRC AND THE CVMA PET FOOD CERTIFICATION PROGRAM

NUTRIENT	NRC† (1985)	NRC‡ (1974)	CVMA‡ (1987)	CMVA§ (1987)
Protein (%)	10.51‖			
Arginine (%)	0.50			
Histidine (%)	0.18			
Isoleucine (%)	0.36			
Leucine (%)	0.58			
Lysine (%)	0.51			
Met-cys¶ (%)	0.39			
Phe-tyr# (%)	0.72			
Threonine (%)	0.47			
Tryptophan (%)	0.15			
Valine (%)	0.39			
Essential (%)	4.25			
Dispensable (%)	6.26			
Fat (%)	5.00	5.00	5.00	50.00
Linoleic acid (%)	1.00	1.00	1.00	
Minerals				
Calcium (%)	0.59	1.10	1.10	4.00
Phosphorus (%)	0.44	0.90	0.90	
Potassium (%)	0.44	0.60	0.60	
Sodium (%)	0.06	0.44	0.44	
Chloride (%)	0.09	0.66	0.66	
Magnesium (%)	0.04	0.04	0.04	
Iron (mg/kg)	31.90	60.00	60.00	1500.00
Copper (mg/kg)	2.90	7.30	7.30	
Manganese (mg/kg)	5.10	5.00	5.00	
Zinc (mg/kg)	35.6**	50.00††	50.00††	
Iodine (mg/kg)	0.59	1.54	1.54	
Selenium (mg/kg)	0.11	0.11††	0.11	10.00
Vitamins				
A (IU/kg)	3710.00	5000.00	5000.00	37100.00
D (IU/kg)	404.00	500.00	500.00	4000.00
E (IU/kg)	22.00	50.00	50.00	1000.00
K (IU/kg)	0.0‡‡			2000.00
Thiamin (mg/kg)	1.00	1.00	1.00	1000.00
Riboflavin (mg/kg)	2.50	2.20	2.20	44.00
Panto ac§§ (%)	9.90	10.00	10.00	2000.00

Modified from Kronfeld D: *Vitamins and mineral supplementation for dogs and cats,* Santa Barbara, Calif, 1989, Veterinary Practice Publishing Co.

*Expressed as a percentage or amount per kg DM.

†DM basis, 3.67 kcal ME/g.

‡DM basis, 3.5 to 4.0 kcal ME/g.

§Suggested upper limit.

‖Quantities sufficient to supply the minimum amounts of available and indispensable (essential) and dispensable amino acids (in purified diets). Compounding practical foods from natural ingredients (protein digestibility ± 70%) may require quantities representing an increase of 40% or greater than the sum of the amino acids as listed depending on ingredients used and processing procedures.

¶Methionine-cystine.

#Phenylalanine-tyrosine.

**In commercial foods with natural ingredients resulting in elevated calcium and phytate contents, borderline deficiencies were reported from feeding foods with less than 90 mg zinc per kg.

††Recommended allowance of nutrient, based on research with other species.

‡‡Dogs have a metabolic requirement, but a dietary requirement has not been demonstrated using natural ingredients.

§§These vitamins may not be required in the diet except when antimicrobials or antivitamins are present.

TABLE 3-8

NUTRIENT REQUIREMENTS OF DOGS* ACCORDING TO THE U.S. NRC AND THE CVMA PET FOOD CERTIFICATION PROGRAM—cont'd

NUTRIENT	NRC† (1985)	NRC‡ (1974)	CVMA‡ (1987)	CMVA§ (1987)
Niacin (mg/kg)	11.00	11.40	11.40	
Pyridoxine (mg/kg)	1.10	1.00	1.00	50.00
Folic acid (mg/kg)	0.20	0.18	0.18	
Biotin (mg/kg)	0.0‡‡	0.10††	0.10	1.00
B$_{12}$ (μg/kg)	26.00	22.00††	22.00	7.80
Choline (g/kg)	1.25	1.20	1.20	

balanced essential–fatty-acid product, including both gamma-linolenic and eicosapentaenoic acids, can help eliminate allergic skin problems such as pyoderma and dermatitis caused by fleas (Logas, 1994; Miller, 1989).

All dogs require a protein intake of 10 essential amino acids for proper growth and maintenance. These essential amino acids are arginine, histidine, isoleucine, leucine, lysine, methionine, phenylalanine, threonine, tryptophane, and valine (Kronfeld, 1989). A deficiency of just one essential amino acid may lead to major changes in food consumption and metabolic disturbances. Protein intake must be balanced to ensure that all the essential amino acids are being provided at optimum levels.

Feeding a multiple vitamin and mineral supplement along with a high-quality natural diet helps maintain optimum levels of key vitamins and minerals and prevent borderline deficiencies. Many experts believe that giving dogs supplements of vitamins C and E throughout their lives is essential for optimal health. Vitamins C and E play important roles in protecting the cells of the body from pollution, toxic substances, free radicals, and pathogenic agents by helping optimize the body's immune and detoxification systems (Halliwell, 1994). Dosages vary with age, size, health, and performance demands.

Supplements are generally better absorbed when given with meals. Dosages of vitamin C should be decreased if diarrhea occurs and increased during times of sickness or stress, when the need for vitamin C increases.

Mineral deficiencies in growing puppies can cause serious bone and skeletal problems. Proper balance and intake of calcium and phosphorus are critical. The calcium/phosphorus ratio of 1.2:1.0 to 1.4:1.0 in dogs is generally considered ideal for maximal assimilation and use. Avoiding excesses of both calcium and phosphorus in the diet is important. With the optimum ratio, vitamin-D requirements are minimized. Excessive amounts of vitamin D may lead to serious renal and skeletal problems (National Research Council, 1985).

As with the cat, a zinc deficiency in the dog can lead from general lethargy to severe growth retardation, skin lesions, and conjunctivitis. Diets that provide 60 mg of

zinc per kilogram of dry ingredient appear to meet maintenance requirements, but the necessary level can rise by 50% to 100% during gestation, lactation, and times of higher work loads (National Research Council, 1985).

Table 3-9 gives the nutrient levels found in a representative supplemental vitamin-mineral product for dogs. Such products provide adequate amounts of the essential nutrients without causing excesses or imbalances. Additional nutritional supplements can be added as required by special health problems or circumstances.

Preventive Nutrition for the Geriatric Dog and Cat

As dogs and cats age, their nutritional needs may vary according to their overall health and condition. Good dietary management can contribute to the well-being and optimal performance of older animals. An inadequate diet can contribute to obesity, poor digestion, suboptimal immunity, and a number of degenerative conditions, such as degenerative joint disorders, cancer, and cardiovascular, gastrointestinal, and renal problems that tend to increase in frequency as animals get older (Goldston, 1989; Hoskins, 1992). Kidney and liver diseases are a frequent cause of illness and death in both dogs and cats.

Older animals tend to become more sedentary as the reserve capacity of the body decreases, and total caloric intake should be reduced to avoid obesity. Poor nutrition in older animals can lead to increased sickness, delayed wound healing, hypoalbuminemia, cachexia, and inferior hair coats (Hoskins, 1992). Goldston (1995) gives a comprehensive overview of the structural and metabolic changes associated with aging in the dog and cat and the corresponding disease conditions that can result (Table 3-10).

Monitoring of the animal's overall condition by physical examinations and laboratory testing should indicate whether the current diet is adequate. A high-quality diet should be emphasized and excessive food intake avoided. Dogs and cats should receive adequate protein (approximately 30% of available energy) to maintain proper weight and body protein reserves (Kronfeld, 1983). Ade-

TABLE 3-9

TYPICAL QUALITY CANINE VITAMIN AND MINERAL SUPPLEMENT: RECOMMENDED DAILY FEEDING PROGRAM

SUPPLEMENT	AMOUNT	SUPPLEMENT	AMOUNT
Vitamin A (fish liver oil)	900 IU	Methionine	7.5 mg
Vitamin D_3 (fish liver oil)	75 IU	Inositol	3.75 mg
Vitamin E (DL-alpha-tocopherol acetate)	7.5 IU	Lecithin	7.5 mg
		Linoleic acid	37.5 mg
Vitamin C (ascorbic acid)	18.75 mg	Desiccated beef liver	1125 mg
Niacinamide	7.5 mg		
Paraaminobenzoic acid (PABA)	3.75 mg	**AMINO ACIDS†**	
Riboflavin (B_2)	3.75 mg	Lysine*	40.2 mg
Thiamine (B_1)	7.5 mg	Methionine*	18.3 mg
Pyridoxine (B_6)	3.75 mg	Leucine*	55.1 mg
Vitamin B_{12}	3 µg	Isoleucine*	31.5 mg
Folic acid	3 µg	Valine*	39.4 mg
Biotin	3 µg	Tryptophan*	9.8 mg
Vitamin K	3 µg	Threonine*	28.2 mg
d-Pantothenic acid (*d*-calcium pantothenate)	7.5 mg	Phenylalanine*	38 mg
		Arginine	42.6 mg
Carrot powder	1.5 mg	Histidine	13.7 mg
Xanthophyll	1.5 mg	Tyrosine	26.9 mg
Cobalt (carbonate)	60 µg	Cystine	7.9 mg
Iodine (kelp)	60 µg	Serine	34.1 mg
Potassium (citrate)	375 µg	Glutamic acid	76.1 mg
Zinc (gluconate)	1.5 mg	Alanine	42 mg
Magnesium (oxide)	37.5 mg	Aspartic acid	58.4 mg
Copper (gluconate)	4.5 µg		
Iron (hydex)	1.5 mg	**DIGESTIVE ENZYMES (ENTERIC COATED)**	
Iron (peptonate)	3 mg	Pepsin	2.25 mg
Phosphorus (tricalcium phosphate)	37.5 mg	Papain	2.25 mg
Calcium (tricalcium phosphate)	75 mg	Bromelin	2.25 mg
Selenium (yeast)	5.25 µg	Protease enzymes	2.25 mg
Chromium (yeast)	5.25 µg	Ox bile	3.75 mg
Choline (bitartrate)	7.5 mg	Lipase enzymes	3.75 mg
Betaine HCl	7.5 mg		

Courtesy VetriScience Laboratories, Essex Jct, Vt, 1996.
*Essential amino acid.
†From dessicated beef liver.

quate fat in the diet improves palatability, supplies essential fatty acids, and enhances absorption of fat-soluble nutrients, but too much fat contributes to obesity. A high-quality, commercially prepared pet food formulated specifically for the geriatric pet or a balanced, specially prepared diet made from fresh ingredients is especially important for improved longevity and wellness in older animals.

Supplementation of nutrients as a preventive measure can help maintain adequate levels of essential nutrients. Digestive enzymes may increase absorption of nutrients from foods and prevent gastrointestinal problems. Nutritional supplements such as vitamin C, coenzyme Q_{10},

DMG, and L-carnitine may enhance immune function, improve overall physical performance, and reduce the incidence and severity of age-related illness. Goldston and Hoskins (1995) especially recommend adequate intake of vitamins A, B_1, B_6, B_{12}, and E because of possible modifications in the digestive system. They also recommend increased intake of unsaturated fatty acids and zinc to maintain a healthy skin and coat. Keeping an older animal lean and a good preventive nutritional program are important for long-term health. Good dietary and nutritional management can enhance the older animal's quality of life and delay the onset of possible disease conditions associated with aging.

TABLE 3-10

NUTRITION AND NUTRITIONAL DISORDERS: STRUCTURAL AND METABOLIC CHANGES ASSOCIATED WITH AGING

BODY PART OR SYSTEM	CHANGES
Oral cavity	Dental calculus, periodontal disease, loss of teeth, oral ulcers, gingival hyperplasia
Digestive system	Altered liver and pancreatic functions; altered intestinal digestion and absorption; altered esophagus, stomach, and colon motility
Endocrine system	Decreased function of thyroid glands or pancreatic islet cells, hyperplasia or tumors of pituitary or adrenal glands, neoplasia of pancreatic islet cells
Integument	Loss of elasticity; thickened skin; dry, thin hair coat; altered function of sebaceous glands; graying of muzzle; brittle nails; hypersensitivity
Cardiovascular system	Structural alterations in heart and blood vessels
Genitourinary system	Reduced renal function, blood flow, and glomerular filtration rate; prostate gland hypertrophy; hyperplasia; squamous metaplasia; cysts; neoplasia
Musculoskeletal system	Loss of muscle mass and tone, brittle bones, degenerative joint disease, disturbed gait
Nervous system and special senses	Reduced reactivity to stimuli; altered memory; diminished visual acuity; lessened ability to heal, taste, perceive, and smell
Metabolism	Reduced sensitivity to thirst; reduced thermoregulation, physical activity, and rate of metabolism

Modified from Goldston R, Hoskins J: *Geriatrics and gerontology of the dog and cat,* Philadelphia, 1995, WB Saunders.

Preventive Nutrition for the Horse

The horse is a nonruminant herbivore, in whom fermentation occurs in the cecum and gut. Nutrient and energy requirements for the horse and pony are derived from forage and concentrated grains and vary greatly according to function and breed. The quality of forage from either pasture or dried hay greatly influences nutritional status and thus affects preventive nutrition. Tables 3-11 and 3-12 present the estimated requirements and recommendations for dietary nutrients for the horse (National Research Council, 1989).

Research in the field of equine nutrition has demonstrated that many health problems occurring throughout the horse's life span can be prevented or ameliorated by proper nutrition and a balanced feeding program (Hintz, Cymbaluk, 1994). Veterinarians, trainers, and equine nutritionists have debated the benefits of using equine nutritional supplements regularly. Many experts believe that supplementation is the key to a successful feed-management program in many instances.

Veterinarians generally agree on the value of supplementing the horse's diet when a deficiency is suspected or confirmed. The challenge lies in determining the horse's actual nutritional problem. Important considerations are biochemical individuality, physiologic state, and environmental factors that can influence possible deficiencies. Studying the NRC guidelines and doing a feed analysis are only part of the answer, mainly because of the large variation among groups of horses and seasonal crops. Some feel that a horse who is fed a high-quality, balanced ration does not require any special supplementation. Others believe that the use of supplements has provided improved nutrient levels needed for optimal growth, maintenance, reproduction, and performance. The goal of preventive nutrition is to raise the nutritional status and well-being of the horse.

Veterinarians often recommend equine nutritional supplements as an adjunct to therapy or a means of enhancing the nutritional status of growing foals, breeding stock, and high-performance horses. The fundamental purpose behind using a general supplement is to provide the horse with an array of essential vitamins, trace minerals, amino acids, and other food factors that may be in short supply in the basic feed ration (which may itself vary seasonally) or during times of increased demands. Borderline deficiencies or marginal levels of nutrients may be common in large numbers of horses as a result of poor farming practices, environmental conditions such as air and water pollution, and deficiencies in the local soils that, over the long term, can produce poor growth, suboptimal performance, slower recovery from heavy workouts or competition, and increased convalescent times. Many horse owners are aware that nutritional supplementation can be used as a form of preventive maintenance. Because subclinical deficiencies are generally not accompanied by physical signs, supplementation compensates for them and can prevent serious health problems later.

Although the general use of an equine multiple vitamin and mineral supplement may seem like a hit-or-miss

TABLE 3-11

DAILY NUTRIENT REQUIREMENTS OF HORSES (600-KG MATURE WEIGHT)

ANIMAL	WEIGHT (KG)	DAILY GAIN (KG)	DE (MCAL)	CRUDE PROTEIN (G)	LYSINE (G)	CAL-CIUM (G)	PHOS-PHORUS (G)	MAGNE-SIUM (G)	POTAS-SIUM (G)	VITAMIN A (10³ IU)
MATURE HORSES										
Maintenance	600		19.4	776	27	24	17	9.0	30.0	18
Stallions (breeding season)	600		24.3	970	34	30	21	11.2	36.9	27
Pregnant mares										
9 months	600		21.5	947	33	41	31	10.3	34.5	36
10 months			21.9	965	34	42	32	10.5	35.1	36
11 months			23.3	1024	36	44	34	11.2	37.2	36
Lactating mares										
Foaling to 3 months	600		33.7	1711	60	67	42	13.1	55.2	36
3 months to weaning	600		28.9	1258	44	43	27	10.4	39.6	36
Working horses										
Light work	600		24.3	970	34	30	21	11.2	36.9	27
Moderate work	600		29.1	1164	41	36	25	13.4	44.2	27
Intense work	600		38.8	1552	54	47	34	17.8	59.0	27
GROWING HORSES										
Weanling, 4 months	200	1.00	16.5	825	35	40	22	4.3	13.0	9
Weanling, 6 months										
Moderate growth	245	0.75	17.0	850	36	34	19	4.6	14.5	11
Rapid growth	245	0.95	19.2	960	40	40	22	4.9	15.1	11
Yearling, 12 months										
Moderate growth	375	0.65	22.7	1023	43	36	20	6.4	20.7	17
Rapid growth	375	0.80	25.1	1127	48	41	22	6.6	21.2	17
Long yearling, 18 months										
Not in training	475	0.45	23.9	1077	45	33	18	7.7	25.1	21
In training	475	0.45	32.0	1429	60	44	24	10.2	33.3	21
Two years, 24 months old										
Not in training	540	0.30	23.5	998	40	31	17	8.5	27.9	24
In training	540	0.30	32.3	1372	55	43	24	11.6	38.4	24

From National Research Council: *Nutrient requirements of horses,* Washington, DC, 1989, National Academy Press.
DE, Dose equivalent.

approach, the benefits of using a basic nutritional supplement are apparent over time. Because repeated analysis of the horse's basic feed ration can be expensive and certain marginal deficiencies are difficult to detect, the following criteria should be reviewed to determine whether such supplementation would be beneficial to a horse's health and performance.

First, sufficient knowledge of equine dietary needs during different stages of growth and physiologic states is es-

sential to proper feed management. After consulting the NRC nutritional guidelines for the horse (National Research Council, 1989), the practitioner should review the nutritional variability relative to the breed, style of work or performance, and local soil conditions (particularly selenium levels). Several well-documented books about equine nutrition have been published, including *Horse Nutrition: A Practical Guide* (Hintz, 1983). With knowledge and experience a veterinarian can identify horses that will

TABLE 3-12

OTHER MINERALS AND VITAMINS FOR HORSES AND PONIES (ON A DRY-MATTER BASIS)

	ADEQUATE CONCENTRATIONS IN TOTAL RATIONS				
	MAINTENANCE	PREGNANT AND LACTATING MARES	GROWING HORSES	WORKING HORSES	MAXIMUM TOLERANCE LEVELS
MINERALS					
Sodium (%)	0.10	0.10	0.10	0.30	3*
Sulfur (%)	0.15	0.15	0.15	0.15	1.25
Iron (mg/kg)	40	50	50	40	1000
Manganese (mg/kg)	40	40	40	40	1000
Copper (mg/kg)	10	10	10	10	800
Zinc (mg/kg)	40	40	40	40	500
Selenium (mg/kg)	0.1	0.1	0.1	0.1	2.0
Iodine (mg/kg)	0.1	0.1	0.1	0.1	5.0
Cobalt (mg/kg)	0.1	0.1	0.1	0.1	10
VITAMINS					
Vitamin A (IU/kg)	2000	3000	2000	2000	16000
Vitamin D (IU/kg)†	300	600	800	300	2200
Vitamin E (IU/kg)	50	80	80	80	1000
Vitamin K (mg/kg)	‡				
Thiamin (mg/kg)	3	3	3	5	3000
Riboflavin (mg/kg)	2	2	2	2	
Niacin (mg/kg)					
Pantothenic acid (mg/kg)					
Pyridoxine (mg/kg)					
Biotin (mg/kg)					
Folacin (mg/kg)					
Vitamin B$_{12}$ (μg/kg)					
Ascorbic acid (mg/kg)					
Choline (mg/kg)					

Modified from National Research Council: *Nutrient requirements of horses,* Washington, 1989, National Academy Press.
*As sodium chloride.
†Recommendations for horses not exposed to sunlight or to artificial light with an emission spectrum of 280-315 nm.
‡Blank space indicates that data are insufficient to determine a requirement or maximum tolerable level.

benefit from a balanced, comprehensive equine supplement.

Other basic considerations that can be used to help determine the need for a feed supplement are as follows:

- The horse's overall condition and expected level of performance
- The quality, quantity, and variety of the horse's diet
- Special risk categories.

Overall Condition and Expected Performance Levels

No one knows a horse better than does its owner. The owner's assistance is invaluable when the veterinarian is completing the subjective areas of the health examination,

such as mood, overall behavior, and the animal's ability to recover from strenuous exercise, injury, and illness. Frequently either overlooked or ignored completely, subtle changes in any area can indicate nutritional deficiencies. The combination of the subjective and clinical evaluations is important in determination of supplement use. Any sudden or gradual departure from normal performance or condition may suggest a nutritional factor as a possible cause.

Diet and Feeding Program

Evaluation of the overall feeding program for specific nutrient imbalances can reveal potential nutritional problems. Many young foals, for instance, are apt to suffer from an improper calcium/phosphorus ratio or some other imbalance in the diet because of an inadequate feeding program. A well-chosen supplement often helps correct a poor calcium/phosphorus ratio, which is essential for proper bone growth and reproduction. Alfalfa hay is relatively high in calcium, whereas grain tends to be high in phosphorus. Grass hay is often low in both. With the right supplement, the horse's basic ration can be enhanced to the NRC-suggested 1.5:1.0 calcium/phosphorus ratio (National Research Council, 1989).

Recently experts have questioned the NRC requirements for certain minerals such as zinc, manganese, and copper. Studies at Ohio State University have indicated that some currently recommended ratios for these minerals may be suboptimum, resulting in increased incidence of developmental orthopedic diseases (including epiphysitis) in young horses, in which such deficiencies are most readily apparent (Knight, 1985). Ohio State University recommends a zinc/copper ratio of approximately 3:1, which varies from the NRC guidelines of 4:1 (National Research Council, 1989). Some have suggested that the maintenance requirements for zinc to copper in the mature horse may be closer to the 3:1 ratio (Pagan, 1994).

A proper supplement must be balanced, with no excesses or deficiencies of key nutrients in the formula that could cause an imbalance in the horse's overall nutrient intake. A good supplement should provide from 10% to 30% of the basic vitamins and minerals in the horse's daily intake.

Risk Categories

A number of reports indicate that certain classes of horses, based on work pattern, gender, and age, require special nutritional attention (Ralston, 1988, 1994). In these cases, feed supplements have been found effective in restoring function and improving performance. Summaries of some of these special-risk categories follow.

High-performance horses

Horses that are involved in regular heavy workouts, endurance training, and race competition benefit from supplementation according to many trainers and veterinarians. Stress and heavy exercise can result in nutritional losses of vitamins C and E and certain key minerals such as chromium and molybdenum (Ralston, 1994). Optimal performance requires strict attention to total nutritional intake. Some nutrients that promote energy and endurance are L-carnitine, DMG, and coenzyme Q_{10}. Other nutrients that support joints and connective tissue such as Perna mussel, glycosaminoglycans, and cartilage products can be recommended for this group of horses.

Sick or injured horses

Horses that experience frequent health problems generally respond well to nutritional supplementation. Injured horses appear to recover faster on a good supplement program including antioxidants, which reduce inflammation and promote healing. A high-quality supplement should provide antioxidants, chelated minerals, key vitamins, and amino acids to enhance the immune system. Because a sick horse may not eat regularly, the supplement becomes an even greater source of much-needed nutrition. A direct-fed probiotic and digestive enzymes may be especially helpful during such times of stress.

Geriatric horses

As horses age, especially beyond 18 years, they tend to take longer to recover from certain health problems. Proper nutrition is one way to keep older horses healthy. Routine examination can help reveal health problems before they become serious. Weight loss is a common problem as horses age and may indicate chronic dental disease, digestive problems, or inadequate diet. If the horse is free of other health considerations, the diet can be improved by adding some fat for energy (unsaturated fatty acids) along with increased protein. A B-complex supplement may enhance the breakdown and assimilation of fats and protein from the diet. A digestive enzyme or probiotic product can help improve the digestive process and the assimilation of nutrients. Gum problems, poor hair coat, inflammation problems, hoof cracks, and degenerative joint problems can be helped by adding certain nutritional products to the diet (see Chapter 4).

Older horses have lower serum values for vitamin C compared with those of younger horses (Ralston, 1988). This may be caused by increased stress, decreased synthesis, or impaired absorption. Research suggests that supplementation with key nutrients is beneficial, leading to increased activity, alertness, and responsiveness. Nutrients that support joints, connective tissue, hoof, and coat conditions are especially important. These include Perna mussel, glycosaminoglycans, sulfur-containing amino acids, and biotin.

Brood mares

Nutritional demands are higher for the brood mare, particularly those who produce foals yearly. Vitamin and mineral requirements can range from 50% to 200% higher than for nonbreeding stock (National Research Council, 1985). This class of horse definitely needs supplemental support, especially minerals, protein, and key vitamins.

Juvenile stock

Mineral deficiencies can be a significant problem in foals and yearlings. Bridges (1988) and Gabel (1987) have observed a growing incidence of growth-related bone and joint abnormalities in juvenile horses. Their studies show that foals commonly have imbalances and deficiencies in several trace minerals, including copper, zinc, and manganese. The researchers also discovered a direct correlation between low copper levels in the blood and the development of specific growth-related skeletal abnormalities (Bridges, 1984, 1990) that were aggravated by high dietary zinc intake. Foals whose mothers are malnourished during pregnancy are especially vulnerable. Proper supplementation is vital for this group of horses to provide adequate levels of minerals and maintain the proper mineral ratios supported by current research.

Table 3-13 presents a balanced, broad-spectrum nutritional supplement that could improve the overall dietary intake of many horses. The nutrients in the supplement must be balanced and in reasonable dosage, and their use should not lead to any significant excess of any single nutrient.

Questions and Possible Controversies Regarding Nutritional Supplements

Many veterinarians ask the following questions about nutritional supplementation:

1. Why are nutritional supplements needed when an animal's diet is balanced and complete according to the NRC guidelines?

We cannot assume that a particular animal's diet contains all the essential nutrients and accessory food factors needed for good health and performance when compared

TABLE 3-13

QUALITY EQUINE VITAMIN AND MINERAL SUPPLEMENT: RECOMMENDED DAILY FEEDING PROGRAM*

SUPPLEMENT	AMOUNT LEVELS/lb	AMOUNT LEVELS/oz	SUPPLEMENT	AMOUNT LEVELS/lb	AMOUNT LEVELS/oz
Vitamin A	200,000 IU	12,500 IU	**ELECTROLYTES**		
Beta-carotene	8 mg	0.5 mg	Calcium	6000 mg	375 mg
Vitamin D$_3$	12,000 IU	750 IU	Magnesium	2000 mg	125 mg
Vitamin E	2000 IU	125 IU	Potassium	3000 mg	188 mg
Vitamin C	2000 mg	125 mg	Sodium chloride	3850 mg	240 mg
Folic acid	20,000 μg	1250 μg			
Thiamine	400 mg	25 mg	**AMINO ACIDS**		
Riboflavin	400 mg	25 mg	Methionine	6600 mg	413 mg
Niacin	200 mg	12.5 mg	Lysine	5000 mg	312 mg
Niacinamide	200 mg	12.5 mg	Aspartic acid	2000 mg	125 mg
Pyridoxine	400 mg	25 mg	Arginine	2550 mg	159 mg
Cyanocobalamin	3000 μg	188 μg	Cystine	1095 mg	68 mg
Pantothenic acid	400 mg	25 mg	Glycine	900 mg	56 mg
Biotin	32,000 μg	2000 μg	Histidine	645 mg	40 mg
Para-aminobenzoic acid (PABA)	400 mg	25 mg	Isoleucine	1050 mg	66 mg
Inositol	400 mg	25 mg	Leucine	3380 mg	211 mg
Choline	1600 mg	100 mg	Phenylalanine	1450 mg	91 mg
Lecithin	400 mg	25 mg	Threonine	1160 mg	73 mg
Phosphorus	4000 mg	250 mg	Tryptophane	322 mg	20 mg
Iodine	6000 μg	375 μg	Valine	1450 mg	91 mg
Iron	600 mg	37.5 mg			
Copper	200 mg	12.5 mg	**DIGESTIVE ENZYMES**		
Manganese	400 mg	25 mg	Papain	400 mg	25 mg
Zinc	600 mg	37.5 mg	Pepsin	400 mg	25 mg
Selenium	2000 μg	125 μg	Amylase (enteric coated)	400 mg	25 mg
Cobalt	5 mg	0.31 mg	Lipase (enteric coated)	400 mg	25 mg
			Cellulase (enteric coated)	400 mg	25 mg

Courtesy VetriScience Laboratories, Essex Jct, Vt, 1996.
*Number of ounces used depends on individual horse; see supplement label.
†Formulated with wheat germ oil and linseed meal.

with the NRC guidelines. The NRC guidelines address the average need for an animal in a specific group and should be used only as general guidelines, not to address nutritional need for individual animals. Biochemical individuality suggests that two animals may have very different nutritional requirements because of a variety of factors. The nutritional content of the animal's daily intake varies considerably, and individual nutrients in the diet have varying degrees of bioavailability. Because of these factors, nutritional supplementation can optimize the total nutritional intake and cover potential deficiencies that may be present.

2. What about the possibility of overdosing on nutritional supplementation and getting a toxic response to a particular supplement if given in too high a dose?

Overdosage of a single nutrient and subsequent nutritional overload are possible, although nutritional supplements are many times safer than drugs because the body can metabolize and dispense with most nutrient excesses without problems. The key exceptions may be with vitamins A and D and certain key minerals such as selenium and iron that can give a toxic response when taken in high, prolonged doses. These nutrients need to be monitored closely to avoid excesses. A balanced mineral intake is important to prevent certain absorption problems. Most nutritional supplements make allowances for these potential problems. The vast majority of nutritional imbalances and excesses are caused by the basic diet, not supplements. Nevertheless, the supplement should be carefully integrated into the total feeding program to avoid single nutrient excesses.

3. What about the lack of double-blind studies to confirm the benefits of a particular supplement in disease management? How do you separate the hype from correct nutritional claims?

Certain nutritional products receive an inordinate amount of publicity, and specific nutrients lack double-blind studies. Because of nutrient synergy, or the teamwork concept, single nutrients do not lend themselves to the drug-study approach. However, a growing body of scientific evidence and clinical studies correctly establishes the role and function of nutrients and food factors in the healing and regenerative process. Increased awareness of these clinical and nutritional studies in the literature, coupled with a greater knowledge and understanding of biochemistry, allows the veterinarian to separate the hype from sound scientific evidence. In the long run, only the actual clinical use of nutritional supplements will establish the validity and effectiveness of the program.

4. What about the problem of absorption of certain nutrients that have large molecular weights?

Certain supplements such as Perna mussel, glycosaminoglycans, and cartilage products do contain ground substances of extremely large molecular weight that may not immediately appear to be absorbed across the mucosal membrane. The actual process involved in the digestion and uptake of nutrients like these is not completely understood, but studies do show these supplements to be biologically active and beneficial in certain areas. Although these large molecules are probably digested to some degree, studies show that many retain their essential characteristics and therapeutic properties after systemic absorption (Billings, 1992; Gardner, 1988; Sanderson, Walker, 1993). The lymphatic system may also be involved in the uptake of such nutrients.

Summary

Preventive nutrition recognizes and compensates for deficiencies of key nutrients that can eventually lead to multiple and possibly irreversible health problems. Nutritional research in the cat, dog, and horse has identified many connections between deficiencies and health problems, but more studies are needed. Correct and balanced nutrition is the foundation for good health in the cat, dog, and horse. For maximal effectiveness, feed management must allow for the biochemical individuality of each animal. With proper knowledge, evaluation, and assessment, an optimal dietary program can be formulated. This formulation may include nutritional supplementation for borderline deficiencies that may not be evident. The combination of basic and preventive nutrition is a safe, effective approach that both reduces potential health problems and optimizes the well-being of the animal.

References

Amella M and others: Inhibition of mast-cell histamine release by flavonoids and bioflavonoids, *Planta Med* 51:16, 1985.

Ashmead D: Tissue transportation of organic trace minerals, *Appl Nutr* 22:42, 1970.

Beisel W: Single-nutrient effects on immunological functions, *JAMA* 245:53, 1981.

Berge J: Polyascorbate (C-Flex®) an interesting alternative for problems on the support and movement apparatus in dogs: clinical trial of Ester-C® ascorbate in dogs, *Norwegian Vet J* 102:579, Aug/Sept 1990.

Bhatia SK and others: Influence of diet on the induction of experimental autoimmune disease, *Proc Soc Exp Biol Med*, 1997 (in press).

Billings PC and others: Distribution of Bowman Birk protease inhibitor in mice following oral adminstration, *Cancer Lett* 62:191, 1992.

Blackburn G, Grant J, Young V, editors: *Amino acids—metabolism and medical applications*, Littleton, Mass, 1983, John Wright.

Bliznakov EG, Casey A, Premuzic E: Coenzyme Q$_{10}$: stimulants of the phagocytic activity in rats and immune response in mice, *Experientia* 26:953, 1970.

Bliznakov EG: Immunological senescence in mice and its reversal by coenzyme Q$_{10}$, *Mech Ageing Dev* 7:189, 1978.

Bridges C, Womak J, Harris E: Considerations of copper metabolism in osteochondrosis of suckling foals, *J Am Vet Assoc* 185:173, 1984.

Bridges C, Harris E: Cartilaginous fractures induced experimentally in foals with low copper diets, *JAMA* 193:215, 1988.

Bridges C, Moffitt P: Influence of variable content of dietary zinc on copper metabolism of weanling foals, *Am J Vet Res* 51:275, 1990.

Brown MG, Park JF: Control of dental calculus in experimental beagles, *Lab Animal Care* 18(5):527, 1968.

Brown M, editor: *Present knowledge in nutrition*, Washington, DC, 1990, International Life Sciences Institute.

Burton A, Anderson F: Decreased incorporation of ^{14}L-glucosamine relative to ^{3}H-N-acetyl glucosamine in the intestinal mucosa of patients with inflammatory bowel disease, *Am J Gastroenterol* 78:19, 1983.

Bush MJ, Verlangieri AJ: An acute study of the relative gastro-intestinal absorption of a novel form of calcium ascorbate, *Res Commun Clin Pathol Pharmacol* 57(1):137, 1987.

Case LP, Carey DP, Hirakawa DA: *Canine and feline nutrition: a sourcebook for companion animal professionals*, St Louis, 1995, Mosby.

Communicable Disease Report: Cryptosporidium in water supplies: the second Badenoch report, *CDR Weekly* 5(46)245, 1995.

Conney AH and others: Metabolic interaction between L-ascorbic acid and drugs, *Ann NY Acad Sci* 92:115, 1961.

Cutler R: Antioxidants and aging, *Am J Clin Nutr* 53:3735, 1991.

Dabrowska H and others: The effect of large doses of vitamin C and magnesium on stress responses in common carp, *Cyprinus carpio*, *Comp Biochem Physiol Act* 99(4):681, 1991.

Egelberg J: Local effect of diet on plaque formation and development of gingivitis in dogs. I. Effect of hard and soft diets, *Odontol Rev* 16:31, 1965a.

Egelberg J: Local effect of diet on plaque formation and development of gingivitis in dogs. III. Effect of frequency of meals and tube feeding, *Odontol Rev* 16:50, 1965b.

Facino R: Free radical scavenging action and anti-enzyme activities of procyanidines from *Vitis vinifera:* a mechanism for their capillary protective action, *Arzneim-Forsch* 44:592, 1994.

Folkers K, Yamamcria Y, editors: *Biomedical and clinical aspects of coenzyme Q*, ed 5, New York, 1986, Elsevier.

Fox AD and others: Effects of glutamine-supplemented enteral diet on methotrexate-induced enterocolitis. *JPEN* 12:325, 1988.

Fox AD and others: Reduction of severity of enterocolitis by glutamine-supplemented enteral diets, *Surg Forum* 38:43, 1987.

Frankel RA, McGarry J, editors: *Carnitine biosyntheses, metabolism and functions*, New York, 1980, Academic Press.

Fujioka T and others: Clinical study of cardiac arrhythmias using a 24-hour continuous electrocardiographic recorder (5th report): anitarrhythmic action of coenzyme Q$_{10}$ in diabetics, *Tohoku J Exp Med* 141 (suppl):453, 1983.

Fuortes L, McNutt LA, Lynch C: Leukemia incidence and radioactivity in drinking water in 59 Iowa towns, *Am J Public Health* 80(10):1261, 1990.

Gabel A, Knight D, and others: Comparison of incidence and severity of developmental orthopedic disease on 17 farms before and after adjustment of ration, *Proc Am Assoc Equine Pract* 33:163, 1987.

Gabor M: Pharmacologic effects of flavonoids on blood vessels, *Angiologica* 9:355, 1972.

Gannon J, Kendall R: A clinical evaluation of *N,N*-dimethylglycine (DMG) and diosopropylammonium dichloroacetate (DIPA) on the performance of racing greyhounds, *Canine Pract* 9:7, 1983.

Gardner ML: Gastrointestinal absorption of intact proteins, *Annu Rev Nutr* 8:329, 1988.

Goldston R, Hoskins J: *Geriatrics and gerontology of the dog and cat*, Philadelphia, 1995, WB Saunders.

Goldston R: Geriatrics and gerontology, *Vet Clin North Am* 19:1, 1989.

Graber C and others: Immunomodulating properties of dimethylglycine in humans, *J Infectious Dis* 143:101, 1981.

Gross WB: Effects of ascorbic acid on stress and disease in chickens, *Avian Dis* 36(3):688, 1992.

Halliwell B: Free radicals and antioxidants: a personal view, *Nutr Rev* August, 1994, p. 52.

Harless SJ, Turbes CC: Choline loading: specific dietary supplementation for modifying neurologic and behavioral disorders in dogs and cats, *Vet Med Small Anim Clin*, 77(8):S1, 1982.

Hayes K: Nutritional problems in cats: taurine deficiency and vitamin A excess, *Can Vet J* 23:2, 1982.

Henderson L: Vitamin B$_6$. In Olson R and others, editors: *Present knowledge in nutrition*, ed 5, Washington, 1984, Nutritional Foundation.

Hintz H: *Horse nutrition: a practical guide*, New York, 1983, Arc.

Hintz H: Vitamin C for horses, *Equine Practice* 10:5, 1988.

Hintz H, Cymbaluk N: Nutrition of the horse, *Annu Rev Nutr* 14:243, 1994.

Hoskins J: Nutritional disorders of the aging dog and cat. In Morgan RV, editor: *Handbook of small animal practice*, ed 2, New York, 1992, Churchill Livingstone.

Huber TL, Wilson RC, McGarity SA: Variations in digestibility of dry dog foods with identical label guaranteed analysis, *JAAHA* 22:571, 1986.

Hurley LS, Everson GJ: Delayed development of righting reflexes in offspring of manganese-deficient rats, *Proc Soc Exp Biol Med* 102:360, 1959.

James T, McKay CM: A study of food intake, activity, and digestive efficiency in different-type dogs, *Br Vet J* 139:361, 1950.

Jensen N: Amino acid chelates: their mechanisms of action and key aspects of preparation, *J Appl Nutr* 31:24, 1979.

Jepson MM and others: Relationship between glutamine concentration and protein synthesis in rat skeletal muscle, *Am J Physiol* 355:E166, 1988.

Kamikawa T and others: Effects of coenzyme Q$_{10}$ on exercise intolerance in chronic stable angina pectoris, *Am J Cardiol* 56:247, 1985.

Kaul TN, Middleton E, and Ogra P: Antiviral effect of flavonoids on human viruses, *J Med Virol* 15:71, 1985.

Kendall PT, Blaza SE, Smith PM: Influence of the level of feed intake and dog size on the apparent digestiblity of dog foods, *Br Vet J* 139 (4): 361, 1983.

Kendler B: Gamma-linolenic acid: physiological effects and potential medical applications, *J Appl Nutr* 39:79, 1987.

Kent GP and others: Epidemic giardiasis caused by a contaminated public water supply, *Am J Public Health* 78(2):139, 1988.

Kishi T and others: Bioenergetics in clinical medicine: studies on coenzyme Q and diabetes mellitus, *J Med* 7:307, 1976.

Kitamura N and others: Myocardial tissue level of coenzyme Q$_{10}$ in patients with cardiac failure. In Folkers K, Yamamura Y, editors: *Biomedical and clinical aspects of coenzyme Q*, vol 4, Amsterdam, 1984, Elsevier,

Knight D and others: Correlation of dietary mineral to incidence and severity of metabolic bone disease in Ohio and Kentucky, *Proc Am Assoc Equine Proct* 31:445, 1985.

Kronfeld D: Geriatric diets for dogs, *Compend Contin Educ Pract Vct* 5:136, 1983.

Kronfeld D: *Vitamins and mineral supplementation for dogs and cats*, Santa Barbara, Calif, 1989, Veterinary Practice.

Langsjoen PerH, Langsjoen PetH, Folkers K: Long term efficacy and safety of coenzyme Q10 therapy for idiopathic dilated cardiomyopathy, *Am J Cardiol* 65:521, 1990.

Lehninger A, Nelson D, Cox M: *Principles of biochemistry,* New York, 1993, Worth.

Levine S and others: Effects of a supplement containing *N,N*-dimethylglycine (DMG) on the racing standardbred, *Equine Pract* 4:11, 1982.

Levine S, Kidd P: *Antioxidant adaptation: its role in free radical pathology,* San Leandro, Calif, 1985, Biocurrents Allergy Research Group.

Lewis L, Morris M, Hand M: *Small animal nutrition III,* Topeka, 1994, Mark Morris Institute.

Logas D, Kunkle GA: Double-blinded crossover study with marine-oil supplementation containing high-dose eicosapentaenoic acid for the treatment of canine pruritic skin disease, *Vet Dermatol* 5(3):99, 1994.

Lowry K, Baker D: Effects of storage, carbohydrate composition, and heat processing on protein quality and amino acid bioavailability of commercial enteral product, *J Food Science* 54:1024, 1989.

MacDonald ML and others: Essential fatty acid requirements of cats, *Am J Vet Res* 45:1310, 1984.

Machlin LJ, Bendich A: Free-radical tissue damage: protective role of antioxidant nutrients, *FASEB J* 1(6):441, 1987.

Machlin L, Sauberlich H: New view on the function and health effects of vitamins, *Nutr Today* Jan-Feb 1994, p 25.

Machlin LJ: Critical assessment of the epidemiological data concerning the impact of antioxidant nutrients on cancer and cardiovascular disease, *Crit Rev Food Sci Nutr* 35(1-2):41, 1995.

Matsushima T and others: Protection by coenzyme Q10 of canine myocardial reperfusion injury after preservation, *J Thorac Cardiovasc Surg* 103:945, 1992.

McKee JS, Harrison PC: Effects of supplemental ascorbic acid on the performance of broiler chickens exposed to multiple concurrent stressors, *Poult Sci* 74(11):1772, 1995.

Middleton E, Drzewieki G: Naturally occurring flavonoids and human basophil histamine release, *Int Arch Allergy Appl Immunol* 77:155, 1985.

Miller W and others: Clinical trial of DVM derm caps in the treatment of allergic diseases in dogs: a nonblinded study, *J Am Animal Hosp Assoc* 25:163, 1989.

Morris J, Rogers Q: Assessment of the nutritional adequacy of pet foods through the life cycle, *J Nutrition* 124:2520S, 1994.

Mortvedt JJ, Giordano PM, Lindsay WW: *Micronutrients in agriculture,* 1972, Soil Science of America.

Nakano K, Suzuki S: Stress-induced change in tissue levels of ascorbic acid and histamine in rats, *J Nutr* 114(9):1602, 1984.

National Research Council: *Nutrient requirements of dogs,* Washington, DC, 1985, National Academy Press.

National Research Council: *Nutrient requirements of cats,* Washington, DC, 1986, National Academy Press.

National Research Council: *Nutrient requirements of horses,* Washington, DC, 1989, National Academy Press.

Newsholme EA, Parry-Billings M: Properties of glutamine release from muscle and its importance for the immune system, *JPEN* 14 (suppl 4): 63, 1990.

Pagan J: Advancing the science of equine nutrition, *The Horse,* p 12, July 1995.

Pagan J, Duren S, Jackson S, Balancing micronutrients, *Equus* 206:27, 1994.

Pagan J, Duren S, Jackson S: Risky rations, *Equus* 208:33, 1995.

Pardue S, Thaxton J: Ascorbic acid in poultry: a review, *World Poult Sci Assoc* 107:123, 1986.

Pearce F, Befus AD, Bienenstock J: Mucosal mast cells. III. Effect of quercetin and other flavonoids on antigen-induced histamine secretion from rat intestinal mast cells, *J Allergy Clin Immunol* 73:819, 1984.

Pion PD and others: Myocardial failure in cats associated with low plasma taurine, a reversible cardiomyopathy, *Science* 237:764, 1987.

Pound AW, Horn L, Lawson TA: Decreased toxicity of dimethylnitrosamine with carbon tetrachloride, *Pathology* 5:233, 1973.

Ralston S: Equine clinical nutrition: specific problems and solutions, *Pract Vet* 10:356, 1988.

Ralston S: Therapeutic nutrition for specific equine syndromes, *Vet Clin Nutr* 1:31, 1994.

Reap E, Lawson J: Stimulation of the immune response by dimethylglycine, a nontoxic metabolite, *Lab Clin Med* 115:481, 1990.

Reynolds RD: Vitamin supplements: current controversies, *J Am Coll Nutrition* 13(2):118-126, 1994.

Rivers JP: Essential fatty acids in cats, *J Small Animal Proct* 23:563, 1982.

Roe D: *Drug-induced nutritional deficiencies,* Westport, Conn, 1978, Avi.

Roe D: Nutrient and drug interactions. In Olson R, Broquist H, Chichester C, and others, editors: *Present knowledge in nutrition,* ed 5, Washington, DC, 1984, Nutritional Foundation.

Roe D: Effect of drugs on vitamin needs, *Ann NY Acad Sci* 669:156, 1992.

Rose WC: The amino acid requirements of adult man, *Nutr Abst Rev* 27 (3):631, 1957.

Sanderson IR, Walker WA: Uptake and transport of macromolecules by the intestine: possible role in clinical disorders (an update), *Gastroenterology* 104:622, 1993.

Schalch W, Weber P: Vitamins and carotenoids—a promising approach to reducing the risk of coronary heart disease, cancer and eye diseases, *Adv Exp Med Biol* 366:335, 1994.

Schroeder H: Losses of vitamins and trace minerals resulting from processing and preservation of foods, *Am J Clin Nutr* 24:562, 1971.

Shils M, Olson J, Moshe S, editors: *Modern nutrition in health and disease,* ed 8, Philadelphia, 1994, Lea & Febiger.

Sies H, Stahl W: Vitamin E and C, beta-carotene, and other carotenoids as antioxidants, *Am J Clin Nutr* 62:1315S, 1995.

Sies H, Wendel A: *Function of glutathione,* New York, 1978, Springer-Verlag.

Simpson J, Anderson R, Markwell P: *Clinical nutrition of the dog and cat,* London, 1993, Blackwell Scientific.

Smith AH and others: Cancer risks from arsenic in drinking water, *Environ Health Perspect* 97:259, 1992.

Souba WW, Smith RJ, Wilmore DW: Glutamine metabolism by the intestinal tract, *JPEN* 9:608, 1985.

Sousa CA and others: Dermatosis associated with feeding generic dog food: 13 cases (1981-1982), *J Am Vet Med Assoc* 192:676, 1988.

Sousa CA: Nutritional dermatoses. In Nesbit GH: *Dermatology: contemporary issues in small animal practice,* ed 9, New York, 1987, Churchill Livingstone.

Stocker R, Frei B, Sies H, editors: *Oxidative stress: oxidants and antioxidants,* London, 1991, Academic Press.

Thomsett L, Lloyd D: Essential fatty acid supplementation in the treatment of canine atopy, *Vet Dermatol* 1:41, 1989.

Verde M, Piquer J: Effect of stress on the corticosterone and ascorbic acid content of the plasma of rabbits, *J Appl Rabbit* 9:181, 1986.

Verlangieri A, Bush M: An acute study on the relative gastro-intestinal absorption of a novel form of calcium ascorbate, *Res Comm Chem Pathol Pharmacol* 57:137, 1987.

Verlangieri AJ, Fay MJ, Bannon AW: Comparison of the anti-scorbutic acitivity of L-ascorbic acid and Ester-C in the non-ascorbate synthesizing osteogenic disorder Shiongi (ODS) rat, *Life Sci* 48(23): 2275, 1991.

Welbourne TC: Enteral glutamine spares endogenous glutamine in chronic acidosis, *JPEN* 17:23S, 1993.

White P: Essential fatty acids: use in management of canine atopy, *Compendium* 15:451, 1993.

Wilkinson EG and others: Bioenergetics and clinical medicine. VI. Adjunctive treatment of periodontal disease with Coenzyme Q$_{10}$, *Res Commun Chem Pathol Pharmacol* 14:715, 1976.

Willett WC: Diet and health: what should we eat? *Science* 264:532, 1994.

Williams RJ: *Biochemical individuality,* New York, 1956, Wiley.

Williams RJ: *Nutrition against disease: environmental prevention,* New York, 1971, Pitman.

Williams RJ, Kalita DK, editors: *A physician's handbook on orthomolecular medicine,* New York, 1977, Pergamon.

Zentec J, Meyer H: Normal handling of diets—are all dogs created equal? *J Small Animal Pract* 36:354, 1995.

Zierler S and others: Bladder cancer in Massachussetts related to chlorinated and chloraminated drinking water: a case-controlled study, *Arch Environ Health* 43(2):195, 1988.

Chapter 4

Therapeutic Nutrition for the Cat, Dog, and Horse

ROGER V. KENDALL

Scientific and clinical studies have demonstrated that a wide variety of nutrients, food factors, and natural products can be used effectively and safely to enhance the healing process from injury or disease (Werbach, 1988). Nutritional intervention as part of the healing process dates back to ancient times: Hippocrates is quoted as saying "Let your food be your medicine." The advent of modern drugs, vaccines, and antibiotics has overshadowed the role that nutrients play in regenerating damaged tissue, enhancing metabolic functions, potentiating the immune response, reducing inflammatory responses, and aiding in the overall healing process. Research and clinical observations reveal that combining modern veterinary medicine with therapeutic nutrition may give better patient response than does either approach alone.

This chapter outlines the scientific rationale and approach of nutritional therapy and then discusses nutrients and other natural food factors that can play a major therapeutic role in the treatment of various disease conditions.

Nutrients Versus Drugs as Therapeutic Agents

Nutrients are a natural part of the cellular environment. The use of nutrients as part of a therapeutic program for promoting healing and regeneration is based on an understanding of the wide role that macronutrients and micronutrients play in cellular physiology and nutritional biochemistry (Brady, 1994). Therapeutic nutrition enhances healing by providing the cells with a better environment for regeneration and overcoming the myriad of stresses caused by injury or disease. Historically, vitamins and essential minerals were considered only as agents used to reverse or cure the condition associated with their deficiency in the diet; however, clinical research now suggests that many disease conditions have nutritional or environmental components that, when properly managed, help potentiate the healing response (Shils, Olsen, Moshe, 1994). Vitamins have many other functions besides simply preventing the deficiency disease associated with their essential nature. For example, vitamin C may enhance immune function (Delafuente, Prendergast, Modigh, 1986), neutralize free radicals (Halliwell, 1994), lower elevated cholesterol and triglyceride levels in the blood (Howard, Meyers, 1995; Simons, 1992), detoxify some harmful metabolites and environmental pollutants (Ginter, 1989), counteract allergic responses (Bielory, Gandhi, 1994; Kodama, Kodama, 1995), act as an antiinflammatory agent, reduce cataract incidence (Seddon and others, 1994), counter stress, and aid in the treatment of degenerative joint disease and cancer (Anderson, 1984; Bendich, Langseth, 1995; Cohen, Bhagavan, 1995). Many published studies show the involvement of vitamin C in the prevention and treatment of many disease processes (Gaby, Singh, 1991). Vitamin C works in concert with many other nutrients to promote healing and recovery from disease. Research continues to demonstrate the healing potential of a wide variety of nutrients, such as coenzyme Q_{10}, vitamin E, L-carnitine, the essential fatty acids, glucosamines, shark cartilage, and potent antioxidants, including proanthocyanidins.

Properly administered, drugs play an important role in veterinary practice. Drugs are effective in the treatment of disease, but they are usually foreign to the body, and the pharmaceutical mode of action differs from that of nutritional therapy. Nutrients support and correct normal cellular metabolic pathways, whereas drugs may block or interfere with biochemical adaptation processes related to the disease. Drugs ameliorate a disease symptom by acting as analgesics, antiinflammatory agents, and antimicrobials, for instance, by blocking an enzymatic pathway, modifying cell membranes, or changing a physiologic process. Aspirin works as an antiinflammatory and analgesic agent by blocking the action of the enzyme cyclooxygenase, which is involved with the formation of the prostaglandins that are part of the inflammatory response. Aspirin is also well known to cause gastroduodenal lesions in dogs, depending on the dosage regimen (Johnston and others, 1995). Drugs are usually fast-acting but can exhibit potentially toxic side effects on the body, especially when used over an extended time. Drugs generally treat symptoms and modify disease conditions, but they fail to potentiate healing by dealing with the basic cause.

Nutrients can function as therapeutic agents (Machlin, Sauberlich, 1994; Werbach, 1988). Although nutrients tend to work more slowly than drugs, in the long run they enhance metabolic processes and help restore function and balance to the body. Nutrients can contribute important metabolites to cellular regeneration, improve the flow of energy, potentiate immune function, detoxify or neutralize cellular toxins, and improve enzymatic activity. Nutrients contribute to the optimal functioning of the cell during times of stress and disease and aid the body in the healing and regeneration process through natural means (Shils, 1994). With few exceptions, nutrients are generally free of side effects. Whereas drugs treat symptoms, nutrients can be used to correct the cause of a health problem, reduce symptoms, and help the body rebuild healthy tissue. Nutritional products can be used with drug therapy. Such a complementary approach usually brings faster, more effective results because the nutrients contribute to the healing process and the improvement of health over the long term. The potential therapeutic use of some nutritional products against various health and disease conditions in the dog and cat are listed in Table 4-1; products for the horse are listed in Table 4-2.

TABLE 4-1

SUGGESTED NUTRITIONAL THERAPIES FOR THE DOG AND CAT

CONDITION	SUPPLEMENT	DAILY DOSE RANGE*
Geriatric dog or cat	B complex	
	B_1, B_2, B_6	5-30 mg
	Folic acid, B_{12}	10-100 µg
	Vitamin C	250-4000 mg
	Vitamin E	50-200 IU
	Coenzyme Q_{10}	20-100 mg
	Primrose oil	500-2000 mg
	Fish oil	250-1000 mg
	Digestive enzymes	4-160 mg
	Dimethylglycine	24-100 mg
	Zinc	1-15 mg
Allergic dermatitis; atopy	Vitamin C	500-6000 mg
	Digestive enzymes	4-160 mg
	Primrose oil	1000-3000 mg
	Fish oil	500-1500 mg
	Proanthocyanidin complex	10-200 mg
	Vitamin E	50-400 IU
	Dimethylglycine	50-250 mg
	Vitamin A	500-10,000 IU
Canine degenerative joint disease; disk and spinal disorders	Perna mussel	300-1500 mg
	Glucosamine sulfate	250-1500 mg
	Bovine tracheal cartilage	500-2000 mg
	Vitamin C	500-6000 mg

A multiple vitamin/mineral product is recommended for all the conditions listed.

This nutrient and supplement list is not necessarily complete for a given condition. The table is meant to be a general guideline and therefore should be changed or modified based on the veterinarian's assessment of individual cases. The actual dose range recommendations are presented only as a general guide for the veterinarian.

*Actual daily dose depends on species variation, weight, age, physiologic state, and other dietary considerations. Actual daily dose should be divided and given in smaller portions, 2 or 3 times daily if possible. Veterinarians should contact manufacturers or suppliers for more exact loading dosage and maintenance program information.

TABLE 4-1

SUGGESTED NUTRITIONAL THERAPIES FOR THE DOG AND CAT—cont'd

CONDITION	SUPPLEMENT	DAILY DOSE RANGE*
Canine degenerative joint disease—disk and spinal disorders—cont'd	Sulfated minerals:	
	Manganese	2-15 mg
	Magnesium	24-300 mg
	Zinc	5-30 mg
	Silicon	2-10 mg
	Vitamin B_6	5-60 mg
Canine heartworm disease	Coenzyme Q_{10}	20-150 mg
	Vitamin C	500-6000 mg
	Vitamin E	100-400 IU
	Proanthocyanidin complex	10-200 mg
	L-Carnitine	200-2000 mg
Canine seizures	Betaine HCl	100-300 mg
	Dimethylglycine	50-500 mg
	Taurine	200-1000 mg
	Proanthocyanidin complex	10-200 mg
Cardiovascular disorders:	Vitamin C	500-6000 mg
Dilated cardiomyopathy	Vitamin E	50-400 IU
Congestive heart failure	Coenzyme Q_{10}	20-100 mg
Myocarditis	L-Carnitine	500-1000 mg
	Taurine	100-1000 mg
	Selenium	5-50 μg
	Fish oil	250-1000 mg
	Dimethylglycine	50-250 mg
Colitis—inflammatory bowel disease	*N*-Acetyl glucosamine	250-1500 mg
	Glutamine	250-3000 mg
	Lactobacillus acidophilus	20-500 (million microorganisms)
	Proanthocyanidin complex	10-200 mg
	Dimethylglycine	50-250 mg
	Vitamin C	250-3000 mg
Chronic diarrhea	*N*-Acetyl glucosamine	250-1500 mg
	Digestive enzymes	4-200 mg
	Lactobacillus acidophilus	20-500 (million microorganisms)
	Glutamine	250-3000 mg
Chronic illness	Vitamin C	500-6000 mg
	Vitamin E	100-400 IU
	Proanthocyanidin complex	20-200 mg
	Digestive enzymes	10-200 mg
Connective tissue disorders:	Vitamin C	500-6000 mg
Arthritis	Perna mussel	300-1500 mg
Hip dysplasia	Glucosamine sulfate	250-1500 mg
Sprains	Proanthocyanidin complex	10-200 mg
	Glycosaminoglycans	100-1000 mg
	Primrose oil	250-1000 mg
Demodicosis	Vitamin C	500-6000 mg
	Digestive enzymes	4-160 mg
	Proanthocyanidin complex	10-200 mg
	Primrose oil	250-1500 mg
	Dimethylglycine	50-250 mg
	Vitamin A	500-10,000 IU

Continued.

TABLE 4-1

SUGGESTED NUTRITIONAL THERAPIES FOR THE DOG AND CAT—cont'd

CONDITION	SUPPLEMENT	DAILY DOSE RANGE*
Diabetes mellitus	Chromium	50-300 μg
	Vitamin C	500-6000 mg
	Digestive enzymes	4-160 mg
	N-Acetyl glucosamine	200-1500 mg
	Proanthocyanidin complex	10-200 mg
Feline hyperthyroidism	B complex vitamins	
	B_1, B_2, B_6	2-10 mg
	Vitamin C	500-4000 mg
	Coenzyme Q_{10}	10-60 mg
	Primrose oil	250-1000 mg
Feline immunodeficiency virus	Vitamin C	500-6000 mg
	Proanthocyanidin complex	5-30 mg
	Coenzyme Q_{10}	20-100 mg
	Dimethylglycine	50-200 mg
Feline leukemia	Vitamin C	500-6000 mg
	Vitamin E	50-400 IU
	Coenzyme Q_{10}	20-100 IU
	Dimethylglycine	50-250 mg
Food intolerance	Pantothenic acid	20-150 mg
	Proanthocyanidin complex	10-200 mg
	B complex vitamins	
	B_1, B_2, B_6	4-40 mg
	Folic acid	50-200 mg
	Digestive enzymes	4-160 mg
Lyme disease	Vitamin C	500-6000 mg
	Fish oil	250-1500 mg
	Perna mussel	250-1500 mg
	Vitamin E	50-400 IU
	Vitamin A	500-10,000 IU
Neoplasia:	Shark cartilage	5-40 g
Vascular tumors	Coenzyme Q_{10}	20-100 mg
Melanoma	Vitamin C	1000-10,000 mg
	Dimethylglycine	50-500 mg
	Proanthocyanidin complex	10-200 mg
Periodontal disease	Coenzyme Q_{10}	10-100 mg
	Vitamin C	500-6000 mg
	Bioflavonoid complex	200-1500 mg
Cataracts	Glutathione	50-250 mg
	Vitamin C	500-4000 mg
	Coenzyme Q_{10}	20-100 mg
	Proanthocyanidin complex	20-200 mg
	Vitamin E	50-400 IU
	Dimethylglycine	100-400 mg

TABLE 4-2

SUGGESTED NUTRITIONAL THERAPIES FOR THE HORSE

CONDITION	SUPPLEMENT	DAILY DOSE RANGE*
Geriatric horse	Yeast culture	
	Digestive enzymes	50-200 mg
	Vitamin C	5-10 g
	Dimethylglycine	750-3000 mg
	Proanthocyanidin complex	1-2 g
	B complex	
	B_1, B_2, B_6	25-75 mg
	Folic acid, B_{12}	200-1500 µg
Digestive disorders:	Direct-fed microbials	250-400 (billion microorganisms)
Colitis	Glutamine	10-40 g
Salmonellosis	Digestive enzymes	50-200 mg
Chronic diarrhea	*N*-Acetyl glucosamine	1-2 g
Enterotoxemia		
Hoof, haircoat, and skin disorders:	Biotin	10-30 mg
Allergic dermatitis	Unsaturated fatty acids	5-15 g
	Sulfur amino acids	
	Methionine	1-10 g
	Cysteine	1-5 g
	Vitamin B_6	10-100 mg
	Silicon	30-100 mg
	Zinc	600-1200 mg
	Dimethylglycine	750-3000 mg
	Vitamin A	25,000-75,000 IU
Degenerative joint disorders:	Perna mussel	4-12 g
Osteochondrosis	Glycosaminoglycans	1-2 g
Osteochrondritis	Vitamin C	1-10 g
Dissecans physitis	Glucosamine sulfate	2-3 g
	Proanthocyanidin complex	1-2 g
	Chelated minerals	Check diet
	Digestive enzymes	50-200 g
Osteoarthritis:	Perna mussel	4-12 g
Ring-bone	Glycosaminoglycans	1-2 g
sesamoiditis	Vitamin C	5-10 g
osselets	Proanthocyanidin complex	1-2 g
splints	Glucosamine sulfate	2-3 g
Bone spavins	Shark cartilage	6-30 g
Podotrochilitis (navicular disease)	Chelated minerals	Check diet
	Digestive enzymes	50-200 mg
Soft-tissue disorders:	Perna mussel	4-12 g
Synovitis (bone spavins)	Vitamin C	5-10 g
Tendonitis	Dimethylglycine	750-3000 mg
Muscular disease:	Vitamin E	125-1000 IU
Rhabdomyolysis (early)	Selenium	Not to exceed 1 mg daily
Azoturia (white muscle disease)	B complex	
	B_1, B_2, B_6	25-200 mg
	Dimethylglycine	1-3 g

This nutrient and supplement list is not necessarily complete for a given condition. The table is meant to be a general guideline and therefore should be changed or modified based on the veterinarian's assessment of individual cases. The actual dose range recommendations are presented only as a general guide for the veterinarian.

*Actual daily dose varies depending on weight of animal, age, physiologic state, and other dietary considerations. Actual daily dose should be divided and given in smaller portions, 2 or 3 times daily if possible. Veterinarians should contact manufacturers or suppliers for more exact loading dosage and maintenance program information.

Continued.

TABLE 4-2

SUGGESTED NUTRITIONAL THERAPIES FOR THE HORSE—cont'd

CONDITION	SUPPLEMENT	DAILY DOSE RANGE*
Respiratory disorders:	Proanthocyanidin complex	2-4 g
Rhinopneumonitis influenza	Vitamin C	5-10 g
Pleuritis	Dimethylglycine	1500-3000 mg
Exercise-induced pulmonary hemorrhage	Bioflavonoids	1-3 g
Chronic obstructive pulmonary disease	Vitamin A	25,000-75,000 IU
Asthma		
Poor performance	Trace minerals	Check diet
	B complex	25-75 mg
	B_1, B_2, B_6	400-2000 mg
	Folic acid, B_{12}	5-10 g
	Amino acids	4-10 g
	Lysine	1-3 g
	Branch-chain AA	3-10 g
	(leucine, isoleucine, valine)	1-5 g
	Dimethylglycine	1-3 g
	Vitamin C	3-10 g
	L-Carnitine	1-5 g

Safety Considerations

Although practical in treating some animal diseases short term, drugs can have negative effects on the animal because of contraindications and side effects when used long term. For instance, the side effects of corticosteroids and nonsteroidal antiinflammatory drugs (NSAIDs) in the treatment of chronic degenerative joint diseases are well documented (Stanton, Bright, 1989; Wallace, Zawie, Garrey, 1990). These drugs generally make arthritic dogs more comfortable by reducing pain and inflammation but do little to arrest the degenerative process itself. This is in contrast to the supportive treatment offered by Perna mussel, glucosamines, glycosaminoglycans, vitamin C, and other therapeutic nutrients.

In her book *Drug-Induced Nutritional Deficiencies,* Daphne Roe (1978, 1984) reviews nutritional disorders caused by drug use. Roe (1992) states that various drugs can lead to an increase in nutrient requirements and cause specific vitamin deficiencies when neither the diet nor supplementation compensates for the additional demands. Drugs can induce impaired absorption, increase excretion, decrease transport and utilization, and have a negative effect on the storage of many nutrients. For example, long-term use of oral diuretics, including the thiazides, chlorthalidone, and furosemide, can lead to increased excretion of potassium, magnesium, and zinc (Lim, Jacob, 1972; Wester, 1975). The antibiotic neomycin can cause increased excretion of potassium, calcium, and vitamin B_{12} (Jacobson, Faloon, 1961). Although the risk factor of drug-nutrient interactions is often overlooked, the prac-titioner should be aware of these interactions. (Box 4-1 shows other drug-related interactions.)

The incorporation of nutritional supplements in therapy is generally without side effects and generally safe over long-term use. This is because the nutrients being used are native to the body and can be metabolized safely, without the formation of harmful or toxic by-products. Higher levels of certain nutrients, such as vitamins A and D, selenium, and iron should be monitored carefully to ensure that no imbalances or excesses occur (Shils, Olsen, Moshe, 1994). Some dietary and nutritional adjustments may be required if high doses of a particular nutrient are to be used to prevent imbalances and absorption problems. For example, excessive zinc can block copper absorption; therefore copper may need to be added to the diet when zinc is being administered (Shils, Olsen, Moshe, 1994).

The Use and Effectiveness of Nutritional Therapy

The effectiveness of therapeutic nutritional programs depends on several factors. These include the nature of the health problem, the nutritional status of the animal, the nutrients and dosages used, and the experience and nutritional expertise of the health care provider. Many products are available to the veterinarian today to use in practice, but literature references that give nutritional protocols or treatment programs for specific disease conditions are lacking. Manufacturers of nutritional products cannot provide therapeutic protocols for their products because the products

*M*INERAL *D*EPLETION *C*AUSED BY *D*RUGS

DRUG OR DRUG GROUP	MINERALS DEPLETED
Diuretics	
Thiazide (e.g., hydrochlorothiazide)	Potassium, magnesium, zinc
Loop (e.g., furosemide)	Potassium, magnesium, zinc, calcium
Glucocorticoids (e.g., prednisone)	Calcium, potassium
Chelating agents (e.g., penicillamine)	Zinc, copper
Cancer chemotherapeutic agents (heavy metal) (e.g., cisplatin)	Magnesium, zinc
Ethanol	Potassium, magnesium, zinc
Laxatives (e.g., phenolphthalein)	Potassium, calcium
Antacids (e.g., aluminum hyroxide)	Phosphate

*V*ITAMIN *A*NTAGONISTS

FOLACIN ANTAGONISTS
Methotrexate
Pyrimethamine
Triamterene
Trimethoprim

VITAMIN B$_{12}$ ANTAGONISTS
Nitrous oxide

VITAMIN B$_6$ ANTAGONISTS
Isoniazid
Hydralazine
Cycloserine
Levodopa

VITAMIN K ANTAGONISTS
Coumarin anticoagulants (warfarin)

Modified from Roe D: Nutrient and drug interactions. In Olson R et al, editors: *Present knowledge in nutrition,* ed 5, Washington, DC, 1984, Nutritional Foundation.

are marketed for nutritional purposes only. Also, funds for large-scale clinical trials for nutritional products that have no patent protection are scarce. In spite of these limitations, many veterinarians have studied the available literature and have established specific nutritional protocols based on years of clinical and field experience in dealing with various animal health problems. Unlike drug use, in which dosage is standardized, the dosage of a particular nutritional product may vary widely depending on the animal's condition, age, and overall nutritional status.

Nutritional therapy depends less on administering a "correct dose" than does drug therapy, which must be given at the lowest effective dose to prevent toxic side effects. Experience has shown that better results are often obtained when higher or "loading" dosages are used initially to saturate the tissues and optimize the animal's uptake and use of the nutritional product. Excess of the nutritional supplement is generally metabolized or eliminated without problems. At first, enzymatic activity associated with the nutritional product may be low because of lack of substrate availability, but activity increases as equilibrium is established over several days or weeks of administration. Once beneficial effects are maximized (usually from 3 to 6 weeks after initial administration), the dosage usually can be reduced to a lower maintenance level. This is especially true for long-term management of degenerative joint problems.

Nutritional therapy may be generally more successful when a combination of nutritional products is used to boost and enhance various metabolic pathways of the body. The "teamwork," or synergy, concept means that a combination of nutrients as part of the program, including the use of a broad-spectrum, multiple vitamin and mineral product, can be expected to give a better overall response. This approach increases nutrient level availability, which provides additional balanced support for regeneration and healing.

Nutritional therapy may not give the fast or dramatic relief of symptoms that drugs often show, but the use of nutrients and supplements can bring more stable and long-lasting results over the long term. As part of the total therapeutic package, the nutritional program does not just cover symptoms but may work to reverse the basic cause of the health problem, and this regenerative process takes time to accomplish.

Nutrients With Therapeutic Applications

Vitamins and Minerals

The use of vitamin and mineral products in preventive nutrition has primarily focused on overcoming deficiency states and the health problems associated with them. Because most, if not all disease states and degenerative conditions have a nutritional component, vitamins and minerals can also function as therapeutic agents against many diseases and health problems. When supplied in balanced, optimum levels, vitamins and minerals optimize metabolism, promote antioxidant activity (Halliwell, 1994), potentiate immune function (Beisel, and others, 1981; Dreizen, 1979; Sherman, Hallquist, 1990; Susanna, 1982), and decrease inflammatory processes (Shils, Olsen,

Moshe, 1994). All of these areas contribute to the healing response, whether it involves infection, allergy, arthritis, cardiovascular disease, degenerative joint disorder, inflammatory bowel disease, diabetes, or cancer.

Vitamin C

Extensive work has been published on vitamin C and its role in both preventive and therapeutic applications (Pauling, 1976; Sauberlich, 1994). Vitamin C is required for many fundamental processes, including the production of collagen, carnitine, hormones, epinephrine, and cortisone. It is involved in electrolyte transport, strengthening of vascular walls, free-radical quenching, immune enhancement, and antiviral activity. Increased intake has been linked to the successful treatment of many conditions in animals, including the following:

- Allergies (food and environmental)
- Stress
- Atherosclerosis
- Cancer
- Infections (bacterial and viral)
- Cardiovascular disease
- Hepatitis
- Periodontal disease
- Osteoarthritis
- Wounds and physical trauma

Although dogs, cats, and horses produce vitamin C, during times of extreme stress, injury, infection, and allergic and degenerative conditions, other animals may be unable to produce adequate amounts of ascorbic acid to compensate for these conditions (Verde, Piquer, 1986). Supplementation may be helpful in treating allergies (Johnston, Martin, Cai, 1992; Johnston, Retrum, Srilakshmi, 1992), dermatitis, degenerative joint disorders, diabetes mellitus (Eriksson, Kohvakka, 1995; Sinclair and others, 1994), cataracts, hip dysplasia (Berge, 1990), and urinary tract infections, and may help in cancer prevention (Alcain, Buron, 1994; Block, 1991, 1992).

Hip dysplasia has been linked specifically with vitamin C deficiency in German shepherds (Belfield, Zucker, 1981). In a 5-year study, eight litters of German shepherd puppies from parents with the disease were evaluated. The pregnant bitch was given from 2 to 4 g of vitamin C daily before whelping, and the puppies were administered increasing amounts of vitamin C as they grew older, ranging from 100 mg to 2000 mg daily over a 2-year period. All dogs in the study were reported to be devoid of dysplasia problems.

A study in Norway was conducted using a polyascorbate form of vitamin C (Ester-C) in dogs exhibiting clinical symptoms of chronic joint, skeletal, and muscle inflammation (Berge, 1990). Over 100 dogs in the group were administered 90 mg of polyascorbate per kilogram of body weight in divided doses daily for over 6 months. Ailments that showed major improvement after 6 weeks included hip dysplasia, arthropathies, spondylosis, and intervertebral disk disease.

Older horses (20 years or older) have been shown to have lower plasma vitamin C levels. Oral supplementation with ascorbic acid in older horses caused significant increases in plasma concentration when daily doses from 4.5 to 20 g were administered (Ralston, 1988). Rhabdomyolysis (tying-up syndrome) brought on by intensive exercise results in high free-radical levels compared with anaerobic activity. Ralston (1994) reports that antioxidant vitamins such as E and C may significantly reduce the possibility of muscle cell damage caused by free radicals and hypoxia. Horses with pituitary adenomas may also benefit from the daily administration of 10 g of vitamin C.

Vitamin E

Vitamin E as an antioxidant vitamin has many applications in animal health and therapy. It helps prevent cardiovascular disease, cataracts, inflammatory conditions, myopathies, skin diseases (Abbey, 1995), and cancer (Das, 1994). Vitamin E is used to treat steatitis in cats (Lewis, Morris, Hand, 1994) and enhances muscle and endurance in working animals. It has also been shown effective in combination with selenium in treating some cases of rhabdomyolysis that occurs early in exercise (Ralston, 1994). Deficiencies of vitamin E and selenium have been linked to nutritional myopathies such as white muscle disease (WMD) (Merck, 1991). Vitamin E is essential to immune function and has been shown to increase disease resistance (Tengerdy, 1990).

Vitamin E deficiency may be involved in equine motor neuron disease because affected horses have shown very low plasma and adipose vitamin E levels. Another disease that may be helped by vitamin E is equine degenerative myeloencephalopathy, a diffuse degenerative disease of the spinal cord and brainstem. Vitamin E (6000 IU per day) is recommended to reduce the incidence of EDM in young horses from affected blood lines or to improve the condition of the affected animals. Response to vitamin E may be related to an increased antioxidant activity in the horses (Hintz, Cymbaluk, 1994).

Vitamin A

Vitamin A and its precursor beta-carotene are beneficial for skin diseases and the immune system (Shils, Olsen, Moshe, 1994). Like vitamins C and E, vitamin A is an antioxidant that may help prevent cancer, retard aging, and protect the body from damage caused by pollutants and chemicals (Halliwell, 1994). Although recent studies dispute the benefits of beta-carotene for cancer prevention, vitamin A is useful therapeutically for eye diseases (cataracts, glaucoma, and conjunctivitis), dermatitis, and immune dysfunctions (Shils, Olsen, Moshe, 1994). Vitamin A can exert toxicity at high levels, and care must be used to prevent overdosing. Dogs and horses can derive vitamin A activity from beta-carotene; cats, however, cannot convert beta-carotene into vitamin A, and adequate amounts must be supplied in their diet (National Research Council, 1989).

B vitamins

B complex vitamins can be beneficial for several health problems, including acute stress, allergies, and infections. B vitamins are essential for energy production, growth, and a healthy immune system (Shils, Olsen, Moshe, 1994).

Biotin supplementation has been shown to be especially beneficial to horses with poor hoof conditions, such as dry, brittle walls resulting in cracking, and impaired growth. Enhanced growth rates and hoof hardness were achieved at a daily dose between 7.5 mg and 15 mg, with greater improvement seen at the higher dose (Buffa and others, 1992). Combining biotin with sulfur containing amino acids such as methionine, cysteine, and taurine enhances the effectiveness of the nutritional program.

Minerals

Minerals (essential and trace), their amounts, and ratios to one another are an important part of therapeutic nutrition. For example, zinc has been found beneficial to dogs and cats with skin problems, such as demodicosis, poor-quality coats, and allergic skin conditions (Broek, Thoday, 1986). Clinically, trace mineral supplementation can be very beneficial in improving the health of cats and dogs in the following ways:

- May encourage darker, thicker coats
- Reduces inflammation and scratching
- Reduces flakiness of skin
- Enhances appetite and physical activity in older animals

A combination of selenium supplementation and vitamin E administration has been used against white muscle disease. Selenium is essential as a cofactor for glutathione peroxidase, which neutralizes hydrogen peroxide and fatty acid hydroperoxides. Selenium levels in serum from myopathic animals also have been found to be low, along with reduced activity of glutathione peroxidase (*Merck Veterinary Manual*, 1991).

Amino Acids and Derivatives

Amino acids are constituents of proteins that serve many biologic functions in the body, including the production of enzymes, hormones, immunoglobulins, neurotransmitters, and structural proteins found in muscle, tendons, hair, and skin (Brady, 1994). Deficiencies of protein or amino acids in the diet are quickly manifested in the animal through loss of muscle mass, overall poor appearance, and loss of activity. Injury, illness, or extreme stress can lead to muscle wasting as the animal goes into a negative nitrogen balance (Lewis, Morris, Hand, 1994). Sup-

plementation with amino acids can be beneficial to the animal to help maintain muscle mass during such times. The branched-chain amino acids valine, leucine, and isoleucine and glutamine are especially helpful in this regard (Blackburn, Grant, Young, 1983).

Other amino acids and derivatives that are not essential to protein production have also been found to have beneficial therapeutic properties. They include L-carnitine, glutamine, dimethylglycine, and taurine.

L-Carnitine

L-Carnitine is required for the transport of long chain fatty acids across mitochondrial membranes of the cell. This is essential to the process of converting fatty acids into energy via β oxidation and the citric acid cycle. The mitochondria are the energy-producing organelles of the cell in which adenosine triphosphate (ATP) and other important metabolites are produced. The body produces carnitine from lysine and methionine in the presence of vitamins C, B_1, and B_6. If the level of L-carnitine is deficient, the number of potential health risks increases, including a buildup of triglycerides in the blood, decreased exercise tolerance, and myocardial disease (Shils, Olsen, Moshe, 1994). The breakdown of fatty acids is the critical source of energy for the heart, and without adequate carnitine to transport the fatty acids into the mitchondria, myocardial insufficiencies may result. Research strongly suggests that L-carnitine may be beneficial in both small and large animals for some cardiovascular problems (Keene, Panciera, Atkins, 1991; McEntee and others, 1995).

A recent report suggests that myocardial concentrations of L-carnitine are quite low in dogs suffering from dilated cardiomyopathy (McEntee and others, 1995). A Labrador suffering from dilated cardiomyopathy showed rapid and substantial clinical, electrocardiographic, and echocardiographic improvements after 2 months of treatment with L-carnitine (50 mg/kg tid). In addition to improved myocardial function, improved appetite and exercise tolerance were reported. The study suggests that L-carnitine supplementation may improve altered myocardial lipid metabolism associated with some cardiac diseases, including initial endocardiosis, ischemic heart disease, congestive heart failure, and dilated cardiomyopathy.

Glutamine

Glutamine is a primary energy source for the mucosal cells of the digestive tract (Windmueller, Spaeth, 1978). During stress periods such as with inflammatory bowel disease the biologic need for glutamine increases dramatically as the body replaces the injured mucosal cells (O'Dwyer and others, 1989). Recent work has shown supplementation with glutamine for inflammatory bowel disease to be especially beneficial (Belli and others, 1988; Yoshimura and others, 1993; Weir and others, 1993). Glutamine also can be useful as a supplement to reduce loss of muscle mass during times of injury, stress, or high-endurance activities.*

Dimethylglycine

Dimethylglycine (DMG) is a versatile metabolic enhancer that has been used in the equine and small animal fields for over 20 years to improve performance and enhance recovery from several health problems. DMG was first used in the early 1970s to enhance equine performance and stamina. Studies revealed that DMG could enhance oxygen usage, prevent lactic acid buildup, and improve muscle metabolism (Meduski and others, 1980). Track studies have demonstrated that DMG enhances stamina and endurance in both racing greyhounds and standardbred horses (Livine and others, 1982; Gannon, Kendall, 1983). DMG can be considered an antistress nutrient that improves the cardiovascular system and reduces recovery time from vigorous physical activity .

Studies have shown that DMG can improve the immune response in both animals and humans (Graber and others, 1981; Lawson, Reap, 1990). These studies show that DMG potentiates both humoral and cell-mediated immunity when administered orally. DMG may potentiate other aspects of the immune system, including interferon production (Lawson, Reap, 1990). Depressed immunity is associated with some degenerative diseases; therefore DMG, when used in combination with other therapies, may offer increased recovery from these diseases by boosting immune responses.

DMG seems to benefit some conditions, including seizures (Roach, Carlin, 1982), respiratory and allergic problems, and inflammation. A recent study at Clemson University indicates that DMG has an antiinflammatory effect in an induced arthritis model in rats (Kendall, Lawson, 1994).

DMG reduced the incidence of arthritis in a group of rats given DMG compared with the controls, but it also afforded reversal of the inflammatory condition in some experimental animals who had previously been induced with arthritis. More work in this area is currently being conducted.

Taurine

Taurine is an essential nutrient in the cat's diet (National Research Council, 1986). Inadequate taurine can result in retinal degeneration, reproduction problems, and dilated cardiomyopathy (Simpson, Anderson, Markwell, 1993). Studies of taurine supplementation in cats with congestive heart failure and feline dilated cardiomyopathy have demonstrated clinical and functional improvement after taurine supplementation of between 500 and 1000 mg per day (Pion and others, 1992).

---

*Caldwell, 1989; Hammarqvist and others, 1989; MacLennan and others, 1987; Marliss and others, 1971; Newsholme, Parry-Billings, 1990; Rennie and others, 1986; Roth and others, 1982; Stehle and others, 1987.

Essential Fatty Acids

A growing body of scientific literature that supports the use of essential fatty acids (EFAs) in the management of skin problems in dogs and cats (Merchant, 1994; White, 1993). The role of EFA in seborrhea and atopic skin disorders is presently undergoing extensive study (Lloyd, Thomsett, 1989; Logas, Kunkle, 1994; Miller and others, 1989).

Signs of EFA deficiency have been reported in cats and dogs. Although they can obtain both linoleic acid (LA) and γ-linolenic acid (GLA) from the diet to make the necessary subsequent conversions (Kendler, 1987), consuming poor-quality or low-fat diets can lead to an essential fatty acid deficiency (Fig. 4-1).

To further complicate matters, the cat cannot convert GLA from LA because of the absence of the Δ-5-desaturase activity and therefore requires dietary sources of this essential fatty acid (Hassam, Rivers, Crawford, 1977). In addition to their role in producing healthy skin and coat, EFAs also play a fundamental role in cutaneous inflammation caused by an allergic response mediated by eicosanoids. Eicosanoids are products of the C_{20} polyunsaturated fatty acids that originate from dihomo-γ-linolenic acid ($DGLA_{20:3\ n-6}$), arachidonic acid ($AA_{20:4\ n-6}$), and eicosapentaenoic acid ($EPA_{20:5\ n-3}$) (see Fig. 4-1). DGLA and AA are omega-6 fatty acids derived from vegetable and meat sources, whereas EPA is an omega-3 fatty acid derived primarily from marine sources. Besides being a major structural component of all cell walls, these C_{20} fatty acids are precursors to regulatory lipids such as prostaglandins (PG) and leukotrienes and thromboxanes, which mediate the inflammatory response in most tissues, including the skin. The PGs generated from the three series of C_{20} fatty acids have opposing functions: namely the PGs from arachidonic acid are proinflammatory, whereas the PGs from DGLA and EPA are antiinflammatory. These three series of fatty acids compete for the same enzymes, Δ-5 desaturase, Δ-6 desaturase, and elongase, needed for the formation of their eicosanoid (Kendler, 1987).

The mechanism of action associated with inflammation and dermatitis may be partly understood as resulting from an imbalanced or abnormal EFA metabolism. The therapeutic application of the EFAs for dogs and cats balances the ratios of the three series of fatty acids in the diet. Fatty acids can compete for and block the activity of the metabolic enzymes involved in the production of the proinflammatory products from arachidonic acid, thereby ameliorating the condition (Bond, Lloyd, 1992; Logas, Beale, Bauer, 1994; Scarff, Lloyd, 1992).

GLA is the precursor to DGLA; nutritional products that contain GLA include evening primrose, borage, and black currant oils. EPA of the omega-3 series is derived from fish oil. Because of the inhibitory competition that the omega-3 (GLA) and omega-6 (EPA) fatty acids exert on the arachidonic acid inflammatory cascade, products

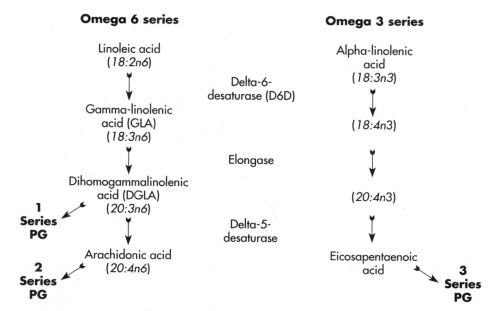

Fig. 4-1 Outline of prostaglandin formation from essential fatty acids. (From Kendler B: Gamma-linoleic acid: physiological effects and potential medical applications, *J Applied Nutr* 39:79, 1987.)

that contain both series are likely to maximize antiinflammatory eicosanoid production from arachidonic acid, especially in pruritus associated with allergic skin disease.

Flea and food allergies and bacterial skin infections should be responsive to EFA supplementation, reducing the pruritus and dermatitis that accompany these conditions. Results may be evident after a few weeks, but in most cases, 6 to 8 weeks of specific therapy may be required. The use of antihistamines, NSAIDs, and immunotherapy may also be required to keep the animal comfortable (White, 1993). The most effective dose of omega-6, omega-3, or a combination of the two series is not specifically known, and more research is needed to establish the best program.

The clinical use of EFAs in veterinary practice certainly extends beyond the treatment of skin disorders. Other areas of potential use for EPA include cardiovascular disease (Capron, 1993), arthritis (Carmichael, 1982), cancer therapy (see Chapter 7), and renal disease (Holub, 1995; Logas, Beale, Bauer, 1991). As more work is done in the veterinary field, more detailed protocols will be forthcoming that will employ both omega-3 and omega-6 fatty acids as natural therapeutic agents.

Coenzyme Q10

Over the past 20 years, many research articles, clinical studies, several books, and major reviews have been published on the essential cofactor, coenzyme Q_{10} (Folkers, Yamamcria, 1986). The biologic and therapeutic aspects of this nutrient have found interest in veterinary practice

because of its beneficial effects for several disease conditions.

Coenzyme Q_{10} is a lipid-soluble benzoquinone that is produced naturally in mammals. It is an essential component of the mitochondrial respiratory chain of the cell and plays a major role in the production of ATP. Coenzyme Q_{10} is involved in the electron transport from reduced flavin-linked dehydrogenase to oxygen (Lehninger, Nelson, Cox, 1993). The coenzyme seems to control the flow of oxygen within individual cells and may reduce the impact of hypoxia (ischemia) to the heart. Coenzyme Q_{10} plays a nonspecific antioxidant role in cellular metabolism and specifically works to reduce free-radical damage caused by peroxidation of fatty acids (Sugiyama and others, 1980).

The principal area of clinical use for coenzyme Q_{10} is for cardiovascular disorders such as cardiomyopathy and myocardial ischemia (Ishiyama and others, 1976, Morisco and others, 1993). Other potential veterinary uses would include periodontal disease, immune dysfunction, and decreased physical performance (Folkers, Yamamcria, 1986). Coenzyme Q_{10} levels decrease with age, especially in the heart and liver. Coenzyme Q_{10} supplementation increases the energy and exercise tolerance in older animals and may be effective in correcting the age-related decline in the immune system (Bliznakov, Casey, Premuzic, 1970).

One recent human study showed that congestive heart failure responds well to coenzyme Q_{10} supplementation (Morisco and others, 1993). Studies with animals show that coenzyme Q_{10} reduces the size of the infarct resulting from an acute coronary occlusion and protects the myocardium against induced cardiomyopathy and myocarditis (Hara, 1981; Kishimoto and others, 1984).

Periodontal and gum disease responds well to coenzyme Q_{10} therapy. Significant improvement can be seen in 1 to 2 weeks with coenzyme Q_{10} supplementation, including a decrease in inflammation, redness, bleeding, pocket depth, sensitivity to pain, and looseness of teeth (Wilkinson, 1976).

Proanthocyanidin Complex

Proanthocyanidins belong to a large group of naturally occurring plant polyphenolic compounds that have multiple health and therapeutic applications. Other terms that can be used to refer to these structures include *procyanidins, bioflavonoids, flavonoids,* and *pycnogenols.*

One primary action of these naturally occurring compounds is their antioxidant effects against lipid peroxidation (Affany, Salvayre, Blaze, 1987; Das, Ratty, 1986). Another important biochemical function of proanthocyanidins is their ability to inhibit lipooxygenase, an enzyme that is needed to convert arachidonic acid into leukotrienes (Tarayre, Lauresserques, 1977), which are potent mediators of inflammation and allergic responses. Proanthocyanidins have been shown to inhibit two key enzymes, cyclic adenosine monophosphate (cAMP) phosphodiesterase and transport ATPases, which work in concert to effect histamine release from mast cells and basophils (Beretz, Anton, Stoclet, 1978; Fewtrell, Gomperts, 1977). The potential use of these bioflavonoids to inhibit allergic responses and asthma attacks is well documented (Clark, Mackay, 1950; Davies, Moodley, 1982; Gabor, 1986; Schoenkerman, Justice, 1952; Yoshimoto and others, 1983). Proanthocyanidins have important clinical application in blocking inflammatory responses in some conditions (Gupta and others, 1971; Villar, Gasco, Alcaraz, 1984; Fourie, Snyckers, 1984).

Proanthocyanidins and related bioflavonoids have shown anticancer activity (Wei and others, 1990) and the ability to potentiate the immune response, including enhancement of T-lymphocyte activity and modulation of neutrophil and macrophage responses (Berg, Daniel, 1988).

The free-radical scavenging action and antienzyme activity of proanthocyanidins has recently been studied (Facino, 1994). The proanthocyanidins isolated from a grape seed extract exhibited potent antioxidant activity against reactive oxygen species in a lipid peroxidation model. In a second part of the study the proanthocyanidins inhibited the activity of xanthine oxidase activity, the enzyme that can induce the oxyradical cascade. In addition, proanthocyanidins were shown to inhibit the proteolytic enzyme activity of collagenase, elastase, glycosidases, hyaluronidase, and β-glucuronidase. These enzymes are involved in the destruction of the main structural components of the extravascular matrix: collagen, elastin, and

hyaluronic acid (Facino, 1994). This research demonstrates a potential therapeutic role for proanthocyanidin complex in animals afflicted with osteoarthritis and other joint and connective tissue disorders.

Proanthocyanidin complex can be isolated from many natural products, including fruits, seeds, and other plant material. Two commercial sources include extracts from pine bark and from grape seed. Pycnogenol® is a trade name for one such proanthocyanidin product on the market.

Glucosamine and Related Compounds

Glucosamine and the related products, glucosamine sulfate and *N*-acetyl glucosamine, have found use as nutritional antiosteoarthritic agents by helping protect and regenerate connective tissue and cartilage in affected joints. *N*-Acetyl glucosamine has shown promise in the treatment of inflammatory disorders including inflammatory bowel disease, Crohn's disease, and colitis (Burton, Anderson, 1983). These compounds are amino sugars produced from glucose and the amino acid glutamine. Glucosamines are the building blocks of glycosaminoglycans (GAG) and proteoglycans. These large polysaccharide structures are incorporated into connective tissues, joint constituents, and mucous membranes. GAGs include chondroitin sulfates and hyaluronic acid, which combine with various fibrous proteins such as collagen to form the extracellular matrix that holds cells together. These molecules are responsible for the gelatinous nature of cartilage. The GAGs allow cartilage to hold water and act as a shock absorber, providing it with the ability to withstand compression forces without breaking (Lehninger, Nelson, Cox, 1993).

Besides providing an organized structure for joints with their supporting tendons, ligaments, and synovial fluid, these amino sugars are important in the production of glycoproteins that make up the structure and support functioning of the mucous membranes of the digestive, respiratory, and genitourinary tracts. This mucous membrane layer, rich in glycoproteins, not only protects the digestive tract from the action of digestive acids and enzymes, but also controls the passage of molecules into and out of the gut. The mucosal cell lining has a very high cell turnover rate and depends on a steady flow of D-glucosamine (for which glutamine is a precursor) for replacing the glycoproteins.

Research indicates that individuals with inflammatory bowel disease have a turnover rate of gastrointestonal (GI) mucosal cells that is 3 times greater than that of healthy patients. These patients were also found to be unable to perform the early acetylation step necessary to produce *N*-acetyl glucosamine. Because *N*-acetyl glucosamine is essential in the production of glycoproteins, this inability exacerbates the patient's condition (Burton, Anderson, 1983).

A deficiency of *N*-acetyl glucosamine can lead to further damage to the intestines, including greater permeability, or a "leaky gut" syndrome. This allows a variety of disease conditions, including allergies, autoimmune disorders, microbial infections, and malabsorption (see Chapter 28). Tissue injury and inflammation can become worse unless repair can be facilitated. Supplemental *N*-acetyl glucosamine can help support glycoprotein synthesis. This amino acid can be readily absorbed and incorporated into the mucosal layer of the gut where damage can be repaired, thereby potentially reducing symptoms associated with inflammatory bowel disease in cats such as vomiting and diarrhea (Burton, Anderson, 1983).

Glucosamine sulfate has been shown in several studies to be efficacious against numerous degenerative joint disorders and osteoarthritis (D'Ambrosio and others, 1981; Reichelt and others, 1994; Tapadinhas, Rivera, Bignamini, 1982; Vaz, 1982). D-Glucosamine and glucosamine sulfate are readily absorbed and can be used for GAG synthesis in the chondrocytes of the joints (Roden, 1956; Karzel, Domenjoz, 1971). Increased D-glucosamine levels have been shown to stimulate GAG and collagen syntheses in the chondrocytes and fibroblasts (Grevenstein and others, 1991). The reversal of damaged osteoarthritic joints by glucosamine salts has been seen in several studies conducted in Europe on humans and animals. In humans, an oral dosage of 500 mg of glucosamine sulfate 3 times daily was effective over a 4- to 10-week period. Results included reduced joint pain, tenderness, and joint inflammation as compared with a control group. Joint mobility and function increased with physical activity (Pujalte, Llavore, Ylescupidey, 1980). In one study, glucosamine sulfate was compared with ibuprofen and found to be more effective over the long term. Initially, ibuprofen was more effective in reducing inflammation than the glucosamine sulfate, but over a longer time the glucosamine salts were more effective in reversing cartilage degradation and reducing inflammation and pain (Muller-Fabender and others, 1994). Examination of cartilage biopsies by electron microscopy revealed actual repair of the damaged cartilage matrix (Drovanti, Bignamini, Rovati, 1980).

Both glucosamine sulfate and glucosamine HCl (a salt of D-glucosamine) are effective in treating degenerative joint disease, although the principal studies have focused on glucosamine sulfate. The body eventually converts D-glucosamine into glucosamine sulfate. These nutrients are showing great promise in veterinary practice, although controlled studies are incompleted. One study has reported the pharmacokinetics, organ distribution, metabolism, and excretion of D-glucosamine in dogs and humans (Setnikar, Giacchetti, Zanolo, 1991). Glucosamine products can be used for many cartilage and disc degeneration conditions, including osteoarthritis, hip dysplasia, spondylitis, osteochondritis, and nonspecific arthritic conditions. The direct benefit appears to be protective and restorative, leading to less pain and inflammation and greater mobility.

Shark and Bovine Cartilage

Shark cartilage has received intense interest from both health practitioners and the general public for its potential use against many types of cancer. The Food and Drug Administration (FDA) has approved a few clinical studies after evaluating the results of smaller cancer studies and case histories that showed a significantly high percentage of reversal in terminally ill cancer patients who were treated with shark cartilage. Pharmaceutical-grade shark cartilage products have been available since 1990.

Work on bovine cartilage began in the 1960s when physician John Prudden began using specially prepared bovine cartilage on several degenerative conditions, including osteoarthritis, rheumatoid arthritis, psoriasis, glaucoma, and cancer (Prudden, Balassa, 1974).

Prudden (1985) reported on several studies using bovine cartilage prepared from pepsin-digested calf trachea (Catrix) that was administered in both oral and injectable forms.

The product was found beneficial in treating patients with both osteoarthritis and rheumatoid arthritis, resulting in reduced pain and inflammation and increased joint mobility. Good results have been noted using bovine cartilage on dogs suffering from degenerative disk and spinal disorders. Psoriasis and ulcerative colitis may respond well to bovine cartilage therapy according to some clinicians (Brown, Weiss, 1988; Prudden, Balassa, 1974).

Catrix also showed promising results in both in vitro and in vivo cancer studies. In cancer patients, bovine cartilage was given orally (9 g/day) or by subcutaneous injection. The studies revealed that the product exerted an inhibitory response on some cancer types and halted the growth of solid tumors in a significant number of patients (Prudden, 1985).

In the mid-1980s, research showed a greater therapeutic potential for shark cartilage than bovine cartilage against certain cancers. The earlier work on bovine cartilage by Folkman (1971) demonstrated that it contained an angiogenesis inhibitor that prevented or reduced the growth of new blood vessels (Langer and others, 1976). Folkman and Langer and others found that bovine cartilage caused inhibition of vascularization around implanted tumors when infused into rabbits or mice.

Later, investigation of shark cartilage found it to be 1000 times more potent than bovine cartilage in inhibiting angiogenesis (Langer and others, 1983). Several controlled studies using implanted tumors in animals showed shark cartilage to be effective in shrinking tumor masses and preventing the growth of new blood vessels around tumor sites (Lee, Langer, 1983; Oikawa and others, 1990). Tumors that are unable to develop their own vascular systems fail to grow, resulting in tumor necrosis.

Bovine and shark cartilage may contain other compounds that slow tumor invasiveness such as inhibitors to collagenase (Moses, Sudhalter, Langer, 1990; Murray and others, 1986). Tumors secrete the enzyme collagenase, which degrades surrounding host tissue, allowing the tumors to spread.

Both bovine and shark cartilage contain GAGs, which have antiinflammatory properties. GAGs can be used by the body to help regenerate connective tissue and therefore repair damaged joints. A growing body of scientific evidence shows that GAGs are effective in treating various types of arthritis, cardiovascular disease, and immune dysfunctions. Both bovine and shark cartilage have been used in the treatment of osteoarthritis in humans, horses, dogs, and cats.

The veterinarian Jacques Rauis administered a dose of 750 mg of shark cartilage per 5 kg of body weight to 10 dogs suffering from lameness caused by secondary osteoarthritis. The osteoarthritic condition followed either joint fractures (2 cases), hip dysplasia (4 cases), spondylopathy (2 cases) or rupture of the cruciate ligament (2 cases), and the diagnosis was confirmed by x-ray examination. The study lasted 21 days, and no other treatment was given. Final evaluation indicated reduced swelling and sensitivity, less pain, and greater mobility in 8 of the 10 animals. All of the dogs reverted to their original states once the administration of shark cartilage ended. When administration of shark cartilage (at 50% of the original dose) was reinstituted, the dogs improved rapidly. This study concluded that shark cartilage appears to work on both the inflammation and angiogenesis associated with osteoarthritis in dogs (Lane, 1992). Cartilage products seem to work well in combination with other modalities in the treatment of some connective tissue and joint problems in both large and small animals.

Glycosaminoglycan (GAG) Products

GAG products have found wide application in clinical nutritional therapy, including the treatment of degenerative joint diseases in large and small animals (Boulay, 1995; Jones, 1988).

Shark and bovine cartilage, Perna canaliculus, and chondroitin sulfate products all contain these GAGs, which are part of the proteoglycan structure that form cross-linkages with collagen within cartilage and other connective tissue. Their presence in the connective tissue gives elasticity and greater resiliency to the extracellular matrix (Lehninger, Nelson, Cox, 1993).

GAGs are composed of repeating disaccharide units in which one of the two monosaccharides is always either N-acetylglucosamine or N-acetylgalactosamine and the other, in most cases, is glucuronic acid. In some GAGs, one or more of the hydroxyl group of the amino sugar is esterified with a sulfate group. The combination of the sulfate and carboxylate groups of the uronic acid residues gives these structures an extremely high density of negative charge. As a result, these large molecular complexes spread out, producing a large volume by interacting with water molecules. This association with water imparts compression-resisting strength to the articular cartilage. When this compression-resisting property and elasticity is diminished or lost as a result of ongoing stress, the cartilage can be subjected to injury and physical breakdown (Lehninger, Nelson, Cox, 1993).

Five GAGs that have relevance to connective tissue are chondroitin 4-sulfate, chondroitin 6-sulfate, keratin sulfate, dermatan sulfate, and nonsulfated hyaluronic acid. Hyaluronic acid contributes to the viscosity of synovial fluid and lubricates the synovial membranes. Along with the other GAGs, hyaluronic acid provides greater flexibility, elasticity, and tensile strength to the articular cartilage and tendons.

Osteoarthritis, or degenerative joint disease, is a progressive deterioration of the synovial joint and bone structure caused by abnormal stress or injury. It is characterized by joint pain, inflammation of the synovial membrane, and loss of the articular cartilage as a result of a breakdown of the proteoglycans in the cartilage matrix. As the disease progresses, synovitis and joint enlargement occur, leading to a decrease in joint motion and abnormal changes within the joint. Space between the collagen fibers increases, and lysosomal enzymes such as collagenase and gelatinase are released, causing further deterioration. Release of free-radical mediators also contributes to major cartilage degradation. The severity of the disease appears to correlate with the loss of GAG content within the joint and surrounding tissues (Boulay, 1995).

Effective treatment of the affected joints should center on decreasing the inflammation, enhancing cartilage synthesis by the chondrocytes, and reducing the degradation of the surrounding cartilage matrix by the lysosomal enzymes. GAGs appear to stabilize the joint in these three areas and prevent the progressive development of the disease. In contrast, administering antiinflammatory drugs will help reduce the inflammation but will do little to improve the healing of the articular cartilage (Boulay, 1995).

GAGs can exert a potent antiinflammatory action on the connective tissue and act directly in the structural repair process. They can provide the chondrocytes with increased availability of chondroitin sulfates and hyaluronic acid precursors, which can not only increase synovial fluid viscosity in the joints but can give a metabolic boost in the natural synthesis of the extracellular matrix. GAG supplementation can have a positive effect on enhancing production of the proteoglycans and connective tissues and thereby slow down and reverse the destructive process. The exact mechanism by which this stimulation of connective tissue growth is achieved is not fully understood.

A partially synthetic polysulfated GAG product, Adequan®, has been approved by the FDA for use on noninfectious degenerative joint disease in horses. This injectable product has been shown effective in inhibiting the actions of cathepsin and hyaluronidase enzymes that contribute to cartilage degradation. This may indicate that orally administered glycosaminoglycans act in the same way to block the destructive activity of these enzymes.

GAG products work to reduce inflammation and pain, help normalize synovial fluid viscosity, and promote the repair of cartilage. At the same time, these products may retard the degradative process caused by the release of the proteolytic enzymes. GAGs can be used effectively in combination with other modalities to promote regeneration and healing of degenerative joint disease in horses and small animals.

Perna Mussel

Perna canaliculus is a marine bivalve mussel produced commercially in New Zealand. An orally administered product of this mussel has been used to treat degenerative joint disorders for over 20 years in both the medical and veterinary fields. Analysis of the Perna mussel shows that it is approximately 60% protein, 25% complex carbohydrates, and 2% to 4% fat. It also contains a broad spectrum of natural vitamins, chelated minerals, and nucleic acids. Approximately 10% of the complex carbohydrate is present as GAG products (Miller, Wu, 1984).

Published work from nearly 20 years ago has shown the Perna mussel to be beneficial in treating arthritis and other inflammatory conditions (McFarlane, 1975; Rainsford, Whitehouse, 1980; Miller, 1981). Two major studies conducted in Scotland and France used human patients suffering from osteoarthritis and rheumatoid arthritis, to demonstrate the Perna mussel's effectiveness in this area (Gibson and others, 1980; Audeval, Bouchacourt, 1985). In one study involving 86 patients with arthritis (31 osteoarthritis and 55 rheumatoid arthritis), Gibson and associates (1980) reported that 67% of the patients with rheumatoid arthritis and 35% of the patients with osteoarthritis received significant benefit after 3 to 6 months. In a second study involving 53 patients with radiologically confirmed osteoarthritis of the knee, 40% of the subjects showed improvement. Areas of improvement in both studies included reduced pain and inflammation and greater joint mobility. Other areas of possible use include inflammatory skin conditions, low sperm motility, and degenerative conditions related to aging. Anecdotal reports by many practicing veterinarians suggest clinical efficacy in treating degenerative joint disease and connective tissue disorders in horses and dogs.

Several studies have linked the Perna mussel's antiinflammatory effect to the presence of certain protein structures (Couch and others, 1982). The Perna mussel contains multiple biologically active agents, including the GAGs and an antihistaminic substance (Kosuge and others, 1988).

Earlier work had shown the Perna mussel to contain an inhibitor of prostaglandin synthesis; this may also help to explain the observed antiinflammatory effect (Miller, Wu, 1984).

Recent work by Lawson and Belkowski has confirmed the potential benefits of the Perna mussel as an antiinflammatory agent (Lawson, Belkowski, 1996). The work shows that Perna mussel has the potential to reverse the degenerative process of rheumatoid arthritis in mice and rats. The study demonstrated that a daily intake of Perna mussel suppressed the development of arthritis in the collagen II–induced model as well as reduced the severity of the inflammation in those animals already afflicted with the disease. One group of mice showed a 50% to 60% reduction in the severity of inflammation compared with that of controls.

The exact mechanism of the way Perna mussel works in controlling and preventing arthritis in laboratory animals has not been clearly shown. The unique combination of complex proteins, GAGs, amino acids, nucleic acids, and naturally chelated minerals may work to give a synergistic, biologic effect that helps repair articular cartilage and prevent further deterioration. Earlier material on the value of GAGs in the area of degenerative joint disease is relevant to this discussion. The Perna mussel may enhance the regenerative capabilities of the chondrocytes that regulate and produce the chondroitin sulfates and hyaluronic acid needed by the joint and connective tissue. The product appears to improve joint lubrication, ease joint pain, and improve mobility and range of motion in the affected joints. Other benefits for Perna mussel include reduced inflammation and improved connective tissue elasticity. As an oral nutritional product, Perna has been shown beneficial in the area of degenerative joint disorders and problems associated with aging in the horse, dog, and cat.

Direct-Fed Microbials (Probiotics)

Proper functioning of the GI system is essential to maintain good health in animals and maximize performance. Illness, injury, and excessive stress can alter the normal microflora population, pH value, and digestive processes in the gut. Such changes may contribute to further ill health and delayed healing. Direct-fed microbials, also referred to as *probiotics,* are beneficial microbial preparations that have experienced a resurgence in use over the past few years. *Lactobacillus bulgaris* and *L. acidophilus* were the earliest recognized microbials used in nutritional therapy for diseases relating to an improperly functioning gastrointestinal GI tract. Under normal and healthy conditions, beneficial microorganisms form a symbiotic relationship with the host, and potentially pathogenic microbes are suppressed. Beneficial bacteria can supply nutrients to the host, aid in digestion, and produce better food conversion (Friend, Shahani, 1984; Kung, 1994; Shahani, Ayebo, 1980).

The discovery of penicillin in the 1940s overshadowed the use of "friendly," or beneficial, bacterial strains as a means of altering the intestinal environment. Antibiotic therapy used in eliminating pathogenic bacteria also has the effect of eliminating beneficial bacteria in the gut. Such reduction in the friendly bacteria predisposes an animal to other possible disease processes. The problem of excessive use of antibiotics led to many pathogenic bacterial strains becoming immune to the very antibiotics used to treat them. As a result, interest in the use of beneficial bacteria was renewed.

The goal of introducing probiotics into a preventive or therapeutic program is to counter the negative consequences that stress, illness, or use of antibiotics have on the GI tract. Examples of stress that can alter an animal's normal microflora populations in the gut are feed changes, poor nutrition, birthing, weaning, close housing, shipping, exposure to pathogenic microorganisms or viruses, weakened immune system, and an extensive work or exercise schedule. Such stress responses can lead to a decrease in food intake, and without adequate energy sources, beneficial microflora populations decline. Subsequently, the pH of the GI tract rises and pathogenic bacterial populations increase. Direct-fed microbials can reestablish the beneficial bacteria that in turn lower the intestinal pH, making the GI environment less favorable for pathogenic organisms such as bacteria, yeasts, and fungi (Kung, 1994).

Probiotics have been used to improve overall performance. One study examined the effects of probiotic supplementation on cardiorespiratory, hematologic, and biochemical parameters for racing thoroughbreds in training. The results of the study suggested that some aerobic metabolic parameters improve during race training in horses fed the probiotic product (Art and others, 1994).

Beneficial bacteria found in direct-fed microbial products help keep disease-causing microorganisms in check by producing antibacterial agents and enzymes that act on and kill many pathogenic bacteria and viruses (Gilbert and others, 1983; Kovacs and others, 1994; Shahani, Valkil, Kilara, 1977; Spencer, Chesson, 1994). Beneficial bacteria also help neutralize the toxins produced by pathogenic bacteria and produce a wide range of B- vitamins and beneficial enzymes (Kung, 1994).

Research on direct-fed microbials has led to the development of microorganisms that are more specific in their function and impact on the GI tract. These specific direct-fed microbials benefit the host animal by being more compatible than the generalized microbials. Also, specific strains are known to have different modes of action. For instance, *L. acidophilus* produces lactic acid to reduce the gut pH and acts as a colonizer, *L. casei* acts to lower oxidation processes, and *L. lactis* acts on hydrogen peroxide, amylase, and protease enzymes (Kung, 1994).

A variety of products are available commercially, and the practitioner should become familiar with them to choose a good product. One recent study found that commercial probiotics may not contain the microbial species listed on the label or may contain no viable cultures at all; in fact, only 2 of 13 products matched the labeled specifications qualitatively and quantitatively (Hamilton-Miller, 1996).

In short, direct-fed microbials have been found to be extremely beneficial in helping restore and maintain health under a variety of conditions. The reintroduction of probiotics into an animal's diet offers the veterinarian not only a natural and effective therapy for diseases relating to GI distress but also an opportunity to establish a stable, healthy gut environment that aids in disease prevention.

Digestive Enzymes

Digestive enzymes play a very important role in maintaining health and proper functioning of the body. Physical situations in which supplemental digestive enzymes may improve digestion and help animals recover from disease also exist.

The two major classes of enzymes in the body are metabolic enzymes, which serve as catalysts to all cellular reactions, and digestive enzymes, which break down proteins, fats, carbohydrates, and cellulose so that an animal may absorb and use the nutrients found in foods. Digestive enzymes are produced by the salivary glands, stomach, pancreas, and liver and secreted into the digestive tract (Brady, 1994).

Digestive enzymes are specific and selective in their digestive capability according to the type of substances and bonds they break in various biomolecules. For example, proteases work on proteins, lipases break down fat, and amylases digest carbohydrates. Some enzymes are secreted in their active form; others are zymogens, which are enzymes that are activated in the stomach or small intestine. In the normal healthy animal, effective digestion takes place effectively as a result of hormonal response to food intake or on signals from the brain that trigger secretion of the enzymes and digestive juices (Brady, 1994).

Physical situations may occur in which the digestive process can be inhibited such that foods are not adequately and completely digested. Illness, intense stress, food intolerance, allergy, and use of drugs such as antibiotics can lead to disturbances of GI function, which result in poor digestion and insufficient enzyme production. At these times the use of a broad-spectrum digestive enzyme product can supplement the normal enzymatic activity of the body and improve the uptake of needed nutrients for energy and building up the body.

The use of selective digestive enzymes in feeding programs may also enhance the feed efficiency. Kung (1994) reports the use of common enzymes as feed additives and discusses their potential application. A cellulase enzyme complex containing multiple enzymes has been developed to improve breakdown of cellulose and high-fiber foods. The use of phytases can facilitate breakdown of phytic acid and improve the use of phosphorus.

Enzyme therapy has been found useful in other diverse conditions. One recognized use is as an analgesic after exercise or for soft tissue trauma. Baumuller (1990) found that human athletes experienced reduced convalescent time, speedier recovery to complete mobility, and reduced pain and swelling when treated with an oral enzyme supplement. Another study evaluated enzyme therapy as a treatment for several pain conditions induced in experimental animals. Papain, a protease, was as effective as acetylsalicylic acid as an analgesic and antiinflammatory agent in a variety of situations (Emele, Shanaman, Winbury, 1966). Bromelain, a hydrolytic protease derived from pineapple stems, was found to inhibit metastasis of implanted lung carcinoma in mice (Batkin, Taussig, Sekerezes, 1988).

Enzymes have immune-modulating properties and have been used in the treatment of cancer and AIDS.

Proteases may have the ability to remove or digest immune complexes (Nakazawa, Emancipator, Lamm, 1985; Stauder and others, 1988) and induce the production of tumor necrosis factor by peripheral blood mononuclear cells (Desser, Rehberger, 1990).

Studies involving the use of digestive enzymes on dogs, cats, and horses are limited, but the use of such products in conditions as diverse as subclinical maldigestion, autoimmune disease, cancer, and a variety of other inflammatory conditions may be beneficial. Digestive enzymes may be especially important to the older animal whose digestive capability may be reduced. Animals under stress or that are experiencing health problems may benefit from the inclusion of digestive enzymes in their diets.

Summary

Using nutrients and nutritional supplements to aid in the healing process is fundamental to the way the body functions and is certainly not a new concept. Therapeutic nutrition is a practical approach that can be incorporated into any clinical condition or disease protocol.

Although there are no officially established guidelines for implementing therapeutic nutrition in veterinary practice, many veterinarians are including the aforementioned approaches in their practices. Therapeutic nutrition is based on the idea that if the body is provided with a better nutritional environment, healing will occur at a higher level of efficacy. The rational use of nutritional products and specific nutrients is based on a combination of clinical and nutritional research, clinical experience, and the availability of high-quality, safe, and dependable nutritional products.

Because nutrients work better in combination with other nutrients, the classic double-blind study on single nutrients is less feasible. In most cases, nutritional products are not protected by patents and therefore the money to carry out such studies for FDA approval is not available. The bottom line to any nutritional protocol must lie with the veterinarian's knowledge and acceptance of available nutritional evidence that such an addition will have beneficial effects on the healing process. Over time, vet-erinarians should see improved results within their patients as a result of incorporating nutritional products in their practices.

The use of nutrients in clinical practice is not meant to replace the use of drugs and surgery, but to work synergistically with the best protocols and tools at the veterinarian's disposal. If properly incorporated into the veterinary practice, the use of therapeutic nutrition can bring about superior results. Knowing the specifics of the timing of and the ways to use nutritional products takes patience, study, and clinical experience.

REFERENCES

Abbey M: The importance of vitamin E in reducing cardiovascular risk, *Nutr Rev* 53:28, 1995.

Affany A, Salvayre R, Blaze L: Comparison of the protective effect of various flavonoids against lipid peroxidation of erythrocyte membranes induced by cumene hydroperoxide, *Fundamental Clin Pharmacol* 1:45, 1987.

Alcain FJ, Buron MI: Ascorbate on cell growth and differentiation, *J Bioenerg Biomembr* 26:393, 1994.

Anderson R: The immunostimulatory, antiinflammatory and antiallergic properties of ascorbate, *Adv Nutr Res* 6:19, 1984.

Art T and others: Cardiorespiratory, haematological and biochemical parameter adjustments to exercise: effect of a probiotic in horses during training, *Vet Res* 251:361, 1994.

Audeval B, Bouchacourt P: Controlled double-blind study with placebo of the mussel extract of Perna canaliculus (green-lipped mussel) in arthritis of the knee, *Gazette Medicale* 93:111, 1986.

Batkin S, Taussig SJ, Sekerezes J: Antimetastatic effect of bromelain with or without its proteolytic and anticoagulant activity, *J Cancer Res Clin Oncol* 114:507, 1988.

Baumuller M: Therapy of ankle joint distortions with hydrolytic enzymes—results from a double blind clinical trial, Proceedings of the twenty-fourth World Congress of Sports Medicine, Amsterdam, 1990.

Beisel W and others: Single nutrient effects on immunologic functions, *JAMA* 245:53, 1981.

Beisel W: Single nutrients and immunity, *Am J Clin Nutr* S35:417, 1982.

Belfield W, Zucker M: *How to have a healthy dog: the benefits of vitamin and minerals for your dog's life cycle,* New York, 1981, New American Library.

Belli D and others: Chronic intermittent elemental diet improves growth failure in children with Crohn's disease, *Gastroenterol* 94:603, 1988.

Bendich A, Langseth L: The health effects of vitamin C supplementation, *J Am Coll Nutr* 14:124, 1995.

Beretz A, Anton R, Stoclet J: Flavonoid compounds are potent inhibitors of cyclic AMP phosphodiesterase, *Experientia* 34:1054, 1978.

Berg P, Daniel P: Effects of flavonoid compounds on the immune response. In *Plant flavonoids in biology and medicine,* 1988, Alan R. Liss.

Berge J: Polyascorbate (C-Flex): an interesting alternative for problems on the support and movement apparatus in dogs: clinical trial of Ester-C ascorbate in dogs, *Norweg Vet J* 102:579, 1990.

Bielory L, Gandhi R: Asthma and vitamin C, *Ann Allergy* 73:89, 1994.

Blackburn G, Grant J, and Young V, editors: *Amino acids—metabolism and medical applications,* Littleton, Mass, 1983, John Wright.

Bliznakov EG, Casey A, Premuzic E: Coenzyme Q10: stimulants of the phagocytic activity in rats and immune response in mice, *Experientia* 26:953, 1970.

Block G: Vitamin C and cancer prevention: the epidemiologic evidence, *Am J Clin Nutr* 53:270S, 1991.

Block G: Vitamin C, cancer, and aging, *Age* 16:55, 1992.

Bond R, Lloyd DH: A double-blind comparison of olive oil and a combination of evening primrose oil and fish oil in the management of canine atopy, *Vet Rec* 131:558, 1992.

Boulay J and others: Medical therapy of osteoarthritis in dogs, *Veterinary Exchange Compendium* 17(suppl):13, 1995.

Brady T: *Nutritional biochemistry,* New York, 1994, Academic.

Broek A, Thoday K: Skin disease in dogs associated with zinc deficiency: a report of five cases, *J Small Anim Pract* 27:313, 1986.

Brown RA, Weiss JB: Neovascularization and its role in the osteoarthritic process, *Ann Rheum Dis* 4:881, 1988.

Buffa E and others: The effect of dietary biotin supplement on equine hoof, horn growth rate and hardness, *Equine Vet J* 6:472, 1992.

Burton A, Anderson F: Decreased incorporation of 14-C glucosamine relative to 3-H-*N*-acetyl glucosamine in the intestinal mucosa of patients with inflammatory bowel disease, *Am J Gastroenterol* 78:19, 1983.

Caldwell MD: Local glutamine metabolism in wounds and inflammation, *Metabolism* 38(suppl): 34, 1989.

Capron L: Marine oils and prevention of cardiovascular diseases, *Revue Praticien* 43:164, 1993.

Carmichael J: Uses of nutritional precursors of prostaglandin E_1 in the management of rheumatoid arthritis and chronic coxsackie infection. In Horrobin D, editor: *Clinical uses of essential fatty acids,* Westmount, Que, 1982, Eden Press.

Clark W, Mackay E: Effect of flavonoid substances on histamine toxicity, anaphylactic shock, and histamine-enhanced capillary permeability to dye, *J Allergy* 1:133, 1950.

Cohen M, Bhagavan HN: Ascorbic acid and gastrointestinal cancer, *J Am Coll Nutr* 14:565, 1995.

Couch R, and others: Antiinflammatory activity in fractionated extracts of the green-lipped mussel, *N Z Med J* 95:805, 1982.

D'Ambrosio E and others: Glucosamine sulphate: a controlled clinical investigation in arthrosis, *Pharmatherapeutica* 2:504, 1981.

Das S: Vitamin E in the genesis and prevention of cancer: a review, *Acta Oncologica* 33:615, 1994.

Das N, Ratty A: Effects of flavonoids on induced non-enzymatic lipid peroxidation. In *Plant flavonoids in biology and medicine,* vol. 1, New York, 1986, Alan R. Liss.

Davies R, Moodley I: Antiallergic compounds, *Pharmacol Ther* 17:279, 1982.

Delafuente JC, Prendergast JM, Modigh A: Immunologic modulation by vitamin C in the elderly, *Int J Immunopharmacol* 8:205, 1986.

Desser L, Rehberger A: Induction of tumor necrosis factor in human peripheral-blood mononuclear cells by proteolytic enzymes, *Oncol* 47:475, 1990.

Dreizen S: Nutrition and the immune response: a review, *Int J Vitamin Res* 49:220, 1979.

Drovanti A, Bignamini A, Rovati A: Therapeutic activity of oral glucosamine sulfate in osteoarthritis: a placebo-controlled double blind study, *Clin Ther* 3:260, 1980.

Emele JF, Shanaman J, Winbury MM: The analgesic-antiinflammatory activity of papain, *Arch Int Pharmacodyn* 159:126, 1966.

Eriksson J, Kohvakka A: Magnesium and ascorbic acid supplementation in diabetes mellitus, *Ann Nutr Metab* 39:217, 1995.

Facino R: Free radical scavenging action and antienzyme activities of procyanidines from *Vitis vinifera:* a mechanism for their capillary protective action, *Arzneim-Forsch* 44:592, 1994.

Fewtrell C, Gomperts B: Effects of flavor inhibitors of transport ATPases on histamine secretion from rat mast cells, *Nature* 265:635, 1977.

Folkers K, Yamamcria Y, editors: *Biomedical and clinical aspects of coenzyme Q,* ed 5, New York, 1986, Elsevier.

Folkman J: Tumor angiogenesis: therapeutic implications, *N Engl J Med* 285:1182, 1971.

Fourie T, Snyckers R: A flavone and antiinflammatory activity from the roots of *Rhus undulata, J Natural Products* 47:1057, 1984.

Friend BA, Shahani KM: Nutritional and therapeutic aspects of *Lactobacilli, J Applied Nutr* 36:125, 1984.

Gabor M: Antiinflammatory and antiallergic properties of flavonoids. In *Plant flavonoids in biology and medicine,* vol 1, New York, 1986, Alan R. Liss.

Gaby S, Singh V: *Vitamin C—vitamin intake and health: a scientific review,* New York, 1991, Marcel Dekker.

Gannon J, Kendall R: A clinical evaluation of *N,N*-dimethylglycine (DMG) and diisopropylammonium dichloroacetate (DIPA) on the performance of racing greyhounds, *Canine Pract* 9:7, 1983.

Gilbert and others: Viricidal effects of *Lactobacillus* and yeast fermentation, *Appl Environ Microbiol* 46:452, 1983.

Gibson R and others: Perna canaliculus in the treatment of arthritis, *Practitioner* 224:955, 1980.

Ginter E:. Ascorbic acid in cholesterol metabolism and in detoxification of xenobiotic substances: problem of optimum vitamin C intake, *Nutrition* 5:369, 1989.

Graber C and others: Immunomodulating properties of dimethylglycine in humans, *J Infect Dis* 143:101, 1981.

Grevenstein J and others: Cartilage changes in rats induced by papain and the influence of treatment with *N*-acetylglucosamine, *Acta Orthop Belg* 57:157, 1991.

Gupta M and others: Antiinflammatory activity of taxifolin, *Jpn J Pharmacol* 21:377, 1971.

Halliwell B: Free radicals and antioxidants: a personal view, *Nutr Rev* 52:253, 1994.

Hamilton-Miller JMT: "Probiotic" remedies are not what they seem (letter), *Br Med J* 312:55, 1996.

Hammarqvist F and others: Addition of glutamine to total parenteral nutrition after elective abdominal surgery spares free glutamine in muscle, counteracts the fall in muscle protein synthesis, and improves nitrogen balance, *Ann Surg* 209:455, 1989.

Hara H: Experimental study on the effect of co Q10 administration to isoproterenol-induced cardiomyopathy of rats, *Kuruma Med J* 28:125, 1981.

Hassam A, Rivers J, Crawford M: The failure of the cat to desaturate linoleic acid: its nutritional implications, *Nutr Metab* 21:321, 1977.

Hintz H, Cymbaluk N: Nutrition of the horse, *Ann Rev Nutr* 14:243, 1994.

Holub B: The role of omega-3 fatty acids in health and disease, Proceedings of the thirteenth annual American College of Veterinary Medicine, May, 1995.

Howard PA, Meyers DG: Effect of vitamin C on plasma lipids, *Ann Pharmacother* 29:1129, 1995.

Ishiyama and others: A clinical study on the effect of coenzyme Q10 on congestive heart failure, *Jpn Heart J* 17:32, 1976.

Jacobson E, Faloon W: Malabsorptive effects of neomycin in commonly used doses, *JAMA* 175:187, 1961.

Johnston CS, Martin LJ, Cai X: Antihistamine effect of supplemental ascorbic acid and neutrophil chemotaxis, *J Am Coll Nutr* 11:172, 1992.

Johnston CS, Retrum KR, Srilakshmi JC: Antihistamine effects and complications of supplemental vitamin C, *J Am Dietetic Assoc* 92:988, 1992.

Johnston S and others: The effect of misoprostal on aspirin-induced gastroduodenal lesions in dogs, *J Vet Int Med* 9:32, 1995.

Jones W: Feeding mucopolysaccharides, *Equine Sports Med News* June p 8, 1988.

Karzel K, Domenjoz R: Effects of hexosamine derivatives and uronic acid derivatives on glycosaminoglycan metabolism of fibroblast cultures, *Pharmacology* 5:337, 1971.

Keene B, Panciera D, Atkins G: Myocardial L-carnitine deficiency in a family of dogs with dilated cardiomyopathy, *J Am Vet Med Assoc* 198:647, 1991.

Kendall R, Lawson J: Treatment of arthritis and inflammation using *N,N*-dimethylglycine, US Patent 5,026,728, 1994.

Kendler B: Gamma-linolenic acid: physiological effects and potential medical applications, *J Applied Nutr* 39:79, 1987.

Kishimoto C and others: The protection of coenzyme Q10 against experimental viral myocarditis in mice, *Jpn Circ J* 48:1358, 1984.

Kodama M, Kodama T: Vitamin C and the genesis of autoimmune disease and allergy, *In Vivo* 9:231, 1995.

Kosuge T and others: Isolation of an antihistaminic substance from green-lipped mussel (Perna canaliculus), *Chem Pharm Bull* 34:4825, 1988.

Kovacs-Zamborsky M and others: Data on the effects of the probiotic "Lacto Sace," *Acta Vet Hung* 42:3, 1994.

Kung L: Direct-fed microbial and enzyme food additives. In *Direct-fed microbial, enzyme and forage additive compendium,* 1994.

Lane W: *Sharks don't get cancer,* Garden City, NY, 1992, Avery.

Langer R and others: Isolation of a cartilage factor that inhibits tumor neovascularization, *Science* 193:70, 1976.

Langer R, Lee A: Shark cartilage contains inhibitors of tumor angiogenesis, *Science* 221:1185, 1983.

Lawson J, Belkowski S: Effect of Perna mussel in collagen (II)-induced arthritis, 1996 (submitted for publication).

Lawson J, Reap E: Stimulation the immune system by dimethylglycine, a nontoxic metabolite, *J Lab Clin Med* 115:481, 1990.

Lee A, Langer R: Shark cartilage contains inhibitors of tumor angiogenesis, *Science* 221:1185, 1983.

Lehninger A, Nelson D, Cox M: *Principles of biochemistry,* New York, 1993, Worth.

Lewis L, Morris M, Hand M: *Small animal nutrition,* ed 3, Topeka, 1994, Mark Morris.

Lim P, Jacob E: Magnesium deficiency in patients on long-term diuretic therapy for heart failure, *Br Med J* 3:620, 1972.

Livine S and others: Effect of a nutritional supplement containing *N,N*-dimethylglycine (DMG) in the racing standardbred, *Equine Pract* 4:11, 1982.

Lloyd D, Thomsett L: Essential fatty acid supplementation in the treatment of canine atopy, *Vet Dermatology* 1:41, 1989.

Logas D, Beale KM, Bauer JE: Potential clinical benefits of dietary supplementation with marine-liver oil, *J Am Vet Med Assoc* 199:1631, 1991.

Logas D, Kunkle GA: Double-blinded crossover study with marine oil supplementation containing high dose eicosapentaenoic acid for the treatment of canine pruritic skin disease, *Vet Dermatol* 5:99, 1994.

Machlin L, Sauberlich H: New view on the function and health effects of vitamins, *Nutr Today,* Jan-Feb, p 25, 1994.

MacLennan PA, Brown RA, Rennie MJ: A positive relationship between protein synthetic rate and intracellular concentration in perfused rat skeletal muscle, *FEBS Lett* 215:187, 1987.

Marliss EB and others: Muscle and splanchnic glutamine and glutamate metabolism in postabsorptive and starved men, *J Clin Invest* 50:814, 1971.

McEntee K and others: Clinical electrocardiographic and echocardiographic improvements after L-carnitine supplementation in a cardiomyopathic Labrador, *Canine Pract* 20:12, 1995.

McFarlane S: Green mussel and rheumatoid arthritis, *N Z Med J* p 569, 1975.

Meduski J and others: Reduction in lactic acid in rabbits given dimethylglycine, Pacific Slope Biochemical Conference, July 1980, University of California, San Diego.

Merchant S: Advances in veterinary dermatology, *Compendium* 16:445, 1994.

Merck veterinary manual, Rahway, NJ, 1991, Merck.

Miller T: Antiinflammatory effects of mussel extract, *N Z Med J* p 23, 1981.

Miller T, Wu H: In vivo evidence for prostaglandin inhibitory activity in New Zealand green-lipped mussel extract, *N Z Med J* 97:355, 1984.

Miller W and others: Clinical trial of DVM derm caps in the treatment of allergic disease in dogs: a nonblinded study, *J Am Animal Hosp Assoc* 25:163, 1989.

Morisco C and others: Effect of coenzyme Q10 in patients with congestive heart failure, *Clinical Invest* 71:S134, 1993.

Moses MA, Sudhalter J, Langer R: Identification of an inhibitor of neovascularition from cartilage, *Science* 248:1408, 1990.

Muller-Fabender H and others: Glucosamine sulfate compared to ibuprofen in osteoarthritis, *Osteoarthritis Cartilage* 2:61, 1994.

Murray JB and others: Purification and partial amino acid sequence of a bovine cartilage derived collagenase inhibitor, *J Biol Chem* 261:4154, 1986.

National Research Council: *Nutrient requirements of horses,* Washington, DC, 1989, National Academy.

Nakazawa M, Emancipator SN, Lamm ME: Proteolytic enzyme treatment reduces glomerular immune deposits and proteinuria in passive Heymann nephritis, *J Exp Med* 164:1973, 1986.

Newsholme EA, Parry-Billings M: Properties of glutamine release from muscle and its importance for the immune system, *JPEN* 14(suppl 4):63, 1990.

O'Dwyer S and others: Maintenance of small bowel mocosa with glutamine-enriched parenteroal nutrition, *JPEN* 13:579, 1989.

Oikawa T and others: A novel angiogenic inhibitor derived from Japanese shark cartilage. I. Extraction and estimation of inhibitory activities toward tumor and embryonic angiogenesis. *Cancer Lett* 51:181, 1990.

Pauling L: *Vitamin C: the common cold and the flu,* San Francisco, 1976, WH Freeman.

Pion P and others: Response of cats with dilated cardiomyopathy to taurine supplementation, *J Am Vet Med Assoc* 201:275, 1992.

Prudden J: The treatment of human cancer with agents prepared from bovine cartilage, *J Biol Resp Modif* 4:1, 1985.

Prudden J, Balassa L: The biological activity of bovine cartilage preparations, *Semin Arthr Rheum* 4:287, 1974.

Pujalte J, Llavore E, Ylescupidey F: A double-blind clinical evaluation of oral glucosamine sulfate in the basic treatment of osteoarthrosis, *Curr Res Med Opin* 7:110, 1980.

Rainsford K, Whitehouse M: Gastroprotective and antiinflammatory properties of green-lipped mussel (Perna canaliculus) preparation, *Drug Res* 30:2128, 1980.

Ralston S: Equine clinical nutrition: specific problems and solutions, *Pract Vet* 10:356, 1988.

Ralston S: Therapeutic nutrition for specific equine syndromes, *Vet Clin Nutr* 1:31, 1994.

Reichelt A and others: Efficacy and safety of intramuscular glucosamine sulfate in osteoarthritis of the knee: a randomised, placebo-controlled, double-blind study, *Arzneimittelforschung* 44:75, 1994.

Rennie MJ and others: Characteristics of glutamine carrier in skeletal muscle have important consequences for nitrogen loss in injury, infection, and chronic disease. *Lancet* i:1008, 1986.

Roach E, Carlin M: *N,N*-Dimethylglycine for epilepsy, *N Engl J Med* 307:1081, 1982.

Roden L: Effect of hexosamines on the synthesis of chontroitin sulphuric acid in vitro, *Ark Kami* 10:345, 1956.

Roe D: *Drug-induced nutritional deficiencies,* Westport, Conn, 1978, Avi.

Roe D: Nutrient and drug interactions. In Olson R and others: *Present knowledge in nutrition,* ed 5, Washington, DC, 1984, The Nutritional Foundation.

Roe D: Effect of drugs on vitamin needs, *Ann NY Acad Sci* 669:156, 1992.

Roth E and others: Metabolic disorders in severe abdominal sepsis: glutamine deficiency in skeletal muscle, *Clin Nutr* 1:25, 1982.

Sauberlich H: Pharmacology of vitamin C, *Annu Rev Nutr* 14:371, 1994.

Scarff DH, Lloyd DH: Double-blind, placebo-controlled, crossover study of evening primrose oil in the treatment of canine atopy, *Vet Rec* 131:97, 1992.

Schoenkerman B, Justice R: Treatment of allergic disease with a combination of antihistamine and falavonoid, *Ann Allergy* 10:138, 1952.

Seddon JM and others: The use of vitamin supplements and the risk of cataract among US male physicians, *Am J Public Health* 84:788, 1994.

Setnikar I, Giacchetti C, Zanolo G: Pharmacokinetics of glucosamine in the dog and man, *Arzneimittelforschung* 36:729, 1991.

Shahani KM, Ayebo AD: Role of dietary *Lactobacilli* in gastrointestinal microecology, *Am J Clin Nutr* 33:2448, 1980.

Shahani K, Vakil J, Kilara A: Natural antibiotic activity of *Lactobacillus acidophilis bulgaricus II, Cultured Dairy Products J* 12:8, 1977.

Sherman A, Hallquist N: *Present knowledge in nutrition,* ed 6, Washington, DC, International Life Sciences Institute. 1990.

Shils M, Olson J, Moshe S, editors: *Modern nutrition in health and disease,* ed 8, Philadelphia, 1994, Lea and Febiger.

Simons JA: Vitamin C and carcdiovascular disease: a review, *J Am Coll Nutr* 11:107, 1992.

Simpson J, Anderson R, Markwell P: *Clinical nutrition of the dog and cat,* London, 1993, Blackwell Scientific.

Sinclair AJ and others: Low plasma ascorbate levels in patients with type 2 diabetes mellitus consuming adequate vitamin C, *Diabetic Med* 11:893, 1994.

Spencer RJ, Chesson A: The effects of *Lactobacillus* spp. on the attachment of enterotoxigenic *Escherichia coli* to isolated porcine enterocytes, *J Appl Bacteriol* 77:215, 1994.

Stanton M, Bright R: Gastroduodenal ulceration in dogs: retrospective study of 43 cases and literature review, *J Vet Int Med* 3:238, 1989.

Stauder G, and others: The use of hydrolytic enzymes as adjuvant therapy in AIDS/ARC/LAS patients. *Biomed Pharmacother* 42:31, 1988.

Stehle P and others: Effects of parenteral glutamine peptide supplements on muscle glutamine loss and nitrogen balance after major surgery, *Lancet* i:231, 1987.

Sugiyama A and others: Antioxidant effect of coenzyme Q10, *Experimentia* 36:1002, 1980.

Susanna CR: Effects of nutritional status on immunological function, *Am J Clin Nutr* 35:1202, 1982.

Tapadinhas MJ, Rivera IC, Bignamini AA: Oral glucosamine sulphate in the management of arthrosis: report on a multicentre open investigation in Portugal, *Pharmatherapeutica* 3:157, 1982.

Tarayre J, Lauresserques H: Advantages of a combination of proteolytic enzymes, flavonoids and ascorbic acid in comparison to non-steroidal antiinflammatory agents, *Arzneimittelforschung* 27:1144, 1977.

Tengerdy R: The role of vitamin E in immune response and disease resistance, *Ann NY Acad Sci* 587:2433, 1990.

Vaz AL: Double-blind clinical evaluation of the relative efficacy of ibuprofen and glucosamine sulphate in the management of osteoarthritis of the knee in out-patients, *Curr Med Res Opin* 8:145, 1982.

Verde M, Piquer J: Effect of stress on the corticosterone and ascorbic acid content of the plasma of rabbits, *J Appl Rabbit* 9:181, 1986.

Villar A, Gasco M, Alcaraz M: Antiinflammatory and antiulcer properties of hypoaletin-8-glucoside, a novel plant flavonoid, *J Pharm Pharmacol* 36:820, 1984.

Wallace M, Zawie D, Garrey M: Gastric ulceration in the dog secondary to the use of nonsteroidal antiinflammatory drugs, *J Am Anim Hosp Assoc* 26:467, 1990.

Wei H and others: Inhibitory effects of apigenin, a plant flavonoid, on epidermal ornithine decarboxylase and skin tumor promotion in mice, *Cancer Res* 50:499, 1990.

Weir C and others: The effect of activity in chronic glutamine-supplemented elemental diet on disease colitis model, *JPEN* 17:345, 1993 (abstract).

Werbach MR: *Nutritional influences on illness,* New Canaan, Conn, 1988, Keats.

Wester P: Zinc during diuretic treatment, *Lancet* 1:578, 1975.

White P: Essential fatty acids: use in management of canine atopy, *Compendium* 15:451, 1993.

Wilkinson EG and others: Bioenergetics and clinical medicine. VI. Adjunctive treatment of periodontal disease with coenzyme Q10, *Res Commun Chem Pathol Pharmacol* 14:715, 1976.

Windmueller H, Spaeth A: Identification of ketone bodies and glutamine as the major respiratory fuels in vivo for postabsorptive rat small intestine, *J Biol Chem* 253:69, 1978.

Yoshimoto T and others: Flavonoids: potent inhibitors of arachidonate-5-lipoxygenase, *Biochem Biophysic Res Comm* 116:612, 1983.

Yoshimura K and others: Effect of enteral glutamine administration on experimental inflammatory bowel disease, *JPEN* 17:235, 1993 (abstract).

SELECTED READINGS

Beisel W: Single nutrients and immunity, *Am J Clin Nutr* 35(suppl):417, 1982.

Bridges C, Moffitt P: Influence of variable content of dietary zinc on copper metabolism of weanling foals, *Am J Vet Res* 51:275, 1990.

Colgan M: *The new nutrition: medicine for the millennium,* San Diego, 1994, CI.

Gabel A and others: Comparison of incidence and severity of developmental orthopedic disease on 17 farms before and adjustment of ration, *Proc Am Assoc Equine Pract* 33:163, 1987.

Huber M, Bill R: The use of polysulfated glycosaminoglycans in dogs, *Compendium* 16:501, 1994,

Leibovitz B: Polyphenols and bioflavonoids, *Townsend Letter Doctors* Apr-May 1994.

Miller H: Medical management of chronic pruritus, *Compendium* 16:449, 1994.

Morrison L, Schjeide O: *Coronary heart disease and the mucopolysaccharides (glycosaminoglycans),* Springfield, Ill, 1974, Charles C Thomas.

Plan P: Myocardial failure in cats associated with low plasma taurine: a reversible cardiomyopathy, *Science* 237:764, 1987.

Schroeder H: Losses of vitamins and trace minerals resulting from processing and preservation of foods, *Am J Clin Nutr* 24:562, 1971.

Chapter 5

Pet Food Preservatives and Other Additives

W. JEAN DODDS

Definition of Therapeutic Modality

Food preservatives and other additives are essential dietary components that maintain the freshness and ensure the balance and completeness of diets for humans and animals. In the international commercial pet-food industry, issues arise about the efficacy, safety, and cost of these preservatives and additives, especially certain antioxidants used to maintain shelf-life. The goal is to prevent spoilage of pet foods, with its attendant deleterious effects on health, while balancing concerns about the potential adverse effects of synthetic chemicals. For a holistic approach to health, fresh, wholesome, well-balanced foods composed of natural ingredients are preferable to commercial diet formulas, which are primarily cereal-based and include a wide array of additives intended to provide "complete nutrition." A multibillion-dollar pet-food industry has evolved over the past several decades to fill the need for convenient, readily available, and wholesome foods for pets in modern society. We are now entering a period in which fundamental issues of nutritional balance and the public preference for more natural sources of ingredients, additives, and supplements have begun to change the face of the industry.

History

Food additives used for purposes of preservation, enhanced palatability, appearance, and ripening have been incorporated into human foods for centuries. Issues surrounding their use remain controversial today (Fennema, 1987). Much of the current information about diets has evolved from nutrition research conducted by biochemists focusing on the mechanisms of mammalian metabolism. Over the past 50 years, researchers have elucidated the roles of vitamins, minerals, fatty acids, and amino acids so that food or supplements rich in these substances could be introduced into human and animal diets (Berdanier, 1994; Roudebush, 1993). Only in the last one to two decades, however, has this knowledge been transferred to the international commercial pet-food industry (Cargill, 1993; Cargill, Thorpe-Vargas, 1994; Dodds, Donoghue, 1994; Roudebush, 1993; Slater, Scarlett, 1995).

Commercial pet foods available today offer an extensive assortment of diets for a wide variety of species, including companion, laboratory, farm, zoo, and aquatic animals. Developed for animals at all stages of life and for every nutritional need, these diets are products of a self-regulated industry in North America and most of the developed western world. These foods generally provide inexpensive and excellent nutrition (Dodds, Donoghue, 1994; Roudebush, 1993). Nevertheless, the last decade has seen increased concern about the increasing use of chemical preservatives, supplements, and other additives; the public is confused by the many options available and is relying more and more on veterinary and animal health-care professionals for advice. Additionally, the increasing number of veterinary prescription diets designed for specific health and disease conditions has necessitated more input from health professionals. This rapid change in the pet-care industry has generated controversy and concerns about the benefits and risks of relying primarily on stored, processed foods.* This chapter reviews the scientific and experiential literature surrounding these issues and focuses on the necessity for and potential adverse effects of commercial pet-food preservatives and additives.

---

*Ackerman (1993); Burger (1994); Burkholder (1995); Cargill (1991, 1993); Cargill, Thorpe-Vargas (1994); Devey and others (1995); Dodds (1991); Dodds, Donoghue (1994); Donoghue (1993); Heanes (1990); Henderson (1995); Roudebush (1993); Scanlan (1995); Schmoling (1995); Slater, Scarlett (1995); Tribby (1995); Wilcox (1993).

Scientific Basis and Literature Review

The beneficial and potentially adverse effects of preservatives and other additives used in pet foods need to be addressed in the broader context of overall animal health and longevity (Dodds, 1991, 1994). This focus is especially important today because of apparent increases in the number of humans and animals with disease states affecting immune function and thyroid metabolism. In fact, because of their genetic implications and the effects of the environment on those of susceptible genotype, autoimmune or immune-mediated diseases are a major threat to humans and animals throughout the world.[*] Furthermore, thyroid dysfunction is currently the most common endocrine problem of dogs and cats, and it has increased in frequency over the last decade. Genetic, nutritional, and environmental factors have created a similar situation for humans (Arthur, Nichol, Beckett, 1993; Berry, Larsen, 1992; Sinha, Lopez, McDevitt, 1990).

Nutritional Factors Influencing Immunity

Wholesome nutrition is the key to maintaining a healthy immune system and resistance to disease. Nutrition plays a significant role in disease and disease prevention in the following examples: alkalinity in diets for miniature schnauzers with calcium oxalate bladder or kidney stones; use of etretinate, a vitamin A derivative, in cocker spaniels and other breeds with idiopathic seborrhea; management of diseases such as diabetes mellitus and the copper-storage disorder prevalent in breeds like the Bedlington terrier, West Highland white terrier, and Doberman pinscher; wheat-sensitive enteropathy in Irish setters; and treatment of vitamin B_{12} deficiency in giant schnauzers (Dodds, Donoghue, 1994). Other examples include the vitamin K–dependent coagulation defect manifested in Devon rex cats following vaccination; hip dysplasia appearing in puppies fed excessive calories; development of osteochondritis dissecans in dogs fed high levels of calcium; and the induction of hypercholesterolemia in inbred sled dogs fed high-fat diets (Dodds, Donoghue, 1994).

Zinc, selenium, vitamin E, vitamin B_6 (pyridoxine), and linoleic acid are important nutrients for immune function.[†] Deficiencies of these ingredients impair both circulating (humoral) and cell-mediated immunity. This requirement for essential nutrients not only increases during periods of rapid growth and reproduction but also may increase in geriatric individuals, when immune function and nutrient bioavailability wane. Excessive supplementation

of any nutrient can lead to significant clinical problems, many of which resemble the respective deficiency states of these ingredients (Burk, 1983; Diplock, 1976; Tengerdy, 1989; Turner, Finch, 1991).

Nutrition and Thyroid Metabolism

Because animals with autoimmune thyroid disease have generalized metabolic imbalance and often have associated immunologic dysfunction, their exposure to unnecessary drugs, toxins, and chemicals should be minimized and their nutritional status optimized. Experience has shown that families of dogs susceptible to thyroid and other autoimmune diseases show generalized improvement in health and vigor when fed premium cereal-based diets preserved naturally with vitamins E and C (without the addition of synthetic antioxidant preservatives). Fresh, home-cooked vegetables with herbs, low-fat dairy products, and meats such as lamb, chicken, and turkey can be added as supplements. Challenging the immune system of animals susceptible to these disorders with polyvalent modified-live vaccines has been associated with adverse effects in some cases (see Chapter 41).

Nutritional factors can significantly influence thyroid metabolism (Ackerman, 1993; Arthur, Nichol, Beckett, 1993; Berry, Larsen, 1992; Kohrle, 1992). Iodine deficiency is the classical example that develops when individuals eat cereal grain grown on iodine-deficient soil. This lack of iodine impairs thyroid metabolism because iodine is an essential component of thyroid hormones. Another important link has recently been shown between selenium deficiency and hypothyroidism (Arthur, Nichol, Beckett, 1993; Berry, Larsen, 1992; Corvilain and others, 1993). As with iodine, cereal grain crops grown on selenium-deficient soil contain relatively low levels of selenium. Although commercial pet-food manufacturers compensate for any fluctuations in basal ingredients by adding vitamin and mineral supplements, they find it difficult to meet the metabolic needs of so many different breeds of animals with varying genetic backgrounds (Berdanier, 1994; Cargill, 1993; Cargill, Thorpe-Vargas, 1993, 1994; Dodds, Donoghue, 1994).

The selenium/thyroid relationship has important clinical implications. Although blood levels of total and free thyroxine (T_4) rise in selenium deficiency, this effect is not transmitted to the tissues, as the elevated or unchanged blood levels of the regulatory thyroid stimulating hormone (TSH) demonstrate (Berry, Larsen, 1992; Kohrle, 1992). Selenium-deficient individuals showing clinical signs of hypothyroidism could be overlooked, therefore, because blood levels of the T_4 hormones appear normal (Ackerman, 1993). The role of selenium is further complicated by the fact that synthetic antioxidants used to preserve pet foods can change the bioavailability of vitamin A, vitamin E, and selenium and alter cellular metabolism by inducing or lowering cytochrome P-450, glutathione peroxidase (a

---

[*]Alexander, Peck (1990); Berdanier (1994); Burkholder, Swecker (1990); Sinha and others (1990); Tengerdy (1989); Turner, Finch (1991).
[†]Boxer (1986); Burkholder, Swecker (1990); Corwin, Gordon (1982); Harris and others (1980); Hayes and others (1970); Lehmann and others (1988); Mino and others (1985); Remillard (1995); Sheffy, Schultz (1979); Tengerdy (1989); Turner, Finch (1991).

selenium-dependent enzyme), and prostaglandin levels.* Manufacturers of many of the premium pet foods began adding the synthetic antioxidant ethoxyquin as a preservative in the late 1980s. Its effects and those of the other synthetic preservatives discussed below could be detrimental over time (Cargill, 1993; Cargill, Thorpe-Vargas, 1993, 1994). Using foods preserved with natural antioxidants such as vitamins E and C or feeding only home-cooked fresh, natural ingredients is a logical way to minimize this potential risk (Cargill, Thorpe-Vargas, 1994; Dodds, Donoghue, 1994).

Food Additives

The benefit and risks of pet-food additives have recently been reviewed (Burger, 1994; Roudebush, 1993). Although all food preservatives are additives, not all additives are preservatives. Food additives include the preservatives (antioxidants, discussed later in this chapter; antimicrobials; and preventives of food discoloration); humectants; color, flavor, and palatability enhancers; emulsifying agents and stabilizers/thickeners; and miscellaneous additives (Roudebush, 1993). The purpose of these additives is to provide or maintain desirable attributes in food, such as color, flavor, texture, stability, and resistance to spoilage (Roudebush, 1993).

Antioxidants

This subject is discussed at length later in the chapter.

Antimicrobial preservatives

Soft-moist pet foods and treats with a high moisture content often contain antimicrobial preservatives to inhibit bacterial putrefaction or mold formation.

Examples include citric, hydrochloric, sorbic, fumaric, pyroligneous, propionic, and phosphoric acids; sodium nitrite; sodium and calcium propionate; and potassium sorbate (Roudebush, 1993).

Humectants

Cereal-based dry pet foods have low moisture content and are resistant to microbial spoilage. Because semi-moist pet foods contain 25% to 50% moisture, humectants must be added to reduce water availability (and subsequent microbial growth) and also prevent water loss after processing to help retain the soft, pliable texture of foods (Roudebush, 1993). Examples of humectants include sorbitol, corn syrups, sucrose, dextrose, and cane molasses. Propylene glycol, which was once used in semi-moist cat foods, is no longer designated "generally recognized as safe" (GRAS) by the federal Food and Drug Administration (FDA) and European Community (EC) because of its

tendency to increase Heinz body formation and decrease erythrocyte survival time (Burger, 1994).

Coloring and emulsifying agents

Coloring agents of natural and synthetic bases are added to enhance consumer appeal. The carotenoids and iron oxide serve as natural colors, whereas additives such as the azo (coal-tar derivatives) and nonazo dyes impart artificial colors. The latter category can be used only if it is listed as safe by federal FDA regulations (Roudebush, 1993). Nitrites, bisulfites, and ascorbates are color protectants used to prevent discoloration.

Emulsifying agents act as stabilizers or thickeners of pet foods. These include gums (hydrocolloids), glycerin, glycerides, and modified starch, which are used to prevent separation of ingredients and create the gravy or sauce for canned pet foods (Roudebush, 1993). Food gums include natural extracts of seaweed, seed and microbial gums, exudate gums from trees, and chemically modified plant cellulose. Modified cellulose and vegetable gums are typically sprayed on the surface of dry dog foods along with the animal digests discussed below.

Flavor and palatability enhancers

Commercial pet foods contain both natural and synthetic flavor and palatability enhancers. Dry foods tend to be less palatable than moist foods, especially to cats. Phosphoric acid is commonly sprayed on dry cat foods to improve palatability, and animal digests made by controlled enzymatic degradation of animal tissues enhance the flavor of dry dog foods. The latter digests usually come from poultry, fish, liver, and beef lungs (Roudebush, 1993). Other additives include spices, onion, garlic, and certain flavorful extracts.

Miscellaneous Additives

These pet-food additives include polyphosphates, which improve condition and texture, retain natural moisture and meat protein, reduce oxidation, and promote better color development. Yucca plant extracts are touted as a way to reduce fecal odor, although they have been approved only for use as a flavoring agent for human foods and not for use in pet foods (Roudebush, 1993).

Controversial Issues

Pet-food additives must conform to the FDA regulations pertaining to general use of food additives or must be composed of ingredients that have the federal GRAS designation (Roudebush, 1993). Some pet-food additives not covered by the preceding classifications are permitted by informal review. Nevertheless, significant controversy remains about the safety of additives, especially the synthetic antioxidants used to prevent spoilage (Cargill, 1991; Dodds, 1991, 1994; Dodds, Donoghue, 1994; Fennema, 1987).

*Combs (1978); Kagan and others (1986); Kim (1991); Langweiler and others (1983); Meydani and others (1991); Parke and others (1972); Rossing and others (1985).

Effects of Synthetic Antioxidants

Synthetic antioxidants such as butylated hydroxyanisole (BHA) and butylated hydroxytoluene (BHT) have been used as preservatives in human and animal foods for more than 30 years (Cargill, 1991). During this period a more potent chemical antioxidant,1,2-dihydro-6-ethoxy-2,2,4-trimethylquinoline (ethoxyquin), was also used to a limited extent. More recently, ethoxyquin has become the preferred antioxidant for preserving the premium commercial dog and cat foods (Cargill, 1993; Cargill, Thorpe-Vargas, 1993). Many pet-food manufacturers have chosen ethoxyquin because of its excellent antioxidant qualities, high stability, and reputed safety. However, ongoing controversy surrounds the question of its safety when regularly fed at permitted amounts. The only long-term feeding trials in dogs were completed 30 years ago and were medically and scientifically flawed by today's standards. Furthermore, no feeding trials have been conducted that address the safety of this preservative in cats (Cargill, Thorpe-Vargas, 1993). These safety questions appear to pertain primarily to genetically susceptible breeds of inbred or closely linebred animals. Toy breeds of dogs may be at particular risk because they eat proportionately more food (and therefore preservatives) for their size to sustain their metabolic needs (Cargill, 1993; Cargill, Thorpe-Vargas, 1993; Dodds, Donoghue, 1994).

Ethoxyquin exerts its antioxidant effect after being absorbed by the gastrointestinal tract (Skaare, Nafstad, 1979). Body functions dependent upon oxidation, especially those involving peroxides, are transiently reduced (Kagan and others, 1986; Kahl, 1984; Kim, 1991; Parke, Rahim, Walker, 1972; Rossing, Kahl, Hildebrand, 1985), although continuous exposure to this potent antioxidant in preserved foods poses the risk of chronic low-level effects. Other downstream effects can be predicted such as decreases in prostaglandins and other eicosanoids (thromboxanes in platelets and leukotrienes in leukocytes) (Meydani and others, 1991). Synthesis of hormones such as progesterone, estrogen, and testosterone can be impaired and could thereby alter reproductive performance in males and females (Steele, Jeffery, Diplock, 1974). Because ethoxyquin has also been shown to cross the placenta, developing fetuses would be continuously reexposed in their closed amniotic environment until birth. Effects of ethoxyquin on other steroid hormones, such as the glucocorticoids and aldosterone, could alter responses to stress and kidney function. Synthetic antioxidants are substrates for cytochrome P-450, which affects hydroxylation of foreign substances and drugs (Rossing, Kahl, Hildebrand, 1985). A consequence of the body's diminished ability to hyroxylate is its reduced capacity to detoxify and excrete toxic and pharmacologic compounds (Kahl, 1984).

Imbalances of essential vitamins and minerals could occur when synthetic antioxidants disrupt the body's natural antioxidant system (Combs, 1978; Hayes, Rousseau, Hegsted, 1970; Langweiler, Sheffy, Schultz, 1983; Leong, Brown, 1992; March, Biely, Coates, 1968). Ethoxyquin simulates vitamin E in vivo and can apparently raise hepatic levels of vitamin A severalfold. In doing so, it lowers the bioavailability and tissue requirements for both vitamin E and selenium.* These are troublesome biologic effects because vitamin A is essential for many biochemical pathways, including thyroid metabolism, and vitamin E and selenium are critical to maintain integrity of the immune system (Corwin, Gordon, 1982; Tengerdy, 1989; Turner, Finch, 1991). Because the clinical signs of toxicity and deficiency for these important nutrients are similar, any observed clinical effects could be related to excess or deficiency states or both (Burk, 1983; Diplock, 1976; Sheffy, Schultz, 1979; Tengerdy, 1989). Pet-food manufacturers have begun to address these concerns by lowering the levels of ethoxyquin added to the finished products from 120 to 150 ppm (the legal limit) to as low as 20 to 40 ppm. An important consideration, however, is the cumulative antioxidant load, because use of BHA or BHT to preserve the animal fat sources in these foods is additive to the ethoxyquin incorporated into the finished product.

Antioxidants also exert both toxic and protective effects on biomembranes (Kagan and others, 1986; Parke, Rahim, Walker, 1972). The lipid bilayer of the cell membrane is not disturbed by natural antioxidants such as tocopherols (vitamin E) and ubiquinols that contain hydrocarbon tails whereas synthetic antioxidants devoid of hydrocarbon tails can exert toxic and destructive effects on the membrane (Kagan and others, 1986, 1990; Rossing, Kahl, Hildebrand, 1985). Examples include effects on erythrocyte membranes, which induce red cell hemolysis; on sarcoplasmic reticular membranes, which inhibit calcium transport; and on platelet membranes, which inhibit calcium ion–dependent platelet aggregation (Diplock, 1976; March, Coates, Biely, 1969). Because antioxidants are substrates for cytochrome P-450, oxidative hydroxylation occurs, which produces a relatively short half-time in biomembranes and the body (Rossing, Kahl, Hildebrand, 1985; Kagan and others, 1986). Although this makes synthetic antioxidants 10 to 20 times more potent as inhibitors of lipid peroxidation, side effects from the changes in membrane function can have important biologic consequences (Kagan and others, 1986, 1990).

Naturally occurring antioxidants (such as tocopherol and ascorbic acid) are also used in pet foods and have become more popular in response to consumer and professional queries about the effects of feeding chemical antioxidants to pets over long periods (Cargill, Thorpe-Vargas, 1993, 1994; Dodds, Donoghue, 1994). Although these natural preservatives are more expensive than synthetic antioxidants and somewhat less effective because of their shorter protectant effect, proponents of natural antioxidants believe their safety outweighs these drawbacks.

---

*Cargill, Thorpe-Vargas (1993, 1994); Combs (1978); Kim (1991); Nafstad, Skaare (1978); Skaare and others (1977).

The focus of this discussion is on concerns about ethoxyquin, but the other commonly used synthetic antioxidants apparently have similar effects (Fennema, 1987; Roudebush, 1993). Pet foods in which chemical antioxidants are not added at the time of final processing often contain ingredients (such as animal tallow or other fats and oils) that are preserved with such antioxidants. Thus claims made about the use of "all-natural" antioxidant preservatives need to be investigated to determine whether they apply to the raw materials (Burger, 1994; Dodds, Donoghue, 1994; Roudebush, 1993).

Synthetic Antioxidants and Cancer

Synthetic antioxidants (BHA, BHT, propyl gallate, and ethoxyquin) have been linked to inducing, promoting, and protecting against a variety of cancers, although some experts disagree.* The increased levels of cytochrome P-450 and glutathione peroxidases induced by these chemicals result in higher levels of the reactive hydrogen peroxides and oxygen radicals that affect cellular metabolism (Burk, 1983; Pearson and others, 1983; Rossing, Kahl, Hildebrand, 1985). These potentially harmful activated oxygen molecules are counterbalanced during normal cellular metabolism by a complex natural antioxidant defense system that includes the glutathione peroxidase enzymes, catalase, superoxide dismutase, and vitamins C and E (Boscoboinik and others, 1991; Prestera and others, 1993; Rose, Bode, 1993). Oxidative stress occurs in the body following impairment of the balance between free radical fluxes and the antioxidant defense system. This imbalance plays an important role in the initiation and promotion of oncogenesis and may contribute to genetic instability and an increase in mutations (Prestera and others, 1993; Rose, Bode 1993). Exposure to increased oxidative stress includes the genetic consequences of a rising number of chromosomal aberrations (DNA breakage) and genetic mutations. Induced hyperoxia, ascorbic acid, and ethoxyquin have been shown to potentiate the clastogenic effect (breaking of DNA/RNA) and increase the number of chromosomal aberrations in ovarian cells. However, simultaneous administration of a mutagen and ethoxyquin has also been shown to reduce the clastogenic effects of the mutagen (Renner, 1984).

Ethoxyquin, BHA, and BHT are the most commonly used synthetic antioxidants (Cargill, 1993; Wilcox, 1993). They have been shown to increase not only the toxicity of other chemicals but also their mutagenicity, sensitivity to radioactivity exposure, and tumor yield from chemical carcinogens (Ito and others, 1986; Manson, Green, Driver, 1987). Production of reactive oxygen species, particularly those of hydroxy-radicals, appears to be a critical determi-

nant. It is tempting to speculate that the rising incidence of leukemias, lymphomas, hemangiosarcomas, and chronic immunosuppressive disorders among companion animals is due at least partially to the widespread use of chemical antioxidants and other additives in commercial pet foods. In genetically predisposed individuals, these environmental chemicals that promote immune suppression or dysregulation and oncogenesis may contribute to the failure of immune surveillance mechanisms protecting the body against the vast array of infectious and other agents that induce immunologic or neoplastic change (Dodds, 1994).

Other Food Additives

Numerous adverse reactions to a variety of human- and pet-food additives have been reported for many years (Burger, 1994; Fennema, 1987; Roudebush, 1993). A diverse group of symptoms has been implicated, including nausea, vomiting, diarrhea, abdominal cramping and pain, headache, provocation of asthma, chronic allergic symptoms, inhalant dermatitis, and behavioral disorders (Roudebush, 1993). The additives most commonly incriminated include sulfites, monosodium glutamate, tartrazine, azo and nonazo dyes, benzoates (allowed in human foods only), parabens, gums, and spices. Benzoic acid and benzoates are not permitted by the FDA and EC in any animal feeds because of their toxicity in cats, a species that cannot efficiently detoxify this chemical (Burger, 1994). Similarly, propylene glycol has been removed from pet foods because it reduces erythrocyte survival time and induces Heinz body formation (without apparent hemolytic anemia) in cats (Burger, 1994). The extent to which these perceived adverse reactions to additives in human and animal foods is real cannot be accurately determined. However, documented reactions do occur, and most are likely to be food intolerances rather than true food allergies or hypersensitivities (Roudebush, 1993).

Incorporation into Conventional Veterinary Practice

The recent escalation of consumer concern about the wholesomeness of pet foods has encouraged the industry to provide ingredients from natural sources as alternatives to the synthetic chemical additives formerly used. Veterinarians should be similarly encouraged to seek and recommend commercial or home-made pet foods and pet-food companies that promote a more holistic approach to food safety. We should not be afraid to challenge the industry with questions about these issues, and we should ask for documentation of the safety and short- and long-term benefits of additives used to prevent spoilage and enhance color, flavor, and palatability. Whereas the marketability of commercial pet foods is a legitimate concern, our professional responsibility to protect the health and longevity of animals should not be diverted.

---

*Cargill, Thorpe-Vargas (1994); Hirose and others (1986); Ito and others (1986); Kahl (1984); Manson and others (1987); Pearson and others (1983); Skaare and others (1977).

Conclusions

The industry needs additional short- and long-term controlled feeding trials that incorporate modern toxicologic, medical, and epidemiologic assessments of synthetic chemical preservatives and other pet-food additives. Also needed is an evaluation of their interactions with other genetic and environmental factors that affect the health and performance of companion animals, with particular emphasis on those that are inbred or closely linebred (Dodds, Donoghue, 1994).

The net result of the concerns summarized in this chapter is a major change in the pet-food industry. Manufacturers of premium pet foods and most newly introduced pet foods have begun using natural antioxidants as the sole source of preservatives and are more conscious of public and industry concerns about the use of additives and other supplements. This change represents a triumph for pet owners who prefer to use natural, fresh, and wholesome ingredients whenever possible.

REFERENCES

Ackerman L: The benefits of enzyme therapy, *Vet Forum* 10(10):45, 69, 1993.

Alexander JW, Peck MD: Future prospects for adjunctive therapy: pharmacologic and nutritional approaches to immune system modulation, *Crit Care Med* 18:S159, 1990.

Arthur JR, Nichol F, Beckett GJ: Selenium deficiency, thyroid hormone metabolism, and thyroid hormone deiodinases, *Am J Clin Nutr Suppl* 57:2365, 1993.

Berdanier CD: The new age of nutrition, *FASEB J* 8:4, 1994.

Berry MJ, Larsen PR: The role of selenium in thyroid hormone action, *Endo Rev* 13:207, 1992.

Boscoboinik D and others: Inhibition of cell proliferation by α-tocopherol, *J Biol Chem* 266:6188, 1991.

Burger IH: Natural food hazards. In Wills JM, Simpson DW, editors: *The Waltham book of clinical nutrition of the dog and cat*, Oxford, 1994, Pergamon.

Burk RF: Biological activity of selenium, *Ann Rev Nutr* 3:53, 1983.

Cargill JC: A look at the ethoxyquin controversy: it's still the consumer's choice, *Dog World* 76(2):14, 1991.

Cargill J: Feed that dog, I-III, *Dog World*, 78(7-9):24-29, 10-16, 14-22, 1993.

Cargill J, Thorpe-Vargas S: Feed that dog (I-IV), *Dog World* 78(10-12):36-42, 28-31, 36-41, 1993; and 79(1-2):18-22, 36-42, 1994.

Combs GF Jr: Influence of ethoxyquin on the utilization of selenium by the chick, *Poult Sci* 57:210, 1978.

Corvilain B and others: Selenium and the thyroid: how the relationship was established, *Am J Clin Nutr Suppl* 57:2445, 1993.

Corwin LM, Gordon RK: Vitamin E and immune regulation. *Ann NY Acad Sci* 393:437, 1982.

Diplock AT: Metabolic aspects of selenium action and toxicity, *CRC Crit Rev Toxicol* 5:271, 1976.

Dodds WJ: Nutritional approach can help enhance immune competence, *DVM Mag* 22(4):15, 1991.

Dodds WJ: Nutritional influences on immune and thyroid function, *Proceedings of the American Holistic Veterinary Medical Association*, p 47, 1994.

Dodds WJ, Donoghue S: Interactions of clinical nutrition with genetics. In *The Waltham book of clinical nutrition of the dog and cat*, Oxford, 1994, Pergamon.

Fennema OR: Food additives—an unending controversy, *Am J Clin Nutr* 46:201, 1987.

Hayes KC, Rousseau JE Jr, Hegsted DM: Plasma tocopherol concentrations and vitamin E deficiency in dogs, *J Am Vet Med Assoc* 157:64, 1970.

Ito N and others: Studies on antioxidants: their carcinogenic and modifying effects on chemical carcinogenesis, *Food Chem Toxicol* 24:1070, 1986.

Kagan V and others: Interfaces of neurones, smoke, and genes, *Arch Toxicol Suppl* 9:302, 1986.

Kagan VE and others: Mechanisms of stabilization of biomembranes by α-tocopherol, *Biochem Pharmacol* 40:2403, 1990.

Kahl R: Synthetic antioxidants: biochemical actions and interference with radiation, toxic compounds, chemical mutagens, and chemical carcinogens, *Toxicology* 33:185, 1984.

Kim HL: Accumulation of ethoxyquin in the tissue, *J Toxicol Environ Health* 33:229, 1991.

Kohrle J: The trace components—selenium and flavonoids—affect iodothyronine deiodinases, thyroid hormone transport, and TSH regulation, *Acta Med Austriaca Suppl* (1) 19:13, 1992.

Langweiler M, Sheffy BE, Schultz RD: Effects of antioxidants on the proliferative response of canine lymphocytes in serum from dogs with vitamin E deficiency, *Am J Vet Res* 44:5, 1983.

Leong VY-M, Brown TP: Toxicosis in broiler chicks due to excess dietary ethoxyquin, *Avian Dis* 36:1102, 1992.

Manson MM, Green JA, Driver HE: Ethoxyquin alone induces preneoplastic changes in the rat kidney whilst preventing induction of such lesions in liver by aflatoxin B$_1$, *Carcinogenesis* 8:723, 1987.

March BE, Biely J, Coates V: The influence of diet on toxicity of the antioxidant 1,2-dihydro-6-ethoxy-2,2,4-trimethylquinoline, *Can J Physiol Pharmacol* 46:145, 1968.

March BE, Coates V, Biely J: Reticulocytosis in response to dietary antioxidants, *Science* 164:1398, 1969.

Meydani M and others: Influence of dietary fat, vitamin E, ethoxyquin, and indomethacin on the synthesis of prostaglandin E$_2$ in brain regions of mice, *J Nutr* 121:438, 1991.

Parke DV, Rahim A, Walker R: Effects of ethoxyquin on hepatic microsomal enzymes, *Biochem J* 130(2):84, 1972.

Pearson WR and others: Increased synthesis of glutathione S-transferases in response to anticarcinogenic antioxidants, *J Biol Chem* 258:2052, 1983.

Prestera T and others: Chemical and molecular regulation of enzymes that detoxify carcinogens, *Proc Natl Acad Sci* 90:2965, 1993.

Renner HW: Antimutagenic effect of an antioxidant in mammals, *Mut Res* 135:125, 1984.

Rose RC, Bode AM: Biology of free radical scavengers: an evaluation of ascorbate, *FASEB J* 7:1135, 1993.

Rossing D, Kahl R, Hildebrand AG: Effects of synthetic antioxidants on hydrogen peroxide formation, oxyferro cytochrome P-450 concentration, and oxygen consumption in liver microsomes, *Toxicology* 34:67, 1985.

Roudebush P: Pet food additives, *J Am Vet Med Assoc* 203:1667, 1993.

Sheffy BE, Schultz RD: Influence of vitamin E and selenium on immune response mechanisms, *Fed Proc* 38:2139, 1979.

Sinha AA, Lopez SM, McDevitt HO: Autoimmune disease: the failure of self-tolerance, *Science* 248:1380, 1990.

Skaare JU, Nafstad I: The distribution of ^{14}C-ethoxyquin in the rat, *Acta Pharmacol Toxicol* 44:303, 1979.

Slater MR, Scarlett JM: Nutritional epidemiology in small animal practice, *J Am Vet Med Assoc* 207:571, 1995.

Steele CE, Jeffery EH, Diplock AT: The effect of vitamin E and synthetic antioxidants on the growth in vitro of explanted rat embryos, *J Reprod Fert* 38:115, 1974.

Tengerdy RP: Vitamin E, immune response, and disease resistance, *Ann NY Acad Sci* 570:335, 1989.

Turner RI, Finch JM: Selenium and the immune response, *Proc Nutr Soc* 50:275, 1991.

Wilcox B: Preservative safety, *Dog Fancy* 24(11):8, 1993.

SELECTED READINGS

Boxer LA: Regulation of phagocytic function by α-tocopherol, *Proc Nutr Soc* 45:333, 1986.

Burkholder WJ, Swecker WS Jr: Nutritional influences on immunity, *Sem Vet Med Surg (Sm Anim)* 5:154, 1990.

Burkholder WJ: Postsurgical nutritional support: response, *J Am Vet Med Assoc* 206:1674, 1995.

Devey JJ, Crowe DT, Kirby R, and others: Postsurgical nutritional support, *J Am Vet Med Assoc* 206:1673, 1995 (letter).

Dodds WJ: Estimating disease prevalence with health surveys and genetic screening. *Adv Vet Sci Comp Need* 39:29, 1995.

Donoghue S: Preservatives: friend or foe? *AKC Gaz* 110(3):18, 1993.

Gilbert PA, Griffin CE, Rosenkrantz WS: Serum vitamin E levels in dogs with pyoderma and generalized demodicosis, *J Am Anim Hosp Assoc* 28:407, 1992.

Harris RE, Boxer LA, Baehner RL: Consequences of vitamin E deficiency on the phagocytic and oxidative functions of the rat polymorphonuclear leukocyte, *Blood* 55:338, 1980.

Heanes DL: Vitamin A concentrations in commercial foods for dogs and cats, *Austr Vet J* 67:291, 1990.

Henderson TR: Comments about vitamins, nutraceuticals, and dietary enzymes, *J Am Vet Med Assoc* 207:31, 1995 (letter).

Hirose M and others: Combined effects of butylated hydroxyanisole and other antioxidants in induction of forestomach lesions in rats, *Cancer Lett* 30:169, 1986.

Lehmann J, Rao DD, Canary J:. Vitamin E and relationships among tocopherols in human plasma, platelets, lymphocytes, and red blood cells, *Am J Clin Nutr* 47:470, 1988

Mino M, Kasugai O, Nagita A: Relationship between red blood cell and liver tocopherol concentration after administration and depletion of vitamin E, *Int J Vit Nutr Res* 55:47, 1985.

Read MA: Flavonoids: naturally occurring antiinflammatory agents, *Am J Pathol* 147:235, 1995.

Nafstad I, Skaare JU: Ultrastructural hepatic changes in rats after oral administration of ethoxyquin (EMQ), *Toxicol Lett* 1(5-6):295, 1978.

Remillard RL: Omega-3 fatty acid supplementation in inflammatory disease, Perspectives Sept/Oct p 20, 1995.

Riis RC and others: Vitamin E deficiency retinopathy in dogs, *Am J Vet Res* 42:74, 1981.

Sakanashi T and others: Vitamin E deficiency has a pathological role in microcytolysis in cardiomyopathic Syrian hamsters, *Biochem Biophys Acta* 181:145, 1991.

Scanlan N: Comments about vitamins, nutraceuticals, and dietary enzymes, *J Am Vet Assoc* 207:30, 1995.

Schmoling GR: Comments about vitamins, nutraceuticals, and dietary enzymes, *J Am Vet Med Assoc* 207:30, 1995 (letter).

Scott DW, Sheffy BE: Dermatosis in dogs caused by vitamin E deficiency, *Comp Anim Pract* 1(4):42, 1987.

Skaare JU, Nafstad I, Dahle HK: Enhanced hepatotoxicity of dimethylnitroasamine by pretreatment of rats with the antioxidant ethoxyquin, *Toxicol Appl Pharmacol* 42:19, 1977.

Tribby MD: Vitamins, nutraceuticals, and dietary enzymes, *J Am Vet Med Assoc* 206:1113, 1995 (letter).

Chapter 6

Glandular Therapy, Cell Therapy, and Oral Tolerance

ALAN E. LEWIS, ALLEN M. SCHOEN

The 1980s saw a surge of interest, in both the scientific and the lay communities, in "folk" and traditional medicine and ethnopharmacology (the study of indigenous medicinal substances). No longer dismissed as superstitions, the medical practices of ancient and traditional cultures began to be regarded as a valuable legacy based on thousands of years of experience. Traditional medicine is now considered a promising source for research in medicinal materials, and new evidence for the efficacy of traditional practices is accumulating rapidly.

Along with this general interest in traditional medicine is an interest in one form of traditional medicine: glandular therapy. Glandular therapy—also known as *tissue therapy, organotherapy,* and *cell therapy*—is the use of animal tissues to produce biologic effects in humans. Whole animal tissues or special extracts of tissues are used for health maintenance, rejuvenation, and treatment of mild functional health problems.

Specific animal tissues are used to tonify the corresponding tissues of the user, resulting in beneficial physiologic changes and healing. Thus, proponents claim, use of liver tissue benefits the user's liver, use of adrenal tissue supports the user's adrenal system, and so on. Initially, this idea seems attractive but scientifically unsound. Skeptics may question the reasons for consumption of particular tissues in the treatment of corresponding tissues in the user. By what mechanism do these materials act, and what evidence supports the claim that they are absorbed and utilized by the user's body?

Scientific developments of the past two decades have provided partial answers to these questions. According to current research, glandular materials have tissue-specific activity and contain physiologically active substances capable of exerting significant biologic and therapeutic effects in humans. This chapter briefly reviews the history of glandular and cellular therapy, the emerging scientific rationale for oral tolerance, and selected current findings in experimental and clinical uses of glandular derivatives.

Historical Background

The idea that glandular materials have specific nutritive and medicinal virtues is ancient. Paul Niehans (1960), pioneer of contemporary cell therapy, makes the following observation:

> Cellular therapy [injections of tissues from young animals] has its roots in the oldest traditions of medicine. The conviction that the administration of the organs of young animals has a strengthening and curative effect is found at the very beginnings of the art of healing. In the oldest medical document we possess, the papyrus of Eber, preparations manufactured from animal organs are mentioned. In 1400 BC the Hindu doctor Susrata recommended Hindus suffering from impotence to eat the sex glands of tigers . Homer relates that Achilles ate the bone marrow of lions in order to increase his strength and his courage. In the *Materia Medica* of Aristotle and of Pliny the Elder, there are allusions to extracts of organs used in medical therapy. In the third century, Chinese doctors prescribed human placenta as a tonic.

Ancient Egyptian medicine employed animal tissues and secretions, and Ayurvedic (Indian) writings of some hundreds of years BC mention the therapeutic use of glandular materials (Harrower, 1916). Paracelsus, the celebrated sixteenth-century physician, developed a "doctrine of signatures" claiming that "like cures like"; in other words, the heart heals the heart, the kidney heals the kidney, and so on (Uhlenbruck, 1967). The value of glandular tissues was probably known prehistorically, because the liver, thymus, kidney, brain, and other organs are the portions of wild animals most prized by aboriginal hunter/gatherers (O'Dea, 1988).

Scientific endocrinology did not emerge until the mid-nineteenth century, with the understanding that a system of ductless glands secretes minute quantities of materials (hormones) that exert profound effects on distant tissues. This discovery was followed by a period of uncritical, almost wild enthusiasm for the therapeutic use of glandular materials and other tissues (Harrower, 1916). Shortly after the turn of the century, this fad lost momentum and rational glandular therapy—then called *organotherapy*—began to be incorporated into mainstream medicine. This period, particularly the 1920s and 1930s, was the golden age of glandular therapy. A variety of tissue concentrates and crude extracts was available from several reputable suppliers, and a large literature developed on the clinical uses of glandular materials. Organotherapy was used for many functional disorders, and thousands of clinical reports documenting the success of this form of therapy were published (Harrower, 1916, 1939). The glandular preparations of this period were usually crude extracts or tablets of whole gland concentrates.

In the mid-twentieth century a new form of organotherapy emerged in Europe, *cell therapy*. This treatment consisted of injecting fresh animal cells into the subject's system and was believed to rejuvenate the corresponding cells of the recipient. Cell therapy developed a modest but persistent following among clinicians in Europe (Popov, 1977; Uhlenbruck, 1967).

Why Glandular Therapy Has Remained in the Background

Medicine in the first half of the twentieth century was characterized by relatively primitive laboratory and clinical techniques. Apart from their hormone content, organotherapeutic preparations and fresh animal cells were used without any evidence of efficacy. Published clinical studies amounted to little more than collections of anecdotes. Although these weaknesses do not invalidate early investigations of glandular therapy, they have kept many contemporary researchers from taking the issue seriously. These unqualified claims led to the reactive assumption that glandular or cellular therapy was not only unproved but unprovable and inherently unscientific.

Analytic methods improved greatly during the middle of this century, and many of the important hormones were discovered and isolated from glandular tissues, such as cortisone from adrenal tissue and thyroxine from thyroid tissue. The biomedical community was quick to ascribe all clinical results of glandular or cellular therapy to the presence of small quantities of hormones, which came to be regarded as the only active constituents of glandular materials. Advanced chemical methods allowed the pharmaceutical industry to produce large quantities of synthetic hormones. The gentle, physiologic action of whole glands or crude extracts was abandoned for the fast, pharmacologic action of inexpensive synthetic hormones. This was

the age of so-called wonder drugs, when both physicians and patients came to expect dramatic and immediate results from medications. These quick results, however, were later associated with problems, such as the diabetes, myopathies, and immune depression of corticosteroid (cortisone) therapy and the development of antibiotic-resistant strains of bacteria following promiscuous use of antibiotics.

Until very recently, little scientific proof existed to support the action of glandular materials. Anyone who used or promoted glandular substances was faced with several questions for which there were no satisfactory answers. The principal challenge to oral glandular or cell therapy has been the lack of evidence that intact glandular materials can be absorbed from the gastrointestinal tract. Skeptics suggested that because glandular materials degraded into simple compounds (e.g., amino acids, fatty acids) by the digestive apparatus, they were not essentially different from dried meat or protein tablets. Moreover, even if complex, potentially tissue-specific compounds were absorbed or instilled, no evidence proved that these materials could exert specific effects on the intended target organs, particularly when animal-derived tissues were used in the treatment of human tissues. Finally, the efficacy of glandular therapy might be due simply to the presence of small quantities of known hormones available in pure form elsewhere. These questions are slowly yielding to a growing body of scientific research.

Absorption of Large Molecules

For many decades, scientists believed that all ingested food materials (proteins, fats, and carbohydrates) are broken down into their smallest molecular constituents before absorption. According to this theory, proteins are broken down into free amino acids, fats into free fatty acids and glycerol, and carbon hydrates into glucose.

Many studies have challenged this thesis over the last 15 years, demonstrating that large, high–molecular-weight molecules (macromolecules) can be absorbed. Since the early 1970s, researchers have demonstrated that an array of large hormones, enzymes, and peptides are absorbed intact or nearly intact across the gut wall (Baintner, 1986; Gardner, 1984, 1988; Hemmings, 1978).

These scientists have found that a small but significant portion of dietary protein macromolecules, even relatively large ones, pass into circulation either whole or partially degraded. For example, extensive dye and radioactive tagging studies show that the proteolytic enzymes bromelin and chymotrypsin—formerly believed to be much too large for absorption—are, in fact, absorbed intact (Ambrus, 1966; Miller, 1968). Large antigenic proteins can cross the gut wall and induce significant immunologic reactions (*Lancet*, 1978). Nonprotein macromolecules such as dextran, heparin, and bacterial polysaccharides can also be absorbed intact (Baintner, 1986).

The absorption of small peptides (e.g., dipeptides and tripeptides) is generally more efficient than that of larger molecules (Humphrey, Ringrose, 1986). However, some reports indicate that molecules of higher mass are actually absorbed more efficiently than smaller molecules (Baintner, 1986). Quantification of macromolecular absorption has proved difficult because the absorbed materials are taken up rapidly and in large quantity by peripheral tissues (i.e., they disappear rapidly from the blood) (Gardner, 1988). Because of these paradoxical findings, scientists cannot make meaningful generalizations about the relationship of molecular size or peptide chain length to the efficiency of macromolecule absorption.

With his concept of "distributed digestion," W.A. Hemmings has proposed that large quantities of intact proteins and peptides (of whatever size) are absorbed and that peripheral tissues are actually the major organs of digestion (Gardner, 1988). If this hypothesis is even partially correct, the practice of clinical nutrition will change significantly. The possibility that macromolecule absorption subserves an important role in normal physiology is echoed by Baintner (1986), who suggests that "the absorption of antigens is a kind of communication between gut lumen and body. Its physiologic role may be the maintenance of the tone of gut-associated lymphatic tissue and the control of the gut flora." More research is needed to develop these intriguing hypotheses.

In sum, these findings are significant for the practice of glandular therapy. Large, potentially tissue-specific (or otherwise physiologically active) molecules can be taken up into circulation and may subsequently exert significant biologic effects. A leading figure in this research subspecialty, M.L.G. Gardner (1984, 1988), makes the following conclusion:

> Developments over the last 15 years have shown beyond doubt that this classical hypothesis of protein absorption, namely that proteins are hydrolyzed to amino acids within the lumen of the alimentary tract and that only free amino acids are absorbed by the intestinal transport systems, is untenable. . . . Biologically or pharmacologically active peptides arising during protein digestion may reach peripheral tissues (including the central nervous system) in active form, and the effects may be profound.

Tissue-Specific Activity of Glandular Materials

European researchers in cellular therapy have performed many basic biologic studies that indicate specific effects of the injected cells on target tissues and organs. Studies using stained or radioactively-tagged cells (both methods allow the researcher to trace the movement and distribution of the injected cells) have shown an active accumulation of the injected cells or their constituents by the target tissues, as predicted (Stein, 1967a). Furthermore, laboratory studies show a more rapid uptake of the corresponding injected cells or cell fragments occurs in traumatized organs than in normal organs (Neumann, 1967). This accelerated uptake of specific cellular materials by actively healing glands may reflect an increased physiologic requirement for precisely those materials supplied by tissue supplements.

Other studies have shown tissue-specific effects of injected or implanted tissues on the corresponding tissues of the recipient (Stein , 1967b). For example, thyroid cells given to animals pretreated with thyroid-damaging chemicals resulted in demonstrably accelerated regeneration of the damaged thyroids. Liver extracts infused into animals induced liver growth in the test animals (Starzyl and others, 1979). Corroborative studies in humans have been performed, although the results are more difficult to quantify because, of course, the subjects are not available for posttherapy dissection and tissue analysis. In any event, the clinical results, including correction of numerous functional complaints and occasionally dramatic revitalization, speak for themselves (Kment, 1967; Popov, 1977; Schmid, Stein, 1967).

As with every empirically deduced method of therapy, cellular therapy was not spared the accusation of being deficient in theoretical foundation. Critics may at one time have been justified in cautioning against this form of therapy, given its wide and uncritical use. Fortunately, such scruples are no longer necessary. Modern research has produced so much new and valuable information on this subject that we are obligated to learn appropriate ways in which it can be used.

Whole Glandular Materials as Sources of Peptides and Oligopeptides

Apart from tissue-specific rejuvenative activity, the results of glandular or cell therapy can be ascribed in part to the hormone content of these materials—particularly the peptide hormones. Excellent evidence suggests that many peptide hormones (and peptides with hormonelike activity) are absorbed when given orally, although larger doses are sometimes necessary to produce demonstrable effects. Orally administered hypothalamic peptides such as thyrotropin-releasing hormone (TRH) (Haigler, 1972; Yokohama, 1984), luteinizing hormone-releasing hormone (LH-RH), and the posterior pituitary hormone vasopressin (Gardner, 1984} are absorbed in significant quantities.

In the case of TRH, the oral route of administration may be not only effective but superior to other routes: oral TRH produces a more prolonged stimulation of thyroxine release than intravenous TRH. Intravenous TRH produces a faster activation of the pituitary-thyroid axis, but the effect is short-lived (Haigler, 1972). The use of low-dose, oral TRH, as it occurs naturally in hypothalamic tissue concentrates, may be a useful physiologic approach to endocrine modification.

The fact that these small peptides (3, 10, and 9 amino acids in the chains of TRH, LH-RH, and vasopressin, respectively) are active on oral administration is not surprising in light of current knowledge regarding macromolecule absorption. However, even the relatively huge polypeptide hormone insulin (51 amino acids) can be absorbed on oral administration under some circumstances (Gardner, 1984). The theoretic basis of glandular and cellular therapy is bolstered greatly by this direct evidence that intact, physiologically active peptide hormones (even large peptides) can be absorbed in this way.

Partially degraded peptide hormones—hormone fragments or oligopeptides—can also exert significant hormonal activity by an indirect mechanism. By competing with endogenous peptide hormones for sites on peptidases (peptide-degrading enzymes), small exogenous peptides can have a "peptide-sparing" action (LaBella, 1985). In other words, exogenous peptides (such as those from whole glandular materials) that may or may not have hormonal activity of their own can inhibit the degradation and thus prolong the activity of endogenous peptides.

The biologic activity of peptide hormones does not always depend on the presence of the entire hormone. In the case of parathyroid hormone, for example, a chain of only 27 of the molecule's 84 amino acids appears to be required for biologic activity (Brewer, 1974). Manberg (1985) makes the following observation:

> Perhaps it is in part these peptide-sparing and oligopeptide effects that are responsible for the remarkably prolonged action of administered peptide hormones. For example, dramatic and lasting results have been noted with even a single, small dose of TRH (thyrotropin-releasing hormone) in the treatment of depression (Garbutt, 1984). One paradox of peptide research has been the apparent dissociation between the plasma levels of peptides and their observed durations of action. It is difficult to understand how a single dose of a compound that is completely cleared from the system within less than an hour can nevertheless exert long-lasting effects spanning days. It is clear that we are far from a complete understanding of the mode of action of these drugs.

Whole Glandulars as Sources of Enzymes

Probably the most well-known and widely accepted form of glandular therapy is the use of pancreas substance or concentrate in the treatment of exocrine pancreatic insufficiency. This practice has not been considered endocrine therapy proper because the effect of the enzyme supplements is strictly local to the gut. However, evidence suggests that intact digestive enzyme molecules secreted by the pancreas are reabsorbed lower in the gut and taken back to the pancreas for storage and rerelease (Liebow, Rothman, 1975). This phenomenon is described as *enteropancreatic circulation* of digestive enzymes and analogous to the enterohepatic circulation of bile acids. Supple-

mentation with enzyme-rich pancreas concentrates thus not only assists digestion at the time of administration, but may exert a lasting, postabsorptive effect on pancreatic enzyme reserves.

The enzyme content of raw glandular materials may promote the production of hormones endogenously in the user. Adrenal tissue, for example, contains enzymes that convert the steroid precursor cholesterol into steroid hormones such as cortisone (Friedman, 1956). In this case the use of whole, raw glandular materials may promote the formation of corticosteroids endogenously. This formation could occur locally in the gut (particularly if the glandular material was taken with cholesterol-containing foods) or, if Hemmings' "distributed digestion" hypothesis (described previously) is correct, systemically. The substance of other steroid-producing glands (gonads and ovaries) probably contains enzymes that convert precursor materials into their respective steroid hormones.

Because all truly raw (non–heat–treated) glandular materials contain a complement of enzymes necessary for converting appropriate substrate into hormones, this phenomenon may be general to other glands and tissues. Perhaps all glandulars provide either intact enzymes, apoenzymes, or other enzyme fragments that encourage the endogenous synthesis of hormones or other biologically active molecules from precursor materials. The small quantities of preformed hormones in glandular materials would thus be supplemented by an accelerated endogenous synthesis of those hormones.

Whole Glandulars as Sources of Active Lipids and Steroids

Whole glandular materials—those prepared in a manner that preserves the lipids—are rich in biologically active, lipid-soluble materials, including small quantities of the steroid hormones of the adrenal cortex, gonads, and ovaries. However, the known steroid hormones are not the only factors of interest. New medicinal applications are continually being developed for a diversity of fat-soluble compounds, and more often than not the glandular structures are the richest natural sources of these substances. Coenzyme Q_{10}, for example, has recently attracted attention as a rejuvenative and therapeutic food factor; the richest natural sources of this vital coenzyme are tissues such as the heart, liver, kidney, and spleen (Bliznakov, Hunt, 1987).

Specialized phospholipids such as phosphatidylcholine, phosphatidylserine, and others have been proposed as therapeutic agents for neurologic and other diseases (Horrocks and others, 1986); these phospholipids are found in the brain, liver, and other glands. These glands are sources of highly unsaturated omega-3 fatty acids, which are now thought to play a vital role in the development and maintenance of the central nervous system.

Even in the early years of organotherapy, practitioners recognized that the full clinical efficacy of several glandular materials required the presence of the lipid fractions. Biologically active lipids from the adrenals, gonads, thyroid, spleen, pancreas, and pituitary were recognized as contributing to the activity of glandular preparations (Harrower, 1916).

Adrenal Androgens and the Case for Crude Glandulars over Pure Hormones

The adrenal androgens (such as DHEA) are an excellent example of the potential medicinal properties of the lipid-soluble fractions of whole glandulars. The medicinal significance of this class of hormones did not become evident until the last 10 to 15 years, although other corticosteroids had been in use for several decades. In contrast, the devolution of adrenal therapy from crude preparations (containing a diversity of hormones and hormone precursors) to the pure, synthetic hormones provides an instructive example of the way medically important substances can be overlooked in the rush to obtain the active fraction of a whole tissue.

Shortly after the first of the cortical hormones (cortisone and deoxycorticosterone) were isolated and synthesized, it became fashionable to use these pure preparations instead of the crude adrenal cortex extracts (ACE) that had been available in the past. In fact, the traditionalists who preferred the crude ACE over the synthetic imitations were ridiculed by mainstream practitioners who believed they were resisting a significant medical advance. Eventually even the U.S. Food and Drug Administration joined the fray, insisting that ACE manufacturers withdraw the product because the synthetic hormones had been "proved" to have all the therapeutic activity of the extracts and were more reliable. As far as demonstrable glucocorticoid and mineralocorticoid activity was concerned (two of the three major classes of corticosteroid activity), the synthetics were as potent as the extracts. However, ACE users persisted, knowing from clinical experience that another substance was active in the whole glandular extract—something with effects beyond those of the synthetics.

The medicinal significance of the third group of corticosteroids—the adrenal androgens—did not begin to be recognized until the late 1970s and early 1980s. Arthur Schwartz and his group at Temple University in Philadelphia showed that DHEA (dehydroepiandrosterone), the prototypical adrenal androgen, has dramatic metabolic and therapeutic effects. DHEA suppresses the development of spontaneous breast cancer in animals and antagonizes the effects of some chemical carcinogens and tumor promoters. Supplemental DHEA protects animals against obesity, diabetes, autoimmune phenomena, and viral infection (Merrill, Harrington, Sunderland, 1989; Schwartz and others, 1981). Women with subnormal plasma DHEA are at in-

creased risk of developing breast cancer (Schwartz and others, 1981). Research has shown that plasma DHEA levels are depressed in people infected with HIV and are greatly depressed in people with acquired immunodeficiency syndrome (AIDS) (Merrill and others, 1989); these findings suggest a role for supplemental DHEA in the prevention or management of HIV-related illness. (Note, in contrast, that other adrenal steroids such as cortisone—in large doses—can actually cause diabetes and obesity and depress the immune response to viruses and cancer.)

Of course, DHEA and other adrenal androgens are found naturally in ACE and other crude adrenal preparations. The traditionalists have been vindicated, and the arrogant assertion that all medicinal activity of cortical preparations is attributable to the better-known steroids stands discredited. Researchers should now concern themselves with learning whether other substances like DHEA remain to be discovered or, if discovered, merit scientific evaluation of their medicinal activity. Meanwhile, the crude preparations are certainly more suitable for common, nonpathologic health problems calling for gentle endocrine support—not metabolism-deranging hormonal replacement. Pure hormones are to glandular therapy as pure sugar is to nutritional therapy; sugar supplies one necessary nutrient but provides it in a form that is unnecessarily (and often unhealthfully) refined and concentrated.

Quantitative Considerations: Clinical Adequacy of Low-Dose Hormones

As far as recognized hormones are concerned, their quantities in glandular materials may be too small to have significant clinical effects. However, low, supplementary doses of hormones (i.e., doses that supplement the body's usual production of that hormone) are often all that is required, at least for the common, functional health problems that concern the general practitioner. Although appropriate in endocrine pathology or for special pharmacologic purposes, the high, replacement-level doses that have been used conventionally (i.e., doses that meet or exceed the body's usual production) are otherwise excessive and unnecessary.

Only small doses of TRH are required for therapeutic effects, and peptides in general have an enigmatic effectiveness characterized by the prolonged activity of even single doses (see the discussion on peptides). However, the efficacy of low-dose hormone therapy is not limited to the peptide hormones.

For example, a trend in rheumatology favors the use of very low doses of corticosteroids for the control of rheumatic pain and inflammation (Buchanan, Stephens, Buchanan, 1988). The doses used amount to only a few milligrams—enough to supplement the body's natural daily production of cortisone but not enough to induce pituitary-adrenal axis suppression or many other side effects of excess corticosteroids. The doses used for the treatment of rheumatic pain and inflammation are similar to the amounts that occur naturally in adrenal concentrates or extracts.

In his book *Safe Uses of Cortisone*, W.M. Jeffries (1981) documented the successful use of supplementary doses of corticosteroids for mild hypoadrenia and its associated functional health problems. Again, the steroid doses in question modestly supplement the endogenous secretion, thus lifting the total circulating steroids to a level that offers freedom from the symptoms of hypoadrenia.

Another example is the use of very low doses of thyroxine (thyroxine supplementation) to correct low-grade hypothyroidism and prevent the development of frank hypothyroidism (Tibaldi, Barzel, 1985). Slow, age-related deterioration of thyroid function, as indicated by elevated thyroid-stimulating hormone levels, is a common clinical finding. These individuals may be considered euthyroid and "normal" by most conventional standards, but they are subtly deficient in thyroxine. Rather than waiting years for overt hypothyroidism to develop, very small doses of thyroxine (doses that supplement the body's natural production) can correct the deficiency and prevent the emergence of serious illness:

> [Supplementary thyroxine] may bring about the resolution of subtle subclinical abnormalities and prevent the development and progression of the insidious and nonspecific physical and mental changes that are reported to precede the obvious clinical symptoms and signs of hypothyroidism (Tibaldi, Barzel, 1985).

Most, if not all, other hormones given in small quantities (as they occur in whole source materials or crude extracts) can probably serve in the same supplementary capacity and be a useful adjunct to nutritional and other physiologic therapy of functional health problems. The provision of supplementary levels of preformed hormones probably contributes to the clinical effects of whole glandular preparations.

Whole Glandulars: Tomorrow's Pharmaceutical Advances—Today

Whole glandular materials provide not only the active substances that have been identified but a variety of hormones, hormonelike materials, hormone fragments, and other substances with biologic activity. This fact is significant because medicinal research is continually uncovering new biologically active entities with therapeutic potential. Because the commercial development of these substances could take decades, whole glandular therapy is the only practical way to take advantage of these research findings today.

For example, two biologically active peptides have been isolated from the thymus, and no fewer than 10 thymic fractions (complexes of polypeptides not yet precisely characterized) with demonstrable biologic activity exist (Goldstein, 1981; Wara, 1981). Biomedical researchers will spend years evaluating the biologic properties of these thymic fractions, and pharmaceutical scientists will spend years more in clinical testing and scale-up for industrial production. (This lengthy evaluation is required by government regulations.)

Of course, even when these concentrated, purified materials become available, still more years will elapse before the long-term side effects, if any, are known. The use of large quantities of one pure substance can create an imbalance in the body—a relative "deficiency" of other and equally important factors. Meanwhile, whole glandular materials or cells provide small, potentially salutary quantities of these substances, both known and unknown, and in naturally occurring proportions.

All the research mentioned has used animal gland tissues, extracts, hormones, and cells; that is, species variation in the molecular composition of hormones and cell constituents is apparently not a limiting factor for glandular therapy in most instances. Indeed, although synthetic versions have become available, popular peptide hormones such as insulin and thyroxine are commonly derived from animals (usually hogs or cattle). Other newer peptides such as calcitonin and thymus hormones are derived from animal glands.

New Hormones and Bioactive Peptides: Research and Outlook

Peptide hormones and other natural tissue extracts are being investigated intensively in laboratories around the world. New thymus, parathyroid, pituitary, and hypothalamic hormones have been identified in the past decade, and no end to these discoveries is in sight. These new compounds have great therapeutic, preventive, and rejuvenative potential.

The thymic (thymus-derived) hormones are of special interest today as a potential treatment for AIDS and other immunodeficient states. For example, Richard Schulof (1986) and his group at the George Washington University Medical Center reported that thymic fractions can restore some aspects of depressed immunity in patients with AIDS and may have long-term value in preventing the progression from HTLV-III seropositivity to frank AIDS.

Many clinical studies and several major review articles have appeared documenting the biologic and therapeutic activity of the thymic factors (Goldstein, 1981; Wara, 1981). Various thymic peptides and extracts are being used to correct congenital immune deficiencies (Rubenstein, 1979) and depressed immunity in patients with cancer and patients infected with herpes virus (Tovo, 1980).

A group of Hungarian researchers has isolated a simple peptide, glutaurine (γ glutamyl-taurine), from parathyroid glands. This peptide profoundly enhances immune status, may participate in the metabolism of vitamin A, and antagonizes the immunodepressant effects of corticosteroids (Feuer, 1978). The research team has found that glutaurine restores the activity of "natural killer" cells—the lymphocytes responsible for killing tumor cells and microbes—in patients with cancer and depressed activity of natural killer cells (Lang, 1983).

Pituitary and hypothalamic hormones are an active area of research. Most pituitary hormones are "releasing factors"—hormones that induce the release of hormones from other glands in the body. Hypothalamic hormones are also usually releasing factors, except that they act as releasing factor–releasing factors: they induce the pituitary to release its releasing factors.

TRH is a good example of releasing-factor activity. Hypothalamic TRH stimulates the release of thyrotropin (TSH) from the pituitary. TSH, in turn, stimulates the release of thyroxine from the thyroid. TRH is used as a diagnostic agent for testing pituitary and thyroid "reserve" (the ability of these glands to respond to stimuli). However, TRH appears to have great therapeutic potential apart from its diagnostic uses (Holaday, 1984). As previously discussed, TRH is active when taken orally (Haigler, 1972) and can be effective in very low doses.

Animal-derived TRH is being used experimentally as an antagonist of opiates and other depressants and in the treatment of shock and depression (Faden, 1984; Garbutt, 1984; Gold, 1977). Because TRH has significant cholinergic effects, it has been suggested as a treatment for Alzheimer's disease (which is caused in part by acetylcholine deficiency) (Yarbrough, 1985). If it is given soon enough, TRH may limit the degree of paralysis following spinal cord injury.

Other hormones and hormonelike factors from the spleen, liver, prostate, bone, brain, gut, and other tissues have been identified. Many laboratories are now testing these substances for quality and quantity of biologic activity. The results of this research promise a renewed and expanded scientific rationale for the organotherapy of yesteryear and the glandular and cellular therapy of today.

Recent Advances in Cell Therapy

Cell therapy is defined as the injection of healthy cellular material into the body to promote physical regeneration (Allen, Solorzano, 1993). It is used to stimulate healing, counteract the effects of aging, and treat numerous degenerative conditions such as arthritis, Parkinson's disease, atherosclerosis, and cancer (Allen, Solorzano, 1993). Although cell therapy is used worldwide, especially in Europe, it is not approved in the United States.

Paul Niehans (1960), a specialist in organ transplants, originally developed cell therapy in 1931. Broadly defined, cell therapy includes the use of human blood transfusions and bone marrow transplants; for the purposes of this discussion, it refers to cellular material from organs, fetuses, and embryos of animals (Allen, Solorzano, 1993). Results

of studies on cell therapy are discussed in the previous section on tissue-specific activity of glandular materials.

More recent developments include therapeutic immunology and bionutritional therapy. In therapeutic immunology, cell extracts are administered along with antibodies raised in animals (Allen, Solorzano, 1993). It appears to be similar to the vaccination approach to regeneration. Dr. Stephan, the developer of therapeutic immunology, states "cells of various organs, glands, and other body parts are taken from specially raised animals who are free of disease and healthy. The cells are placed in solution and filtered to remove unwanted protein elements and then introduced into another (secondary) mammal" (Allen, Solorzano, 1993). The injected antigens produce antibodies that appear in its bloodstream and are measured (Allen, Solarzano, 1993). When antibodies reach the desired level, blood is taken, the serum is separated, and the antibodies are prepared and tested for purity and efficacy. The preparations are administered over an extended period to assist in regenerating components of the immune system (Allen, Solorzano, 1993).

Bionutritional therapy uses cells, cell extracts, and antibodies combined with nutrients and ATP to promote cellular and tissue regeneration (Allen, Solorzano, 1993). The mixture is placed under the tongue. This method appears to prevent side effects (Allen, Solorzano, 1993).

Cell therapy, therapeutic immunology, and bionutritional therapy have been used successfully on more than 30,000 human patients. Conditions treated include arthritis; cardiovascular disorders; and urogenital, respiratory, and viral conditions (Allen, Solorzano, 1993). In a study on 72 patients with arteriosclerosis who were treated with a mixture of placenta, liver, and testes, 58 showed marked improvement. Cholesterol levels were lowered significantly, and walking distance improved (Schmid, 1967).

Oral Tolerization

Oral tolerization is a term recently coined to define the process of turning off patients' rejection of their own tissues by feeding them small amounts of a protein directly or indirectly involved in the attack by the immune system (Weiner and others, 1994). Examples include feeding insulin to patients with diabetes or a protein from the myelin sheath to patients with multiple sclerosis. The protein may be administered in a capsule. With no apparent side effects, the technique seems safe; in fact, the Food and Drug Administration has sanctioned studies on humans (Weiner and others, 1994).

Oral Tolerance

Oral tolerance describes the exogenous administration of antigen to the peripheral immune system via the gastrointestinal tract (Weiner and others, 1994). It is a form of antigen-driven peripheral immune tolerance (Weiner and others, 1994) that has been found to be clinically effective in the treatment of both human and animal autoimmune diseases such as multiple sclerosis, rheumatoid arthritis, and uveitis (Weiner and others, 1994). No apparent toxicity or decreases in T cell autoreactivity have been found. One of the first attempts at oral tolerization may have been practiced by Native Americans who are thought to have fed their children Rhus leaves to prevent them from becoming sensitized to poison ivy (Dakin, 1829).

Oral tolerance, the observation that orally fed antigens can suppress immune responses, was first described in 1911, when systemic anaphylaxis in guinea pigs was prevented by previous feeding of proteins from hens' eggs (Wells, 1911). In the past 20 years, much research has focused on the use of oral tolerance in the treatment of various autoimmune diseases, including insulin-dependent diabetes. Restoration of peripheral (i.e., extrathymic) tolerance with oral antigen administration is based on three concepts. The first is that gut mucosa contains immunologically active lymphoid tissue known as *gut-associated lymphoid tissue (GALT)*. The second is that two related subclasses of helper T cells exist, Th1 and Th2. Th1 cells are predominantly involved in priming and sustaining cell-mediated immune responses. They tend to be pathogenic in autoimmune disease. Th2 cells tend to suppress Th1 immune responses and are required to restore or maintain tolerance (Weiner, 1995).

The third concept on which oral tolerance is based is called *bystander suppression*. Oral tolerization is believed to be triggered in an antigen-specific manner, but it suppresses nonspecifically in the local environment of the diseased organ (Weiner, 1995). Identification of the target autoantigens in autoimmune diseases may not be necessary; oral administration of a protein capable of inducing Th2 cells to secrete suppressive cytokines at the target organ may be sufficient.

Three proposed mechanisms of action explain antigen-driven tolerance: clonal deletion, clonal anergy, and active suppression (Kroemer, 1992; Miller, 1992). This section of the chapter reviews the research and mechanisms of action of oral tolerance as developed by Weiner (Weiner and others, 1994). A comprehensive discussion of these concepts is reviewed in the *Annual Review of Immunology* (Weiner and others, 1994).

Gut-associated lymphoid tissue consists of discrete lymphoid nodules know as *Peyer's patches,* perivillous intraepithelial lymphocytes and lymphocytes scattered throughout the lamina propria (Weiner and others, 1994). Peyer's patches contain T and B lymphocytes, macrophages, dendritic cells, and a germinal center with B lymphocytes. Peyer's patches are one of the primary areas in the GALT where specific immune responses are generated. Peyer's patches are a major source of IgA-producing B cells. They have also been identified as a site where regulatory cells that mediate the active suppression component of oral tolerance are generated (MacDonald, 1983;

Mattingly, 1984; Santos and others, 1993). Th2-type responses may also be generated in Peyer's patches.

No evidence suggests that the perivillous intraepithelial lymphocytes participate in oral tolerance induction, although they do have a role in the gut's immunologic defenses. The lamina propria lymphocytes appear to have cytokine profiles similar to those of Peyer's patch T cells. They have a ratio of CD4/CD8 cells similar to the Peyer's patch (Brandtzaeg, 1989).

Mechanism of Action

The three main mechanisms of antigen-driven oral tolerance are active suppression, antigen-driven bystander suppression, and clonal anergy (Kroemer, 1992; Miller 1992). With appropriate dose manipulation, administration of a self-antigen to an animal may engage GALT and restore peripheral tolerance. Most studies have shown that active suppression is the primary mechanism (Moat, 1987). The primary factor that determines the form of peripheral tolerance to develop following oral antigen administration is that low doses of antigen favor the generation of active suppression or regulatory cell-driven tolerance, whereas high doses of antigen favor anergy-driven tolerance (Weiner and others, 1994). These forms of oral tolerance are not mutually exclusive and may occur simultaneously. The use of oral tolerance to treat autoimmune diseases is critically dependent on which of these two mechanisms is triggered.

Active suppression is a critical mechanism for oral antigen-driven tolerance. Low doses of orally administered autoantigens have been shown to suppress experimental autoimmune diseases via the generation of regulatory cells that suppress both in vitro and in vivo via the secretion of downregulatory cytokines (Miller and others, 1992). After feeding antigens such as sheep red blood cells, transferable suppression mediated by T cells from Peyer's patches, mesenteric lymph nodes and spleen has been found (Guatam, Chikkala, Battisto, 1990).

Antigen-driven bystander suppression suggests that activation of suppressor pathways may induce tolerance not only against the antigen used but also against cellular reactivity to other local antigens (Weiner and others, 1994). The tolerogen may determine the area where activation occurs but does not limit the targets of the activated cells and their cytokines (Weiner, 1995). Cells from guinea pigs' myelin basic protein (MBP) that are fed to animals have been shown to suppress proliferation of an ovalbumin (OVA) line across a transwell (Miller and others, 1991). The reverse was also found. The soluble factor responsible for the suppression was the cytokine TGF-b. Suppression is mediated by OVA-specific regulatory cells that migrate to the draining lymph node and secrete TGF-b on encountering OVA, thus inhibiting the generation of the MBP-specific immune response generated in the lymph node (Weiner and others, 1994). Clinically, autoimmune disease is believed to result from a loss of tolerance to antigens such as collagen and pancreatic B cells. However, additional proteins in the organ under attack can also serve as autoimmune targets.

Anergy has only recently been proposed as a mechanism for oral tolerance (Melamed, Friedman, 1993; Whitacre and others, 1991). *Anergy* is defined as "a state of T-lymphocyte unresponsiveness characterized by absence of proliferation, IL-2 production, and diminished expression of IL-2R" (Schwartz, 1990). The induction of anergy depends on antigen dosage and frequency of feeding (Friedman, Weiner, 1993).

Neonatal Tolerance

Administration of antigens to neonates has been shown to induce tolerance in some cases, although it may also result in immune priming for both humoral and cell-mediated immune responses. Tolerance may occur when the same antigens are fed to adult animals (Hanson, 1981; Strobel, Ferguson, 1984). Some researchers have suggested that immaturity of the immunoregulatory network associated with oral tolerance and sensitization to autoantigens via the gut in the neonatal period may contribute to the pathogenesis of autoimmune diseases (Weiner and others, 1994).

Treatment of Organ-Specific Autoimmune Diseases in Animals

Oral tolerance may be used in the treatment of autoimmune conditions in both humans and animals (Weiner and others, 1994). Oral tolerance has been shown to suppress autoimmunity in animals in the treatment of uveitis (Nussenblatt and others, 1990), diabetes (Zhang and others, 1991), adjuvant arthritis (Zhang and others, 1990), myasthenia gravis (Wang, Qiao, Link, 1993), and autoimmune encephalomyelitis in the rat (Higgins, Weiner, 1988). Collagen-induced arthritis in rats was suppressed by feeding type II collagen (Nagler-Anderson and others, 1986; Thompson, Staines, 1986). In the treatment of autoimmune uveitis, low doses of antigen were found to favor suppression, whereas high doses were found to induce unresponsiveness or anergy (Gregerson, Obritsch, Donoso, 1993).

Oral tolerance was used successfully in the treatment of autoimmune diabetes in NOD mice. Porcine insulin was administered orally at a dosage of 1 mg twice a week for 5 weeks and then weekly until 1 year of age (Zhang and others, 1991). The severity of the lymphocytic infiltration of pancreatic islets was reduced by oral administration of insulin, and the onset of diabetes was delayed. A decreased incidence of diabetes was observed in animals followed for 1 year (Zhang and others, 1991). Orally ad-

ministered insulin had no metabolic effect on blood glucose levels. Another point of interest is that splenic T cells from animals treated orally with insulin adoptively transferred protection against diabetes, which suggests that oral insulin generates active cellular mechanisms that suppress disease.

Oral tolerance has also been found to protect against chronic immune complex–mediated nephritis and immune complex disease (Devey, Bleasdale, 1984). Oral tolerance may also be useful in downregulating alloreactivity associated with transplantation (Weiner and others, 1994). In humans a double-blind study on the treatment of multiple sclerosis (MS) with oral administration of bovine myelin for 1 year demonstrated a significantly decreased incidence of major MS attacks compared with a control group taking a placebo (Weiner and others, 1993).

Veterinary Applications

A small number of U.S. veterinarians have been using glandular therapy in their practices for decades. Anecdotal evidence shows promising results in the use of glandular and cell therapies for various conditions. Oral freeze-dried concentrates of liver, kidney, heart, thyroid, collagen, bone, spleen, adrenal, pituitary, and other tissues have been used to treat degenerative conditions with some success. The positive results associated with use of oral tolerization in the treatment of various immune-mediated diseases such as uveitis and rheumatoid arthritis have significant implications in the treatment of companion animals with similar conditions. This area of veterinary medicine should be explored further through both laboratory studies and clinical efficacy trials.

Contraindications, Side Effects, and Controversies

Live cell or glandular therapy has given rise to concerns about sterility, potential transmission of viruses from one species to another, and immune reactions in the organ or cells. A process whereby the cellular material is freeze-dried seems to have resolved these problems. The freeze-drying process regulates sterility and allows for cell material to be conserved for a longer time. The cellular material contains lesser amounts of foreign protein, substantially reducing rejection risk (Allen, Solorzano, 1993). If freeze-dried whole cells are used, the cell surface is still present and may be antigenic, although this is rare. A process of ultrafiltration is now being used to remove the cell surface coat and its antigenic material and thereby reduce the risk of rejection. The use of freeze-dried cell ultrafiltrates allows for better quality control and prolonged storage (Allen, Solorzano, 1993).

The source of the animal tissues must also be addressed. Bovine spongoencephalopathy virus, which recently infected cattle in the United Kingdom, is but one source of potential interspecies viral transmission that must be prevented. Further studies ensuring that such viruses are not transmitted is essential when using organ tissues from one species to treat another. One solution adopted by a number of glandular supply companies is to use tissues only from countries and herds or flocks known to be free of such diseases. One company (PHP) uses only certified, organically raised lamb tissue from New Zealand that is free of pesticides, hormones, and viruses. The tissues are also byproducts of another industry (i.e., the lambs are not sacrificed specifically for this use), which is an important ethical consideration.

Cell therapy is not recommended for patients with severe kidney disease, liver failure, or acute infectious and inflammatory processes. Patients who experience an allergic reaction to the test injection should not receive treatment. The bionutritional therapy approach, which uses oral drops, may be safer and more efficacious for these conditions.

Bioethical considerations should be considered when using the body parts of one animal to treat another. Responsible veterinarians emphasize the importance of humane treatment of donor animals before using these therapies.

The concerns of sterility and transmission have been addressed. Therapeutic modes of action have been proposed and some documented. Further research is required to document modes of action and specific indications.

Future Implications

New approaches to glandular and cell therapy, such as oral tolerization, therapeutic immunology, and bionutritional therapy, offer exciting possibilities in the use of glands, tissues, and organs from healthy animals to assist in the regeneration of degenerative, diseased organs in other animals. Further research should enhance the development of this field in veterinary medicine.

Orally administered autoantigens may play a significant role in the treatment of organ-specific inflammatory autoimmune disease in both humans and animals. With the advantages of being orally administered, nontoxic, and antigen specific, this therapy may be the latest, most specific development in the field previously known as *glandular therapy*. The use of orally administered autoantigens may also substantiate the concept of "like cures like," a basic tenet of homeopathy. Potential applications of oral tolerization in veterinary medicine include the possible treatment of immune-mediated uveitis, rheumatoid arthritis, degenerative myelopathy, and other immune-mediated diseases. This therapy would be particularly valuable in veterinary medicine because of the ease of administration. Research on the treatment of autoimmune disease must explore these therapeutic avenues.

REFERENCES

Allen T, Solorzano H: Cell therapy. In *Alternative medicine: the definitive guide,* Purallup, Wash, 1993, Future Medicine.

Ambrus JL: Absorption of exogenous and endogenous proteolytic enzymes, *Clin Pharmacol Ther* 8:362, 1966.

Antigen absorption by the gut, *Lancet* ii: 715, 1978.

Baintner K: *Intestinal absorption of macromolecules and immune transmission from mother to young,* Boca Raton, Fla, 1986, CRC Press.

Bliznakov EG, Hunt GL: *The miracle nutrient: coenzyme Q₁₀,* New York, 1987, Bantam Books.

Brandtzaeg P: Overview of the mucosal immune system, *Curr Topics Microbiol Immunol* 146:13, 1989.

Brewer HB: Recent studies on the chemistry of human, bovine, and porcine parathyroid hormones, *Am J Med* 56:759, 1974.

Buchanan WW, Stephens LJ, Buchanan HM: Are "homeopathic" doses of oral corticosteroids effective in rheumatoid arthritis? *Clin Exper Rheumatol* 6:281, 1988.

Dakin R: Remarks on a cutaneous affection produced by certain poisonous vegetables, *Am J Med Sci* 4:98, 1829.

Devey ME, Bleasdale K: Antigen feeding modifies the course of antigen-induced immune complex disease, *Clin Exp Immunol* 56:637, 1984.

Faden AI: Opiate antagonists and thyrotropin-releasing hormone. II. Potential role in the treatment of central nervous system injury, *JAMA* 252:1452, 1984.

Feuer L: Effect of glutaurine on vitamin A and prednisolone-treated thymus cultures. *Acta Morphol Hung* 26:75, 1978.

Friedman R: Cholesterol metabolism, *Annu Rev Biochem* 25:613, 1956.

Friedman A, Weiner HL: Induction of anergy and/or active suppression in oral tolerance is determined by frequency of feeding and antigen dosage, PNAS USA, 1993.

Garbutt JC: A dramatic behavioral response to thyrotropin-releasing hormone following low-dose neuroleptics, *Psychoneuroendocrinol* 9:311, 1984.

Gardner MLG: Intestinal assimilation of intact peptides and proteins from the diet: A neglected field? *Biol Rev Camb Philos Soc* 59:289, 1984.

Gardner MLG: Gastrointestinal absorption of intact proteins, *Annu Rev Nutr* 8:329, 1988.

Gold PW: Pituitary thyrotropin response to thyrotropin-releasing hormone in affective illness, *Am J Psychiatry* 134:1028, 1977.

Goldstein AL: Current status of thymosin and other hormones of the thymus gland, *Recent Prog Horm Res* 37:369, 1981.

Gregerson DS, Obritsch WF, Donoso LA: Oral tolerance in experimental autoimmune uveoretinitis: distinct mechanisms of resistance are induced by low versus high dose feeding protocols, *J Immunol* 151:5751, 1993.

Guatam SC, Chikkala NF, Battisto JR: Oral administration of the contact sensitizer trinitrochlorobenzene: initial sensitization and subsequent appearance of a suppressor population, *Cell Immunol* 125:437, 1990.

Haigler ED: Response to orally administered synthetic thyrotropin-releasing hormone in man, *J Clin Endocrinol Metab* 35:631, 1972.

Hanson DG: Ontogeny of orally induced tolerance to soluble proteins in mice, *J Immunol* 127:1518, 1981.

Harrower HR: *An endocrine handbook,* Glendale, Calif, 1939, Harrower Laboratory.

Harrower HR: *Practical hormone therapy-a manual of organotherapy for general practitioners,* New York, 1916, American Medical.

Hemmings WA: Transport of large breakdown products of dietary protein through the gut wall, *Gut* 19:715, 1978.

Higgins P, Weiner HL: Suppression of experimental autoimmune encephalomyelitis by oral administration of myelin basic protein and its fragments, *U Immunol* 140:440, 1988.

Holaday JW: Protirelin (TRH): a potent neuromodulator with therapeutic potential, *Arch Int Med* 144:1138, 1984.

Horrocks LA and others, editors: Phospholipid research and the nervous system. In *Phospholipid research and the nervous system,* Berlin, 1986, Springer Verlag.

Humphrey MJ, Ringrose PS: Peptides and related drugs: a review of their absorption, metabolism and excretion. *Drug Metab Rev* 17:283,1986.

Jeffries WM: *Safe uses of cortisone,* Springfield, Ill, 1981, Charles C Thomas.

Kment A: The objective demonstration of the revitalization effect after cell injections. In Schmid F, editor: C*ell research and cellular therapy,* Thoune, Switzerland, 1967, Ott.

Kroemer G, Martinez AC: Mechanisms of self-tolerance, *Immunol Today* 13:401, 1992.

LaBella FS: Administered peptides inhibit the degradation of endogenous peptides: the dilemma of distinguishing direct from indirect effects, *Peptides* 6:645, 1985.

Lang, I: Glutaurine enhances the depressed NK cell activity of tumor patients, *Immunol Comm* 12:519, 1983.

Liebow C, Rothman SS: Enteropancreatic circulation of digestive enzymes, *Science* 189:472, 1975.

MacDonald T: Immuno-suppression caused by antigen feeding. II. Suppressor T cell mask Peyer's patches B cell priming to orally administered antigen, *Eur J Immunol* 13:138, 1983.

Manberg PJ: Problems in the development of neuropeptides as psychotherapeutic drugs. In Lal H, LaBella F, Lane J, editors: *Endocoids,* New York, 1985, Alan R Liss.

Mattingly JA: Immunological suppression after oral administration of antigen. III. Activation of suppressor-induced cells in the Peyer's patches, *Cell Immunol* 86:46, 1984.

Melamed D, Friedman A: Direct evidence for anergy in T lymphocytes tolerized by oral administration of ovalbumin, *Eur J Immunol* 23:935, 1993.

Merrill CR, Harrington MG, Sunderland T: Plasma dehydroepiandosterone levels in HIV infection, *JAMA* 261:1149, 1989 (letter).

Miller JM: The absorption of proteolytic enzymes from the gastrointestinal tract, *Clin Med* 10:35, 1968.

Miller A, Lider O, Weiner HL: Antigen-driven bystander suppression following oral administration of antigens, *J Exp Med* 174:791, 1991.

Miller J, Moraham G: Peripheral T cell tolerance, *Ann Rev Immunol* 10:51, 1992.

Miller A and others: Suppresssor T cells generated by oral tolerization to myelin basic protein suppress both in vitro and in vivo immune responses by the release of TGF-b following antigen-specific triggering, *Proc Natl Acad Sci USA* 89:421, 1992.

Moat AM: The regulation of immune responses to dietary protein antigens, *Immunol Today* 8:93, 1987.

Nagler-Anderson C and others: Suppression of Type II collagen–induced arthritis by intragastric administration of soluble type II collagen, *Proc Natl Acad Sci USA* 83:7443, 1986.

Neumann KH: The influence of tissue injections on experimental liver damage. In Schmid F, editor: *Cell research and cellular therapy,* Thoune, Switzerland, 1967, Ott.

Niehans P: *Introduction to cellular therapy,* New York, 1960, Pageant Books.

Nussenblatt RB and others: Inhibition of S-antigen induced experimental autoimmune uveoretinitis by oral induction of tolerance with S-antigen, *J Immunol* 144:1689, 1990.

O'Dea K: The hunter-gatherer lifestyle of Australian aborigines: implications for health. In McLean A, Wahlquist ML, editors: *Current problems in nutrition, pharmacology, and toxicology,* London, 1988, John Libbey.

Popov IM: Cell therapy. *J Internat Acad Preventive Med* 3:74, 1977.

Rubenstein A: In vivo and in vitro effects of thymosin and adenosine deaminase on adenosine deaminase-deficient lymphocytes, *N Engl J Med* 300:387, 1979.

Santos LMB and others: Oral tolerance to myelin basic protein induces TGF-b secreting T cells in Peyer's patches, *J Immunol* 150:811: 1993.

Schmid F: *Cell therapy: a new dimension of medicine,* Thoome, Switzerland, 1993, Ott.

Schmid F, Stein J: Preface to the first edition. In Schmid F, editor: *Cell research and cellular therapy,* Thoune, Switzerland, 1967, Ott.

Schulof RS: Phase I/II trial of thymosin fraction 5 and thymosin alpha one in HTLV-III seropositive subjects, *J Biol Response Mod* 5:429, 1986.

Schwartz RH: A cell culture model for T-lymphocyte clonal anergy, *Science* 248:1349, 1990.

Schwartz AG and others: Dehydroepiandnosterone: an anti-obesity and anti-carcinogenic agent, *Nutr Cancer* 3:46, 1981.

Starzyl T and others: Growth-stimulating factor in regenerating canine liver, *Lancet* i:127, 1979.

Stein J: Objective demonstration of the organ-specific effectiveness of cellular preparations. In Schmid F, editor: *Cell research and cellular therapy,* Thoune, Switzerland, 1967a, Ott.

Stein J: Specific effect of implanted endocrine tissues. In Schmid F, editor: *Cell research and cellular therapy,* Thoune, Switzerland, 1967b, Ott.

Strobel S, Ferguson A: Immune responses to fed protein antigens in mice: systemic tolerance or priming is related to age at which antigen is first encountered, *Pediatr Res* 18:588, 1984.

Thompson HSG, Staines NA: Gastric administration of type II collagen delays the onset and severity of collagen-induced arthritis in rats, *Clin Exp Immunol* 64:581, 1986.

Tibaldi J, Barzel US: Thyroxine supplementation: method for the prevention of clinical hypothyroidism. *Am J Med* 79:241, 1985.

Tovo PA: Thymus extract therapy in immunodepressed patients with malignancies and herpes virus infections, *Thymus* 2:41, 1980.

Uhlenbruck P: Introduction. In Schmid F, editor: *Cell research and cellular therapy,* Thoune, Switzerland, 1967, Ott.

Wang ZY, Qiao J, Link H: Suppression of experimental autoimmune myasthenia gravis by oral administration of acetylcholine receptor, *J Neuroimmunol* 44:209, 1993.

Wara DW: Thymic hormones and the immune system, *Adv Pediatr* 28:229, 1981.

Weiner H: Oral tolerance: mobilizing the gut, *Hosp Pract,* p 53, Sept 1995.

Weiner H and others: Double-blind pilot trial of oral tolerization with myelin sheath antigens in multiple sclerosis, *Science* 259:1321, 1993.

Weiner H and others: Oral tolerance: immunologic mechanisms and treatment of animal and human organ-specific autoimmune disease by oral administration of autoantigens, *Annu Rev Immunol* 12:809, 1994.

Wells H: Studies on the chemistry of anaphylaxis. III. Experiments with isolated proteins, especially those of hen's egg, *J Infect Dis* 9:147, 1911.

Whitacre C and others: Oral tolerance in experimental autoimmune enccephalomyelitis. III. Evidence for clonal anergy, *J Immunol* 147:2155, 1991.

Yarbrough GG: The therapeutic potential of thyrotropin-releasing hormone (TRH) in Alzheimer's disease (AD), *Prog Neuropsychopharmacol Biol Psychiatry* 9:285, 1985

Yokohama S: Intestinal absorption mechanisms of thyrotropin-releasing hormone, *J Pharmacobiodyn* 7:445, 1984.

Zhang J and others: Suppression of diabetes in NOD mice by oral administration of porcine insulin, *Proc Natl Acad Sci USA* 88:10252, 1991.

Zhang J and others: Suppression of adjuvant arthritis in Lewis rats by oral administration of type II collagen, *J Immunol* 145:2489, 1990.

Chapter 7

Nutritional Approaches to Cancer Therapy*

GREGORY K. OGILVIE

For generations people have suspected that nutrients are important for the prevention, control, and treatment of malignancies (Ogilvie, Moore, 1995a, 1995b; Ogilvie, Vail, 1992, 1996; Shein and others, 1976). Once dominated by legend, folklore, and emotional testimony, the field of nutritional therapy for cancer patients is rapidly maturing as a science. Nutrients are used in veterinary medicine both to support the cancer patient's energy needs and to serve as specific therapeutic tools. Most traditional veterinarians accept the use of nutrients as anticancer agents because many excellent examples in the literature show that compounds derived from nature, including nutrients, can be effective as anticancer compounds. For example, vincristine and vinblastine are derived from the periwinkle plant, found in gardens throughout the world. Taxol and taxol analogs are present in yew trees, and doxorubicin is produced from a common soil bacterium. The belief that a single nutrient or set of nutrients is effective when used alone for the treatment of cancer is naive. However, some experts are optimistic that one or more nutrients can be effective in preventing certain types of malignancies in people and animals. Some of the nutrients under investigation in human medicine are noted in Table 7-1; these data may provide direction for interventional studies to prevent cancer in pets. The most promising area is in cancer prevention.

Micronutrients are most effective for the treatment of cancer when used with traditional therapies such as surgery, chemotherapy, radiation therapy, and biologic-responsive modifiers. Nutrients are termed *adjuvant therapeutics* when they are used in conjunction with other anticancer treatments for an enhanced anticancer effect. The objectives of adjuvant nutrition for the treatment of cancer are as follows (Buzby, Steinberg, 1981; Ogilvie, Vail, 1996; Theologides, 1979; Vail, Ogilvie, Wheeler, 1990):

- Prevention or reversal of cancer cachexia
- Reduction of toxicity from chemotherapy and radiation therapy
- Reduction of the side effects of cancer therapy, such as oral mucositis, alopecia, constipation, and nausea
- Enhancement of patient recovery from surgery and radiation therapy
- Enhancement of the immune defense mechanisms against oncogenesis
- Reduction of the metastatic process
- Protection of the immunocompromised and genetically vulnerable cancer patient from the carcinogenic effects of chemotherapy and radiation therapy
- Reduction of the risk for recurrence of malignant disease

Cachexia is a diverse metabolic consequence of cancer that is profoundly important; this paraneoplastic syndrome is also an important target for nutritional therapy. Cancer cachexia, a common manifestation of a wide variety of malignancies in people and pets, is a complex paraneoplastic syndrome of progressive involuntary weight loss that occurs even in the face of adequate nutritional intake (Ogilvie, Moore, 1995b; Ogilvie, Vail, 1992, 1996; Shein and others, 1976). Humans with cancer cachexia have a decreased quality of life, a decreased response to treatment, and a shortened survival time when compared with those who have similar diseases but do not exhibit clinical or biochemical signs associated with this condition (Buzby, Steinberg, 1981; Landel, Hammond, Mequid, 1985; Theologides, 1979). Growing evidence suggests that cancer cachexia is a critical problem in the

*Supported in part by Grant #2 CA 29582 from the National Cancer Institute. Its contents are solely the responsibility of the authors and do not necessarily represent the official views of the National Cancer Institute.

TABLE 7-1

CHEMOPREVENTIVE AGENTS

AGENT	TARGET SITES
SINGLE AGENTS	
Retinoids (vitamin A, tretinoin, isotretinoin, fenretinide)	Many
Beta-carotene	Many
Tamoxifen	Breast
Calcium	Colon
Finasteride	Prostate
α-Tocopherol	Many
Selenium	Skin, esophagus
Ascorbic acid	Esophagus, stomach, colon, cervix
N-acetylcysteine	Oral/GI system, lung, breast, colon, bladder
NSAIDs (aspirin, sulindac, piroxicam, ibuprofen)	Colon, bladder, skin, breast
	Esophagus, cervix
DFMO	Oral/GI system, lung, skin, breast, bladder, colon
Dithiolthiones (Oltipraz)	Oral/GI system, lung, skin, breast, colon, bladder
Glycyrrhetinic acid	Colon, skin, breast
Carbenoxolone	Colon, breast
DHEA analogs (fluasterone)	Oral/GI system, lung, skin, colon, breast
Curcumin	Oral/GI system, lung, skin, colon, breast
Protease inhibitors	Oral/GI system, lung, colon
Polyphenols (ellagic acid)	Skin, colon, bladder, esophagus, breast
Organosulfur compounds (S-allyl-1-cysteine)	Skin, cervix, colon, esophagus, lung
Fumaric acid	Lung, breast, liver
Phenhexyl isothiocyanate	Breast, lung
COMBINATIONS	
Vitamin A/beta-carotene	Lung, oral/GI systems
Vitamin A/N-acetylcysteine	Lung, oral/GI systems
α-tocopherol/beta-carotene	Lung, oral/GI systems
DFMO/piroxicam	Colon
Fenretinide/tamoxifen	Breast
Fenretinide/Oltipraz	Lung, bladder
Fenretinide/beta-carotene	Lung
Fenretinide/DFMO	Bladder
DFMO/Oltipraz	Bladder

NSAIDs, nonsteroidal antiinflammatory drugs; *DFMO*, difluoromethylornithine; *DHEA*, dehydroepiandrosterone; *GI*, gastrointestinal.

majority of veterinary cancer patients (Ogilvie, Moore, 1995b; Ogilvie, Vail, 1992, 1996). The metabolic alterations associated with cancer cachexia occur before any overt clinical signs associated with this phenomenon are ever identified. The end-stage of cancer cachexia is weight loss that is caused not only by primary effects of the tumor such as compression or infiltration of the alimentary tract but also possibly related to therapy (e.g., chemotherapy-induced anorexia, nausea, or vomiting) or the alteration of metabolic pathways comprising this paraneoplastic syndrome (Ogilvie, Moore, 1995b; Ogilvie, Vail, 1992, 1996). Recent research suggests that many tumor-bearing animals have metabolic alterations

that require not only special methods for delivering nutrients but also specific types of fluid and nutrient support (Bray, Campfield, 1975; Ogilvie, Moore, 1995a; Ogilvie, Vail, 1990, 1996).

This chapter is divided into three main parts and designed to be used in conjunction with Chapters 3 and 4. First, an understanding of the way nutrients can be effectively used to treat patients with cancer requires that the reader become aware of changes the body undergoes during malignant processes. Then, some of the better-studied anticancer or cancer preventive nutrients are reviewed, followed by some data about the use of nutrients in patients with cancer.

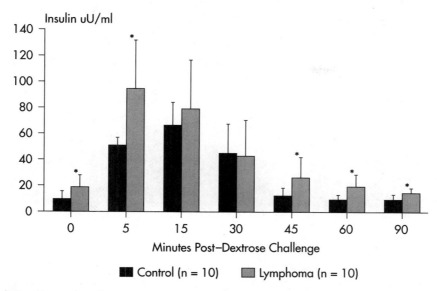

Fig. 7-1 Serum insulin concentrations in dogs with and without lymphoma before and after IV administration of 500 mg/kg dextrose. Asterisks (*) indicate values from dogs with lymphoma that differ significantly (P <0.001) from control dogs at the same time. (From Vail DM and others: Alterations in carbohydrate metabolism in canine lymphoma, *J Vet Intern Med* 4:11, 1990.)

Clinical and Metabolic Consequences of Cancer

General

Three phases are associated with cancer cachexia (Ogilvie, Vail, 1990, 1992, 1996). The first phase is the preclinical "silent" phase, wherein the patient does not exhibit any clinical signs of disease but biochemical changes such as hyperlactatemia, hyperinsulinemia, and alterations in amino acid profiles are evident (Ogilvie, Vail, Wheeler, 1992; Vail and others, 1990). During the second phase the patient begins to exhibit weight loss, anorexia, and lethargy. These patients are more likely to exhibit side effects associated with chemotherapy, radiation therapy, immunotherapy, and surgery. Owners may suggest that their pet is "aging" rapidly and is less active. The third and final phase of cancer cachexia is an accentuated form of the second phase marked by debilitation, weakness, and biochemical evidence of negative nitrogen balance such as hypoalbuminemia. In this third phase the attending clinician observes that the patient is losing carbohydrate and protein stores within the body. Loss of fat depots occurs in this third and final stage of the disease. These patients are literally wasting away because of the physical effects of the malignancy and the resulting cancer-induced alterations in metabolism. Nutritional therapy must begin early in all cancer patients, before the third phase occurs.

Metabolism

Carbohydrate Metabolism

Perhaps the most dramatic metabolic alterations in animals with cancer occur in carbohydrate metabolism. Abnormalities have been documented in peripheral glucose disposal, hepatic gluconeogenesis, insulin effects, and whole-body glucose oxidation and turnover (Chlebowski, Heber, 1986; Ogilvie, Vail, Wheeler, 1992; Vail and others, 1990). These abnormalities often exist before clinical evidence of cachexia is present. For example, when dogs with lymphoma and without clinical evidence of cachexia were evaluated with a 90-minute intravenous glucose tolerance test, lactate and insulin concentrations were significantly higher when compared with controls (Vail and others, 1990) (Figs. 7-1 and 7-2). The hyperlactatemia and hyperinsulinemia did not improve when these dogs achieved remission with doxorubicin chemotherapy (Ogilvie, Vail, Wheeler, 1992) (Fig. 7-3). Metabolic alterations result in part because tumors preferentially metabolize glucose for energy by anaerobic glycolysis, forming lactate as an end product (Heber and others, 1986; Ogilvie, Vail, 1992). To convert lactate to glucose by way of the Cori cycle, the host must then expend necessary energy, resulting in a net energy gain by the tumor and a net energy loss by the host (Dempsey, Mullen, 1985; Heber and others, 1986; Vail and others, 1990).

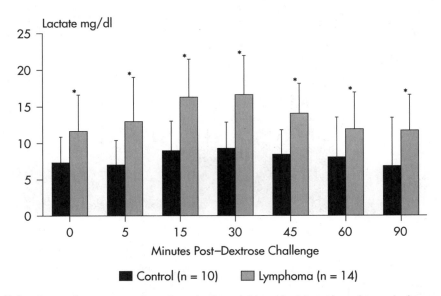

Fig. 7-2 Serum lactate concentrations in dogs with and without lymphoma before and after IV administration of 500 mg/kg dextrose. Asterisks (*) indicate values from dogs with lymphoma that differ significantly (P < 0.001) from control dogs at the same time. (From Vail DM and others: Alterations in carbohydrate metabolism in canine lymphoma, *J Vet Intern Med* 4:11, 1990.)

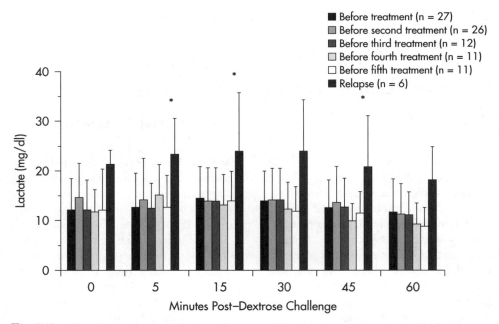

Fig. 7-3 Blood lactate concentrations in dogs with and without lymphoma before and during IV infusion of lactated Ringer's solution. Asterisks (*) indicate values from dogs with lymphoma that differ significantly (P < 0.05) from controls at the same time. Plus sign (+) indicates values that differ significantly (P < 0.05) from preinfusion baseline values within the same test group. (From Vail DM and others: Exacerbation of hyperlactatemia by infusion of lactated Ringer's solution in dogs with lymphoma, *J Vet Intern Med* 4:228, 1990.)

These alterations in metabolism are not restricted to dogs with lymphoma. For example, after a 12-hour fast, blood samples were obtained from 90 dogs with previously untreated nonhematopoietic malignancies (e.g., osteosarcoma, mammary adenocarcinoma, pulmonary bronchogenic adenocarcinoma) before and 5, 15, 30, 45 and 60 minutes after an intravenous challenge with 500 mg/kg dextrose (Ogilvie and others, 1995a). Samples were assayed for glucose, lactate, and insulin concentrations. The mean of all time points during the intravenous glucose tolerance test for lactate (12.9 mg/dl) and insulin (62.9 microunits/ml) concentrations in untreated dogs with nonhematopoietic malignancies in this study were significantly higher than controls (lactate, 9.7 mg/dl; insulin, 31.7 microunits/ml). This hyperlactatemia and hyperinsulinemia did not improve when a subset of dogs in this study were surgically rendered free of all observable evidence of cancer. The results indicate that carbohydrate metabolism is altered in dogs with a variety of nonhematopoietic malignancies and these abnormalities do not improve when the disease is surgically eliminated.

Researchers are only now beginning to understand the clinical significance of alterations in carbohydrate metabolism. A recent report documents the degree to which infusion of lactated Ringer's solution (LRS) in dogs with lymphoma worsens hyperlactacidemia (Vail and others, 1990). During that study, researchers found that blood lactate concentrations of relatively healthy, well-hydrated dogs with lymphoma were significantly elevated before, during, and after LRS was infused at a relatively modest rate (4.125 ml/kg/hr) compared with the levels of dogs in a control group. This LRS-induced increase in lactate concentration may place a metabolic burden on the host to convert lactate back to glucose, further exacerbating the energy demands on the host. This consequence may be even more important for septic, critically ill patients with cancer who require more intensive fluid therapy. Another logical assumption is that glucose-containing fluids likely increase hyperlactatemia, as demonstrated by elevation in these parameters during a glucose tolerance test. Additional studies are under way to determine the clinical significance of lactate-containing fluids to critically ill dogs with cancer. Until further information is known about the effects of hyperlactatemia on critically ill animals with cancer, glucose- or lactate-containing fluids should be avoided unless specifically indicated.

The inability of some tumor-bearing animals to tolerate parenteral administration of glucose may affect the dietary management of the patient with cancer. A logical conclusion is that diets high in simple carbohydrates may increase the total amount of lactate produced and the need for the host to utilize excessive energy for conversion of lactate. This increase in lactate may have long-term detrimental effects on animals with cancer.

To test this hypothesis in the dog, researchers evaluated a group of dogs with lymphoma to determine whether a diet high in simple carbohydrates is detrimental (Ogilvie and others, 1995c). In this study, 22 dogs with high-grade lymphoblastic lymphoma received an intravenous glucose tolerance test (IVGTT) and diet tolerance test (DTT) with concurrent evaluation of glucose, insulin, and lactate concentrations and analysis of fasting lipid and amino acid profiles. The dogs were randomized into a blind study and fed isocaloric amounts of a high-fat or high-carbohydrate diet before and after remission was attained with up to 5 doses of doxorubicin chemotherapy (30 mg/m² IV). Of the 22 dogs in the study, 17 achieved complete remission. Of the dogs randomized to receive the high-fat diet, 9 of 10 (90%) achieved complete remission. Of the dogs ran-

domized to receive the high-carbohydrate diet, 8 of 12 (66.6%) achieved complete remission. Groups of dogs showed no significant differences with respect to age, sex, body weight, dietary intake, and performance scores. Amino acid levels, lipid profiles, and glucose, lactate, and insulin concentrations from the IVGTTs were not statistically different by diet, evaluation period, or the time the sample was acquired during each timed test, using 2-way ANOVA for repeated measures. Comparing the dogs fed the high-carbohydrate diet with those fed the high-fat diet, researchers found that the median glucose level obtained from the latter group during the DTT was significantly (P < 0.05) lower when the dogs were in remission at the time of the second dosage of chemotherapy and then higher at the time of the third, fourth, and fifth chemotherapy treatments. The median lactate level from the dogs fed the high-carbohydrate diet was significantly higher than the level from the dogs fed the high-fat diet at the time of the second and third chemotherapy sessions. The median insulin level from the group fed the high-carbohydrate diet was significantly higher than the insulin values from the group fed the high-fat diet. Dogs fed the high-fat diet were also more likely to go into remission. This study showed that diet was effective in influencing response to therapy and select aspects of carbohydrate metabolism.

✗ Clinical Importance

Cancer induces significant alterations in carbohydrate metabolism. Simply speaking, carbohydrates feed the cancer at the expense of the host. Therefore oral and parenteral administration of simple carbohydrates seems to be contraindicated because it may induce significant increases in lactate and insulin levels. Fluids containing lactate should also be avoided until more is known about the metabolic consequences associated with the administration of these types of fluid in the cancer patient.

Protein Metabolism

Research has shown that cancer results in decreased body muscle mass and skeletal protein synthesis, with altered nitrogen balance and a concurrent increase in skeletal protein breakdown, liver protein synthesis, and whole-body protein synthesis (Bozzetti, Pagnoni, Del Vecchio, 1980; Dempsey, Mullen, 1985; Heber and others, 1986). Because tumors use energy stores at the expense of the host, tumors often preferentially use amino acids for energy via gluconeogenesis.[*] The use of amino acids for energy by the tumor becomes clinically significant for the host when protein degradation and loss exceed synthesis.

---

[*]Bozetti, Pagnoni, Del Vecchio (1980); Chory, Mullen (1986); Heber and others (1986); Kurzer, Meguid (1986); Langstein, Norton (1991); Oram-Smith, Stein (1977); Teyek and others (1986).

This effect can cause alterations in many important body functions, such as immune response, gastrointestinal function, and surgical healing (Kurzer, Meguid, 1986; Langstein, Norton, 1991).

In one study, amino acid analyses were performed on the plasma of 32 dogs with cancer and 8 normal dogs in a control group (Ogilvie, Moore, 1995a; Ogilvie, Vail, 1990). With regard to the 25 amino acids evaluated, tumor-bearing dogs had significantly lower plasma concentrations of threonine, glutamine, glycine, valine, cystine, and arginine and significantly higher levels of isoleucine and phenylalanine. The results did not differ between the different types of tumors represented.

Compared with controls, dogs with nonhematopoietic malignancies have different amino acid profiles. The fact that these alterations do not normalize after the cancer is surgically eliminated suggests that cancer induces long-lasting metabolic changes resulting from resetting of the body's metabolic "set point." This effect may be caused by the elaboration of specific cytokines, such as tumor necrosis factor or toxhormone.

Providing high-quality dietary amino acids or protein may be critical for the veterinary patient with cancer. A high-quality protein diet that is highly bioavailable may be ideal. Arginine and glutamine may have valuable therapeutic purposes (Barbul and others, 1981; Brennan, 1977; Heyman and others, 1991; Tachibana and others, 1985). Arginine stimulates lymphocyte blastogenesis, and its addition to total parenteral nutrition solutions has been shown to decrease tumor growth and metastatic rate in some rodent systems (Barbul and others, 1981; Tachibana and others, 1985). Some amino acids may decrease toxicity associated with chemotherapy. For example, glycine has been shown to reduce cisplatin-induced nephrotoxicity (Ogilvie, Moore, 1995a; Ogilvie, Vail, 1996).

Clinical Importance

The host and cancer cells compete for amino acids. If the diet does not provide these amino acids, the malignant process takes them from the host. Therefore high-quality, moderate amounts of proteins should be provided. Specific amino acids such as arginine and glutamine can greatly benefit the host by enhancing the immune system and reducing gastrointestinal toxicity.

Fat Metabolism

The loss of fat primarily accounts for weight loss occurring in cancer cachexia; the fact that human beings and animals with cancer have dramatic abnormalities in lipid metabolism is therefore not surprising (Dewys, 1982; McAndrew, 1986; Ogilvie and others, 1994). The decreased lipogenesis and increased lipolysis observed in humans and rodents with cancer cachexia result in increased levels of free fatty acids, very-low-density lipoproteins, triglycerides, plasma lipoproteins, and hormone-dependent lipoprotein lipase activity, whereas levels of endothelial-derived lipoprotein lipase decrease (McAndrew, 1986). Lipid profiles in dogs with lymphoma were recently studied to determine whether alterations similar to those reported in other species were present (Ogilvie and others, 1994). When compared with healthy controls, dogs with lymphoma had significantly higher concentrations of the cholesterol concentrations associated with very-low-density lipoprotein (VLDL-CH) and total triglyceride (T-TG), as well as the triglyceride concentrations associated with very low density lipoprotein (VLDL-TG), low-density lipoprotein (LDL-TG), and high-density lipoprotein (HDL-TG). Significantly lower levels of cholesterol concentrations associated with high-density lipoprotein (HDL-CH) were also noted. HDL-TG and VLDL-TG concentrations from dogs with lymphoma were significantly increased above pretreatment values after the dogs failed to achieve remission and developed overt signs of cancer cachexia. These abnormalities did not normalize when clinical remission was obtained.

The clinical significance of the previously mentioned lipid parameters in dogs with lymphoma is not known; however, abnormalities in lipid metabolism have been linked to a number of clinical problems, including immunosuppression, which correlates with decreased survival in affected humans (Heber and others, 1986; McAndrew, 1986). Dietary therapy may lessen the clinical impact of the abnormalities in lipid metabolism. In contrast to carbohydrates and proteins, some tumor cells have difficulty using lipid as a fuel source while host tissues continue to oxidize lipids for energy (Shein and others, 1986). This difference has led to the hypothesis that diets relatively high in fat, compared with diets high in simple carbohydrates, may benefit animals with cancer. Further research may reveal that the type of fat, rather than the amount, may be of greater importance. In one study, mean nitrogen intake, nitrogen balance, in vitro lymphocyte mitogenesis, time for wound healing, prevalence of wound complications, and duration of hospitalization were significantly better in 85 surgical patients fed an omega-3 fatty acid supplement when compared with controls (Daly and others, 1991; Tisdale, Brennan, Fearon, 1987).

Clinical Importance

Significant alterations occur in the lipid metabolism of dogs with cancer. Because many malignant cells cannot efficiently utilize lipids for energy, this nutrient source appears to be a logical choice for feeding the host. Specific types of fats, such as n-3 fatty acids, have been shown to reduce many metabolic alterations seen in the patient with cancer. In addition, n-3 fatty acids may have anticancer effects and reduce the adverse effects associated with radiation therapy.

Energy Expenditure

According to standard dogma, cancer cachexia may in part be caused by a negative energy balance secondary to decreased energy intake or altered energy expenditure (Dempsey and others, 1984; Lawson and others, 1982). Many investigators originally observed alterations in basal metabolic rate (BMR) and resting energy expenditure (REE) in human patients with cancer cachexia and associated these changes with derangements in carbohydrate, protein, and lipid metabolism (Dempsey and others, 1984; Lawson and others, 1982). Because the thyroid gland and its constitutive hormones are intimately involved in the control of energy homeostasis (Premachandra, 1981; Sestoft, 1980), researchers have speculated that changes in thyroid function and thyroid hormone concentrations may play a role in altering energy states in tumor-bearing cachectic individuals. Abnormally high concentrations of active thyroid hormone may play a significant role in the hypermetabolic state often found in individuals suffering from cancer cachexia. However, this hypothesis did not hold true in a recent investigation of thyroid function in tumor-bearing dogs (Vail, Panciera, Ogilvie, 1994). In this study of 83 dogs, serum concentrations of thyroxine (T_4), 3,5,3′-triiodothyronine (T_3), free thyroxine (fT_4), and free 3,5,3′-triiodothyronine (fT_3) were compared among tumor-bearing dogs with and without chronic weight loss and nontumor-bearing dogs with and without chronic weight loss. Diminished serum concentrations of T_4, T_3, and fT_3 occurred in dogs in proportion to the degree of weight loss associated with their disease state and regardless of their tumor-bearing status. These declines are apparently related to abnormal nutritional state or severity of illness rather than to a tumor-related phenomenon.

Recently, studies were initiated to determine whether animals with cancer have altered energy expenditure and whether healing from surgery causes an increase in energy utilization. These studies determined the energy use by indirect calorimetry, wherein the animal breathes into a mask that draws the respiratory gases into a machine to determine precisely the amount of oxygen consumed and the amount of carbon dioxide produced by metabolic processes. These data are essential to provide nutritional support for these animals, especially those receiving enteral or parenteral nutritional therapy. The following paragraphs outline some of these pivotal studies.

Indirect calorimetry is a method by which REE is estimated from measurements of oxygen consumption and carbon dioxide production is evaluated to provide information about nutrient assimilation, substrate utilization, thermogenesis, the energetics of physical exercise, and the pathogenesis of diseases such as cancer.[*] Indirect

calorimetry was performed on 22 dogs with lymphoma who were randomized into a blind study and fed isocaloric amounts of either a high-fat or a high-carbohydrate diet before and after chemotherapy (Ogilvie and others, 1995b). Surprisingly, during the initial evaluation period, resting energy expenditure (REE/kg 0.75) was significantly lower than in 30 tumor-free controls. Six weeks after the start of the study, REE/kg 0.75 was significantly lower in both groups of dogs with lymphoma when compared with the controls and the pretreatment values of the dogs with lymphoma. Dogs fed the relatively high-fat diet maintained a more normal energy expenditure than dogs fed a diet relatively high in carbohydrates.

According to reports, energy expenditure and caloric requirements increase in tumor-bearing animals and humans in comparison with those of healthy individuals (Ogilvie and others, 1995b). To determine whether this occurs in dogs, researchers compared apparently resting, healthy, client-owned dogs (N = 30) with a group of apparently resting, client-owned dogs with nonhematopoietic malignancies before (N = 46) and 4 to 6 weeks after (N = 30) surgical removal of all gross evidence of tumors (Ogilvie and others, 1995). The following parameters were determined using an open-flow indirect calorimetry system: rate of oxygen consumption (VO_2/kg: ml/min/kg; VO_2/kg 0.75: ml/min/kg 0.75), energy expenditure (EE/kg: kcal/kg/day; EE/kg 0.75: kcal/kg 0.75/day), and respiratory quotient, or VCO_2/VO_2 (RQ). Surgical removal of the tumor did not significantly (P > 0.05) alter any parameter when all dogs were assessed as a single group or subdivided into the following groups: carcinomas (N = 16 pre, N = 10 post) and sarcomas (N = 29 pre, N = 20 post), osteosarcomas (N = 21 pre, N = 17 post), and mammary adenocarcinomas (N = 6 pre and post). The values obtained from the dogs in any group before treatment were not significantly different from those of controls. These data suggest that energy expenditure (54.4 + 16 kcal/kg/day; 125 + 19 kcal/kg 0.75/day) and presumably caloric requirements of dogs with nonhematopoietic malignancies are not different from those obtained from healthy client-owned dogs (53.9 + 16 kcal/kg/day; 116 + 32 kcal/kg 0.75/day). Furthermore, these parameters do not change significantly when the tumor is removed surgically and the patient is reassessed after 4 to 6 weeks. These data may be useful in planning nutritional therapy for dogs with nonhematopoietic malignancies.

Energy expenditure and caloric requirements have been reported to increase in animals with and without cancer who are recovering from surgery. A study was performed to determine whether this increase also occurs in dogs. Energy expenditure was determined using an open-flow indirect calorimetry system on a group of 40, apparently resting, client-owned dogs who had been given general anesthesia for the following surgical procedures: ovariohysterectomy (N = 10), orchiectomy (N = 10), localized malignant tumor resection (N = 10), and repair of a major

---

[*]Delarue and others (1990); Dempsey and others (1986); Ferrannini (1988); Fredrix and others (1991); Hansell, Davies, Burns (1986); Quebbeman, Ausman, Schneider (1982); Walters and others (1993); Zyliez and others (1990).

orthopedic problem (N = 10) (Ogilvie and others, 1995a). Each dog was evaluated before and after surgery (0, 1, 2, and 3 days after surgery and then at the time of suture removal more than 14 days later) and compared with apparently resting, normal, client-owned dogs (N = 30). The following parameters were evaluated: rate of oxygen consumption (VO_2/kg: ml/min/kg; VO_2/kg 0.75: ml/min/kg 0.75), energy expenditure (EE/kg: kcal/kg/day; EE/kg 0.75: kcal/kg 0.75/kg/day), and respiratory quotient, or VCO_2/VO_2 (RQ). Surgery and anesthesia did not significantly (P > 0.05) alter any of these parameters at any time in any group. Dogs in all groups did not differ significantly from each other. In addition, none of the pretreatment parameters assessed in any of these groups was significantly different from controls. These data suggest that unlike what has been reported elsewhere, the energy expenditure of dogs that undergo anesthesia and surgery for malignant and nonmalignant conditions does not increase from baseline values or in comparison with normal, client-owned pet dogs. These data may be valuable in planning nutritional therapy for dogs recovering from anesthesia and surgery.

Clinical Importance

Each patient with cancer should be assessed individually to determine the appropriate amount of nutrients. However, most of these patients apparently do not have substantially increased requirements for kcal in comparison with normal animals. In addition, surgery for elective and nonelective procedures apparently does not increase the energy requirements.

Select Nutrients with Preventive or Therapeutic Potential

The following paragraphs contain some examples of nutrients and some situations in which their preventive or therapeutic effects have been shown. Because there are few studies in veterinary medicine, studies involving rodents or human cancer patients are used as models for animal disease. A list of chemopreventive agents is outlined in Table 7-1.

Vitamins

Retinoids, beta-carotene, and vitamins C, D, and E all appear to influence the growth and metastasis of cancer cells through a variety of mechanisms.* Some of these mecha-

---

*Bertram, Kolonel, Meyskens (1987); Boutwell (1988); Chance and others (1993); Hong and others (1990); Lamm and others (1994); Li, Sartorelli (1992); Mirvish (1986); National Academy of Sciences (1982, 1989); Pirisi and others (1992); Quillan (1993); Wargovich and others (1991); Weisburg (1991); Yen and others (1992).

nisms include selected receptor-mediated antiproliferative activities. Studies show that these vitamins bind their cytosolic receptors and then translocate the bound complex to the nucleus, where the receptors can mediate gene regulation. Other effects from the vitamins result from their antioxidant hormone and immune modulatory capabilities.

The scientific community has found it difficult to evaluate vitamins as anticancer agents because the studies that show a positive effect are often complex and difficult to unravel. For example, in one study (Lamm and others, 1994), 65 patients with biopsy-confirmed transitional cell carcinoma of the bladder were enrolled in a randomized comparison of intravesicular BCG with and without percutaneous administration of the same drug. In addition, these patients were randomized into two groups, one receiving multiple vitamins in the recommended daily allowances (RDA) and one receiving RDA multivitamins plus 40,000 units of vitamin A, 100 mg of vitamin B_6, 2000 mg of vitamin C, 400 units of vitamin E, and 90 mg of zinc. The addition of percutaneous BCG did not significantly lessen tumor recurrence. Recurrence after 10 months was markedly reduced in the patients receiving megadose vitamins. The 5-year estimates of tumor recurrence are 91% in the RDA arm and 41% in the megadose arm (P = 0.0014). The overall recurrence rate of the patients was 24 of 30 (80%) in the RDA arm and 14 of 35 (40%) in the megadose arm (P = 0.0011). This study suggests that megadoses of vitamins are helpful in the treatment of bladder tumors in humans. It also illustrates the difficulty in determining the most effective treatment when so many agents are used together.

Retinoids

In humans, 13-cis retinoic acid prevents secondary tumors in patients treated for squamous cell carcinoma of the head and neck (Pirisi and others, 1992; Quillin, 1993; Weisburg, 1991). Transretinoic acid produces a high percentage of complete remissions in patients with acute promyelocytic leukemia.

Potent modulators of growth and differentiation, retinoids can reverse the effects of cervical human papillomavirus infection (Pirisi and others, 1992). Retinoic acid suppresses human papillomavirus–mediated transformation associated with cervical cancer and inhibits the expression of the human papillomavirus-16 oncogenes (Pirisi and others, 1992). Retinoids appear most effective when combined with other agents. For example, when used in the adjuvant treatment of retinoblastoma, a childhood cancer, 1,25-dihydroxycholecalciferol and retinoic acid resulted in translocation of bound receptor vitamin complexes to the nucleus, which leads to the regulation of the neuroblastoma gene (Yen and others, 1992). The potential value of using retinoic acid for the treatment of melanoma cannot be overlooked. Melanoma in mice has been successfully treated with retinoid by up-regulating protein kinase C production (Niles, Loewy, 1989).

A recent study evaluated the synthetic retinoids isotretinoin and etretinate in the treatment of dogs with intracutaneous cornifying epitheliomas (ICE), other benign skin neoplasias, and cutaneous lymphoma (White and others, 1993). The study used 24 dogs. All tumors were diagnosed by histologic examination. Ten dogs with multiple (at least five) benign skin tumors (seven with ICE, one each with inverted papillomas, sebaceous adenomas, and epidermal cysts) were treated with isotretinoin (N = 7) and/or etretinate (N = 5). Twelve dogs with cutaneous lymphoma were treated with isotretinoin, and two dogs with cutaneous lymphoma were initially treated with etretinate. Successful treatment with isotretinoin was achieved in one dog with ICE, one with inverted papillomas, and one with epidermal cysts. Partial improvement with isotretinoin was seen in two dogs with ICE. Successful treatment was achieved with etretinate in four dogs with ICE (Norwegian elkhound was the predominant breed with ICE). Remission was achieved in six of the fourteen dogs with cutaneous lymphoma. Adverse effects developed in seven of the twenty-four dogs, so treatment was stopped in two dogs.

Clinical Importance

Retinoids, either alone or in combination with other agents, appear to have the potential for regulating cancer cells. Specific studies in human and veterinary medicine suggest that retinoids alone or with other agents can be effective in the treatment of certain types of malignancies.

Vitamin C

Vitamin C has been studied continuously over the last several decades as an antioxidant and agent for reducing conditions such as colds, cardiovascular disease, and cancer. Vitamin C has the greatest potential in the prevention of malignant disease; however, some researchers have suggested that vitamin C may also be useful in the treatment of certain types of cancers (Mirvish, 1986). Water-soluble vitamin C has been widely reported to inhibit nitrosation reactions and prevent chemical induction of cancers of the esophagus and stomach (Quillin, 1993; Weisburg, 1991). Processed foods high in nitrates and nitrites, such as bacon and sausage, are often supplemented with vitamin C to reduce the carcinogenic capability of the resultant nitrosamines.

A human cell line that was resistant to vincristine was established from a cell line derived from small cell lung cancer. The resistant cell line was pretreated with ascorbic acid, which resulted in potentiation of the vincristine effects. Sensitive cell lines were not affected (White and others, 1993). The growth inhibition caused by vincristine treatment in the ascorbic acid–free medium was decreased in the resistant and sensitive lines. These findings suggest that an ascorbic acid–sensitive mechanism may be involved in drug resistance in this cell line, which differs from the phosphoglucoprotein-mediated or multiple drug–resistance mechanisms. Therefore ascorbic acid may be one therapeutic alternative for overcoming a drug resistance in some cancer cells.

Clinical Importance

Vitamin C has been extensively studied and is reported to be somewhat effective in the prevention of certain diseases, including colds, cardiovascular disease, and cancer. Despite the extensive amount of research on this particular vitamin, little direct data exist to prove its efficacy.

Vitamin E

Like vitamin C, lipid-soluble vitamin E (or α-tocopherol) can inhibit nitrosation reactions, but it also has a broad capacity to inhibit mammary tumor carcinogenesis and colon carcinogenesis in rodents (Quillin, 1993). Research indicates that vitamin E mediates its activity by influencing a variety of cell functions, including free-radical scavenging, which can prevent oxidative damage possibly leading to cell death (Branda, 1991). In addition to having chemopreventative properties, vitamin E may have potentially therapeutic efficacy against certain malignancies (Kline and others, 1990; Kline, Cochran, Sanders, 1990; Kline, Sanders, 1989). Vitamin E reportedly has antiproliferative activity, which involves the binding of the vitamin to salicylic receptors, followed by translocation to the nucleus, where DNA binds on the domains of receptors that mediate gene regulatory events (Kline and others, 1990; Kline, Cochran, Sanders, 1990; Kline, Sanders, 1989). Retrovirus-induced tumorigenesis involves transformation of normal cells into tumor cells. Evidence suggests that vitamin C may normalize the immune system by interacting with macrophages, T-lymphocytes, and retroviral-induced infections.

In a cooperative study by the Comparative Oncology Unit at Colorado State University and the Harvard School of Public Health, Department of Dental Medicine, the effect of injecting D,L-α tocopherol and beta-carotene directly into dogs with a variety of oral malignancies was evaluated. Researchers studied a total of 12 dogs who received weekly injections of this combination for the mediation of tumor cell growth. This study resulted in two dogs achieving a complete remission (50% reduction in the original size of the tumor—both soft tissue sarcomas) and minor reduction in tumor size in two other cases. No direct evidence of tumor cytolysis emerged in this study. Additional studies have been initiated in humans at Harvard School of Public Health. The results are pending at this time.

✗ Clinical Importance

The antioxidants D,L-α tocopherol, beta-carotene, and ascorbic acid may have some value in preventing or working as an adjuvant treatment for some malignancies in dogs and cats. The optimum effective dosage is not known at this time. Additional studies are essential to better understand the value of these vitamins.

Minerals

Minerals suggested as chemopreventive or anticancer agents that are also valuable nutrients include copper, zinc, magnesium, calcium, lead, iron, potassium, sodium, arsenic, iodine, and germanium. Selenium has been one of the most widely studied minerals associated with the development of cancer (Ip, 1981; Jacobs, Griffin, 1979; Jacobs, Jansson, Griffin, 1977; Shamberger and others, 1973; Vernon, 1984). Low serum selenium levels have been seen in human patients with gastrointestinal cancer (Shamberger and others, 1973). In rodents, dietary supplementation of selenium has been shown to inhibit colon, mammary gland, and stomach carcinogenesis (Ip, 1981; Jacobs, Jansson, Griffin, 1977). An additional study is essential to determine whether alteration of selenium levels is valuable in the treatment of veterinary and human cancer patients.

Iron transferrin and ferritin have been linked to cancer risk and cancer cell growth (Torti, Torti, 1993). Lung, colon, bladder, and esophageal cancers in humans are strongly linked with increases in serum iron and transferrin saturation. Many tumor cells require iron for growth. Therefore some researchers have suggested that the increased use of iron by the tumor depresses the serum iron levels in human cancer patients. Mice with low levels of iron have slow tumor growth compared with those who do not have altered iron levels. The mechanism for which iron influences tumor growth is unknown. In humans, low levels of zinc in blood and diseased tissue have been observed in esophageal, pancreatic, and bronchial cancers. In laboratory animals, zinc deficiency appears to enhance carcinogenesis.

✗ Clinical Importance

Some minerals have been associated with the regulation of malignant processes and therefore may be of value in the treatment of malignant conditions. Another possibility is that the disease process results in altered levels of the minerals and these minerals may not play a direct role in carcinogenesis over the malignant process.

Amino Acids

Several amino acids have been associated with the control of cancer. Methionine has been observed in several tumor cell lines and used as a basis for inhibiting tumor growth (Stern, Hoffman, 1986). Replacement of methionine with its precursor, homocysteine, results in methionine–dependent tumor cells locked into late S and G_2 phases of the cell cycle, improvement of the therapeutic index, and an increased percentage of tumor cells that are sensitive to chemotherapy. In addition, L-asparaginase inhibits asparagine; this leads to an induction of complete remissions of up to 80% of dogs and cats with lymphoma (Asselin and others, 1989). Therefore asparagine is essential, at least for the short term, for tumor cell growth. Another area of research focuses on the restriction of tyrosine and phenylalanine, which has been reported to suppress melanoma cell growth in tissue cultures and rodent systems (Meadows and others, 1982; Meadows, Oeser, 1983). The administration of tyrosine and phenylalanine increases the survival of melanoma tumor–bearing mice and increases the effectiveness of levodopa against melanoma. Glutamine also reduces the gastrointestinal toxicity of some chemotherapeutic agents and prevents radiation-induced enteritis (Ogilvie, Moore, 1995a; Ogilvie, Vail, 1996). In addition, arginine may enhance the effects of the immune system, which might have anticancer effects (Barbul and others, 1981; Tachibana and others, 1985).

✗ Clinical Importance

Several amino acids have been associated with positive clinical effects in the cancer patient. Of specific interest is arginine, which may enhance certain aspects of the immune system, and glutamine, which may help maintain the health of the gastrointestinal tract. The potential value of glutamine is especially evident in work that demonstrates its effectiveness in decreasing chemotherapy-induced vomiting and diarrhea.

Protease Inhibitors from Soybeans

A great deal of information suggests that soybean-derived Bowman-Birk inhibitor (BBI) can inhibit or suppress carcinogenesis both in vivo and in vitro.* Research has shown that extracts of BBI inhibit carcinogenesis in several animal model systems, including colon- and liver-induced carcinogenesis in mice, anthracene–induced cheek-pouch carcinogenesis in hamsters, lung tumorigenesis in mice, and esophageal carcinogenesis in rats (Messadi and others, 1986; St. Clair and others, 1990; Weed, McGandy, Kennedy, 1985). BBI concentration has been shown to inhibit metastasis and weight loss associated with radiation-induced thymic lymphoma in mice (Billings, Habres, Kennedy, 1990). Irradiated rodents treated with dietary BBI concentration have fewer deaths,

---

*Billings, Habres, Kennedy (1990); Kennedy (1990); Messadi and others (1986); St. Clair and others (1990); Weed, McGandy, Kennedy (1985); Witschi, Kennedy (1989).

a lower average grade of lymphoma, and larger fat stores than controls. Therefore this protease inhibitor from soybeans may be an important adjunct to cancer chemotherapy protocols and prevention of secondary cancers.

Soybeans also contain the isoflavones genistein and daidzein. Although these weak estrogen agonists are recognized as potentially useful in the prevention of human breast cancer, their usefulness may be limited to only the first 6 to 9 months of life in dogs and cats (Peterson, Barnes, 1991; Troll, Frenkel, Wiesner, 1990).

Clinical Importance

BBI may be useful in the prevention and treatment of specific malignant diseases, but further studies are needed.

Therapeutic Enzymes

Enzymes have substantial therapeutic potential, although approval in the United States is limited. L-Asparaginase is probably the most valuable therapeutic modality for the treatment of lymphoma and leukemia in animals and humans (Asselin and others, 1989). Oral enzyme preparations are used in the treatment of chronic pancreatic insufficiency and disaccharidase deficiency. Several enzyme preparations are available in Europe for oral adjuvant treatment of cancer and other diseases. Of those, the brands Wobenzyme and Mulsal contain a similar mixture of enzymes. Recent studies report efficacy in the treatment of cancer patients, but researchers do not fully understand the mechanism by which these enzymes work. One hypothesis is that they eliminate pathogenic immune complexes. Therefore enzymes may indeed be useful in the adjuvant treatment of cancer. One available product has the following formulation: pancreatin, papain, chymotrypsin, lipase, rutin.*

Clinical Importance

L-Asparaginase and other enzymes have been shown to be useful in the treatment of cancer in combination with other, traditional anticancer treatments.

Garlic in Cancer Prevention and Treatment

Epidemiologic studies have suggested a correlation between high garlic consumption and reduced risk of cancer development (Wargovich and others, 1991). Each garlic extract and several garlic and thioalkyl compounds have been shown to inhibit the activation of carcinogens and the bonding of polyarene thiol epoxide to DNA bases, which causes DNA lesions and initiates a chemically induced carcinogenic process. Garlic and the thioalkyl compounds inhibit carcinogen-induced aberrations in the cell nucleus. Garlic extracts also have an antipromotion effect in animals exposed to carcinogens. Moreover, garlic exerts direct cytolytic effects against human breast cancer cells that were cultured and human melanoma cells. The concentrations of garlic used in these studies exert no effect on normal cells. Pretreatment of rodents with garlic protects them against subsequent induction of tumors caused by a variety of carcinogens.

Clinical Importance

Growing data suggest that garlic may be valuable in preventing or treating some malignancies. However, no definitive studies demonstrate the safety and efficacy of garlic for the prevention or treatment of cancer in human or veterinary medicine.

Tea

Although dogs and cats seldom acquire the taste for tea, compelling data suggest that both green and black teas have anticancer properties (Khan and others, 1992; Wang and others, 1992a, 1992b). Green tea extracts contain catechin, and black tea contains the fermentation products theoflavins and theorubigins. These active agents inhibit cancer-promoting agents, protect against oxidative damage, and enhance antioxidant enzymes. Black tea also appears to have soothing properties that reduce the discomfort associated with radiation–induced oral mucositis. The tannic acid and other ingredients have astringent and local anesthetic properties when the oral cavity of affected dogs is lavaged 2 to 3 times daily.

Clinical Importance

Provocative data from epidemiologic studies suggest that certain ingredients in tea may be valuable in the treatment of cancer. However, further research is necessary before this link can be established.

Eicosanoids and Cancer

One recent study has shown that omega-3 fatty acids, arginine, and RNA can help improve the immune system, metabolic status, and clinical outcomes of human cancer patients (Dempsey, Mullen, 1985). As Daly and others have noted (1991), 85 surgical patients with upper gastrointestinal cancer were randomized to receive either a supplemental diet high in omega-3 fatty acids and arginine or a control diet. The mean nitrogen intake and nitrogen balance were significantly better in the group that

---

*Wobenzyme, Mucose Pharma GmbH. Similar products include Mulsal, Wobe-mugos, and AE-Mulsin.

was given the omega-3/arginine diet. In vitro lymphocyte mitogenesis was significantly improved in the group that received the supplemented diet. Time for wound healing, the prevalence of wound complications, and the duration of hospitalization were significantly less in the group receiving the omega-3/arginine supplemented diet.

Omega-3 fatty acids have also been shown to inhibit tumorigenesis and the spread of cancer in animal models, and they are the basis of compelling work in the prevention and treatment of cancer in humans (Ramesh and others, 1992). As a general rule, n-3 fatty acids (e.g., eicosapentaenoic acid, docosahexaenoic acid) inhibit tumor growth. Metastases are enhanced by the n-6 fatty acids (e.g., linoleic acid, gamma-linolenic acid). In vivo studies have shown that eicosapentaenoic acid has selective tumoricidal action but does not harm normal cells.* Essential fatty acids containing n-3 fatty acids have been shown to reduce radiation-induced damage to the skin of pigs (Hopewell and others, 1992). This effect appears to be specific to normal, not malignant cells. Studies are under way to determine whether this phenomenon can reduce morbidity in dogs receiving external beam radiation therapy.

The secretion of tumor necrosis factor-α (TNF-α), interleukin-1β (IL-1β), interleukin-1α (IL-1α), and interleukin-2 is reduced with the administration of n-3 fatty acids. This effect may be important because IL-1 and TNF are known to be important mediators of cachexia and the metastatic process. Indeed, TNF and IL-1 promote, rather than restrict, tumor growth; these cytokines may actually act as tumor growth factors (Endres and others, 1989; Gelin and others, 1991; Hopewell and others, 1992; Kumar and others, 1992). This phenomenon is surprising because ongoing clinical trials are evaluating use of TNF as a therapy for cancer. Studies suggest, however, that endogenous amounts of TNF enhance metastases, whereas pharmacologic levels may be therapeutic (Orosz and others, 1993).

Investigators have shown that eicosapentaenoic acid has not only antitumor effects but also anticachectic effects, which result in part because protein degradation decreases without an effect on protein synthesis (Beck, Smith, Tisdale, 1991). One of the hallmarks of cancer cachexia in dogs with lymphoma is hyperlactatemia. Recently, diets with n-3 fatty acids have been shown to ameliorate endotoxin–induced lactic acidosis in guinea pigs (Pomposelli and others, 1989). This finding may be extremely important because hyperlactatemia is a significant problem in dogs with lymphoma. Indeed, in a study recently completed at Colorado State University, hyperlactatemia was reversed and eliminated in dogs with lymphoma. Further studies are essential to determine whether

dogs with nonhematopoietic malignancies benefit from this effect. Determining whether the n-3 supplemented diets improve quality of life and response to therapy is also important.

Clinical Importance

Eicosanoids of the n-3 series, but not the n-6 series, may be of value in correcting some metabolic alterations of cancer patients. In addition, n-3 fatty acids appear to have anticancer and antimetastatic effects. Many fish oils (such as menhaden fish oil) contain n-3 fatty acids, and commercially formulated sources are also becoming available.

Nutritional Support for the Veterinary Patient with Cancer

The ideal method of addressing cancer cachexia is to eliminate the underlying neoplastic condition, but because this is often impossible, efforts to provide nutritional support become increasingly important. Specific recommendations for nutritional support of patients with neoplastic disease should be based on estimates of caloric requirements, the patient's current and past nutritional status, and knowledge of the underlying disease. Not all patients with cancer are candidates for nutritional support. In human medicine, clinical judgment based on past, present, and anticipated nutrient intake and needs; physical examination with attention to body condition; and a working knowledge of underlying disease mechanisms is the best measure of nutritional status and the need for nutritional support. In light of this fact, the simplest, most reliable method of assessment in veterinary patients is clinical judgment. As with any treatment modality, serial assessment of nutritional status and subsequent modifications in nutritional support are indicated as the patient's status changes.

For veterinary patients with cancer who do not yet need intensive enteral therapy, many practitioners are finding some success with the "paleolithic diet," which involves home-prepared meals based on many of the previous guidelines. In general, these diets contain high-quality protein sources and restricted amounts of simple carbohydrates. The data are changing so rapidly that a general diet is difficult to recommend, but the practitioner should strive for balance, using multivitamin/mineral and antioxidant supplements as a base from which to design a nutritional protocol. In addition, n-3 fatty acids supplied as 8% of the caloric needs on a dry-matter basis, additional glutamine, arginine, and fiber are recommended.

Enteral dietary therapy has proved to be a practical, cost-effective, physiologic, and safe modality that may abate or eliminate cancer cachexia. Several studies have failed to document the possibility of increasing tumor

---

*Begin and others (1985, 1986); Dippenaar, Booyenes (1982); Holian, Nelson (1992); Jenski and others (1993); Lowell, Parnes, Blackburn, (1990); Mengeaud and others (1992); Pascale and others (1993); Plumb, Luo, Kerr (1993); Ramesh and others (1992); Roush and others (1991).

growth by enhancing the nutritional status of the host. Enteral dietary support of the patient can result in weight gain, as well as increased response to and tolerance of radiation, surgery, and chemotherapy. Other factors that improve with enteral nutritional support include thymic weight, immune responsiveness, immunoglobulin and complement levels, and the phagocytic ability of white blood cells (Boutwell, 1988). Although the optimal diet formulation is still unknown, the guidelines described in the following paragraphs may apply.

As a general rule, mature dogs and cats with functional gastrointestinal tracts who either have a history of inadequate nutritional intake for 3 to 7 days or have lost at least 10% of their body weight over a 1- to 2-week period are candidates for enteral nutritional therapy. Veterinarians should remember that the current standard of allowing 3 or more days of inappetence to pass before considering nutritional support may not be appropriate for feline patients, who have relatively higher metabolic rates. For example, daily adenosine triphosphate (ATP) turnover in an 80 kg man at rest is roughly 60% of body weight versus 136% in a 3.5 kg cat, and humans have approximately twice the energy storage capabilities per unit of metabolic body size. In fact, most experts believe in the earlier implementation of nutritional support in feline patients, when such support is clearly indicated.

All methods to encourage food consumption, including the use of chemical stimulants, should be attempted first (Mirvish, 1986; National Academy of Sciences, 1986; Ogilvie, Moore, 1995b; Wargovich and others, 1991) (Fig. 7-4). Enhancing the palatability of food is the simplest way to increase voluntary intake. Offering a variety of food from freshly-opened cans and warming it to body temperature may help. Appetite stimulants of the benzodiazepine family (diazepam, oxazepam) used at low doses orally or intravenously may, when used in conjunction with a variety of foods, result in consumption of nearly 25% of total daily requirements in responsive cats. This measure is usually reserved for short-term appetite stimulation of patients likely to recover quickly.

Additional procedures, such as the use of feeding tubes, may be necessary to ensure that these animals consume their total caloric needs. Many other pharmacologic compounds have undergone or are undergoing scientific scrutiny for their potential to reduce or abate the metabolic alterations occurring in patients with cancer. Carefully controlled studies of human patients with cancer suggest that cyproheptadine, corticosteroids, and nandrolone decanoate have little or no impact on objective indexes of nutritional status or clinical outcome. Megestrol acetate has been proved beneficial in patients with significant gastrointestinal morbidity. Several studies recently reviewed by Chlebowski (1991) have shown that the clinical use of megestrol acetate has resulted in substantial increases in weight gain in humans with cancer; the clinical utility of this drug for the treatment of cancer cachexia in veterinary patients remains to be determined.

Routes of Enteral Feeding

After veterinarians decide to provide nutritional support, they must choose an appropriate method of feeding. Enteral feeding should always be considered before total parenteral nutrition (TPN) unless it is contraindicated because the gastrointestinal tract is unable to digest or assimilate nutrients in adequate quantities. A vast body of basic and clinical literature supports the superiority of enteral routes. Although parenteral nutrition is a useful tool, maintenance of mucosal integrity in the gut and of the complex neuroendocrine network that orchestrates nutrient digestion, absorption, and metabolism is paramount and best served by enteral nutrition. Additionally, enteral feeding tends to be more cost-effective and is associated with fewer complications. A number of enteral feeding routes are commonly used in veterinary patients. Access to the gastrointestinal tract should be achieved with a feeding tube that is as far proximal as possible to maximize normal digestion, thus minimizing complications associated with bypassing normal digestive processes. Anticipated duration of nutritional support, patient tolerance, overall expense, and familiarity of hospital staff with a specific tube type should also be considered when choosing a feeding site.

Nasogastric tube feeding is one of the most common methods used for short-term nutritional support of dogs and cats (Heyman and others, 1991; Mirvish, 1986; Ogilvie, Vail, 1992; Reddy, Cohen, 1986; Wargovich and

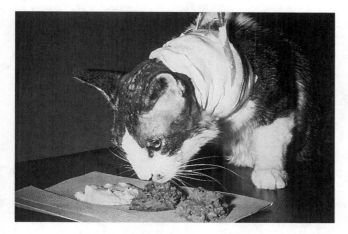

Fig. 7-4 All methods to encourage food consumption, including feeding a variety of highly palatable, aromatic foods; uniformly warming the food to just below body temperature; and administering chemical stimulants should be tried before starting enteral support. Avoid foods that contain onion powder because this ingredient may cause Heinz body anemia. The optimal pharmacologic agent for use in the veterinary patient with cancer is unknown; however, megestrol acetate has been shown to result in substantial weight gain in humans with cancer.

others, 1991) (Fig. 7-5). The use of small-bore silastic or polyurethane catheters has minimized complications associated with this delivery system. To decrease any discomfort associated with the initial placement of the catheter, the veterinarian may tranquilize the patient by instilling lidocaine into the nasal cavity (with the nose pointing up). The tube is lubricated and passed to the level of the thirteenth rib in dogs and the ninth rib in cats (Boutwell, 1988). In cats the tube should be bent dorsally over the bridge of the nose and secured to the frontal region of the head with a permanent adhesive. In dogs the permanent adhesive or suture should be used to secure the tube to the side of the face that is ipsilateral to the intubated nostril.

Esophagostomy tube feeding is an excellent method for providing short- or long-term enteral feeding without the need for placement of the endoscopy tube. The patient is first positioned in lateral recumbency. A carmalt is placed in the esophagus below the larynx and dorsal to the jugular and directed outward so that directed outward to "poke" it slightly pushes out the skin from the esophagus. An incision is made over the instrument, and the carmalt is then extended through the skin. The tip of a large red-rubber feeding tube is pulled through the skin and into the esophagus. The tip of the tube is placed into the esophagus two thirds of the way down until it is slightly above the cardia. The tube is then sutured into place.

Gastrostomy tubes are increasingly used in veterinary practice for animals that need nutritional support longer than 7 days (Mirvish, 1986; National Academy of Sciences, 1989; Ogilvie, Moore, 1995b; Reddy, Cohen, 1986; Wargovich and others, 1991) (Fig. 7-6). These tubes can be placed surgically or with endoscopic guidance (Mirvish, 1986; National Academy of Sciences, 1989; Ogilvie,

Moore, 1995, Reddy, Cohen, 1986). If surgery is chosen, a 5 ml balloon-tipped urethral catheter is usually placed (e.g., Foley catheter, Bardex, Murray Hill, NJ) or a "mushroom-tipped" de Pezzer proportionate-head urologic catheter (Bard Urological Catheter, Bard Urological Division, Covingtion, GA). The reader is referred to other sources for a detailed description of this surgical procedure (Jacobs, 1991; Mirvish, 1986; Ogilvie, Vail, 1990; Reddy, Cohen, 1986). Many veterinarians consider endoscopically placed gastrostomy tubes ideal for their cancer patients.

The percutaneous placement of a gastrostomy tube by endoscopic guidance is quick, safe, and effective (Jacobs, 1991; Mirvish, 1986; Ogilvie, Moore, 1995; Reddy, Cohen, 1996). A specialized 20-French tube (e.g., Dubhoff PEG, Biosearch, Summerville, NJ; Bard Urological Catheter, Bard Urological Division, Covingtion, GA) is used in both dogs and cats. First, the stomach is distended with air from an endoscope placed into the stomach. Once the stomach is distended, an area just caudal to the last left rib below the transverse processes of the lumbar vertebrae is depressed. The clinician, viewing the stomach lining by nylonendoscopy, locates this area. With the IV catheter in place and the target area located by the endoscopist known, a polychloride sleeve is positioned over the needle and inserted through the skin and into the stomach. The first portion of a 5-foot-long piece of 8-pound nylon test filament or suture is introduced through the catheter into the stomach and then caught by a biopsy snare passed through the endoscope. The attached nylon and endoscope are then pulled up the esophagus and

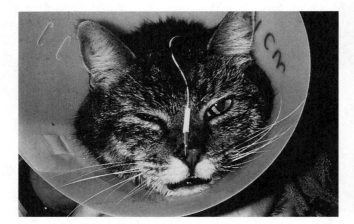

Fig. 7-5 Nasogastric tube feeding is an excellent short-term method for initiating nutritional support. Liquid nutrients must be used in this type of feeding method. Another option is esophagostomy tube feeding, which allows the use of blended food that may benefit anorectic animals. Note that most cats require an Elizabethan collar to prevent them from scratching the catheter.

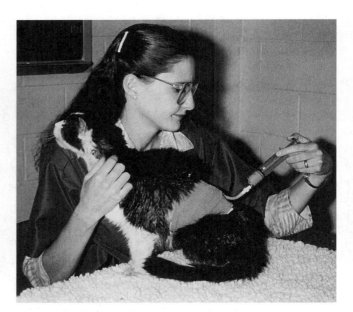

Fig. 7-6 Gastrostomy tube feeding is an excellent method for short- or long-term nutritional support. Blended foods can easily be given to most patients. These gastrostomy tubes can be placed during surgery or with a fiberoptic endoscope. They are well tolerated by most patients.

through the oral cavity. The end of the gastrostomy tube opposite the mushroom tip is trimmed to create a point that will fit inside another polyvinylchloride catheter after the stylet is removed and discarded. This second polyvinylchloride catheter is then placed over the nylon suture so that the narrow end points toward the stomach. The free end of the nylon, which has just been pulled out of the animal's mouth, is then sutured to the end of the tube. The catheter-tube combination is then pulled from the end of the suture located outside the abdominal wall until the pointed end of the IV catheter comes down the esophagus and out the abdominal wall. The tube is then grasped and pulled until the mushroom tip is adjacent to the stomach wall (as viewed by endoscopy). To prevent slippage, the middle of a 3- to 4-inch piece of tubing is pierced completely through both sides, positioned over the feeding tube so that it is adjacent to the body wall, and then glued or sutured securely in place. The tube is capped and bandaged in place. An Elizabethan collar is recommended. Once the tube has been in place for 7 to 10 days, the tube just below the bumper is severed to allow the mushroom tip to fall into the stomach. Removal of this piece by endoscopy may be necessary in all but very large dogs.

Needle catheter jejunostomy tubes should be considered for dogs and cats with functional lower intestinal tracts that will not tolerate nasogastric or gastrostomy tube feeding (Jacobs, 1991; Mirvish, 1986; Ogilvie, Moore, 1995a; Reddy, Cohen, 1986) (Fig. 7-7). This method is especially valuable in patients with cancer who have undergone surgery to the upper gastrointestinal tract. In the procedure for placement of jejunostomy tubes the distal duodenum or proximal jejunum is located and isolated by surgery (Jacobs, 1991; Mirvish, 1986; Ogilvie, Moore, 1995; Reddy, Cohen, 1986). A purse-string suture of 3-0

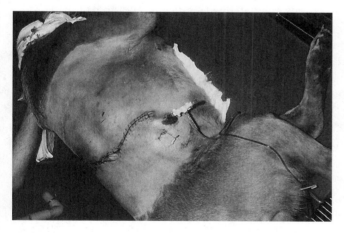

Fig. 7-7 Jejunostomy tube feeding is an excellent method of providing nutrients while bypassing the stomach. Fluid nutrients are used in this feeding method. Note that this patient has had extensive surgery to resect the upper portion of the gastrointestinal tract; nutritional support was essential for this animal's rapid recovery.

nonabsorbable material is placed in the antemesenteric border of the isolated piece of bowel. A 5-French polyvinyl nasogastric infant feeding tube is passed through a small incision in the skin and abdominal wall, through a piece of omentum (referred to as an *omental patch*), and then into the lumen of the bowel through a small stab incision in the center of the area encircled by the purse-string suture. An ideal placement site is in the bowel, 20 to 30 cm from the enterostomy site or neoplastic lesion. The purse string is tightened and secured around the tube. The loop of bowel with the enterostomy site is then secured to the abdominal wall with four sutures that will be cut 7 to 10 days later, after the tube is removed and feeding is complete. This method has complications similar to those of the gastrostomy tube, including peritonitis, diarrhea, and cramping.

Enteral Feeding Formulations

The type of nutrients to be used depends largely on the type of enteral tube and the status of the patient. Blended canned pet foods may be adequate for feeding by gastrostomy tubes; enteral feeding products for humans are easily administered through nasogastric and jejunostomy tubes (Jacobs, 1991; Mirvish, 1986; Ogilvie, Moore, 1995; Reddy, Cohen, 1986). In any case, feeding is usually not started until 24 hours after the tube is placed. Once feeding begins, the amount of nutrients is gradually increased over several days and administered frequently in small amounts or continuously to allow the animal to adapt to this method of feeding. Regardless, the tube should be aspirated 3 to 4 times a day to ensure that no excessive residual volume is present in the gastrointestinal tract and flushed periodically with warm water to prevent clogging.

Additional research is necessary to determine whether recent studies are correct in claiming that standard texts overestimate the caloric requirements of normal dogs, including those with cancer (Ogilvie, Vail, 1990; Vail, Ogilvie, Wheeler, 1990). Until such research exists, recommendations for determining the amount of enteral nutrients should be followed (Jacobs, 1991; Mirvish, 1986; Ogilvie, Moore, 1995a; National Academy of Sciences, 1989; Reddy, Cohen, 1986). Briefly, the basal energy requirement (BER) is calculated in kcal/day by multiplying 70 and the animal's weight in kg 0.75 and then multiplying by a factor to derive the illness energy requirement (IER), calculated in kcal/day as nonprotein calories. For normal dogs at rest in a cage the BER is multiplied by 1.25. For those who have undergone recent surgery or are recovering from trauma, the BER is multiplied by 1.2 to 1.6. If the dog is septic or has major burns, the BER is multiplied by 1.5 to 2.0. Although the IER has not been determined for dogs with cancer, it may be high even in the absence of sepsis, burns, trauma, or surgery (Ogilvie, Vail, 1992). The protein requirement is 4 g/kg/day for normal dogs and 6 g/kg/day for dogs who have experienced heavy protein losses. Dogs and cats with renal or hepatic insufficiency should not be given high protein loads (<3 g/100 kcal in the dog; <4 g per 100 kcal in the cat). Because most high-quality pet foods can be put through a blender to form a gruel that can be passed through a large-bore catheter, the IER of the animal is divided by the caloric density of the canned pet food to determine the amount of food to administer. The same calculation can be used for human enteral feeding products; the volume fed may need to be increased if the enteral feeding product is diluted to ensure that it is approximately isoosmolar before it is administered.

Total Parenteral Nutrition (TPN)

Indications for total parenteral nutrition (TPN) are identical to those for enteral nutrition but include the inability of the gastrointestinal tract to retain, digest, and absorb adequate nutrients. The benefit of long-term TPN in patients with cancer is questionable at best. Although the theoretical gains of TPN are similar to those of enteral support, few have been realized to date according to the scientific literature. Metaanalysis of large numbers of clinical trials for TPN in tumor-bearing people has revealed no significant benefit with respect to nutritional parameters, survival, treatment tolerance, and tumor response. Recipients of bone marrow transplants, who appear to enjoy significant improvement with TPN, are an important exception to the rule. At the same time, tumor-bearing patients receiving TPN are much more likely to develop serious systemic infections and slightly less likely to respond to antineoplastic therapy. TPN is recommended for only those cancer patients who are expected to recover from the underlying circumstances (Fig. 7-8). Candidates include patients who have undergone postoperative gastrointestinal surgery, those with chemotherapy-induced anorexia, and those with tumors in which remission or cure is likely. The veterinary literature listed in the References and Selected Reading section contains several excellent reviews of TPN principles and procedures.

The following general rules appear to apply:

- Initiate enteral and parenteral feeding early: do not wait for evidence of overt signs of cachexia before initiating feeding plans.
- Use the gut whenever possible. Enteral therapy is the preferred approach.
- Because the healing process that occurs in most cancer patients is slow, do not remove gastrostomy or jejunostomy tubes prematurely.
- Minimize the use of fluids containing lactate.
- Consider foods that are highly bioavailable, digestible, and palatable.
- Consider foods with relatively low amounts of simple carbohydrates, moderate amounts of proteins from

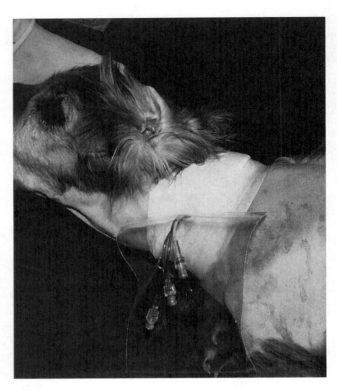

Fig. 7-8 Total parenteral therapy is a valuable tool for supporting the cancer patient when enteral routes cannot be used for whatever reason. TPN requires the use of a dedicated catheter that must be maintained aseptically. Note the small plastic bag over the ports that prevents contamination when the catheter is not in use.

high-quality sources, and moderate amounts of fats; fats of the n-3 fatty acid series may be effective in reducing or eliminating some of the metabolic alterations associated with cancer cachexia. Antioxidants are essential whenever n-3 fatty acids are used.
- Enhanced quantities of arginine and glutamine may help maintain a more normal immune system and gastrointestinal tract.
- Fiber, both soluble and insoluble, is essential to maintain normal bowel health. A diet with adequate amounts of fiber is essential to prevent or treat various problems of the gastrointestinal tract.
- Each patient has unique caloric needs and should therefore be considered individually. In general, cancer patients do not have elevated caloric needs compared with normal animals. Surgery and chemotherapy do not increase caloric needs.
- Plan carefully. Place feeding tubes early (at the time of initial therapy) in high-risk cancer patients. Placing feeding tubes early and then removing them unused is better than not providing nutritional therapy because a feeding tube was not inserted.

REFERENCES

Asselin BL and others: In vitro and in vivo killing of acute lymphoblastic leukemia cells by L-asparaginase, *Cancer Res* 49:4363, 1989.

Barbul A and others: Arginine stimulates lymphocyte immune response in healthy human beings, *Surgery* 90:244, 1981.

Beck SA, Smith KL, Tisdale MJ: Anticachectic and antitumor effect of eicosapentaenoic acid and its effect on protein turnover, *Cancer Res* 51:6089, 1991.

Begin ME and others: Selective killing of human cancer cells by polyunsaturated fatty acids, *Prostaglandins Leukot Essent Fatty Acids* 19:177, 1985.

Begin ME and others: Differential killing of human carcinoma cells supplemented with n-3 and n-6 polyunsaturated fatty acids, *J Natl Cancer Inst* 77:2053, 1986.

Bertram JS, Kolonel LN, Meyskens FL: Rationale and strategies for chemoprevention of cancer in humans, *Cancer Res* 47:3012, 1987.

Billings PC, Habres JM, Kennedy AR: Inhibition of radiation-induced transformation of C3H10T1/2 cells by specific protease substrates, *Carcinogenesis* 11:329, 1990.

Boutwell RK: An overview of the role of diet and nutrition in carcinogenesis. In *Nutrition, growth and cancer*, New York, 1988, Alan R Liss.

Bozzetti F, Pagnoni AM, Del Vecchio M: Excessive caloric expenditure as a cause of malnutrition in patients with cancer, *Surg Gynecol Obstet* 150:229, 1980.

Branda RF: Effects of folic acid deficiency on tumor cell biology. In Jacobs MM, editor: *Vitamins and minerals in the prevention and treatment of cancer*, Boca Raton, Fla, 1991, CRC Press.

Bray GA, Campfield LA: Metabolic factors in the control of energy stores, *Metabolism* 24:99, 1975.

Brennan NF: Uncomplicated starvation versus cancer cachexia, *Cancer Res* 37:2359, 1977.

Buzby GP, Steinberg JJ: Nutrition in cancer patients, *Symp Surg Nutr* 61:691, 1981.

Chance WT and others: Possible role of neuropeptide Y in experimental cancer anorexia. In MM Jacobs, editor: *Diet and cancer: markers, prevention and treatment*, New York, 1993, Plenum.

Chlebowski RT: Nutritional support of the medical oncology patient, *Hematol Oncol Clin North Am* 5:147, 1991.

Chlebowski RT and others: Influence of nandrolone decanoate on weight loss in advanced non–small cell lung cancer, *Cancer* 58:183, 1986.

Chlebowski RT, Heber D: Metabolic abnormalities in cancer patients: carbohydrate metabolism, *Surg Clin North Am* 66:957, 1986.

Chory ET, Mullen JL: Nutritional support of the cancer patient: delivery systems and formulations, *Surg Clin North Am* 66:1105, 1986.

Daly JM and others: Enteral nutrition with supplemental arginine, RNA and omega-3 fatty acids: a prospective clinical trial, Abstract, 15th Clinical Congress, American Society for Parenteral and Enteral Nutrition, *Journal of Parenteral and Enteral Nutrition* 15:19S, 1991.

Delarue J and others: Effect of chemotherapy on resting energy expenditure in patients with non-Hodgkin's lymphoma, *Cancer* 65:2455, 1990.

Dempsey DT and others: Energy expenditure in malnourished patients with colorectal cancer, *Arch Surg* 121:789, 1986.

Dempsey DT and others: Energy expenditure in malnourished gastrointestinal cancer patients. *Cancer* 53:1265, 1984.

Dempsey DT, Mullen JL: Macronutrient requirements in the malnourished cancer patient, *Cancer* 55:290, 1985.

Dewys WD: Pathophysiology of cancer cachexia: current understanding and areas of future research, *Cancer Res* 42:722, 1982.

Dippenaar N, Booyenes J: The reversibility of cancer: evidence that malignancy in melanoma cells is gammalinolenic acid deficiency dependent, *S Afr Med J* 62:505, 1982.

Endres S and others: The effect of dietary supplementation with N-3 polyunsaturated fatty acids on the synthesis of interleukin-1 and tumor necrosis factor by mononuclear cells, *N Eng J Med* 320:265, 1989.

Ferrannini E: The theoretical basis of indirect calorimetry: a review, *Metabolism* 37:287, 1988.

Fredrix EWHM and others: Resting energy expenditure in patients with non–small cell lung cancer, *Cancer* 68:1616, 1991.

Gelin J and others: Role of endogenous tumor necrosis factor and interleukin-1 for experimental tumor growth and the development of cancer cachexia, *Cancer Res* 51:415, 1991.

Hansell DT, Davies JWL, Burns HJG: The relationship between resting energy expenditure and weight loss in benign and malignant disease, *Ann Surg* 203:240, 1986.

Heber D and others: Pathophysiology of malnutrition in the adult cancer patient, *Cancer* 58:1867, 1986.

Heyman SN and others: Protective action of glycine in cisplatin nephrotoxicity, *Kidney Int* 40(2):273, 1991

Holian O, Nelson R: Action of long-chain fatty acids on protein kinase C activity: comparison of omega-6 and omega-3 fatty acids, *Anticancer Res* 12:975, 1992.

Hong WK and others: Prevention of secondary primary tumors with isotretinoin in squamous cell carcinoma of the head and neck, *N Engl J Med* 323:796, 1990.

Hopewell JW and others: The modulation of radiation-induced damage to pig skin by essential fatty acids, *Cancer Res* 3:703, 1992.

Ip C: Factors influencing the anticarcinogenic efficacy of selenium in dimethylbenzanthracene-induced mammary tumorigenesis in rats. *Cancer Res* 41:2638, 1981.

Jacobs MM, editor: *Vitamins and mineral in the prevention and treatment of cancer*, Boca Raton, Fla, 1991, CRC Press.

Jacobs MM, Griffin AC: Effects on selenium on chemical carcinogenesis: comparative effects on antioxidants, *Biol Trace Elem Res* 1:2, 1979.

Jacobs MM, Jansson B, Griffin AC: Inhibitory effects of selenium on 1,2-dimethylhydrazine and methylazoxymethanol acetate induction of colon tumors, *Cancer Lett* 2:133, 1977.

Jenski LJ and others: Omega-3 fatty acid modification of membrane structure and function. I. Dietary manipulation of tumor cell susceptibility to cell and complement mediated lysis, *Nutr Cancer* 19:135, 1993.

Kennedy AR: Effects of protease inhibitors and vitamin E in the prevention of cancer. In Prasad KN, Meyskens FL, editors: *Nutrients and cancer prevention*, Clifton, NJ, 1990, Humana Press.

Khan SG, Kartiyar SK, Agarwal R, Mukhtar H: Enhancement of antioxidant and phase II enzymes by oral feeding of green tea polyphenols in drinking water to SKH-1 hairless mice: possible role in cancer prevention, *Cancer Res* 52:4050, 1992.

Kline K and others: Vitamin E effects on retrovirus-induced immune dysfunction, *Ann NY Acad Sci* 587:294, 1990.

Kline K, Cochran GS, Sanders BG: Growth inhibitory effects of vitamin E succinate on retrovirus-transformed tumor cells in vitro, *Nutr Cancer* 14:27, 1990.

Kline K, Sanders BG: Modulation of immune suppression and en- hanced tumorigenesis in retrovirus tumor challenged chickens treated with vitamin E, *In Vivo* 3:161, 1989.

Kumar GS and others: Effect of n-6 and n-3 fatty acids on the prolif- eration of human lymphocytes and their secretion of TNF and IL- 2 in vitro, *Nutr Res* 12:815, 1992.

Kurzer M, Meguid MM: Cancer and protein metabolism, *Surg Clin North Am* 66:969, 1986.

Lamm DL and others: Megadose vitamins in bladder cancer: a double blind clinical trial, *J Urol* 151:21, 1994.

Landel AM, Hammond WG, Mequid MM: Aspects of amino acid and protein metabolism in cancer-bearing states, *Cancer* 55:230, 1985.

Langstein HN, Norton JA: Mechanisms of cancer cachexia, *Hematol Oncol Clin North Am* 5:103, 1991.

Lawson DH and others: Enteral versus parenteral nutritional support in cancer patients, *Cancer Treatment Report* 65:101, 1981.

Lawson DH and others: Metabolic approaches to cancer cachexia, *Ann Rev Nutr* 2:277, 1982.

Li J, Sartorelli CA: Synergistic induction of the differentiation of WEH1-38 D+ myelomonocytic leukemia cells by retinoic acid and granulocyte colony-stimulating factor, *Leuk Res* 16:571, 1992.

Lowell JA, Parnes HL, Blackburn GL: Dietary immunomodulation: beneficial effects on carcinogenesis and tumor growth, *Crit Care Med* 18:S145, 1990.

McAndrew PF: Fat metabolism and cancer, *Surg Clin North Am* 66:1003, 1986.

Meadows GG and others: Dietary influence of tyrosine and phenylala- nine on the response of B16 melanoma to carbidopalevodopa methyl ester chemotherapy, *Cancer Res* 42:3056, 1982.

Meadows GG, Oeser DE: Response by B16 melanoma-bearing mice to varying levels of phenylalanine and tyrosine, *Nutr Report Int* 28:1073, 1983.

Mengeaud V and others: Effects of eicosapentaenoic acid, gamma- linolenic acid and prostaglandin E1 on three human colon carci- noma cell lines, *Prostaglandins Leukot Essent Fatty Acids.* 47:313, 1992.

Messadi DV and others: Inhibition of oral carcinogenesis by a protease inhibitor, *J of the Natl Cancer Inst* 76:447, 1986.

Mirvish SS: Effects of vitamins C and E on N-nitroso compound for- mation, carcinogenesis, and cancer, *Cancer* 58:1842, 1986.

National Academy of Sciences: *Diet, nutrition and cancer,* Washington, DC, 1982, National Academy Press.

National Academy of Sciences: *Diet and health: implications for reducing chronic disease risk,* Washington, DC, 1989, National Academy Press.

Niles RM, Loewy BP: Induction of protein kinase C in mouse melanoma cells by retinoic acid, *Cancer Res* 49:4483, 1989.

Ogilvie GK and others: Alterations in lipoprotein profiles in dogs with lymphoma, *J Vet Intern Med* 8:62, 1994.

Ogilvie GK and others: Alterations in select aspects of carbohydrate, lipid and amino acid metabolism in dogs with non-hematopoietic malignancies, *Am J Vet Res,* 1995a (in press).

Ogilvie GK and others: Effect of anesthesia and surgery on energy ex- penditure determined by indirect calorimetry in dogs with malig- nant and non-malignant conditions, *J Vet Intern Med,* 1995b (in press).

Ogilvie GK and others: Treatment of dogs with lymphoma with adri- amycin and a diet high in carbohydrate or high in fat, *Am J Vet Res,* 1995c (in press).

Ogilvie GK, Moore AS: Nutritional management. In *Managing the vet- erinary cancer patient: a practice manual,* Trenton, 1995a, Veterinary Learning Systems.

Ogilvie GK, Moore AS: Nutritional Support. In *Managing the veteri- nary cancer patient: a practice manual.* Trenton, 1995b, Veterinary Learning Systems.

Ogilvie GK, Vail DM: Advances in nutritional therapy for the cancer patient, *Vet Clin North Am Small Anim Pract* 20:4, 1990.

Ogilvie GK, Vail DM: Unique metabolic alterations associated with cancer cachexia in the dog, *Curr Vet Therapy* 11:433, 1992.

Ogilvie GK, Vail DM, Wheeler SJ: Effect of chemotherapy and remis- sion on carbohydrate metabolism in dogs with lymphoma, *Cancer* 69:233, 1992.

Ogilvie GK, Vail DM: Metabolic alterations and nutritional therapy for the veterinary cancer patient. In Withrow SJ, MacEwen EG: *Clin- ical veterinary oncology,* Philadelphia, 1996, WB Saunders.

Oram-Smith JC, Stein TP: Intravenous nutrition and tumor host pro- tein metabolism, *J Surg Res* 22:499, 1977.

Orosz P and others: Enhancement of experimental metastasis by tumor necrosis factor, *J Exp Med* 177:1391, 1993.

Pascale AW and others: Omega-3 fatty acid modification of membrane structure and function. II. Alteration by docosahexaenoic acid of tu- mor cell sensitivity to immune cytolysis, *Nutr Cancer* 19:147, 1993.

Peterson G, Barnes S: Genistein inhibition of the growth of human breast cancer cells: independence from estrogen receptors and multi- drug resistance gene, *Biochem Biophys Res Commun* 179:661, 1991.

Pirisi L and others: Increased sensitivity of human keratinocytes im- mortalized by human papillomavirus type 16 DNA to growth con- trol by retinoids, *Cancer Res* 52:187, 1992.

Plumb JA, Luo W, Kerr DJ: Effect of polyunsaturated fatty acids on the drug sensitivity of human tumor cell lines resistant to either cis- platin or doxorubicin, *Br J Cancer* 67:728, 1993.

Pomposelli JJ and others: Diets enriched with n-3 fatty acids ameliorate lactic acidosis by improving endotoxin-induced tissue hypoperfu- sion in guinea pigs, *Ann Surg* 213:166, 1989.

Premachandra BN, Perlstein IB, Williams K: Circulating and tissue thy- roid hormones in relation to hormone action: pathophysiologic sig- nificance. In Fotherby K, Palde Druyter SB, editors: *Hormones in normal and abnormal human tissues,* vol 2, Berlin, NY, 1981, De Gruyter.

Quebbeman EJ, Ausman RK, Schneider TC: A re-evaluation of energy expenditure during parenteral nutrition, *Ann Surg* 195:282, 1982.

Quillin P: An overview of the link between nutrition and cancer. In Quillin P, Williams RM: *Adjuvant nutrition cancer treatment,* Ar- lington Heights, Ill, 1993, Cancer Treatment Foundation.

Ramesh G and others: Effect of essential fatty acids on tumor cells, *Nu- trition* 8:343, 1992.

Reddy BS, Cohen LA, editors: *Diet, nutrition, and cancer: a critical eval- uation, vol 2, Micronutrients, nonnutritive dietary factors and cancer,* New York, 1986, CRC Press.

Roush GC and others: Modulation of the cancer susceptibility mea- sure, adenosine diphosphate ribosyl transferase (ADPRT), by dif- ferences in n-3 and n-6 fatty acids, *Nutr Cancer* 16:197, 1991.

St. Clair W and others: Suppression of DMH-induced carcinogenesis in mice by dietary addition of the Bowman-Birk protease inhibitor, *Cancer Res* 50:580, 1990.

Sestoft L: Metabolic aspects of the calorigenic effect of thyroid hor- mone in mammals, *Clini Endocrinol* 13:489, 1980.

Shamberger RJ and others: Antioxidants and cancer. I. Selenium in the blood of normals and cancer patients, *J Natl Cancer Inst* 50:867, 1973.

Shein PS and others: Cachexia of malignancy, *Cancer* 43:2070, 1976.

Shein PS and others: The oxidation of body fuel stores in cancer pa- tients, *Ann Surg* 204:637, 1986.

Stern PH, Hoffman RM: Enhanced in vitro selective toxicity of chemotherapeutic agents for human cancer cells based on a metabolic defect, *J Natl Cancer Inst* 76:629, 1986.

Tachibana K and others: Evaluation of the effect of arginine-enriched amino acid solution on tumor growth, *J Parent Enter Nutr* 9:428, 1985.

Teyek JA and others: Improved protein kinetics and albumin synthesis by branched chain amino acid-enriched total parenteral nutrition in cancer cachexia, *Cancer* 58:147, 1986.

Theologides A: Cancer cachexia, *Cancer* 43:2004, 1979.

Tisdale MJ, Brennan RA, Fearon KC: Reduction of weight loss and tumour size in a cachexia model by a high fat diet, *Br J Cancer* 56:39, 1987.

Torti FM, Torti SV: Cytokines, iron homeostasis and cancer. In Jacobs MM, editor: *Diet and cancer: markers, prevention, and treatment*, New York, 1993, Plenum Press.

Troll W, Frenkel K, Wiesner R: Protease inhibitors as anticarcinogens, *J Natl Cancer Inst* 73:1245. 1984.

Vail DM and others: Exacerbation of hyperlactatemia by infusion of lactated Ringer's solution in dogs with lymphoma, *J Vet Intern Med* 4:228, 1990.

Vail DM, Ogilvie GK, Wheeler SL: Metabolic alterations in patients with cancer cachexia, *Compend Contin Educ Pract Vet* 12:381, 1990.

Vail DM, Panciera D, Ogilvie GK: Thyroid hormone concentrations in conditions of chronic weight loss in dogs with special reference to cancer cachexia, *J Vet Intern Med* 8:122, 1994.

Vernon LN: Selenium in carcinogenesis, *Biochem Biophys Acta* 738:203-110, 1984.

Walters LM and others: Repeatability of energy expenditure measurements in normal dogs by indirect calorimetry, *Am J Vet Res* 54:1881, 1993.

Wang ZY and others: Inhibition of N-nitrosodiethylamine and 4-(methylnitrosamino)-1-(3-pyridyl)-1-butanone-induced tumorigenesis in A.J mice by green tea and black tea, *Cancer Res* 52:1943, 1992a.

Wang ZY and others: Protection against benzo(a)pyrene and *N*-nitrosodiethylamine-induced lung and forestomach tumorigenesis in A/J mice by water extracts of green tea and licorice, *Carcinogenesis* 13:1491, 1992b.

Wargovich MJ and others: Chemoprevention of gastrointestinal cancer in animals by naturally occurring organosulfur compounds in allium vegetables. In Jacobs MM, editor: *Vitamins and minerals in the prevention and treatment of cancer*, Boca Raton, Fla, 1991, CRC Press.

Weed H, McGandy RB, Kennedy AR: Protection against dimethylhydrazine-induced adenomatous tumors of the mouse colon by the dietary addition of an extract of soybeans containing the Bowman-Birk protease inhibitor, *Carcinogenesis* 6:1239, 1985.

Weisburg JH: Interactions of nutrients in oncogenesis, *Am J Clin Nutr* 53:2265, 1991.

SELECTED READING

Allen TA: Specialized nutritional support. In Ettinger SJ, editor: *Textbook of veterinary internal medicine*, ed 3, Philadelphia, 1989, WB Saunders.

Copeland EM, Daly JM, Dudrick SJ: Nutrition as an adjunct to cancer treatment in the adult, *Cancer Res* 37:2451, 1977.

Donohue S: Nutritional support of hospitalized patients, *Vet Clin North Am Small Anim Pract* 19(3):475, 1989.

Lippert AC, Fulton RB, Parr AM: A retrospective study of the use of total parenteral nutrition in dogs and cats, *J Vet Intern Med* 7:52, 1993.

McGeer AJ, Detsky AS, O'Rourke K: Parenteral nutrition in cancer patients undergoing chemotherapy: a meta-analysis, *Nutrition* 6:478, 1990.

Remillard RL, Thatcher CD: Parenteral nutritional support in the small animal patient, *Vet Clin North Am Small Anim Pract* 19:1287, 1989.

Sonnenschein EG and others: Body conformation, diet, and risk of breast cancer in pet dogs: a case-control study, *Am J Epidemiol* 133(7):694, 1991.

Wheeler SL, McGuire BM: Enteral nutritional support. In Kirk RW, editor: *Current veterinary therapy X.* 1989, pp 30-36.

White SD and others: Use of isotretinoin and etretinate for the treatment of benign cutaneous neoplasia and cutaneous lymphoma in dogs, *J Am Vet Med Assoc* 202(3):387, 1993.

Witschi H, Kennedy AR: Modulation of lung tumor development in mice with the soybean-derived Bowman-Birk protease inhibitor, *Carcinogenesis* 10:2275, 1989.

Yamashita Y, Kawada S, Nakano H: Induction of mammalian topoisomerase II dependent DNA cleavage by nonintercalative flavonoids genistein and omega-3 fatty acids, *Biochem Pharmacol* 39:737, 1990.

Yen A and others: Coupled down-regulation of the RB retinoblastoma and c-Myc genes antecedes cell differentiation: possible role of RB as a "status-quo" gene, *Europ J Cell Biol* 57:210, 1992.

Zyliez Z and others: Metabolic response to enteral food in different phases of cancer cachexia in rats, *Oncology* 47:87, 1990.

Chapter 8

Orthomolecular Medicine: A Practitioner's Perspective*

WENDELL O. BELFIELD

In modern times, most people in the medical sciences conceptualize vitamins and minerals as substances to prevent nutritional deficiency diseases. Recently, clinical investigators have discovered that these same nutrients, at quantities beyond minimum levels, do more than prevent deficiency diseases. This chapter addresses the effects of high levels of vitamins and minerals on viral diseases and degenerative conditions, biochemical changes in tissues, and free radicals and oxidation of cells.

The earliest recorded evidence of a nutritional deficiency in animals or humans appeared in 1753 in the book *A Treatise on Scurvy,* by John Lind. Lind described sailors dying of scurvy at sea and theorized that the cause was a lack of fresh food. He recommended that the sailors eat limes in addition to their normal ration, thereby preventing scurvy. Lind's theory was proved when seafarers adopted this practice and scurvy deaths decreased. About 400 years later, in 1928, Dr. Albert Szent-Györgyi, a Hungarian physician, discovered ascorbic acid, the substance in the limes that prevents scurvy.

Good health can be fostered only through good nutrition. Pets must rely on their owners, who in turn must rely on the pet food industry. This industry relies on the National Research Council (NRC) for nutritional requirements. For the most part, the recommendations of the NRC are based on preventing deficiency diseases such as scurvy and beri-beri. Many nutrition experts question the reason that these experts have not attempted to determine the optimum amounts of nutrients and their effects during the stresses of pregnancy and disease. A minimum amount of nutrients may have been adequate to maintain good

health 50 or 100 years ago, but today the contamination of the environment and the chemical additives in some commercial pet diets lessen the likelihood that minimum nutrition will maintain good physical and mental health. Many scientists think that the National Academy of Sciences should reevaluate nutritional recommendations in light of present-day conditions (Reynolds, 1994).

Veterinary Practitioners' Perspective on Orthomolecular Medicine

In 1968 the late Linus Pauling (PhD and two-time Nobel Prize winner) used the term *orthomolecular,* which by definition means *right molecule.* During a conversation, he defined it as follows:

> Orthomolecular medicine is the preservation of health and the treatment of disease by the provision of the optimum molecular constitution of the body, especially the optimum concentration of substances that are normally present in the human body and are required for life.

"Our physical bodies are made up of water, fat, protein, carbohydrates, and similar substances," notes Jonathan Wright (1990), explaining a basic principle of orthomolecular medicine. "Therefore it's logical to expect that if something is wrong with our bodies, proper manipulation of the elements of which they are made will be a major factor in reestablishing health."

As early as the sixteenth century, the French astrologer and physician Nostradamus enjoyed a greater cure rate than his colleagues in part because he incorporated ground rose petals, which we now know contain vitamin C, into his remedies. Although the use of vitamins and minerals to treat conditions not recognized as classic nutrient deficiencies probably began early this century, strong clinical studies did not appear until the 1950s. Abram Hoffa and Humphrey Osmond treated schizophrenics with high doses

*NOTE: This chapter represents the clinical experience of a pioneer in the field of orthomolecular medicine. The reader is reminded that, although the opinions expressed may not be scientifically supported or referenced as such, they may serve as a valuable starting place for the clinical practice of therapeutic nutrition.

of vitamin B_3 (niacin) and dramatically improved recovery rates. Their studies showed that niacin in combination with standard medical therapy doubled the number of recoveries in a 1-year period. Increasing interest in the treatment of many conditions using high-dose vitamin therapy has led to important research findings.

Basic Principles of Orthomolecular Medicine

Most physicians and veterinarians believe that a balanced diet will provide all required nutrition. Orthomolecular physicians recognize that variability in food quality, such as that caused by soil depletion, and the presence of biochemical individuality among patients are critical determinants of nutritional need.

Biochemical Individuality

The concept of biochemical individuality is based on the work of Roger J. Williams. Williams realized that individuals are unique because each has specific nutritional needs or requirements. As previously noted, the minimum levels for nutrients established by the government, or recommended daily allowances (RDA), may prevent severe deficiency diseases, but orthomolecular physicians and veterinarians claim that these levels do not provide for optimal health, and people and domestic animals may require levels higher than the RDAs.

The Principles of Orthomolecular Medicine

In 1987, Richard Kunin, of San Francisco, California, summarized the principles of orthomolecular medicine (Goldberg, 1993):

- Nutrition comes first in medical diagnosis and treatment, and nutrient-related disorders are usually curable once nutritional balance is achieved.
- Biochemical individuality is the norm in medical practice; therefore universal RDA values are unreliable nutrient guides. Many people require an intake of certain nutrients far beyond the RDA suggested range (often called *megadose*), because of their genetic disposition or the environment in which they live.
- Drug treatment is used only for specific indications and always with consideration of the potential dangers and adverse effects.
- Environmental pollution and food adulteration are an inescapable fact of modern life and are a medical priority.
- Blood tests do not necessarily reflect tissue levels of nutrients.
- Hope is the indispensable ally of the physician and the absolute right of the patient.

Megavitamin Therapy: How Does It Work?

Megavitamin therapy treats disease by attempting to supply optimal concentrations of substances normally found in the body. These nutrients may be supplied orally or parenterally, and the dosages are frequently much higher than conventional recommendations—hence the term *megavitamin therapy*. As with any substance that exerts physiologic effects, therapeutic effects must be weighed against possible side effects. Vitamins A and D have well-recognized toxicity potential. Vitamin E, in high doses, may contribute to coagulation problems. High levels of selenium, iron, and zinc must be used with caution when they are taken over long periods. Still, most vitamins, especially those that are water soluble, are extremely safe for long-term use at high levels (*Alternative medicine: expanding medical horizons*, 1992).

Possible Indications for Orthomolecular Supplementation

Physicians and veterinarians commonly use vitamins and minerals in the treatment of certain diseases. These include folic acid in the prevention of human neural-tube defects and the treatment of cervical dysplasia, magnesium sulfate in the treatment of human heart attack, and vitamin E to treat feline steatitis. Newer techniques include the use of EFA to reduce inflammation and pathology in cardiovascular, renal, musculoskeletal, dermatologic, and immune-mediated disorders; chromium and vanadium to manage some forms of diabetes; and vitamin E to treat liver disease.

The Future of Orthomolecular Medicine

Most veterinary practitioners receive nutritional training that concentrates on balancing rations, with some attention to the functions of vitamins and minerals in metabolic processes. Use of micronutrients to treat diseases other than deficiency conditions is not introduced into most academic curricula.

Abram Hoffer, a pioneer in orthomolecular medicine, made the following statement:

It takes approximately 40 years for innovative thought to be incorporated into mainstream thought. I expect and hope that orthomolecular medicine, within the next 5 to 10 years, will cease to be a specialty in medicine and that all physicians will be using nutrition as an essential tool in treating disease (Goldberg, 1993).

Although veterinary professionals have shown some interest, most resist the idea that vitamins and minerals can be administered to animals for treatment, prevention, and control of seemingly unrelated disease. Health care professionals and the general public tend to associate vitamin and mineral therapies with specific quantities of food for daily consumption. However, the quantities of vitamins and minerals necessary to treat, prevent, and control diseases discussed in this chapter far exceed the small amounts consumed as food in the diet. Fortunately, chemists can extract vitamins and minerals from natural sources. These nutrients can then be administered and consumed in concentrated amounts. A few tablets of vitamins and minerals are equivalent to a bushel of fruits or vegetables.

Many physicians are not fully aware of specific properties of certain nutrients influencing disease processes. Practitioners should know five important facts about the nutrients they administer to patients: (1) quality, (2) quantity, (3) source, (4) compatibilities, and (5) form.

- *Quality* standards have been established by the U.S. government and are described in *The United States Pharmacopoeia (USP)*. This text guarantees that the nutrient listed meets the quality standards set forth by the U.S. government.
- *Quantity:* The quantity of nutrients is extremely important: more does not necessarily mean better. Each disease process has its own specific quantity requirement; a few milligrams plus or minus can determine success or failure in treating and preventing a disease.
- *Sources:* The sources of vitamins and minerals must be considered because the wrong source can lead to serious consequences. A classic example is the use of beta-carotene, a source of vitamin A. This vitamin-A source is not available to felines because they are not able to convert this provitamin into vitamin A. Vitamins A and E in their natural states are fat-soluble; when administered in megaquantities they can eventually become toxic. The preferred sources are water-soluble (palmitate) vitamin A and water-miscible vitamin E. Several sources of vitamin C exist: ascorbic acid and the nonacid mineral forms, such as sodium ascorbate and calcium ascorbate. The practitioner should know the specific differences.
- *Compatibility:* Compatibility of ingredients is usually a concern for manufacturers; however, even they sometimes combine incompatible nutrients. Some nutrient sources can inhibit the effectiveness of other nutrients. Ferrous sulfate, a common source for iron, can minimize the action of vitamin E.
- *Form:* Vitamin and mineral supplements are supplied as liquids, crystals, tablets, capsules, and injectables. The practitioner must identify the form that provides optimal utilization. In some instances, especially if the gastric mucosa is irritated, the oral administration of a harsh, compact tablet can perpetuate the mucosal irritation, resulting in incomplete use of the nutrients. Time-release preparations are of little value if large

levels of vitamins and minerals are required to treat, prevent, or control a disease process.

The U.S. government requires only a list of nutrients and quantities on nutritional product labels. The qualities, sources, and compatibilities determine whether the product is efficacious; the label information does not offer the necessary information for consumers to select the most effective product. Also, consumers should select products from manufacturers with impeccable reputations.

Vitamin Therapies

Definition of Therapeutic Modality

Exogenous vitamins and minerals in prescribed quantities can be effective therapeutic agents in the treatment, prevention, and control of specific disease processes. Among these nutrients are antioxidant vitamins and minerals, such as alpha-tocopherol (vitamin E), vitamins A and C, and zinc. In human medicine, these nutrients show great promise in preventing cancer and cardiovascular disease and improving immune function in older people (Block, 1991; Florence, 1995; Kline and others, 1989; Knight, 1995). These findings can be used for new therapeutic approaches to some veterinary problems.

History

This author first described the use of vitamin C in the treatment of viral disease in 1967 (Belfield, 1967). Leveque supported these results 1 year later in a paper titled "Ascorbic Acid in the Treatment of Canine Distemper Complex" (1968). Another paper described a vitamin-mineral protocol to effectively prevent and control feline leukemia (Belfield, 1983). The concept that exogenous nutrients such as vitamin C, a liver metabolite in dogs and cats, can be administered for the treatment, prevention, and control of diseases (Box 8-1) is viewed with skepticism by the academic community because of a lack of controlled studies. Many small animal practitioners have found it necessary to seek new avenues to solve veterinary problems encountered in practice that have yet to be solved by veterinary researchers.

Antioxidant Research

Although research in antioxidant therapies has shown impressive results, it has not been conducted in veterinary systems. The therapies presented in this chapter are based on research conducted mainly in human medicine using animal models.

Vitamin E is a lipophilic membrane antioxidant that functions as a chain-breaking antioxidant, interrupting chain propagation of free radical–mediated peroxidation of biologic molecules and membranes by scavenging free

PHYSIOLOGIC EFFECTS OF ASCORBIC ACID

Detoxification of histamine
Phagocytic functions of leukocytes
Metabolism of drugs
Formation of nitrosamine
Tubulin function
Expression of acetylcholine receptor
Leukotriene biosynthesis
Lipid metabolism
Tetrahydrofolate reduction
Immunity
Cancer
Diabetic complications
Cataract formation
Periodontal disease
Rheumatoid arthritis
Infections

Modified from Padh H: Vitamin C: newer insights into its biochemical functions, *Nutr Rev* 65:70, 1991.

TABLE 8-1

DAILY PRODUCTION OF ASCORBATE IN ANIMALS

ANIMAL	ASCORBATE PRODUCTION
	MG/KG BODY WEIGHT PER DAY
Snake	10
Tortoise	7
Mouse	275
Rabbit	226
Goat	190
Rat	150
Dog	40
Cat	40
Monkeys, apes, humans	0

From Levine M: New concepts in the biology and biochemistry of ascorbic acid, *N Engl J Med* 314:892, 1986.

radicals. Vitamin E may also act as a membrane stabilizer. As an antioxidant, vitamin E is more effective when directed against the radicals on the outside of the membranes rather than those within the bilayer (Florence, 1995; Takahashi, Tsuchiya, Niki, 1989). Vitamin E has also been shown to be a biomodulator of immune function in studies of retrovirus-infected chickens and retrovirus-transformed tumor cells (Kline and others, 1989).

Certain antioxidants are function specific. As an example, lipid peroxidation is prevented by ascorbic acid in guinea pig tissue both in vivo and in vitro. In ascorbic acid deficiency, lipid peroxidation occurs progressively in guinea pig tissues, despite the presence of adequate levels of antioxidants, such as alpha-tocopherol, GSH, protein thiols, and the presence of scavenging enzymes such as superoxide dismutase (SOD), catalase, and glutathione peroxidase. Therefore all antioxidants are not effective in every oxidative situation (Chakraborty and others, 1994).

Vitamin A deficiency has been associated with greater susceptibility to infection. Vitamin A is critical in the development of T and B lymphocytes. Insufficient vitamin A levels cause a reduction in cell-mediated immune function and decreased specific antibody responses to immunization. Marginal deficiencies decrease responses to vaccines and production of antigen-specific antibodies.

Suboptimal Compensatory Feedback and Ascorbic Acid

Compared with the aquatic life amphibians faced, the transition to terrestrial existence meant excessive oxidative stress in hot, dry climates, with much higher oxygen tension. This change coincided with the evolutionary emergence of amphibians' ability to synthesize ascorbic acid (Padh, 1991).

A mechanism that evolved in mammals is a feedback system that increases the liver's production of ascorbate during increased stress (Subramanian, 1973). This protective mechanism once contributed greatly to survival and is still present in many mammals today. For example, a rat increases its daily ascorbic acid synthesis tenfold when under stress (Levine, 1986). Exceptions to this rule are humans and guinea pigs, who cannot produce ascorbic acid.

Present-day birds are living examples of the kidney-to-liver transfer of ascorbic acid synthesis. The older species of birds are kidney producers. As we go up the evolutionary ladder, we find birds producing ascorbic acid in both their kidneys and livers. The most recent species of birds are solely liver producers (Burton, 1972).

For decades, veterinarians have supposed that mammals capable of synthesizing their own ascorbic acid produce enough each day to satisfy their requirements. This is far from the truth, especially during periods of stress. Table 8-1 details the wide variation among species. Mere endogenous production is no assurance of optimal production. Dogs and cats, as noted in Table 8-1, appear to be particularly low producers. The classic signs of frank clinical scurvy normally do not appear in mammals capable of making their own ascorbic acid. However, under very severe stresses the signs of scurvy may appear. Nearly 50 years ago the severe stresses of Antarctic cold, a heavy workload, and a lack of fresh food caused husky dogs to become listless and develop swollen, hemorrhagic gums. These scorbutic symptoms readily cleared with the provi-

TABLE 8-2

ENZYMES STIMULATED BY ASCORBIC ACID

PROCESS	ENZYME	MONO/DIOXYGENASE	METAL ION
Collagen synthesis	Prolyl-4-hydroxylase	Di-	Fe^{2+}
	Prolyl-3-hydroxylase	Di-	Fe^{2+}
	Lysyl hydroxylase	Di-	Fe^{2+}
Carnitine biosynthesis	6-*N*-trimethyl-L-lysine hydroxylase	Di-	Fe^{2+}
	γ-Butyrobetaine hydroxylase	Di-	Fe^{2+}
Metabolism of pyrimidine and its nucleotide in fungi	Thymine 7-hydroxylase	Di-	Fe^{2+}
	Pyrimidine Deoxyribonucleoside 2'-hydroxylase	Di-	Fe^{2+}
Cephalosporin synthesis	Deacetoxycephalosporin C synthetase	Di-	Fe^{2+}
Catabolism of tyrosine	4-Hydroxyphenyl pyruvate hydroxylase	Di-	Fe^{2+}
Norepinephrine biosynthesis	Dopamine β-monooxygenase	Mono-	Copper
Conversion of inactive precursors to active hormones	Peptidylglycine α-amidating monooxygenase	Mono-	Copper

From: Padh H: Cellular functions of ascorbic acid, *Biochem Cell Biol* 68:1166, 1990.

sion of fresh seal meat containing ascorbic acid (Burton, 1972) (Table 8-2).

Free Radicals and Antioxidants: Their Role in Illness

Halliwell (1995) describes free radicals as follows:

Electrons in atoms and molecules occupy regions of space termed *orbitals,* each of which holds a maximum of two electrons. A free radical is any species capable of independent existence that contains one or more unpaired electrons; that is, electrons alone in an orbital. Radicals react with other molecules in several ways. If two radicals meet, they can combine their unpaired electrons and join to form a covalent bond (a shared pair of electrons). A free radical might donate its unpaired electron to another molecule, causing a reduction reaction. A free radical might take an electron from another molecule, thereby oxidizing it.

"Activated oxygen species (AOS) include both oxygen free radicals and nonradical species such as single oxygen and hydrogen peroxide. These nonradical AOS can be as dangerous as free radicals if liberated in biologic systems" (Florence, 1995). Sources of free radicals are shown in Box 8-2.

Defenses Against Free Radicals

Antioxidants, or free radical scavengers, defend normal cells against damage by AOS. Maximum life-span potential (MLP) correlates to antioxidant potential when antioxidant potentials of tissues and serum from various mammalian species are compared. Humans have the best antioxidant defenses of any mammal, possibly the reason for our long life-span potential. Antioxidants include enzymes such as catalase and superoxide dismutase and mo-

BOX 8-2

*S*OURCES OF *F*REE *R*ADICALS

Electron transport chain
Phagocytosis
Oxidant enzyme (e.g., xanthine oxidase)
Autoxidation (e.g., epinephrine)
Redox drugs (e.g., paraquat)
Tobacco
Sunlight and ionizing radiation

TABLE 8-3

SOME ANTIOXIDANTS AND THEIR ACTIONS

SUBSTANCE	ACTION
Ascorbic acid	Destroys nitrosamines and many free radicals
Alpha-tocopherol	Destroys lipid peroxides
Beta-carotene	Destroys singlet oxygen
Catalase	Destroys hydrogen peroxide
Superoxide dismutase	Destroys superoxide radical
Glutathione peroxidase	Destroys hydrogen peroxide and lipid peroxides

lecular antioxidants such as ascorbic acid (vitamin C) and alpha-tocopherol (vitamin E) (Table 8-3).

Components of the antioxidant defense system function synergistically; a deficiency of one causes the others to be less effective. For example, vitamins C and E have a complementary relationship. Vitamin C is water soluble and does not enter the cell membrane, whereas vitamin E is lipophilic and intercalated in the membrane bilayer. Vitamin E reduces membrane lipid peroxide molecules to convert them to the free lipid, and a vitamin E free radical is formed. Extracellular vitamin C then reacts with the vitamin E radical chroman group to regenerate vitamin E. Vitamin E is protected and continues to prevent the potential cascade of lipid peroxidation in cell membranes. One vitamin E molecule protects 1000 lipid molecules (Florence, 1995).

A Nutritional Approach to Feline Leukemia Prevention and Control

Feline leukemia virus (FeLV) is an exogenous retrovirus transmitted primarily by saliva. FeLV and FeLV-related complications may be the most prevalent cause of death in domestic cats (Gandolfi, 1991). FeLV is often present in the blood and bone marrow and shed in the saliva, urine, feces, milk, and nasal secretions of some infected cats. The virus is spread by both horizontal and vertical transmission modes (Cotter, 1991).

This discussion is confined to an alternative approach to the control and prevention of FeLV through immunotherapy. Although people once believed leukemia vaccines would reduce infections, the verdict is still out on the efficacy of the present vaccines (Gandolfi, 1991). Control of FeLV infection is still best effected by routine testing and isolation of infected cats (Cotter, 1991).

Controversial Issues

In the past, veterinarians routinely recommended euthanasia for cats who tested positive for FeLV. (Because false positives can occur when using in-house tests, in-house testing should be done for screening only.) Cats testing positive and exhibiting signs of illness should be given a guarded prognosis, but the prognosis is better for FeLV detected in routine screening of healthy cats. "The median survival time for healthy FeLV-positive cats is approximately 2 years, with 20% still alive 3 years after the first positive test results" (Cotter, 1991).

This author has experienced success with a nontraditional protocol in households with FeLV-positive cats, contrary to the conventional approach of isolating the viremic cats from FeLV-negative cats to control transmission of the virus. Viremic and unvaccinated FeLV-negative cats on the nutritional protocol described later have been permitted to cohabitate, with no spread of infection (Belfield, 1983). All (more than 100) FeLV-positive cats became negative through daily oral administration of a crystalline vitamin-mineral supplement. (The only cats not accounted for are those belonging to clients who relocated and those that died of unrelated causes.) This supplement consists of vitamin C as sodium ascorbate with other essential antioxidants (alpha-tocopherol and vitamin A) with a support of many significant vitamin and minerals.* This regimen has been used with great success for many cats.

Practical Theory and Applications: Supplemental Protocol

The protocol consists of 750 mg of sodium ascorbate (buffered vitamin C), 750 IU (International Units) vitamin A, and 75 IU of vitamin E.* This combination of vitamins, in conjunction with other essential supplemental nutrients in crystalline form, is mixed once daily into a wet ration. The first patient on whom this protocol was attempted was a 1-year-old intact female Persian who had recently tested positive for FeLV using the immunofluorescent antibody test (IFA). The subject was retested 9 weeks later, and the IFA test was negative for FeLV. The FeLV was suspected to be transient and eliminated from the subject through natural means. Researchers chose older subjects who were known to have been viremic for a minimum of 1 year, with an average duration of 2 years. The average age of the subjects was 2½ years, most were of mixed parentage, and the group included both sexes.

Observations

All subjects testing positive for more than 1 year but less than 2 years tested negative approximately 6 months later. Those viremic for more than 2 years but less than 3 years tested negative for FeLV between 9 and 12 months later. Those testing positive for FeLV 3 years or more tested negative after 2 years (Table 8-4).

---

*Mega C Plus, Orthomolecular Specialties, 3091 Monterey Rd., San Jose, CA 95111-3204; mailing address: P.O. Box 32232, San Jose, CA 95152-2232.

TABLE 8-4

SAMPLE RESULTS OF MEGAVITAMIN PROTOCOL ON FeLV-POSITIVE CATS

CAT NO.	AGE AT POSITIVE TEST (YEARS)	AGE AT FIRST NEGATIVE TEST (YEARS)	FOLLOW-UP NEGATIVE TEST (YEARS)
1	1.5	2	3
2	2.5	3.5	4
3	4	7	7

The exceptions to the results in Table 8-4 were older cats who were viremic most of their lives, stray cats with no history of FeLV testing, and feral cats. These cats were on the nutritional regimen 3 to 5 years before testing negative to IFA and ELISA antigen tests; they numbered approximately 15. Since the nutritional protocol was begun in 1977, hundreds of previously positive cats have tested negative for FeLV.

Cats that displayed signs of chronic illness caused by immunosuppression became devoid of symptoms. Queens with a history of infertility, abortion, or fetal resorption gave birth to normal, healthy litters. Fading kitten syndrome was eliminated. Other chronic secondary diseases, such as stomatitis, abscesses, and upper respiratory tract infections, were eliminated.

Feline leukemia virus may become latent in bone marrow, resulting in false negatives by ELISA and IFA. Although not every cat was given a bone marrow test for FeLV, several were assessed for the possibility of false negatives to antigen tests. Those FeLV negatives were then included in the results. The bone marrow test, in conjunction with the IFA or ELISA, is essential to determine conclusively whether a cat is in fact negative.

Practical Theory and Applications

The role of antioxidants in the treatment, prevention, and control of infectious diseases has provoked curiosity among some medical practitioners. As previously noted, a great deal of information is available, and it is the responsibility of practitioners to explore even obscure avenues to help their patients. One strategy for improving survival from infectious disease is to enhance cell-mediated immunity. Vitamins A, C, and E are known to increase CD4 numbers as well as CD4/CD8 ratios and lymphocyte responsiveness to the mitogen PHA (Penn and others, 1991). Phagocytes mediate the innate immunologic response by releasing products that damage invading microorganisms. These products include proteins such as lysozyme, peroxidases, and elastase and reactive oxygen species such as superoxide, hydrogen peroxide, hypohalous acid, and hydroxyl radical (Rosen and others, 1995). Increased production of interferon (Scott, 1982), an integral part of the mechanism that interferes with viral propagation because of its direct virucidal action, is one effect of the antioxidant vitamin C. Vitamin E interrupts the chain propagation of free radical–mediated peroxidation of biologic molecules and membranes by scavenging radicals and is considered a membrane stabilizer. The fact that vitamin E scavenges radicals at or near the surface of the membranes (Takahashi and others, 1989) makes this antioxidant an early adversary of the pathogen.

The role played by the antioxidant vitamin E in acquired immunodeficiency syndrome (AIDS) has generated interest among researchers. Like FeLV, AIDS is a clinical disorder caused by a retrovirus infection and represents the end point in a progressive sequence of immunosuppressive changes. Wang briefly summarizes the literature with regard to immunologic, nutritional, and other pathologic modifications caused by AIDS and the properties of immunoenhancing, antioxidant activity, and undernutrition-restoration of vitamin E supplementation. The report states that these abnormalities in AIDS resemble those that are stimulated or restored by intake of high doses of vitamin E (Wang, Watson, 1993).

Treatment may be lifelong if the subjects' immune susceptibility is genetically linked or chronically influenced by other factors, such as the environment. In other words, these cats may become FeLV positive if the protocol is discontinued; the cat reverts to its previous immune-deficient state, rendering it susceptible to symptoms of FeLV.

The ability to prevent and control a retrovirus such as FeLV through natural immunotherapy is significant because the body contains and maintains the necessary defenses to prevent the development and replication of the most deadly virus of felines. This nutritional protocol is also effective against FIP and FIV viruses. In most cases, treatment, prevention, and control of viruses through nutritional supplementation require time for the body to respond to the nutritional supplements because of the biochemical changes necessary for positive results.

Pet owners are becoming more knowledgeable about the role of nutrition in preventing diseases. Practitioners should further explore the role nutrition plays in disease processes. Natural immunotherapy through nutritional supplementation can be another weapon in the practitioner's arsenal to prevent and control FeLV. At present, no other natural, economical, and efficacious treatment exists for this deadly disease.

Skin Allergies

In most small animal practices, among the most perplexing and stubborn conditions to treat are skin allergies. Because these allergies are triggered by the animal's environment, the practitioner must address this factor for successful treatment of the disease. The major symptom, pruritus, can be triggered by exposure to pollen, foods, house dust, and insect bites. One therapeutic approach is to optimize immune function through immunotherapy, increase cortisol production in the adrenal cortex, and produce antihistaminic effects.

Traditional Medical Theory

Inappropriate immune responses to exogenous substances or autogenous substances produce allergic or autoimmune diseases, respectively.

Two types of hypersensitivity reactions commonly observed in practice are immediate hypersensitivity and anaphylaxis, mediated by IgE. Canine and

feline atopy, some parasite hypersensitivities, food allergies, and drug reactions are examples of type I reactions. Type IV reaction, or cell-mediated hypersensitivity, is mediated by sensitized T lymphocytes that release cytokines when stimulated by certain antigens. Allergic contact dermatitis and some parasite hypersensitivities are examples of type IV reactions (White, Ihrke, 1983).

Conventional Veterinary Therapies

Conventional therapy currently centers on allergen avoidance, topical therapies, fatty-acid and vitamin E supplementation, and antihistamines and steroids.

Food allergy dermatitis is not common in cats (White, Ihrke, 1983). In general, food-allergy dermatitis is more common in dogs. Symptomatic treatment with prednisone and use of elimination diets are recommended for control of the food hypersensitivity.

Chemicals found in the environment often act as haptens, uniting with the dermal collagen to produce a complete antigen. These chemicals may include detergents, topical medications, metals, and natural or synthetic fibers. Treatment should include removing the offending substance from the environment of the sensitive individual. Palliative treatment may then lead to resolution of the problem. Corticosteroid administration for 3 to 5 days may ameliorate signs of reexposure.

Intradermal skin testing is the diagnostic test of choice for environmental allergies. When appropriate immunotherapy is administered and used in conjunction with avoidance, shampoo therapy, fatty acids, and low doses of prednisone and antihistamine, hyposensitization is effective in 50% to 80% of cases (Scott, Miller, Griffin, 1995). Prolonged use of corticosteroids is not recommended for control of skin allergies. However, some clients insist the animal be given "the shot that stops the scratching," and more often than not the clinician obliges. A life of avoidance, shampoo therapy, fatty acids, prednisone, and antihistamines is not pleasant for the patient or the owner.

A Nutritional Approach to the Treatment, Prevention, and Control of Skin Allergies

For any therapy to be successful the patient must be on a hypoallergenic diet—that is, one free of chemicals normally used as preservatives, potentially offending ingredients, and impurities. Some veterinarians recommend a premium lamb and rice diet that contains lamb as the only protein source, rice as the carbohydrate source, and either lamb fat or a vegetable oil rich in omega-6 as the fat source.*

Recently, raw meat diets have come in vogue. Use of this diet is discouraged for several reasons. First, some animals are unable to digest raw meat diets; this can be manifested by vomiting. Second, no regulatory controls exist for animal foods at all government levels. Third, the risk of bacterial contamination can lead to serious gastrointestinal consequences and even death.

Decreased blood cholesterol levels can indicate malabsorption of foods (Sodikoff, 1995). Although low blood cholesterol is not seen at pathologic levels, it may be an indication that the animal is not thoroughly assimilating its ration. When animals are fed a cooked ration for several days, blood cholesterol levels return to within normal range.

Many chemicals are incorporated into some commercial pet foods as preservatives, others to add color, and still more as emollients. According to many veterinarians, a steady diet of such chemicals can cause pathologic conditions in various body systems over time.

Before initiating the vitamin-mineral protocol, the practitioner should perform a complete blood profile (chemistry and hematology), including cortisol and thyroid function evaluation. Because antioxidants used in the treatment can create changes in these hormones, observed increases should not be confused with Cushing's or thyroid disease. If a patient has been on antioxidants (e.g., vitamin A, vitamin E, selenium) and the cortisol and TSH levels are elevated, the antioxidants should be discontinued for 3 weeks and the patient retested. If the patient has these conditions, this protocol is not recommended.

The basis for this therapy is to (1) optimize immune function through immunotherapy, (2) prevent the insult and destruction of cells of the integument, (3) optimize adrenal function, and (4) detoxify histamines. Crystalline sodium ascorbate preparation* is administered to bowel-tolerance level to improve immune function and detoxify histamines.

INITIAL DOSE

Small dogs and cats	750 mg
Medium dogs (25 to 50 lb)	1500 mg
Large dogs (50 to 100 lb)	3000 mg

This preparation is mixed daily into a moist ration. Every third day, increase dosage by $1/8$ teaspoonful for small canines and felines and $1/4$ teaspoonful for medium and large dogs. When stool loses its cylindric form, decrease the dosage one increment dose and remain at this level; this is the bowel-tolerance level. At this level, the stool should maintain its cylindric form.

A combination of alpha-tocopherol, vitamin A, and selenium is also administered daily with the ration.†

---

*California Natural Dog Food, Natura Pet Products, 1171 Homestead Rd., No. 275, Santa Clara, CA 95050-5478.

*Mega C Plus, Orthomolecular Specialties, 3091 Monterey Rd., San Jose, CA 95111-3204; mailing address: P.O. Box 32232, San Jose, CA 95152-2232.
†Vital Tabs, Orthomolecular Specialties, 3091 Monterey Rd., San Jose, CA 5111-3204; mailing address: P.O. Box 32232, San Jose, CA 95152-2232.

DAILY DOSAGE

Small dogs and cats:	800 IU vitamin E
	10,000 IU vitamin A
	20 µg selenium
Medium dogs (25 to 50 lb):	1600 IU vitamin E
	20,000 IU vitamin A
	40 µg selenium
Large dogs (50 to 100 lb):	2400 IU vitamin E
	30,000 IU vitamin A
	60 µg selenium

Every patient on this protocol in my practice has shown great improvement. The total elimination of corticosteroids, antihistamines, tranquilizers, and hormones is often possible. This is not a "quick-fix" cure or treatment; the body requires approximately 6 weeks to adjust to this biochemical change. The challenge is for the practitioner to assure the pet owner that the protocol will be effective (Fig. 8-1).

When the patient is asymptomatic, supplementation with a maintenance protocol is continued.

VITAMIN C (SODIUM ASCORBATE) COMPOUND:

Small dogs and cats	750 mg
Medium dogs (25 to 50 lb)	1500 mg
Large dogs (50 to 100 lb)	3000 mg

VITAMIN E, A, AND SELENIUM COMBINATION:

Small dogs and cats	100 IU vitamin E
	1250 IU vitamin A
	2.5 µg selenium

Larger animals are similarly maintained at one fourth of the starting dose. Practitioners must remember that immunologically stressed animals regress under stress conditions. When this regression occurs, the symptoms may resurface and the patient must return immediately to the initial treatment protocol.

Inflammatory Bowel Disease (IBD)

Traditional Medical Theory

Tams (1988) describes inflammatory bowel disease as follows:

> *Inflammatory bowel disease (IBD)* is a general term that applies to various disease processes manifested as inflammation of the bowel. The inflammatory reaction is characterized by infiltration of the mucosa by various populations of inflammatory cells, which can include lymphocytes, plasma cells, eosinophils, and neutrophils. The four substances that seem to be the most common causes of chronic intestinal disease in the dog and cat are food, antigens, bacteria, and parasites.

If the cause is not determined, the condition is referred to as *idiopathic IBD.*

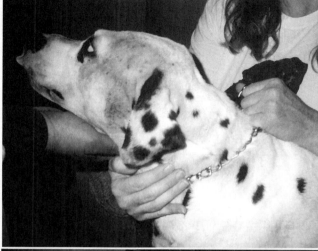
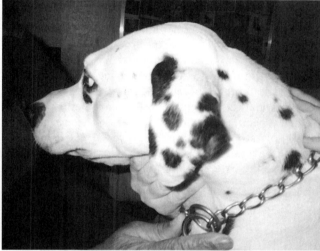

Fig. 8-1   This 8-year-old intact male dalmatian with a chronic allergic dermatitis responded to the vitamin/mineral protocol in 12 days. The patient remains on the protocol indefinitely.

Cats with IBD may exhibit vomiting, diarrhea, or both. Weight loss and small bowel type of diarrhea usually accompany disease of the small intestine. Large bowel disease may manifest as less voluminous diarrhea without weight loss (Tams, 1988). A proper diagnosis of IBD must be made based on intestinal biopsy. In this chapter the therapeutic aspects of this disease are emphasized rather than the pathologic ones.

Conventional Therapy

Idiopathic IBD may be treated with corticosteroids, metronidazole, or a combination of agents (Tams, 1988). Many patients respond to elimination diets; homemade diets are preferred for better control of the ingredients, as well as for the relative lack of artificial flavorings and other extraneous materials (Willard, 1995).

A lifetime of medications and elimination diets is expensive and stressful for the patient and owner. Drugs may be tolerated well, but the duration of tolerance is variable.

Controversial Issues

Inflammatory cells (plasma cells, lymphocytes, eosinophils, and neutrophils) are present in the lamina propria in patients with IBD (Willard, 1995). Because IBD has an inflammatory component, a logical assumption is that the pathology of free radicals may play a part in the clinical symptoms commonly observed.

Practical Theory and Applications: Vitamin-Mineral Therapy

The combination of the antioxidants alpha-tocopherol, vitamin A, and selenium is effective in the treatment of IBD. The clinician should insist on a good diet—that is, one free of chemical preservatives. Vitamin C (sodium ascorbate, ascorbic acid) should not be a part of the protocol because of its cholinergic effect on the intestinal tract. As previously mentioned, the bowels tolerate specific levels of vitamin C, but beyond these levels soft stools or diarrhea can occur. IBD patients tend to have a low threshold or tolerance for vitamin C–induced diarrhea.

DAILY ORAL DOSAGE

Medium dogs (25 to 50 lb)	800 IU vitamin E
	1000 IU vitamin A
	20 μg selenium
Large dogs (51 to 100 lb)	1200 IU vitamin E
	3000 IU vitamin A
	30 μg selenium

In general, small dogs and cats do not tolerate antioxidants in tablet form. The compactness of the tablet may act as a gastric irritant and often precipitates vomiting. For these sensitive patients a liquid vitamin E (400 IU) and selenium (25 μg) are administered PO bid.*

Most IBD patients respond to this nutritional therapy within 2 days to 2 weeks. Then the patient can be placed on the same antioxidant maintenance dosage described for skin allergy therapy. The patient is recommended to remain on the protocol indefinitely, but the owner may exercise discretion. Because this condition is an allergy by some definitions, the patient may regress during stress and exhibit IBD symptoms. Should regression occur, the initial therapeutic protocol must be instituted.

---

*Vital Liquid, Orthomolecular Specialties, 3091 Monterey Rd., San Jose, CA 5111-3204; mailing address: P.O. Box 32232, San Jose, CA 95152-2232.

Epilepsy: A Manifestation of Hypersensitivity

Parker (1979) defines *epilepsy* as follows: "*Epilepsy* is defined as repeated seizures; thus any dog having repeated seizures can be described as epileptic." Animals with seizures from brain tumors or acute encephalitis are not classified as epileptics. Traumatized animals with seizures may exhibit posttraumatic epilepsy; when the acute problem persists longer than a few weeks, it is called *epilepsy* (Parker, Small, 1979). Manifestations of idiopathic epilepsy usually occur between 1 and 3 years of age (Gerard, Conarck, 1991).

Scientific Basis and Research

Because the subject of seizures is quite involved, this chapter deals only with idiopathic epilepsy. The clinician must be satisfied with diagnosis by elimination in cases in which the cause of seizure is labeled *idiopathic*. An unknown number of idiopathic cases are genetic and therefore not acquired (Parker, Small, 1979).

Some authors have associated idiopathic epilepsies with hypersensitivities. Textbooks describe hypersensitivities involving skin, the respiratory and gastrointestinal tracts, eyes, and ears. The administration of vitamin C with phenytoin was shown to eliminate seizures in a 20-pound dog (Belfield, Stone, 1975). Vitamin C was believed to enhance phenytoin. The recommended dosage for phenytoin with a 1-gram dose of sodium ascorbate caused ataxia in the subject, indicating an overdose of the central nervous system (CNS) depressant. The recommended dosage of phenytoin was diminished by half to prevent ataxia and seizures. In 1994, I applied a vitamin-mineral protocol employed in hypersensitivity cases to an Australian shepherd with severe epilepsy (10 seizures daily). Within a few weeks the patient improved remarkably. Until recently, the literature was devoid of information supporting the theory that epilepsy may be managed nutritionally.

Some evidence indicates that nutrition and nutritional supplementation can control and prevent epilepsy in dogs (Collins, 1994). Weber and others have suggested that a deficiency in glutathione peroxidase produces seizures. In their study, four children with intractable seizures, repeated infections, and intolerance to anticonvulsants showed evidence of glutathione peroxidase deficiency. Two children had low intracellular enzyme activity but normal blood selenium and high plasma glutathione peroxidase concentrations. The other two had low intracellular glutathione peroxidase activity with low circulating glutathione peroxidase and selenium concentrations. The clinical state of the children improved after discontinuation of anticonvulsant medication and administration of selenium (Weber, 1991). The investigators concluded that glutathione peroxidase deficiency may be a cause of childhood seizures. The first two patients appeared to have a primary deficiency of the intracellular enzyme, whereas the other two may have had a disturbance of selenium resorption or transport (Weber, 1991).

Collins (1994) attributes epilepsy in dogs to possible food hypersensitivities. Some patients experienced a reduction in seizures when diets were changed and resumption of seizures when the seizure-producing diet was fed. Collins associates some dermatologic conditions accompanied by possible concurrent seizures with food allergies. He recommends a diet of boiled lamb and rice, prepared using distilled water and glass cooking vessels, to eliminate allergens causing the seizures.

Collins (1994) makes the following conclusion:

> An immunochemical basis for many nervous system pathologic responses is becoming increasingly apparent. Findings that short-lived vasoactive neurotransmitters and neuromodulator molecules that have long been known to mediate inflammation and immediate hypersensitivity also profoundly affect neurons have provided a view into the fascinating world of immunoneuroregulation. Given the complexity of the nervous system, practitioners should recognize the possibility of aberrations mediated by immune responses and mediators released in this process. This is not to suggest that all idiopathic disease entities should be considered allergic; however, the diagnostician should consider the possibility of allergic or immune-mediated disease.

One approach to idiopathic epilepsy is to administer anticonvulsant drugs. These drugs are often administered in combination when individual drugs are ineffective. These "drug cocktails" may cause impaired liver function, drug tolerance, and behavior changes. Because of the risks associated with these drugs, practitioners must determine whether the seizures are hypersensitivity related.

Anecdotal evidence suggests that skin and blood allergy testing is of little value. Elimination diets are somewhat valuable because they provide temporary relief. However, the animal often becomes sensitive to other allergens because of genetic susceptibility. Elimination diets must be taken a step further. Because the target is the immune system, the most logical approach is to optimize immune response—hyperactivity may result in the generation of free radicals, causing oxidation of cells. When the antioxidants vitamins A and C and the trace mineral selenium are introduced, the oxidative process is suppressed and the recovery process is initiated.

Practical Theory and Applications: Nutritional Protocol

Thus far, I have instituted nutritional therapy in two patients. Physical examination and blood chemistry profiles indicated no abnormalities. Typical treatment protocol includes oral administration of a combination of phenobarbital (1/8 gr to 1 gr bid or tid) and phenytoin (2 mg/kg/day to 80 mg/kg/day tid or bid). Because the half-life of phenytoin is comparatively short, maintenance of effective CNS suppression (by use of phenobarbital) is critical. This combination is administered orally to disrupt the seizure pattern. The same combination of nutrients previously discussed in skin allergies is also administered. When the patient has been free of seizures for at least 2 weeks, the phenytoin portion of the combination is reduced by half. If the patient remains seizure free for a second 2-week period, the phenytoin is decreased to one fourth of the original dosage. At the end of 6 weeks with no seizures, the phenytoin is discontinued.

Phenobarbital is decreased within the same time frame as the phenytoin. If seizures recur, the process starts over again with the full phenytoin and phenobarbital combination. The nutritional protocol remains at the therapeutic level. Cessation of seizures takes approximately 2 months. The therapeutic level of nutrients must be maintained for 30 days after the last seizure, after which the patient may receive maintenance dosages.

Although these patients have not suffered relapses, allergies typically recur during stress periods (estrus, travel, pregnancy). If allergies recur, the process must begin again. Currently the duration without seizures averages 2 years. The initial time frame between seizure episodes in the first subject, a 5-year-old intact Australian shepherd female, was 10 days. For a period of 3 to 5 days, 3 to 10 grand mal seizures occurred within a 24-hour period. The second subject was a male intact golden retriever having mild seizures bimonthly. These seizures occurred at intervals of 2 days to 2 weeks.

This nutritional approach is valuable because it lessens the need for extensive drug use. Because the aim of this approach is to prevent and control allergic reactions, immune function can be improved through natural immunotherapy.

Other Observations

Increased serum glutamic pyruvic transaminase (SGPT) and blood urea nitrogen (BUN) levels on blood chemistry analysis with no involvement of microorganisms can be reduced to normal with the administration of antioxidant vitamins A and E and selenium in dosages previously mentioned. These levels may indicate potential liver and kidney problems. Acanthosis nigricans responds to therapeutic levels through the oral administration of the previously mentioned trio of antioxidants (vitamins A and E and selenium). Because increases in thyroid hormone levels may occur with the administration of these antioxidants, these increased levels may contribute to the success of the therapy.

Canine Hip Dysplasia (CHD)

Hip dysplasia, long considered an inherent birth defect, may be an easily controlled biochemical condition in many breeds of dogs. The lesion in canine hip dysplasia (CHD) may be caused by insufficient collagen synthesis resulting in poor osteogenesis, chondrogenesis, and myogenesis. If insufficient amounts of ascorbate (vitamin C) exist in affected dogs, these animals may have difficulty synthesizing sufficient collagen to maintain joint stability.

In October, 1976, I published a controversial paper describing a nutritional approach to preventing CHD. Then, as now, development of CHD was assumed to be hereditary. The study examined eight litters of pups from dysplastic German shepherd parents or parents that had produced dysplastic offspring. No signs of CHD appeared in the progeny when the bitches were administered megadoses of ascorbate during pregnancy and the pups were maintained on a similar regimen until adulthood (Belfield, 1976).

Scientific Basis and Research

Vitamin C is required for development of connective tissue such as muscle, cartilage, and bone.

Vitamin C deficiency, or scurvy, affects these connective tissues. The scorbutic patient exhibits defects in fracture repair and wound healing, whereas infants with scurvy exhibit impaired bone formation and disruption of dentition. These defects are assumed to be related to known requirements for ascorbic acid in collagen production (Franceschi, 1992; Leboy and others, 1992; Russell, Manske, 1991). Padh (1991) makes the following statement:

> Collagen synthesis is an elaborate process of protein synthesis, posttranslational modifications, protein secretion, and extracellular matrix formation. Collagen is a unique animal protein. In a variety of cell types, ascorbate increases transcription, translation, and stability of mRNA for procollagen. Ascorbate also stimulates secretion of procollagen for the formation of extracellular matrix. This suggests that each step in collagen synthesis, hydroxylation, and secretion is efficiently regulated by the rest of the process.

Synthesis of glycosaminoglycans associated with collagen fibers increases 30% to 90%, and deposition into the extracellular matrix increases 80% in the presence of ascorbic acid (Kao and others, 1990).

Myogenesis: the Development and Formation of Muscle

Ascorbic acid is necessary for myogenesis because ethyl-3,4-dihydroxybenzoate, an ascorbic acid antagonist, blocks myotube formation, collagen synthesis, and myosin light chain–mRNA induction. This inhibition is reversed with excess ascorbic acid (Franceschi, 1992).

Osteogenesis: the Development and Formation of Bone

Ascorbic acid is essential for type I collagen matrix, alkaline phosphatase, osteocalcin accumulation, and mineralization of bone (Franceschi, 1992; Leboy and others, 1992; Russell, Manske, 1991).

Traditional Medical Theory

CHD is a polygenic, multifactorial heritable disease (Tomlinson, McLaughlin, 1996).

> Osseous development is a developmental phenomenon orchestrated by synchronous bone and muscle maturation. Normal or nearly normal osseous development of the cartilage model for the acetabulum and femoral head takes place during this period, and, with time, the hip will stabilize. This potential for normal osseous development is greatest at birth and gradually decreases as the animal approaches maturity (Fox and others, 1987).

Controversial Issues

Control of CHD relies on a threefold approach: (1) selective breeding, (2) conservative therapy, and (3) medical and surgical therapies.

Selective breeding

Although breeding dogs with normal hips improves hip conformation only in resulting litters, this strategy has not, on a wider scale, improved this widespread problem. Still, dogs used for breeding should have excellent hips according to OFA or PennHip criteria.

Conservative therapy

Conservative therapy for dogs with radiographically visible hip dysplasia includes moderate exercise (consisting only of short leash walks until 15 months of age) and weight control (Tomlinson, McLaughlin, 1996).

Medical and surgical therapy

Dogs with clinical signs of osteoarthritis may require medical or surgical intervention. Drug therapies include nonsteroidal antiinflammatories such as aspirin, meclofenamic acid, carprofen, and phenylbutazone. Corticosteroids should not be routinely used in treating osteoarthritis. Polysulfated glycosaminoglycan (PSGAG) may induce synthesis of cartilage matrix (Tomlinson, McLaughlin, 1996). Surgical approaches include varus osteotomy, pelvic osteotomy, total hip replacement, excision arthroplasty, biceps sling augmentation to femoral head osteotomy, and pectenotomy (Fox and others, 1987).

In general the previous conventional solutions to CHD are extensive and expensive. No significant progress has occurred since CHD was first reported in 1945 (Schnelle, 1945). The selective breeding approach has not eliminated this crippling disease: Dysplastic parents are producing normal progeny, and nondysplastic parents are producing dysplastic offspring. Although parents selected for breeding may be free of CHD, have excellent hips, and be two generations removed, they still can produce dysplastic offspring if they carry the genes. The genetic theory has not been conclusively proved as the sole cause of CHD, however. Some evidence suggests that one cause of CHD is biochemical (i.e., caused by inadequate collagen synthesis that adversely affects myogenesis, chondrogenesis, and osteogenesis). In recent years, scores of scientific papers support the role of vitamin C in collagen synthesis.

Ligament laxity, possibly secondary to poor collagen synthesis, may also contribute to hip dysplasia (Fig. 8-2). The reason that only the coxofemoral joint is affected as a result of poor collagen synthesis is not yet fully understood. The pectineus muscle begins at the iliopectineal eminence and ends on the medial branch of the linea aspera above the distal end of the femur. In the young, developing dog the femur grows and develops at a normal rate, and the development of the pectineus muscle is not commensurate with femoral development. This uneven development may be primarily the result of poor myogenesis and atrophy. Because of the origin and insertion of the pectineus, a stress tension develops that causes the head of the femur to separate from the acetabulum, resulting in subluxation.

Bardens and Hardwick (1968) conducted a study to establish the involvement of the pectineus muscle in CHD. Hips of 4-month-old pups were palpated under a general anesthetic to determine ligament laxity in predisposed pups. In those pups displaying ligament laxity in both hips, the pectineus tendon was excised in only one hip and the other remained attached as a control. When the pups reached maturity, they showed subluxation of the hip in which the pectineus muscle remained intact. The other hip was normal where the pectineus tendon had been excised. This study suggests the involvement of the pectineus muscle in CHD.

In the 1990 "Iams Abstracts" the director of the Orthopedic Foundation for Animals made the following announcement: "Mass selection (breeding only normal dogs) has succeeded in increasing the number of normal dogs at a rate of 1.7% to 2.5% per year in a number of breeds and has improved the radiographic phenotype of the normal subjects by increasing the number of 'excellent' classifications of phenotype." These percentages are impressive, but the statistics fail to include factors such as new therapeutics, preventive nutritional protocols, and integrity in certification of individual dogs. Some breed lines have decreased in number by sterilization, euthanasia, and the reputation of CHD in the line. Nutritional interventions might change the fate of these breeds.

Researchers have documented the pathology involved in CHD for decades and have not yet explained its genetic component. Because collagen synthesis is essential

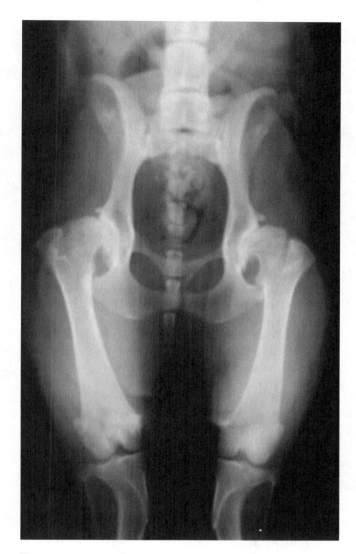

Fig. 8-2 This radiograph is of a 13-year-old altered female springer spaniel. CHD with severe osteoarthritis is evident. The fissures between the trochanter major and heads of both femurs and the medial curvature of the proximal ends of the tibias are attributed to poor collagen synthesis, resulting in poor osteogenesis. This dog was subjected to a life of poor and inadequate diets.

for optimal muscle, bone, and cartilage formation, researchers have logically hypothesized that the genes involved in CHD contribute to normal bone, cartilage, and muscle formation. If the genetic component for CHD is related to ascorbate metabolism, new control strategies through nutritional supplementation may become possible.

Practical Theory and Applications

As previously noted, vitamin C is essential for the synthesis of collagen, which is essential for myogenesis, chondrogenesis, and osteogenesis. For good or adequate collagen synthesis, a good body pool of vitamin C must be established. Because cells rely on a specific vitamin C transporter to maintain intracellular stores of this nutrient, loss of transport function can lead to certain pathologies of connective tissue, even under conditions in which serum levels of vitamin C are considered adequate (Franceschi, 1992). Researchers are not able to determine the precise quantities of vitamin C required to ensure optimum collagen synthesis. One strategy is to administer vitamin C, per os, to bowel-tolerance levels.

Protocol

The ascorbate regimen begins with the pregnant bitch. This protocol is extremely important because a healthy pregnancy fosters healthy progeny. The protocol is designed to address large breeds of dogs (50 to 100 pounds of body weight). The initial dose is 3000 mg of sodium ascorbate compound daily in moist food for 3 days.* If the stools remain firm, increase the ascorbate level 750 mg every third day, until stools begin to lose their cylindric form. The dose is then reduced by 750 mg to return the stools to their normal form; this is known as *bowel tolerance level*. The maximum dosage of ascorbate should not exceed 10,000 mg daily.

Newborn pup
For the first 5 days, each pup receives 66 mg of ascorbate-collagen mixture per os by dropper daily.*

BEFORE WEANING:

5 to 10 days old:	100 mg per os
10 days to weaning:	132 mg per os

AFTER WEANING:

Weight-pounds	*Ascorbate* (mg)
8 to 20	750 to 1500
20 to 50	Bowel tolerance
50 to 100	Bowel tolerance

The clinician should avoid excessive doses because this can cause diarrhea in the animal. If the initial dose of ascorbate causes soft stools, withhold vitamins for 2 to 3 days or until stools become firm and begin at a lower level. Some individuals will require time to adjust to these levels of ascorbate.

Other joint diseases that have proved responsive to optimal collagen synthesis are arthritis, osteochondritis dissecans, and Legg-Calvé-Perthes disease. Because these conditions involve cartilage pathology, improving or maintaining good chondrogenesis may improve the prognosis and comfort level for these patients.

Feline Nonspecific Gingivitis

Traditional Medical Theory

Nonspecific gingivitis and stomatitis in the cat are often extremely refractory to treatment. Clinical signs include chronic inflammation, vesiculation, and ulceration of the oral mucosa. Several organisms have been isolated, including spirochetes, *Fusiformis* genera, *Bacteroides,* and *Actinomyces,* but the etiology is not clear. The significance of the presence of these microorganisms is unclear. Calcivirus is often present in affected cats, and FeLV and FIV also predispose cats to repeated and persistent episodes of stomatitis and gingivitis (Gruffydd-Jones, Evans, Gaskell, 1983).

Treatment may include long-term antibacterial therapy; corticosteroids, clindamycin, and metronidazole afford some success. In severe cases, removal of affected (or all) teeth may provide some relief.

Controversial Issues

Prolonged administration of antibiotics and corticosteroids can be detrimental to the patient. A major problem with this condition is the constant introduction of new organisms. The oral cavity is constantly bombarded with bacteria as the animal grooms itself and eats foods that have been in contact with contaminated soil. Although antibiotics and steroids may control microorganisms and inflammation, they may also inhibit the healing process.

Practical Theory and Applications

The theory, applications, and protocol previously discussed in the section on feline leukemia also apply to this condition. Administration of vitamins A, C, and E may improve cell-mediated immunity by mobilization of leukocytes and increased phagocytosis. The degenerative changes of gum tissue in feline nonspecific gingivitis may be caused by pathologic oxidative processes, and vitamins E and A, in combination with the trace mineral selenium, may help ameliorate the damage caused by gingivitis.

The oral administration of clindamycin (50 to 75 mg bid for 3 to 4 weeks) is recommended. The gum tissues improve while the antibiotic is being administered but probably do not heal completely. Some veterinarians recommend including with the antibiotic therapy 400 IU vitamin E and 25 μg selenium per orum bid with meals. Because their mouths are very sensitive, cats may resist the administration of tablets or capsules; vitamin E and selenium in liquid form are easily administered if mixed in the daily ration.* To improve immune function,

---

*Mega C Plus, Orthomolecular Specialties, 3091 Monterey Rd., San Jose, CA 95111-3204; mailing address: P.O. Box 32232, San Jose, CA 95152-2232.

*Vital Liquid, Orthomolecular Specialties, 3091 Monterey Rd., San Jose, CA 5111-3204; mailing address: P.O. Box 32232, San Jose, CA 95152-2232.

sodium ascorbate compound is administered to bowel tolerance.*

Although the antibiotic controls bacterial replication, it does nothing to prevent recurrent infections and correct the underlying immunologic disorder. Vitamins A and E and selenium can complement and complete the therapy by healing involved tissues. In most cases, repetition of the antibiotic therapy is unnecessary. I have treated 40 cases, with successful results. About half of these patients were referred from other clinics because the clients rejected dental extractions. The patient should remain on a maintenance regimen as a preventive measure.

This protocol should be incorporated into a small animal practice because it offers an alternative to dental extractions. The client should be made aware of good dental hygiene and the necessity for routine teeth cleaning.

Feline Struvite Urolithiasis

A syndrome characterized by urethral obstruction in the male and dysuria with or without hematuria in both sexes has been given various names in the veterinary literature, including *cystitis–urethral obstruction complex, feline urethral obstruction, feline urolithiasis, feline urolithiasis syndrome, urethroadenocystitis, feline urinary retention, retention cystitis* (Finco, 1983), and, more recently, *feline urologic syndrome* (FUS) and *feline lower urinary tract disease* (FLUTD). Recent clinical research indicates that naturally occurring FLUTD may result from causes that may be single, multiple, and interacting, and the clinical signs may include hematuria, dysuria, pollakiuria, and urethral obstruction (Osborne, Lulich, Polzin, 1994).

Osborne, Lulich, and Polzin (1994) provide the following explanation:

> FLUTD is suspected to involve viral agents. Some researchers hypothesize that interstitial cystitis may be a component in some patients. Urinary tract inflammation that occurs without concomitant crystalluria results in nonobstructive dysuria and hematuria. Alternatively the presence of risk factors that promote crystal growth in urine may result in the formation of classic matrix-poor uroliths.

Definition of Therapeutic Modality

Recent literature supports the hypothesis that organisms may play a role in FLUTD. Struvite urolithiasis can sometimes be controlled with the daily administration of cranberry extract. Recent data suggest that cranberry juice inhibits the adherence of bacteria to mucosal surfaces. Cranberry juice and the urine produced by mice fed a cranberry beverage inhibited adherence of *Escherichia coli* to

uroepithelial cells by about 80%. Two compounds in cranberry juice may inhibit lectin-mediated adherence of *E. coli* to mucosal cells: One is fructose, common to many fruit juices, and the other is a nondialyzable polymeric compound that inhibits adhesins associated with pathogenic strains of *E. coli*. This compound was isolated from cranberry and blueberry juices but was not found in grapefruit, orange, guava, mango, and pineapple juices (Avorn and others, 1994).

The oral administration of cranberry extract powder in tablet form may be useful in the treatment, prevention, and control of canine and feline magnesium ammonium phosphate crystals and uroliths. Buffington and others (1985) reported the effects of feline urine pH as a factor in the formation of feline struvite crystals. These researchers determined that struvite uroliths did not necessarily emanate from magnesium compounds. Osborne, Lulich, and Polzin (1994) hypothesize that inflammatory disorders, possibly caused by organisms, may be a cause for struvite uroliths.

History

Several studies have been conducted on urinary acidification by oral administration of cranberry juice to determine its effects on bacteriuria and pyuria in older women. However, no studies on record indicate that cranberry juice or extract can prevent the formation of struvite uroliths.

Scientific Basis and Research

The scientific rationale for this nutritional protocol is based on studies conducted by Buffington and others (1985) and Taton, Hamar, and Lewis (1984) demonstrating that lowering the urine pH level to 6.5 or lower prevents and dissolves struvite uroliths. The addition of 1.5% ammonium chloride to an experimental ration containing 0.44% magnesium oxide inhibited urolith formation and dissolved preformed uroliths (Taton, Hamar, Lewis, 1984). Moreover the work of Osborne and others suggests that diet modification can minimize risk factors associated with struvite crystalluria (Osborne, Lulich, Polzin, 1994).

Traditional Medical Theory

FLUTD is the most common urologic disease for which cats are presented for veterinary services. The most common symptom is pollakiuria with or without hematuria. Anatomic factors predispose male cats to outflow obstruction, a potentially lethal situation. Many studies have been conducted to elucidate etiologic factors important in the formation of struvite ($MgNH_4PO_4$-$6H_2O$), the crystalline material associated with most cases of FLUTD.

As previously noted, Buffington and others and Taton, Hamar, and Lewis recognized the involvement of diets

---

*Mega C Plus, Orthomolecular Specialties, 3091 Monterey Rd., San Jose, CA 95111-3204; mailing address: P.O. Box 32232, San Jose, CA 95152-2232.

in the formation of struvite crystals. Osborne and others have offered another possible etiology in the potential involvement of inflammatory disorders as a cause of FLUTD.

Controversial Issues

Urinary acidifiers such as DL-methionine, ascorbic acid, and ethylenediamine dihydrochloride; ammonium chloride may be effective. Methenamine is sometimes used, but its safety is suspect. Methylene blue and products containing it are contraindicated because of the potential for Heinz body formation and hemolytic anemia in cats (Harvey, Kornick, 1976).

No known effective and safe urinary acidifiers can be administered on a daily basis for an indefinite time without the potential for adverse side effects and the need for dosage adjustments. The oral administration of ascorbic acid is sometimes successful; however, it is associated with adverse side effects such as gastric upset, flatulence, and diarrhea. (These symptoms can be attributed to the low pH level of 2.0.) Ammonium chloride is an effective urinary acidifier, but frequent dosage adjustments are necessary to maintain a urine pH level of 6.5.

Cranberry extract has proved a safe and effective acidifier that can be administered orally daily for an indefinite period without adverse side effects. Whether its mode of action is hippuric acid excretion or the nondialyzable polymeric compound with its bacteriostatic properties or a combination of the two is not clear. Because the form of the cranberry is a concentrated extract, greater amounts can be administered, resulting in greater concentrations in the urine. Cranberry juice, being more dilute, is less concentrated in urine and less likely to be effective.

The term *vitamin C* is used to include all forms of vitamin C, even those mineral ascorbates with a pH of 7.4. Sodium ascorbate, a buffered form of ascorbic acid, is particularly recommended. This buffered form of vitamin C tends to be better tolerated in the gut in gram doses.

Veterinarians should note that side effects associated with gram doses of ascorbic acid have been reported. Ascorbic acid has been implicated in the formation of oxalate calcium. Studies attempting to document this phenomenon remain contradictory; nevertheless, vitamin C should not be administered to animals with a history of oxalate stone formation.

Pet food manufacturers are now acidifying feline diets and recommending these diets for all cats. Because only 0.8% of the total cat population in the United States has signs of FLUTD (Sherding, 1988) this may be an extreme measure. Cats not afflicted with FLUTD are compromised by this regimen and can develop calcium oxalate uroliths. Only cats with FLUTD should receive urine acidifiers.

Practical Theory and Applications

Acidification of urine and antimicrobial treatment are clearly helpful in the prevention of struvite crystals and uroliths. In human studies, subjects received 300 ml of cranberry juice daily through oral administration. This form of cranberry is impractical in veterinary medicine because of the obvious difficulty of administering juice to a cat. A 250-mg tablet of cranberry extract powder that can be easily administered orally by pilling or mixed into wet food is therefore recommended.*

Diets containing protein of animal origin usually cause production of acid urine. A high-level, good-quality protein diet in combination with the cranberry extract protocol is recommended.† The recommended dosage for the cranberry extract is 250 mg bid for 5 to 10 days, then 250 mg daily maintenance. Some patients may require a total of 750 mg in divided daily doses. The practitioner can titrate the cranberry acidity with diagnostic litmus strips or sedimentation or identify crystals by microscopic examination of the urine. Dissolution of crystals can be expected within 24 hours. This protocol has been 100% effective in my experience, and the patient may remain on the regimen indefinitely with no adverse effects.

References

Alternative medicine: expanding medical horizons: a report to the National Institutes of Health on Alternative Medical Systems and Practices in the United States. Prepared under the auspices of the Workshop on Alternative Medicine, Chantilly, Va, September 14-16, 1992.

Avorn J and others: Reduction of bacteriuria and pyuria after ingestion of cranberry juice, *JAMA* 271(10):751, 1994.

Bardens JW, Hardwick H: New observations on the diagnosis and cause of canine hip dysplasia, *Vet Med Small Anim Clinician* 63:238, 1968.

Belfield WO: Vitamin C in the treatment of canine and feline distemper complex, *Vet Med Small Anim Clinician* ** :345, 1967.

Belfield WO: Chronic subclinical scurvy and canine hip dysplasia, *Vet Med Small Anim Clinician* 71(10):1401, 1976.

Belfield WO: An orthomolecular approach to feline leukemia prevention and control, *J Int Acad Prev Med* 8(3):40, 1983.

Belfield WO, Stone I: Megascorbic prophylaxis and megascorbic therapy: a new orthomolecular modality in veterinary medicine, *J Int Acad Prev Med* 11:25, 1975.

Block G: Epidemiologic evidence regarding vitamin C and cancer, *Am J Clin Nutr* **:1310S, 1991.

Buffington CA and others: Feline struvite urolithiasis: magnesium effect depends on urinary pH, *Feline Pract* 15(6):29, 1985.

Burton ARC: Scurvy in the Antarctic, *Lancet* 1146, 1972.

Chakraborty S and others: Ascorbate protects guinea pig tissues against lipid peroxidation, *Free Radic Biol Med* 16:417, 1994.

---

*Carpon, Orthomolecular Specialties, 3091 Monterey Rd., San Jose, CA 95111-3204; mailing address: P.O. Box 32232, San Jose, CA 95152-2232.
†Innova, Natura Pet Products, 1171 Homestead Rd., No. 275, Santa Clara, CA 95050-5478.

Collins JR: Seizures and other neurologic manifestations of allergy, *Vet Clin North Am Small Anim Pract* 24:735, 1994.

Cotter S: Management of healthy feline leukemia virus–positive cats, *JAMA* 199:1470, 1991.

Florence TM: The role of free radicals in disease, *Aust N Z J Ophthalmol* 23:3, 1995.

Fox SM and others: Osteotomy and hip replacement: key treatments for dysplastic dogs, *Vet Med* 82(7):709, 1987.

Franceschi RT: The role of ascorbic acid in mesenchymal differentiation, *Nutr Rev* 50(3):65, 1992.

Gandolfi RC: Vaccination against the feline leukemia virus: a complicated endeavor, *Vet Med* 86(3):290, Mar 1991.

Gerard VA, Conarck CN: Identifying the cause of an early onset of seizures in puppies with epileptic parents, *Vet Med* 86(1):1060, 1991.

Goldberg B: *Alternative medicine,* Puyallup, Wash, 1993, Future Medicine.

Gruffydd-Jones, Evans RJ, Gaskell CJ: Nonspecific gingivitis and stomatitis. In *Feline Medicine,* American Veterinary, 1983.

Halliwell B: Oxygen radicals, nitric oxide and human inflammatory joint disease, *Ann Rheumatic Dis* 54:505, 1995.

Harvey JW, Kornick HP: Phenazopyridine toxicosis in the cat, *JAVMA* 169:327, 1976.

Kao J and others: Ascorbic acid stimulates production of glycosaminoglycans in cultured fibroblasts, *Exper Mol Pathol* 53:1, 1990.

Kline K and others: Vitamin E modulation of retrovirus-induced immune dysfunctions and tumor cell proliferation: vitamin E biochemistry and health implications, *Ann N Y Acad Sci* 570:470, 1989.

Knight JA: Diseases related to oxygen-derived free radicals, *Ann Clinl Lab Sci* 25(2):111, 1995.

Leboy PS and others: Ascorbic acid induction of chondrocyte maturation: bone and mineral, *J Orthop Res* 17:242, 1992.

Leveque JI: Ascorbic acid in the treatment of canine distemper complex, *Vet Med Small Anim Clinician* 997:1000, 1968.

Levine M: New concepts in the biology and biochemistry of ascorbic acid, *N Engl J Med* 892:902, 1986.

Melman SA: Skin deep: organize diagnosis and treatment of allergy, pyoderma, seborrhea, *Vet Product News* 7(5):18, 1995.

Osborne CA, Lulich J, Polzin D: Feline lower urinary tract disease, *DVM Mag* 25(10):13, 1994.

Padh H: Vitamin C: newer insights into its biochemical functions, *Nutr Rev* 49(3):65, 1991.

Parker AJ, Small E: *Canine medicine,* ed 4, vol 2, Modern Veterinary Textbook Series, American Veterinary, 1979.

Penn ND and others: The effects of dietary supplementation with vitamins A, C, and E on cell-mediated immune function in elderly long-stay patients: a randomized controlled trial, *Age and Aging* 20:169, 1991.

Reynolds RD: Vitamin supplements: current controversies, *J Am Coll Nutr* 13:118, 1994.

Rosen GM and others: Free radicals and phagocytic cells, *FASEB J* 9:200, 1995.

Russell JE, Manske PR: Ascorbic acid requirement for optimal flexor tendon repair in vitro, *J Orthop Res* 714:719, 1991.

Schnelle GB: *Radiology in canine practice,* Evanston, Ill, 1945, North American Veterinarian.

Scott DW, Miller WH, Griffin CE: *Small animal dermatology,* ed 5, Philadelphia, 1995, WB Saunders.

Scott JA: Biochemical similarities of ascorbic acid and interferon, *J Ther Biol* 98:235, 1982.

Sherding RG, editor: *The cat: diseases and clinical management,* 1988, Churchill.

Sodikoff C: *Laboratory profiles of small animal diseases,* ed 2, St Louis, 1995, Mosby.

Subramanian N: Detoxication of histamine with ascorbic acid, *Biochem Pharmacol* 22:1671, 1973.

Takahashi M and others: Mode of action of vitamin E as antioxidant in membranes as studied by spin labeling: vitamin E biochemistry and health implications, *Ann N Y Acad Sci* 570:521, 1989.

Tams TR: Inflammatory bowel disease: an important cause of vomiting and diarrhea in cats. Paper presented at Kal Kan 12th Annual Symposium, p 19, Oct 1988.

Taton GF, Hamar DW, Lewis LD: Urinary acidification in the prevention and treatment of feline struvite urolithiasis, *JAMA* 182:437, 1984.

Tomlinson J, McLaughlin R, Jr: Canine hip dysplasia: developmental factors, clinical signs, and initial examination steps, *Vet Med* 91(1):26, 1996.

Wang Y, Watson RR: Is vitamin E supplementation a useful agent in AIDS therapy? *Prog Food Nutr Sci* 17:351, 1993.

Weber GF: Glutathione peroxidase deficiency and childhood seizures, *Lancet* 337:1443, 1991.

White SD, Ihrke: Immune-mediated diseases, *Feline Medicine,* ed 1, American Veterinary, 1983.

Willard MD: Nutritional therapy should play role in treatment of chronic bowel disorders, DVM, *The News Mag Vet Med* 26(6):4S, June 1995.

Wright J: Dr. *Wright's guide to healing with nutrition,* New Canaan, Conn, 1990, Keats.

SELECTED READINGS

Bendich A: Physiological role of antioxidants in the immune system, *J Dairy Sci* 76:2789, 1993.

Fleet JC: New support for a folk remedy: cranberry juice reduces bacteriuria and pyuria in elderly women, *Nutr Rev* 52(5):168, 1994.

Geesin JC, Gordon JS, Berg RA: Retinoids affect collagen synthesis through inhibition of ascorbate-induced lipid peroxidation in cultured human dermal fibroblasts, *Arch Biochem Biophys* 278(2):350, 1990.

Kurtz TW, Al-Banar HA, Morris RC, Jr: "Salt-sensitive" essential hypertension in men, *N Engl J Med* 317:1043, 1987.

Padh H: Cellular functions of ascorbic acid, *Biochem Cell Biol* 68:1166, 1990.

Pinnell SR, Murad S, Darr D: Induction of collagen synthesis by ascorbic acid, *Arch Dermatol* 123:1684, 1987.

Shaw DH: Lower urinary tract infections: how they arise and how the body combats them, *Vet Med* **:344, 1990.

Trentham DE and others: Effects of oral administration of type II collagen on rheumatoid arthritis, *Science* 296:1727, 1993.

Physical Medicine

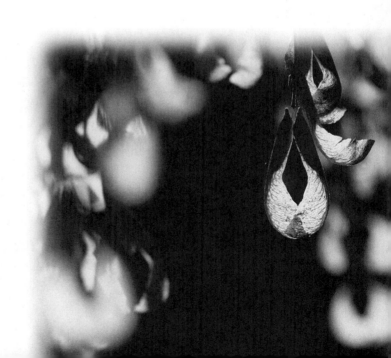

Chapter 9

Traditional Chinese Medical Theory

JOHN B. LIMEHOUSE, PRISCILLA A. TAYLOR

Definition

Acupuncture is one of the oldest methods of Chinese therapy. The term *acupuncture* comes from the Latin words *acus*, meaning "needle," and *pungere*, meaning "to pierce." This method involves piercing the skin with slender needles at predetermined foci called *acupuncture points* to prevent or treat disease. Stimulation of these points by modern methods includes needling, injection, ultrasound, laser, ultraviolet, magnetic induction, and electrical stimulation.

Western and Chinese Medicine— A Comparison

Although the basic concepts and conceits of Western and Chinese medicine differ widely, both disciplines address the same physical disorders. Each school embodies concepts that are foreign to the other. Traditional Chinese medicine (TCM) considers neither the endocrine nor peripheral nervous systems, and Western medicine has no format for diagnoses of diseases caused by "external pathogenic factors" such as Heat, Cold, Wind, or Damp. However, practitioners of both types use their training to achieve the same goal—the optimal health of the patient (Kaptchuk, 1983).

The difference between the two approaches has been compared to the difference between the mindset of a mechanic versus that of a gardener. The doctor of Western medicine is trained to detect specific diseases or disorders in the patient—to assess where the body has malfunctioned and repair or replace the damaged part. The practitioner of TCM strives to view the patient and the disease in terms of their relationship to each other and then helps the body return to a balanced state, thereby "tending the garden" rather than "fixing the machine."

Yin-Yang Theory

Health can be defined as a state of harmony that exists between the body and its internal and external environment. When such a state of harmony exists, the organism is said to have adapted successfully to its internal and external environment so that it can carry on its functions. Factors that influence the external environment include nutrition, climate, and geophysical and electromagnetic forces. The internal factors include hereditary influences, the neuroendocrine system, and the emotional state. According to this concept, health is not an absolute but a relative state of being.

Disease arises when an imbalance occurs within the internal environment or between the internal and external environment. Illness usually results from several causes working together and overloading the homeostatic mechanisms of the body. The early Chinese explained this relationship as the *Yin-Yang* theory, which is based on the philosophical principle of two polar complements of *Qi*, or *Ch'i* (pronounced *chee*). The theory of *Yin* and *Yang* is derived from centuries of observing nature and describes the way in which phenomena naturally group in pairs of opposites. All phenomena in the universe may be placed in either the *Yin* or the *Yang* category. Balance or equilibrium is maintained by the mutual antagonism as well as mutual dependence of opposing forces. *Yin* exists by virtue of *Yang*, and *Yang* exists by virtue of *Yin*.

The interdependent relation of *Yin* and *Yang* means that each of the two aspects is the condition for the other's existence and neither of them can exist in isolation. For instance, without daytime there would be no night. Hence, it can be seen that *Yin* and *Yang* are at once in opposition and in interdependence; they rely on each other for existence, coexisting in a single entity. The movement and change of a thing are the result not only of the opposition and conflict between

Yin and *Yang* but also of their relationship of interdependence and mutual support (Beijing, Shanghai and Nanjing Colleges of Traditional Chinese Medicine, 1980).

In medicine the concept of interdependence of *Yin* and *Yang* is widely used in physiology, pathology, and treatment. Blood and *Qi*, two fundamental elements of the human body, provide an example: in relation to each other, Blood is *Yin* and *Qi* is *Yang*. *Yin* is related to fluids in the body, which includes all water and blood. *Yang* is related to the metabolism in the body.

The Concept of *Qi*

Qi is the force or energy that controls harmony in the human body. It is the "Vital Force" or "Life Energy" that activates and maintains the life process. This energy is derived from our environment through such processes as nutrition and respiration, converted into an absorbable form by certain organs, and stored in the body and distributed throughout the system by other organs. Basically, everything that exists is defined by its *Qi*. It is matter on the verge of becoming energy; it is energy on the verge of becoming matter; it is tangible and it is intangible. *Qi* denotes function, process, and change. *Qi* is necessary to digest food, but the food itself creates the growth. *Qi* is responsible for movement and movement produces *Qi*, but *Qi* is not movement.

Basic Functions of *Qi*

Promotion
Qi is the source of all movement in the body (Stiteler, 1984) and is in all parts of the body at all times. It flows to the organs, muscles, and joints of the body in four primary movements: ascending, descending, entering, and exiting. When this movement stops, life ceases.

Protection
The outer defense of the body, *Qi* prevents pathogenic influences from entering. When disease develops in the body, *Qi* becomes active and fights to destroy the pathogen and restore balance.

Transformation
Each organ has its own share or source of *Qi* and functions to transform it into a substance available to the body. Spleen *Qi* transforms food into energy, Lung *Qi* transforms air into oxygen, and the *Qi* of the Chest transforms Food *Qi* into Blood.

Retention
Qi holds organs in their place and thereby prevents hernias and prolapses. By holding fluids in their place, it keeps blood in the vessels and prevents hemorrhage. This function also keeps the pores open or closed as necessary, thus

regulating normal sweat production. It prevents excess fluid loss from incontinence or enuresis.

Warming
Qi is vitality or "creative life." It is the fire that ignites metabolism and is closely related to the adrenal glands. This *Qi* produces heat and therefore controls the temperature of the body.

Nourishment
The nutrient substance *Ying Qi* circulates in the blood vessels, thereby nourishing the body (Xinnong, 1987).

Types of *Qi*

Different types of *Qi* exist, depending on its location in the body and its function. These different aspects of activity allow it to be called by different names: Organ *Qi*, Channel *Qi*, Nutritive *Qi*, Defensive *Qi*, Gathering *Qi*, and Prenatal *Qi*.

Organ *Qi*
Each of the internal organs has its own *Qi*, which is the basis of its activity and physiologic functions.

Channel, or meridian, *Qi*
Channel, or meridian, *Qi* flows through the meridians and is controlled by needles at acupuncture points. The sensation felt when a needle is inserted and manipulated is this *Qi* being stimulated.

Nutritive *Qi*
Nutritive *Qi* forms the blood and flows in the vessels, nourishing the entire body.

Defensive *Qi*
The Chinese call Defensive *Qi Wei Qi*. This *Qi* flows outside the vessels and is described as bold and uninhibited. It functions near the exterior, just underneath the skin and above the muscles, and is mainly evident in the shoulder region and at the back of the neck. It provides resistance against disease.

Gathering *Qi*
Gathering *Qi* is the *Qi* of the chest. It regulates the heartbeat and respiration.

Prenatal, or original, *Qi*
Prenatal, or original, *Qi* is basically limited to a set amount supplied at birth. It is depleted throughout life by illness, drugs, excess sex, and alcohol. This *Qi* is mainly stored in the kidneys.

Qi is a mixture of opposing forces: *Yin* (the passive or negative force) and *Yang* (the active or positive force). The totally balanced system has equal amounts of *Yin* and *Yang*. Neither can exist in isolation: some *Yin* always exists in *Yang* and some *Yang* in *Yin* (Fig. 9-1). Each is necessary for the other, yet each opposes the other. For example, for life to exist (as we know it on our planet), a balance of sunlight and darkness is necessary. (Table 9-1 shows some other examples of *Yin-Yang*.)

Yin-Yang is dynamic and seldom in exact balance. For example, in winter, darkness exceeds daylight (*Yin* is predominant) and in the Summer, daylight exceeds darkness (*Yang* is predominant). Equal amounts of *Yin* and *Yang* (night/day) occur only at the equinoxes (March 21 and September 23). The limits of *Yin* and *Yang* are seen at the winter solstice (December 21), when *Yin* is maximal (relative to *Yang*) and the summer solstice (June 21), when *Yang* is maximal (relative to *Yin*). This transformation of *Yin* to *Yang* and *Yang* to *Yin* is a natural, universal phe-

nomenon. *Yin* predominates at certain times, and *Yang* predominates at other times, in dynamic cycles.

Modern medicine easily accepts the idea of duality and relativity. We know that homeostasis in the body is maintained by mutually antagonistic but mutually dependent systems. For instance, besides the opposites listed in Table 9-1, health also requires the balance (harmony) of *Yin/Yang*: for example, sleep/wakefulness; flexor/extensor muscles; sensory/motor systems; calcitonin/parathyroid hormone. We also know that an excess or deficiency of any one of these can lead to an imbalance in the system and may eventually lead to disease. Thus the TCM concept of *Yin-Yang* is not as foreign as it may seem at first glance.

Pathology of *Qi*

In TCM, pathologies are called *disharmonies* or *disorders* of *Qi*. The primary disharmonies are deficiency, stagnation, rebellion, and collapse of *Qi* (Kaptchuk, 1983).

Deficient *Qi*

Deficient *Qi* occurs when an organ does not contain sufficient energy. If deficiency occurs in the Spleen or Stomach, a digestive problem results. Poor digestion indicates a Spleen *Qi* deficiency. *Qi* deficiencies may manifest as fatigue, shortness of breath, weak voice, poor appetite, enuresis, and weakness of any organ. Deficiency is usually caused by a chronic illness, old age, poor nutrition, or congenital weakness.

Stagnant *Qi*

Normally, *Qi* circulates smoothly throughout the entire body without any blockages. If a disturbance occurs because of trauma, pathogens, or emotions, the flow is blocked. *Qi* stagnation can progress into Blood and Fluid

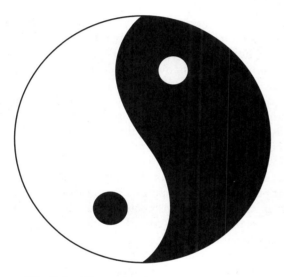

Fig. 9-1 The traditional *Yin-Yang* symbol.

TABLE 9-1

EXAMPLES OF YIN AND YANG (STATES OF RELATIVE OPPOSITES)

YIN	YANG	YIN	YANG
Water	Fire	Water	Steam
Ice	Water	Cold	Hot
Solid	Gas	Female	Male
Passive	Active	Material	Nonmaterial
Slow	Fast	Dark	Bright
Night	Day	Winter	Summer
Moon	Sun	Downward	Upward
Precipitation	Evaporation	Inner	Outer
Below waist	Above waist	Ventral	Dorsal
Medial	Lateral	Inhibition	Excitation
Relaxation	Contraction	Parasympathetic	Sympathetic
Hypo (deficient)	Hyper (excess)	Chronic	Acute

Stagnation, which is manifested in the body as cysts, clots, and even tumors. *Qi* stagnation in the lungs is a form of asthma in which the air does not move and is therefore stagnant. The main symptoms of *Qi* stagnation are distention, swelling, dyspnea, and local pain.

Rebellious *Qi*

When the normal pattern of *Qi* movement is in an ascending or descending direction and the reverse occurs, this change indicates rebellious *Qi*. Rebellious *Qi* is associated with nausea, vomiting, belching, and hiccups.

Collapse of *Qi*

When *Qi* deficiency has progressed to the point at which the organ or meridian can no longer perform its basic functions, collapse of *Qi* exists. This condition may be limited to gross physical abnormalities—hernias or prolapses secondary to collapse of Spleen *Qi*—or may even mean death if the condition progresses to collapse of *Yang*.

Blood

Formation and Function

Relative to *Qi*, Blood is more *Yin*. It flows primarily through vessels and is pumped by the heart to circulate throughout the whole body. According to TCM, blood is primarily produced in the chest by the function of the *Qi* from the Lungs and Spleen but is also produced in bone marrow. Certain organs are intimately related to Blood. Along with the Heart, which controls the movement of Blood, the Spleen holds Blood in the vessels, and the Liver stores and distributes it. Blood has three primary functions: to nourish, maintain, and moisten. These functions affect the skin, body hair, tendons, bones, organs, channels, and other tissue relying on the Blood for nutrition.

Relationship Between *Qi* and Blood

In TCM, *Qi* and Blood are the two basic, classic elements of all physiologic activity. *Qi* denotes function and helps make the Blood. Blood nourishes the organs that make the *Qi*. Therefore, we see that they complement and depend on each other; they are different from each other, yet they are inseparable. An ancient Chinese saying explains their relationship as follows:

> *Qi* is the commander of Blood. Where *Qi* goes, the Blood must follow. Blood is the Mother of *Qi*. Where the *Qi* is, Blood is already there (Institute of Acupuncture and Moxibustion, 1982).

Blood Disorders

Disorders or disharmonies of the Blood are deficiency and stagnation.

Blood deficiency

Insufficient Blood results from either hemorrhage or lack of production. Generally, Blood deficiency is a chronic condition usually accompanied by anemia, but not all deficiencies of Blood involve anemia. Characteristic symptoms include insomnia, palpitations, dizziness, dry skin, contracted tendons, and dry or lifeless hair.

Blood stagnation

Blood stagnation is caused by an obstruction in the flow of Blood or the accumulation of Blood in a local area. The obstruction is usually caused by trauma and characterized by signs such as bruises, lumps, painful swellings, blood clots, and stabbing pain at the point of stagnation.

Meridian Theory

As the pathways by which *Qi* and Blood circulate in the body, meridians form the basis of acupuncture. They are not physically visible, but their existence and distribution throughout the body have been amply demonstrated by the measurement of neuroelectric potentials. The meridian system unifies all parts of the organism, connecting the internal organs with the external body, and maintaining harmony and equilibrium.

The organs of the body are divided into six *Yin* and six *Yang* organs, collectively referred to as the *Zang-fu* organs. In TCM, organs are always discussed with reference to their function as well as their specific structure. Because *Yang* organs are those containing smooth muscle, they are subject to spastic conditions such as colic. They function to absorb nutrients and eliminate waste products. *Yin* organs process the absorbed nutritive substances and store metabolic products; thus an individual's health depends on the function of these organs. (*Yin* and *Yang* organs are listed in Box 9-1.)

BOX 9-1

Yin and *Yang* Organs of the Body

YANG ORGANS (HOLLOW ORGANS OF THE BODY)	
Stomach	ST
Small intestine	SI
Large intestine	LI
Gallbladder, including bile ducts	GB
Urinary bladder, including ureter and urethra	BL
Triple heater	TH

YIN ORGANS (SOLID ORGANS OF THE BODY)	
Liver	LIV
Spleen—pancreas	SP
Kidney	KI
Heart	HT
Lungs	LU
Pericardium or heart constrictor	

BOX 9-2

Summary of Different Types of Points or Classifications of Points

Alarm Points (*Mu* Points): Alarm points are located on the ventral part of the abdomen. An alarm point exists for each of the 12 *Zang fu* organs, but it may or may not lie on the same meridian for which it serves as the alarm point. Alarm points are used in both diagnosis and treatment. Sensitivity at an alarm point indicates a problem with the organ or meridian for which it is named (see Fig. 9-2 and Table 9-2).

Association Points (*Shu* Points): Association points can be the most important points in acupuncture diagnosis. These points are also named for the organ or meridian that they treat. All association points are located on the Bladder meridian along the back, about two finger widths on either side of the dorsal midline, lateral to the dorsal spinal processes. A painful response to light pressure indicates an acute condition, whereas pain from deep pressure indicates a chronic condition of that meridian or corresponding organ (see Fig. 9-3 and Table 9-2).

Tonification Points: These are used to increase or stimulate the energy flow on the corresponding meridians or to stimulate the organs themselves.

Sedation Points: Sedation points are used to selectively decrease energy level in a specific meridian or organ.

Source Points: These points, always located in the carpal or tarsal area, are often used in treatment of organ disease or dysfunction. They act to augment the action of the tonification and sedation points and are extremely powerful (see Table 9-2).

Luo Points (Connection Points): These points connect meridians: a *Yin* meridian is connected to a *Yang* meridian via the *Luo* Point. When stimulated, it permits the direct transfer of energy *(Qi)* from one meridian to its counterpart (e.g., Lung/Large Intestine, Spleen/Stomach, Heart/Small Intestine, Kidney/Bladder, Pericardium/Triple Heater, Liver/Gallbladder) (see Table 9-2).

Horary Points (Element Points): Five elements are found in TCM. Each meridian has a horary point for each of the elements. When the points are stimulated during the time of day at which the meridian receives its greatest energy, the effects are enhanced. *Qi* travels throughout the body in a circadian rhythm. Beginning with the Lung, which receives its maximum energy at 4:00 AM, *Qi* moves through a different organ every 2 hours until it reaches the Liver at 2:00 AM (see Fig. 9-4).

Accumulation Points (*Xi*-Cleft Points): These points represent the location on the meridian at which energy is greatest. They are responsive in acute cases and are used for sedation (see Table 9-2).

Trigger Points or Local Points: These points are apparent only when a localized pathologic process is occurring. They may or may not lie directly on an established meridian. Acupuncture or acupressure can be applied directly to these points to treat the area involved.

Extra Points: These points are not found on meridians but do have special effects, usually on nearby areas.

Auricular Points (Ear Points): Such points are used for auricular acupuncture. These points on the ear correspond to different parts of the body and can be used either in place of or in addition to points on the primary meridians.

Master Points: Six master points can be used in treating conditions in certain areas (see Table 9-3).

Special Action Points: These points are used solely for their influential effects (see Table 9- 4). (See Table 9-2 for a complete list of the command, alarm *[Mu]*, association *[Shu]*, *Luo*, and accumulation *[Xi*-Cleft] points.)

The meridian system comprises the 12 regular meridians, each one corresponding to one of the 12 *Zang-fu* organs. In addition, eight extra, nonpaired channels exist, with different pathways than the 12 regular meridians, that do not connect directly with the *Zang-fu* organs. Of these eight extra meridians, only two are considered major because only they have points not found on any other meridian. These two channels, the *Du* (or Governing Vessel) and *Ren* (or Conception Vessel), along with the 12 regular meridians, comprise the 14 major meridians used in contemporary acupuncture. Other collateral meridians, connecting other areas of the body, also exist, and their use is indicated in specific conditions.

Meridian theory assumes that channels can be used diagnostically as well as therapeutically. Disorders of the organs may be manifested peripherally via the meridians, and resolution of the imbalance in the meridian treats the root cause (Kaptchuk, 1983).

Acupuncture Points

Along the meridians are *acupuncture points,* or *acupoints.* These points range in size from 1 mm to 25 mm and can be located by their electrical conductivity, which differs from that of surrounding tissue. Acupoints are used both to diagnose and to treat conditions. When palpated, the points may be sensitive if *Qi* is imbalanced (i.e., a deficiency of *Yang* and an excess of *Yin* or an excess of *Yang* and a deficiency of *Yin*.)

Classic acupuncture theory recognizes about 365 acupuncture points located on the surface meridians. With the inclusion of miscellaneous points and new points used in ear acupuncture and other recent methods, the total has risen to at least 2000 points that may be used. In practice, however, a typical doctor's repertoire would include only 150 points (Kaptchuk, 1983, p 80).

Each acupuncture point has a defined and specific function based on the response of the body. Some points may be used singly, but it is more common to use several points, treated simultaneously, to achieve the desired effect. A typical treatment may involve the use of as few as one to as many as 20 acupuncture points. (Box 9-2 summarizes the different types or classifications of points.)

The Five Phases

The theory of the Five Phases is based on the idea that everything in the universe is the product of the movement and change of five basic elements: Wood, Fire, Earth, Metal, and Water. In TCM, this theory has had a major influence on diagnosis, treatment, pathology, and physiology. In Chinese philosophy the interaction of the five elements explains the nature of all phenomena. These elements are not actual matter but concepts. This conceptual basis has caused problems for Western doctors trying to incorporate Chinese theory into a practice that emphasizes matter.

Cycles

Placing these Phases on a circle makes it easier to visualize laws that govern the five elements (Fig. 9-5). Two distinct cycles of the elements are used in diagnosis and treatment: the *Sheng* cycle and the *Ko* cycle.

The Sheng cycle

The *Sheng* cycle is one of creation or production (Fig. 9-6). A certain phase creates another to its right in a clockwise fashion, which produces the next one, and so on around the circle. Therefore Fire produces Earth, Earth produces Metal, Metal produces Water, Water produces Wood, and Wood produces Fire. More specifically, when Fire burns, it produces ashes, which then go into Earth. From the Earth we receive ore, which is made into Metal. Metal at high temperatures becomes molten or liquid, which gives off steam, thus producing Water. Wood is produced from this Water, much as vegetation needs water or moisture to grow. When burned, this Wood gives off Fire, thus completing the Creative, or *Sheng*, Cycle. Commonly used terms are *Mother* and *Son*. The promoting element represents the Mother, and the one it promotes represents the Son. According to these terms, Wood is the Mother of Fire and Fire is the Son of Wood.

The Ko cycle

The *Ko* cycle is one of control or destruction (Fig. 9-7). Everything created in nature can be destroyed. Destruction is nature's way of keeping things in balance so that nothing can become harmful by being too powerful. Wood restrains Earth, Earth restrains Water, Water restrains Fire, Fire restrains Metal, and Metal restrains Wood. For example, Wood destroys Earth when its roots erupt through the Earth's surface and its leaves shadow or cover the ground. Earth destroys Water by damming the flow of Water through the Earth or absorbing it into the ground. Water destroys Fire in an obvious way. Fire destroys Metal by melting it. Metal destroys Wood by cutting into it or chopping it down. Other cycles represent disruptions, but that information is not pertinent to this discussion.

In TCM the Five Elements are used to categorize organs, tissues, senses, colors, seasons, and emotions (Table 9-5). Early in the development of Chinese medicine the Five Element theory was used to explain physiologic and pathologic processes in the body. The meridians and organs interact in a particular way when one part of the body is diseased. According to the Five Element theory, other tissues may become involved because of the Creation *(Sheng)* Cycle or Destruction *(Ko)* Cycle. For example, when the Liver has a disease, this disease can be transmitted to the Heart. In this instance the Mother is affecting the Son. When a disease of the Liver affects the Spleen, it may be described as Wood dominating Earth. These pathologic influences can also be expressed in clinical, Western terms.

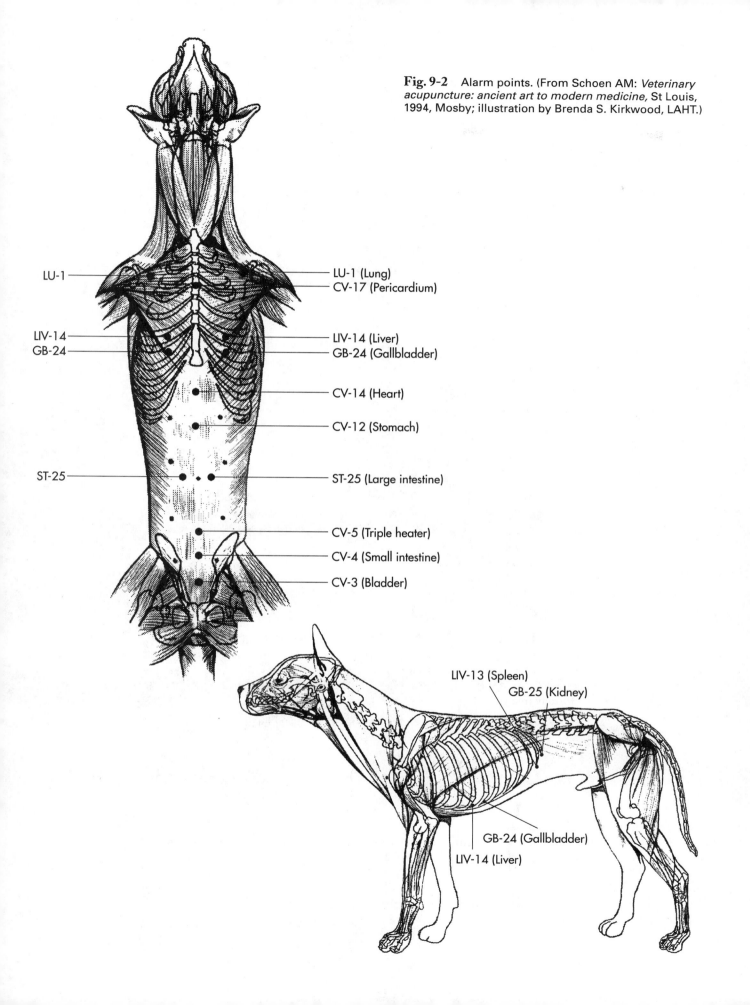

LU-1

LIV-14
GB-24

ST-25

LU-1 (Lung)
CV-17 (Pericardium)

LIV-14 (Liver)
GB-24 (Gallbladder)

CV-14 (Heart)

CV-12 (Stomach)

ST-25 (Large intestine)

CV-5 (Triple heater)

CV-4 (Small intestine)

CV-3 (Bladder)

Fig. 9-2 Alarm points. (From Schoen AM: *Veterinary acupuncture: ancient art to modern medicine,* St Louis, 1994, Mosby; illustration by Brenda S. Kirkwood, LAHT.)

LIV-13 (Spleen)
GB-25 (Kidney)

GB-24 (Gallbladder)

LIV-14 (Liver)

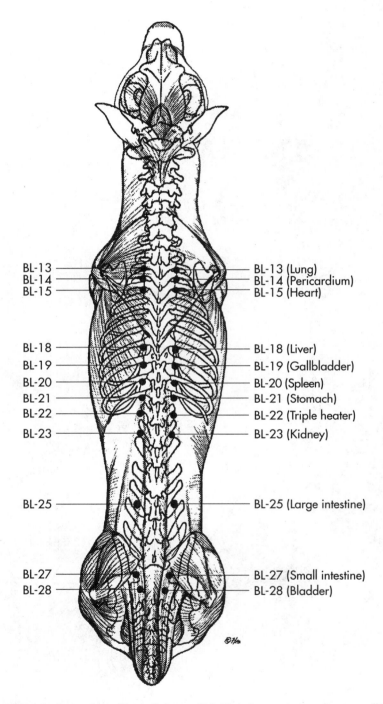

BL-13 — BL-13 (Lung)
BL-14 — BL-14 (Pericardium)
BL-15 — BL-15 (Heart)

BL-18 — BL-18 (Liver)
BL-19 — BL-19 (Gallbladder)
BL-20 — BL-20 (Spleen)
BL-21 — BL-21 (Stomach)
BL-22 — BL-22 (Triple heater)
BL-23 — BL-23 (Kidney)

BL-25 — BL-25 (Large intestine)

BL-27 — BL-27 (Small intestine)
BL-28 — BL-28 (Bladder)

Fig. 9-3 Association points. (From Schoen AM: *Veterinary acupuncture: ancient art to modern medicine,* St Louis, 1994, Mosby; illustration by Brenda S. Kirkwood, LAHT.)

TABLE 9-2

COMMAND AND SPECIAL ACTION POINTS

	METAL		EARTH		FIRE		WATER		FIRE		WOOD	
	LU	LI	ST	SP	HT	SI	BL	KI	PC	TH	GB	LIV
Wood	11	3	43	1	9	3	65	1	9	3	41	1
Fire	10	5	41	2	8	5	60	2	8	6	38	2
Earth	9	11	36	3	7	8	40	3	7	10	34	3
Metal	8	1	45	5	4	1	67	7	5	1	44	4
Water	5	2	44	9	3	2	66	10	3	2	43	8
Source	9	4	42	3	7	4	64	3	7	4	40	3
Luo	7	6	40	4	5	7	58	4	6	5	37	5
Xi-Cleft	6	7	34	8	6	6	63	5	4	7	36	6
Mu	LU-1	ST-25	CV-12	LIV-13	CV-14	CV-4	CV-3	GB-25	CV-17	CV-5	GB-24	LIV-14
Shu	BL-13	BL-25	BL-21	BL-20	BL-15	BL-27	BL-28	BL-23	BL-14	BL-22	BL-19	BL-18

TABLE 9-3

MASTER POINTS

MASTER POINTS	REGION
LI-4	Face and mouth
LU-7	Head and neck
PC-6	Chest and cranial abdomen
BL-40	Back and hips
ST-36	Abdomen and gastrointestinal
SP-6	Caudal abdomen and urogenital

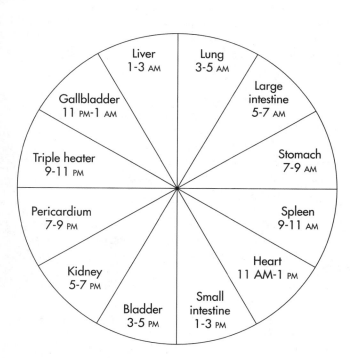

Fig. 9-4 The circadian (Chinese) clock.

TABLE 9-4

INFLUENTIAL POINTS

SPECIAL ACTION POINTS	INFLUENCES
BL-11	Bone
BL-12	Wind and trachea
BL-17	Blood and diaphragm
GB-34	Tendons
GB-39	Marrow
CV-17	*Qi*
LU-9	Arteries
CV-12	*Yang* organs
LIV-13	*Yin* organs
ST-40	Phlegm

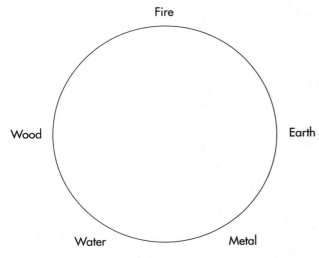

Fig. 9-5   The Five Phases.

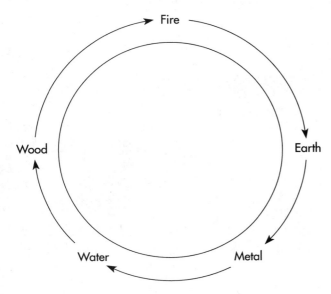

Fig. 9-6   The *Sheng* cycle.

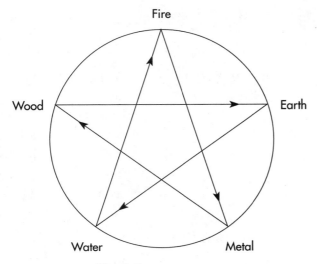

Fig. 9-7   The *Ko* cycle.

Treatment using the *Sheng* cycle

Specific points on each meridian correspond to each of the Five Phases, and points representing each of the Five Elements appear on each meridian (Table 9-6). These points are referred to as *command points* and are used clinically in the *Sheng* cycle according to the theory of the "Mother-Son Law." This law states the following:

> In a deficiency condition, tonify the Mother; in an excess condition, sedate the Son.

Clinical examples

Azotemia; chronic renal disease: This signifies a Kidney deficiency (Water) and is treated by tonifying the Mother point (Metal) on the Kidney meridian (KI-7).

Syncope; irregular, weak pulse: This indicates a Heart deficiency (Fire) and is treated by tonifying the Mother point (Wood) on the Heart meridian (HT-9).

Hyperthyroidism with cardiomyopathy: This is an excess condition of the Heart (Fire) and is treated by sedating the Son point (Earth) on the Heart meridian (HT-7).

Feline urologic syndrome with crystalluria: An excess condition of the Bladder (Water), feline urologic syndrome is treated by sedating the Son point (Wood) on the Bladder meridian (BL-65).

Treatment using the *Ko* cycle

The same principles of tonification and sedation are followed when using the Ko cycle, but the theory (law) is as follows: *In an excess, tonify the Grandparent; in a deficiency, sedate the Grandparent.* In this situation, the "Grandparent" is the element that restrains or destroys.

Clinical examples

Convulsions: This condition indicates Liver excess (Wood), which is treated by tonifying the Metal point on the Liver meridian (LIV-4).

Canine infectious tracheobronchitis: This indicates a Lung excess (Metal) and is treated by tonifying the Fire point on the Lung meridian (LU-10).

Treatment using both the *Sheng* and the *Ko* cycles

In an excess, sedate the Son and tonify the Grandparent; in a deficiency, tonify the Mother and sedate the Grandparent.

Clinical examples

Convulsions: This condition indicates Liver excess and is treated by sedating the Fire point and tonifying the Metal point on the Liver meridian (LIV-2 and LIV-4, respectively).

Chronic renal disease: This indicates a Kidney deficiency. Treat by tonifying the Metal point and sedating the Earth point on the Kidney meridian (KI-7 and KI-3, respectively).

Many practitioners use the Five-Element theory successfully in treating conditions involving internal organs

TABLE 9-5

CLASSIFICATION BY THE FIVE ELEMENTS

	WOOD	FIRE	EARTH	METAL	WATER
Yin Organ	Liver	Heart	Spleen/pancreas	Lung	Kidney
Yang Organ	Gallbladder	Small Intestine	Stomach	Large Intestine	Bladder
Tissue	Tendons	Blood vessels	Flesh	Skin	Bones
Sense organ	Eyes	Tongue	Mouth	Nose	Ears
Sense	Sight	Speech	Taste	Smell	Hearing
Season	Spring	Summer	Indian Summer	Fall	Winter
Emotion	Anger	Joy	Worry/obsession	Grief	Fear
Expression	Shouting, sighing	Laughing	Singing	Crying	Groaning
Taste	Sour	Bitter	Sweet	Pungent	Salty
Color	Green	Red	Yellow	White	Blue/black

TABLE 9-6

CLASSIFICATION BY THE EIGHT CONDITIONS

	YANG	*YIN*
Location	Exterior	Interior
Quality	Heat'	Cold
Quantity	Excess	Deficiency

or joints and tendons along the meridians. When using this approach, practitioners should realize the limitations. These theories were developed at various stages of Chinese history and are incomplete. For this reason, the Five-Element theory cannot fully explain all organ functions, but it can be used for making analogies and broad generalizations. Although the terms *Yin* and *Yang* are still used today in general practice, reference to the organs by their corresponding elements is becoming less common. For greater clarity the organs are referred to by their own names.

The Role of External Pathogenic Factors in Disease

TCM views disease or dysfunction as a reflection of the imbalance between the Defensive *Qi* of the body and the invasion or influence of one or several environmental factors. These environmental influences, variously referred to as *pernicious evils* or *external pathogenic factors,* are considered the true causes of disease, capable of causing direct injury to the body. The analysis of the influence of these pathogens is extremely significant in determining appropriate treatment.

The six external pathogenic factors—Wind, Cold, Summer Heat, Dampness, Dryness, and Heat—are nat-ural phenomena that can invade a body already in a state of disharmony or imbalance. If Defensive *Qi* is adequate, the illness remains superficial and recovery is rapid. However, when the pathogen is stronger than the patient's defenses, more severe illness involving the organs may result.

Each factor has specific characteristics. Wind is associated with constant movement; Cold with contraction and immobility; Summer Heat with extreme heat and dehydration; Dampness with heaviness and turbidity; Dryness with dehydration, especially of the respiratory system; and Heat with fever, inflammation and eruptions of the skin, and constipation. Each factor is more common at specific times of the year, depending on local climate. Wind invasion is most common during the spring, Cold during the winter, and Heat primarily during the summer months. Pathogens may appear individually or in combination (i.e. invasion of Damp-Heat or Cold-Damp). Treatment is directed at resolving the existing imbalance and strengthening the Defensive *Qi.*

Illnesses caused by the invasion of external pathogenic factors are usually acute in onset and characterized by aversion to the climatic condition causing the syndrome. Pathogenic factors may also arise internally, manifesting similar signs in a subacute or chronic state. Ultimately, pathogenic factors may be viewed as models for disease processes that resemble or mimic specific aspects of nature.

Eight Conditions

TCM uses several methods to diagnose disease, including the Five-Phases theory, the theory of meridians and collaterals, the theory of *Qi* and Blood, the theory of *Yin* and *Yang* organs *(Zang-fu),* and differentiation of disease according to the Eight Conditions. Combinations of these theories can be used to refine or expand on the diagnosis and disease process. For the experienced doctor, diagnosis depends on understanding the cause or causes of the disease. Without an understanding of the Eight Conditions, most of TCM is incomprehensible. Modern Chinese acupuncture and herbalism use this system more than any of the others.

The Eight Conditions are expressed as opposites: *Yin* and *Yang,* internal and external, cold and hot, and deficiency and excess. Based on a primary consideration of *Yin* and *Yang* pathology, these principles allow further identification of the location, quality, and quantity of the pathogenic factor (see Table 9-6).

Characteristics of each subdivision become useful when using this aspect of TCM in diagnosis. *Yin* and *Yang* are general terms that usually incorporate the other six conditions, because Exterior, Heat, and Excess are *Yang,* and Interior, Cold, and Deficiency are *Yin. Interior* and *exterior* refer to the depth and location of the disease and are useful in identifying the exogenous etiology as well as the course of development. Pathogens rarely invade the interior without first passing through the exterior. *Heat* and *cold* describe the quality or nature of the disease and the activity or reaction of the body and provide clues as to whether warming or cooling herbs should be used in treatment. Finally, the terms *excess* and *deficiency* indicate the relative strength of the pathogen versus antipathogenic *Qi (Wei Qi).* If the *Wei Qi* is strong or compromised, the strength of the antipathogenic factor itself and the presence of either hypofunction or hyperfunction of the *Zang-Fu* organs involved must be considered. One of the most important conditions in classifying disease, this differentiation between excess and deficiency determines whether the treatment should involve stimulating or sedating.

The Eight Conditions are seldom expressed singularly; TCM practitioners rarely speak of a simple *"Yang"* or "Cold" condition. More commonly, these principles are considered together to describe the condition at hand. For example, the dog who has a fever and a harsh, loud, productive cough with yellow mucus is described as exhibiting a Lung *Yang* excess with Heat signs. The elderly cat with failing kidneys who moves slowly, meows weakly, and seeks heat shows a pattern characteristic of a Kidney *Yin* deficiency with Cold.

Clinical Examples

Case 1: An elderly dog exhibits generalized weakness, polyuria/polydipsia, lethargy, and loss of hearing.

TCM DIAGNOSIS: Loss of hearing (ears) is associated with the Kidneys, and decreased hearing indicates decreased Kidney energy. The Kidney is also responsible for maintenance of the bones and marrow. (In TCM, *marrow* refers to the brain as well as the bone marrow.) Weakness and lethargy indicate a deficiency condition; as other signs refer to the Kidney, this pattern is characteristic of Kidney *Yin* deficiency.

TREATMENT PRINCIPLE: Tonify Kidney and marrow; build *Yin.*

POINTS: BL-17, BL-23, BL-52, GB-25, KI-3, SP-6.

Case 2: A male dog exhibits hematuria and stranguria.

TCM DIAGNOSIS: The presence of hematuria and stranguria may indicate Heat and Dampness, respectively. This pattern is characteristic of Damp Heat in the Bladder.

TREATMENT PRINCIPLE: Eliminate the Damp and Heat.

POINTS: CV-3, BL-20, BL-28, BL-39, BL-40, SP-6, KI-3, KI- 6.

When treating diseases using the Eight Conditions, the doctor must have a working knowledge of the action and use of each acupuncture point. Some points stimulate one area of an organ, whereas other points sedate the same area. Some relieve excess Heat, whereas others relieve the pain from excess Cold conditions. The novice practitioner can select and use some basic formulas or groups of points. A proficient doctor abandons formulas, practicing acupuncture by determining the cause of the imbalance and then restoring the body's balance by selecting points according to their indication. Formulas can be found in the many human-oriented books marketed to the Western doctor and are a good way to start using acupuncture in practice while developing knowledge and proficiency. Use of these formulas in the treatment of common diseases helps bridge the gap between the Western and Eastern approaches.

TCM and Chinese Herbs

The Eight Conditions and Five Phases are also used in prescribing Chinese herbal formulas. Used with acupuncture, appropriate Chinese herbs can greatly benefit patients. The eight basic therapeutic methods used in Chinese herbal medicine are sweating, vomiting, purging, harmonizing, warming, clearing, reducing, and tonifying (Bensky, Barolet, 1990). Herbs are classified by their inherent characteristics: energy, taste, action, properties, meridian attribution, and therapeutic category (Dharmananda, 1992) and prescribed accordingly. As such, a formula may be chosen to disperse Cold, Heat, Dampness, or Wind or relieve stasis or stagnation in an organ or meridian. Combinations of herbs are used to normalize rebellious *Qi* and to harmonize and fortify the *Zang-fu* organs. Once the TCM diagnosis has been made, the herbs may be used in their raw form (mixed by the practitioner) or obtained as "patent herbs" (already combined and available commercially).

The concurrent use of acupuncture and Chinese herbal therapy allows a complete approach to patient care using TCM, and careful study of both modalities is warranted by the interested practitioner.

*R*EFERENCES

Beijing, Shanghai, and Nanjing Colleges of Traditional Chinese Medicine: *Essentials of Chinese acupuncture,* Beijing, 1980, Foreign Language Press.

Bensky D, Barolet R: *Chinese herbal medicine: formulas and strategies,* Seattle, 1990, Eastland Press.

Dharmananda S: *Chinese herbology: a professional training program,* Portland, 1992, Institute for Traditional Medicine.

Institute of Acupuncture and Moxibustion: Class notes, Beijing, 1982, the Institute.

Kaptchuk T: *The web that has no weaver,* Chicago, 1983, Contemporary Books.

Stiteler S: Personal communication, 1984.

Xinnong C, editor: *Chinese acupuncture and moxibustion,* Beijing, 1987, Foreign Language Press.

Chapter 10

Small Animal Acupuncture: Scientific Basis and Clinical Applications

SHELDON ALTMAN

Traditional Chinese Medicine

Acupuncture, in the Eastern view, is part of a complete medical system called *traditional Chinese medicine (TCM)*. This system embraces acupuncture, moxibustion, massage, breathing exercises, nutrition, herbal medicine, and even philosophy of life. The theory of TCM is that living creatures are a microcosm within a macrocosm. In simpler terms, humans and animals are a small part of the infinite universe and are subject to the same laws that govern the rest of the living and (according to Western philosophy) nonliving cosmos. The same laws that affect the Earth, the heavens, the seasons, and other physical aspects of our environment also affect our physiology, emotions, and health. According to TCM, an understanding of health begins with an understanding of nature and the laws that govern it. A person who follows the laws of nature properly will enjoy good health, a long life, contentment, and good fortune (Monte, 1993). Examination of a patient is conducted according to TCM techniques, with the aim of discovering an imbalance in the distribution or magnitude of life energy *(Qi)* within the patient's body (diagnosis). The aim of treatment is to rebalance the body's energy system (therapy). The ultimate goal is to discover the cause of the imbalance (etiology) and eliminate it from the environment or help the patient overcome the pathologic factor if reencountered (preventive medicine).

The Occidental Viewpoint

In the hands of many Western practitioners, acupuncture is a method of eliciting a physiologic response by stimulating specific anatomic loci. Diagnosis of pathology is done by conventional means, using physical examination, laboratory examination, radiology, ultrasonography, and other modern diagnostic techniques. The result is a conventional diagnosis. The practitioner then selects points that are known to have a beneficial effect on the malady being treated. Many formularies are available to guide practitioners in the selection of points for treating human and animal diseases and pathologic conditions. Some of the most common applications of acupuncture are to relieve pain, cause autonomic nerve responses, and, occasionally, induce surgical analgesia.

Definition of Acupuncture

Acupuncture is derived from the Latin words *acus,* meaning *needle,* and *punctura,* meaning *to prick.* In the narrowest sense, acupuncture is the insertion of very fine needles (Fig. 10-1) into specific predetermined points on the body to produce physiologic responses. In addition to needles, many other methods are used to stimulate acupuncture points. These include acupressure, moxibustion, cupping, heat, and cold applied to acupuncture points as well as ultrasound, aquapuncture, electrostimulation, implantation, and the use of lasers.

The specific points used, the depth to which the needles are inserted, the type of stimulation applied to the needles (prescription), and the duration of each treatment session (dosage) vary according to the condition being treated. In humans, most acupuncture points are described as lying on "meridians" or "channels" that connect loci having functional relationships. According to traditional Oriental philosophy, the acupoints communicate with the body organs and tissues through these channels (Altman, 1989). There are 361 traditional acupuncture points lo-

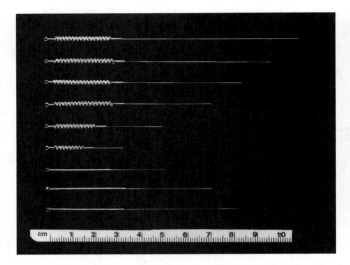

Fig. 10-1 Typical stainless-steel acupuncture needles. (From Ettinger SJ, Feldman EC: *Textbook of veterinary internal medicine,* ed 3, Philadelphia, 1989, WB Saunders.)

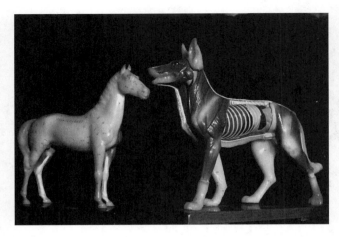

Fig. 10-2 Plastic figures of the horse and dog available from China, showing the location of traditional acupuncture points. (From Ettinger SJ, Feldman EC: *Textbook of veterinary internal medicine,* ed 3, Philadelphia, 1989, WB Saunders.)

cated on the channels or meridians. Some of these occur bilaterally, bringing the total of channel acupoints to 670. In addition, other points exist that lie outside these channels, including the 133 acupuncture points in the ear (Huang, 1974), bringing the total number of points to over 1000. A handbook published in Hong Kong (Lee-kin, 1985) describing acupuncture points in dogs and cats lists 32 single points and 40 bilateral points, for a total of 112 selection possibilities. Several other charts have been published with numbers of points varying between these two extremes (Altman, 1981a; Janssens, 1984; Klide, Kung, 1977; Shores, 1975; Weinstein, 1975; Young, 1978).

There are two schools of thought on the location and nomenclature of acupuncture points in veterinary medicine. The most common approach is to transpose the human points onto animal anatomy. The second approach is to use traditional points derived from Chinese charts. Plastic figures of the horse and dog showing the location of traditional points are available from China (Fig. 10-2).*

Each acupuncture point has specific actions when stimulated. When points are used in combination with other points, the results may be altered. An analogy can be made to playing musical notes. If single notes are played, the tone is plain, direct, and easily recognized. The addition of other notes produces major, minor, or other chords, giving a completely different quality of sound to the original note. Sometimes the wrong combination of notes creates discord. Similarly, simultaneous stimulation of points in harmony can enhance specific actions beyond the capabilities of single-point excitation. In other cases, effects can be obliterated or medical problems exacerbated by improperly combining acupoints (Altman, 1989).

---

*China National Machinery Import & Export Corp., Tientsin Branch, 14 Chang The Road, Tientsin, China.

History

Origins

Acupuncture is one of the oldest forms of medical treatment. Acupuncture-like therapy is thought to have existed in India 7000 years ago. In the Orient, acupuncture has been used as a preventive and therapeutic modality for several thousand years. Stone and fish-bone needles were used in China during the Stone Age, an estimated 3000 years BC. Bamboo, jade, copper, iron, gold, silver, and now primarily stainless steel have been used for the manufacture of needles as technology and the use of various metals and alloys developed (Chuan, 1990; Hsu, Peacher, 1977; Wei-kang, 1975). Published sometime between 400 and 200 BC, the *Huang Ti Nei Ching,* or *Yellow Emperor's Classic of Internal Medicine,* is one of the oldest known documents on TCM. Considered the basis of TCM, this work describes the Oriental philosophy of anatomy, physiology, pathology, diagnosis, and treatment of maladies of that time. For example, it states that blood flows continuously throughout the body, controlled by the heart. This was written 2000 years before William Harvey made the same discovery for Western medicine in 1628. The *Huang Ti Nei Ching* lists 365 traditional points for humans, illustrates nine basic types of needles, and provides indications and contraindications for acupuncture points.

Other books and commentaries were published in China during the following centuries as the medical knowledge of the *Huang Ti Nei Ching* was passed from generation to generation. New knowledge and experience accumulated along the way. These books provided more information on pain therapy and treatment of disease using acupuncture and moxibustion (the heating of acupuncture points by the burning of an herb, *Artemisia vulgaris,* on the points), yet the basic concepts of point and channel anatomy and therapy have remained virtually identical to those described in the *Huang Ti Nei Ching*. TCM divided medical professionals into four distinct disciplines: physicians, surgeons, veterinarians, and dietitians. Because training and practice often overlapped, a single practitioner might practice all or several of these disciplines. Until Occidental medical philosophies were introduced during the Ching dynasty (1644 to 1911), TCM was the exclusive form of therapy practiced in China. Included in TCM are acupuncture, moxibustion, *Tuei-Na* (manipulative therapy or massage), *Qi-Gung* (breathing exercises), *Shu-Shieh* (nutrition and diet), and herbal medicine (Mok, 1984).

The Chinese government banned the practice of TCM in 1929 because of the growing popularity and influence of Western medicine and surgery. Most of the populace ignored the ban, however. The practice of TCM became somewhat clandestine, but practitioners were readily available. During the days of the Red Revolutionary Army in China, Mao Tse-Tung's troops were stricken severely with malaria. Military paramedics had run out of Atabrine and quinine to treat the soldiers, and they were no longer able to fight effectively. Mao's army appeared close to defeat, which meant the failure of Mao's revolution. According to legend, Mao was approached by TCM practitioners who offered to treat the soldiers, with the following condition: If Mao's forces were victorious, TCM would occupy a place of honor in the new order. Acupuncturists then began to treat the troops and returned them to duty within 3 days. This demonstration apparently convinced Mao of the effectiveness of acupuncture. When he came to power, he insisted that Chinese physicians study both TCM (including acupuncture) and modern Western medicine. He ordered that the old and new medical modalities be given equal status in training, research, and practice under the new government. He stated emphatically that "Chinese Medicine and Pharmacology are a great treasure house and efforts should be made to explore them and raise them to a higher level" (Wei-kang, 1975). Today, modern Western medicine and acupuncture are practiced together in China and other Oriental countries. An estimated 1,300,000 paramedical personnel, 100,000 pharmacists, 200,000 nurses, 250,000 medical doctors, 150,000 veterinarians, and 700,000 paraveterinary personnel have received training in acupuncture. Research in acupuncture has been conducted in China, Taiwan, Russia, Italy, Romania, France, Germany, Japan, Korea, Portugal, Switzerland, the United States, and Canada, among other countries.

The Use of Acupuncture in Veterinary Medicine

Veterinary acupuncture is probably almost as old as acupuncture itself. A treatise on the use of acupuncture on Indian elephants, estimated to have been written 3000 years ago, has been discovered in Sri Lanka (Concon,

1979). Shun Yang (also called Pao Lo), who lived about 480 BC, was the first full-time practitioner of Chinese veterinary medicine on record. He is considered the father of the profession in China. A rock carving from the Han dynasty (about 200 BC) shows soldiers using arrows to perform acupuncture on their horses to stimulate them before battle. Government veterinarians and paraveterinary medical personnel have treated cows, horses, pigs, and chickens from the Chow dynasty (2303 BC to 221 BC) to the present in China (Altman, 1977a). Japan's history of veterinary acupuncture seems to end in the middle 1800s, when Western medicine was introduced (Joechle, 1975).

The Introduction of Acupuncture in the West

Visits by Jesuits to Macao and Chao Ch'ing, Kuantung Province, in 1582 and to Beijing (Peking) in 1600 established the first recorded communication between China and the West. P.P. Harvieu, a French Jesuit, published the first European work on acupuncture in 1671. Since that time, France has had a strong and steady history in the use of acupuncture. Veterinary acupuncture was used there in the 1700s and early 1800s and was revived again during the past 40 to 50 years (Janssens, 1981; Joechle, 1975, 1978). In 1836, French veterinary literature documented the treatment of an ox with acupuncture. (The feverish and paraplegic bovine had 30 3-inch needles implanted, with the help of a mallet, in what appears to be the Bladder channel. The needles remained in place for 48 hours.) In 1943 M. and C. Lavergne cited cures for animal lameness in the *Abstract of Acupuncture* (Klide, Kung, 1977). In the 1950s and 1960s, several theses on veterinary acupuncture were written at the National Veterinary School in Alfort, France.

Edward Jukes, of the Westminster Medical Institution, introduced human acupuncture to England in 1821. In 1822 and 1828, J.M. Churchill published books containing some case histories of patients treated with acupuncture. The first English report on veterinary acupuncture was published in 1828 in *The Veterinarian* by the British Veterinary Association. This journal was the forerunner of the *Veterinary Record* (Jaggar, 1992).

The Ludwig Boltzmann Acupuncture Institute has helped promote human and veterinary acupuncture in Austria. Veterinarians Oswald Kothbauer and Ferdinand Brunner, members of the institute, were active in gathering information and disseminating it to other veterinarians.

Acupuncture appears to have been introduced to the United States in the nineteenth century. In 1893, Sir William Osler, author of the textbook *The Principles and Practice of Medicine*, mentioned acupuncture as a treatment for lumbago. In 1926 the first article on acupuncture appearing in a medical journal, "Cases Illustrative of the Remedial Effects of Acupuncture," was published in the *North American Medical and Surgical Journal* (Jaggar, 1994; Klide, Kung, 1977). Acupuncture did not seem to make much of an impression outside Asian-American communities until President Richard Nixon visited China in the early 1970s. The press entourage accompanying Nixon was exposed to acupuncture, and the writers were for the most part favorably impressed. Their articles generated public interest and curiosity (Reston, 1971).

In the late 1960s, David Bresler was completing work on a Ph.D. in psychology at the University of California in Los Angeles (UCLA). He had already completed a B.A. in biology and an M.A. in psychology. Bresler became intrigued with acupuncture while pursuing an interest in *Tai Qi Chuan,* a Chinese system of physical exercises designed especially for martial arts and meditation. He apprenticed himself to a Chinese Master Acupuncturist, Gim Shek Ju, and began the process of becoming a certified acupuncturist. Bresler was initially convinced that the effects of acupuncture were produced through some sort of hypnotic process. He believed that his background in psychology would be a good platform for the investigation of acupuncture's mode of action. As his knowledge increased, Bresler's belief that hypnosis accounted for the effects of acupuncture began to falter. He decided to see if acupuncture would work on animals. If so, placebo or psychologic mechanisms could be discounted. Along with two fellow students, Steven Rosenblatt and Bill Prensky, he initiated an informal research project treating pets and animals belonging to relatives and friends. Their results showed promise, and the researchers then tested their treatments on horses. Positive responses to these treatments led to a deeper involvement in basic and clinical research. The researchers petitioned the UCLA Medical School, where Dr. Bresler was a faculty member, to underwrite a research program in acupuncture. In 1972 a core group of medical doctors and research scientists from the departments of anesthesiology, psychiatry, and psychology was formed to conduct clinical and basic research studies on the therapeutic efficacy of acupuncture. In 1973, after more than 18 months of hard work and in spite of heavy resistance, Dr. Bresler and his group received approval to begin clinical trials in human patients. Thus the Acupuncture Project, under the sponsorship of the Department of Anesthesiology, was born (Bresler, 1982).

Dr. Bresler and an anesthesiologist, Dr. Norman Levin, began the initial work at UCLA. Although UCLA administrators allowed the clinical studies to begin, they did not allocate funds to support the research. To finance the project and related research, Dr. Bresler and his colleagues formed the National Acupuncture Association. This group recruited other professionals and began lecturing and teaching courses in acupuncture. Stipends, proceeds, and honorariums were donated to UCLA. In addition, the Center for Integral Medicine was formed to generate income through courses in acupuncture and other alternative therapies. These funds were also donated to UCLA, with the stipulation that they be used to support acupuncture research.

At first the research was conducted on a private and informal basis. Then, in March 1973, the outpatient department, known as the UCLA Acupuncture Clinic, was opened. The project became the largest ongoing clinical investigation of acupuncture in the United States at the time. Throughout its existence, the project was financially self-sufficient and self-supporting. Except for a few National Institute of Health grants and other grants, research activities and operations of the outpatient clinic were funded by patient charges and donations. The volume of activity was approximately 150 to 200 patient visits per week. Most patients were treated twice a week for chronic pain problems. The average patient received a course of 10 to 12 treatments. In the first 3½ years of the project, over 3000 people were treated. After approximately 3 years the clinic enlarged its scope and became the Pain Control Unit, augmenting the research and use of acupuncture with that of other modalities to treat pain. The project ended activities in 1980, after administering nearly 80,000 acupuncture treatments (Bresler, 1979).

In the UCLA Acupuncture Project the types of problems treated in humans were approximately as follows: 20% to 25% headache, 40% low back pain, 15% various forms of arthritis, and the remainder a wide range of miscellaneous problems. Of the patients treated, those with osteoarthritis responded best. Other conditions showing positive responses included musculoskeletal pain, soft tissue injury, and headaches. Poorest response occurred in peripheral neuropathies, rheumatoid disease, phantom limb pain, and causalgia.

From a staff beginning with Dr. Bresler and Dr. Levin, the roster grew to include 55 people. Personnel at various times included five or six physicians, anesthesiologists, psychiatrists, neurologists, orthopedists, psychologists, and dentists and one or two veterinarians, certified acupuncturists, biofeedback therapists, nutritionists, kinesiologists, electrophysiologists, registered nurses, medical and acupuncture assistants, medical students, residents and interns, and administrative support employees. The staff reported that acupuncture was an effective tool in relieving many kinds of musculoskeletal pain, such as that caused by arthritis, bursitis, tenosynovitis, and vertebrogenic disease. Other findings were that large joints responded better than smaller joints (e.g., shoulder bursitis and tenosynovitis were more rapidly and successfully treated than elbow epicondylitis, and phalangeal arthritis had the least successful response). In general, if muscle spasm was a major component of the pain problem, rapid and dramatic relief was often attained. Headaches, both tension and migraine, responded well to the acupuncture treatments. After a full course of treatment, headache recurrence was eliminated or diminished. Acupuncture for temporomandibular joint (TMJ) dysfunction was particularly effective. Although treatment of peripheral neuropathy, trigeminal neuralgia, postherpetic neuralgia, phantom limb pain, and causalgia was not as successful in some cases, many people were helped significantly. Most experienced diminished intensity and frequency of pain, and some enjoyed the complete abolishment of pain.

The acupuncturists had varied backgrounds. Chinese, Japanese, Korean, and American practitioners performed acupuncture at various times. No statistics were recorded on the difference of response in patients treated by acupuncturists using traditional methods of prescribing treatment (e.g., pulse diagnosis, five elements, eight principles, seven emotional factors, six exogenous factors) versus the "recipe" or "cookbook" approach, but the results showed no significant differences. Surprisingly enough, a slight but significant inverse correlation existed between expectations and results of treatment—that is, the more pessimistic people often responded better than the optimists. Dr. Bresler rationalized this phenomenon as follows: People who were influenced by reports of good results and came in expecting that one or two treatments would miraculously cure them were disappointed if complete remission of symptoms did not occur rapidly. They were more critical in evaluating benefits because their expectations were so high. On the other hand, those who had lower expectations were surprised when they experienced results and were impressed with a lower level of response. An approximation of the clinical results showed that about 25% showed major improvement, becoming asymptomatic or nearly so; 50% showed significant improvement but not total resolution; and 25% derived little if any benefit. Sequelae were rare, with minor discolorations or small hematomas the usual problems encountered. In an evaluation made after 20,000 treatments, one case of auricular chondritis, one case of pneumothorax, and one case of dysesthesia that lasted 2 days were reported. Patients were warned about possible sequelae to acupuncture and were told that a temporary exacerbation of symptoms might occur. (Some of the research findings of UCLA Acupuncture Research Project are included in Box 10-1) (Bresler, Katz, Kroening, 1975b).

At first the medical staff at UCLA regarded the project with curiosity. A bell-shaped curve evolved, with approx-

---

BOX 10-1

RESEARCH FINDINGS OF *UCLA* ACUPUNCTURE RESEARCH PROJECT

ACUPUNCTURE ANALGESIA FOR SURGERY

Electroacupuncture was used successfully as the sole analgesic for various orthopedic, obstetric, and surgical procedures. The main advantage was low morbidity. The disadvantage was that it was less efficient and reliable than more conventional anesthetic techniques. The best use seemed to be in controlling postoperative pain and nausea.

USE OF ACUPUNCTURE IN TREATING CHRONIC PAIN

In an initial study, 410 patients with intractable pain were treated with acupuncture and evaluated for 6 months following the completion of therapy. Subjective and functional pain indexes, activity levels, and subsequent medical requirements were used to evaluate the level of success in treatment. About 50% of the patients showed statistically significant improvement. Except for some functional variables related to sleep patterns, no significant relapses occurred in the 6-month follow-up period. Prognostic variables that proved significant included age, diagnosis, surgical history, and number of treatments given. Younger patients did better than older ones. Patients with osteoarthritis, myofascial pain, musculoskeletal pain, and headache showed more improvement than those with rheumatoid arthritis, neuralgias, and chronic postsurgical pain syndromes. The patients who had undergone surgery for pain-related problems before acupuncture therapy did not respond as well and showed a greater degree of pain recurrence than those who had not undergone surgery. There was also a positive relationship between the number of treatments and the success of therapy. Those patients who received more than 10 treatments responded better than those who had fewer than 10 treatments. Other variables, such as gender, race, marital status, duration of illness, and the ethnic background of the acupuncturist did not seem to be significant in the success of treatment.*

ACUPUNCTURE THERAPY IN SENSORY-NEURAL HEARING LOSS

Audiometric evaluations showed no statistically significant improvement, although 40% of the patients subjectively reported anecdotal evidence of improvement.

---

*From Bresler DE, Katz RL, Kroening RJ: *Review of research findings of the UCLA Research Project,* Los Angeles, 1975, UCLA Acupuncture Research Project; Levin N. Acupuncture in acute and chronic pain problems, *Anesthesiol Rev,* p 10, Jan 1976. *Continued.*

BOX 10-1

RESEARCH FINDINGS OF *UCLA* ACUPUNCTURE RESEARCH PROJECT—cont'd

ACUPUNCTURE FOR COMPULSIVE DISORDERS

Used to treat obesity and tobacco and drug addiction, acupuncture helped reduce physiologic need but not psychologic craving for the addictive substance. Acupuncture can be a valuable adjunctive modality to psychotherapy, but is less effective if used alone.

ACUPUNCTURE THERAPY IN BRONCHIAL ASTHMA

This study was undertaken to get more measurable data than the sometimes subjective evaluations in pain relief studies. Through spirometry and plethysmography, more objective results could be obtained. This experiment was done as a double-blind placebo controlled study. To study effects in acute bronchial asthma, bronchospasm was induced using methacholine. The subjects were divided into the following five groups:

1. Patients treated with nebulized Isuprel
2. Patients receiving nebulized saline (placebo control)
3. Patients receiving traditional acupuncture
4. Patients receiving placebo acupuncture (control)
5. Patients receiving no treatment (control)

The group receiving nebulized Isuprel showed the most rapid and effective relief of bronchospasm. Traditional acupuncture was not quite as effective as the Isuprel. A longer latency period occurred between the beginning of treatment and the onset of desired results, but the effects of acupuncture lasted longer and had fewer side effects. Nebulized saline was significantly less effective than Isuprel or traditional acupuncture, but more effective than placebo acupuncture or the absence of treatment. There was no significant difference between the placebo acupuncture and the nontreated groups.†

EXPERIMENTAL EVALUATION OF AURICULAR DIAGNOSIS

Forty patients were medically examined to determine areas of the body where there was musculoskeletal pain. Then each patient was draped so that the investigator could not visibly detect any physical problems. The investigator had no prior knowledge of the patient's history or physical condition; he just examined the exposed ear for areas of tenderness or increased skin electroconductivity. The concurrence of the medical examination diagnosis and the auricular acupuncture point diagnosis was 75.2%. The results supported the hypothesis that distinct areas of the ear correspond to specific anatomic portions of the body, and that there is a somatotropic organization of the body represented on the human auricle (i.e., the existence of acupuncture points distant to sites of pathology and related anatomic structures and the validity of auricular diagnosis).‡

---

†From Tashkin DP and others. Comparison of real and simulated acupuncture and isoproterenol in methacholine induced asthma, *Ann Allergy* 39:379, 1977.
‡From Oleson RD, Kroening RJ, Bresler DE. Diagnostic accuracy of examining electrical activity at ear acupuncture points for assessing areas of the body with musculoskeletal pain, *Pain Abstracts* 1:185, 1978.

---

imately 25% welcoming the investigations, calling them "fascinating" and "interesting." About 50% of the staff members were indifferent. The remaining 25% were resolutely opposed, considering the modality as "quackery, having no place at a reputable institution such as UCLA." Over the course of the study, acceptance of the project by physicians in the Los Angeles area increased significantly. At first the project met with resistance, especially from orthopedic surgeons. Intractable patients were referred to the project, sometimes in sincerity but often with the probable intention to challenge the acupuncture staff.

When many of these patients responded to treatment, the referring physicians sent more and better-quality cases and then began to appear as patients themselves. Public acceptance was much faster than that of the medical community. Media coverage and public speaking engagements by staff members helped publicize the project. Satisfied patients enthusiastically referred new patients to the project. The demand for evaluation and treatment was such that, at times, patients had to wait 4 to 6 weeks for an appointment (Bresler, 1979).

Members of the initial group of National Acupuncture

Association members also helped interested veterinarians found the National Association for Veterinary Acupuncture (NAVA). Dr. Bresler acted as an advisor to the fledgling organization. Acupuncturists John Ottaviano, Sang Hyuck Shin, and Bobby Klein performed the acupuncture treatments for clinical studies on animals. Wolfgang Joechle, D.V.M., advised on the protocols and analyzed data. The veterinary staff consisted of Richard Glassberg, D.V.M., Horace Warner, D.V.M., Michael Gerry, D.V.M., and Alice DeGroot, D.V.M. I was fortunate enough to participate in both the UCLA Acupuncture Project and the National Association for Veterinary Acupuncture after the hard work of organizing and launching the organizations had been completed. NAVA conducted veterinary clinical research, provided classes for veterinarians interested in acupuncture, and, from 1973-1978, operated a facility for treating animals referred by veterinarians and the general public.

The Acupuncture Research Project was important because it showed the skeptical American medical community that acupuncture is a valuable clinical tool in the treatment of pain and other medical problems. It served as an important source of information on acupuncture. The project was a starting point for experimentation and basic research into the efficacy and efficiency of acupuncture use in treating problems in both human and animal subjects. It aided in the formation of NAVA, which became the focus and inspiration for veterinary acupuncture in the western part of the United States. At that time the International Veterinary Acupuncture Society (IVAS) was performing a similar function for veterinarians in the eastern and central parts of the country.

The Organization of Veterinary Acupuncture in the United States

In early 1973 the California Veterinary Medical Association (CVMA) appointed a committee to study veterinary acupuncture. The committee enlisted the aid of the UCLA Acupuncture Project to translate Chinese, German, and French veterinary literature and set up clinical field trials. Six southern California veterinarians offered the use of their clinics 1 day a week so that a large-scale study could be undertaken. This also gave local veterinarians the opportunity to observe the treatments and gain experience in acupuncture techniques.

The California Board of Examiners in Veterinary Medicine became concerned about the sudden interest in this controversial modality generated by the project. They were afraid that the studies would be used for less-than-professional goals and that greed would generate "quackupuncturists." They therefore ruled that any further trials were to be conducted only in a facility exclusively for nonprofit acupuncture treatment of animals. They also stipulated that the project be under the direction of a school of veterinary medicine. In compliance with these stipulations

a nonprofit organization, the National Association for Veterinary Acupuncture (NAVA), was formed. A veterinary hospital was leased for acupuncture treatment of animals. The Dean of the School of Veterinary Medicine at the University of California at Davis appointed a faculty committee to supervise and coordinate the activities of the acupuncture project. Until 1978, NAVA conducted research, treated clinical cases, and conducted courses in acupuncture for veterinarians. By that time acupuncture had become an accepted modality available in conventional veterinary practices (*Guide to Acupuncture for Animals*, 1978*). Many of the NAVA members became active members of the International Veterinary Acupuncture Society (IVAS).

In April 1974, the Acupuncture Society of America, Inc., presented the seminar "Acupuncture for the Veterinarian" in the eastern United States. Two Japanese acupuncturists addressed approximately 35 veterinarians. Many veterinarians present were motivated to found IVAS. Since 1975, IVAS has been the primary organization for veterinary acupuncturists in the United States and now has many international members. The IVAS conducts regular courses, seminars, and international veterinary acupuncture congresses and is responsible for the accreditation of veterinary acupuncturists in the United States and internationally. Publications of the IVAS include the *Veterinary Acupuncture Newsletter* (quarterly, since 1975), the *International Journal on Veterinary Acupuncture* (semiannually, since 1990), and proceedings of their annual meetings (Jaggar, 1992, 1994).

Various state veterinary societies and State Boards of Veterinary Examiners have investigated the use and possible abuse of veterinary acupuncture. Chapters on acupuncture are now included in reputable veterinary medical texts (Altman, 1989, 1995; Clifford, 1986; Klide, 1992) and journals, mainstream publishing companies are publishing veterinary acupuncture textbooks (Schoen, 1992, 1994), and the American Veterinary Medical Association (AVMA) has changed its recommendations on veterinary acupuncture. In a policy statement approved by the AVMA House of Delegates in 1980, the following Guidelines on Acupuncture were approved (AVMA Directory, 1987):

> The AVMA has grave concern about acupuncture, regarding it as experimental. The public must be protected from those who make claims for acupuncture that are not based on adequate controlled experiments or documented research. Veterinarians must be aware of their legal responsibilities when acupuncture is used. The administration of an acupuncture needle should be regarded as a surgical procedure under the state veterinary practice acts.

In January 1986 the AVMA's Alternate Therapies Study Committee began a 2-year study on the safety and

---

*Guide to acupuncture for animals, a publication by NAVA, is available by writing R. Glassberg, D.V.M., 1905 Sunnycrest Dr., Fullerton, CA 92635.

efficacy of procedures and regimens differing from traditional forms of veterinary medicine and surgery. One modality studied was acupuncture. The committee was charged with reporting its findings to the Council on Veterinary Service. This body was asked to determine the appropriateness of a given modality as an alternative form of therapy in veterinary medicine and then make recommendations to certify or accredit practitioners in the approved modalities (JAVMA, 1986). The ad hoc committee recommended that the guidelines on acupuncture be changed to read as follows:

> Veterinary acupuncture and acutherapy are considered valid modalities, but the potential for abuse exists. These techniques should be regarded as surgical and/or medical procedures under state veterinary practice acts. It is recommended that extensive educational programs be undertaken before a veterinarian is considered competent to practice acupuncture. There is a need to establish criteria for competency assessment (Minutes, 1987).

The concern of the AVMA has been shared by veterinarians who perform acupuncture. IVAS was formed in 1974 to promote "excellence in the practice of veterinary acupuncture as an integral part of the total veterinary health delivery system. The Society endeavors to establish uniformly high standards of veterinary acupuncture through its educational programs and accreditation examination. IVAS seeks to integrate veterinary acupuncture and the practice of western veterinary science. . ." (The IVAS, 1974*). For certification, IVAS requires at least 120 hours of accredited class instruction, passing of a comprehensive examination, and submission of five detailed case reports. IVAS has drafted a code of ethics that details the general duties of its member practitioners, the commitment of practitioners to the patient and to the profession, the ethics of the practitioner in commercial undertakings, and the relationship of the practitioner to the general public in making public statements, advertising, and professing education, training, and experience.

Today, most published reports on veterinary acupuncture come from France, Austria, China, Belgium, Australia, Taiwan, and the United States. The most complete reviews of the literature to date have been compiled by Phillip A. Rogers, M.R.C.V.S., who has become a liaison for veterinary acupuncturists around the world (Rogers, 1966—present, 1974; Rogers and others, 1977).

Does Acupuncture Really Work?

Clinical Evidence of Efficacy

Clinical studies and experimental reports indicate that acutherapy is a safe and effective modality for specific con-

ditions if used properly and competently. In 1979 after an interregional seminar held in Beijing (Peking), the World Health Organization (WHO) published its views on acupuncture. WHO concluded that "acupuncture is clearly not a panacea for all ills; but sheer weight of evidence demands that acupuncture must be taken seriously as a clinical procedure of considerable value." A provisional list of 40 human diseases lending themselves to acupuncture treatment was compiled (Bannerman, 1980). In veterinary medicine, many reproductive disorders, musculoskeletal problems, pulmonary and gastrointestinal disorders, neurologic disorders, and dermatologic diseases in many species have been treated with considerable success.*

Clinical reports on the successful treatment of reproductive disorders, intervertebral disk syndrome†, musculoskeletal problems (Buchli, 1976; Janssens, 1976a; Schoen, 1983, 1986, 1992, 1994), dermatologic conditions (Bullock, 1978; Waters, 1992, 1994), pain therapy (Clifford, Lee, 1978; Janssens, 1976d), neurologic disorders (Joseph, 1992, 1994; Klide, 1984; Stefanatos, 1984), and anesthetic emergencies (Altman, 1979; Janssens and others, 1979) in dogs have been published (Altman, 1981b; Joechle, 1977). In cats, arthritis, nerve paralysis, and eczema have been treated (Rogers, 1976—present). Acupuncture analgesia has been used in small animal surgery, but it is not likely to gain popularity in view of more practical conventional anesthetic techniques (Janssens, 1982; Lee and others, 1976; O'Boyle, Vajda, 1973; Wright, McGrath, 1981; Young, 1979).

Research Findings

Controlled studies under laboratory conditions have shown that acupuncture can elicit various physiologic changes. Some interesting effects reported are changes in uterine contraction, gastrointestinal changes‡, cardiovascular changes§, transient changes in hemograms and immune responses (Brown and others, 1974b; Rogers, Bossey, 1981), and analgesic effects.

How Does Acupuncture Work?

The clinical and experimental results of acupoint stimulation indicate that acupuncture produces physiologic responses and therapeutic effects. For over 4000 years, acupuncture has been used as an effective medical proce-

---

*The IVAS brochure is available by writing IVAS at P.O. Box 1478, Longmont, CO 80502-1478.

*Altman (1981b); Feng (1981); Gideon (1977); Joechle (1975, 1977); Kussaari (1983); Lakshmipathi and others (1984); Rogers (1974, 1977); White, Christie (1974).
†Buchli (1975); Janssens (1976a, 1976b, 1982, 1983, 1985, 1989, 1992, 1994); Janssens, De Prins (1989); Still (1987, 1988, 1989).
‡Clifford, Lee (1979); Lee (1975); O'Conner, Bensky (1975); Rogers and others (1977); Smith, (1994).
§Chin, Ching (1974); Clifford, Lee (1979); Lee, Lee (1979); Lee and others (1974, 1975); Rogers and others (1977); Smith (1994).

dure on a large portion of the world's population, which may make it the most thoroughly field-tested technique known to medicine. How are these effects mediated? What biophysical mechanisms are involved in the acupuncture process?

Explanations of the mechanisms of acupuncture vary widely. The proposals include traditional Oriental meridian theories, gate-control and multiple-gate-control theories, reflex stimulation, neurophysiologic interference theories, holographic and dermatome theories, autonomic nervous system input theories, biochemical reactions, and many psychologic and hypnosis theories (Bresler, Kroening, 1976). Research in the UCLA Acupuncture Research Project seemed to indicate that a combination of at least three factors was necessary to obtain successful therapeutic results in humans:

1. Immune-inflammatory reaction due to the physical act of traumatizing tissue as it is stimulated, causing a generalized response
2. Peripheral neural stimulation at the acupuncture points, modulating central neural regulation and causing more specific responses
3. Psychologic support (Bresler, Kroening, 1976)

The effectiveness of acupuncture on animals and the lack of response to placebo acupuncture undermined the validity of psychologic and hypnosis theories and the need for psychologic support.

Modern Theories

Neurologic theories

Probably the most popular theories of acupuncture are neurologic explanations.

GATE THEORY   The gate theory is one approach used to explain the analgesic effects of acupuncture (Melzack,

Wall, 1965). When the large myelinated A-beta or delta afferent nerve fibers that conduct touch and pressure sensations are stimulated, impulses from small unmyelinated C nerve fibers that carry pain sensations are blocked from passing a hypothetic "gate" located in the substantia gelatinosa of the spinal cord. As a result, the pain impulses cannot be transmitted higher in the central nervous system (CNS) and no perception of pain occurs (Levin, 1976). Acupuncture points may be areas where many large touch and pressure receptor fibers and small unmyelinated pain receptor fibers converge. Both sets of afferents synapse with neurons carrying impulses to the brain. These impulses are recognized as pain. Both afferents also synapse with interneurons, which can inhibit the input of these peripheral nerves to the neurons carrying the impulses higher in the CNS. In effect, an "accelerator-and-brake" effect is present. The pressure and touch afferents facilitate the interneurons, acting as accelerators. The pain afferents inhibit the interneurons, acting as brakes. Increased stimulation of the touch and pressure afferents produces blockage of pain impulses coming to the synapse with the neurons that compose the pain pathway to the brain. Stimulation of the acupuncture points increases input over the large afferents, thus producing an analgesic effect (Fig. 10-3) (Latshaw, 1975).

One flaw of this explanation is that cells of the substantia gelatinosa are believed to terminate in the medulla. This raises the following question: How can needles placed in the extremities produce analgesia to areas supplied by cranial nerves? Multiple-gate theories have been suggested as possible solutions, with the second gates thought to exist in either the thalamus or the brainstem. The thalamic-gate theory (Man, Chen, 1973) suggests that activation of large A-beta fibers by peripheral needling causes impulses to ascend to the thalamic level, causing the reticular and limbic systems to shut the gate on pain sensations ascending

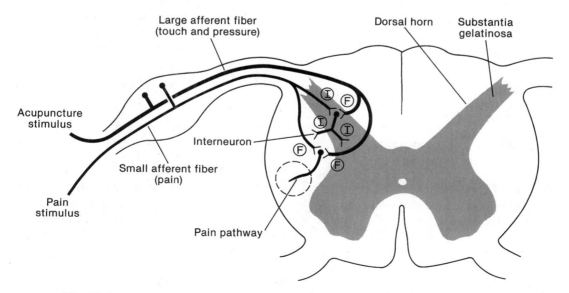

Fig. 10-3   Acupuncture stimulus producing analgesic effect. (From Ettinger SJ, Feldman EC: *Textbook of veterinary internal medicine*, ed 3, Philadelphia, 1989, WB Saunders.)

through the spinothalamic and bulbothalamic tracts. The brainstem theory postulates the existence of a brainstem central biasing mechanism, or reticular activating system, that controls transmission information being received through the integumental sensory afferents (Bresler and others, 1980). The central biasing mechanism theory has also been used to explain the way stimulation of a point innervated by one nerve tract can provide pain relief at a site innervated by a completely different nerve complex (Levin, 1976). The gate theory leaves unanswered two questions: Why does the analgesic effect last for 30 to 60 minutes after discontinuing stimulation when used for surgical analgesia, and why can chronic pain be eliminated after multiple acupuncture treatments?

Some experts propose the theory of memory banks in pain-receiving cells. According to this theory, chronic pain represents the storage of the original pain sensation in these memory banks after the injury has been healed. Some examples cited are phantom limb pain and phantom dental causalgia in humans. Acupuncture is said to produce an amnesia effect in the memory banks of pain-receiving cells, thus diminishing or obliterating chronic pain. These memory banks in pain-receiving cells may be activated or deactivated by weather or barometric pressure conditions, which is the reason that some chronic pain seems to be weather-affected (Concon, 1979).

INHIBITORY SURROUND Another neurologic theory used to explain the way acupuncture analgesia works using points supplied by nerve complexes unrelated to the site of pathology is the cortical inhibitory surround hypothesis. According to this theory, a peripheral stimulus is mediated through afferent pathways and projected onto the cerebral cortex. When a site of focal excitation is elicited in the cortex, the area immediately surrounding it is inhibited. Thus, if a point or combination of points (whose cortical projection sites are adjacent to the cortical projection site of an area causing pain) are stimulated, the resulting inhibition surrounding the stimulated cortical areas could obliterate or diminish the pain interpretation at the cortical level (Bresler, Kroening, 1976).

Autonomic Theories

Another approach to explaining the mechanisms of acupuncture has been the investigation of the autonomic nervous system (Clifford, Lee, 1979). Studies using rabbits have demonstrated that the ability to produce acupuncture analgesia in the nasal area is lost if the sympathetic chains are surgically interrupted (Loony, 1974). In support of the autonomic nervous system theory, acupuncture points often do correspond with Head's areas of referred pain (Toyama, Nishizwa, 1972). According to Head's postulate, "the cutaneous pain felt in visceral disease is located in the areas where sensory nerves enter the spinal cord at the same segmental levels which supply nerves to the viscera concerned." Cutaneous stimulation by needles may be transmitted to the internal viscera through somatovisceral neu-

ronal synapses in the spinal cord. During the process of such excitation, either the parasympathetic or sympathetic components of the visceral nerves seem to be selectively stimulated and the function of the autonomic nervous system is regulated (Fig. 10-4) (Toyama, Nishizwa, 1972). The ancient Chinese stated that external acupuncture points and channels were connected to internal organs. They spoke of tonifying or sedating points or organs. In classical Oriental terms, tonification may have referred to activating the sympathetic nervous system and sedation may have referred to parasympathetic activation (Altman, 1977).

Humoral Theories

A humoral factor seems to be involved in acupuncture and has been demonstrated in cross-circulation experiments in rats (Lung and others, 1974). In these experiments, 36 rats were subjected to 10 to 20 minutes of acupuncture stimulation. When analgesia was achieved, blood was allowed to circulate from the analgesic donor rats to paired recipients. Of the rats that did not receive acupuncture directly, 27 had significant increases in pain threshold and the remaining nine did not. Donors and recipients all returned to normal control levels after acupuncture was discontinued. No analgesic effects occurred in a control group of 19 pairs of rats. Studies have also demonstrated that the effect of acupuncture can be reversed with naloxone (Cheng, Pomeranz, 1980; Ha and others, 1981; Mayer and others, 1975). This suggests that acupuncture causes the release of a substance or substances that are neutralized by narcotic-antagonistic drugs. A series of methionine- or leucine-linked molecules synthesized in the brain have been isolated. These compounds, enkephalins and endorphins, may be the humoral factors involved in acupuncture. They appear to fit the requirements for a humoral explanation of the effects of acupuncture: They are produced endogenously; there is evidence that they increase after acupuncture stimulation; they have physiologic effects resembling morphine (e.g., they attach to opiate receptors, are analgesic in effect, and are antagonized by naloxone); and they are rapidly destroyed (Rogers, 1976; Wong, Cheng, no date).

Combination Theory

The combination theory links the neurologic and humoral concepts and describes acupuncture phenomena as follows: Nerve impulses caused by peripheral acupuncture stimuli are transmitted to the subcortical layer of the cerebrum by afferent A-delta myelinated nerve fibers. From the cerebrum the impulses are transmitted to the thalamus, and from the thalamus to the pituitary gland. Beta lipotropin is stored in the anterior pituitary gland. When the acupuncture-activated stimulus arrives, the beta lipotropin is acted on by two enzymes: proenkephalinase to release enkephalins and proendorphinase to release endorphins. Enkephalin is then transmitted through A-delta

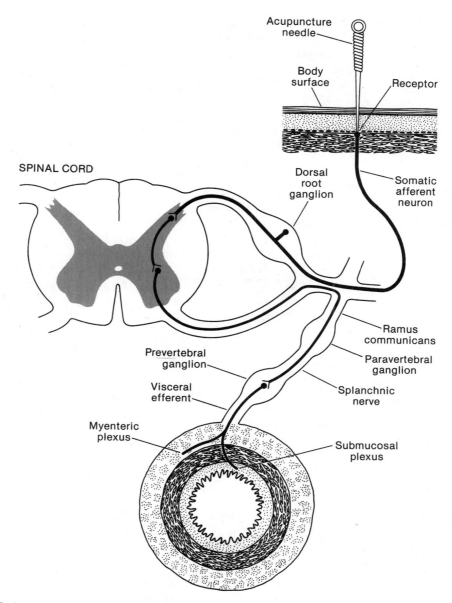

Fig. 10-4   Parasympathetic or sympathetic components of the visceral nerves seem to be selectively stimulated, and the function of the autonomic nervous system is regulated. (From Ettinger SJ, Feldman EC: *Textbook of veterinary internal medicine,* ed 3, Philadelphia, 1989, WB Saunders.)

myelinated nerve fibers to interneurons in the dorsal horn of the spinal cord, in the substantia gelatinosa. There it acts as a neurotransmitter, or neuromodulator, to block release of substance P (a peptide neurotransmitter associated with the transmission of pain impulses) caused by afferent C-unmyelinated nociceptor messages coming from the site of pain stimulus. Because this release of substance P is blocked, no pain messages reach the pain-receiving cells in the dorsal horn of the spinal cord in the substantia gelatinosa. At the same time, endorphin is transmitted through efferent A-delta fibers to interneurons in the medulla oblongata, medial thalamus (nucleus centralis medialis, nucleus parafascicularis, and nucleus centralis lateralis), and cerebral cortex. At these sites the endorphins block the release of substance P caused by impulses com-

ing in from afferent C-unmyelinated nerve fibers arising at the site of noxious stimuli. Therefore no pain messages reach the pain-receiving cells in the medulla oblongata, medial thalamus, and cerebral cortex. When acupuncture analgesia ends, enzyme enkephalinase destroys enkephalins, and enzyme endorphinase destroys endorphins, returning the system to normal so that new pain signals can be received if further injury should occur (Fig. 10-5).

Bioelectrical Theory

After 15 years of studying factors that initiate and control healing mechanisms, another group of researchers has described a complete control system that is separate from the nervous system but works in conjunction with it (Reich-

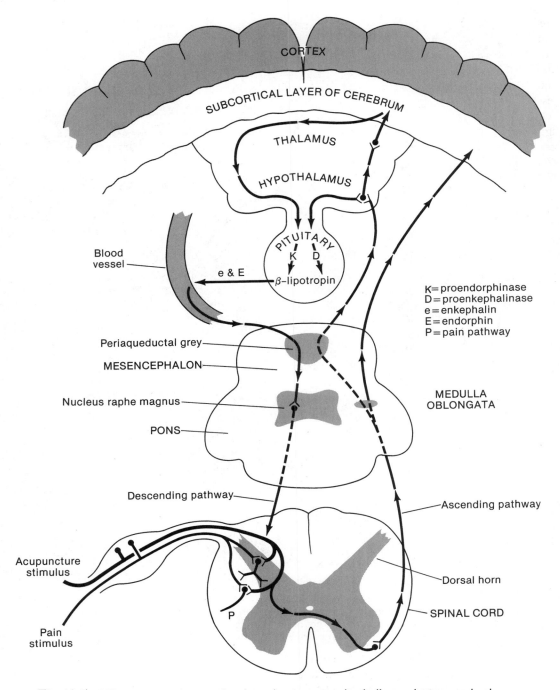

Fig. 10-5 When acupuncture analgesia ends, enzyme enkephalinase destroys enkephalins and enzyme endorphinase destroys endorphins, returning the system to normal, so that new pain signals can be received if further injury should occur. (From Ettinger SJ, Feldman EC: *Textbook of veterinary internal medicine,* ed 3, Philadelphia, 1989, WB Saunders.)

manis and others, 1975). The system is essentially a primitive data transmission and control mechanism whose prime function is sensing injury and starting the healing process, then stopping the process when healing is complete. The system works on DC electronic signals generated and distributed by the perineural cells—that is, Schwann cells peripherally, and satellite and glial cells centrally. The system could be compared to a computer network with peripheral transmission lines and central integrating areas. The output or control system has been studied for its effects on growth processes; the input portion of the system indicates that damage or injury has been received.

In the transmission of DC signals, resistance, capacitance, and inductance reduce the magnitude of the signal as the transmission distance increases. Booster amplifiers in the system are needed to restore signal strength. The acupuncture meridians are comparable to DC communication channels, and the acupuncture points to booster amplifier locations. A metallic needle inserted into these amplifier points could alter the signal itself or the system's ability to transmit signals (Becker, Selden, 1985). The theories of these researchers have been supported by their data on the electrical properties demonstrated at acupuncture points (higher conductance, lower resistance, organized field patterns, and differences in potential) (Becker and others, 1976; Bergsman, Woolley-Hart, 1983; Brown and others, 1974b; Reichmanis and others, 1975, 1976, 1979).

No single theory seems to explain all the effects of acupuncture. A combination of the preceding theories or undiscovered physiologic phenomena may be responsible for the action of acupuncture therapy. My opinion is that the mechanism involved depends on the particular point used—that is, certain points or groups of points work through one set of mechanisms and other points are mediated by other physiologic reactions, depending on anatomic site, type of innervation, and the nature, magnitude, and duration of the stimulus. The magnificent biologic machines that we and our animal patients inhabit may have built-in reset buttons and adjustment controls that we can use if we learn the ways they work (Altman, 1989).

The Theories of Traditional Chinese Medicine

The basis for traditional Chinese medicine (TCM) is the theory that a life energy *(Qi)*, consisting of positive *(yang)* and negative *(yin)* components, flows through the body in channels. These conduits are close to the surface at specific points on the body: the acupuncture points. Each channel is believed to correspond to a particular organ, from which energy is either generated or stored at a particular time of day. In contemporary thinking, *Qi* can be compared to electronic energy, the channels to printed circuits, the internal organs to generators and storage batteries, the *yin* and *yang* energy polarities to the negative and positive electrical polarities, and the body itself to an electronically operated machine. Imbalances in the energy levels between the positive *(yang)* and negative *(yin)* polarity or impairment of flow through the channels allows pathologic processes to function. Imbalances or blockages can be produced by external factors (wind, cold, summer heat, excessive dampness, excessive dryness, and excessive heat), emotional factors (joy, anger, melancholy, worry, grief, fear [e.g., prolonged tension or stress], fright [e.g., sudden and drastic upset]), and miscellaneous pathogenic factors (irregular food intake, too much or too little physical stress and exertion, traumatic injuries, and impaired circulation) (Xinnong, 1987). Adjustment of energy levels through stimulation of specific acupuncture points or a combination of points reestablishes a homeostatic condition and allows healing to occur. Various laws are used to explain pathology, selection of therapy, and prevention of recurrence. The study of traditional Oriental medicine is intricate but fascinating and provides insight into the powers of observation and astuteness of the early practitioners.

Current Uses of Acupuncture in Small Animal Medicine

Indications

Two large-scale clinical studies on animal acupuncture in California indicated that the most common causes for acupuncture referral in small animal practice were, in decreasing order of frequency: (1) paresis, paralysis, and pain in small dogs, usually resulting from intervertebral disk syndrome or trauma; (2) large dog paresis or paralysis syndromes resulting from neural compression caused by type II disk protrusions, spondylopathies and spinal instabilities, spondylolisthesis and cauda equina syndrome, and degenerative myelopathy; (3) pain caused by hip dysplasia and resulting coxofemoral osteoarthritis; (4) other arthritic pain syndromes; (5) miscellaneous conditions not responding to conventional therapy, including allergy and dermatitis, lick granulomas, central nervous system disorders (ataxia, chorea, epilepsy), chronic respiratory diseases, gastrointestinal problems, osteochondritis dissecans, traumatic peripheral nerve injuries, and miscellaneous pain syndromes (Altman, 1981b; Joechle, 1977).

Precautions

The most important contraindication for acupuncture is treatment before an adequate diagnosis has been made. An honest, objective, and diligent attempt to determine the etiology of the condition is necessary before treatment begins. This precaution is critical because acupuncture may mask or alter clinical signs (e.g., pain and neurologic syndromes), making accurate diagnosis more difficult later. Acupuncture might also delay treatment of a life-threatening condition (e.g., neoplasia) until it is too late to save the patient. Elimination of pain may encourage the animal to be too active, thus hindering healing of the original condition or even making it worse.

Certain precautions should be observed before using acupuncture therapy. If possible, acupuncture should not be performed in the following circumstances: immediately after a heavy meal; on a fatigued subject; on a subject that is extremely frightened, angry, or emotional; on pregnant animals, especially if points below the umbilicus are to be used; if the subject has just been bathed or is going to be bathed within a short time after treatment; if injections of atropine, narcotics, narcotic antagonists, or corticosteroids* have been used; or if the animal cannot be comfortably re-

---

*This is a controversial subject. I occasionally inject low doses of corticosteroids into acupuncture points.

strained and observed throughout the treatment period. The practitioner must be careful to avoid traumatizing underlying internal structures and inadvertently producing thermal burns with moxibustion and electrical shock or electrolytic burns with electroacupuncture (Altman, 1981a). In addition, practitioners should not insert needles in animals with severe blood dyscrasias or clotting deficiencies or into areas where local malignancies or skin infections are present.

Sequelae

Sequelae seldom occur when acupuncture is performed by a knowledgeable practitioner. However, some adverse effects can occur. The most common problem is exacerbation of the condition being treated, especially in pain cases. The worsening is usually short-lived (less than 24 to 48 hours) and frequently not a poor prognostic sign. The problem is commonly caused by "overacupuncturing": Too many points were used, wrong points were selected, too much stimulation was applied, or needles were left in place too long. Correcting these procedures in future sessions usually resolves the problem. Other sequelae that may occur are as follows: bent or broken needles; "needle-lock" or "frozen needles" (needles caught in tissue, usually because of muscle spasms or becoming tangled in fascia, which makes them difficult to remove); injury to vital organs such as the heart, liver, kidneys, and spleen; hematomas; pneumothorax; infections; nausea; vomiting; and, in one instance, syncope (Chu and others, 1979; Rogers, 1981).

Techniques and Instrumentation

Physiologic events take place when acupuncture points are stimulated. The specific stimulus, strength of excitative action, and duration of stimulation all affect the body's response. The methods of applying the stimuli vary considerably, from a method as simple as application of finger pressure to a method as complex as electronic stimulation, wherein such variables as wave form, amplitude, frequency, and patterns of stimuli can be adjusted to achieve different results (Altman, 1994).

Methods of Stimulation

Acupressure

Acupressure, or transdermal pressure therapy, was probably one of the earliest forms of point therapy. We unconsciously practice it on ourselves every time we rub a painful place or scratch a pruritic area. The early Chinese physicians described eight different forms of therapeutic massage (Bresler and others, 1976): thrusting, grasping, pressing, rubbing, rolling, pinching, rubbing between the palms, and tapping. Acupressure can be described as finger pressure applied to the body surface in a general pattern or at designated points or locations (Siciliano, 1980). Many styles of acupressure are in current use, among them *Shiatsu, Do-In, Jun Shin Do Jitsu,* and *Tsubo* therapy.

Shiatsu is thumb-pressure massage, usually using double thumb pressure in an overall body pattern. *Do-In* is seldom used in animal treatment because it relies on a self-treatment technique to relieve headache, indigestion, cramping, and dizziness. In performing *Jin Shin Do Jitsu,* the practitioner holds consecutive sets of two points simultaneously. *Tsubo* therapy is similar to *Shiatsu* in the use of thumb pressure, but attention is given to specific groups of points with interrelated therapeutic properties, and points are treated for a longer period of time. In veterinary medicine, acupressure is used rarely, mostly to relieve muscle spasm and alleviate pain. It can be taught to owners to augment veterinarian-applied acupuncture.

Cupping and vacuum therapy

Negative pressure can be applied to points by the ancient technique of cupping. Three types of cups are available. One type is made of bamboo and has a small mouth and base and a slightly enlarged midsection. The other two types are globular, small-mouthed pots made of clay and glass (Silverstein and others, 1975). A combustible solution such as alcohol is applied to the interior of the cup and ignited. The cup is then placed firmly over the point. As the fire in the cup consumes oxygen, a vacuum is created that pulls the skin into the cup. In China, cupping is used regularly in humans and sometimes in large animals. Because of the risk of iatrogenic burns, this modality is not popular among veterinarians in the United States.

Needles

The *Huang Ti Nei Ching* describes nine traditional types of needles. Today, 25- to 34-gauge filiform stainless-steel needles, ½ to 2 inches (1.25 to 5 cm) long, are most commonly used in small animal treatments (see Fig. 10-1). The size of the animal and the location of the points being treated determine the length of the needles used. Shorter needles (½ inch, or 1.25 cm) are used in small breeds and in points over bony areas such as the head, face, and distal limbs and in areas where body cavities might be penetrated, such as the abdomen and lateral thorax. Medium needles (1 inch, or 2.5 cm) are used paravertebrally along the dorsal midline and in the upper thighs. Longer needles (1½ to 2 inches, or 3.75 to 5 cm) are used around the hip joints and popliteal fossae of large canine breeds. Cats can usually be treated using only ½-inch (1.25-cm) needles. The needles are solid and flexible, with a smooth shaft. If examined under a microscope, the point appears rounded and pencil-like. High-quality needles are flexible enough to bend to at least a 90-degree angle without breaking and then be straightened to their original shape without kinking. The needles of highest quality are manufactured in China, Korea, and Japan. Disposable presterilized needles are available, but because the standard needles can be straightened, sharpened, honed, autoclaved, and reused many times, they may be more economical. The proper techniques for inserting needles to the correct depth and at the proper angle, applying the appropriate manipulation to the needles while in situ, and removing the needles are more difficult than they initially appear. Proper training and extensive practice are necessary before a practitioner should treat animal patients.

Temperature variation

USE OF HEAT   Moxibustion is described in the *Huang Ti Nei Ching*, which suggests that it is probably almost as old as acupuncture itself. Moxa is the Chinese name for the powdered leaves of the mugwort, *Artemisia vulgaris.* The leaves of this medicinal herb are cured, dried, and ground in a mortar. The remaining pale-yellow fiber is sifted to separate the moxa "wool" from the stems. For direct moxibustion, the moxa wool, or "punk," is rolled into the shape of a tiny cone and placed directly on the acupuncture point being treated. It is then ignited and allowed to burn down toward the skin. The cone is removed with forceps before it can cause a thermal burn. The procedure is repeated several times, producing a local area of intense erythema over the acupuncture point. A base of bland ointment can be applied to the shaved skin before placement of the moxa cones. The ointment helps the cone adhere to the skin and protects the skin from injury.

Indirect moxibustion is much more common. The moxa can be obtained prerolled into a cigar-shaped stick and wrapped in a specially treated paper. (In ancient times, the moxa was rolled and sealed in mulberry bark.) The moxa stick is ignited and then moved slowly back and forth over an acupuncture point or over a needle inserted into an acupuncture point. The procedure is carried out until the skin becomes slightly erythematous. Practitioners using both direct and indirect moxibustion must be careful not to burn the patient or singe surrounding hair. These techniques are particularly effective in treating chronic pain problems.

Another method of using heat to stimulate acupuncture loci is the use of infrared lamps. The lamps are placed at a distance of 18 to 24 inches from the body surface to heat needles already in place. Special electronic thermal devices have been developed specifically for acupoint stimulation. Irritant blister pastes for further stimulation of these areas have been used in large animals, but their use in small animals is discouraged.

USE OF COLD   Cryotherapy is effective in many acute pain conditions. Ice cubes, dry ice, prepackaged chemical coolants, and ethyl chloride spray have been used. The stimulation of acupuncture points with cold is not advocated for chronic pain conditions.

Ultrasound

Sonapuncture, the ultrasonic stimulation of acupuncture loci, has been advocated because it is noninvasive and shortens the treatment time. Only 10 to 30 seconds per point are required; small sound heads or probes as small as ¼ inch (5 mm) in diameter are available.

Aquapuncture

Injection of solutions into acupuncture points is rapid, easily accomplished in most cases, and sometimes the only way to treat an animal who can be restrained for a very short time only. In small animals a 25-gauge ½- to 1-inch (1.25- to 2.5-cm) hypodermic needle can be used. Examples of substances suggested for injection include distilled water, electrolyte solutions (preferably hypotonic or hypertonic), vitamins (especially B_{12} and C), antibiotics, herbal extracts, local anesthetics, analgesics (e.g., phenylbutazone), and steroidal and nonsteroidal antiinflammatory agents. Amounts injected range from 0.25 cc to 2 cc, depending on the site of injection and size of the animal. A dermojet can also be used for aquapuncture. It is held approximately ½ inch (1.25 cm) from the skin and, when activated, sprays a high-pressure jet of solution into the top layers of skin, producing a wheal.

Electroacupuncture

Electronic devices have been developed to augment the stimulation given to acupuncture points (Fig. 10-6). Some devices are attached to inserted needles to deliver electronic stimulation percutaneously. Others use an electroconductive medium and probes to pass the stimulus transcutaneously to underlying nerve structures. The electronic stimulation is more intense than manual manipulation of needles and usually causes more profound effects. Its use is almost essential in producing acupuncture analgesia for surgery. Most of the better machines are battery-powered to prevent the danger of electrocution, AC rather than DC to prevent the danger of electrolysis burns, and small enough to be easily portable. Many different types of electrostimulators are available. The better ones have the following characteristics: They are operated by transistor, cell, or rechargeable battery packs; they have a pulse generator that produces the frequency and pulse shape of the current; they possess frequency and pulse control knobs to regulate the pulse generator; and they have a current con-

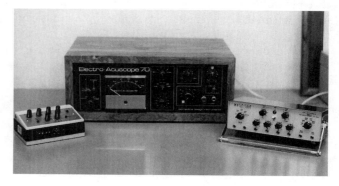

Fig. 10-6   Electroacupuncture machines. (From Ettinger SJ, Feldman EC: *Textbook of veterinary internal medicine,* ed 4, Philadelphia, 1995, WB Saunders.)

trol to modulate the amplitude of the current going to the body (Chan, 1974). Electroacupuncture is commonly used in both human and animal acupuncture in Europe and the United States.

Implantation

A more prolonged stimulation of acupuncture points is achieved by implanting various materials into the loci. The most familiar examples are press needles or staples in the ears of humans to treat certain addictions, smoking, and obesity. These implantation techniques are seldom used in small animals. Sutures can also be buried at acupoints to provide long-term therapy. Catgut and stainless-steel sutures have been used. The most common implantation technique in small animals is the use of metallic beads around the hip joints to treat chronic pain resulting from hip dysplasia–induced osteoarthritis (Durkes, 1994). Under general anesthesia and aseptic conditions a large-gauge (14-gauge) hypodermic needle is inserted into the proper acupuncture points. Several small gold beads are inserted through the lumen of the needle. A stylet is passed down the lumen of the needle to keep the beads in place as the needle is withdrawn. Then the hypodermic needle and stylet are withdrawn (in that order), leaving the beads permanently in the deeper tissues. In addition to treating chronic hip pain, the technique has been used to treat epilepsy in dogs (Klide and others, 1984).

Laserpuncture

The use of low-intensity lasers to stimulate acupuncture points is popular among many veterinary practitioners, particularly those who work with horses. This practice began in 1973. Advocates of laser therapy cite successful results in the treatment of pain, inflammatory conditions, and neurogenic disorders and the enhancement of healing in wounds, burns, ulcers, tendons, and bones (Basko, 1983; Jaggar, 1982). The term laser is derived by combining the first letters of *L*ight *A*mplification by *S*timulated *E*mission of *R*adiation. Laser therapy has been described as "a form of intense light therapy using various frequencies and wave lengths which promote positive physiologic changes within cells that support the living organism in healing and reducing or eliminating pain" (Basko, 1983). The two types of lasers most commonly used in acupuncture are the red light emitters (wave length of 632 to 650 nm, generated by either a helium-neon gas tube or a laser-simulating diode device) and the infrared light emitters (wave length 902 nm, generated by a gallium-arsenite diode). The red light penetrates to a depth of 0.8 to 15 mm, and the infrared light penetrates to a depth of 10 mm to 5 cm. The detractors of laserpuncture claim that very little penetration of tissues takes place with the emissions from low intensity, or "cold," lasers—at least not enough to cause physiologic changes.

The advantages claimed for laser acupoint therapy are noninvasiveness, asepsis, freedom from pain, minimal re-

straint requirements, and short treatment time. The disadvantages are the cost of laser units (except for some small hand-held units), limitations in treating large areas, and insufficient data about the optimal parameters used to produce specific effects (e.g., wavelength, time of exposure, intensity of energy, frequency of light emissions, and frequency of treatment) (Jaggar, 1982). Researchers have made the following claims about the effects of laser biostimulation effects: increased phagocytosis, increased tissue granulation, increased collagen synthesis, increased vascularization, increased acetylcholine release, increased production of T- and B-lymphocytes, increased synthesis of serotonin, inhibition of prostaglandin effects on tissues (e.g., pain, inflammation, and vasoconstriction), stimulation and release of beta endorphins, and increased synthesis of ketosteroids and hydroxycorticosteroids (Basko, 1983).

Acupuncture Points

Description

TCM categorizes acupuncture loci into two main groups: those lying on the 14 channels and those not on these 14 channels (designated extra points). The points have traditional Chinese names but are more commonly characterized in the United States and Europe by an alpha-numeric designation that shows the particular channel on which the point is located and the number of the point on the channel (e.g., *BL-60* refers to the sixtieth point on the Bladder channel). The points are further classified according to action as *source, connecting, accumulating, association, alarm, master, action, trigger, terminal, tonification, and sedation points*. Further exploration of these categories is beyond the scope of this chapter.

Acupuncture points have been classified into four groups based on their relationship to neural structures. Type I corresponds to known anatomic entities (e.g., the motor points of muscles),* type II corresponds to the focal meeting of superficial nerves in the sagittal plane, type III points lie over the superficial nerves or nerve plexuses, and type IV lie over the Golgi tendon organs at the muscle-tendon junction (Hwang, Egerbacher, 1994). Some physical attributes of acupoints are a lower electrical skin resistance than that of surrounding skin, a higher thermographic register than surrounding skin, and local tenderness on palpation. Most acupoints lie in anatomic depressions and are located by using relationships with anatomic landmarks, proportional measurements using anatomic descriptions and maps, palpation (points usually feel like small indentations or nodules under the skin), and

---

*Motor point: "1. the point at which a motor nerve enters a muscle. 2. Any point on the skin over a muscle at which the application of galvanic stimulation will cause contraction of a corresponding muscle." From *Dorland's Illustrated Medical Dictionary,* ed 26, Philadelphia, 1994, WB Saunders.

electronic point finders. The point finders are used to locate the areas of lower electrical resistance or higher conductance on the skin. Unfortunately, interference by hair or skin moisture can sometimes produce false readings.

Selection of Points

Practitioners must first learn the anatomic locations of acupuncture points. Next, they must learn the physiologic consequences of stimulating each point individually and in combination with other points. Then, after making a diagnosis and determining that acupuncture is indicated, practitioners must select the points to be used (prescription), establish the duration of the therapy session, and choose the type of stimulus (dosage). In TCM, several laws are used to determine these parameters (Wei-Ping, 1974) (Box 10-2).

Expected Results

In acute problem cases, treating the animal every 2 to 3 days usually causes steady improvement until the desired results are achieved. If the animal is treated only once weekly, the improvement seems to peak at the third or fourth day and then decrease; at the next treatment the condition is only slightly better than when therapy was last given. At each treatment, however, improvement peaks a little higher and wanes more slowly, until progress becomes steady. In chronic cases, improvement is usually achieved more slowly and may vary at each treatment session until the desired effects are seen. Exacerbation of signs may be seen after treatment, but this effect is usually temporary.

In two large-scale clinical evaluations, acceptable improvement was seen in 50% to 63.4% of the cases treated (Altman, 1981; Joechle, 1977). This does not seem to be an especially high response level until one considers that most of the cases were presented because they were refractory to more conventional therapies.

Attitudes Toward the Use of Acupuncture

Reasons for Past Nonacceptance

Acupuncture has elicited responses ranging from apathy to antagonism. Only recently has the veterinary community expressed real enthusiasm. Several reasons may account for the lack of widespread popularity. The use of foreign or unfamiliar terms, such as *"yang," "yin," "Qi,"* and

---

BOX 10-2

TCM LAWS FOR DETERMINING PARAMETERS OF ACUPUNCTURE

Yi Pan Yun Yong Fa: Local points used in combination with major distal points (e.g., mandibular pain can be treated with needles in the jaw plus needles in the toes on related meridians).

Tan Hseuh Tu Yung Fa: Use of only a single point known to have a specific action for a specific malady (e.g., a point on the midline directly between the eyes is used for treating epilepsy).

Shuang Hsueh Ping Yong Fa: Use of two symmetric points (e.g., treating points bilaterally for a more intense effect).

Szu Chih Hsiang Ying Fa: Use of points on all four extremities.

Lien Suo Ping Chen Fa: Use of a chain of points on the same extremity for more profound effects.

Nei Wai Hu Ying Fa: Use of two points at the same level on a body part, usually head or trunk, one point located anteriorly, the other posteriorly (e.g., one needle at the foramen magnum, the other in the nasal philtrum to treat brain disorders).

Lun Huan Chiao Ti Fa: Encircling a point (e.g., using points surrounding a burn).

Hsun Ching Ch'u Hsueh Fa: Use of points at the distal part of a meridian to treat disorders at the proximal end and vice versa (e.g., the use of a point on the hand to treat epistaxis, because the distal end of the meridian terminates next to the nares).

Piao Li Hsiang P'ei Fa: The relationship between an exterior point and an internal organ, probably by stimulating a somatovisceral reflex.

Tui Cheng Ch'u Hsueh Fa: The application of known and well-proven formulas. This method is used by novice Oriental practitioners and by most Occidental practitioners.

Alarm Points and Associated Points: Use of specific alarm points or associated points for diagnosis and treatment of disorders of internal organs or disorders located along the related channels (e.g., McBurney's point for appendicitis in humans).

The Five-Element Theory: Use of traditional oriental laws of the relationships between channels.

"meridian," sometimes makes a new modality less attractive to the medical community. Some early investigators, who claimed fantastic results and provided little clinical or research data to support them, created poor first impressions. A community of professionals habituated to controlled studies, scientific investigations, and hard facts found this anecdotal support unacceptable. A few advocates adopted a mystical tone in presenting their findings, which many veterinarians disliked. In fact, many approaches to acupuncture have been presented in an unscientific manner, one that is unpalatable to veterinarians with a sound scientific education. The lack of an all-inclusive physiologic explanation made others hesitant to accept the validity of acupuncture. To those able to overcome these hurdles came the further problem of limited access to information and educational opportunities. The many hours of study and considerable commitment in class time, financial expense, and travel associated with acupuncture have discouraged other veterinarians. Many practitioners also have misgivings about the way acupuncture is perceived by colleagues and clients.

Present Resurgence of Interest

Fortunately, in spite of these obstacles, a greater acceptance of veterinary acupuncture is gradually occurring. Media interest has led to client interest. Client interest has caused veterinarians to seek the help of veterinary acupuncturists. The favorable results obtained have stimulated the curiosity and interest of veterinary organizations. Articles and papers on veterinary acupuncture are now being accepted by more veterinary journals. Local, regional, state, national, and international meetings, seminars, and conventions have featured speakers on acupuncture. However, regard for the rights of the pet-owning public and concern for the image of the veterinary profession have prompted the American Veterinary Medical Association and several state associations to designate ad hoc committees to investigate the validity of acupuncture therapy and the credentials of those professing to practice this modality. This involvement benefits the public, which is entitled to competent service; the profession, because the reputation of veterinary medicine will be upheld; and veterinary acupuncturists, who will be compelled to maintain a high level of proficiency to earn the respect and trust of the general public and veterinary professionals.

Sources of Information and Education

IVAS presents courses composed of four intensive 4-day sessions at regular intervals. The courses feature lectures by a faculty of American, European, and Asian experts; literature reviews; hand-out materials; and live demonstrations with opportunities for hands-on training. The annual courses provide at least 120 hours of class time. Information regarding the courses and the organization can be obtained by writing to the current executive director.*

Two-day introductory courses are sometimes offered to individuals or organizations. IVAS can also be of aid in recommending such courses.

Legal and Ethical Implications of Acupuncture

Legal briefs in the Journal of the American Veterinary Medical Association (Hannah, 1977a, 1977b) indicate that the use of acupuncture constitutes the practice of veterinary medicine and/or surgery and that nonveterinarians practicing acupuncture on animals are probably in violation of local practice acts, unless special provisions exist for the treatment of an animal by a nonveterinary acupuncturist under the direction and control of a licensed veterinarian. No regulations exist, however, to ensure the competence of a licensed veterinarian to practice acupuncture on animal patients. Eventually, for protection of the public and the reputation of the profession, provisions may be necessary to ensure that veterinarians or accredited nonveterinary acupuncturists under veterinary supervision are indeed educated and qualified in the practice of acupuncture on animals (Altman, 1977a). Ideally the profession will soon accept the certification of an organization such as the IVAS, or a College of Veterinary Acupuncturists will be formed to examine and accredit candidates as other specialty boards accredit diplomates.

REFERENCES

Altman S: Acupuncture: a modern look at an ancient art, *California Vet* 31:6, 1977a.

Altman S: Acupuncture: taking a closer look, *MVP* 58:1003, 1977b.

Altman S: Acupuncture as an emergency treatment, *Calif Vet* 33:6, 1979.

Altman S: *An introduction to acupuncture for animals,* Monterey Park, Calif, 1981a, Chan's Corporation.

Altman S: Clinical use of veterinary acupuncture, *VM/SAC* 76:1307, 1981b.

Altman S: Acupuncture therapy in small animal practice. In Ettinger SJ, ed: *Textbook of veterinary internal medicine,* ed 3, Philadelphia, 1989, WB Saunders Co.

Altman S: Techniques and instrumentation. In Schoen AE: *Veterinary acupuncture: ancient art to modern medicine,* St Louis, 1994, Mosby.

Altman S: Acupuncture therapy in small animal practice. In Ettinger SJ, Feldman EC, editors: *Textbook of veterinary internal medicine,* ed 4, Philadelphia, 1995, WB Saunders.

AVMA Directory, Schaumberg, Ill, 1987, AVMA.

Bannerman RH: World Health Organization viewpoint on acupuncture. Reprinted in *Am J Acup* 8:231, 1980.

Basko IJ: A new frontier: laser therapy, *Calif Vet* 37:17, 1983.

Becker RO, Selden G: *The body electric,* New York, 1985, William Morrow.

---

*Executive Director, International Veterinary Acupuncture Society, P.O. Box 1478, Longmont, CO 80502-1478.

Becker RO and others : Electrophysiological correlates of acupuncture points and meridians, *Psychoenergetic Systems* 1:105, 1976.

Bergsman O, Woolley-Hart A: Differences in electrical skin conductivity between acupuncture points and adjacent skin areas, *Am J Acup* 1:27, 1983.

Bresler DE: *Free yourself From pain*, New York, 1979, Simon and Schuster.

Bresler DE: Personal communication, 1982.

Bresler DE, Katz RL, Kroening RJ: *Acupuncture and chronic pain: a comprehensive follow up evaluation*, Los Angeles, 1975a, UCLA Acupuncture Project.

Bresler DE, Katz, RL, Kroening, RJ: Review of research findings of the UCLA Research Project, Los Angeles, 1975b, UCLA Acupuncture Research Project.

Bresler DE, Kroening RJ: Three essential factors in effective acupuncture therapy, *Am J Chin Med* 4:81, 1976.

Bresler DE and others: *Acupuncture for control and management of pain*, Pacific Palisades, Calif, 1976, Center for Integral Medicine.

Bresler DE and others: *Traditional and contemporary theories of acupuncture. II. Contemporary theories of acupuncture: acupuncture, acupressure, and TENS for pain control*, Pacific Palisades, Calif, 1980, Center for Integral Medicine.

Brown ML and others: The effects of acupuncture on white blood counts, *Am J Chin Med* 2:383, 1974a.

Brown ML and others: Acupuncture loci: techniques for location, *Am J Chin Med* 2:67, 1974b.

Buchli R: Successful acupuncture treatment of a cervical disc syndrome in a dog, *VM/SAC* 70:1302, 1975.

Buchli R: Acupuncture treatment of post-myositis syndrome, *VM/SAC* 71:465, 1976.

Bullock J: Acupuncture treatment of canine lick granuloma, *Calif Vet* 32:14, 1978.

Chan P: *Electroacupuncture: its clinical applications in therapy*, Los Angeles, 1974, Chan's Corporation.

Cheng RS, Pomeranz BH: Electroacupuncture is mediated by stereospecific opiate receptors and is reversed by antagonists of type 1 receptors, *Life Sci* 26:631, 1980.

Chin DTJ, Ching K: A study of the mechanisms of the hypotensive effect of acupuncture in the rat, *Am J Chin Med* 2:413, 1974.

Chu LSW and others: *Acupuncture manual: a western approach*, New York, 1979, Marcel Dekker.

Chuan Y, editor: *Handbook on Chinese veterinary acupuncture and moxibustion*, Bangkok, 1990, FAO Regional Office for Asia and the Pacific.

Clifford DH: Acupuncture in veterinary medicine. In Kirk RW, editor: *Current veterinary therapy IX, small animal practice*, Philadelphia, 1986, WB Saunders.

Clifford DH, Lee MO: Trends in acupuncture research. I. Acupuncture in the control of pain, *VM/SAC* 73:1513, 1978.

Clifford DH, Lee MO: Trends in acupuncture research. II. Acupuncture and the autonomic nervous system, *VM/SAC* 74:35, 1979.

Concon AA: Energetic concepts of classical Chinese acupuncture, *Am J Acupunct* 1:66, 1979.

Durkes TE: Gold bead implants. In Schoen AM, editor: *Veterinary acupuncture: ancient art to modern medicine*, St Louis, 1994, Mosby.

Feng K: A method of electro-acupuncture treatment for equine intestinal impaction, *Am J Chin Med* 9:174, 1981 (Translated and edited by Hwang YC).

Gideon L: Acupuncture: clinical trials in the horse, *JAVMA* 170:220, 1977.

Ha H and others: Naloxone reversal of acupuncture analgesia in the monkey, *Exp Neurol* 73:298, 1981.

Hannah H: Legal brief: more about acupuncture, *JAVMA* 171:44, 1977a.

Hannah H: Veterinary medicine and acupuncture, *JAVMA* 170:802, 1977b.

Hsu H-Y, Peacher WG: *Chen's history of Chinese medical science*, Taipei, 1977, Modern Drug.

Huang HL: *Ear acupuncture: a complete text by the Nanking army ear acupuncture team*, Emmaus, Penn, 1974, Rodale.

Hwang, YC, Egerbacher M: Anatomy and classification of acupoints. In Schoen AM, editor: *Veterinary acupuncture: ancient art to modern medicine*, St Louis, 1994, Mosby.

Jaggar DH: A review of the low intensity laser and its application to acupuncture. Proceedings of the eighth Annual International Veterinary Acupuncture Conference, IVAS, Ft. Mitchell, Ky, 1982.

Jaggar DH: Basic introduction to veterinary acupuncture. In Schoen AM, editor: *Probs Vet Med* 4(1):1, Mar 1992.

Jaggar DH: History and concepts in veterinary acupuncture. In Schoen AM, editor: *Veterinary acupuncture: ancient art to modern medicine*, St Louis, 1994, Mosby.

Janssens LA: Acupuncture therapy for the treatment of chronic osteoarthritis in dogs: a review of 61 cases, *VM/SAC* 71:465, 1976a.

Janssens LA: Acupuncture treatment for thoracolumbar disc hernia in the dog: preview results. Paper presented at the twelfth Annual International Congress of Veterinary Acupuncture, Pa, Sept 1976b.

Janssens LA: The investigation and treatment of canine thoracolumbar disc disease: a personal view on the practical approach in a one-person veterinary practice. Paper presented at the twelfth Annual International Congress of Veterinary Acupuncture, Pa, Sept 1976c.

Janssens LA: Myofascial pain syndrome in dogs: the treatment of trigger points: a review of 41 cases. Paper presented at the twelfth Annual International Congress of Veterinary Acupuncture, Pa, Sept 1976d.

Janssens LA: An overview: veterinary acupuncture in Europe, *Am J Acupunct* 9:151, 1981.

Janssens LA: Practical possibilities of acupuncture analgesia in small animal practice. Proceedings of the eighth annual International Veterinary Acupuncture Conference on Veterinary Acupuncture, *IVAS* 33, Ft. Mitchell, Ky, 1982.

Janssens LA: Acupuncture treatment for canine thoracolumbar disk protrusions: a review of 78 cases, *VM/SAC* 78:1580, 1983.

Janssens LA: *Acupuncture points and meridians in the dog*, Antwerp, 1984, Blondian.

Janssens LA: The treatment of canine cervical disc disease by means of acupuncture: a review of 32 cases, *J Small Anim Pract* 26:203, 1985.

Janssens LA: Canine disc disease: a survey of acupuncture therapy. In Janssens LA, editor: *Some aspects of small animal acupuncture*, Brussels, 1989, Belgian Acupuncture Society.

Janssens LA: Acupuncture for the treatment of thoracolumbar and cervical disc disease in the dog. In Schoen AM, editor: *Probs Vet Med* 4(1):107, 1992.

Janssens LA: Acupuncture for thoracolumbar and cervical disc disease. In Schoen AM, editor: *Veterinary acupuncture: ancient art to modern medicine*, St Louis, 1994, Mosby.

Janssens L, De Prins EM: Treatment of thoracolumbar disc disease in dogs by means of acupuncture: a comparison of two techniques, *J Am Anim Hosp Assoc* 25:169, 1989.

Janssens L and others: Respiratory and cardiac arrest under general anesthesia: treatment by acupuncture of the nasal philtrum, *Vet Rec* 105:273, 1979.

Joechle W: Acupuncture in veterinary medicine: fact, fraud, or hoax? *Pract Vet* July/Aug, p 4, 1975.

Joechle W: How effective is acupuncture: a report by the National Association for Veterinary Acupuncture, *Calif Vet* 31:22, 1977.

Joechle W: Veterinary acupuncture in Europe and America: past and present, *Am J Acupunct* 6:149, 1978.

Joseph R: Neurologic evaluation and its relation to acupuncture for neurologic disorders. In Schoen AM, editor: *Probs Vet Med* 4 (1):98, 1992.

Joseph R: Acupuncture for neurologic disorders. In Schoen AM, editor: *Veterinary Acupuncture: Ancient Art to Modern Medicine,* St Louis, 1994, Mosby.

Klide A: Acupuncture therapy for the treatment of intractable idiopathic epilepsy in 5 dogs. Proceedings of the 10th Annual International Conference on Veterinary Acupuncture, *IVAS* 55, Austin, Tx, 1984.

Klide AM: Use of acupuncture for the control of chronic pain and for surgical analgesia. In Short CE, Van Poznack A, editors: *Animal pain,* New York, 1992, Churchill Livingstone.

Klide AM, Kung SH: *Veterinary Acupuncture,* Philadelphia, 1977, University of Pennsylvania Press.

Klide AM and others: Acupuncture therapy for the treatment of intractable, idiopathic epilepsy in 5 dogs. Proceedings of the tenth Annual International Conference on Veterinary Acupuncture, *IVAS* 1984.

Kussaari J: Acupuncture treatment of aerophagia in horses, *Am J Acupunct* 11:363, 1983.

Lakshmipathi OR and others: Caesarean section in an ewe under acupuncture anesthesia, *Am J Acupunct* 12:161, 1984.

Latshaw WK: Current theories of pain perception related to acupuncture, *JAAHA* 2:449, 1975.

Lee DC, Lee MO: Endorphins, naloxone, and acupuncture, *Calif Vet* 33:24, 1979.

Lee DC and others: Cardiovascular effects of acupuncture in anesthetized dogs, *Am J Chin Med* 2:271, 1974.

Lee GTC: A study of electrical stimulation of acupuncture locus *Tsusanli* (ST-36) on mesenteric microcirculation, *Am J Chin Med* 2:53, 1975.

Lee GTC and others: Acupuncture anesthesia used in rabbit abdominal operations, *Am J Acupunct* 4:149, 1976.

Lee MO and others: Cardiovascular effects of acupuncture at *Tsusanli* (ST-36) in dogs, *J Surg Res* 18:51, 1975.

Lee-kin: *A handbook of acupuncture treatment for dogs and cats,* Hong Kong, 1985, Hong Kong Medicine and Health (Translated by Tinshen).

Levin N: Acupuncture in acute and chronic pain problems, *Anesthesiol Rev,* p 10, Jan 1976.

Loony GL: Autonomic theory of acupuncture. Proceedings of the second World Symposium on Acupuncture and Chinese Medicine, *Am J Chin Med* 2:332, 1974.

Lung CH and others: An observation of the humoral factor in acupuncture analgesia in rats, *Am J Chin Med* 2:203, 1974.

Man PL, Chen CH: Mechanism of acupunctural anesthesia: diseases of the nervous system. In Woods W: Relief of localized pain by transcutaneous electrostimulation, *Am J Acupunct* 3:137, 1973.

Mayer DJ and others: Antagonism of acupuncture analgesia in man by Naloxone, *Brain Res* 121:368, 1977.

Melzack R, Wall P: Pain mechanisms: a new theory, *Science* 150:971, 1965.

Minutes of meeting of AVMA Alternate Therapies Committee, Chicago, Ill, Jan 20-21, 1987.

Mok M: Medicine: East meets West, *Int J Chin Med* 1:1, 1984.

Monte T, editor: *World medicine: the East West guide to healing your body,* New York, 1993, Jeremy P Tarcher/Perigree.

New committee studies alternate therapies, *JAVMA* 188:669, 1986.

O'Boyle MA, Vajda GK: Acupuncture anesthesia for abdominal surgery, *MVP* 56:705, 1973.

O'Conner J, Bensky D: A summary of research concerning the effects of acupuncture, *Am J Chin Med* 3:377, 1975.

Oleson RD, Kroening RJ, Bresler DE: Diagnostic accuracy of examining electrical activity at ear acupuncture points for assessing areas of the body with musculoskeletal pain, *Pain Abstracts* 1:185, 1978.

Reichmanis M and others: Electrical correlates of acupuncture points, *IEEE Transactions on Biomed Engineering,* p 553, Nov 1975.

Reichmanis M and others: DC skin conductance variation at acupuncture loci, *Am J Chin Med* 4:69, 1976.

Reichmanis M and others: Laplace plane analysis of impedence on the H. Meridian, *Am J Chin Med* 7:188, 1979.

Reston J: Now about my operation in Peking, *The New York Times,* p 1, July 26, 1971.

Rogers PAM: Success claimed for acupuncture in domestic animals: a veterinary news item, *Irish Vet J* 28:182, 1974.

Rogers PAM: The primitive nervous systems and enkephalins, *Am J Chin Med* 4:410, 1976.

Rogers PAM: Personal communication, 1976—present.

Rogers PAM: Serious complications of acupuncture . . . or acupuncture abuses? *Am J Acupunct* 9:347, 1981.

Rogers PAM, Bossey J: Activation of the defense systems of the body in animals and man by acupuncture and moxibustion, *Acupunct Res Q* 5:47, 1981.

Rogers PAM and others: Stimulation of the acupuncture points in relation to analgesia and therapy of clinical disorders in animals, *Vet Ann* 17:258, 1977.

Schoen AM: Critical evaluation of veterinary acupuncture therapy for chronic arthropathies. Proceedings of the ninth Annual International Conference on Veterinary Acupuncture, *IVAS,* p 73, 1983.

Schoen AM: An introduction to veterinary acupuncture, mechanisms of action, indications, and clinical applications. Proceedings of the fifty-third annual meeting of AAHA, p 374, 1986.

Schoen AM: Acupuncture for musculoskeletal disorders. In Schoen AM, editor: *Probs Vet Med* 4(1):88, 1992a.

Schoen AM, editor: Veterinary acupuncture, *Probs Vet Med* 4:1, March, 1992b.

Schoen AM: Acupuncture for musculoskeletal disorders. In Schoen AM, editor: *Veterinary acupuncture: ancient art to modern medicine,* St Louis, 1994, Mosby.

Schoen AM, editor: *Veterinary acupuncture: ancient art to modern medicine,* St Louis, 1994, Mosby.

Shores A: Canine acupuncture chart, 1975 (self-published).

Siciliano FR: Acupressure technique for pain control. Paper presented to Center for Integral Medicine, Pacific Palisades, Calif, Jan 1980.

Silverstein ME and others: *Acupuncture and moxibustion: a handbook for the barefoot doctors of China (a translation),* New York, 1975, Schocken Books.

Smith FWK: The neurophysiological basis of acupuncture. In Schoen AM, editor: *Veterinary acupuncture: ancient art to modern medicine,* St Louis, 1994, Mosby.

Stefanatos J: Treatment to reduce radial nerve paralysis, *VM/SAC* 79:67, 1984.

Still J: Acupuncture treatment of thoracolumbar disc disease: a study of 35 cases, *Companion Animal Pract* 2:19, 1988.

Still J: Analgesic effects of acupuncture on thoracolumbar disc disease in dogs, *J Small Animal Pract* 30:298, 1989.

Still J: Acupuncture treatment of type III and IV thoracolumbar disc disease, *Mod Vet Pract* 7:35, 1987.

Tashkin DP and others: Comparison of real and simulated acupuncture and isoproterenol in methacholine induced asthma, *Ann Allergy* 39:379, 1977.

Toyama P, Nishizwa M: The physiological basis of acupuncture therapy, *J Nat Med Assoc,* p 397, Sept 1972.

Waters KC: Acupuncture for dermatological disorders. In Schoen AM, editor: *Probs Vet Med* 4(1):194, 1992.

Waters KC: Acupuncture for dermatological disorders in dogs and cats. In Schoen AM, editor: *Veterinary acupuncture: ancient art to modern medicine,* St Louis, 1994, Mosby.

Wei-kang F: *The story of Chinese acupuncture and moxibustion,* Peking, 1975, Foreign Language Press.

Wei-Ping W: *Chinese acupuncture,* Wellingsborough, England, 1974, Health Service Press, (Translated by Chancellor PM from the French edition by Lavier J).

Weinstein W, editor: *Veterinary acupuncture, vol 2, Dog,* North Hollywood, Calif, 1975, Eastwind.

White SS, Christie M: Traditional acupuncture and tetanus in the horse, *Am J Acupunct* 12:359, 1974.

Wong J, Cheng R: *The science of acupuncture therapy,* self-published, no date.

Wright M, McGrath CJ: Physiologic and analgesic effects of acupuncture in the dog, *JAVMA* 178:502, 1981.

Xinnong C, editor: *Chinese acupuncture and moxibustion,* Beijing, 1987, Foreign Languages Press.

Young HG: *Atlas of veterinary acupuncture charts,* ed 2, Thomasville, Ga, 1978, Oriental Veterinary Acupuncture Specialties.

Young HG: Regional analgesia in dogs with electro-acupuncture, *Calif Vet* 33:11, 1979.

Chapter 11

Equine Acupuncture

PEGGY FLEMING

Equine acupuncture has recently experienced an enormous surge in popularity in the United States. From prestigious race tracks to the show grounds of top hunter-jumper events, veterinarians can be found practicing this ancient art on some of the best performance horses in the country. Curiously, this surge in popularity has surpassed that of the human acupuncture field. The discrepancy may partly result from the inherent "needlephobia" of the American public but probably has more to do with the enormous clinical response of the equine species to this modality.

As many ways exist to practice equine acupuncture as ways to practice conventional equine medicine. In fact, most equine acupuncturists in the United States practice methods far different from those used in China. Much of this disparity stems from the incorporation of Japanese perspectives by the early pioneers of American equine acupuncture. For example, the Japanese method of needling is gentler than that used by the Chinese.

Another reason for the methodologic differences is the use of acupuncture with chiropractic and homeopathy in many equine holistic practices. In the United States, acupuncture is an adjunct to not only the aforementioned modalities but also shoeing techniques, saddle fit, and advanced nutrition. Moreover, in China, acupuncture is used in the treatment of farm animals, whereas U.S. practitioners focus on performance athletes.

This chapter focuses on the most popular styles of equine acupuncture currently used in the United States. Some equine acupuncturists believe that only the Chinese methodology is appropriate and derive their treatment approach from points detailed by the ancient masters. Most veterinarians in the United States have adopted acupuncture practices similar to those used for humans, locating points on the human and transposing them to the horse. This method is somewhat controversial because of obvious variations in anatomy (such as rib number) and tremendous anatomic differences in the extremities. Despite this controversy, clinical trials over the past two decades by experienced equine practitioners have proved the merit of these techniques.

History of Equine Acupuncture

Historical evidence shows that equine acupuncture has been performed for over 3000 years (Rogers, 1988). In fact, the field of veterinary acupuncture began with the treatment of horses because of their importance in an economy based on war and agriculture. A sculpture from the Tang dynasty (580-590 AD) shows a soldier performing acupuncture on the shoulder of a horse, and literature dating to the tenth century describes acupuncture therapy for equine heatstroke (Schoen, 1994). During the Ming dynasty, Jesuit priests compiled a reference book on equine acupuncture and brought it to Europe. This collection, entitled *The Treatise on Horses,* later became the basis of modern Chinese veterinary medicine.

Today, Chinese veterinary acupuncturists combine traditional Chinese and Western medicines. The most popular text on acupuncture in China today is *Traditional Chinese Veterinary Acupuncture* (Klide, Kung, 1977). This textbook is a compilation of points used by the ancient masters that are clinically effective in certain conditions.

In America, equine acupuncture began in 1974, when a small group of veterinarians invited two Japanese acupuncturists to the United States to share information about this curious subject. This group became the International Veterinary Acupuncture Society (IVAS). Today, this not-for-profit organization educates veterinarians in traditional Chinese medicine (TCM) through certification courses and yearly conventions. Before 1988 the American Veterinary Medical Association viewed acupuncture as strictly experimental. Today, it views acupuncture as a valid modality but strongly recommends extensive training for veterinarians who practice this form of medicine.

Concepts of Acupuncture

TCM views disease as a state of imbalance between two polarities: *Yin* (i.e., negative, cold, deficiency) and *Yang* (i.e., positive, hot, excess). All elements of nature can be placed in one of these two categories, and the balance of life relies on both the dependence and antagonism of these two extremes. In Western medicine, this concept is illustrated by the sympathetic *(Yang)* and parasympathetic *(Yin)* systems. If one system is underactive, the opposing system appears in excess. If balance does not exist, disease occurs. This concept extends beyond the internal body. Health is also related to the balance of the organism with its environment (nutrition and climate). This philosophy contrasts with that of Western medicine, which concentrates on a singular cause of disease. A striking analogy has been made comparing an acupuncturist and a Western practitioner with a gardener and a mechanic respectively (Beinfield, 1991). Whereas the gardener considers many factors as relevant to the health of his plant (e.g., the amount of sunlight, the proximity of one plant to another, and the amount and type of fertilizer), the mechanic searches only for the dysfunctional part.

Qi is a fundamental concept in Chinese culture. In simple terms, it is energy, or more appropriately, matter on the verge of becoming energy. *Qi* is the source of metabolism within the body. It functions to maintain the normal equilibrium that maintains health. Because *Qi* includes the immune system, it protects the body from external attack. *Qi* also has a structural role, holding everything in its proper place (e.g., it keeps the blood in the vessels and the organs within the abdomen). For example, a horse that is deficient in *Qi* may exhibit lethargy, limb edema, and prolapse of an organ.

Acupuncture Points and the Meridian System

According to TCM, *Qi* flows throughout the body along paths called *meridians,* or *channels.* Along these channels are acupuncture points, foci of neural terminals and vascular bundles with the unique characteristic of increased electrical conductivity. These loci act as capacitors that can be manipulated to influence the flow of *Qi* along the respective channel.

The body contains 14 basic meridian pathways, 12 of which are named after organ systems because each of these meridians communicates with its associated organ, according to Chinese medical theory. Treatment of acupuncture points on these meridians influences the corresponding organs. This phenomenon conforms to the neurophysiologic concepts of viscerosomatic and somatovisceral reflexes. Research in horses has substantiated this theory (Schoen, 1994).

The 12 organ meridians are divided into pairs of six *Yin* and six *Yang* organs. According to TCM, the *Yang* organs are similar in function to their Western counterparts and are involved in absorption of nutrients and elimination of wastes. The *Yin* organs are more involved in the consequent use of the *Qi* derived from these processes and are therefore more involved in the balance of energy necessary to maintain homeostasis. The names of these paired *Yin-Yang* meridians are as follows: the Lung (LU) and Large Intestine (LI), the Pericardium (PC) and Triple Heater (TH), the Heart (HT) and Small Intestine (SI), the Spleen (SP) and Stomach (St), the Liver (LIV) and Gallbladder (GB), and finally the Kidney (KI) and Bladder (BL).

To those unfamiliar with TCM, *triple heater* is a foreign word. TCM does not view organs as simply anatomic viscera but extends the definition to include complex functions that extend beyond the scope of Western medical concepts. This is especially true for the *Yin* organs. For example, in TCM the liver plays the same role in detoxification as it does in Western medicine, but it is also deeply involved in immune function and the health of the eye, hooves, and muscles. The triple heater is comparable to the endocrine system. The Chinese divide the body into three sections (the chest, middle abdomen, and lower abdomen) and discovered that the triple heater ties the function of these three sections together.

When attempting to understand these seemingly foreign perceptions of anatomy, Westerners must realize that the Chinese developed the idea of homeostasis and negative feedback principles long before Western medical science existed. TCM perceives symbolic interrelationships between these organ systems. A philosophic and somewhat poetic culture influenced their understanding of health and disease. Their terminology, adopted long before neurophysiologic concepts existed, is often confusing. To understand these unfamiliar but useful concepts, neophytes are advised to temporarily relinquish their own paradigms and maintain an open mind.

TCM defines each organ pair in terms of a natural element, which symbolizes the neurophysiology of that organ system. The Liver and Gallbladder are associated with the element of wood, which represents expansion and growth (e.g., the spring growth of a forest). Symbolically the Liver functions in directing and collecting the blood. This directorial role also assures the smooth flow of emotion and consistent behavior. The Liver (wood) sends energy to the Heart (fire) (Fig. 11-1). In other words, the Liver is involved in directing blood to the heart. The Liver also regulates the smooth flow of *Qi* and is therefore comparable to the sympathetic nervous system, which produces excitation. If Liver energy in a horse is excessive, the horse may seem agitated. If the Liver is weak and unable

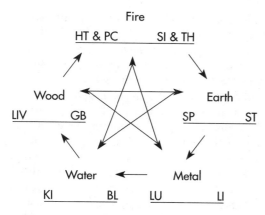

Fig. 11-1 The five-element cycle.

to distribute the blood evenly, the horse may develop a syndrome such as azoturia.

The Heart and Small Intestine are symbolized by the element fire. The Heart warms the entire body. This warmth includes not only circulation but also the soundness of the spirit. The term *spirit* here is not synonymous with the Christian concept but instead refers to an animal's connection to its external surroundings. In Western medical terms, this connection could relate to the function of the cerebral cortex. When the Heart functions properly, a horse is tranquil, alert, and responsive. When the Heart is weak, the horse seems anxious, as if he is unable to comprehend his environment.

The Spleen and Stomach are symbolized by the Earth. The Earth represents nourishment through agriculture. In Chinese medicine, unlike Western medicine, the major function of the Spleen is to supply nourishment derived from food. The Spleen can also be compared to gravity. In other words, it helps the body maintain shape and form by transferring energy and mass from one part of the body to another. It accomplishes this task by regulating metabolism, distributing moisture, and preserving the uprightness of muscles and viscera. A horse with a weakened Spleen may exhibit lethargy, lack of movement (lower metabolism), limb edema, and organ prolapse.

The Lung and Large Intestine are symbolized by the element metal. As a metal gate protects a city, the Lung protects the entranceway to the body and manages external security by controlling the skin. The Lung is involved in the regulation of perspiration and the ability to vasodilate or vasoconstrict according to environmental influences. In other words, the Lung allows adaptation. The Lung also transmutes air into *Qi*. This *Qi* is sent downward by the Lung to the muscles and skin. In addition, the Lung controls the dispersal of moisture downward and outward and is therefore involved in urine regulation. A horse with weakened Lung *Qi* may exhibit continual respiratory infections, scanty urine output, and shortness of breath.

The functions of the Kidney and Bladder are symbolized by the element water. As water is necessary to sustain life, the Kidney is involved in reproduction, specifically in the quality of genetic information passed from generation to generation. Consequently the Kidney supports the reproductive organs and reproductive activity of the animal. The ancient Chinese called this *Essence Qi*. Because the Kidney also governs the function of the hypothalamus, pituitary, and adrenal gland, it is the fulcrum of the basic mechanisms essential to life.

The Kidney also controls the growth of the animal from birth to maturation. For example, the quality of bone formation in a growing foal is strongly influenced by this organ. Similarly, the kidney also influences aging of the older horse. In TCM, premature aging (e.g., early arthritis, fragility of bone, loss of sperm quality, and infertility) is mainly caused by a weakened Kidney *Qi*. Another important function of the Kidney and Bladder is fluid metabolism, which involves not only urine but also tears, mucus, sweat, synovial fluid, cerebrospinal fluid, and plasma. The Kidney also acts synergistically with the Lung. The Kidney takes the *Qi* from the Lung and anchors it downward, allowing deep inhalation. Many cases of asthma have been successfully treated with acupuncture by treating the Kidney instead of the Lung.

All organ networks are interconnected and interdependent (see Fig. 11-1). Excessive activity in one results in the weakening and hyperactivity of others. The circular phase of this five-element relationship is called the *Sheng* cycle, in which one element nourishes another. This cycle is also compared to the relationship between mother and son. The cycle within the circle is called the *Ko* cycle. Here, each organ sets limits on the other, ensuring that no organ system oversteps its bounds. Diseases of excess usually migrate from one organ to another along the *Ko* cycle, whereas diseases of deficiency migrate along the *Sheng* cycle. These physiologic concepts compose the Chinese interpretation of homeostasis. As previously explained, TCM defines disease as disorder in relationships, not as a singular entity. For example, if the Liver system is in excess (as might result with overmedication), it may have too strong an effect on the Spleen and Stomach (wood dominates over earth). This condition could manifest as bloating in the stomach, nausea, loose stools, and inappetence.

Neurophysiology: The Science Behind the Symbolism

Acupuncture has inspired a great deal of research, particularly relating to its pain-controlling properties. Many American scientists were amazed when the first reports of surgical-level analgesia were sent from China and began to investigate the mechanisms behind acupuncture.

As mentioned previously, acupuncture points are areas of concentrated nerve bundles and vessels with the unique property of increased electrical conductance. One author conducted histologic examinations on the acupuncture points of cows and concluded that these points (found by the use of ohmeters) are organized around sites where cutaneous nerves enter the dermis and nerves and vessels enter the fascia (Egerbacher, 1994).

When a needle is inserted into an acupuncture point, a stimulus is transmitted along the spinal cord via afferent peripheral nerve fibers, following pathways used for pain transmission (Kendall, 1989a). The first theory about the way acupuncture blocks pain, called the *gate theory*, was based on the hypothesis that the stimulation of fast-acting A-delta fibers would block sensory input from the slow-conducting C-fibers (the conductors of pain) to the substantia gelatinosa of the spinal cord (Kendall, 1989a). Several studies involving nerve blocks support this theory (Dong, Zheng, 1985).

Ancient acupuncturists mapped these channels by stimulating a point and asking their patients to describe the path of their reaction. The Chinese call this propagation of nervous stimuli *De Qi*. They discovered that interruption of this pathway at any point between the acupuncture point and the brain can decrease the effectiveness of the treatment (Chen, 1981). Research has since shown that this response depends on an intact spinal cord to propagate or reflect nociceptive and proprioceptive dorsal root interactions. These interactions are achieved by eliciting descending control mechanisms.

Research also suggests that the brain plays a role in acupuncture analgesia (Pan and others, 1984). Naloxone, an opioid antagonist, can reverse acupuncture analgesia, and the effects of enkephalins and beta-endorphins increase in the brain after electroacupuncture (Pan and others, 1984). Other studies have shown that serotonin also affects acupuncture analgesia (Zhong and others, 1989). When the serotonin inhibitor pCPA was injected in rats, it did not greatly suppress analgesia produced by electroacupuncture. The injection of naloxone produced similar results. However, if both antagonists were given simultaneously, analgesia was significantly reduced, leading researchers to suspect that an important relationship exists between the two substances (Han, Terenius, 1982).

The release of endorphins and serotonin found in the bloodstream after acupuncture analgesia suggests a humoral mechanism for acupuncture. Research has shown that after acupuncture, serotonin concentrations increase 40% in the systemic circulation and that beta-endorphins and cortisol levels have been found to rise in horses (Bossut and others, 1983). Endorphins are not only analgesic but also involved in the decrease of peristalsis, the increase in vasodilation, the production of adrenocorticotropic hormone (which results in a release of cortisone), and the release of growth hormone (Xie, 1982). Research has also shown that acupuncture can enhance immunity by increasing levels of white blood cells, interferon, antibodies, and immunoglobulins (Chao, Loh, 1987). Acupuncture also affects the ovary and thyroid, as shown by rises in luteinizing hormone and thyroid hormones following treatment (Xie, 1982).

The autonomic nervous system plays an important role in acupuncture. The Bladder channel is a meridian pathway lateral to the spine. Special-function acupuncture points named *back-shu*, or *association points*, are located along this meridian at the level of the intervertebral spaces. According to ancient acupuncture texts, the circulating Qi of the organs passes through these points; disease in these organs can be detected by palpation of tenderness at the association points. When considering the neurophysiologic explanations for such a phenomenon, note that these points are located at the same level as their related organs. For example, the Lung, Pericardium, and Heart association points are all located at the level of the cranial thorax, whereas the Kidney association point is at the level of the kidneys.

Autonomic efferent nerves innervate and regulate various viscerae. For example, the cardiac sympathetic nerve emerges from the cranial thoracic levels of the spinal cord, and parasympathetic innervation to the Bladder emerges from the pelvis. Somatic sensory stimulation has been shown to produce autonomic reflex responses (Kendall, 1989a).

Research has also shown that certain regions on the surface of the body react to pathologic changes of organs (O'Connor, Bensky, 1988). These reactive sites were found by probing with an instrument along the surface of the skin. (Fig. 11-2 shows the location of these zones (Head's zones) and demonstrates that the Lung and Stomach association points are located at the most sensitive sites within areas corresponding to the same organs in the illustrated zones.)

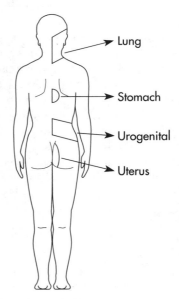

Fig. 11-2 Head's zones: surface regions reactive to organ disease. (Modified from Schoen AM: *Veterinary acupuncture: ancient art to modern medicine,* St Louis, 1994, Mosby.)

Studies have revealed the segmental nature of this somatovisceral reflex. Acupuncture points PC-6 and ST-36 are known to exert strong influences over the Heart and Stomach respectively. Research has also shown that the somatovisceral afferents from these points and the respective organs overlap in the dorsal horn gray matter (Kendall, 1989b).

As mentioned previously, stimulation of an acupuncture point elicits a sensation along the channel known as *De Qi.* Therefore the acupuncture response appears to have a bioelectric basis. Researchers have suggested that acupuncture points act as DC power sources along a current propagated by the cells of the nervous system. Acupuncture points are positively charged in relation to their surroundings. Some experts hypothesize that insertion of a needle into an acupuncture point changes the electrical charge in the tissue by causing a capacitive flow of current to equalize the potential difference between the skin and needle, which results in a physiologic alteration (Nordenstrom, 1987).

Other research has suggested that a sodium ion exchange potentiates the acupuncture phenomenon. The core of this theory is that pain results from local hypoxia secondary to vasoconstriction, which leads to local sodium depletion. This sodium depletion causes affected cells to burst and release inflammatory mediators. Researchers have demonstrated that the injection of sodium is more effective than traditional needling (Takasek, 1983).

The Primary Acupuncture Points of the Horse*

In human acupuncture the meridian system forms the basis of therapy. The system comprises 12 paired channels, each of which corresponds to one of the Chinese, or *Zang-fu,* organ systems. In addition, there are two unpaired channels, the *Du* (Governing Vessel) and the *Ren* (Conception Vessel). This meridian system not only balances the internal organs with the external body but also helps maintain homeostasis. According to TCM, disease occurs when one meridian is depleted and another excessive. Located along these meridians, each acupuncture point is named according to its position along the channel. Each locus has a specific action. One point may strengthen the channel, whereas another may weaken it. A desired effect can be achieved by using one or more of these points in an acupuncture formula that balances the meridians.

Chinese veterinary acupuncture does not acknowledge that these meridians exist in animals as they do in humans. Acupuncture points in current use were compiled by the ancient masters, who reported reliable results for certain

disease states in humans. Therefore TCM diagnoses cannot be made for animals with the level of complexity achieved in human acupuncture.

Attempting to adopt these acupuncture techniques to treat their patients, equine acupuncturists began transposing human acupuncture points to horses. This allowed the use of meridian therapy for the horse. This concept, popularized by the Japanese, focuses on finding meridian deficiencies and excesses, balancing them through the use of specific points, and restoring health in the process. Listed below are the 14 major meridians and a few important acupuncture points used to treat most conditions in the horse. Where applicable, the more important traditional Chinese points found on or near the relevant meridians are noted. The focus of this chapter, however, is on the transposition system. For a detailed account of the Chinese points as well as the transpositional points, please refer to *Veterinary Acupuncture: Ancient Art To Modern Medicine,* edited by Allen Schoen.

Acupuncture Point Nomenclature

1. *Alarm points:* Diagnostic points named for the organ they affect; sensitivity at a point may indicate a disorder in the corresponding organ system
2. *Association points:* Diagnostic points located on the Bladder meridian, named according to the organ-meridian system with which they are associated; pain with light palpation indicates acute disease, whereas pain with deep palpation indicates a chronic condition
3. *Diagnostic points:* When sensitive to palpation, these points reflect disease in the associated structure
4. *Sedation points:* Points used to decrease energy flow of the meridians to which they correspond
5. *Tonification points:* Points used to increase energy flow of the meridians to which they correspond
6. *Master points:* Points used for their powerful effect on the structures with which they are associated
7. *Influential points:* Points used for their influential effect on the structures with which they are associated

Acupuncture Meridians of the Forelimb

The lung and large intestine meridians

The Lung meridian begins at the level of the third rib on the pectoral muscle. It courses dorsally up the chest, then ventrally to the cranial aspect of the axilla along the biceps tendon. From there it courses down the medial edge of the radius to end on the caudomedial aspect of the coronary band.

The *Yang* meridian paired with the Lung is the Large Intestine. It begins proximal to the craniomedial aspect of the coronary band of the forelimb and continues up the medial aspect of the pastern and metacarpus. Crossing

---

*Much of this material is derived from Schoen AM: *Veterinary acupuncture: ancient art to modern medicine,* St Louis, 1994, Mosby.

over the carpus, it continues laterally up the radius to the elbow, shoulder, and neck and over the larynx, ending at a location lateral to the ventral border of the nares.

LUNG 1 (LU-1)
Location: At the level of the third rib, in the center of the chest, in the depression over the transverse pectoral muscle

Indication: Sensitivity at this point indicates lung dysfunction, cough, and pain in the chest, shoulder, and forearm

LUNG 5 (LU-5)
Location: On the lateral side of the biceps tendon, at the level of the cubital crease

Indication: This point is the sedation point of the lung and indicates cough of excess and acute pharyngitis

LUNG 7 (LU-7)
Location: Just proximal to the medial styloid process of the radius

Indication: Master point for conditions of the head and neck; indicates neck pain, facial paralysis, and cough

LUNG 11 (LU-11)
Location: On the caudomedial aspect of the coffin joint of the front limb

Indication: Epistaxis, laminitis, sidebone, pneumonia, throat disorders, immunostimulation

LARGE INTESTINE 1 (LI-1)
Location: On the medial aspect of the coffin joint of the front limb cranial to Lung 11.

Indication: Hoof problems, diseases of the fetlock, fever

LARGE INTESTINE 4 (LI-4)
Location: Just distal to the head of the second metacarpal bone

Indication: Master point for the head and neck, motor point for the forelimb, mouth pain, immunostimulation, fever

LARGE INTESTINE 11 (LI-11)
Location: In the transverse crease of the elbow, in the depression created when the elbow is flexed

Indication: Eliminates heat in the body; elbow, pharyngeal, abdominal, and ophthalmic pain; immunostimulation

LARGE INTESTINE 16 (LI-16)
Location: Just dorsal to the point of the shoulder, at the intersection of the cranial margin of the scapular muscle and the dorsocaudal margin of the brachiocephalic muscle.

Indication: Forelimb pain, pneumonia, diagnostic point for fetlock problems

LARGE INTESTINE 18 (LI-18)
Location: At the level of the ventral aspect of the mandible, on the cranial border of the cleidomastoid muscle

Indication: Diagnostic point for hoof problems, pharyngitis

LARGE INTESTINE 20 (LI-20)
Location: On the lateral border of the dilator naris lateralis, caudal to the nares

Indication: Rhinitis, lung congestion, fever, sunstroke, sinusitis, influenza

Pericardium and triple heater meridians

The Pericardium meridian begins on the chest at Pericardium 1 at the level of the fifth intercostal space just level with the elbow. This channel courses caudomedially down the forelimb to end at the back of the hoof between the bulbs of the heel.

The paired *Yang* meridian to the Pericardium is the Triple Heater. Beginning with TH-1 on the front of the coffin joint of the forelimb, it courses dorsally toward the head. Its path includes the front of the cannon bone and carpus and the lateral aspect of the elbow, shoulder, and neck. It terminates on the head, at the level of the eye.

PERICARDIUM 1 (PC-1)
Location: On the chest at the fifth intercostal space at the level of the elbow

Indications: Diagnostic point for foot problems, chest pain

PERICARDIUM 6 (PC-6)
Location: On the medial side of the forelimb, directly cranial to the chestnut

Indications: Master point for the cranial abdomen (chest and stomach disorders), calming point, medial forelimb pain

PERICARDIUM 9 (PC-9)
Location: In the depression between the bulbs of the heel of the forelimb

Indications: Tonification point for the Pericardium meridian; indications include laminitis, navicular disease, tendinitis, fetlock pain

TRIPLE HEATER 1 (TH-1)
Location: On the midline of the front of the forelimb, at the level of the coffin joint

Indications: Laminitis, any hoof disorder, fever, carpal problems

TRIPLE HEATER 5 (TH-5)
Location: 2 cun* dorsal to the top of the carpus, in the groove formed by the lateral digital extensor and the common digital extensor

Indications: Disorders of the tendons, forelimb pain, reproductive disorders

TRIPLE HEATER 9 (TH-9)
Location: Directly distal to the lateral tuberosity of the radius of the forelimb

Indication: Forelimb pain, tendinitis, laminitis, analgesic point.

Equivalent Chinese point: Cheng Zhong—used for same condition as in transpositional system

TRIPLE HEATER 17 (TH-17)
Location: Caudal to the ear, between the mastoid process and the mandible

Indication: Tranquilizing point, wobbler syndrome, facial paralysis

---

*The term *cun* is a Chinese body measurement referring to the width of the seventeenth rib of the horse.

TRIPLE HEATER 21 (TH-21)

Location: In the temporal fossa at the rostromedial corner of the ear base

Indication: Encephalitis, irregular estrous cycles, anhidrosis

Equivalent Chinese point: Cheng Zhong—also used for tetanus and spleen deficiency conditions

TRIPLE HEATER 23 (TH-23)

Location: At the lateral canthus of the eye on the ventral border of the zygomatic process

Indication: Facial paralysis, disorders of the eye, encephalitis

Equivalent Chinese point: Zhuan Nao—same indications

The heart and small intestine meridians

Heart 1 begins in the center of the axilla. From here, this meridian courses distally down the back of the forearm to the level of the carpus, where it turns laterally and ends over the caudolateral aspect of the coffin joint.

The Small Intestine meridian starts cranial to where the Heart meridian ends, on the craniolateral aspect of the coffin joint. It then travels proximally up the forearm, traversing the shoulder, continuing up the neck dorsal to the cervical vertebrae, and ending at the base of the ear.

HEART 1 (HT-1)

Location: In the center of the axilla, at the junction of the trunk and forelimb

Indication: Cardiac dysfunction, shoulder lameness, thoracic limb pain.

HEART 7 (HT-7)

Location: Proximal to the lateral aspect of the accessory carpal bone of the forelimb

Indication: Sedation point for the Heart meridian, calming point, pain in the carpus and shoulder

HEART 9 (HT-9)

Location: Over the caudolateral aspect of the front coffin joint, just cranial to the collateral cartilage

Indication: Tonifies the Heart meridian; indications include laminitis, sidebone, aberrant behavior (particularly in stallions)

SMALL INTESTINE 1 (SI-1)

Location: Over the craniolateral aspect of the coffin joint of the front limb

Indications: Febrile conditions, laminitis, problems along the Small Intestine meridian

SMALL INTESTINE 3 (SI-3)

Location: Just distal to the end of the fourth metacarpal bone on the lateral aspect of the forelimb

Indications: Tonifies the Small Intestine meridian; master point for the neck, shoulder and back; anemia; laminitis; fetlock and carpal problems

SMALL INTESTINE 9 (SI-9)

Location: In the large depression on the lateral aspect of the shoulder, formed by the border of the deltoids and the long and lateral heads of the triceps brachii

Indication: Major point for forelimb pain, diagnostic point for shoulder pain, forelimb paresis

SMALL INTESTINE 16 (SI-16)

Location: Between the second and third cervical vertebrae of the neck

Indications: Diagnostic point for tendinitis, pharyngitis, cervical pain and restriction

SMALL INTESTINE 19 (SI-19)

Location: At the temporomandibular joint, in the fossa created when the mouth is open

Indication: Temporomandibular joint pain, facial paralysis, deafness

Equivalent Chinese point: Shang Guan—same indications

Acupuncture Meridians of the Hindlimb

Three paired meridians exist on the hindlimbs. The *Yin* meridians begin at the level of the hooves and travel medially up the limbs to end on the trunk. The *Yang* meridians begin on the face, travel across the trunk, and course down the medial aspect of the limbs to end at the level of the hooves.

Spleen and stomach meridians

The Spleen meridian begins at the caudomedial aspect of the coffin joint. Traveling medially up the leg, it passes cranial to the tuber coxae. From there, it traverses the chest to a point at the fourth intercostal space, where it turns caudally to end at the tenth intercostal space at the level of the shoulder.

The Stomach meridian begins at the ventral aspect of the orbit of the eye. From there, it travels cranially toward the mouth, switches back across the jaw, extends down the ventral aspect of the neck and abdomen, and courses across the stifle to the craniolateral aspect of the hock. From there it continues down the leg to end on the front of the coffin joint.

SPLEEN 1 (SP-1)

Location: On the caudomedial aspect of the rear coffin joint

Indication: Regulates the function of the spleen, affects allergies, limb edema, organ prolapse, deep-seated chronic conditions

SPLEEN 6 (SP-6)

Location: Directly caudal to the tibia, on the medial aspect of the hindlimb, 2 *cun* cranial to the cranial aspect of the hock

Indications: Master point for reproductive disorders, spleen function, limb edema, gastrointestinal and urinary disorders, immunostimulation

SPLEEN 9 (SP-9)

Location: In a depression on the distal border of the medial condyle of the tibia

Indications: Useful in point formula with SP-6 to benefit function of spleen, stifle problems, reproductive and urinary disorders, infectious diarrhea

SPLEEN 13 (SP-13)

Location: Cranioventral to the tuber coxae

Indications: Stifle problems, pain in the lower lumbar and hip regions

SPLEEN 20 (SP-20)

Location: In the fourth intercostal space, at the level of the elbow

Indications: Diagnostic point for carpal problems, lung and skin disorders

SPLEEN 21 (SP-21)

Location: In the tenth intercostal space at the level of the scapulohumeral joint

Indications: Major point for tonifying the *Yin* of the body, exhaustion with cold limbs, infertility, emphysema.

STOMACH 1 (ST-1)

Location: At the intersection of the medial and middle third of the lower border of the orbit of the eye

Indications: Ophthalmic disorders, facial paralysis

STOMACH 2 (ST-2)

Location: Ventral to the medial canthus of the eye on the bifurcation of the angular vein

Indications: Gastrointestinal pain, ophthalmic disorders, facial paralysis

STOMACH 7 (ST-7)

Location: Just ventral to the zygomatic arch, at the temporomandibular joint

Indication: Facial paralysis, temporomandibular joint pain

Equivalent Chinese point: Xia Guan—same indications

STOMACH 10 (ST-10)

Location: One handbreadth cranial to the point of the shoulder, on the ventral aspect of the brachiocephalic muscle

Indication: Diagnostic point for stifle problems, gastrointestinal disorders, aerophagia, pharyngitis, chronic obstructive pulmonary disease

STOMACH 30 (ST-30)

Location: At the cranioventral border of the tuber coxae

Indication: Major point for stifle problems, hip pain, and infertility

Equivalent Chinese point: Dan Tian

STOMACH 35 (ST-35)

Location: In a depression between the lateral and middle patellar ligaments

Indication: Pain of the stifle and pelvic limb

Equivalent Chinese point: Lu Cao

STOMACH 36 (ST-36)

Location: One finger's width laterally from the distal edge of the tibial crest

Indication: Master point for the digestive system, gastrointestinal disorders, anorexia, lethargy (stimulates *Qi*), immunostimulation, fever, pain in the stifle and hock

STOMACH 45 (ST-45)

Location: On the midline of the hind hooves, over the coffin joint

Indication: Sedation point of the Stomach meridian, stifle problems, laminitis, all hoof problems, gastrointestinal problems

Liver and gallbladder meridians

The Liver meridian begins over the medial aspect of the hind coffin joint (just cranial to SP-1). It courses up the medial aspect of the hindlimb to the inguinal region and ends in the fourteenth intercostal space at the level of the elbow.

The Gallbladder meridian begins at the lateral canthus of the eye and passes just medial to the ear to run down the dorsal aspect of the neck and shoulder. It then travels across the chest, around the coxofemoral joint, and down the lateral aspect of the hindlimb to end over the craniolateral aspect of the coffin joint.

LIVER 1 (LIV-1)

Location: Over the craniomedial aspect of the hind coffin joint

Indication: Myositis, allergies, laminitis, overexertion

LIVER 3 (LIV-3)

Location: Just cranial to the head of the second metatarsal bone

Indication: Liver function, gynecologic and ophthalmic disorders, hock pain

Equivalent Chinese point: Pal Hyal

LIVER 4 (LIV-4)

Location: Medial to the cunean tendon of the hock, over the saphenous vein

Indication: Hock and fetlock pain

Equivalent Chinese point: Qu Chi

LIVER 8 (LIV-8)

Location: Just caudal to the medial epicondyle of the femur

Indication: Tonification point of the liver meridian, stifle pain, caudal abdominal pain, uterine prolapse

LIVER 13 (LIV-13)

Location: Distal end of the eighteenth rib

Indication: Diagnostic point for spleen dysfunction (alarm point), myositis, laminitis, reproductive disorders, abdominal pain

LIVER 14 (LIV-14)

Location: In the fourteenth intercostal space at the level of the elbow

Indication: Diagnostic point for liver dysfunction (alarm point) myositis, laminitis, ophthalmic disorders, hepatitis

GALLBLADDER 1 (GB-1)

Location: On the transverse facial vein, just caudal to the lateral canthus

Indication: Ophthalmic disorders, anhidrosis, heatstroke

Equivalent Chinese point: Tai Yang

GALLBLADDER 20 (GB-20)

Location: In the large depression just caudal to the occipital condyle

Indication: Neck pain, wobbler syndrome, febrile conditions, encephalitis

Equivalent Chinese point: Feng Men

GALLBLADDER 21 (GB-21)

Location: In a depression located halfway along the cranial edge of the scapula

Indication: Neck, shoulder, and forelimb pain; shoulder paralysis

GALLBLADDER 25 (GB-25)

Location: Caudal to the costochondral junction of the eighteenth rib

Indication: Diagnostic point for kidney imbalance (alarm point), lumbar pain, abdominal pain, kidney disorders

GALLBLADDER 27 (GB-27)

Location: Just caudal to the dorsal edge of the wing of the ilium

Indication: Hock pain, infertility

Equivalent Chinese point: Yan Chi

GALLBLADDER 28 (GB-28)

Location: Halfway along the length of the cranial edge of the iliac spine

Indication: Pain in the lumbar and gluteal region, pain in the hip and stifle

GALLBLADDER 29 (GB-29)

Location: Craniodorsal to the head of the femur

Indication: Major point for hip pain, myositis of the hindlimb, stifle pain

GALLBLADDER 30 (GB-30)

Location: Caudoventral to the greater trochanter of the femur

Indication: Major point for hip pain, myositis of the hindlimb

GALLBLADDER 34 (GB-34)

Location: In a depression craniodistal to the head of the fibula

Indication: Influential point for tendon, muscle atrophy, joint weakness

GALLBLADDER 44 (GB-44)

Location: Over the craniolateral aspect of the coffin joint of the hindlimb

Indication: Problems of the hip, stifle, and hock; laminitis

Kidney and bladder meridians

The Kidney meridian begins in a depression between the bulbs of the heel. It travels caudomedially up the hindlimb to the ventral abdomen to end at the level of the first rib.

The Bladder meridian begins at the medial canthus of the eye. It continues over the skull and past the wings of the atlas, where it traverses the dorsal aspect of the neck and back. At the level of the scapula, this meridian divides into two branches that parallel each other along the length of the spine. These branches join at the popliteal fossa, where the single meridian continues distally along the lateral aspect of the hindlimb to end over the caudolateral aspect of the coffin joint.

KIDNEY 1 (KI-1)

Location: In a depression between the bulbs of the heel of the hindlimb

Indication: Sedation point of the kidney meridian; calming effect on the *Shen*; shock; fever; heel pain

KIDNEY 3 (KI-3)

Location: Between the medial malleolus and the tendo calcaneus

Indication: Arthritis of the hock, kidney and bladder disorders, reproductive dysfunction, paralysis of the pelvic limb

KIDNEY 7 (KI-7)

Location: 2 *cun* proximal to the hock on the cranial border of the tendo calcaneus

Indication: Tonification point of the kidney, reproductive disorders, anhidrosis, hock pain

KIDNEY 10 (KI-10)

Location: Between the semimembranosus and semitendinosus at the level of the popliteal fossa

Indication: Stifle problems, exhaustion

BLADDER 1 (BL-1)

Location: At the medial canthus of the eye

Indication: Ophthalmic disorders, calming point

BLADDER 10 (BL-10)

Location: On the caudal border of the wings of the atlas, 2 *cun* ventral to the mane

Indication: Cervical pain and stiffness, shoulder and back pain, encephalitis

Equivalent Chinese point: Fu Tu

BLADDER 11 (BL-11)

Location: In a depression just cranial to the shoulder blade, 3 *cun* lateral to the dorsal midline

Indication: Influential point for bone healing, neck and back pain, cough and fever

BLADDER 13 (BL-13)

Location: In the eighth intercostal space, 3 *cun* lateral to the dorsal midline of the back

Indication: Association point for the lung, medial front limb pain, chronic obstructive pulmonary disease, respiratory disorders

BLADDER 14 (BL-14)

Location: In the ninth intercostal space, 3 *cun* lateral to the dorsal midline of the back

Indication: Association point for the pericardium meridian; calming effect on shen; cough; lung congestion

Equivalent Chinese point: Fei Zhi Shu—association point for the lung; cough; asthma; overexertion; pneumonia

BLADDER 15 (BL-15)

Location: In the tenth intercostal space, 3 *cun* lateral to the dorsal midline of the back

Indication: Association point for the Heart meridian; cardiac problems; calming effect on the shen; problems along the Heart meridian

Equivalent Chinese point: Ge Shu—diaphragm association point, asthma, spasm of the diaphragm

BLADDER 18 (BL-18)

Location: In the thirteenth intercostal space, 3 *cun* lateral to the midline

Indication: Association point for the Liver; hepatitis, toxicity, myositis, laminitis, ophthalmic disorders, tendinitis, back soreness

Equivalent Chinese point: Gan Zhi Shu—associate to the Liver; icterus, indigestion, conjunctivitis, keratitis

BLADDER 19 (BL-19)

Location: In the fifteenth intercostal space, 3 *cun* lateral to the midline of the back

Indication: Association point for the Gallbladder; hip pain, tendinitis

Equivalent Chinese point: Pi Shu—association point for the Spleen; enterospasm, constipation, indigestion, diarrhea

BLADDER 20 (BL-20)

Location: In the seventeenth intercostal space, 3 *cun* lateral to the dorsal midline of the back

Indication: Association point for the Spleen; pain along the Spleen meridian, gastrointestinal and reproductive disorders, edema

Equivalent Chinese point: Da Chang Shu—Large Intestine association point; diarrhea, colic, enteritis, constipation

BLADDER 21 (BL-21)

Location: Caudal to the last rib, 3 *cun* lateral to the midline of the back

Indication: Association point of the Stomach; pain along the Stomach meridian, gastrointestinal disorders

Equivalent Chinese point: Guan Yuan Shu—constipation, abdominal pain, indigestion, dilation of the stomach, gaseous bowel

BLADDER 22 (BL-22)

Location: Between the first and second lumbar vertebrae, 3 *cun* lateral to the midline of the back

Indication: Association point of the Triple Heater meridian; endocrine imbalances, gastrointestinal conditions

Equivalent Chinese point: Xiao Chang Shu—Small Intestine association point; constipation, abdominal pain, gastroenteritis

BLADDER 23 (BL-23)

Location: Between the second and third lumbar vertebrae, 3 *cun* lateral to the dorsal midline of the back

Indication: Association point for the Kidney meridian; strengthens the caudal area of the back; improves water metabolism, infertility, urinary disorders, problems along the Kidney meridian

Equivalent Chinese point: Pang Guang Shu—association point of the Bladder; polyuria, stomach pain, enterospasm, constipation

BLADDER 25 (BL-25)

Location: Between the fifth and sixth lumbar vertebrae, 3 *cun* lateral to the dorsal midline of the back

Indication: Association point for the Large Intestine; pain along the large intestine meridian; sciatica, colic, constipation, diarrhea, fever, rhinitis

BLADDER 27 (BL-27)

Location: Between the first and second sacral vertebrae, 3 *cun* lateral to the midline

Indication: Association point for the Small Intestine; caudal back pain, lower abdominal pain

BLADDER 28 (BL-28)

Location: Between the second and third sacral vertebrae, 3 *cun* lateral to the midline

Indication: Association point for the Bladder, pain along the Bladder meridian, genitourinary disorders

BLADDER 35 (BL-35)

Location: On the proximal end of the muscle groove created by the biceps femoris and the semitendinosus muscles

Indication: Diagnostic point for hock problems, hindlimb pain, sciatica, vaginal and cervical disorders

Equivalent Chinese point: Hui Yang—similiar indications

BLADDER 36-38 (BL-36—38)

Location: Equidistantly spaced 3 *cun* apart along the muscular groove between the biceps femoris and the semitendinosus, beginning with BL-36, 2 *cun* dorsal to the tuber ischii

Indication: Diagnostic points for stifle problems, hindlimb pain, myositis, sciatica

BLADDER 39 (BL-39)

Location: In the depression at the end of the groove created by the biceps femoris and the semitendinosus

Indication: Diagnostic point for hock pain, hock problems, arthritis of the hindlimb

BLADDER 40 (BL-40)

Location: In the popliteal fossa, directly caudal to the stifle joint

Indication: Master point for lower back pain; cooling effect; stifle and hip pain

BLADDER 60 (BL-60)

Location: Between the tuber calcaneis and the lateral malleolus of the hock

Indication: Alleviates swelling, heat, and pain (aspirin point); strengthens the lower back; relieves hock pain

Equivalent Chinese point: Kun Lun—coryza, pain in loin, rump, pelvic limb

BLADDER 62 (BL-62)

Location: In a depression just below the lateral malleolus of the hock

Indication: Used with SI-3 to treat back pain, arthritis of the hock

BLADDER 67 (BL-67)

Location: Over the caudolateral aspect of the coffin joint of the hindlimb

Indication: Tonifies the Bladder meridian, all hoof and back problems, urinary disorders

The conception and governing vessel

Although these extra meridians are not related to the Zang-Fu organs, they are extremely important in treatment of the horse. The Governing Vessel starts between the anus and tail and travels cranially along the midline of the back to end at a point between the upper lip and gum.

The Conception Vessel meridian starts between the genitalia and the anus and travels cranially along the ventral midline to end in the center of the lower lip.

GOVERNING VESSEL 1 (GV-1)

Location: Between the anus and base of the tail

Indication: Low back pain, constipation and diarrhea, rectal prolapse, genitourinary disorders

Equivalent Chinese point: Hou Hai—similiar indications

BAI HUI

Location: In the lumbosacral space

Indication: Connects all the *Yang* meridians; strengthens the hind end; alleviates overexertion and reproductive, respiratory, and gastrointestinal disorders; is the same point in Chinese system

GOVERNING VESSEL 4 (GV-4)

Location: Between the second and third lumbar vertebrae

Indication: Strengthens the *Yang*; alleviates hindquarter pain, kidney imbalance, genitourinary disorders

GOVERNING VESSEL 14 (GV-14)

Location: Between the seventh cervical vertebra and the first thoracic vertebra

Indication: Cervical problems, back pain, fever, heatstroke, cold, dermatitis, convulsions

Equivalent Chinese point: Da Zhui—nasal discharge, fever, cough, back pain

GOVERNING VESSEL 26 (GV-26)

Location: Midway between the ventral border of the nostrils in the center of the upper lip

Indication: Epinephrine point, shock, unconsciousness, facial paralysis, enterospasm

Equivalent Chinese point: Fen Shui

CONCEPTION VESSEL (CV-1)

Location: Between the genitalia and the anus

Indication: Uterine disorders, urinary retention

CONCEPTION VESSEL 12 (CV-12)

Location: On the ventral midline, halfway between the umbilicus and the xiphoid

Indication: Diagnostic point for stomach disorders (alarm point), colic, and diarrhea

CONCEPTION VESSEL 17 (CV-17)

Location: Along the midline at the level of the caudal border of the elbow

Indication: Influential point for respiration and the alarm point for the pericardium; epistaxis, respiratory disorders, anhidrosis

Treatment Techniques

Traditional Versus Modern Needling

As a general rule the Chinese employ a method of stimulation that is considered strong compared with that used in the United States. The more traditional needles are thicker than the Japanese-style needles used in the United States (Xinnong, 1987). The latter are of stainless steel and available in many lengths (0.25 to 8 inches) and several gauges (32- to 36-gauge). Most of these needles are presterilized, disposable, and encased in an insertion tube. The insertion tube is thought to reduce the pain of insertion and make the technique easier for the operator. These needles are particularly useful on the distal limbs, where reduction of pain is essential; 30-gauge, 1.5-inch needles work well for most points. Often larger-gauge needles are necessary in the hip region because of the thickness of the skin.

Another technique used by many equine acupuncturists is called *aquapuncture.* This technique involves injection of a liquid into the acupuncture point with a hypodermic needle. Many substances have been used, including saline, distilled water, procaine, homeopathic agents, vitamin B_{12}, and iodine in oil (Mackay's solution). Aquapuncture is popular for several reasons. First, acupuncture needles can be more difficult and time consuming to insert than aquapuncture needles. Second, horses have a strong skin-twitch reflex, which makes maintaining acupuncture needles difficult in certain points. Finally, traditional acupuncture poses the risk of a displaced needle being lost in the patient's stall.

The amount of fluid injected varies depending on the discretion of the acupuncturist. Some use as little as 1 ml, whereas others use up to 40 ml (Yu, Hwang, 1990). The size of the hypodermic needle can vary from 20- to 25-gauge.

Moxibustion

Moxibustion is a method whereby a cone or cylinder of an herb *(moxa)* is burned on or near the skin at acupuncture points. Useful for animals in weakened conditions, moxibustion stimulates circulation of *Qi* (Xinnong, 1987). According to Chinese medicine, most musculoskeletal conditions are caused by a blockage of *Qi* along the involved meridian pathway; therefore moxibustion is an important treatment for such conditions.

The easiest moxa to use in equine acupuncture is a stick that resembles a large cigar. The moxa stick is lit at one end and held about half an inch from the surface of the skin. Moxa can also be applied to the top of an acupuncture needle to increase the effectiveness of treatment. Moxibustion is contraindicated in acute inflammatory and infectious conditions.

Electrical Acupuncture

Electrical acupuncture is a variation of transcutaneous electrical neural stimulation (TENS) using electrodes placed on specific acupuncture points. This technique is often used in treating equine musculoskeletal disease and impaction colic. The advantages are that the effects appear to last longer than those of simple needling and the degree of accuracy in needle placement is less critical.

Most units permit modulation of the intensity and frequency of the stimulus. A low frequency is indicated for chronic pain, whereas a high frequency is useful for acute pain and muscle spasm. Many machines offer a compromise between high and low frequencies in the form of a "dispense and disperse" mode. On this setting the frequency alternates between high and low, and the patient is less likely to develop a tolerance to the stimulation, which increases the effectiveness of the therapy. The duration of treatment usually varies from 10 to 30 minutes depending on the condition and tolerance of the patient.

Chinese Medical Diagnosis of the Horse

At first glance a traditional Chinese examination resembles a Western examination. Both are based on four factors: looking (observation), listening (auscultation), asking (history taking), and touching (palpation). The difference between the two types of examination lies in the emphasis on the subsequent results.

Using the results obtained from the four factors, an acupuncturist must first determine if the disorder represents a deficiency or an excess. If the condition is one of deficiency, the patient must be tonified (i.e., points are used to strengthen the involved meridians and the *Qi* of the horse). For example, in a deficiency disorder, specific signs are accompanied by exhaustion, depletion, and motor retardation; in an excess disorder, symptoms may include heat, spasm, increased fluid production, nervousness, and overexcitement.

The second step is to determine the quality of *Yin* (cooling ability, fluid production) and *Yang* (warming ability, moving ability, metabolism). If the *Yin* is deficient, the patient may show dryness and appear unduly warm (anhidrosis). Points are then chosen to improve the *Yin* of the body. If the *Yang* is deficient, the patient may demonstrate an inability to stay warm with concomitant lethargy (as in hypothyroidism), and *Yang* tonification points might be added to a point formula.

The third step is to identify the meridians (musculoskeletal disorders) or Zang-fu organs (internal disorders) that are involved. This is determined by comparing the presenting signs with response to palpation of the 12 meridians and pulses.* Equine acupuncture places greater emphasis on meridian palpation because of the difficulty in evaluating pulses.

Diagnostic Palpation in the Horse

Acupuncture palpation is an art form requiring skills that take time to master. These skills involve palpation of the acupuncture points along each meridian using either finger pressure or an object such as a needle cap. Response to light pressure indicates an excess, acute, or superficial

---

*In human acupuncture diagnosis the state of the meridians is reflected in the quality of the pulse on the radial arteries. The pulse is taken at 12 locations, 6 on each wrist, 3 superficial, and 3 deep, corresponding to the internal organs. For a more detailed description, refer to Schoen AM: *Veterinary acupuncture: ancient art to modern medicine.*

condition *(Yang)*, whereas a reaction to deep pressure usually indicates a state of deficiency *(Yin)*.

The examination begins at the neck. BL-10 and GB-20 are palpated to determine dysfunction in the cervical spine. This step is important because trigger points often result from chiropractic problems (rotation of the atlas is common in horses because of the use of halters and fixed ties). These trigger points make an evaluation of the meridians more difficult and often obscure the presence of discrete, painful diagnostic points until chiropractic adjustments are performed.

LI-18 is reactive when a problem exists below the coronary band. Coupled with PC-1 and CV-17, pain in these regions is a reliable indicator of hoof problems. Tendon problems are often manifested as sensitivity at SI-16. However, pain at this point may also be caused by chiropractic disorders of the second or third cervical vertebra. Often sensitive in performance horses, LI-16 reacts strongly when forelimb pain is present. As a general rule, a large region around LI-16 is usually painful, and the more distal the loci of pain, the more distal the problem on the forelimb (Snader, 1982). In fact, knee problems are reflected by pain occurring closer toward the region of LI-17. When coupled with pain at SP-20, this point is often a reliable diagnostic indicator for problems in this joint. TH-15, located on the cranial border of the scapula at the junction of its dorsal edge and the scapular cartilage, is an important diagnostic point for problems on the lateral aspect of the suspensory or check ligament (Snader, 1982). The final diagnostic point found on the neck is ST-10. This point is often painful when stifle problems are present.

The most important part of the examination is the palpation of the back *shu*, or association, points. Pain at these points can reflect pain along the associated meridian or organ. Once again, the importance of differentiating pain at these points caused by traumatic chiropractic malalignments cannot be overstated. Although BL-13 is an important diagnostic indicator for respiratory disorders or medial forelimb pain, it can become tender simply from an improperly fitting saddle.

BL-14 (Pericardium *shu* point) and BL-15 (Heart *shu* point) are often sensitive when the patient is overly anxious. This sensitivity is due to the role of the Pericardium and the Heart in protecting the shen. If BL-13, -14, and -15 are all reactive, particularly on the right side, the horse may be a bleeder. Further tests should then be performed to verify this finding (Rogers, Cain, 1987).

BL-18 (Liver association point) may be painful in any conditions overseen by the Liver, including the state of the muscles, tendons, hooves, and eyes and the presence of allergies. Because BL-19 (Gallbladder association point) is the paired meridian to the Liver, it usually reacts for the same reasons. BL-19 may also become sensitive when problems such as hip and lateral hock pain arise along its meridian pathway.

BL-20 (Spleen association point) is often painful in disorders involving circulation (it usually reacts in bleeders, for instance) and digestion. Along with BL-21, ST-10, and BL-36, -37, and -38, BL-20 may reflect stifle problems. BL-21 (Stomach association point) is often reactive in chronic digestive disorders and dental problems.

BL-22 (Triple Heater association point) is a major diagnostic point for most endocrine disorders, particularly those related to the ovary. A mare with this condition often experiences pain along the ipsilateral path of the Triple Heater as it courses down the neck. These mares often appear to be suffering from shoulder pain.

BL-23 (Kidney association point) often reacts in patients suffering from urinary disturbances or reproductive disorders. Along with BL-35, BL-39, and BL-18, it is used in the diagnosis of hock problems.

In addition to disorders of the Large Intestine, BL-25 (Large Intestine association point) also becomes reactive in horses with problems of the opposite front limb. Apparently, caudal to the umbilical cord the association point–meridian relationship goes from ipsilateral to contralateral (Snader, 1982).

This contralateral relationship is also related to the Small Intestine association point BL-27. Tenderness at this point can reveal problems of the posterior aspect of the opposite forelimb (flexor tendinitis).

Because BL-28 is the association point of the Bladder meridian , it is important in the treatment and diagnosis of problems of the spinal column. Of course, this point may also become sensitive when problems arise along the lateral aspect of the hindlimb or the Bladder.

Some equine acupuncturists use the alarm points to assess disorders in the associated organs. Because the position of these points in horses is still controversial, this topic is not discussed here.

Acupuncture Point Selection

Acupuncture can be used alone or with other alternative modalities. In China, TCM comprises not only acupuncture but also herbalism, massage, and chiropractic manipulation. In fact, most organ disorders are treated primarily with herbs, with acupuncture serving as a secondary form of therapy. Musculoskeletal disorders, on the other hand, are treated primarily with acupuncture, massage, and chiropractic.

A horse's response to therapy can be rapid, usually much faster than that of humans. A marked clinical improvement is often apparent after one treatment. In chronic disease, however, multiple treatments are often necessary before the patient responds. The patient should generally respond after four treatments. If no response is evident by then, the case should be reevaluated. A good schedule for most horses is one or two treatments per week for a month, tapering off to one treatment a month; of course, this frequency varies depending on the case.

Because all aspects of a disease must be considered in determining a treatment protocol, a look at the underlying causes in terms of prevention is also necessary. The acupuncturist must examine all predisposing factors surrounding the problem. In organ disease, this workup includes an evaluation of the feeding program, toxicities in the environment (automatic fly-spray systems), the effect of previously administered drugs, and emotional stress. In musculoskeletal disease the acupuncturist must consider the integrity of the spinal column (e.g., malalignment of the sacroiliac joint can cause abnormal weight bearing on the stifle), shoeing and hoof balance, improper saddle fit, poor footing, inappropriate training schedules, unskilled riders, and the use of hot walking machines (which can put stress on the cervical spine).

Treatment of Musculoskeletal Disorders

In TCM, most musculoskeletal disorders are grouped according to a syndrome termed *Bi*. In simple terms, *Bi* means obstruction. Several types of *Bi* exist, and specific formulas are made depending on the characteristics of the pain. In wandering *Bi* the pain may change in location rapidly (for instance, Lyme's disease). GB-39 is used for hindlimb problems, whereas TH-5 is used for *wandering Bi* of the forelimb. *Painful Bi* is characterized by severe pain aggravated by cold. ST-36 is useful for this condition. Arthritis worsened by damp weather is categorized as *fixed Bi*. Use of SP-6 can improve this condition. Infectious arthritis is an example of *febrile Bi*, in which the symptom of heat predominates. LI-4 is an excellent point for this condition. Finally, *bony Bi* reflects the end stages of degenerative arthritis characterized by bony proliferation. A useful point might include BL-11 (master point for bone).

Besides the preceding considerations, additional approaches may be used in the selection of points in a formula for treating musculoskeletal disease. Points are chosen according to the same dermatome as the problem area, tender points, points cranial and caudal, proximal and distal, and lateral and medial to the area. In addition, the acupuncturist may employ the back *shu* points as well as any appropriate master points. The number of needles used per treatment should normally be fewer than 10 because the effect of each needle diminishes as the number of needles increases (Snader, 1982). (Table 11-1 summarizes some of the more common acupuncture point prescriptions useful in equine musculoskeletal disorders.)

Treatment of Internal Organ Disease

After gathering information through the traditional procedure of observation, auscultation, olfaction, questioning, and palpation, the veterinarian creates a paradigm, using the five-element theory and a concept called the *eight-principle approach.*

These principles are the paired opposites of *Yin* and *Yang:* Interior and Exterior (Is the disease deep within the body or at the exterior?); Heat and Cold (Is the patient chilled or showing signs of fever?); and Excess and Deficiency (Are the involved organs in a state of hy-

TABLE 11-1

POINT PRESCRIPTIONS FOR EQUINE MUSCULOSKELETAL DISORDERS

CONDITION	SUGGESTED POINT FORMULAS
Cervical pain	GB-20, BL-10, TH-16, SI-16, LI-16, BL-11, GB-21
Back pain	SI-3, BL-62, BL-40, BL-18, Bai Hui, BL-35, BL-28
Shoulder pain	SI-9, SI-10, TH-13, SI-3, LI-11, LI-4, LI-1, SI-1, LU-1
Elbow pain	LI-10, LI-11, SI-8, TH-10, LI-4, TH-5
Carpal pain	TH-1, TH-5, BL-13, LI-17, LI-4, BL-11, PC-6, LI-1
Bucked shins	TH-1, BL-23, BL-11, BL-23, SI-9
Medial splint	LU-11, LI-4, BL-11, BL-13, BL-23, SI-9
Tendinitis	PC-9, SI-9, TH-5, BL-18, BL-19, GB-34, BL-14, BL-15
Fetlock pain	LI-1, LI-16, BL-25, BL-23, LU-1, SI-9
Laminitis	PC-9, PC-1, SI-9, HT-3, TH-1, LU-7, BL-18, BL-23
Navicular	PC-9, PC-1, SI-9, BL-11, BL-23, BL-18, HT-3
Pelvic pain	Bai Hui, BL-27, BL-28, BL-35, BL-40, GB-28, GB-29, GB-30
Stifle pain	BL-20, BL-21, BL-27, BL-36, BL-37, BL-38, LIV-8, SP-9, KI-10
Hock pain	BL-18, BL-19, BL-23, BL-35, BL-39, BL-60, BL-62, ST-45, LIV-4
Azoturia	BL-18, BL-19, BL-23, BL-28, BL-40, BL-62, ST-36, LIV-1, LIV-3
Facial paralysis	LI-4, LU-7, ST-7

perfunction or hypofunction?). For example, a horse with shipping fever who shows symptoms of a high fever; rapid, loud breathing; and strong agitation is suffering from a Lung *Yang* Excess. In contrast, the elderly horse with chronic arthritis; infertility; and dry, flaky skin is showing symptoms of a Kidney *Yin* Deficiency. (The Kidney dominates reproduction and bone formation.)

As mentioned previously, Chinese herbs are considered more important than acupuncture in treating organ disease. The paradigms are primarily designed to help the practitioner select the appropriate herbal formula. For example, certain herbs are cooling (used for Heat conditions), whereas others promote warmth (used for Cold conditions). Acupuncture is then used for supportive measures. (Table 11-2 shows some common traditional Chinese paradigms designed for horses.)

Treatment for Gastrointestinal Disorders

Several studies show the effectiveness of acupuncture on gastrointestinal motility (Matsumoto, Hayes, 1973). In a study done on postoperative ileus in horses, vitamin B_{12} was injected into ST-36, followed by electroacupuncture. Recovery from ileus occurred within 48 hours.

Other studies have shown the efficacy of acupuncture in the treatment of diarrhea (Hwang, Jenkins, 1988), colic (Xiaoma, 1988), and impaction (White and others, 1984). In a study on equine impaction, electroacupuncture was performed on the Chinese points *Guan Yuan Shu*, located caudal to the eighteenth rib on the longissimus dorsi. The

success rate was 97.8 %. Acupuncture also appears to be effective in the treatment of aerophagia when concomitant gastrointestinal signs are present. One author reported a good success rate using ST-9 and ST-10 with electroacupuncture (White and others, 1984). (Box 11-1 shows some of the more common point formulas used to treat gastrointestinal disease in the horse.)

Treatment for Reproductive Disorders

As with gastrointestinal disease, the use of acupuncture without the use of herbs is often ineffective in treating reproductive disorders, although some evidence suggests otherwise. In one study, 35 mares were treated for a variety of reproductive disorders. After use of *Bai Hui* and BL-26 (located lateral to the lumbosacral space), 77% showed a significant improvement (Tominaga, 1985). (Box 11-2 shows some recommended point formulas for equine reproductive disorders.)

Treatment for Respiratory Disorders

The lungs sit in the upper portion of the body and are considered closely related to the first line of defense. They filter pathogens and pollutants during respiration and are the organs most sensitive to the external environment. If the lungs cannot withstand these external attacks, they respond by producing phlegm. This phlegm blocks the dispersion of *Qi* from the Lung and creates congestion. Acupuncture not only improves the direct physiology of the Lung but also enhances the immune system.

TABLE 11-2

TRADITIONAL CHINESE MEDICAL DIAGNOSIS OF ORGAN DYSFUNCTION

TCM DIAGNOSIS	WESTERN DIAGNOSIS	SYMPTOMS
Lung *Yang* excess	Bleeder	Loud, nonproductive cough with blood-tinged discharge, coarse breathing
Lung *Yin* deficiency	Chronic COPD	Weak respiration, weak cough with dry sound, difficult exhalation
Kidney *Yang* deficiency	Infertility	Frequent urination, infertility, cold limbs, weakness of back and hindlimb
Kidney *Yin* deficiency	Infertility	Low-grade fever; scanty, yellow urine; infertility; dry skin
Spleen *Qi* deficiency	Sterile bowel	Poor appetite, loose stools, edema, prolapse of uterus
Stomach *Yin* deficiency	Ulcers	Blood in stools, dry skin and mucous membranes, low-grade fever
Spleen heat	Enteritis	Loose manure with foul odor; fever; scanty, yellow urine; inappetence
Liver *Yin* deficiency	Irregular estrus	Irritability, irregular estrous cycles, pain behind ribs, dry skin
Liver *Qi* stagnation	Indigestion	Sour regurgitation, inappetance, poor energy level until exercised
Heart *Yin* deficiency	Dysrhythmias	Restlessness, palpitations, low-grade fever

COPD, chronic obstructive pulmonary disease.

BOX 11-1

POINT FORMULAS USED TO TREAT GASTROINTESTINAL DISEASE IN THE HORSE

Indigestion	PC-6, ST-45, BL-20, BL-21, ST-2
Ulcer	ST-36, PC-6, BL-18, BL-21, BL-20, ST-1
Proximal enteritis	ST-36, PC-6, ST-1, BL-21
Sterile bowel	SP-6, SP-9, BL-20, ST-36, SP-1
Impaction	BL-2, BL-21, BL-25, ST-36, Bai Hui
Flatulent colic	BL-27, ST-36, LIV-3, BL-25, SI-1, LI-1
Cribbing	ST-9, ST-10, BL-21, ST-45, BL-17

BOX 11-2

RECOMMENDED POINT FORMULAS FOR REPRODUCTIVE DISORDERS IN THE HORSE

Anestrus	BL-23—26 (10-cm needles and moxibustion), BL-54, SP-6, ST-36, Bai Hui, GV-1 (25 cm toward sacrum)
Ovarian cysts	BL-21—23, BL-26—28, Bai Hui, BL-39, ST-36, SP-6
Metritis	BL-26—28 (10-cm needles and moxibustion), BL-35, GV-1—2, SP-6, Bai Hui
Infertility	BL-11, BL-22—28, BL-35, GV-1—2, SP-6, KI-7, LIV-3, Bai Hui, ST-36
Retained placenta	BL-26, BL-60, BL-67
Labor induction	SP-6, ST-36, LI-4, CV-2
Milk letdown	ST-36, GB-21, ST-41

Acupuncture has also proved effective in the treatment of pharyngitis, chronic obstructive pulmonary disease, and exercise-induced pulmonary hemorrhage (Rogers, Cain, 1987). When treating any respiratory disorder, veterinarians should carefully evaluate all symptoms to arrive at a correct Chinese diagnosis. (The points listed in Box 11-3 serve only as a guide; most points should be chosen according to the energy status of the patient.)

Conclusion: Acupuncture Versus Western Medicine

After finishing this chapter, the reader should appreciate the differences in the philosophies of traditional Chinese and Western medicines. Trained in a science based on dou-ble-blind studies, Western researchers attempt to verify TCM concepts, forgetting that by doing so they lose the essence of these ancient theories. For example, according to TCM, laminitis may be treated by several contradictory methods depending on the Chinese diagnosis. An older pony may have a Kidney *Yin* deficiency, whereas the overstressed racehorse may be suffering from Liver *Qi* stagnation. To the Western practitioner focusing merely on the symptom of laminitis, the horse and pony suffer from the

---

BOX 11-3

RECOMMENDED POINT FORMULAS FOR RESPIRATORY DISORDERS IN THE HORSE

Influenza	LU-1, LU-2, LU-7, LU-11, LI-4, LI-11, LI-16, LI-18, LI-20, GB-20, GB-21, BL-13, GV-14, TH-5
Sinusitis	LI-4, LI-11, LI-20, BL-13, BL-18, BL-25, ST-2, ST-9, ST-10, GV-26, LU-7, PC-6
Pharyngitis	LU-5, LU-7, LU-11, LI-1, LI-11, LI-18, PC-6
Pneumonia	BL-13, BL-14, BL-15, GV-14, GB-21, LI-4, LI-11
COPD	BL-13—15, LU-1, LU-7, LU-9, ST-36, GV-14, GV-20
Bleeder	BL-13—15, BL-20, Bai Hui, BL-18, GV-26

same disease; to the acupuncturist, treating both patients identically would ultimately lead to the demise of one. Investigating the effect of a general group of points on a group of horses suffering from laminitis would be difficult, if not impossible; each case must be evaluated individually because, according to TCM, the horses do not have the same disease. Therefore clinical efficacy trials may be the only true way to evaluate the effectiveness of this modality.

The need for further research is unquestionable. Unfortunately, most available research funds are allocated to commercial pharmaceutic development because acupuncture is not lucrative. Most research heretofore has focused on the neurophysiologic effects of acupuncture on pain, but underlying TCM principles must still be respected. Thoughtful consideration of these concepts often determines the success or failure of a case. Although we cannot explain all effects of acupuncture, we should not ignore thousands of years of clinical efficacy.

REFERENCES

Beinfield H: *Between heaven and earth,* New York, 1991, Ballantine.

Bossut DFB and others: Plasma cortisol and β-endorphins in horses subjected to electroacupuncture for cutaneous analgesia, *Proc Intl Vet Acup Soc* 4:501, 1983.

Chao WK, Loh WP: The immunologic responses of acupuncture stimulation, *Acupunct Electrother Res* 12:282, 1987.

Chen GB: Role of nervous system of human body with regard to acupuncture analgesia, *Acupunct Electrother Res* 6(1):7, 1981.

Dong QS, Zheng RT: *The relationship between acupuncture analgesia and the afferent fibers of group III and IV acupuncture research,* Beijing, 1985, Foreign Language Printing House.

Egerbacher M: Anatomy and physiology of selected bovine and canine acupuncture points. In Schoen AM: *Veterinary acupuncture: ancient art to modern medicine,* St Louis, 1994, Mosby.

Han JS, Terenius I: Neurochemical basis of acupuncture analgesia, *Am J Pharmacol Toxicol* 22:193, 1982.

Hwang YC, Jenkins EM: Effect of acupuncture on young pigs with induced enteropathogenic *Escherichia coli* diarrhea. *Am J Vet Res* 49: 1641, 1988.

Kendall DE: Part I. A scientific model for acupuncture, *Am J Acupunct* 17(3):251, 1989.

Kendall DE: Part II. A scientific model for acupuncture, *Am J Acupunct* 17(4):343, 1989.

Klide AM, Kung SH: *Veterinary acupuncture,* Philadelphia, 1977, University of Pennsylvania.

Matsumoto T, Hayes MF: Acupuncture electric phenomenon of the skin and postvagotomy gastrointestinal atony, *Am J Surg* 125:176, 1973.

Nordenstrom BEW: An electrophysiologic view of acupuncture of capacitive and closed circuit currents and their clinical effects in the treatment of cancer and chronic pain, *Am J Acupunct* 17(2):105, 1987.

O'Connor J, Bensky D: *Acupuncture: a comprehensive text,* Seattle, 1988, Eastland.

Pan XP and others: Electroacupuncture analgesia and analgesic action of NAGA, *J Tradit Chin Med* 4(4):273, 1984.

Rogers PAM: *A brief history of acupuncture and the status of veterinary acupuncture outside mainland China: Course in Veterinary Acupuncture,* Oslo, IVAS, 1988.

Rogers PAM, Cain M: Clinical acupuncture in the horse. Proceedings of the 13th Annual Meeting, *IVAS,* 1987.

Schoen AM: *Veterinary acupuncture: ancient art to modern medicine,* St Louis, 1994, Mosby.

Snader M: Clinical acupuncture diagnosis in the horse. Proceedings of the 13th Annual Meeting, *IVAS,* 1982.

Takasek K: Revolutionary new pain theory and acupuncture treatment procedure based on a new theory of acupuncture mechanism, *Am J Acupunct* 11(4):305, 1983.

Tominaga T: The therapeutic effect of acupuncture of reproductive disorders and lameness in horses, *Bull Japanese Soc Vet Acupunct Moxibust* 4:2, 1985.

White S and others: *Electropuncture in veterinary medicine: an original translation,* San Francisco, 1984, Chinese Materials Center Publications.

Xiaoma W: Electroimpulse acupuncture treatment of 110 cases of abdominal pain as a sequela of abdominal surgery, *J Tradit Chin Med* 8:269, 1988.

Xie QW: Endocrinological basis of acupuncture, *Am J Chin Med* 9(4):298, 1982.

Xinnong C: *Chinese acupuncture and moxibustion,* Beijing, 1987, Foreign Language Press.

Yu C, Hwang YC: *Handbook on Chinese veterinary acupuncture and moxibustion,* Bangkok, 1990, FAO/APHCA Publication.

Zhong XH and others: Correlation between endogenous opiate-like peptides and serotonin in laserpuncture analgesia, *Am J Acupunct* 17(1):39, 1989.

SELECTED READING

Bossut D, Page E: Preliminary study of the treatment of paralytic ileus in horses by electroacupuncture. Proceeding of the Annual Meeting, *IVAS,* 1984.

Jang JH: Ear acupuncture for hypotonia in GI exam, *Am J Res* 147:862, 1986.

Kothbauer O: Diagnostic acupuncture points in the horse. Proceedings of the Eighth Annual Meeting, *IVAS,* 1982.

Lee GTC: A study of electrical stimulation of acupuncture locus, Su-SanLi (ST36) on mesentric microcirculation, *Am J Chin Med* 2:53, 1974.

Chapter 12

Chiropractic Care

SHARON WILLOUGHBY

Health care for animals is an evolving science. Our veterinary predecessors used the accepted therapies and treatment protocols of their day. A veterinarian in the early 1900s offers an interesting viewpoint on therapeutics.

> "Give me mercury, iodine, quinine, and the lancet and I will combat disease with it." To which the author says: "Give me aconite, iodine, iron, mineral acid, soda, creosote, and a few others and I will not only combat but successfully cure and overcome disease" (McClure, 1901).

Veterinary shelves are now stocked with many antibiotics, corticosteroids, synthetic hormones, and other pharmaceuticals that have been developed in the last 50 years. Significant progress has been made in surgical procedures. Growth in the understanding of disease and therapeutics is vital to the survival of a health profession.

One result of this growth in the medical field is the rapid influx of therapeutic modalities such as acupuncture, botanical medicine, homeopathy, and chiropractic into animal health care. These health care systems represent divergent philosophies on health and disease and unique therapeutic approaches such as adjustment of the spine and insertion of needles into acupuncture points. Preconceptions and prejudice about these alternative therapies must be set aside to allow serious investigation into the potential benefits for the animal patient. The veterinary profession should not consider modern pharmaceutic and surgical interventions the only valid approaches for the care of sick and injured animals.

Chiropractic and other modalities are integral parts of the holistic trend in animal health care. A holistic philosophy stresses the integration of external and internal influences on the organism. Holistic therapies are designed to intervene at the appropriate level and to work with, not against, the inborn homeostasis of the organism. This differs from "allopathic" philosophy, which treats symptoms, sometimes in isolation from the entire health picture of the animal. Conventional veterinary medicine is not purely allopathic. The natural evolutionary path for animal health care is toward holism. For example, veterinary practitioners no longer believe that antibiotic therapy should be administered without consideration of the animal's immune response, nutritional condition, and environmental stress.

Chiropractic offers tremendous potential in animal health care. It belongs in the health care spectrum with medicine, surgery, acupuncture, homeopathy, and other such modalities. Chiropractic care does not encompass the entire study of health and disease, but it does offer alternative explanations for disease and provides complementary approaches. Chiropractic philosophy is based on the relationship of the spinal column to the nervous system and the role of the spinal column in biomechanics and movement.

Animal Chiropractic History

Spinal manipulation has been practiced on humans for centuries in many cultures. The Chinese were practicing spinal manipulation as early as 2700 BC. Hippocrates used spinal manipulation, and his maxim, "Look well to the spine for the cause of disease," is often quoted by chiropractors. The earliest English text on bonesetting, an early form of chiropractic, was published in 1656 (Wardwell, 1992). Although chiropractic is one of the most frequently used forms of alternative therapy for humans in the United States, the application to animals has been haphazard and sporadic. The use of chiropractic on animals was attempted as a curiosity by early chiropractors. The developer of chiropractic, B.J. Palmer, claimed to have run a veterinary clinic as part of his chiropractic school and research facility. He made the following observation:

In the early days of chiropractic we maintained a veterinarian [sic] hospital where we adjusted the vertebral subluxations of sick cows, horses, cats, and dogs, etc. We did this to prove to ourselves that the chiropractic principle and practice did apply (Palmer, 1944).

Few records of this activity have survived. The profession of chiropractic was fighting for survival against the medical establishment, and veterinary chiropractic was frowned on by mainstream chiropractic practitioners. Dr. Palmer explained the situation as follows:

Many doctors of chiropractic think that we should "soft-pedal" this animal application of Chiropractic. They fear the public might call them "horse-doctors" (Wardwell, 1992).

Many chiropractic publications carried articles describing chiropractic success on animals. In 1923 *The Fountain Head News*, a Palmer School publication, published a letter entitled "Pigs have backbones with Subluxations that Adjustments Work On." This article describes the apparently successful treatment of two paretic pigs (*Fountain Head News*, 1923). Although chiropractors have probably been adjusting animals for decades, the development of veterinary chiropractic has been impeded by the lack of a distinct historical foundation.

In recent years the beginning of a veterinary chiropractic profession is evident in the organization of courses designed to teach veterinary chiropractic techniques and in the elementary clinical research into these techniques. Most of the work in veterinary chiropractic is extrapolated from the human chiropractic profession, both in technique and in functional theories to explain the clinical results. Applications in clinical practice over the last decade have demonstrated the potential benefits of veterinary chiropractic. Unfortunately, clinical results are often considered anecdotal and discounted by established professionals.

Until recent years the veterinary profession has ignored the possibilities of chiropractic care for animal patients, preferring to take a position similar to that of other medical physicians. As recently as 1963 the American Medical Association relegated chiropractic practices to the Committee on Quackery, whose mission was to be the "containment and, ultimately, the elimination of chiropractic" (Wardwell, 1992). The American Veterinary Medical Association (AVMA) has only recently (1995) chosen to take a serious look at chiropractic care for animals.

Definition of Chiropractic

Chiropractic comes from the Greek words, *cheir*, which means *hand*, and *praxis*, which means *practice*, or *done by hand*. A drugless form of therapy, chiropractic is based on manual spinal manipulation. Modern definitions of chiropractic include the following:

. . . that science and art which uses the inherent recuperative powers of the body and deals with the relationship between the nervous system and the spinal column, including its immediate articulations, and the role of this relationship in the restoration and maintenance of health (Homewood, 1962).

Chiropractors focus on the interactions between neurologic mechanisms and the biomechanics of the spine, basing theories of disease manifestations on these interactions. Therapy is directed at the vertebral column to alter the progression of the disease process. Before attempting chiropractic, conventionally trained practitioners must rethink the importance of the nervous system in the health of the organism and the subsequent functional interplay between the central nervous system and the spinal column. Most conventional practitioners fail to comprehend the significance of this neurologic hierarchy, despite the increasing amount of scientific research indicating the activity of complex neurologic mechanisms.

Subluxations

Chiropractors have created a terminology that is unique to their profession. The vertebral lesions described by early chiropractors were called subluxations to designate contiguous vertebrae that displayed an abnormal positional relationship. The early use of the word *subluxation* was consistent with that of the medical author Hieronymous, whose definition of a subluxation in 1746 was characterized by "...lessened motion of the joints, by slight change in the position of the articulating facets..." (Leach, 1986). Currently a subluxation is defined by chiropractic as a "disrelationship of a vertebral segment in association with contiguous vertebrae resulting in a disturbance of normal biomechanical and neurological function" (Homewood, 1962). Modern chiropractic theorists have substituted the phrases "vertebral subluxation complex (VSC)" or "segmental dysfunction (SDF)" to describe the neurologic and biomechanic manifestations of these vertebral lesions (Leach, 1986).

The term *subluxation* is commonly used by chiropractors and veterinarians, but each profession defines it differently. This difference can create confusion and ill will in the veterinary medical community unless the definition is well understood. Veterinarians define subluxation as being "a partial dislocation less than a luxation," and most view this "subluxation" as nearer to a dislocation than to "a slight change in articular surfaces." This understanding of subluxation differs from that of chiropractors. Whereas a chiropractor might use the term *subluxation* to include concepts such as the effects of nociceptive sensations on the lateral spinothalamic tract and the dorsal horn cells, a veterinarian may assume that the chiropractor is talking only about a partial dislocation. Similar misunderstandings have hampered scientific inquiry into the science of chiropractic. However, the veterinarian can no longer afford to dismiss chiropractic as an "unscientific cult" without further inquiry into the rationale and scientific basis of chiropractic.

The conventionally trained veterinary practitioner must put aside preconceptions and study the significant research of the chiropractic profession, as well as that of the scientific community, on the complex functions of the nervous system. The veterinarian would be well advised to study texts such as *Chiropractic Theories* by Robert Leach, in which the scientific basis of chiropractic is discussed. The purpose of the book, as stated by Dr. Leach, is to have "testable hypotheses systematized in some manner that can be used as a platform for scientific inquiry" (Leach, 1986).

Pathophysiology of Subluxations

Chiropractic is based on the same anatomic and physiologic facts used by all medical practitioners. Essentially the same basic science textbooks are used in veterinary, medical, and chiropractic schools. The same anatomic, physiologic, and pathologic research is analyzed. From this common foundation, several current therapies have arisen to explain the subluxation complex and the effects of spinal adjustments. The theories discussed in the following section are chosen because they have significant experimental validation (Leach, 1986).

Facilitation hypothesis

The facilitation hypothesis states that subluxations produce a lowered threshold for firing in spinal cord segments. Subluxations result in afferent bombardment to the central nervous system from pathologically altered tissues surrounding the vertebral misalignment. The afferent input to each segment of spinal cord is largely composed of nonmyelinated C fibers or nociceptors. This nociceptor stimulation can create spinal lesions that may affect dorsal horn cells, autonomic fibers, the lateral spinothalamic tract, and other components of the complex neurologic system. The result can be clinical findings such as localized tenderness, muscle spasm, trigger points, or muscle hypoxia (Leach, 1986). Trigger points are hard, nodular, hyperirritable structures within muscle or fascia and generally occur in stable anatomic sites.

Somatoautonomic dysfunction

The somatoautonomic dysfunction hypothesis is based on the theory that autonomic responses are initiated by altered neurologic functions present in subluxations. When the adaptive mechanisms of the nervous system fail as a result of strong or long-lasting stimuli, the resulting aberrant somatoautonomic reflexes may be associated with several visceral disorders affecting functions such as heart rate, bronchial smooth muscle, and gastrointestinal tract function (Leach, 1986).

Nerve compression

The nerve compression hypothesis states that pressure on spinal nerve roots is caused by a subluxation, or misaligned vertebra, altering normal transmission of nerve energy. This pressure may arise from intervertebral foraminal encroachment, nerve root traction, axoplasmic transport block, or changes in the amplitude and velocity of the action potential. Chiropractic researchers agree that the explanation of "bone out of place" is too simplistic physiologically and believe that ischemia and edema may instead be the major causes of spinal nerve dysfunction (Leach, 1986).

Compressive myelopathy

The compressive myelopathy hypothesis theorizes that vertebral subluxations, particularly those in the cervical region, may compress or irritate the spinal cord. The cord can be affected by ischemia from spinal arterial spasm or even directly (by an upward translocation of the odontoid) (Leach, 1986).

Fixation

The fixation hypothesis is based on the theory that a subluxated vertebra may be in normal or abnormal position yet still fixed within its normal biomechanical range of motion. This fixation includes the involvement of paraspinal musculature and kinesthetic receptors, creating somatic bombardment of spinal pathways with somatic and autonomic reflex facilitation (Leach, 1986).

Vertebrobasilar arterial insufficiency

The vertebrobasilar arterial insufficiency hypothesis maintains that the vertebral arteries are constricted in subluxations, especially when passing through the transverse foramina of the upper cervical spine. This interference causes vascular insufficiency, or ischemia, to the spinal cord or the structures of the cranium (Leach, 1986).

Axoplasmic aberration

The axoplasmic aberration hypothesis maintains that intracellular movement of proteins, glycoproteins, or neurotransmitters in nerve cell processes is altered by irritation or blockages created by subluxations. In addition, altered axoplasmic transport may result in toxic levels of proteins, creating clinical symptoms of pain and numbness in peripheral nerves (Leach, 1986).

Neurodystrophic hypothesis

The neurodystrophic hypothesis states that neurologic dysfunction is stressful to the viscera and other body structures and that this lowered tissue resistance can modify the immune response. This theory, contrary to traditional veterinary ideas, proposes an interaction between the central nervous system and immunity. The work of Selye, however, has demonstrated neuroendocrine-immune connections in the response of the organism to stress (Selye,

1956). Mechanisms proposed by other researchers include a connection between the thymus and the CNS, norepinephrine immunomodulation, and a connection between the hypothalamus and immune responses (Leach, 1986).

Adjustment versus Manipulation

Chiropractors identify subluxations of the spine during clinical examination and then proceed to correct these lesions by specifically adjusting the involved segments. A spinal adjustment has specific characteristics that distinguish it from spinal manipulations. An adjustment is a specific physical action designed to restore the biomechanics of the vertebral column and indirectly influence neurologic function. Haldeman (1992) defines it as a "passive, carefully regulated thrust or force delivered with controlled speed, depth and magnitude to articulations at or near the end of the passive or physiological range of motion."

An adjustment is characterized by a specific force applied in a specific direction to a specific vertebra. It is a short-lever maneuver, with a contact taken directly on the involved vertebral segment. Adjustments are high-velocity procedures designed to deliver maximal force with minimal tissue damage. The adjustment is unique to the chiropractic profession and requires a great deal of skill to control the depth, direction, speed, and amplitude of the procedure.

Manipulations are not characterized by specificity to vertebral segments and often distribute force to multiple segments, as in traction and mobilization procedures. Furthermore, manipulations are generally characterized as long-lever and are delivered with slow velocity. A chiropractic practitioner may use a combination of short-lever, long-lever, and nonthrust techniques in clinical practice. However, the distinct nature of the spinal adjustment distinguishes the chiropractor from the manipulator or the physical therapist.

Basic Chiropractic Therapeutic Rationale

Chiropractic does not pretend to encompass the entire spectrum of health and therapy for the animal patient. It focuses on problems resulting from neurologic or biomechanic origin that can be affected by changing physiologic and pathologic mechanisms. A simple example is muscular back pain caused by vertebral subluxations. Although muscle pain and trigger points may be the clinical findings, the cause of aberrant muscle activity may originate in facilitated spinal segments.

A traumatic fracture of the femur is a pathologic condition not directly amenable to chiropractic therapy, although a chiropractic examination is indicated because the traumatic incident capable of fracturing a bone such as the femur might also have caused secondary trauma to the vertebral column. The health of the animal depends on proper repair of the femur, as well as restoration of vertebral function. To the chiropractor, therefore, the causes of disease are subluxations that interrupt neurologic function, disrupt homeostasis, and alter kinesthetic functions of the spine.

Most veterinarians tend to use similar medical therapeutic regimens, surgical customs, and treatment options. Chiropractic systems, however, range from those favoring active movement of the joints between vertebral segments to those using low-force techniques. Different systems may favor one particular region over another, such as upper cervical-specific techniques or chiropractic systems that treat the entire vertebral column. Theories on the mechanism of subluxations and the role of adjustments differ among chiropractic systems. For example, one system emphasizes the role of cerebrospinal fluid in spinal column function, and another concentrates on the potential neurologic pathology at the intervertebral foramen.

This lack of agreement on technique and treatment may contribute to the suspicion with which the veterinary community regards chiropractic. Chiropractic, however, is a young profession with rapidly evolving and complex theories. The medical community has misinterpreted and dismissed the therapeutic rationales of chiropractic for most of the last century. Dismissing chiropractic because of early claims and inaccuracies is as unfair as dismissing Western medicine because of its historical use of bloodletting. Chiropractic has survived its first century with the current medical and scientific literature rapidly providing substantiation for the physiologic and pathologic basis of its theories.

Skills of the Practitioner

The basic treatment modality of the chiropractor is spinal adjustment. Adjustments are specific according to spinal segment, force expended, and timing of the adjustive thrust. To those unfamiliar with chiropractic care the treatment regimen may appear to be a randomly ordered, simplistic series of forces applied to the spine. This is no more accurate than the belief that a medical injection is random or simple. A syringe is loaded with a specifically selected agent, such as a vaccine or an antibiotic, aimed at a specific anatomic target, such as a muscle or vein, and accompanied by a rationale for the subsequent effect in the body. An adjustment is directed at a specific vertebral segment, and a specific force and depth of application are used, with a specific rationale for the desired effect of the adjustment. The apparent simplicity of both procedures should not mislead the observer about the training, experience, and clinical judgment of the practitioner.

Chiropractic practice entails a specific set of mental and physical skills different from those generally used in veterinary practice. The physical skills of palpation and adjusting are first acquired through professional education and then developed by continual practice into skilled procedures. The following section discusses the basic skills necessary in veterinary chiropractic practice.

Anatomic Knowledge

All medical practitioners must understand the anatomy of the tissue or organ targeted by their therapeutic modalities. The physician must be familiar with the structures in the thoracic cavity visualized on radiograph. Before performing surgery, the surgeon must be familiar with the ligamentous structures in the coxofemoral joint. Before performing an adjustment, the chiropractor must understand the specific articular relationships in the vertebral column. The chiropractor must be able to visualize vertebral structures in a three-dimensional context, understanding accurately the orientations of joint surfaces. One of the most important anatomic features in the context of adjusting technique is joint surface orientations. Chiropractic adjustments produce vertebral movement along the plane line of joints. It would be counterproductive to apply forces to a joint that would cause jamming of the articular surfaces. A veterinary chiropractor must become familiar with all the articular surfaces and types in the spinal column of each species to which chiropractic will be applied. For example, the joints between lumbar vertebra five and lumbar vertebra six in the horse consist of two synovial zygopophyseal joints, one synarthrodial intervertebral joint, and two synovial intertransverse joints. The zygapophyseal joints are characterized by a sagittally curved surface and classified as *trochoid joints*. The partially movable intervertebral joint displays a slightly curved surface with an eccentric center of rotation. The intertransverse joints, which are distinctive in the horse, also display a curved articular surface.

Chiropractors divide the spinal column into functional or motor units for a more precise concept of the biomechanics involved in spinal movements, misalignments, and adjustments of subluxated segments. A motor unit consists of two adjacent vertebrae, the intervertebral disk, articular facets, ligaments, tendons, muscles, nerves, and the blood vessels that combine two vertebrae into a movable unit. The practitioner must study each of these motor units individually because each has a different type, number, and joint orientation. For example, a midthoracic motor unit exhibits coronal articular facets, slightly curved intervertebral disk joints, synovial ball-and-socket costovertebral joints, and plane costotransverse joints. The chiropractor must consider seven joints when adjusting the sixth thoracic vertebra of a dog. This chapter does not propose to discuss in depth the relevant anatomy of each motor unit. (Tables 12-1 and 12-2 illustrate the basic anatomic joint characteristics in the vertebral column of horses and dogs.)

The chiropractic practitioner must know the location and orientation of vertebral processes in the animal. This knowledge is necessary to achieve the desired therapeutic result. For example, a practitioner may choose the mammillary process for the contact point on a lumbar vertebra to correct for a rotational misalignment. The relative location of the mammillary process must be identified beneath layers of soft tissue, without direct palpation on this osseous process. The orientation and angulation of spinous processes and the location and angulation of the mammillary processes and transverse processes are important factors in precise adjustment technique.

The chiropractic practitioner must understand the relationships of neurologic components of the vertebral column to determine the potential pathology created by a subluxation (i.e., pain, paresthesia, and autonomic nervous system manifestations) and predict the possible benefits of the adjustment. The intervertebral foramen (IVF) is of particular interest to the chiropractor because its boundaries consist partially of the osseous structure of the vertebrae and partially of ligamentous structures involved in spinal movement. The IVF is the communication portal of the nervous system, with the enclosed spinal nerves carrying the afferent and efferent fibers essential to the coordination of nerve centers and target organs. Foraminal encroachment by surrounding structures could interfere with the relay of neurologic information. (The contents of the IVF are in Table 12-3, and the boundaries are listed in Box 12-1.)

Other anatomic features of the nervous system are important in chiropractic theory, including the flow of cerebrospinal fluid, the meningeal suspension of the spinal cord within the vertebral foramen, the relationships of cranial nerves to vertebral structures, and the proximity of the autonomic chain ganglia to the ventral surface of the column.

The study of vertebral biomechanics necessitates fundamental knowledge of muscular attachments and actions on the vertebrae. Many of the major muscle groups, such as the longissimus and gluteal, have attachments on the vertebral column. Other less well-known intrinsic muscles, such as the multifidis and the rotatores, may be used in a chiropractic examination. Motor nerves form a functional loop with the muscular system; that is, motor fibers incite the muscles to contract, producing movement, and sensory fibers relay proprioceptive and stretch readings back to the central nervous system.

Vertebral Movement

Chiropractic science focuses on the biomechanics of spinal movement and the encompassing nature of this movement. The vertebral column, a jointed structure at the core of every vertebrate, enables movement in a variety of gaits, postures, and stretches. As a mechanical structure the vertebrae move in controlled directions by a complex of levers and pivots restrained by ligaments and activated by muscles (White, Panjabi, 1990). Vertebral movement can be extremely subtle, such as that present during respiration, or very obvious, such as flexion and extension in

CHARACTERISTICS OF EQUINE VERTEBRAL MOTOR UNITS

MOTOR UNIT	ZYGAPOPHYSEAL JOINT	INTERVERTEBRAL JOINT	ANCILLARY JOINTS
Atlantooccipital	Prominent, egg-shaped facets of occiput projecting into deep concave facets of atlas	None	None
Atlantoaxial	Saddle-shaped facets that allow joint with extensive axial rotation	None	Trochoid joint of the dens
Cervical	Plane joints with 45-degree facet angle	Curved surfaces with almost a ball-and-socket orientation, concave on caudal body and convex on cranial body	None
Cervical/thoracic	Plane joints switching from 45-degree angle to coronal orientation	Decreasing concavity/convexity of intervertebral disk plane	Beginning of rib articulations (see below)
Thoracic	Plane joints with coronal orientation	Slightly curved intervertebral disc plane	Curved demifacets on two adjacent vertebrae providing socket for head of rib; plane facet on transverse process for rub tubercle
Thoracolumbar	Coronal plane joints switching to sagittal trochoid surfaces	Slightly curved intervertebral disk plane	
Lumbar	Sagittal trochoid joints	Slightly curved intervertebral disk plane	
Low lumbar	Sagittal trochoid joints	Slightly curved intervertebral disk plane	Curved surfaces join in intertransverse joint
Lumbosacral	Sagittal trochoid joints	Slightly curved intervertebral disk plane, with thick wedge-shaped disk	Curved surfaces join in intertransverse joint
Sacroiliac	Plane synarthrodial joint with 65-degree angle	None	None

the equine gallop. Freedom of movement requires that the organism experience peak flexibility, precise proprioception, maximal muscular response, and an absence of musculoskeletal pain. Horses trained for dressage must be able maintain flexion of the entire vertebral column. The thoracolumbar spine is flexed to "round" the back, resulting in lowering of the hindquarters for forward impulsion. Dressage horses must elevate or flex the cervicothoracic region, shifting the center of gravity to the hindquarters and lightening the forehand. The cervical spinal column is flexed for proper head carriage. Dogs in agility training are required to jump obstacles, which requires flexion and extension of the spinal column. These dogs must bend their bodies around poles, using lateral flexion. Restriction or pain in one or two functional motor units may create minimal gait problems yet markedly restrict spinal movement.

Movement of the spinal column is the result of the sum of movements at individual motor units. The motor unit is the smallest segment of the spine that exhibits biomechanic characteristics and consists of two adjacent vertebrae and their ligaments (White, Panjabi, 1990). The range of motion at each motor unit is relatively small; however, the sum of movement at multiple motor units can be considerable (Stasek, 1987). Furthermore, minimal range of movement at the vertebral level can create exponential movement in the extremities. Consider the movement of a pendulum in a grandfather clock. The point at which the pendulum attaches to the clock does not move in a great arc, but further from the attachment point, at the end of the pendulum, a wide arc is created. Similarly, movement created at the vertebral level in a horse creates a great amount of movement at the hoof (i.e., the end of this living pendulum). A good example of this occurs

TABLE 12-2

CHARACTERISTICS OF CANINE VERTEBRAL MOTOR UNITS

MOTOR UNIT	ZYGAPOPHYSEAL JOINT	INTERVERTEBRAL JOINT	ANCILLARY JOINTS
Anlantooccipital	Prominent, egg-shaped facets of occiput projecting into deep concave facets of atlas	None	None
Atlantoaxial	Saddle-shaped facets that allow joint with extensive axial rotation	None	Trochoid joint of the dens
Cervical	Plane joints with 45-degree facet angle	Slightly curved intervertebral disk plane	None
Cervical/thoracic	Plane joints switching from 45 degrees to coronal	Slightly curved intervertebral disk plane	None
Thoracic	Plane joints with coronal orientation	Slightly curved intervertebral disk plane	Curved demifacet on adjacent vertebrae forming socket for head of rib; plane facet on transverse press for rib tubercle
Thoracolumbar	Coronal plane joints switching to sagittal trochoid surfaces	Slightly curved intervertebral disk plane	None
Lumbar	Sagittal trochoid joint	Slightly curved intervertebral disk plane	None
Low lumbar	Sagittal trochoid joint	Slightly curved intervertebral disk plane	None
Lumbosacral	Sagittal trochoid joint	Slightly curved intervertebral disk plane	None
Sacroiliac	Plane synarthrodial joint with 20-degree angle	None	None

TABLE 12-3

CONTENTS OF INTERVERTEBRAL FORAMEN

STRUCTURE	FUNCTION
Spinal nerve	Radicular nerve with distribution to skin, muscles, and viscera
Recurrent meningeal nerve	Nerve supply to disk, dorsal longitudinal ligament, and meninges; sympathetic function
Dural extension	Dura mater that follows spinal nerve through the IVF and blends with the epineurium of the nerve
Cerebrospinal fluid	Circulates between dural extension and radicular nerve carrying neurotransmitters and neuroendocrines
Intervertebral veins	Carry blood supply from the ventral venous sinus
Spinal artery	Carries blood supply into the vertebral canal
Connective tissue	Areolar and adipose tissues filling in spaces between previous structures
Lymphatic vessels	Lymphatic drainage

when the standardbred moves at a racing pace, using both lateral flexion and axial rotation of the thoracolumbar region. A pendulum-like movement is created in the hindquarters, with the feet traveling in a wide arc created by minimal but critical movements of the spinal column.

Spinal movements are as essential to athletic performance as the movements of the extremities. When motor units are restricted in range of motion, the results are restrictions in the character and range of motion of the extremities, such as stride length. A restricted lumbosacral

BOUNDARIES OF IVF

STRUCTURE
Vertebral notches
Intervertebral disk
Ligamentum flavum
Joint capsule of the articular facet

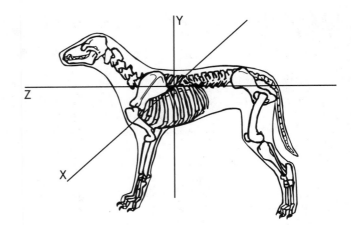

Fig. 12-1 Axes of movement.

joint may result in short stride of a rear leg. Chronic alterations in the biomechanic function of the spinal column can result in degenerative joint disease when extremity joints land repeatedly in abnormal patterns.

The vertebral column undergoes movement in several ranges, including flexion, extension, lateral flexion, axial rotation, compression, tension, vertical glide, and horizontal glide. In some cases, these movements are combined simultaneously into coupled motions.

Flexion-extension

The jointed spinal column can flex and extend around the X-axis (Fig. 12-1). This ability is apparent when horses gallop by folding or flexing the lumbar spinal column and then opening or extending the lower back. The behavior of a motor unit during flexion or extension varies depending on the spinal region. Generally the disk becomes wedged, and the nucleus pulposus moves dorsally in flexion and ventrally in extension. The dorsal annular fibers exhibit tension at flexion, and ventral annular fibers exhibit tension at extension (Kapandji, 1974).

Axial rotation

The jointed column can also rotate around the Z-axis. Here the vertebral body twists along its horizontal axis. The oblique fibers of the annulus are brought into tension. This tension is most pronounced in the central fibers of the annulus, where the fibers are most oblique. The nucleus is strongly compressed during axial rotation. Movements with excessive combinations of flexion and axial rotation tend to tear the annular fibers and drive the nucleus dorsally through these tears (Kapandji, 1974).

Lateral flexion

The jointed column curves around the Y-axis in lateral bending. The intervertebral disk wedges to the side opposite the lateral bend. The nucleus is then driven toward the open-wedge side of the disk, creating tension in the annular fibers (Kapandji, 1974).

Compression/tension

The spinal column is also able to stretch and shorten along the horizontal or Z-axis, altering the overall length of the column. Tension or elongation of the column in-creases the disk height and puts tension on the annular fibers. When the spine shortens, the disk undergoes compression and becomes flatter and wider (Kapandji, 1974). Tension and compression are also part of coupled motions during axial rotation, flexion, extension, and lateral bending. For example, in flexion the dorsal portion of the ligaments in the motor unit undergoes tension as the ventral portion undergoes compression (White, Panjabi, 1990).

Vertical gliding or shear

Forces acting on the spinal column in a vertical direction create movement that tends to separate or shear contiguous vertebrae. Gravity is the most constant vertical shear force acting on the backs of quadrupeds. Excessive shear forces, such as a heavy load on this horizontal column, disrupt the intrinsic resistant properties of spinal ligaments. An example is the overweight dog who develops a lordotic spinal column, which results in ligament damage and subsequent spondylosis.

Horizontal glide or shear

The spine separates in response to horizontal shear or forces that produce an impact on the vertebral column at 90 degrees. Extreme horizontal shear can exceed the capacity of the ligamentous structures to resist.

Coupled movement

Vertebral movement is the result of several joints in a motor unit acting in multiple planes with different axes of motion (Kapandji, 1974). A combination of movements is called a *coupled motion*. Each joint in the motor unit moves in a particular plane according to anatomic characteristics. For example, when the lumbar spine flexes, the upper portion of the disk undergoes tension and the lower portion undergoes compression. The curved lumbar zygapophyseal joints glide and separate along the Z-axis. In the cervical spine, lateral flexion combines with flexion and extension to become circumflexion. In chiropractic technique, this coupled movement is accommodated by using adjustments designed to act on all relevant phases of movement involved in a subluxation complex.

Functional Spinal Regions

When considered as a functional entity, the vertebral column should be divided into regions that differ from those used for purely anatomic categorization. (The functional divisions of the vertebral column are listed in Table 12-4.) Several of these divisions are transition regions between groups of vertebrae that bear similar anatomic characteristics. The vertebrae in transition areas display unique anatomic features and distinct motion characteristics. Spinal pathologies, including the chiropractic subluxation complex, are frequently located in transition regions.

Anatomic Study of the Vertebral Column

Practitioners interested in the study of chiropractic technique must first study vertebral anatomy. Chiropractors must be able to visualize individual vertebrae beneath layers of soft tissues. An understanding of the three-dimensional structure of each vertebra (including orientation and size of processes, joint surfaces, and foramens) is the foundation of this study. The chiropractor must also understand the movement characteristics of coupled segments of jointed vertebrae and the spatial relationships of segmental processes. Finally, to understand the vertebral column as a functional anatomic whole, the chiropractor must understand the way the spinal regions are combined into a unit. The vertebral column should be studied by using nonarticulated vertebrae that can be considered both individually and together. Although helpful, photographs and diagrams are inadequate to familiarize the practitioner with the functional and three-dimensional characteristics of the vertebral column (Fig. 12-2).

The following observations should be made in vertebral anatomic study:

- What are the characteristics of joint facets? Are they curved or flat? In which directions do they face? (The thoracic cranial articular facets are flat plane joints that face cranially, slightly laterally, and dorsally.)
- What is the relationship of the vertebral processes to the joints? (The mammillary process is located dorsal and lateral to the cranial articular facet of the lumbar vertebra.)
- How do the vertebral processes, such as the transverse process and spinous process, compare in different regions? (The spinous processes of the midcervicals are reduced to a bony ridge.)
- How do adjacent vertebrae move along the facet joints and through the disk? (The lumbar zygapophyseal joints move in axial rotation and glide in extension and flexion.)
- What are the characteristics of transition regions? (The cervicothoracic region displays transitions from an angled facet (45 degrees) to a coronal facet, spinous processes are elongating, and transverse processes are rising dorsally.)
- What are the shapes and orientations of the foramina? (The vertebral foramen is larger in the cervical region than in the thoracic, and the cervical intervertebral foramen has an oblique rather than perpendicular orientation to the long axis of the spine.)

Chiropractic Examination Techniques

Patient Observation

All types of physical examination include initial observation of the patient. In a chiropractic examination the subtleties of patient posture, gait, and behavior must be considered at the vertebral level of mechanic and neurologic function. When observing a limping dog, for example, the practitioner should observe the extremity joints without disassociating them from their functional con-

---

TABLE 12-4

TRANSITION REGIONS

		HORSE	DOG
Upper cervical region	Transition region	Occiput, atlas, axis	Occiput, atlas, axis
Cervical		C2, C3, C4, C5	C2, C3, C4, C5
Cervicothoracic	Transition region	C6, C7, T1, T2	C6, C7, T1, T2
Thoracic		T3-T16	T3-T11
Thoracolumbar	Transition region	T17, T18, L1, L2	T12, T13, L1, L2
Lumbar		L3, L4, L5	L3, L4, L5, L6
Lumbosacral	Transition region	L6 and sacrum	L7 and sacrum
Sacral		Sacrum and ilium	Sacrum and ilium

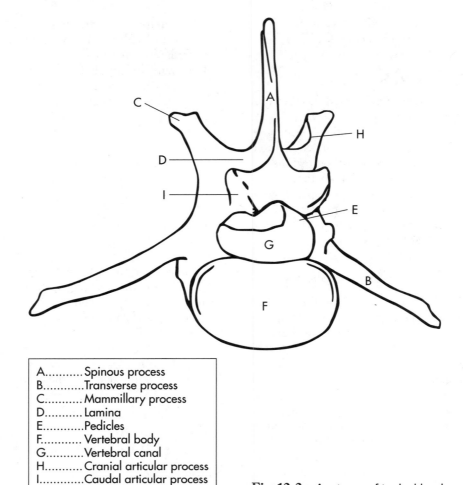

A............Spinous process
B.............Transverse process
C............Mammillary process
D............Lamina
E.............Pedicles
F.............Vertebral body
G............Vertebral canal
H............Cranial articular process
I..............Caudal articular process

Fig. 12-2   Anatomy of typical lumbar vertebra.

nections to the vertebral column. If the dog is shortening the stride length of the right rear leg, chiropractic considerations should include the following:

- Mechanical pathology of the extremity joints: Decreased range of motion in joints as a result of abnormal joint alignments; ligamentous damage, such as spurs, scar tissue, and inflammation; uneven muscular contraction of stabilizing and opposing muscle groups
- Neurologic pathology of the extremity joints: Pain, abnormal proprioception
- Mechanical and neurologic pathology of the sacroiliac joint and lumbosacral joints: Decreased range of motion of joint as a result of abnormal joint alignments; ligamentous damage, such as spurs, scar tissue, or inflammation; uneven muscular contraction of stabilizing and opposing muscle groups
- Neurologic pathology of the lumbar spine: Affected lumbosacral plexus motor nerves, nerves from joint receptors, and pain fibers

The chiropractor does not isolate the observation of extremity joints but considers neurologic and core biomechanic function. The veterinary practitioner must see the animal as a functional whole rather than the sum of its parts.

Chiropractic examination includes observation of the skin, muscle condition, and general attitude. Some types of behavior patterns are related to neurologic problems such as pain. The horse who flattens its ears and bites during saddle placement is indicating that the saddle is causing or aggravating pain. If this behavior changes when the pain is eliminated, the behavior can be attributed to the former neurologic condition.

Static Palpation

A chiropractic spinal examination incorporates static palpation of the topographic processes of the vertebrae. Static palpation findings may be informative, but several precautions are relevant. Without an intimate grasp of normal spinal anatomy, practitioners may make inaccurate assumptions. For example, the anticlinal vertebra (T10) in the dog has a very abbreviated spinous process compared with adjacent segments. Palpation of the spinous process of this vertebra often detects a depression that might be inaccurately interpreted as a ventrally subluxated segment.

Asymmetric processes may occur with no pathology present in the vertebra or motor unit. For example, a spinous process may be twisted away from the exact midline, whereas the vertebral body and the articular joints are in normal apposition. Finally, static palpation does not provide any information about the functional condition of the segment as it participates in its motor units. For example, upon palpation a vertebra may show normal alignment of the spinous process and transverse process, when in fact the segment is restricted in range of motion.

Static palpation is used on vertebral prominences that lie beneath soft tissue. Relying on anatomic knowledge and palpation skills, the examiner compares the relationships between adjacent vertebrae. For example, the relative heights of transverse processes are compared bilaterally on the same vertebra and between adjacent vertebrae. The global relationships of the column are assessed through palpation for such conditions as kyphosis (roach back), scoliosis, and lordosis. Static palpation examination involves the soft tissues that surround the vertebral segments, such as alterations in muscle tone; inflammatory symptoms, such as those produced by heat; and sensory aberrations, such as pain or hypalgesia.

Motion Palpation

A key element in chiropractic examination is evaluation of the active and passive ranges of motion in vertebral motor units. The examiner must assess each joint in all ranges of motion, such as lateral flexion, axial rotation, and flexion/extension. Ranges of joint motion have been divided into several categories (Table 12-5). *Active range of motion* refers to the portion of vertebral movement that is available with voluntary muscle action. When a horse laterally flexes its neck to the right, each motor unit moves to provide maximal global range of motion for the neck. If one cervical joint loses all or part of the active range of motion, muscular contractions fail to produce total active range of movement.

Every joint has an additional range of motion beyond the active range. This is called *passive range of motion*, or *joint play*. Joint play gives elastic and protective properties to joints when they are in the closed-pack position. This range of motion is much more limited than the active range and is not produced by voluntary muscular contraction. It is available only when an external force is applied (as, for example, during examination).

The chiropractor assesses the motor units' active and passive ranges of motion during motion palpation examination. Evaluation of passive and active range of motion considers the expected ranges of motion at each motor unit. These ranges of motion can be expected to vary among species and individual animals and in the presence of degenerative joint disease. For example, the lumbar spine of the cow has limited flexion-extension compared with the same region in the horse. The cervical spine of the older dog would be expected to have less range of motion than that of the puppy. Furthermore, thoracolumbar extension in a dog with spondylosis is less than that in a dog with a healthy column. The practitioner must have sufficient experience in motion palpation to recognize these differences and properly evaluate the motion findings in an examination.

In human chiropractic practice, active range of motion can be easily assessed in cooperative patients who participate actively in the examination. In animal chiropractic, however, motion palpation is more difficult. Animal patients may be uncooperative, actively resisting the examination or activating muscle groups that artificially change range-of-motion findings. Motion palpation of the vertebral column in animals is a difficult skill to perfect.

Chiropractic Adjustments

An alteration in range of motion is an important reason to perform a chiropractic adjustment on a vertebral joint. In chiropractic practice an adjustment is a specific force applied to a specific articulation with a specific vector of application. *Adjustment* can also be defined as follows: "a short-lever, specific, high velocity, controlled forceful thrust by hand or instrument which is directed at specific articulations and designed to restore biomechanical and neurological function" (Haldeman, 1992).

The goal of the adjustment is not to return a vertebra to a specific position but to initiate or activate the homeostatic mechanisms of vertebral kinesthetics. When a restricted joint is moved along its functional plane lines, the innate proprioceptive and restorative mechanisms of the joint are initiated. If the joint ranges are altered by muscular hypertonicity or ligamentous scarring, the subluxation may reappear and may require multiple adjustments. Neurologic reprogramming of muscular contractions and healing of damaged ligaments are not immediate results. The innate homeostatic mechanisms of the body require time to respond to an adjustment. Depending on the severity, duration, and pathology of the subluxation pattern, chiropractic care is generally used in a series of ther-

TABLE 12-5

RANGES OF JOINT MOTION

RANGE	CARTESIAN MOVEMENT
Flexion	Movement around the X-axis
Extension	Movement around the X-axis
Axial rotation	Movement around the Y-axis
Lateral flexion	Movement along the Z-axis
Compression/tension	Translation along the Y-axis
Horizontal shear	Translation along the X-axis
Vertical shear	Translation along the Z-axis

apeutic visits that allow gradual restoration and then maintenance of biomechanic and neurologic function.

Vertebral motor units that are severely damaged with osseous bridging (characteristic of spondylosis) may respond poorly or not at all to adjustments. However, routine radiographic examination does not reveal the amount of vertebral motion present in either normal or in pathologically altered segments. Many cases of spondylosis identified by radiographic examination are restricted in some ranges of vertebral motion. Many vertebral sections that appear normal on radiographs exhibit severe restriction in motion characteristics.

Understanding Adjusting Speed

Chiropractic adjustments are characterized by manual thrusts delivered at high velocity. Understanding the theory behind high-velocity adjustments requires knowing the basic law of physics that governs quantity of force. Force is created by the interplay of mass and acceleration; that is,

$$F = M \times A$$

The chiropractor wishes to increase acceleration during the physical act of the adjustment. This effectively increases the resultant force. The chiropractor can also increase the resultant force to increase the mass during an adjustment. However, increasing the mass may endanger soft tissues surrounding the motor unit. This technique can be compared to driving a nail into a board: A sledge hammer can be used to increase mass, producing the force necessary to drive the nail. However, the sledge hammer may be inappropriately heavy for the type of wood. The same result can be achieved with a lighter-weight hammer head. A carpenter develops the skill to deliver a biomechanically effective force by increasing acceleration with a smaller hammer.

The chiropractor generates higher forces with acceleration, facilitating effective adjustment of large quadrupeds such as the horse. In large animals, sufficient force must be created to move only one vertebral segment along its articular lines. The size of the entire organism is irrelevant to the effective adjustment of one vertebra in one motor unit. The nature of jointed motor units underscores their primary function of movement. This movement is specific along plane lines created by the orientation of facet surfaces and the intrinsic properties of the ligaments. The speed and timing of the adjustment overcome the relative stability of the motor unit against shear forces.

Understanding Short-Lever Techniques

The chiropractor adjusts forces as closely as possible to the joint or joints that display biomechanic aberrations. For example, in the lumbar region a rotational misalignment may be characterized by right zygapophyseal joint fixation. The appropriate choice of vertebral contact points for the adjustment would be the right mammillary pro-

cess. The right mammillary process is just lateral to and slightly superior to the vertebral joint in question. Because the center of rotation of vertebral segments lies within the nucleus pulposus, the resultant lever arm is relatively short between the mammillary process and the nucleus. The combination of high velocity and short lever creates an effective and specific adjustment.

Some long-lever techniques may be used on an extremity, such as the foot, and delivered in a way that generates sufficient leverage to act at the vertebral level. Although sometimes effective, these long-lever techniques require increased application of force at the end of the lever arm. Because the lever arm in question is a leg with multiple joints, the potential exists to damage intermediate extremity joints. For example, pulling the foot of a horse far and high enough forward to affect the sacroiliac joint places the hock and stifle at risk.

Joint Biomechanics

At the end of the passive range of motion is an elastic barrier that consists of the ligamentous structures of the joint. Chiropractors describe the relatively small portion of joint motion beyond the elastic barrier as the *paraphysiologic space*. A chiropractic adjustment is designed to force the joint slightly beyond the elastic barrier and into the paraphysiologic space. Because this paraphysiologic space is relatively small, the depth of adjusting force must be skillfully controlled. At the limit of the paraphysiologic space is the anatomic barrier. This barrier marks the end of the greatest possible range of joint movement (Haldeman, 1992). Movement generated beyond this barrier alters the ligamentous and osseous integrity and may cause a vertebral pathologic condition. An adjustment is applied to restore active and passive ranges of motion by rapidly forcing the joint though the fixed regions of joint motion and temporarily into the paraphysiologic space.

Joint Audibles

Audibles, or joint noises, may be produced during an adjustment. These articular noises are created when an adjustment causes a sudden drop in intraarticular pressure (Haldeman, 1992). The audible alone does not indicate therapeutic success of the adjustment. Therapeutic success is achieved when the affected joint is restored to biomechanic and neurologic function. Often audibles occur immediately after the adjustment, as the animal voluntarily moves spinal regions by stretching or shaking. These voluntary movements may be considered a homeostatic mechanism; the animal instinctively attempts to activate specific muscle groups and move a previously dysfunctional joint. The process of restoring the joint to biomechanic function is initiated by the adjustment and completed by the animal's movements.

Line of Correction

Vertebral motor units have limited ranges of motion that are determined by the facet orientations of the multiple joints involved and the intrinsic stability of the ligamentous structures. For example, the anatomic characteristics of the atlantooccipital joint effectively restrict axial rotation of this motor unit. The atlas and occiput therefore tend to subluxate in lateral flexion malpositions. If the goal of the adjustment is to restore biomechanic function, the movement characteristics of each motor unit must be understood. The adjustment is applied to vertebral segments along articular plane lines. Simply put, the way a motor unit moves out of alignment is the opposite of the way it should be moved to return to its proper position. Because each motor unit presents variations in articular planes and muscular and ligamentous stability, a precise anatomic understanding of each vertebral articulation is necessary. Inappropriate or inaccurate adjustments can cause joint and soft-tissue damage, ranging from pain to ligamentous tears.

Chiropractic Technique

Individual motor units can be adjusted in several ways. Different osseous contacts, such as transverse processes or spinous processes, may be used. Adjustment may be made directly, using the physical skills of the chiropractor, or indirectly, using a small impacting device called an *activator*. Adjustments may vary in the amount of force applied or type of stabilization given to the vertebral segments during the adjustments. An adjustment is generally designed to affect one motor unit at a time, and stabilization is used to prevent the force of the adjustment from affecting other vertebral areas. Stabilization during the adjustment may be brought about by patient position, the adjuster, or an assistant.

The timing of the adjustive thrust also depends on voluntary muscle relaxation around the motor unit. Muscle relaxation in animals is achieved by skillful handling that results in a relaxed and cooperative patient. Anesthetics are contraindicated during adjustments because normal proprioceptive mechanisms are not active and damage may occur in motor units that are chemically relaxed. Anesthetics are also impractical for repeat adjustments.

In an adjustment, after the animal's voluntary muscles relax, the joint is brought to tension by removing joint play or passive range of motion. At the elastic barrier a specific adjusting force is applied in a specific direction determined by articular characteristics. The thrust moves the joint temporarily into the paraphysiologic space, restoring lost active and passive ranges of motion. The motor unit maintains its proper alignment and biomechanic function as the neurologic and biomechanic dysfunction is repaired.

Example of Equine Technique: Rationale and Procedure

A horse has slight muscle atrophy of the left hamstrings, and the tuber sacrale is visibly lower on the left side. During gait analysis the horse exhibits a shortened stride length in the right rear and pulls the left rear medially inside the normal line of progression of footfall. The action of the pelvic region during gait analysis shows a high right hip that does not exhibit normal rise and fall, and the left hip is dropped continuously during movement. Static palpation reveals a trigger point in the right gluteus medius muscle and muscle tenderness in the right hamstring muscles. The right tuber sacrale palpates higher than does the left, and the horse flinches when direct dorsal-ventral pressure is applied to the right tuber sacrale. The sacrum palpates normally. Motion palpation of the right sacroiliac joint reveals fixation.

Sacroiliac joint misalignments may be the result of either sacral or pelvic misalignments. In this case, the right tuber sacrale appears higher and palpates higher. A common subluxation of the ilium is characterized by dorsal, caudal, and medial movement of the ilium along the orientation of the surfaces of the sacroiliac joint. This dorsal misalignment is responsible for the static palpation findings and the observable height differences in the bilateral tuber sacrales. Because the sacrum is in normal position, this subluxation primarily involves the ilium. A critical differential diagnosis is a possible pathologic condition (e.g., a fracture of the left ilial wing) that can also create a low left tuber sacrale.

When the sacroiliac joint is misaligned, fiber endings are stimulated, creating joint pain that can be assessed with manual pressure. Motion palpation reveals that the right sacroiliac joint is not moving properly. Lack of proper movement causes shortened stride of the right rear leg. Because of the movement dynamics of the right rear leg, the left leg compensates by moving more medially under the body. The abnormal concussive forces of these strides can potentially cause problems in the left hock. The shortened right stride may also jeopardize the function of the right stifle, eventually leading to secondary joint involvement. Primary lesions in the hock or stifle may cause compensatory problems at the sacroiliac joint. This possibility emphasizes the importance of looking at the entire horse with regard to biomechanic function.

Restrictions in right sacroiliac movement cause the right hip to be carried high and exhibit little motion. The left hip rises and falls with movement, whereas the right stays high and fixed. Changes in gait have increased the muscular stress on the right gluteals and right hamstrings, with secondary atrophy in the opposite leg. The horse's right leg works harder but more ineffectively.

Further predictions can be made based on movement characteristics. Involvement of the pelvic region tends to prevent the horse from using the hindquarters in impulsion. The horse tends to be heavy in the forehand and often has a pathologic condition in the left forelimb, the leg diagonal to the involved right rear. The horse may also experience difficulty with the right lead in the canter because of problems in the right rear. The lack of normal rolling movement of the pelvis tends to cause the saddle and the rider to shift toward the left side of the horse, further aggravating the condition.

Although this discussion is limited to the right sacroiliac joint, other spinal regions can be involved. The lumbar vertebrae rotate in response to abnormal pelvic alignment and resultant gait changes. When the pelvic region is not working correctly, the upper thoracic regions become fixed as a consequence of an abnormal cranial shift of the center of gravity.

Knowledge of the relevant anatomy is required for adjustment of the right sacroiliac joint. The sacroiliac joint in the horse is a synarthrodial joint with flat plane surfaces that exhibit relatively little range of motion. Many veterinarians mistakenly believe that the sacroiliac joint is immovable. The anatomic classification of this structure as a joint prescribes its function as movement. Although movement is limited, sacroiliac function is essential for transmission of forces from the hindquarters forward along the spine. The facet orientation is approximately 65 degrees from the vertical axis. The sacrum is a ventral wedge beneath the two ilial wings. The adjustment must account for the joint angle and relative joint stability. To create an effective adjustive force, the chiropractor must generate a rapid and concentrated force from muscular contractions of the pectoral and triceps muscles. The chiropractor must be in an elevated position to approach the joint from the dorsal aspect. Because the ilium has moved medially in relation to the sacrum, the chiropracter must work from the medial to the lateral aspect of the joint. In this case, a common technique is to stand on an elevated surface to the left side of the horse. The base of one hand should contact the right tuber sacrale while the other hand supports and stabilizes the contact hand. The contact point of the tuber sacrale provides a convenient position to create a short lever from contact point to joint surface. The vector of the adjustive force is determined by the position of the adjuster on the elevated left side of the horse and the placement of the adjuster's hands, elbows, shoulders, and sternum in alignment with the plane line of the joint. This is accomplished by alignment of the hands and body of the adjuster through the right tuber sacrale, toward the right tuber coxae. Pressure on the sacroiliac joint is used and maintained to remove the available joint play with the hands. A chiropractic thrust is then performed.

Therapeutic Considerations

The veterinary chiropractor faces a formidable dilemma when discussing chiropractic therapy in relation to traditional diagnoses. Chiropractors generally identify and eliminate vertebral subluxations. Therefore the diagnosis made by a chiropractor during therapy is always "vertebral subluxation complex," regardless of the traditional diagnosis. The chiropractor is merely being loyal to the theorized etiologic cause of the neurologic or biomechanic pathology. A dog presented for examination and treatment may be accompanied by a veterinary diagnosis of hip dysplasia, spondylosis, or incontinence. The immediate goal of the chiropractic examination, however, is to identify relevant vertebral subluxations. Despite their apparent disparity, both diagnoses may be based on neurologic manifestations of the same lumbosacral motor unit. The neuropathy manifested by a subluxation varies depending on whether the motor nerve or autonomic nerve portion of the nervous system is affected. Neurologic dysfunction in motor nerves caused by vertebral subluxations may be the factor behind muscle laxity that leads to hip dysplasia. Subluxations may be a critical factor in the instability of motor units and subsequent degenerative joint disease of spondylosis. Subluxations also may result in autonomic nervous system abnormalities that result in problems in the urinary sphincter and bladder. The traditional diagnosis is of secondary importance to the chiropractor and may even be irrelevant.

Some diagnoses of traditional medicine, such as a fractured femur, are obvious and indisputable. Patient history, palpation, and radiographs prove the fracture diagnosis. The therapeutic dilemma arises when a traditional diagnosis is nonspecific, such as hip dysplasia, spondylopathy, and idiopathic epilepsy. In these cases the diagnosis often describes a group of symptoms and does not identify the etiology of the problem. Surrounding these diagnoses are popular and ever-changing theories about the cause of the pathologic condition and its proper treatment. Often the designation of a diagnosis limits the practitioner's ability to determine the etiology, especially if the practitioner focuses only on the symptoms and not on the integrated functional whole. If a dog is diagnosed with hip dysplasia, current veterinary thought assumes a congenital etiology. Considerable effort is made to identify dysplastic dogs in breeding programs, and most medical and surgical procedures are instituted as salvage procedures. Other practitioners, however, consider environmental factors more important than congenital factors in the development of joint laxity. Environmental factors include nutrition, exercise, and joint stresses, including trauma. The chiropractic theories of neurologic dysfunction may offer an alternative etiology for hip dysplasia and other pathologic conditions.

Chiropractors often provide therapeutic regimens for animals diagnosed with so-called incurable or other orthopedic conditions. The chiropractic rationale for these types of therapy is often misunderstood. A dog with a ruptured cruciate ligament may still benefit from chiropractic adjustments after the joint is surgically stabilized. An adjustment may be indicated even if the owner refuses surgical intervention. Limping or carrying the leg in non–weight-bearing position can create secondary compensations at vertebral levels. The chiropractor treating such a patient is attempting to repair the compensatory effects on the vertebral column, not treat the ruptured cruciate ligament. Chiropractic care does not replace the need for proper joint evaluation and surgical intervention in the affected joint. Instead, adjustments are used to correct biomechanic problems related to the primary problem.

Another reason that chiropractic theories are not widely accepted lies in the basic philosophic differences between conventional medicine and chiropractic. Conventional veterinary medicine is often allopathic: a veterinarian treats a vomiting patient with medication to counteract the vomiting, often without considering the organism's ability to heal itself. Chiropractic philosophy is rooted in the concept of homeostasis. In other words, if the organism is operating properly on a neurologic level, it can respond successfully to many external or internal assaults. The practitioner trained according to the tenets of conventional medicine must make a dramatic shift in philosophy to practice chiropractic successfully. An experienced veterinary practitioner who is new to chiropractic may find it difficult to perform a spinal adjustment without considering the use of medications.

In animal health care, all therapies—whether traditional or complementary, medical or chiropractic, surgery or acupuncture—have an appropriate place. The practitioner must recognize the need for a particular therapy and either provide that option or refer the patient to a specialist.

Integration of Chiropractic into Conventional Practice

The integration of veterinary chiropractic into conventional practice requires the veterinary practitioner to make a paradigm shift. The ability to consider the entire patient—that is, the genetic blueprint, the anatomic and physiologic interplay, and the homeostatic mechanisms that are exposed to changing internal and external environments—is important to all holistic modalities. For example, in a holistic practice, prescribing synthetic thyroid hormone to compensate for a low level of thyroid hormone in the blood is not therapeutically responsible without considering the following:

- The time of day, the time of the year, and the environmental conditions when the blood was drawn for the test; these variables can affect metabolic rate and thyroid production
- The integral role of other endocrine glands, such as the pituitary and the adrenals, in hormonal feedback mechanisms
- Factors that influence the hormone system, such as environmental stress
- The health of organs such as the liver that manufacture precursors for thyroxin
- The nutritional availability of the amino acids, minerals, and vitamins involved in production of the precursors and activated forms of thyroxin
- The ability of the animal to use the necessary nutrients in its internal environment

- The presence in the animal's environment of nutritional ingredients (intended or unintended) or toxins that interfere in delivery, absorption, and use of critical nutrients
- Relationships between the neurologic and endocrine system

The treatment protocol for such a patient should include consideration of the consequences of changing the animal's internal environment with a product that directly affects the homeostasis of the hormone system. The introduction of a chemical that produces negative feedback mechanisms may complicate the animal's ability to produce its own thyroxin.

The holistic practitioner must assess traditional therapeutic regimens and diagnoses from a different perspective. Veterinary practitioners cannot easily abandon traditional ideas of cause and effect. The integration of chiropractic requires new ways of thinking about the etiology of disease, the application of therapy, the nature of the nervous system, and the health of the organism.

The practitioner must understand the basic philosophy of a holistic modality. In chiropractic, the integral relationship of the nervous system and the vertebral column must be thoroughly understood and appreciated. Without this knowledge the practitioner will have difficulty understanding the indications and use of chiropractic in animal practice. For example, the preventive role of chiropractic requires that every physical examination, from pediatric to geriatric, include a chiropractic examination.

Role of Chiropractic in Animal Health Care

For the veterinarian who understands the elements of holistic practice and the philosophy of chiropractic, every patient becomes a possible chiropractic patient. Every examination should include a spinal examination, and every treatment protocol should include an adjustment if necessary.

Chiropractic care is ideal for the athletic animal. Athletic performance requires that the organism perform at peak efficiency, free from stiffness and pain. Medical therapies may reduce pain or muscle spasms without addressing their causes. The entire vertebral column is integral in movement. The major locomotion muscles are attached to this highly jointed structure. For example, lack of proper joint function in the lumbar spine limits power from the rear limbs and restricts flexibility. If a human athlete has a stiff and painful lower back, the resulting loss of freedom of movement affects performance ability. Likewise, stiffness and pain in the horse's back impair athletic performance, such as jumping.

Chiropractic is not restricted to the athletic animal. The dog who is severely traumatized when hit by an automobile may require surgical intervention for a fracture and laceration. However, this trauma may also have resulted in spinal problems. Exacerbating these problems are environmental factors: Humans sit on the backs of horses and pull on the necks of dogs, making these areas of the spine vulnerable.

Chiropractic care can be integrated into a conventional practice in several different ways, such as preventive health care, prepurchase examinations of horses, and treatment of animals with back and neck pain or intervertebral disk disease. Many degenerative diseases such as spondylosis may respond to chiropractic adjustments, increasing the quality of life for that animal. The definitive role of chiropractic has not been fully explored in veterinary practice.

Future of Veterinary Chiropractic

The future of chiropractic in animal health care is limited by the lack of serious research and resistance from mainstream professionals. Chiropractic is a diversified and complex field for the human patient, one that offers a great number of benefits that could be explored and extrapolated into animal practice. In the lay literature, information on animal chiropractic has grown rapidly. Clients' acceptance of animal chiropractic, requests for chiropractic services, and understanding of potential benefits to animals are growing.

The veterinary practitioner can choose to see chiropractic as a personally and professionally rewarding service to offer clients. Chiropractic care can become a veterinary practice specialty, just as in orthopedics or neurology. Specialty practices allow a practitioner to concentrate efforts, develop expertise, and accept referrals from other practitioners. As veterinary medicine moves into the twenty-first century, specialty practices will increase and information about health and disease will expand.

Training in Animal Chiropractic

The American Veterinary Chiropractic Association (AVCA) offers the only postgraduate course in veterinary chiropractic.*

The course consists of 150 hours divided into five modules, four of which teach the regional chiropractic techniques of sacropelvic, thoracolumbar, cervical, and extremity adjusting. The fifth integrated module synthesizes the regional work into a global look at veterinary chiropractic therapy and chiropractic case management.

References

Fountain head news, 1923, Davenport, Iowa, Palmer School of Chiropractic.

Haldeman S: *Principles and practice of chiropractic,* Norwalk, Conn, 1992, Appleton and Lange.

Homewood AE: *The neurodynamics of the vertebral subluxation,* 1962, Parker Research Foundation.

Kapandji IA: *The physiology of the joints,* New York, 1974, Churchill Livingstone.

Leach RA: *The chiropractic theories,* Baltimore, 1986, Williams & Wilkins.

McClure R: *American horse, cattle and sheep doctor,* Chicago, 1901, Frederick J. Drake.

Palmer BJ: *It is as simple as that,* Davenport, Iowa, 1944, Palmer College of Chiropractic.

Selye H: *Stress and disease,* New York, 1956, McGraw-Hill.

Stasek TS: *Adams' lameness in horses,* Philadelphia, 1987, Lea & Febiger.

Wardwell W: *Chiropractic: history and evolution of a new profession,* St Louis, 1992, Mosby.

White A, Panjabi M: *Clinical biomechanics of the spine,* Philadelphia, 1990, JB Lippincott.

---

*American Veterinary Chiropractic Association, P.O. Box 249, Port Byron, IL 61275; 309-523-3995, Fax: 309-523-2926.

Chapter 13

*P*hysical Therapy

MIMI PORTER

Physical therapy involves the use of certain physical measures in the treatment and evaluation of disease. The diagnostic applications are limited, but the therapeutic scope is broad. As it is applied to animals, physical therapy follows a veterinary diagnosis and relies on veterinary diagnostics to establish the treatment plan. The appropriate tools and techniques of the physical therapist are selected once the location, type, and extent of the injury are determined. Those tools and techniques include the use of natural, physical modalities such as electricity, light, sound, magnetics, heat, cold, manual techniques, and movement. These modalities affect the blood and lymphatic circulatory system, the muscular system, the nerve network, and the intercell and intracell messenger systems. Injury or disease causes an imbalance in one or more of these systems. The goal of physical therapy is to correct the imbalance as quickly as possible. This approach is especially valuable in sports medicine, where time lost from activity results in impaired performance. An animal is particularly vulnerable to loss of performance ability during recuperation because it cannot exercise isolated body parts while resting the injured area.

Physical therapists look at injury as a process, not an event. Physical therapists are taught to examine muscles for spasms and imbalances in tension, flexibility, and strength. These imbalances in muscle function often lead to acute injury, and they persist in chronic injury.

Goals of Physical Therapy

Whether applied to animals or humans, physical therapy has several fundamental goals. A primary goal is the relief of pain. Several of the tools of the physical therapist are effective in pain relief, without producing negative side effects or completely blocking sensation. Movement is made easier and more comfortable, but the body's natural protective capacity is still intact.

Another goal of physical therapy is to return full range of movement and strength to the injured part. In other words, the injured part should regain full functioning. This point is important because physical therapy is often considered only the application of certain tools to effect a physical change. Exercise, in the form of manual manipulations or controlled activities, is an essential part of successful physical therapy. A specific modality is applied to make the exercise activity more comfortable. For example, electrical stimulation can be applied to spasmodic muscles, reducing the spasmodic tone and allowing for more normal extension and flexion during exercise. Treating soft-tissue contractures or dense connective tissue with ultrasound softens the bonding and allows tissue elongation through stretching exercises. Laser therapy effectively suppresses pain when applied to acupuncture points and prevents muscle imbalances during exercise. Exercise, or controlled movement, is an essential ingredient in most physical therapy sessions.

This chapter discusses the use of some modalities used by the physical therapist and includes protocols developed through personal experience and based on scientific studies. The tools and techniques of physical therapy described in this chapter are electrical stimulation, iontophoresis, ultrasound, heat, cold, and stretching. The physical therapist also uses low-level laser therapy, magnetic fields, and massage. These modalities are discussed in detail elsewhere in this book and are only briefly mentioned here. This chapter is only an overview of the emerging profession of animal physical therapy. *Equine Sports Therapy* (Porter, 1990) contains a more complete discussion of the role of the therapist and in-depth descriptions of the use of the specific modalities and their application to horses.

History of Veterinary Physical Therapy

The written history of the use of physical therapy for animals is relatively recent, although the practice of these techniques is undoubtedly quite old. In 1973, Charles Strong published a book describing the use of electrical stimulation on horses (Strong, 1973). In this book, Strong argues that the treatment *least* likely to bring relief is over-rest; in fact, he advocates rest only throughout the range of movement that is painful. A few years later, Ann Downer, a professor in the school of physical therapy at Ohio State University, published a book describing techniques for selected physical therapy treatments on animals (1978). For many years the idea of physical therapy for animals was dormant. Recently, however, the number of scientific articles on the subject has grown significantly.

A practical foundation for veterinary physical therapy is only now being established in the United States. In 1993 the American Association of Equine Practitioners (AAEP) set guidelines for the practice of physical therapy on horses. The American Veterinary Medical Association (AVMA) has described the modality in more general terms. According to the AAEP, a physical therapist uses noninvasive techniques for the rehabilitation of injuries. *Physical therapy* is defined as including the use of laser, electrical stimulation, magnetic therapy, therapeutic ultrasound, rehabilitative exercise, hydrotherapy, heat and cold, massage, and stretching. The work must be performed under the supervision of a veterinarian following a veterinary diagnosis and in accordance with state practice acts. A need exists for college-level curricula to train people as animal therapists. Such curricula are in the developmental stages now. More training opportunities and research in this area will establish veterinary physical therapy as a legitimate profession.

Theory and Application of Physical Therapy

Electrical Stimulation

The therapeutic use of electrical currents dates back to the ancient Greek and Roman eras. The earliest documented study on electrical stimulation treatments documented the use of the electric ray fish in the treatment for gout (A New Approach to Pain, 1974). The modality has evolved considerably since then. The output from today's electrical units is smooth, comfortable, and suitable for use on animals, unlike past devices that caused shocking or burning sensations.

The therapeutic electric stimulator emits a type of energy with wavelengths and frequencies that can be classified as electromagnetic radiation. The electromagnetic spectrum contains wavelength and frequency outputs of other therapeutic tools, such as magnets and therapeutic lasers. *Wavelength* is defined as the distance between the peak of one wave and the peak of the next wave. *Frequency*

is defined as the number of wave oscillations occurring in 1 second and is expressed in hertz (Hz) units or in pulses per second. The wavelength and frequency of the output determine the biologic effect of electrical stimulation. Wavelength and frequency are adjustable in some units and set by the manufacturer in others. Electrical stimulating currents that affect nerve and muscle tissue have the longest wavelengths and the lowest frequencies of any of the modalities (Fig. 13-1).

Therapeutic electrical stimulators use electrical current to stimulate sensory and motor nerves. They are generally classified as either high-voltage or low-voltage stimulators. High-voltage devices produce wave forms with an amplitude of 150 volts or greater and a relatively short pulse duration of less than 100 ms. This extremely short pulse duration and relatively long interpulse interval make the therapeutic electrical stimulator comfortable. The high peak current allows deep penetration through the tissues, evoking responses in deeper tissue. High-voltage devices produced in the United States are generally direct current devices, but alternating current devices are also available.

Low-voltage devices produce less than 150 volts at very rapid frequencies, often several thousand pulses per second (Prentice, 1986). Low-voltage devices do not have the wide range of application common among the high-voltage units or the ability to penetrate to deep tissue. The primary function of low-voltage devices is to provide sensory stimulation for pain relief. The low-voltage devices are often referred to as *transcutaneous electrical nerve stimulator (TENS) units,* although this term applies to both high- and low-voltage devices because they both conduct their

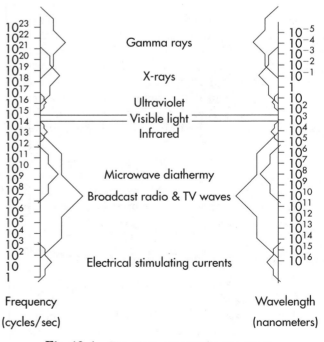

Fig. 13-1 The electromagnetic spectrum.

stimulation through the skin to the sensory and motor nerves.

Electrical stimulators on the market today go by several different names and are categorized according to their intended effects. Besides TENS and high-voltage stimulators, there are MENS (microvoltage currents), EMS (muscle stimulating currents), and interferential currents, which use two different current frequencies that cross in the tissues. Before an electrical stimulating device is chosen, the therapist must have a clear goal for treatment.

Perhaps the most versatile of the therapist's modalities, the therapeutic electrical stimulator is capable of providing pain relief, stimulating absorption in edema, promoting wound healing, and producing muscle contraction for the retardation of atrophy and the reduction of spasm. Many types of portable units are available for use on animals (Fig. 13-2).

Electrical stimulation for pain relief

Electrical stimulators are effective in the relief of pain, whether acute or chronic. For pain suppression, sensory nerves are stimulated, resulting in endogenous opiate discharge and inhibition of nociception. Two approaches to pain relief using electrical stimulation have been outlined. To stimulate the release of endogenous polypeptides such as beta-endorphins, enkephalins, dopamines, and dynorphins, the appropriate acupuncture points are stimulated using a low-frequency current of 2 to 10 pulses per second (Chapman, Bendetti, 1977; Cheng, Pomeranz, 1979). Another approach is to modulate the pain threshold by stimulating the A-delta and C fibers with high-frequency current of 80 to 100 pulses per second. This high level of activity in these peripheral fibers overrides pain transmission in the spinal cord (Klein, Pariser, 1987). The electrodes can be placed on the painful site and specific dermatomes or myotomes corresponding to the painful area. The electrodes can also be placed on the spinal cord segment that innervates the area. For a review of studies on the efficacy of electrical stimulation for afferent fiber activation and a blockade of peripheral nociceptors, see Abram's review (Abram, 1993).

Electrical stimulation for disuse atrophy

Disuse atrophy can be treated with electrical stimulation through protocols designed to stimulate muscle contraction. Electrical stimulation for muscle contraction requires the stimulation of the motor nerve at a motor point. A motor point is a site at which the motor nerve enters the muscle. From the skin surface, motor points are located where the greatest muscle contraction can be elicited with the least amount of current. These sites can be used to create rhythmical muscular contractions for spasm relief or improvement of muscle strength. Electrically induced muscle contractions differ from voluntary contractions in that each time the electrical stimulus is applied, the same motor units respond with the same amount of force. Voluntary muscle contraction activates some motor units while others remain inactive. Because some units are resting while others are firing, voluntary contractions do not lead to muscular fatigue as early in the exercise activity as electrically stimulated contractions (Benton and others, 1980). This effect is useful in stimulating the muscles to prevent atrophy when voluntary movement is limited by pain or immobilization casting.

Stimulators with a wide pulse width (long pulse duration) are used to improve muscle strength. When nerves in the muscle have been damaged or when surgery results in muscle inhibition, motor point stimulation is an effective means of returning the muscle to functionality. Some investigators have evaluated the ability of specific wave forms and frequencies of electrical current to increase muscle strength (Eriksson and others, 1981; Currier, Mann, 1983). One theory suggests that the effectiveness of electrical stimulation to improve strength might be caused by the increased recruitment of motor neurons that previously were not activated because of inhibition. Where pain is present, electrical stimulation can be used to simulate voluntary contraction and thereby maintain more normal levels of oxidative enzymes and blood flow (Eriksson, Haggmark, 1979). The pain relief obtained would aid in more normal movement, further improving muscle strength.

Electrical stimulation effects on blood and lymph circulation

Vascular problems that can be treated with electrical stimulation include arterial disorders such as arteriosclerosis and thrombosis, venous disorders such as chronic venous insufficiency and thrombophlebitis, and microcirculatory disorders such as edema. Many studies have demonstrated an increase in blood flow following electrical stimulation. Currier and others (1986) quantified a 20% increase in muscle blood flow one minute after electrical stimulation began, an increase that continued after stimulation ended. In the 1960s, Doran, Drury, Sivyer

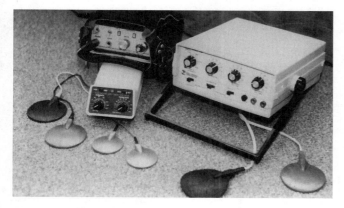

Fig. 13-2 Several different portable electrical stimulation devices.

(1964) conducted studies of venous return and the incidence of postoperative thrombi using radioactive tracers. They found that venous return was decreased significantly when muscle relaxants were used and that venous stasis could be effectively remedied with electrical stimulation.

An unpublished study using horses as subjects examined the effects of blood flow through the common digital artery, a large artery that supplies most of the equine digit with blood (Porter, 1983). A low pulse rate of 16 Hz was used at an intensity just below perception, and blood flow was measured over 25 minutes. During this time the treated limbs showed a twofold increase of blood flow compared with the nontreated limbs. This finding suggests that electrical stimulation of the horse's lower leg over major vessels could improve perfusion of the foot. The results of this experiment support a published report on eight cases of laminitis that were treated with only electrical stimulation. No adjunctive medication or other form of therapy was used. In this study, electrical stimulation was started within 2 hours of the onset of symptoms and applied twice daily for 2-hour sessions. A decrease in the clinical signs of laminitis and rapid return to normal gait was observed (Vasko, Spauchus, Lowry, 1986). Low-voltage TENS devices were used in this study. The use of a high-voltage device would have reduced treatment time, because less time is needed to accumulate sufficient charge in the tissues and effect vascular changes.

Electrical stimulation can be of great benefit to laminitic horses because it reduces pain and increases blood flow to the foot. As laminitis occurs, endotoxins cause arteriospasm and a disruption in the blood flow through the hoof, resulting in extreme pain and eventual death to the oxygen-deprived tissue. Hood and others (1978) reported a decrease in perfusion of the capillaries of the foot resulting from significant arteriovenous shunting during the onset of laminitis. Electrical stimulation has been shown to increase microcirculation, indicating a bypass of the A-V shunt. This effect, along with pain-relieving qualities, makes electrical stimulation a valuable therapeutic tool against laminitis. Electrical stimulation effectively shortens the acute inflammatory process and reduces lameness, hoof temperature, and associated muscle spasm in the upper body. It is far more comfortable and efficient than the traditional use of hot- and cold-water soaks. Combined with appropriate medications, stable management, and hoof care, electrical stimulation is a valuable part of the care of laminitic horses.

Because of its effects on the lymph and vascular systems, electrotherapy is effective in edema reduction. Low-frequency stimulation of 2 to 10 pulses per second produces a marked increase in microcirculation. Increased capillary density in muscle has also been noted after as little as 28 days of intermittent stimulation (Myrhage, Hudlica, 1978).

When electrical stimulation is used to treat edema, dramatic results can be seen. Electrical stimulation is used immediately after the initial period of intertissue bleeding has been suppressed with ice and compression. The suggested protocol includes the use of a stimulator that provides direct current. Using the negative polarity, the practitioner places the active electrode over the site of edema or just distal to it. The practitioner then places the dispersive electrode proximally. The path of the current should flow through the area of edema. Low frequencies (approximately 10 pulses per second) are recommended. The intensity is maintained at a low level to relax the animal. The treatment for edema should begin as soon after veterinary examination as possible. The addition of compression bandaging and cold applications enhances electrical therapy for swelling. Mendel, Wylegala, and Fish (1992) found edema volume in electrically stimulated limbs to be significantly less than in untreated limbs following impact injury. Ice, compression, and electrical stimulation should be used immediately after injury to inhibit edema formation. Too often, prevention is overlooked in injury care for animals. Allowing metabolites to accumulate in the tissues only delays the healing process. The suggested technique for reducing these "waste products of injury" is simple and effective.

Electrical stimulation and wound repair

OPEN WOUNDS   Both open and closed wounds are effectively treated with electrical stimulation. Healing of open, or skin surface, wounds is stimulated by placing the anode, or the positive pole, at the wound site to trigger or enhance the development of a positive electrical potential in the injured area. Without this positive electrical potential the early stages of wound repair do not progress. Dermal cell movement was examined following electrical stimulation and found to be enhanced with anodal current (Harrington, Meyer, Klein, 1974). In a review of recent research, investigators found that therapeutic electrical stimulation débrides necrotic tissue, attracts neutrophils and macrophages, decreases edema, stimulates receptor sites for growth factors, stimulates growth of fibroblasts and granulation tissue, and prevents post–oxygen-radical-mediated damage (Gentzkow, 1993). The therapist can make use of electrically stimulated muscle contractions to débride a deep wound. The electrodes are placed on muscles around the wound, and contractions are elicited to pump out debris. This approach is much less traumatic than scrubbing a wound and removes waste products of injury from deeper within the wound.

Decubitus ulcers, wounds resulting from the pressure of prolonged recumbency, respond well to electrotherapy. Ischemic ulcers, or pressure sores, result when tissue is deprived of oxygen to the point that the blood vessels collapse and dermal cells die from oxygen depletion. Passing electric current through the wound aids in fluid removal and increases tissue oxygenation so white blood cells can attack bacteria. Tissue nutrition increases, and the healing process is stimulated, even though the animal is still recumbent much of the time. Electrical stimulation can be used preventatively by increasing the blood flow through tissues that are in danger of breaking down from constant pressure.

CLOSED WOUNDS   Closed wounds, such as those produced by tendinitis, respond to electrical stimulation. Shortening the recovery time from a tendon injury is important for both humans and animals. However, regaining strength and functionality of the damaged tendon is more essential. Investigation of this matter began in 1982, with a series of "load to breaking" studies applying electrical stimulation to damaged tendons. A significant difference was seen in the breaking strength of treated tendons (Owoeye, 1982; Stanish and others, 1985). Certainly the addition of electrical stimulation can benefit an animal confined to stall or cage rest, which only erodes tendon tensile strength.

A treatment protocol for equine digital flexor tendons includes placing electrodes in the zone of acupuncture points HT-7 and HT-8 to stimulate acupuncture effects and vasodilate the digital vessels. The zone of LI-3, LI-4, and LI-5 is also used to disperse congestion. Applying electrical stimulation to the motor point of the associated muscle augments this treatment by adding pumping muscle contractions to further increase blood flow. Adhesion formation is minimized with early removal of injury metabolites. Early pain and edema reduction allows earlier movement. Increased mobility and reduced edema benefit the intrinsic healing of the tendon. Research indicates that tendon fibers align along lines of electrical force, whether it is the tendon's own *piezo* electric force or externally applied currents (Enwemeka, Spielholz, 1992). Passing electrical current through the tendon longitudinally may aid in parallel fiber alignment.

Because atrophy of collagen fibrils can occur after only 2 weeks of inactivity, electrical stimulation should begin as early as possible after initial first aid. Atrophy is followed by loss of fibril orientation, allowing the development of less functional scar tissue. Fibroblasts are sensitive to low-intensity, low-frequency current and respond as if the tendon is being used. Fibroblast proliferation is enhanced, as is collagen synthesis. The electric current mimics the stress of activity and promotes strengthening.

Injuries to the flexor tendons of the horse's leg caused by load stress range from strain to rupture. A tendon strain involves elongation of the collagen fibers to the point of microfailure. Although disruption of connective cells and fibers occurs, the tendon appears intact on the surface. A rupture results when the load causes tendon fibers to break, resulting in inflammation, edema, and pain. Preventive procedures include reducing the stress before partial rupture begins, providing sufficient rest so that the tendon fibers return to their original length, and conditioning the tendon by slowly progressing stress overload

and stretch. Some evidence suggests that tendinitis has, at least in part, a vascular etiology. Maintaining the intra-tendinous blood supply becomes important with impending injury because tendon fiber fatigue can be repaired in the early stages if the nutritional supply is adequate.

Electrical stimulation has not gained the recognition it deserves in animal physical therapy, perhaps because the variety of treatment options is daunting to the untrained user. When the proper mode of treatment is used, this modality is effective for a wide variety of injury problems.

Iontophoresis

All matter is composed of atoms that contain positively and negatively charged particles called *ions*. These charged particles possess electrical energy and can move about, propelled by an electrical force (Prentice, 1986). Iontophoresis, sometimes called *ion transfer*, uses electrical current to move ions across biologic membranes. When an electrical charge is applied to an ionized drug, a steady drift of positively charged ions moves away from the positive pole and negatively charged ions move away from the negative pole. A mild direct current of 4 milliamps transports the positive or negative ions away from the drug solution into the tissues. Drugs introduced via iontophoresis have been found in deeper tissues because the drug enters tissue fluids and is disseminated. Conditions that can be treated by this method are tendinitis, epicondylitis, bursitis, acute arthritic flare-ups, and musculoskeletal inflammatory conditions (Kahn, 1987).

Advantages of iontophoresis over conventional injection are that the former is painless and sterile. No tissue damage results from the injection of a bolus of fluid or the needle itself. No fluid enters the skin, only the ionized particle of the drug. This method is an improvement over the injection of needles into tendons: Corticosteroid injection has been shown to produce focal areas of necrotizing inflammation, and calcification often develops at the injection site (Pool, 1980). The quantity of corticosteroid delivered by iontophoresis is much less than that normally given by injection. The iontophoresis method delivers 28 µg of medication per gram of tissue, or 100 times less than an injection. It is a safe and painless alternative mode of delivering medications into tissues and may prevent some of the problems associated with injection (Fig. 13-3).

Ultrasound

Ultrasound is a heat-producing modality effective in the postacute stage or in chronic injury. Ultrasound makes use of ultra-high-frequency, 1 MHz sound waves that transfer their energy to the molecules they pass, adding to their oscillatory motion. The increased oscillation results in increased tissue temperature. Heating fibrous structures such as ligaments, tendons, and scar tissue can cause a temporary increase in their extensibility. When combined with

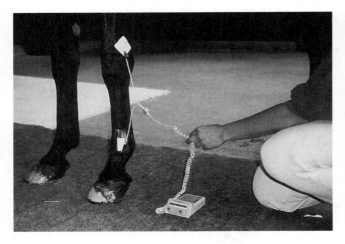

Fig. 13-3   An iontophoresis device.

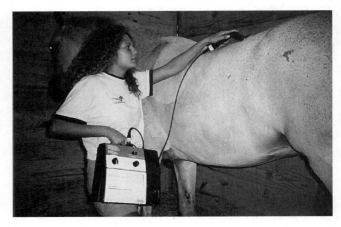

Fig. 13-4   Ultrasound treatment of a horse.

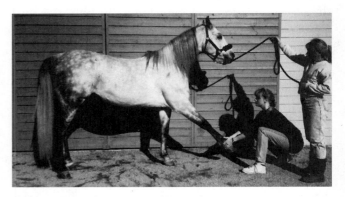

Fig. 13-5   Ultrasound should be followed by range-of-motion exercise.

range-of-motion exercises, ultrasound produces optimal results. Adding gentle flexion and extension exercises after ultrasound as well as other controlled exercise reduces the necessity to break down adhesions and reduce the formation of nonparallel fibers as rehabilitation progresses.

The vibratory frequency of a sound wave affects its absorption into body tissues. *Frequency* refers to the number of vibrations that a molecule in the sound wave undergoes in 1 second. The higher the frequency, the less the sound waves diverge. Audible sound ranges between 16 and 20,000 cycles of vibration per second. Sound waves at this frequency appear to spread out in all directions. Ultrasound waves have a frequency of greater than 20,000 Hz and are well collimated (Ter Haar, 1978). Physical therapy devices produce a beam of sound at a frequency of 1 million cycles per second, or 1 MHz—that is, sufficiently collimated to penetrate to selected target tissues.

Generally, ultrasound is applied for 5 minutes to an area of 5 cm². Treatment is applied directly to the injury site using gel coupling. A transmission medium is essential to effective treatment because air is a perfect reflector of ultrasound. Dampening the hair coat also helps eliminate air. If the hair coat is long, clipping may be necessary. Certainly the skin and hair coat should be clean.

The sound head is kept in contact with the skin and moved in slow sweeps over the skin surface. The skin should not gain appreciable heat during an ultrasound treatment. Ultrasound is absorbed by collagen-dense tissues that lie below the skin surface, making it a valuable tool for the rehabilitation of sports injuries. Tissues with a high fluid content, such as blood and muscle, absorb sound waves better than less hydrated tissues. Nerve has a high coefficient of ultrasound absorption, which expands the treatment possibilities to sounding nerve roots that are associated with peripheral conditions. Accumulation of heat in the skin is a sign that not enough gel is being used or the sound head is not in firm contact, allowing a rebound of the sound waves at the skin-sound head interface (Figs. 13-4 and 13-5).

Heating effects of ultrasound

Ultrasound has traditionally been used for its heating effects. These effects come from mechanical activity in the tissue as sound waves increase molecular motion. Ultrasound waves are compression waves of sound energy that move through tissue. Energy from the ultrasound wave is transferred to the molecules it passes through, adding to their oscillatory motion. The increased molecular oscillation results in an increase in tissue temperature. When the unit is operated in the 100% mode (sometimes called the *continuous mode*), heating effects can be as deep as 4 to 6 cm into the tissues (Lehmann, Delauteur, 1982). Heating deep structures results in increased extensibility of connective tissue so that adhesions, tension, fibrotic muscle, and joint capsule tissue can move through a more normal range of motion. When dense connective tissue limits motion, ultrasound can be used to increase the range. The heating effects of ultrasound on scar tissue render it more susceptible to remodeling by stretch forces. Diagnostic ultrasound often reveals less scar tissue around tendons that have been treated with ultrasound and stretching exercises.

Injury causes guarding muscle contractions that can eventually lead to shortened muscle tissue. Ultrasound renders collagen more malleable, reducing focal areas of stress when stretching is used to regain full range of movement and contractility. Preparing the muscle with ultrasound before stretching allows a more even distribution of stress along the length of the muscle. Early restoration of full range of movement is extremely important in recovery from injury or surgery because it prevents function-limiting adhesion formation and loss of tensile strength.

Prevention of the recurrence of disability is often overlooked in animal medicine. The use of ultrasound and stretching exercises following muscle strains resulted in a recurrence rate of 1%, according to a study using human subjects. The average treatment time of 6 days and a low recurrence rate illustrate the value of this approach over rest and reduced activity (Millar, 1976). A great advantage in the use of ultrasound is that deep structures can be affected without overheating superficial tissues. Elevating the tissue temperature before passive or active stretching enhances the effects of stretching. Preheating connective tissue before it is stretched produces greater residual increase in tissue length with less potential damage (Lehmann, 1970). Heating the deep tissues alters the elastic properties of collagen tissue and its molecular bonding. Deep tissues surrounding a joint are high in collagen. Because it is selectively absorbed by this type of tissue, ultrasound is the ideal modality for prestretch heating.

With a rise in tissue temperature an increase in circulation and changes in nerve conduction velocity are expected. The pain threshold is elevated with therapeutic ultrasound, and metabolic activity is stimulated. These effects make continuous ultrasound an ideal treatment for hoof abscesses and other hoof trauma. Because ultrasound can be applied under water, a warm water soak is a convenient medium of application to the hoof. Water is an excellent conductor of ultrasound, but air is not. Accumulated air bubbles on the sound head and skin surface should be wiped away throughout the underwater treatment. The treatment head should be held parallel to the limb and approximately 1 to 2 cm away.

Ultrasound can be used to deactivate muscular trigger points and acupuncture points. A setting of 0.5 W/cm² is used, and the sound head is moved in a tight, slow circular movement over the area of the point. A 3-minute treatment time is usually sufficient to make the trigger point less tender and irritable. Acupuncture points are areas of the skin surface that have increased electrical conductivity. Scientific measurement of the skin potential before and after ultrasound treatment helps in establishing accurate dosages for animals for this procedure.

Because of its ability to raise deep tissue temperature, ultrasound should not be used by an untrained operator. Heat can build up at tissue interfaces such as the bone and the periosteum, where sound waves are reflected back and forth between the two different tissue types. Other tissue interfaces where sound wave reflection occurs are the nerve and nerve sheath, scar tissue and the tissue surrounding it, muscle and muscle sheath, joint capsule and joint structures, and tendon and tendon sheath. The absence of skin surface heat may cause the unskilled operator to administer too high a dose for too long a time, resulting in burning of the delicate membrane of the sheath.

Ultrasound should never be applied immediately after exercise. Exercise-induced inflammation is increased by the heat produced by ultrasound. The heating effects of ultrasound can benefit the tissues, but if applied in intensities or duration outside the therapeutic window, ultrasound can cause tissue damage.

Nonthermal effects of ultrasound

In recent years the nonthermal benefits of ultrasound have been recognized. These chemical effects are often compared to the chemical reaction that is stimulated when a test tube is shaken. Nonthermal effects of ultrasound are maximized when the pulsed mode of operation is used, minimizing the heating effects. In the pulsed mode the wave train is interrupted at specific intervals, reducing the total number of waves produced in any second of treatment. Breaks in the wave train occur so that heat can be dissipated by circulation. Use pulsed ultrasound when effects other than those associated with tissue heating are desired or when the area to be treated is small and provides little room for sound head movement.

As the sound wave penetrates the tissue, the wave motion causes compression and expansion of the molecules and gas bubbles within the tissue and blood. This action is called *compression* and *rarefaction*. During the compression phase, molecules are compressed. During rarefaction, molecules expand. This pulsation causes changes in cellular activity and membrane permeability. Diffusion changes occur along cell membranes, aiding in the reduction of edema. Changes in membrane permeability of sodium ions could be involved in the altered electrical activity of nerves following ultrasound application, resulting in pain relief.

Movement of the ultrasound wave through the tissues produces cellular responses that could help in the stimulation of tissue repair. During the granulation stage of repair, which begins approximately 3 days after injury, fibroblasts can be stimulated to produce more collagen. Ultrasound has been shown to promote synthesis by allowing the entry of calcium ions that affect cellular activity (Tyson, 1987).

Like the continuous mode the pulsed mode should be used only at prescribed dosages. If the molecular pulsation is too violent (because of ultrasound intensities that are too high), free-radical production and tissue destruction, particularly damage to the vascular endothelial cells, results (Ziskin, Michlovitz, 1986).

Low-intensity ultrasound has been shown to affect the healing strength of tendons (Enwemeka, Rodriguez, Mendosa, 1990). During the remodeling stage, ultrasound applied at 0.5 W/cm² for 5 minutes every day resulted in a significant increase in tensile strength and energy-absorbing capacity of the tendons (Fig. 13-6).

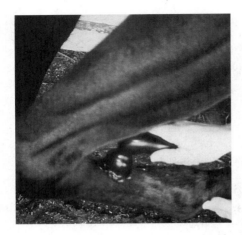

Fig. 13-6   Applying ultrasound to a tendon.

Ultrasound dosage

Ultrasound dosage must be sufficient to create a biologic change without causing overexposure. To arrive at the appropriate dosage, the practitioner should consider the power output intensity (watts), duration of exposure, and size of the surface area over the structures to be treated.

The intensity dosage is determined by the amount of soft tissue in the target area. When using the continuous mode to elevate tissue temperature in an area such as a horse's back or hip, practitioners may choose intensities as high as 1.5 to 2.0 W/cm^2. Lower intensities of 0.5 to 1.0 W/cm^2 are used over areas where less soft-tissue coverage exists and bone is closer to the skin surface. Higher intensities are chosen when the desired effect is tissue heating, such as before stretching exercises. Lower intensities are used for pain reduction, spasm relief, and edema dispersal. Lower intensities still, of 0.3 to 0.5 w/cm^2 of the sound head, are suitable for wound repair, use on small animals, or treatment of the lower leg of the horse.

Duration of treatment depends on the condition treated and the size of the treatment site. The size of the area to be treated is 2 to 3 times the size of the surface of the sound head. An area of this size should be sonated for 5 minutes. If the treatment area must extend over a larger area, it should be subdivided into small treatment areas, each of which is treated for 5 minutes.

Ultrasound is not dangerous if the operator carefully follows the treatment rules and understands the capabilities of this therapeutic modality. An important principle that applies to ultrasound is that too small an amount of energy produces no useful reaction, too much energy destroys tissue, and the appropriate amount of energy provides the desired response.

Therapeutic Heat, Therapeutic Cold, and Compression

The use of cold or heat in some form are age-old therapeutic remedies. In this discussion, *heat* refers to agents that increase the temperature only of superficial tissue. A deep tissue–heating device, therapeutic ultrasound, has been discussed in preceding paragraphs. Cold therapy is most effective if the agent is ice. The effects of cold therapy are augmented by compression. Evenly applied compression should be included as a part of all cold treatments.

Therapeutic heat

Therapeutic heating agents are divided into two categories: those that heat superficial tissues and those that heat deeper tissues. Agents that produce temperature changes in the skin and subcutaneous tissue (to a depth of approximately 1 cm) include hot packs, infrared lamps, electric heating pads, and warm water baths. These agents elevate skin temperature with little change in the temperature of the underlying structures. Increasing the temperature of these devices does not increase their depth of penetration; it only increases the danger of thermal damage to the skin. The effects of heat include increased circulation locally and an analgesic effect. With the application of heat, smooth muscle tone decreases and vessel diameter increases, resulting in increased nourishment of the tissue.

Therapeutic cold

Ice is underused as a therapeutic agent for animals. Once an injury occurs, intertissue bleeding must be stopped quickly to reduce the hematoma size. The inflammatory process must be quickly arrested to inhibit the series of deleterious events that occur in and around the injury—that is, blood and lymph vessel disruption, consequential extravasation of blood, platelet aggregation, and ultimately blood coagulation (Currier, Nelson, 1992).

Cold and compression cause local vasoconstriction and reduction in local tissue metabolism. Both cold and compression are important to quickly reduce intertissue bleeding and edema production. When only cold is used, vasoconstriction is delayed. One study examining the effect of cooling on blood flow found that no reduction of blood flow was seen in the first 5 minutes of cooling. After 10 minutes a maximum reduction of 69% was observed (Thorsson and others, 1985). This delayed reaction in blood flow reduction indicates the importance of compression in quickly stopping intertissue bleeding and effectively reducing the hematoma size and accumulation of edema.

The use of cold and compression for as little as 15 minutes results in vasoconstriction. When the use of cold is prolonged or intense, a cold-induced vasodilation follows the initial period of vasoconstriction. During cold-induced vasodilation, blood flows through arteriovenous anastomoses. This shunting accounts for reduced hemorrhage through damaged capillaries. The decreased tissue temperature slows down metabolic processes in the cell. Because of a decreased need for oxygen and nutrients, the need for capillary exchange is diminished and less volume passes through the capillary bed (Michlovitz, 1986).

Cold therapy, sometimes called *cryotherapy,* is used for musculoskeletal trauma and for postsurgical swelling and pain. A convenient form of application is the ice-cup massage. A Styrofoam cup filled with water and then frozen provides an effective ice-therapy tool. Ice massage is given for up to 20 minutes several times a day and combined with compression wraps. Acupuncture points can be treated with ice massage and are effectively deactivated. Ice massage is far more comfortable than ice immersion, in which the body part is placed in a container of ice and water. Ice massage is more effective than the use of crushed ice packs because the air surrounding the pieces of ice results in uneven application. The least effective form of cold therapy is the application of cold water from a hose. A stream of water directed to the injury site is a common treatment for leg injury because a water hose is a convenient source of cold water. The water is usually colder than the body part being treated, but controlling the water temperature and accuracy is difficult. Also, the massaging effect of the water stream can further damage exposed subdermal cells and capillaries. If this method is employed, the water stream should be slow and gentle and followed by a compression wrap. This labor-intensive method of applying cold to an injury should be replaced with the use of ice and a compression wrap.

Cold stimulates cutaneous afferent nerves that act reflexively on the motor neuron, decreasing its firing and reducing the irritability of the nerve-muscle junction. In this way, cold can be effective therapeutically, beyond first-aid care. The reduction in muscle spasm makes early movement possible and more comfortable. It is often the preferred treatment for managing the early stages of sprains, muscle strains, and contusions. Pain and muscle spasm generally accompany musculoskeletal injuries to some degree. Pain is caused by damage to nerve fibers and pressure on the nerve fibers caused by surrounding edema. Muscle spasm protects an injured part by splinting or bracing it and reducing movement. The spasm causes pressure on nerves, which increases pain. The body responds to this pain by increasing the protective spasm, and the well-known pain-spasm-pain cycle is born. This cycle can be broken through the use of ice massage (Fig. 13-7).

Ice should be applied immediately after injury. Cold reduces swelling and acts as a local anesthetic. Heat is used once bleeding and swelling have stopped, usually after 72 hours. This increases blood flow to the injury and removes waste products from the area. Using heat too soon greatly increases swelling and bleeding into tissues, exacerbating the injury.

Stretching

The purpose of any exercise is to produce certain changes in the tissues—that is, to strengthen, increase endurance for sustained activity, or increase extensibility under stretching stresses. This last aspect of fitness is called *flexibility.* Endurance and strength training is usually in-

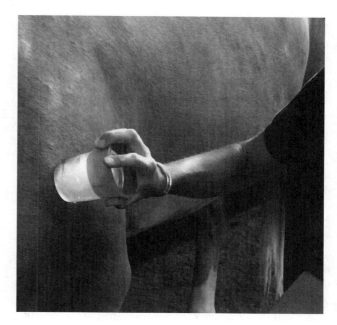

Fig. 13-7   Ice-cup massage.

cluded in conditioning programs, but the capacity of soft tissues to elongate and recoil is often forgotten. Flexibility is a measure of the range of motion of a joint. It can be limited by bone structure or dense connective tissue in the muscles, joint capsule, or tendons. A combination of heating and stretching exercises improves flexibility limited by dense connective tissue in the soft tissues. Looking at the effects of manual stretching on adhesive capsulitis, investigators found that manual stretching was superior to traction in reducing dense connective tissue (Nicholson, 1982). Manually assisted stretching exercises are appropriate for use on animals and give the handler an opportunity for intimate communication with the animal.

Philosophy of stretching

Stretching exercises offer many benefits to animals and their handlers. Used in injury rehabilitation, manual stretching exercises are part of the prescription and should be considered as such. The appropriate type, intensity, and timing of exercise have an impact on its effectiveness. Exercises for flexibility should be done when the soft tissues are warmed up. They should be carried out with the concept of balance in mind—that is, with the handler looking for equality of flexibility in comparable joints. Manually assisted flexibility exercises should be gentle so the animal does not tense his muscles to guard against the discomfort of overstretching sore structures.

Benefits of stretching

Stretching exercises, whether manually assisted or done as an "under-tack" maneuver, provide several benefits. When performed as part of the warm-up routine, they can prevent injury by stretching tight structures to enhance balanced movement. Stretching exercises provide relief

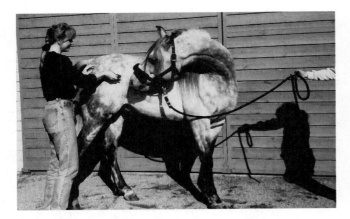

Fig. 13-8 Stretching exercises for the horse.

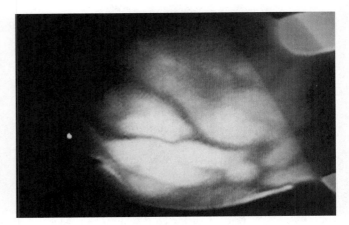

Fig. 13-9 LLLT through a human hand. Note absorption by blood.

from trigger-point pain. In this instance the "more is better" philosophy must be discouraged because excessive stretching can aggravate trigger points and increase pain.

Stretching exercises are an important part of rehabilitation from injury. Repeated, gentle stretching exercises stimulate tissue remodeling with increases in tissue length and reduced muscle spasm. Cartilage nutrition is improved and postoperative fibrosis of periarticular structures is reduced when repeated, gentle range-of-motion movements are manually assisted.

Manual stretching for animals must never exceed their pain-free range. Overstretching a joint or stretching when tissues are cold results in protective muscle contracture and reduces the elongation effects. Overstretching can damage collagen bundles and blood vessels, causing significant inflammation.

Benefits of stretching include improved athleticism, which lessens the possibility of injury. Stretching can be used to reduce strains and tearing of muscle fibers caused by an imbalance in muscle tension. Stretching after exercise reduces postexercise muscle soreness. Less tangible advantages include improved communication with and understanding of the animal. Stretching exercises involve cooperation and harmony of movement between the animal and the therapist, who work as a team in the cycle of stretching and release.

Contraindications for stretching

Manual stretching should be avoided when acute inflammation is present. An acute sprain of a joint or a muscle strain should not be subjected to manual stretching. Ice should be applied and the area rested until the initial inflammatory process ends. At this point, gentle and progressive stretching may prevent loss of mobility resulting from stiffness (Fig. 13-8).

Therapeutic Laser

The use of therapeutic lasers is discussed in more detail elsewhere in the book, but because it is such a useful tool for the veterinary physical therapist, it is briefly mentioned here.

Although therapeutic lasers first appeared on the market only 30 years ago, the computer database MEDLINE lists nearly 2 million journal entries on medical laser. Since 1990, 2500 articles have been listed on low-level laser therapy (LLLT) alone. *LLLT* is the internationally accepted term for lasers that do not cause a thermal reaction. These devices cause a chemical reaction in the cells and do not raise tissue temperature.

Perhaps the most salient question about LLLT is whether the radiation penetrates to a depth sufficient to produce results in the target tissues. Laser emits electromagnetic waves, and these waves (between 600 and 1000 nm) can penetrate tissue. The precise depth of penetration cannot be given because optical properties vary among individuals and tissue type. Depth of penetration depends on the absorption spectra of the tissue (i.e., the wavelengths the tissue molecules will absorb). Wavelengths of up to 700 nm are highly absorbed in pigments such as melanin and carotene, and they are absorbed fairly superficially. Wavelengths from 700 to 1000 nm are primarily absorbed by molecules of blood, myoglobin, hemoglobin, and tissue protein and have deeper penetration (Fig. 13-9).

GaAlAs diode lasers are thought to have the optimal wavelength (830 nm) for peak tissue penetration, with protein being the primary absorbing medium (Baxter, 1994). The volume of photons available is greater when multisource radiation is used, as with cluster units. These multidiode arrays consist of superluminous diodes and sometimes a laser-emitting diode, all operating at one wavelength or within a range of wavelengths (Fig. 13-10). The cross-interference from neighboring diodes increases forward scatter below the dermis (Baxter, 1994).

Therapeutic lasers are designed to be used in contact with the tissue. The beam should be applied perpendicularly to the target. The skin should be compressed slightly to blanch the surface vessels. LLLT is highly absorbed by

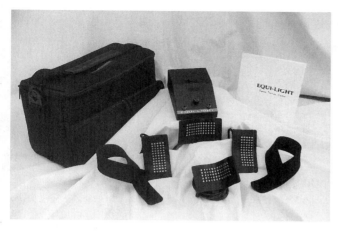

Fig. 13-10 A multidiode LLLT device.

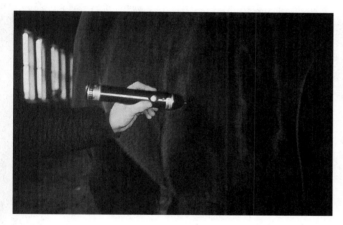

Fig. 13-11 A single-diode LLLT device. LLLT should be applied in contact with the skin at a perpendicular angle, with slight pressure.

blood proteins, so depth of penetration is increased if gentle pressure is applied (Fig. 13-11).

Conclusion

Physical therapy has certain limitations. It also has the potential for doing harm. No modality capable of making physiologic changes is harmless. The veterinary physical therapist is a health-care specialist who should complete advanced training. The use of therapeutic modalities in the treatment of animal injuries by individuals without the appropriate education, professional license, or certification is currently controversial. College-level instruction in the use of therapeutic modalities for animals has not yet been established. Until a course of instruction is available to those who wish to pursue animal physical therapy, no meaningful regulations can be placed upon this practice. Readers are advised to acquaint themselves with the relevant laws of the state in which they wish to practice. This chapter is in no way intended to encourage readers to disregard state law. Until the profession of veterinary physi-

cal therapy is more well established (e.g., with course work leading to a degree and certification), it cannot achieve its full potential benefit to animals.

A list of equipment manufacturers can be found on the World Wide Web at http://www.cybersteed.com or by writing to Equine Therapy, Inc, 4350 Harrodsburg Road, Lexington, KY 40513.

REFERENCES

A new approach to pain, *Emerg Med* 6:240, 1974.

Abram SE: Advances in chronic pain management since gate control, *Reg Anesth* 18:66, 1993.

Baxter D: *Therapeutic lasers,* New York, 1994, Churchill Livingstone.

Benton LA and others: *Functional electrical stimulation: a practical clinical guide,* Downey, Calif, 1980, Rancho Los Amigos Hospital.

Chapman CR, Bendetti C: Analgesia following transcutaneous electrical stimulation and its partial reversal by a narcotic antagonist, *Life Sci* 21:1645, 1977.

Cheng R, Pomeranz B: Electroacupuncture analgesia could be mediated by at least two pain-relieving mechanisms: endorphin and non-endorphin systems, *Life Sci* 25:1957, 1979.

Currier DP, Mann R: Muscular strength development by electrical stimulation in healthy individuals, *Phys Ther* 63:915, 1983.

Currier DP, Nelson RM: *Dynamics of human biologic tissues,* Philadelphia, 1992, FA Davis.

Currier DP, Petrilli CR, Threlkeld AJ: Effects of graded electrical stimulation on blood flow to healthy muscle, *Phys Ther* 66:937, 1986.

Doran FS, Drury M, Sivyer A: A simple way to combat the venous stasis which occurs in limbs during surgical operations, *Br J Surg* 51:486, 1964.

Downer A: *Physical therapy for animals,* Springfield, Ill, 1978, Charles C Thomas.

Enwemeka CS, Rodriguez O, Mendosa S: The biomechanical effects of low-intensity ultrasound on healing tendons, *Ultrasound Med Biol* 16:801, 1990.

Enwemeka CS, Spielholz NL: Modulation of tendon growth and regeneration by electrical fields and currents. In Currier D, Nelson R, editors: *Dynamics of human biologic tissues,* Philadelphia, 1992, FA Davis.

Eriksson E, Haggmark T: Comparison of isometric muscle training and electrical stimulation supplementing isometric muscle training in the recovery after major knee ligament surgery, *Am J Sports Med* 7:171, 1979.

Eriksson E and others: Effect of electrical stimulation on human skeletal muscle, *Int J Sports Med* 2:18, 1981.

Gentzkow GD: Electrical stimulation to heal dermal wounds, *J Dermatol Surg Oncol* 19:753, 1993.

Harrington DB, Meyer R, Klein RM: Effects of small amounts of electric current at the cellular level, *Ann NY Acad Sci* 238:300, 1974.

Hood DM and others: Equine laminitis. I. Radioisotopic analysis of the hemodynamics of the foot during the acute disease, *J Equ Med Surg* 2:439, 1978.

Kahn J: *Principles and practices of electrotherapy,* New York, 1987, Churchill Livingstone.

Klein J, Pariser D: Transcutaneous electrical nerve stimulation. In Nelson R, Currier D, editors: *Clinical electrotherapy,* Norwalk, Conn, 1987, Appleton & Lange.

Lehmann JF: Effects of therapeutic temperatures on tendon extensibility, *Arch Phys Med Rehab* 51:481, 1970.

Lehmann JF, Delauteur BJ: Therapeutic heat. In *Therapeutic heat and cold,* ed 3, Baltimore, 1982, Williams & Wilkins.

Mendel FC, Wylegala JA, Fish DR: Influence of high voltage pulsed current on edema formation following impact injury in rats, *Phys Ther* 72:668, 1992.

Michlovitz S: *Thermal agents in rehabilitation,* Philadelphia, 1986, FA Davis.

Millar AP: An early stretching routine for calf muscle atrains, *Med Sci Sports* 8:39, 1976.

Myrhage R, Hudlica O: Capillary growth in chronically stimulated adult skeletal muscle as studied by intravital microscopy and histological methods in rabbits and rats, *Microvas Res* 116:73, 1978.

Nicholson G: The effects of passive joint mobilization on pain and hypomobility associated with adhesive capsulitis of the shoulder, master's thesis, Birmingham, 1982, Division of Physical Therapy, University of Alabama.

Owoeye IO: The therapeutic effects of galvanic current following rupture of the Achilles' tendon in rats, doctoral dissertation, New York, 1982, New York University.

Pool RR, Wheat JD, Ferraro GL:. Corticosteroid therapy in common joint and tendon injuries, Parts I and II, *Proceedings of AAEP,* p 397, 1980.

Porter M: Electrical stimulation of blood flow through the equine limb, Unpublished manuscript, 1983.

Porter M: *Equine sports therapy,* Wildomar, Calif, 1990, Veterinary Data.

Prentice WE: *Therapeutic modalities in sports medicine,* St Louis, 1986, Mosby.

Stanish WD and others: The use of electricity in ligament and tendon repair, *Phys Sportsmed* 13:109, 1985.

Strong C: *Horse's injuries,* New York, 1973, Arco.

Ter Haar G: Basic physics of therapeutic ultrasound, *Physiotherapy* 64:100, 1978.

Thorsson O and others: The effect of local cold application on intramuscular blood flow at rest and after running, *Med Sci Sports Exercise* 17:710, 1985.

Tyson M: Mechanisms involved in therapeutic ultrasound, *Physiotherapy* 73:116, 1987.

Vasko K, Spauchus A, Lowry A: Laminitis treatment with electrotherapy, *Equine Pract* 8:28, 1986.

Vodovnik L, Miklavcic D, Sersa G: Modified cell proliferation due to electrical currents, *Med Biol Eng Comput* 30:CE21, 1992.

Ziskin M, Michlovitz A:Therapeutic ultrasound. In Michlovitz A, editor: *Thermal agents in rehabilitation,* Philadelphia, 1986, FA Davis.

Chapter 14

Massage Therapy

MIMI PORTER, MARY BROMILEY

In the past 10 years, massage has regained a respected place among physical therapy techniques. The use of massage in rehabilitation and warm-up before sports competition declined during the past 50 years. Two factors played a role in this decline. Electrical stimulation devices that produced smooth, comfortable currents were developed; these devices were used for relaxing specific areas of tension. Also, as athletes began to appreciate the value of warm-up exercise, active warm-up stretching routines and sport-related activity to elevate the heart rate began to replace massage as a precompetition preparation.

Recently developed massage techniques and the use of massage as a therapeutic modality have been subjected to scientific scrutiny. In his book *Beating Muscle Injuries for Horses* (1985), Jack Meagher makes the point that massage can help prevent injury in horses by reducing muscle tension before injury occurs. His success encouraged others, and equine sports massage is now used widely.

Basic Principles of Massage

Massage is used to increase circulation, release scar tissue, balance muscle function, and relax the individual; it is both a preperformance and postperformance therapy. Several basic principles precede the use of massage. The therapist must obtain a complete diagnosis of the patient's health status so that massage is a useful part of total care. The hands-on contact of massage must promote understanding and trust. The therapist must be aware of the animal's response to tactile stimuli. Empathic communication with the animal aids in the success of massage therapy.

Each stroke must have a purpose. Random movements of the hands are ineffective. The strokes of a massage given for sedative purpose should be slow and rhythmic. Special strokes are used to stimulate. Massage requires concentration on each manipulation (Fig. 14-1).

To be successful, massage must be administered skillfully. The massage therapist must be patient, perceptive, and exceptionally sensitive with the hands. The therapist must examine muscle for imbalances in tension, flexibility, strength, and weakness and detect areas of tension and spasm. Imbalances in muscle function often lead to acute injury and are always present in chronic injury. When using massage as a rehabilitative tool, the therapist usually begins at a site away from the area of injury to avoid creating guarding muscle contractions.

Techniques of Massage

The massage therapist should begin with gentle stroking to search for areas of spasm and tenderness and accustom the animal to the therapist's touch. The strokes should be of even pressure and run longitudinally along the muscle, following the direction of hair growth. The initial stroking should be superficial rather than deep to create a sedating effect and prevent protective muscle contractions (Porter, 1990). Gradually increasing the pressure, the therapist begins to work in the direction of venous flow, or toward the heart. Massage oils are rarely used on animals because they may make the fingers slide too quickly. Baby powder is recommended if a lubricant is needed.

Trigger-Point Massage

Trigger-point massage is sometimes called *myotherapy* or *myofascial trigger-point massage*. The therapist begins the massage by examining the musculature for taut bands and other evidence of trauma or imbalance. Associated with trigger points, taut bands are regions in muscle tissue that have an increased resistance to palpation. The trigger point is a zone of maximal tenderness that will react with

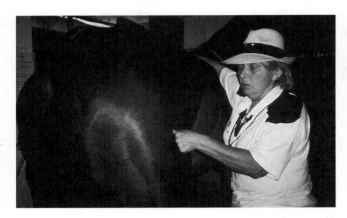

Fig. 14-1 Therapist using massage technique.

a twitch response when pressure is applied. Massaging a trigger point reduces its reactivity and induces relaxation of the muscle.

Manual techniques for deactivating a trigger point include firm digital pressure applied directly to the trigger point, which creates ischemic compression. The elbow is often used to apply pressure. Pressure initially causes ischemia, followed by reactive hyperemia. A massage that involves vigorously rubbing an active trigger point could cause an adverse reaction and increased pain resulting from muscle contractures to guard the area.

Acupressure Massage

Acupressure massage is the use of finger or elbow pressure to deactivate sensitive acupuncture points. These sites are subjected to a penetrating pressure. Acupressure massage is similar to trigger-point massage in technique but different in theory. The treatment approach centers on the Chinese meridian theory, which posits that all organs of the body are connected by a network through which energy flows. A high degree of correlation exists between the location of trigger points and acupuncture points on the skin surface. Tender trigger points correspond to an injury in the underlying muscle and fascia. According to acupuncture theory, specific areas on the skin surface relate to specific organs or remote parts of the body through a system of channels. Systematic pressuring of these points keeps the channels open and maintains the flow of energy.

The fascia has an electrical function. Nodes of facial contraction interfere with electrical conduction and interrupt cell-to-cell communication. Acupressure massage requires accurate location of acupuncture points and an understanding of the interrelationship of these points with their related organs. The equine application of this massage technique is described in *Equine Acupressure* (Zidonis, Soderberg, Pederson, 1991).

Sports Massage

Proponents of sports massage promote it as a way to improve athletic performance. Sports-massage therapists use primarily deep strokes and cross-fiber frictions to increase the efficiency of limb movement. This approach alleviates muscle tension, removes lactic acid, increases the pain threshold, increases flexibility, and stimulates circulation. Few of the claims made for sports massage are based on laboratory studies. One study to determine the physiologic responses during submaximal exercise following a 30-minute sports massage found no differences in specific physiologic measures. The results indicate that massage for 30 minutes immediately before exercise had no effect on cardiovascular measures, such as cardiac output, oxygen consumption, heart rate, blood pressure, and lactic acid responses. Sports massage was not found to improve exercise performance, and a 30-minute massage just before exercise did not provide subjects with increased oxygen flow to the body tissues (Boone, Cooper, Thompson, 1991). This study contradicted the idea that sports massage is a necessary part of sport preparation.

A study on stride frequency in human sprinters after massage reported that preperformance massage did not increase stride frequency. Participants in the study, however, stated that they felt relaxed and better able to cope with physical exertion after massage (Harmer, 1991). A contrasting study on the effects of massage on hamstring muscles reported that range of motion can be significantly improved (Crosman, Chateauvert, Weisberg, 1984). This finding would validate the theory that massage can be used for prevention of injuries such as strains and sprains. Confirming the effects of massage on blood flow, a thermographic study showed increases in skin temperature after massage to areas overlying muscle spasm (Meade and others, 1990).

The benefits of sports massage may not be measurable by standard means. Massage may put the athlete in an appropriate frame of mind for successful competition. No one knows precisely the value for animals of mental relaxation and preparedness before competition. Skilled riders know what their horses need before competition, but these needs cannot be subjected to laboratory analysis.

Craniosacral Therapy, or Energy Work

The craniosacral concept is based on identification by the therapist of the craniosacral rhythm, or the movement of the cerebrospinal fluid in the spinal canal. The body moves in a subtle motion that corresponds to the movement of the cerebrospinal fluid. The strength and synchronicity of the rhythm can be used to diagnose restrictions in the body. The removal of these restrictions is called a *release*. Very little force is used in this type of massage. The theory behind this approach is that a small force over a long time can do more for the body than a strong force over a short time. Some experts believe that a small force produces much less resistance in the patient's body. Deep relaxation is a primary goal of craniosacral therapy. Profound physiologic restoration, called *therapeutic rest,* is thought to occur in deep dreamless sleep or deep relaxation (Upledger, Vredevoogd, 1983).

Ice Massage

The therapeutic effects of cold are described in Chapter 13. Cold lowers cell metabolism and causes vasoconstriction and decreased nerve-conduction velocity, which results in an increased pain threshold. Ice massage involves massaging a block of ice directly on the skin. A convenient method of applying ice massage is to freeze water in a Styrofoam cup, expose a rim of ice by removing the lip of the cup, hold the cup base, and apply the ice massage directly to the injured area for 5 to 10 minutes. Muscle soreness, local edema, arthritis, bursitis, and tendinitis respond to ice massage. Cold penetrates deeply to treat tissues lying deep beneath superficial layers.

Effleurage

The term *effleurage* comes from the French word, *effleurer,* which means to *touch* or *graze.* The technique is used at the beginning and end of every massage session and can link one technique to another. Effleurage uses gliding strokes of firm, even pressure in the direction of venous flow. The goal is to relax the patient and assist venous and lymphatic flow.

Pétrissage

The word *pétrissage,* also derived from French, means *kneading.* With this stroke the skin is lifted and gently squeezed. Pétrissage is used to free adhesions and increase local blood flow by stimulating reactive hyperemia. For treatment of a large area, this stroke is performed with the fists placed over the target area. Pressure is exerted inward, downward, and outward in a grinding or compressing movement. Pétrissage is best done with alternate hands, one pressing downward and inward while the other relaxes.

Tapotement or Cupping

Tapotement and cupping are percussive movements done in a gentle striking motion, using the hypothenar surface of the hand. The rhythmic blows have a stimulative effect on superficial sensory nerves and vasodilate the skin capillaries.

Friction or Deep Cross-Fiber Friction

Friction massage uses compression created by the tip of the index finger and reinforced by the second finger. Pressure is placed firmly over the target area. Short, deep cross-fiber movement produces local eschemia followed by hyperemia. Friction massage is the only massage technique that is performed in a transverse manner across the directional flow of the underlying tissue fibers. The skin moves with the finger as it separates the fibers that form adhesions in the deeper tissues. The muscles of the patient must be relaxed for friction to be successful. Several contraindications to deep friction exist. If the therapist is overly aggressive, tissue cells and capillaries can be damaged. Because it can be uncomfortable and produce tension, friction massage should never be performed over an acute injury.

When an injury occurs, new collagen fibers form transverse adhesions that bind muscle or ligament fibers and restrict range of movement. Deep transverse frictions are believed to prevent adhesion formation and restore tissue mobility when applied to chronic lesions (Cyriax, 1980). Friction massage is controversial because of its potential to cause tissue damage. In a study on the effect of deep transverse friction on the healing of a minor sprain, histologic observations revealed no difference between treated and nontreated ligaments (Walker, 1984).

Passive Movement

Passive range-of-motion exercises are a form of massage because they require hands-on contact by the therapist. These movements of a specific joint are done without voluntary assistance or resistance from the animal. To perform passive movements correctly, the therapist must be aware of the normal range of movement available in the joint to be treated. The body is unable to evoke normal protective mechanisms when no muscle activity is involved; therefore care must be taken not to overstretch the joint during a passive movement. In contrast to assisted stretching exercises, in which the joint is moved gently beyond its normal range, passive movements are performed within the limits of the soft tissue without stretching. Passive movement is performed to improve synovial fluid production in the joints and increase joint mobility.

Contraindications to Massage

Cautions that must be observed when making use of massage include the following:

- Massage should not be performed over bacterially or virally infected lesions.
- The skin over the target tissue must be intact.
- Massage should not be applied to a torn muscle or an acute hematoma. Massage can be very detrimental when injury is in the acute stage.
- Massage should be avoided in the presence of phlebitis or inflammatory arthritis.

- Massage should be avoided in cases of recent high fever or high blood pressure.
- The therapist should have a complete knowledge of the horse's state of health before applying massage.
- Veterinary consultation is required for effective treatment.

*R*EFERENCES

Boone T, Cooper R, Thompson W: A physiologic evaluation of the sports massage, *Athletic Training* 26:51, 1991.

Crosman L, Chateauvert S, Weisberg J: The effects of massage to the hamstring muscle group on range of motion, *J Orthop Sports Phys Ther* 6:168, 1984.

Cyriax J: Clinical applications of massage. In Rogoff JB, editor: *Manipulation, traction, and massage,* Baltimore, 1980, Williams & Wilkins.

Harmer P: The effect of pre-performance massage on stride frequency in sprinters, *Athletic Training* 26:55, 1991.

Meade TW and others: Low back pain of mechanical origin: randomized comparison of chiropractic and hospital out-patient treatment, *Br Med J* 300:1431, 1990.

Meagher J: *Beating muscle injuries for horses,* Hamilton, Mass, 1985, Hamilton Horse.

Porter M: *Equine sports therapy,* Wildomar, Calif, 1990, Veterinary Data.

Upledger JE, Vredevoogd JD: *Craniosacral therapy,* Seattle, 1983, Eastland.

Walker J: Deep transverse frictions in ligament healing, *J Orthop Sports Phys Ther* 6:89, 1984.

Zidonis N, Soderberg M, Pederson S: *Equine accupressure,* Parker, Colo, 1991, Equine Acupressure.

Chapter 15

*T*TEAM Approach

JOYCE C. HARMAN

Linda Tellington-Jones created TTEAM in 1978 after studying with Dr. Moshe Feldenkrais, who formalized a system for teaching physical awareness through the use of nonhabitual movements. Tellington-Jones sought a gentle approach to help horses with behavioral problems. An accomplished horsewoman in all competitive disciplines, she developed from Feldenkrais's work (1972) a systematic method of educating and reeducating horses. Later, she created a series of simple tactile techniques using small, circular hand movements on the body. Many species of animals and even some people have benefited from her work.

Although TTEAM is not technically considered a medical approach, improvements in overall health are not uncommon after animals have been trained using TTEAM techniques. Aware of the connection between body and mind, some researchers suspect that many of these physical improvements may have a mental component, a concept under investigation in the field of psychoneuroimmunology. When an animal is exposed to TTEAM, major changes in behavior and mental awareness occur. Although TTEAM is not yet supported by experimental data, enough clinical and anecdotal information has surfaced to warrant further study and evaluation. This chapter is based on the clinical experience of TTEAM practitioners.

TTEAM exercises are based on common sense. A unique and gentle way of working with animals, TTEAM enhances the human/animal relationship; it also simplifies the veterinarian's work by making animals more docile. As a dramatic example, San Diego Zoo handlers use TTouch, a related approach, as a safety measure before the animals receive veterinary care.

History and Evolution of TTEAM

The basis for TTEAM is in the human bodywork modality called Feldenkrais, which is a way of increasing self-awareness and fluid motion through the use of two different systems: gentle nonhabitual movements and bodywork. The nonhabitual movements, described by Feldenkrais as *awareness through movement* (1972), are often slight and are designed to train the body to avoid posture and movement patterns that interfere with normal body functions. The bodywork, called *functional integration*, uses gentle manipulations and helps guide the body to a new level of awareness without being invasive, as massage sometimes is.

TTEAM was originally known as *TEAM*, which stood for *Tellington-Jones Equine Awareness Method*, but when practitioners began to use the techniques successfully on different species, the words behind the acronym were changed to *Tellington-Jones Every Animal Method*. The name *TTouch* refers to an independent system of circular hand movements applied to the body of the animal. The *TT* stands for Π, which defines a circle. The *T* was added to *TTEAM* to indicate that TTouch was the Tellington Touch (Tellington-Jones, 1992).

Early TTEAM methods primarily involved exercises for teaching horses to focus and learn. These ground exercises have grown into an excellent body-awareness program that can benefit all animals. Using plastic poles that vary in width depending on the size of the animal, the TTEAM practitioner creates patterns on the ground through which the animal walks. A short session can make a major difference in many animals, and regular work can make unfocused and uncoordinated animals responsive, coordinated, and balanced.

Added in 1984, the TTouch system helps bring awareness to various parts of the body. Part of the TTouch effect is to activate all four categories of brain waves in both the performer and recipient of TTouch. In a study using biofeedback on a group of four people and horses, a machine was used to measure the brain waves of distinguished professionals, healers, and business people in England (Cade, 1995). The machine, developed by Maxwell Cade, uses spectral analysis to simultaneously measure 11 different frequencies from each hemisphere.

Alpha waves are midrange waves normally present when a person is relaxed. They are often achieved only when the eyes are closed. Alpha waves appear to have little significance by themselves, but in combination with other waves, they may represent a bridge between the conscious and unconscious minds. Beta waves are involved in the normal waking states of thinking, logic, and problem solving. Overactive beta waves are seen in the fight-or-flight response. Theta waves are dream and sleep waves associated with memories, sensations, and emotions. Delta waves are linked to deep sleep and subconscious states. In the study, subjects who had taken a week-long course in TTEAM showed relatively high theta and delta waves and produced alpha waves when working on horses, whereas people without training produced no alpha waves. The horses registered beta (thinking) and delta (subconscious thought) waves in both hemispheres of the brain during normal resting states. When the TTouch was performed on the horses, all four categories of waves were activated, particularly alpha and some beta (Cade, 1995). When a telemetered unit was used, a higher frequency of brain waves appeared during some patterns of walking.

As TTEAM has evolved, its exercises and bodywork have profoundly affected many species. Single sessions have produced enormous changes in so-called problem cases. Dogs who bit when frightened, cats who could not be handled, zoo animals who did not adapt to captivity, and horses with serious behavioral problems have all responded to treatment. Although not every animal can be cured, many problems stem from communication difficulties between animals and humans. TTEAM helps both: humans learn new, nonthreatening patterns of handling, and animals acquire a new understanding of human expectations.

Originally perceived as a slow process of retraining, TTEAM is now understood to involve rapid change. For example, despite great promise, an Olympic-caliber dressage horse from Germany was so fearful during his few competitions that his chance of ever competing successfully was jeopardized. After four sessions of TTEAM, he won several Grand Prix Specials at top European competitions. He has continued to receive TTEAM periodically, and he now appears focused and attentive to his rider during competitions. Owners of performance dogs have also found that TTEAM enhances their ability. Zoos have used TTouch to help their animals adapt to the stresses of living in confinement, and in the process have become better places for animals to live. Veterinarians have found that if TTouch is incorporated into their practices, animals seem more relaxed and receptive to being handled. People who simply enjoy their animals as pets and companions have found that TTouch adds a new dimension to their relationships.

Some veterinarians mistakenly perceive TTEAM as overly lenient. In general, domineering people become gentler when doing TTEAM, and people who are too permissive with their animals learn to draw clear boundaries and administer appropriate discipline. TTEAM is gentle but not opposed to strong reprimand when necessary. TTEAM practitioners understand the importance of timing, intent, and consistency in the application of discipline.

Tellington-Jones has always strived to teach her techniques to as many people as possible. Although only a few practitioners are qualified to teach the week-long seminars, many practitioners at various levels of qualification offer hands-on workshops to solve training problems and teach basic skills. A list of practitioners and their qualifications can be obtained from the TTEAM office (refer to the end of the chapter for the address). As with any profession, some practitioners are better than others, but the TTEAM organization prosecutes members who violate the principles of the organization and does not support practitioners who attempt to perform medical procedures. Appropriate education of the TTEAM practitioner is essential so that attempts at TTEAM work do not delay necessary veterinary medical attention. Responsible practitioners work with veterinarians, who are best equipped to evaluate their competence.

Basic TTouches and Exercises

TTouch differs from massage because it manipulates only the skin and not the deeper tissues. TTouch is designed to stimulate the nervous system, not just the muscles. Interestingly, an injured limb often improves when the opposite limb is treated by TTouch, a phenomenon also seen with acupuncture treatment. Unlike massage, which should cover most of the body to be effective, TTouch can be effective when used on even a small area of the body. For detailed information concerning TTouch and exercises, please refer to the books and videos listed at the end of the chapter, or contact the TTEAM office for a list of clinics. This chapter is only an introduction to the possibilities of TTEAM.

The basic TTouch circle is made by holding the hand in a relaxed position and touching the body with the thumb and heel of the hand, allowing the first three fingers to rest gently on the skin and letting the last finger follow. The fingers should be relaxed. The skin is then gently pushed around in a circle, beginning at the six o'clock position and completing a circle and one quarter, past six o'clock to eight o'clock. This amounts to 14 hours, using the clock analogy. The circles are done in connected lines along the body: After completing one circle, the hand slides to the next location, always making only one circle at each location. The other hand remains close to the working hand on the animal's body to complete the connection and provide balance for the person. If the practitioner is performing TTouch on another human, the difference between making the circles with both hands and only one hand touching the other person becomes apparent. If the animal or the area being treated is small, using only one or two fingers may be appropriate.

The appropriate pressure is determined using a scale of 1 to 10. The lightest contact possible to move the eyelid in a circle over the closed eye is designated as Level 1; at this level, pressure should not create any indentation of the skin. The practitioner determines Level 3 by making a circle with as much pressure as is comfortable on the practitioner's own eyelid while the eyes are closed; this pressure should make a slight indentation in the skin of the forearm. Level 6 is twice this pressure, and 9 or 10 is about 3 times this pressure. The pressure is adjusted for each animal and for different parts of the body depending on what is comfortable and nonthreatening.

The different techniques used in TTouch are given animal-related names to enhance the learning process for clients. For example, the Raccoon TTouch is quick, gentle, and light, whereas the Bear TTouch is deep and slow. The names of each touch style are described throughout the text (Tellington, Jones, 1992).

The basic circular TTouch (described first) is called the *Clouded Leopard,* its differing pressures named for an animal capable of both softness and strength. The Lying Leopard is gentler and uses the flat part of the fingers. The Raccoon TTouch uses the tips of the fingers and the same pressures as the Clouded Leopard, whereas the Bear TTouch uses the fingernails and a very deep but nonpainful pressure. The Abalone TTouch uses the flat of the hand as if the hand were sticking to the animal's skin, and the Tiger TTouch uses the nails as in the Bear TTouch but with the fingers spread apart to allow each finger to make contact separately.

Several TTouches are done in a linear pattern, generally moving the skin over the underlying connective tissue. In performing the Snail's Pace, the hand is held still and the skin moved with the first and second phalanx. In The Tarantula Pulling the Plow a fold of skin is gently pulled along, going with or across the direction of hair growth. The Lick of the Cow's Tongue is done with a cupped hand, the tips of the fingers and the heel of the hand running along from the abdomen to the top of the back. The Python Lift is done by placing the hands around a leg, back, or other part of the body, gently raising the skin up, holding for 4 seconds, and slowly lowering the skin. The Butterfly often follows the Python Lift, with the thumbs surrounding the legs and gently lifting the skin and muscle proximally around the leg and back down again. The Noah's March is used at the end of a session and consists of firm strokes by the flat of the hand either over the entire body starting on the neck or just over the area being treated.

Two of the TTouch techniques involve the abdomen and back. The Belly Lift is a technique with which every veterinarian, especially equine practitioners, should be familiar. Hands or arms are placed flat under the animal's thorax, just caudal to the elbows. For large animals such as cows, two people can join hands from each side or hold a towel under the animal's abdomen. The chest is gently lifted upward, held for 10 to 15 seconds, then slowly released. The slow release is important and appears to contribute to increased peristalsis, a beneficial effect. The lifts should begin just caudal to the elbow and move slowly toward the rear, with care being taken in the flank area, which is particularly sensitive. Several repetitions can be done at each session. The Back Lift is similar to the Belly Lift, using gentle pressure along the midline to get the back to rise, stretching and relaxing the back muscles. The Badger Rake can also be used, especially on horses; in this maneuver the fingers are gently (or firmly, depending on the sensitivity of the animal) raked across the abdominal muscles beginning on the far side of the belly and continuing partially up the near side.

Gently manipulating the ears has become a staple of the TTEAM bodywork for many reasons. Working on the ears from the base out to the tips appears to stimulate all the acupuncture points in the ear. Because ears contain acupuncture points that affect the whole body, earwork is particularly effective. The tip of the ear is considered a "shock" point similar to the acupuncture point GV-26 at the base of the nostril. (For more information on acupuncture, refer to Chapters 10 and 11.)

Mouthwork can be done on many species of animals. Innervation to the mouth is connected to the limbic system (Halderman, 1992), the part of the brain that controls emotions and learning. Mouthwork is beneficial for a wide variety of problems, especially in horses who frequently bite or nip. The lips and nostrils should be gently manipulated, moving the tissue in soft circles. Next, the hand can be inserted in the patient's mouth along the gums as the gentle, circular motion continues. As the animal relaxes, the practitioner should cover a larger area of the mouth, spending about 10 minutes at each session. Obviously, appropriate caution should be exercised for animals with a history of biting.

Leg exercises are another aspect of TTEAM. The legs are made to perform nonhabitual movements that increase their range of motion and flexibility. Theoretically the movements reprogram the brain to move the body in a different way. The leg exercises are extremely valuable, but because they are difficult, the reader should consult the reference list for detailed information.

Ground Exercises

TTEAM ground exercises are excellent for training (or retraining) the animal's body and mind. They teach focus, eye-foot coordination, and balance. Often when these exercises are initiated, animals who previously paid little attention to their handlers appear to concentrate on each movement. Many supporting exercises can be performed with the basic ground exercises discussed here. If a veterinarian enjoys rehabilitation work, a technician trained in TTEAM exercises may be a valuable addition to the practice.

The Labyrinth is a type of maze excellent for developing balance, coordination, and focus. It is constructed from poles that vary in size depending on the type of animal, from 12-foot poles for horses to pencil-sized rods for cats. The animal is led through the Labyrinth very slowly, often one step at a time in the beginning. The pace is varied a bit to teach balance and focus, but the animal is never allowed to rush through. Facial expressions and body language reveal that the animal is thinking as it goes through the Labyrinth (Fig. 15-1).

Pick-up sticks are a simple way to teach eye-foot coordination, although some animals need to do preparatory exercises first. Basically, appropriately sized poles are arranged in a pile, with enough room between them for the animal's foot to step. The animal walks through the pile one step at a time and is forced to place each foot differently. The Star is another exercise that causes the body to perform different movements on each side. Poles are placed in a curve on a bale of hay (or smaller object) with one end of each pole high on the bale and the other on the ground. As the animal negotiates between the poles, the inside leg must be raised higher than the outside leg.

A tool frequently used as an aid is the Wand. The basic Wand is identical to a 4-foot dressage whip, but because it is used as an extension of the hand, the name

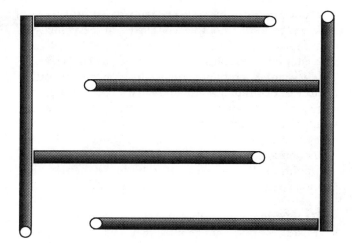

Fig. 15-1 Poles of any material are used to create a maze or labyrinth for the animals to walk through and thereby learn balance and focus. The size of the poles range from 12 feet long for horses to small-diameter plastic pipe for dogs and pencil-thickness rods for cats.

Wand was adopted for a positive connotation. On small animals a shorter (3-foot) Wand may be used, and for animals that are very frightened of being touched, a feather can be used. Animals who are too fearful to be touched often tolerate gentle stroking with the wand before hand contact is made. This technique has been used successfully with zoo animals.

TTEAM incorporates a number of other training devices that have been found successful, gentle, and consistent with the philosophy. Many animals can be trained for improved physical coordination by applying an elastic bandage or rope in a figure-eight shape across the chest and over the back. Ropes across the chest are used to drive horses, rather than traditional bridles and reins. The TTEAM training bit commonly used for horses looks like a common Western curb bit, but it is engineered differently and may help a horse balance itself better while being lunged. Instead of a traditional collar on dogs, a halter is placed over the dog's head. With horses a chain is used across their noses for subtle commands or aids. Many more useful ideas can be implemented depending on the animal's individual needs.

Use of TTEAM in Veterinary Practice

This section describes the incorporation of certain TTEAM exercises and bodywork into veterinary practice. As practitioners become more skilled at TTEAM, they find more uses for TTEAM and observe that their patients are less resistant. Various books and videos provide more complete information, and training seminars are held around the world. The practitioner should contact the TTEAM office for details.

TTEAM works best when the animal and veterinarian trust each other; however, trust can also develop through the use of TTEAM. If the animal seems resistant, anxious, and uncooperative, more work is necessary to develop the necessary trust. An experienced TTEAM practitioner may be consulted to help refine the technique. Beginners should remember to slow down, refocus, and practice regularly.

Equine Practice

The equine practice presents many situations in which a few minutes of TTEAM make life easier for veterinarians and more pleasant for horses. Perhaps the most important exercise for most horses is teaching them to lower their heads for all procedures. Working with horses who are thinking rather than merely reacting is much easier. When their heads are raised and their necks tense, horses are in the fight-or-flight mode and training becomes more difficult. A long chain-lead shank should be woven over the noseband of the halter and snapped to the ring on the cheek-piece of the opposite side of the halter (rather than to the nose ring) to prevent the halter from pulling over the eye. The purpose of the chain is to send a definitive message to the horse by putting pressure on the top of the nose and poll. Whereas the traditional way of attaching the lead rope under the halter encourages the horse to raise its head, the gentle tugs and releases of this method reward the horse for lowering its head. The practitioner should also praise the horse when it relaxes, even momentarily. Beginners should be patient during verbal instruction because horses learn at different rates. However, once the horse has mastered the command "head down," it will remember not to panic when the head is caught or the halter pulled.

Horses often perceive veterinarians as their enemies, and cooperation is often obtained only after a fight, when the horse learns to fear the practitioner. TTEAM may appear time consuming at first because bodywork must often be performed at locations distant from the targeted area to gain the horse's trust. However, in addition to its other merits, TTEAM actually saves time over the long run.

Because veterinarians give injections so frequently, they are encouraged to spend a few minutes using TTouch on the area to be injected and following up afterward with more TTouch. These efforts generally result in a more cooperative horse. After receiving TTouch, even horses who have never been handled can receive injections or have blood drawn relatively quietly. Moreover, performing TTouch for 2 minutes may help prevent swelling and soreness at an injection site.

Deworming some horses (or administering any oral medication) is often difficult. A few minutes spent performing mouthwork and teaching horses to lower their heads can make the situation less stressful. The Lying Leopard should be done on the outside of the lips, and then the hand can be inserted into the lower part of the mouth and slid back and forth over the gums. The upper lip should be handled the same way. When the dewormer is finally introduced, the horse is generally much more receptive. The owner should also be encouraged to practice this technique.

Cleaning sheaths is never a pleasant task, and many horses object strongly. Many mares object when their udders are handled. Many horses have sensitive flanks and abdomens and dislike being touched in these areas. TTouch circles, beginning along the ribs where most horses are comfortable about being touched, may help the animals accept contact at more sensitive areas. The practitioner should move slowly toward the abdomen and back toward the sheath or udder, adjusting the pressure according to the horse's level of comfort. If necessary, a front leg can be lifted to prevent kicking. The circles are done in connected lines, with more time spent at sensitive areas to ensure that the horse is comfortable. The loose skin around the sheath can be worked in a manner similar to the mouthwork described previously. While cleaning the sheath, the practitioner should continue to make gentle, circular movements, preferably with a warm, damp cloth, warmed petroleum jelly, or oil. Although not all horses

find this pleasant, many will become much more manageable.

TTouch can be used anywhere horses object to being touched, including injured areas, which are touched very lightly. Work should begin in an area where the horse is comfortable being touched and slowly moved to the problem area. If the whole body is a problem, wands can be used as an extension of the hands. Generally, horses do not feel threatened when hands are not touching their bodies. The horse should become accustomed to the wand and gradually allow hand contact.

TTouch can also make foal handling less stressful. Two Wands are used for foals that are afraid of being touched. The foal should be stroked with Wands before other restraint is attempted. As the foal relaxes, the practitioner slowly moves closer to touch the foal. TTouch may be ideal as the first contact with the foal.

Some cases of nonsurgical colic may be treated using TTouch earwork alone. Along with earwork, Belly Lifts help increase peristalsis by moving gas or impaction through the intestines and helping to normalize gut function. Horses in endurance rides who have reduced gut sounds and function respond well to Belly Lifts.

Choked horses also tend to respond to earwork and deep TTouch circles done with the fist in the jugular groove. The area around the trachea can be rocked back and forth with a little gentle shaking to loosen the esophagus. Horses that resent having their ears handled may become receptive during distress. When a few minutes are spent working their ears, horses relax and become much less head-shy. Horses in distress and shock also benefit from earwork, and owners may be shown how to treat the ears while practitioners work on the rest of the body.

During rehabilitation from injuries or neurologic disorders, ground exercises can increase coordination. The neural pathways need new input for reestablishment, and TTEAM is an excellent adjunct to other rehabilition techniques. Exercises like the Labyrinth, Star, Pick-up Sticks, and Leg Circles stimulate new neural pathways more effectively than hand-walking or even cavaletti work.

During a difficult birth, Belly Lifts can be an excellent way to start contractions in a fatigued animal without resorting to more forceful techniques. Because the animal is prone during labor, Belly Lifts can be done on one side at a time. Working at the base of the ears, where the Triple Heater meridian is located (see Chapters 10 and 11), and gradually working to the tip of the ear, where the shock point is located, can be effective during a difficult labor. Various TTouches can be used over the abdomen also.

TTEAM for Horse Owners

TTEAM lends itself well to client participation. Veterinarians can give clients exercises for follow-up work. They can also instruct clients over the telephone during emergency situations before help is available. For colic or choke, clients can begin Belly Lifts and earwork as soon as they have called the veterinarian. Taking time to explain or show these techniques to clients is helpful, particularly for clients with many horses or horses with frequent colic problems,. Even clients unfamiliar with TTEAM can be instructed over the phone to perform simple exercises. In an emergency, clients may be upset and should be cautioned to do the exercises slowly.

After suture or surgery, clients can do Raccoon TTouches around the wound to prevent or reduce swelling when they change the bandages. While a bandage or cast is in place, clients can do Lying Leopard TTouches or any of the circular TTouches on the areas above and below the bandage. Python Lifts can be done to improve circulation in the leg. Clients can begin doing the TTouches when the injury occurs if they know the basic circle or Raccoon TTouch. If a leg has been involved, gentle use of the Leg Circles may help preserve joint mobility, even though the horse may be lame. Research has shown that in traditional Chinese medicine, treatment of the opposite leg has an effect on the injured leg. If the injured leg is too painful, the opposite leg can be treated using TTouch circles, Leg Circles and Python Lifts.

Difficult horses may be handled more easily if clients learn about TTEAM and apply it on a regular basis. Whereas rough handling of foals often leads to chiropractic problems, TTEAM can be used safely and effectively from birth onwards and is an excellent way to teach foals basic skills. Adult horses who crowd the handler or run over people can learn self-control with ground exercises. Many chiropractic problems can be prevented when owners convey their expectations in positive ways instead of pulling their horses roughly. Horses with annoying habits such as biting and fussing during handling benefit from regular mouthwork and earwork, particularly during veterinary examinations. Earwork is relaxing, calming many unruly horses.

An unpublished study by veterinarians at the Bitsa Sports Center in Moscow, Russia, measured ACTH levels of horses receiving TTEAM on a regular basis. The 10 horses receiving TTEAM had significantly lower levels of ACTH than the 10 horses not receiving TTEAM. Both groups had the same workload. Many horses are under a great deal of stress, especially during transport and competition, and TTEAM may decrease some common stress-related conditions such as colic and poor performance.

Surgery is another area in which TTEAM can be beneficial. The potential for injury during postanesthetic recovery is great, and the stress-relieving properties of TTEAM are beneficial to many horses during this critical time. Earwork and TTouch (performed anywhere that is safe during the recovery period) may lead to calmer recoveries. Before surgery, earwork, TTouches, and Python Lifts may be useful, especially if the surgery involves the leg.

When euthanasia is necessary, TTouches make the process less upsetting for horse and owner, creating a special bond and a sense of closure. Owners feel that they are contributing to the process and are less inclined to resist it, making the veterinarian's job easier.

Small Animal Practice

Although TTEAM was originally developed for use in horses, its use in small animals has expanded greatly to include handling of difficult pet animals as well as performance animals. Many ideas presented in the equine section also apply to small animals. In a small animal practice a technician knowledgeable about TTEAM can make the clinic work more smoothly. The skilled practitioner can teach the entire support staff the basics of handling difficult animals safely and quietly. After surgery or any other painful procedure, an animal's discomfort can be relieved with TTouches—particularly the Raccoon TTouch around the incision or wound—or gentle Belly Lifts to restore intestinal function after abdominal surgery or trauma. Anyone doing wildlife work or postsurgical rehabilitation will find TTEAM helpful.

Animals that bite when fearful can often be touched easily with the initial use of Wands while the animals are caged or their owners are present. The Wand is used as an extension of the arm, and most animals relax after just a few minutes of stroking, which begins on the least threatening areas. A few minutes of TTouches can change an atmosphere from antagonistic to peaceful. Mouthwork can then be used if the animal seems approachable. If the animal has a serious habit of biting, an experienced practitioner must assist in doing the mouthwork. A towel or cloth may be used for mouthwork as well. If the animal is staying in the clinic, regular work for a few minutes a day can calm previously unapproachable animals.

Nail trimming is often traumatic for everyone involved. TTEAM TTouches may be used, starting on areas that are not threatening or sensitive. The type of TTouch selected depends on the amount of pressure the animal needs and is able to enjoy. The practitioner should work slowly down the leg with Python Lifts and TTouch circles toward the feet; a Wand (or feather) may be used before application of the hands. Animals who usually require tranquilization may become much more cooperative when these techniques are used.

All animals in shock or with serious injuries will benefit from earwork. Trained technicians should begin working the ears as soon as practically possible and continue at every opportunity during the treatment until a positive response is observed. Belly Lifts can be used for abdominal disorders (such as bloating) to normalize intestinal function.

TTEAM may be used for all animals, including birds, reptiles, and wild animals. Wild animals are especially afraid and do not understand human interaction. A few minutes with a feather or Wand can reduce the animal's stress level and increase the chance that treatment will succeed. Both the San Diego Zoo and the Zurich Zoo, among others, have incorporated TTEAM into their programs with much success, and many have subsequently improved overall conditions for the animals with this increased awareness of their needs.

Veterinarians who work in animal shelters can ease the stress, pain, and fear experienced by these animals. Even euthanizing the animals can be done more compassionately with a few minutes of TTouches. If the shelter staff is trained in a few of the basic TTouches and work with the wand, animals that have never been properly handled can become more manageable and more likely to find homes, whereas without TTEAM they might cower in the back of their cages and never be considered for adoption.

TTEAM for Small Animal Owners

Clients can be instructed to use TTEAM both regularly and during emergencies. As with the horse, even clients with no training in TTEAM can be told over the telephone to do earwork on the way into the clinic or TTouches or Belly Lifts on the abdomen. TTEAM can be added to the discharge instructions to speed healing after injuries and surgeries. Clients who prefer holistic treatment generally want to contribute to the healing process, and they enjoy the extra bonding that occurs. The TTouches appear to speed the healing process, especially the Raccoon TTouch around wounds and the various circle touches around bandaged areas. Belly Lifts are excellent for any abdominal trauma or surgery and can be done regularly by the clients at home.

Difficult animals may become more manageable when clients use TTEAM exercises and perform bodywork at home or in a supervised setting. Very difficult animals often need experienced help; regular TTEAM training sessions at the clinic or sponsored by the clinic may be beneficial for both clients, who gain experience in a supervised setting, and clinic staff, whose jobs are made easier by more manageable patients. A poster explaining the basic TTouches or a video on TTEAM may be displayed in the waiting room to reduce patient stress and relieve client boredom. This information encourages clients to use TTouches instead of habitually stroking their animals.

Euthanasia is difficult for everyone involved, and having clients participate in the experience using TTouches is beneficial. Clients feel they are participating and helping the animal through the use of circular touches, earwork, or Belly Lifts, depending on the comfort and response of each animal. The client can do TTEAM at home before bringing the animal into the clinic, or the work can be done in the clinic by the veterinarian and/or the client just before the injection. These techniques help clients deal with their emotions and understand that veterinarians are a caring part of the health care team.

Conclusion

TTEAM can improve the veterinary practice in many ways. The physical and emotional contact often enhances the relationship between the veterinarian, client, and animal. Practically speaking, TTEAM makes the veterinarian's interactions with animals less physically and emotionally challenging. TTEAM encourages people to participate in the healing process, an important aspect of holistic healing. TTEAM also offers owners of abused animals or animals with behavior problems a way to reeducate and socialize these animals .

TTEAM often fosters a special connection between people and animals. People learn positive ways to interact with their animals based on the idea of partnership instead of dominance. Many people find that other aspects of their lives improve as they learn to work with TTEAM. The spiritual side of relationships, as each individual defines it, begins to surface. Various cultures recognize the importance of the circle of healing, a healing energy that TTouch circles represent.

References

Cade M: *High performance mind-mastering brain waves for insight, healing and creativity,* New York, 1995, J Tarcher-Putnam, p 213.

Feldenkrais M: *Awareness through movement,* New York, 1972, Harper & Row.

Halderman S: *Principles and practice of chiropractic,* San Mateo, Calif, 1992, Appleton & Lange.

Tellington-Jones L: *The Tellington touch,* New York, 1992, Viking Penguin.

Selected Readings

Tellington-Jones L, Bruns U: *Introduction to Tellington-Jones equine awareness methods,* Millwood, NY, 1988, Break Through Publications.

Tellington-Jones L: *The touch of magic for horses,* LaQuinta, Calif, 1994a, Thane Marketing (video).

Tellington-Jones L: *The touch of magic for dogs,* LaQuinta, Calif, 1994b, Thane Marketing (video).

Tellington-Jones L, Hood R: *The Tellington TTouch for dogs and puppies,* LaQuinta, Calif, 1994c, Thane Marketing International (video).

Tellington-Jones L, Taylor S: *Getting in TTouch,* Pomfret, Vt, 1995, Trafalgar Press.

*T*TEAM Offices

TTEAM Training USA
PO 3793
Santa Fe, New Mexico 87501-0793
1-800-854-TEAM

TTEAM Training Canada
5435 Rochdell
Vernon, British Columbia
Canada V1B 3E8
604-545-2336
(This office publishes a 30 page quarterly journal.)

Acknowledgments

I would like to thank Linda Tellington-Jones and Kate Riordan for their help in researching this chapter.

Energetic Medicine

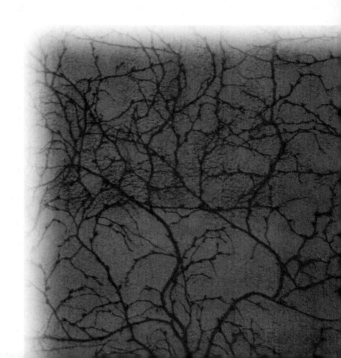

Chapter 16

*I*ntroduction to Bioenergetic Medicine

JOANNE STEFANATOS

Using various forms of energetic frequencies for the diagnosis, prevention, and treatment of disease, energy medicine encompasses many modalities, including acupuncture, homeopathy, low-level laser therapy, and magnetic field therapy. All traditional medical philosophies throughout the world include elements of energy medicine. The principles of energy medicine originate in quantum physics. Bioenergetic medicine is the study of human and animal bodies as dynamic electromagnetic fields existing in an electromagnetic environment. Based on Einstein's theories of quantum physics, these energetic concepts are being integrated into medicine for a comprehensive approach to disease diagnosis, prevention, and treatment.

Newton's Mechanistic Model versus Einstein's Quantum Model of Physics and Their Relationship to Medicine

A brief review of Newton's mechanistic concepts and Einstein's quantum energetic theories of physics is necessary to distinguish the differences between these two models and introduce the concept of energy medicine. Modern medicine currently uses energetic concepts in the study of electroencephalograms (EEGs), electromyograms (EMGs), electrocardiograms (ECGs), nuclear magnetic resonance (NMR) studies, and many other applications.

Founded on the laws of biochemistry and physics, Western medicine views the body essentially as a machine that can be modified and repaired—the body being equal to the sum of its parts. This paradigm in physics and medicine was introduced by Sir Isaac Newton (1642-1727), whose monumental work *The Principia Mathematica* described the laws of motion and gravity that form the physical basis for the mechanistic model of reality. Newton de-scribed the motion of the universe, and his three elementary laws of physics are a cornerstone of modern medicine (Gamow, 1961):

Law I: Every body continues in its state of rest, or of uniform motion in a straight line, unless it is compelled to change that state by forces upon it.

Law II. The change of motion (i.e., of mechanical momentum) is proportional to the motive force impressed and is made in the direction of the right line in which that force is impressed.

Law III. To every action there is always opposed an equal reaction: or, the mutual actions of two bodies upon each other are always equal, and directed to contrary parts.

Newtonian thinking revealed the benefits of a rational, objective approach to nature and life. The mechanistic model viewed the human body as a machine equal to the sum of its parts, with all operations explained in mechanical terms and biochemical equations. Scientists applied the Newtonian model in an attempt to move body function from the realm of the divine and into a mechanistic world that could be understood and manipulated (Capra, 1925). Newton's paradigm was considered dogma from the eighteenth to the nineteenth centuries.

Newton's model of reality saw the body as a machine controlled by the brain and the peripheral nervous system—the ultimate biologic computer. The first Newtonian medical approaches were surgery (removal of diseased parts) and drug therapy. Both surgery and drug therapy target tissues of the body to either strengthen or destroy any aberrantly functioning cells, depending on the need. Therefore both approaches subscribe to the Newtonian view of the human body as an intricate clockwork mechanism of physical organs, chemistry, enzymes, and membrane receptors.

According to Gerber, however, "pharmacology and surgical approaches appear incomplete because they ignore the Vital Force which animates and breathes life into the biomachinery of living systems" (1988). Newtonian thinking assumed that the whole can be predicted by the sum of its parts; unlike machines, however, humans and animals are more than the sum of their parts. Newtonian thinkers saw the universe as an orderly and predictable grand clockwork and the body as a complex machine. Advances in biomedical technology such as mechanical replacements and parts for the organs of the body (for example, artificial heart and hemodialysis machines) have given us a wide range of replacement organs, but knowledge of methods to reverse or prevent many chronic diseases is still lacking. Newtonian philosophy has limited the methods used to bring about healing as well as our perception of the body's ability to heal itself. In fact, contemporary Western medicine has ignored the body's innate ability to heal.

For rising numbers of chronic degenerative diseases in the Western world, chemical medication can offer only palliative treatment and no real cure (Becker, 1990). Some researchers claim that 60% of problems presented daily to primary care physicians defy diagnosis and are assumed to be neurotic or psychosomatic in origin (Goldberg, 1993). Traditional drug therapies pose a serious threat of side effects, along with an alarming increase in iatrogenic diseases. The main emphasis of Western chemical-based medicine is crisis intervention rather than prevention. Convinced that the body is a machine that cannot heal itself, Western medicine offers powerful drugs and mechanical technologies as the only appropiate therapies. This emphasis on disease rather than health has caused growing dissatisfaction among consumers of Western medicine (Goldberg, 1993). Recent studies have confirmed that many of them are willing to explore alternative approaches (Eisenberg, 1993).

Veterinary education has focused primarily on the mechanistic approach to medicine and life in general. If something is broken or malfunctioning, veterinarians simply repair or remove it with medical technology. The molecular theory of disease causation and the notion that mind and matter do not interact are scientific dogma. The biochemical approach of conventional scientific medicine does not recognize the existence of energy fields and the importance of the mind in the healing process.

After the last 45 years of technologic advances and medical research, scientists are still focused upon the microscopic, micromolecular mechanisms behind disease causation. They have only recently begun to study the reasons that people and animals stay healthy. Dissatisfied with the prevailing reductionism of Western medicine, many of these scientists are seeking a holistic approach. As our present knowledge of the universe is expanding beyond Newtonian boundaries, Western medicine is beginning to acknowledge energy phenomena and incorporate the principles of energy medicine.

When Albert Einstein first expounded his theories, they were considered radical. Before his ideas were validated by other scientists, 60 years elapsed. Eventually, however, Einstein's quantum model replaced the Newtonian mechanistic model of humankind and the universe. Einstein believed that each human being is a microcosm, a reflection of the universal macrocosm (Einstein, 1954, 1961). Einstein saw human beings as multidimensional organisms made up of physical and cellular systems in dynamic interplay with complex regulatory energetic fields. He believed the body is more than the sum of its parts and that electricity and magnetism are the basis of life. Fellow physicists began to comprehend the true relationship between matter and energy and effect a transition from the fragmented, Newtonian, mechanistic understanding of health to the more inclusive Einsteinian quantum-mechanical worldview.[*]

Energetic concepts of medicine have been described in all traditional medical philosophies throughout the world. In traditional Chinese medicine (TCM), the primal energy is known as *Qi* (also spelled *Chi* or *Ki*) or life energy force. In Ayurvedic medicine, it is commonly called *Prana;* in homeopathy, it is known as the *Vital Force.* The closest correlate in Western medicine is the bioelectric current measured in electrocardiograms, electromyograms, and electroencephalograms. Because science and medical technology have developed more sophisticated instrumentation, the existence of bioelectricity and electromagnetic fields has been scientifically validated (Barnard, 1969; Becker, 1961b, 1963, 1969; Burr, 1939).

Energetic force creates order in living systems and constantly rebuilds and renews cellular components. When energetic force leaves the body at death, the physical body slowly decays and becomes a disorganized collection of chemicals. Energetic force is unique, distinguishing living from nonliving systems and people from machines. Medical therapies that promote this energy and the body's own healing mechanism should be given primary consideration.

Bioenergetic Medicine

The principles of energy medicine originate in quantum physics. Bioenergetic medicine is the study of human and animal bodies as dynamic electromagnetic fields existing in an electromagnetic environment—the universe. All chronic disease conditions manifest first at the level of energy (Becker, 1985; Tiller, 1971).

The electromagnetic fields (EMF) emanating from bacteria, viruses, and toxic substances affect the cells of the body and weaken its constitution. Immunosuppression is a disorder at the electromagnetic and physical levels that

---

[*]Bohr (1965); de Broglie (1979); Heisenberg (1971); Kuhn (1977); Planck (1968); Popper (1959); Schrodinger (1967).

manifests itself in the body in the form of symptoms (Brown, 1975; Royal, Mayfield, 1983; Tiller, 1971). No antibiotic or drug, no matter how powerful, will save an animal if the vital force of healing is suppressed or lacking. The final destruction of toxins is conducted within the body by the body's own defense systems. A change in energy must precede a change in structure. The ultimate quest of preventive medicine is to find and eliminate the disease before it appears on a clinical and destructive plane. Veterinary medicine is on the verge of reaching a new understanding of biologic processes, medical diagnosis, and therapy that recognizes the electromagnetic environment. Energy medicine is the medicine of the future; it will allow us to return to true preventive medicine—and that will be a quantum leap.

Historical Development of Energy Concepts

The visionary ideas of Einstein, Heisenberg, Bohr, Bohm, and other physicists influenced the move toward a holistic view of matter, energy, and the universe. New conceptions of health and illness have eradicated the traditional separation between science and spirituality. The most important figures in medicine and science have suggested the presence of something that exceeds the power of logic and observation: the timeless quality of spirit. Gerber makes the following observation:

> The unseen connection between the physical body and the subtle forces of spirit holds the key to understanding the inner relations between matter and energy. The spiritual element is a part of existence that must be taken into account if we are to truly understand the basic nature of health, illness and growth (1988).

Western medicine is believed to have begun in 500 BC in ancient Greece with Hippocrates, the father of medicine. From the days of Hippocrates to Paracelsus to Mesmer to Galvani, the biologists and physicists were certain that a life force existed, that all living things have the ability to heal themselves, and that the whole of the body is more than the sum of its parts. Paracelsus believed that thoughts had a physical reality and could produce an action on the physical plane. He recognized the power of thoughts to heal. Paracelsus saw the defect in reductionist philosophy several centuries before the rise of reductionism and built his system of medicine on the legacy of the vital force, which can be traced back from the Greeks to prehistoric man (Becker, 1990).

Luigi Galvani, an obstetrician and anatomist in the late 1700s, researched the electrical nature of the life force and believed he found it when he observed that muscles contract when connected to the spinal cord with metallic wires. He termed this phenomenon *animal electricity,* recognizing that it was produced by the body. Galvani also

discovered direct current, or continuously flowing electrons. He established the relationship between biology and electricity, and animal electricity was believed to be the vital force that thinkers had sought.

Allesandro Volta discovered that animal electricity flowing from injured tissue could be evoked by bringing the contracting muscle into contact with a cut end of the spinal cord itself. This was called the *current of injury,* which refers to the electrical current found in any injured tissue (Becker, Selden, 1985). Volta's work with animal electricity is now called *electrobiology.* Matteucci confirmed that when contact is made with a nerve to stimulate muscle contraction, the electrical action potential precedes the muscle contraction (Becker, Marino, 1982; Becker, Selden, 1985; Geddes, Hoff, 1971). Even in the eighteenth century, experiments showed that millivolt nerve and muscle potentials are measurable.

Nikola Tesla, considered to be the father of electrical engineering, discovered that during the thinking process, cerebral neurons produce waves received by other neurons, which results in the transfer of thought from one person's cerebrum to another. Miller (1977) observed that thoughts produce a moving wave pattern inside an atomic cloud chamber. In 1871, Julius Bernstein explained the nerve impulse. He believed that the ions (charged atoms of sodium, potassium, and chloride) inside the nerve cell differ from outside tissue fluid, a difference that results in the nerve-cell membrane being electricically charged, or polarized. Membrane polarization is the basis for conductance of the nerve impulse. At that time, anatomists working with microscopes discovered that the nerve did not actually contact the muscle because a synaptic gap existed between them. The fact that an electrical-biochemical connection is the basis for energy medicine was not established until 1921, when physiologist Otto Loewi proved that transmission of the nerve impulse across the synaptic gap is also chemical (Becker, 1990). Loewi received the Nobel Prize in 1936.

In the nineteenth century, Michael Faraday discovered that an electrical current can produce a magnetic field, a finding that led to the conversion of magnetism into electricity, an interchange called *electromagnetic (EM) induction.* In 1860, James Clerk Maxwell discovered that electricity could be converted into magnetism, producing electromagnetic oscillations able to travel at the speed of light. In 1887, Heinrich Hertz showed that an oscillating electrical current emitted an electromagnetic wave of invisible radiation (Wolf, 1981). This electromagnetic wave shared characteristics with visible light waves.

Max Planck discovered that matter absorbed heat energy and emitted light energy in "chunks" instead of a continuous wave. Planck's mathematical formula is as follows:

$$E = hf$$

or

(Energy = the frequency of the light emitted (f) × a constant (h)

Using this equation, Planck proved that light waves do not behave in the same way as mechanical waves. The heat energy absorbed by the material or emitted as light energy depends on the frequency of light emitted. (Einstein later called these chunks *quanta* of energy and noted that they carry a definite amount of energy proportional to their frequency, a discovery that heralded the Quantum Age of Physics.)

By the turn of the century the idea that medicine should be based completely on the chemical-mechanistic model was firmly established. In 1909 Paul Ehrlich discovered the "cure" for syphilis in an arsenic compound. Ehrlich called this "a magic bullet," a chemical specifically designed to seek out and destroy the targeted bacterium. He predicted that for the rest of the twentieth century, medicine would discover specific solutions for all diseases. The biologists and physicists reduced life to chemical machinery, believing that each disease had a single cause and therapy and the only valid therapies were surgical or chemical. Not coincidentally, Ehrlich began to believe that science would provide cures for all diseases during the technologic explosion of World War I, when the antibiotic penicillin revolutionized the practice of medicine. At that time, scientists believed that electrical currents administered to the body could have an effect only in strengths high enough to produce shock or burns; electrical force below this level could not affect the body at all.

Bioelectrical Energy

When an organism did not function properly, scientists in the past reasoned that structural defects arising from chemical imbalances were the cause. Physicists postulated that chemical-level homeostasis might depend on a connection with a deeper-level energy structure in the organism but were never able clearly to describe this connection. Currently, experts are becoming increasingly aware of the interaction between chemical states and electromagnetic fields.

Evidence That the Body Has an Electrical-Biochemical Connection

Neuropsychiatric research suggests that small electrical currents between specific brain points give rise to the same behavioral changes observed with certain specific brain-stimulating chemicals (Brown, 1975; Woolridge, 1963). Low-level direct current (DC) between 10 to 12 amp/mm^2 and 10 to 9 amp/mm^2 applied to leukocytes in vitro produces cellular regeneration, whereas greater current densities produce cellular degeneration (Tiller, 1988). Becker's research in limb regeneration in salamanders showed that the control system that started, regulated, and stopped healing is electrical. Becker collaborated with Andrew Bassett of Columbia University to research fracture healing and bone growth in dogs and discovered that large amounts of bone growth surround the negative electrode, whereas resorption of bone occurs at the positive electrode. This fact suggests that negative electrical polarity stimulates growth, and positive polarity inhibits it. Low-level DC currents cause cellular regeneration, tissue repair, and fracture healing (Becker, 1972a; Becker, Murray, 1970). Although scientists do not yet understand the detailed pathways whereby electric and magnetic fields couple into cellular metabolism, they are becoming increasingly confident that energy connections exist.

Davies summarizes the paradigmatic shift as follows:

> It is often said that physics invented the mechanistic-reductionist philosophy, taught it to the biologists and then abandoned it themselves. It cannot be denied that modern physics has a strongly holistic flavor, and that this is due in large part to the influence of quantum theory (Davies,1988).

Einstein upset the Newtonian mechanistic concepts when he discovered that light appeared as waves only if one observed it over fairly long time intervals. He proved that $E = mc^2$, or matter and energy are dual expressions of the same substance. At the quantum level of subatomic particles, all matter is literally frozen, particularized energy fields (frozen light). Light and matter both have frequency characteristics. The higher the frequency of matter, the less density it contains. The energy contained within a particle is equivalent to the product of its mass multiplied by the speed of light squared, and each particle of matter contains an enormous amount of potential energy. Einstein's equation suggests that matter and energy are interconvertible. Einstein believed that human beings and animals are complex biologic mechanisms in dynamic interplay with a series of interpenetrating vital energy fields that interface with physical cellular systems (1954). The body-electric concept is based on the recognition that all matter is energy and all living bodies are dynamic energetic systems.

The first scientist to use high-frequency electromagnetic fields (EMFs) in biologic experiments, Georges Lakhovsky compiled his observations about the effect of electrical and radio waves on living organisms (1970). These fields had a frequency of 150 megahertz with a wavelength of 2 meters. According to Lakhovsky, the nucleus of a living cell can be compared to an electrical oscillating circuit. The nucleus consists of tubular filaments, chromosomes, and mitochondria made of insulating material and filled with a conducting fluid containing all mineral salts found in sea water. These filaments are comparable to oscillating circuits endowed with capacity and self-inductance and therefore capable of oscillating according to a specific frequency. Lakhovsky proved through photographs that "every living being emits radiations; the great majority of living beings are capable of receiving and of detecting waves" (1970).

Equating health with the "oscillating equilibrium" of living cells and disease with "oscillatory disequilibrium,"

Lakhovsky speculated that the living organism and invading microbes engage in a war of radiation. Lakhovsky's theories have since been confirmed by Becker and Selden (1987). Lakhovsky summarizes his theory as follows: "Life is created by radiation; Life is maintained by radiation; Life is destroyed by oscillatory disequilibrium" (1970).

Our Inability to Perceive Energy Does Not Invalidate Its Existence

All animals, including insects and birds, emit radiations. Sensory limitations prevent humans from perceiving the radiations of living beings. However, these radiations have been detected by means of the spectroscope and photographic plate. In 1939, Cremonese made direct photographic records of radiations emitted by human subjects and their saliva and blood specimens. Until that point the growth process could be scientifically explained. However, scientists did not understand the control system that starts this process and regulates it to produce a desired effect. The mitogenic radiation given off by rootlets of growing plants and vegetables has since been linked by Gurwitsch and Frank to the ultraviolet region of the light spectrum. They showed that the growth stimulus is oscillatory in character and associated with a specific wavelength, which confirmed Lakhovsky's theories (Smith, Best, 1989). Experiments by Reiter and Gabor showed that embryonic tissues and malignant tumors possess a high radiation potential varying in intensity according to the rate of growth. Reiter and Gabor succeeded in measuring the wavelength of radiating tissues and modifying the development of se-

lected organisms by subjecting them to a certain range of ultraviolet rays (Lakhovsky, 1939).

Becker demonstrated that the body not only heals itself but can regenerate missing body parts and that the control system to start, regulate, and stop healing is electrical (1990). In his experiments with limb regeneration in frogs and salamanders, Becker suggested electromagnetic energy as the substance regulating limb regeneration, pointing out that the electrical current is negative in polarity during regeneration and positive during scarification healing (Becker, 1990).

Szent-Gyorgyi showed that electrical conduction and semiconduction play an active role in living cells (Szent-Gyorgyi, 1941). After discovering that semiconductance is a property specific to the crystallike structure of proteins constituting the cells, he eventually proved the existence of acupuncture meridians in the body and described their electrical nature, an accomplishment for which he received the Nobel Prize.

Becker demonstrated that DC currents arising from a variety of tissues are propagated along the glial and Schwann cells, which act as semiconductors. Membranes are capacitators, and mitochondria, with their electron transport chains, can be viewed as tiny batteries or electrical power sources (Becker, 1985; Becker, Marino, 1982).

Early experiments with electromagnetic fields caused researchers to shift their focus from physiochemical cellular reactions to biologic systems in continuous interaction with a new frequency realm—that of the bioenergy field (Smith, Best, 1989) (Fig. 16-1).

The diagnostic application of x-rays provided a critical

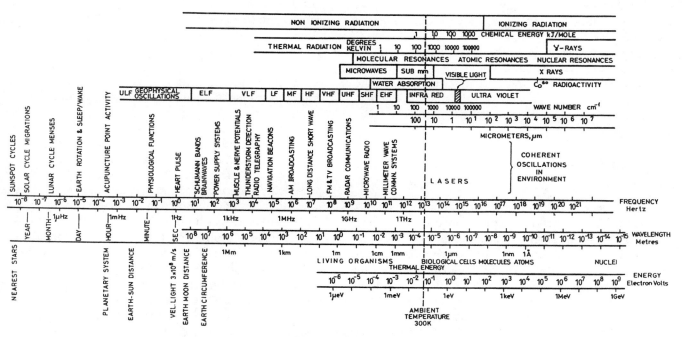

Fig. 16-1 The spectrum of electromagnetic radiation.

look into a previously unseen world within the human body. The development of diagnostic x-ray equipment has increased our understanding of electromagnetic radiation biophysics. The therapeutic application of electricity was not extensively explored until the twentieth century.

George de la Warr made the following observation: "For some time it was thought unlikely that any radiation could exist with a higher energy than gamma rays (they are higher than x-rays), but at length, physicists began to notice something unaccountable was happening to their electroscopes" (Smith, Best, 1989). This phenomenon was determined to be cosmic rays, considered the highest possible form of energy. At the forefront of science today are investigations of the "tachyon," a particle that moves faster than the speed of light (Tiller, 1987b). With the invention of the spectroscope and atomic cloud chamber—the most sensitive physical tool to date—we are able to see "bioenergy" (Karagrulla, 1967; Miller, 1977, 1987; Tiller, 1977).

Björn Nordenstrom is credited with discovering the electrical circulatory system of the body. In the field of radiology, he is the pioneer of percutaneous needle biopsy, radiopaque chemical dyes, and the balloon catheterization used for x-ray examinations of the heart, blood vessels, and lungs. In 1979, after 30 years of research, Nordenstrom published his revolutionary book, *Biologically Closed Electric Circuits: Clinical, Experimental and Theoretical Evidence for an Additional Circulatory System,* which explains how these circuits are switched on by injury, infection, and tumors. Voltages build and fluctuate in intimate association with the blood vessels and guide metabolic processes throughout the body. Nordenstrom's research has led to the successful treatment of lung tumors (1983). Nordenstrom suggests that his findings account for the effects of acupuncture and presents a possible explanation of the healing process.

Even into the twentieth century, few Western scientists were aware of the Chinese and Ayurevedic systems, which developed bioenergy to a sophisticated science long before the onset of Western technologic science. The trend in medicine is clearly toward bioenergetic, or energy, medicine. Evidence of bioenergy continues to accrue.

Bienergetic Interactions: Electrical-Biochemical Interface

Researchers are beginning to recognize the primary role of the Vital Force: energies that animate the living body. Bioenergy must be recognized as different from ordinary electricity because it has a life of its own—a consciousness—apart from electricity. Bioenergy is contained within all living matter and characterized by oscillating pulsation (Lakhovsky, 1970). Bioenergy and electricity act differently than electricity alone. Bionenergy conducts the process of healing and growth from birth to death. It exhibits polarity and can be reflected like light (Becker,

Selden, 1985; Einstein, 1954). Bioenergy can be controlled by the mind and communicated. Because it flows in the direction of higher concentration, it can establish order from disorder, thus promoting healing and regeneration (Becker, Murray, 1970).

Becker investigated the application of electrical currents to stimulate the body's capacity for tissue regeneration. His work suggests that externally applied elecromagnetic fields accelerate bone healing of fractures. When tissue becomes injured, a "current of injury," a DC current, is produced. Becker's experiments with regeneration of a salamander's amputated leg revealed that the outermost cells of the skin across the cut surface grow rapidly. The cut ends of the nerves in the stump grow 2 days later and make an unusual connection with each skin cell, called the *neuroepidermal junction (NEJ)*. Shortly after the formation of the NEJ a mass of primitive cells appears between it and the cut end of the stump. The new limb grows from this mass of embryonic cells, called the *blastema*. These primitive cells derive from mature bone and muscle cells that remained in the stump and returned to an embryonic state.

The control system that starts, regulates, and stops healing is electrical. The current of injury is negative in polarity. Becker found that negative electrical polarity stimulates bone growth, whereas positive electrical polarity inhibits it. The blood cells in the clot that formed at the fracture site were dedifferentiated by the negative electricity at the fracture site, proving that specific extremely small electrical currents can influence the activities of living cells. In the mammal, only certain cells of the bone marrow have this capability. The NEJ is the source of the negative DC electrical current that stimulates sensitive cells in the area to dedifferentiate and form a blastema, which initiates regeneration (Becker, 1990).

Limitations of the Senses

Every living being emits radiation. All matter emits energy through radiation and absorbs energy through gravitation at known frequencies (Lakhovsky, 1970). We experience sound and color by distinguishing between various wavelengths and frequencies. Human ears can distinguish between tones spanning 10 octaves, and the human eye recognizes a range of one octave. Animals are more acute in their perception of sound and light. The canine visual system surpasses the human visual system in the ability to detect motion and differentiate shades of gray (Miller, Murphy, 1995). We can reasonably assume our senses are limited in the perception of other types of radiation as well.

Sensory limitations prevent us from perceiving the radiations of living things and the electromagnetic (EM) waves crossing the atmosphere (Becker, 1990). Bats and homing pigeons have a homing instinct based on their ability to detect EM waves (Keeton, 1971; Walcott, 1979;

Walker, 1984). Radiations from living beings—humans, animals, and plants—have been detected by the use of the spectroscope and Kirlian photographic plate (Becker, 1985; Gerber, 1988). Every living being radiates energy, which is called *photon emission of living cells,* or commonly the *aura* (Boyers, Tiller, 1973).

Everything in nature oscillates (Lakhovsky, 1970). All forces and movements have polarity. When energy flows, it moves from positive (+) to negative (−) to create equilibrium. The body contains a bioelectronic energy system that is both organizational and informational in function. Bioenergetic fields influence patterns of cellular growth and physical processes. At the quantum level of subatomic particles, all matter is frozen light–particularized energy fields (Einstein, Infeld, 1938). Just as light has a particular frequency or frequencies, matter also has frequency characteristics (Einstein, 1954).

All matter is in motion. Einstein described matter as actually energy in a denser form. Every substance contains energy that may be released. When the molecules of a substance undergo dispersion, or a decrease in organization, energy is released. When the molecular structure is so altered, matter is transformed into radiant energy. According to David Bohm, "matter is a kind of condensed or frozen light or energy moving at speeds slower than the speed of light; light energy moves through the universe without end" (1980).

F.A. Popp (1979) identified photons emitted by the cell and suggested that light is an essential part of every cell because cells store and emit light. Light regulates all cellular function. All matter exists in a particular energy dimension because "all is energy." All matter is composed of atoms bonded by energy fields and forces. Atoms join together to form molecules, which form cells, tissues, and organs. On the atomic level, all physiologic and metabolic changes in the body are energy changes.

External toxins such as pesticides, heavy metals, and chemicals and internal toxins such as cellular waste products neutralize the oscillatory movement of cells, weaken them, and sometimes kill them (Lakhovsky, 1970). When damaged by these toxins, cells can no longer oscillate according to their specific frequency for health maintenance. Health is equivalent to oscillatory equilibrium of living cells, whereas disease means oscillatory disequilibrium (Lakhovsky, 1970). Electricity is a major controlling factor in healing.

Bohm made the following observation: "The chief aim of all healing methods should be directed towards the preservation, restoration and regeneration of the electrical potential. It is within the electrical potential of an organism that the key to curing and healing are found" (Wolf, 1988). The electromagnetic radiation spectrum is part of a still larger spectrum that spans an enormous range of frequencies. Humans can see only the narrow band of visible light and are aware of only a small portion of the whole (Fig. 16-2). Some species have senses that detect parts of this spectrum in addition to magnetic fields. Owls and night-flying predatory birds perceive infrared or heat emanation from their prey. Geese become disoriented by extremely-low-frequency (ELF) broadcasts (Becker, 1990). Honeybees are sensitive to UV light and both the direction in which light waves are polarized and their angle of vibration; they are also magnetically sensitized to the Earth's magnetic field (Keeton, 1979).

Bees, ducks, pigeons, dolphins, bacteria, tuna, and humans all contain magnetite crystals, Fe_3O_4, a naturally occurring loadstone. These crystals are responsible for orienting our central nervous system to the geomagnetic field of the Earth (Becker, Selden, 1984). Other species are aware of energy fields and vibrations that humans cannot perceive. Other species are also sensitive to electricity and electromagnetic and magnetic influences, whereas we are not aware of them (Becker, Selden, 1984).

In 1960, Becker noted that the flow of DC current in the brain produces a magnetic field and predicted that it could be observed outside the head if a sufficiently sensitive magnetometer could be invented. In 1970, Brian D. Josephson invented the SQUID (superconducting quantum interference detector) magnetometer. We now know that the brain's magnetic field, called the MEG *(magnetoencephalogram),* can be detected (Cohen, 1972). Studies with the MEG show a vector of DC current running between the front and back of the brain, giving rise to the polarity of the head (Cohen, 1972). Humans, animals, and plants are surrounded by a magnetic field extending out into space from the body (Becker, 1990).

Magnetic Organs

The total-body effects of external fields are mediated through at least two highly specific internal organs: the magnetite "organ" composed of magnetite crystals found in the brain (Dunn and others, 1995; Kirschvink, 1992) and the pineal gland, which is part of the brain. Baker showed that all living beings have a "magnetic organ" in the posterior wall of the ethmoid sinus, in front of the pituitary gland (Becker, Selden, 1988; Walcott, 1979; Walker, 1984). The pineal gland regulates all glands in the body and produces major neurohormones such as melatonin, serotonin, and dopamine. The pineal gland is extremely sensitive to the daily cycle patterns in the Earth's electromagnetic field. The cyclic pattern of sleep-wakefulness depends on the level of melatonin secreted by the pineal gland (Ganong, 1969). Recent research shows that a patient's biocycle is a major determinant of outcome (Preslock, 1984; Semm, 1980).

The Biofield

The first scientific proof that electrodynamic fields influence the growth and functioning of the human organism appeared in 1935, when Burr published *The Electro-*

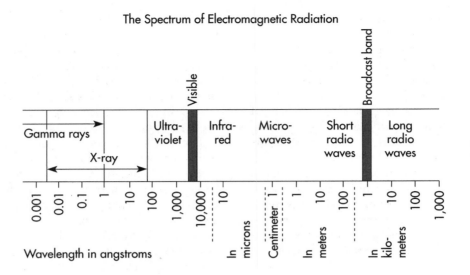

The Spectrum of Electromagnetic Radiation

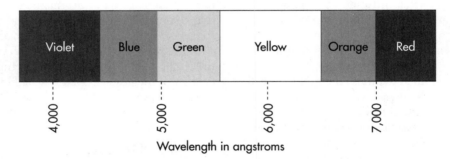

The Visible Spectrum

Fig. 16-2 The visible spectrum.

dynamic Theory of Life, an investigation of the existence of these energy fields and their qualities. He devised a voltmeter to measure the presence and effects of what he termed "L-fields," energy fields that surround, power, and maintain every living system from tiny plants and trees to human beings. Burr found electrical fields around worms, salamanders, humans, mammals, and slime molds. He measured changes in the field potentials and correlated them to growth, regeneration, tumor formation, and drug effects (1972).

Cell division produces low intensities of ultraviolet radiation that may contain information encoded into its modulated wave pattern. Much research comes from Russia, where Semyon and Valentina Kirlian developed a new technique of photography. Kirlian photography uses an oscillator generating between 75,000 and 200,000 electrical oscillations per second. Any living object can be photographed to reveal emanations. The device creates a high-frequency field that causes living things to radiate a bioluminescence on photographic paper. This bioluminescence

is the radiation of the living energy and is similar to the aura (Pierrakos, 1977). The Kirlians photographed healthy and diseased plants and observed a difference in emanations. They speculated that these emanations were from a unified biologic energy field (Dumitrescu, Kenyon, 1983).

Bioenergetics of Animals and the Environment

All matter, living and nonliving, is an electromagnetic phenomenon. The physical world is an atomic structure held together by electromagnetic forces (Becker, 1985). Four fundamental forces are present in the universe: nuclear, electromagnetic, weak interacting, and gravitational. The Earth's electromagnetic field is 0.174 gauss, which varies with the position of the Earth to the sun (Lakhovsky, 1970). Every 8 days the sun's rotation presents the Earth with a different solar magnetic field. This field varies from 1 to 25 hertz (Becker, 1985). Charged particles emitted continuously from the sun at a velocity of 670,000 to 1,600,000 miles per hour compress into a rounded, thin layer on the daylight side of the Earth and sweep into a tail on the night side of the Earth (Becker, 1985). The strongest electromagnetic fields are located at the poles, and the weakest at the equator. The Earth's electromagnetic field causes a positive charge in the morning and a negative charge at night (Lakhovsky, 1970). The Earth's electromagnetic field increases with altitude. Pulsations of extremely low frequency result from the electrodynamic resonating cavity between the Earth's surface and the ionosphere (Becker, 1985).

If any living thing is deprived of the Earth's relatively weak magnetic field for prolonged periods of time, it will become ill and die (Becker, 1985). Magnetism is an intangible force that affects all living systems. The average frequency pulsation is extremely low—approximately 10 hertz but possibly as high as 25 hertz. Humans can continue normal activity in environments up to 58 hertz, but 60 hertz affects our biorhythms, produces stress, and can eventually influence genetic and evolutionary factors. One study found that strong magnetic fields can affect discriminatory learning in mice (Levine, 1994).

Between the Earth's surface and the ionosphere a voltage gradient of about 200,000 volts of static electricity exists, representing a differential of 400 volts between our heads and feet when we are standing outside. This electrostatic field is not constant but contains varying, vertical oscillating waves of a fundamental basic frequency modulated with many harmonics—the whole having a sequence that repeats several times per second. These harmonics extend into the megahertz range and have a regulatory and stabilizing influence on physiologic processes (Tiller, 1977a).

Schumann waves are a natural part of our environment. Schumann resonance between the Earth and ionosphere is in the 3- to 14-hertz range, which encompasses the alpha, beta, and theta ranges of dominant human brain-wave patterns (Tiller, 1977b). Schumann waves are a natural part of our environment. Healthy people and animals can tolerate the absence of Schumann waves, but when ill they require the stabilizing effect these waves impart. NASA uses Schumann wave generators to keep the astronauts in good psychologic condition (Davidson, 1987). The INDUMED magnetic field device developed by Ludwig in 1963 employs magnetic field generators that use iron filament impregnated with trace elements. These generators mimic the natural electron-plasma and Schumann waves, creating an excellent therapeutic aid for all health problems.

Unfortunately, Schumann waves are blocked or reduced by modern building materials, a particular problem in urban areas. We live in the Earth's natural magnetic field, and we have created a vast global network of manmade EMFs.

Electricity is a phenomenon common to all living processes, and all normal and pathologic conditions can be interpreted in electrical terms. Every substance or element has its own electrical wavelength and frequency of vibration (Lakhovsky, 1970). In humans and animals, biologic clocks and circadian rhythms are influenced by a weak 10-hertz electrical field (Becker, 1990). The glands that control the body's biologic rhythms are sensitive to magnetic fields (Brown, 1972). Humans in underground habitats shielding them from the Earth's magnetic field develop abnormal circadian rhythms. Normal body rhythm can be restored with use of a signal that oscillates at the average frequency of the Earth's micropulsation (Wever, 1974).

Muscles and nerves generate electrical currents that subsequently produce magnetic fields, most notably the EMF created by the heart and brain. For optimal health, our bodies must be in electromagnetic harmony with our environment. All brain waves are in the same range as the Earth's micropulsation (1 to 25 hertz). The dominant (alpha) frequency of the EEG in animals is 10 hertz (Wever, 1974). The biomagnetic field is negative in front of the brain and positive at the back of the brain and brainstem. The direct current field of the brain is one billionth of the Earth's field. The body's cells operate at DC current measured in picoamps (1 trillionth of an amp) and nanoamps (1 billionth of an amp). Weak EMFs exert effects at the cell membrane by acting on calcium binding and action potentials for ion transport (Adey, Bawin, Lawrence, 1982).

EMFs are used to promote healing of skin, tendons, and bones. With the application of DC current at a vibration that enhances the normal bioelectric field, accelerated healing of tumors, wounds, and emotional illness is possible. Veterinary medicine seeks to understand the life energies of the body in relation to the energies of the environment. A new paradigm of life, energy, and medicine is emerging as a result.

Body Polarity

All cells are bipolar. Energy is positive, negative, or neutral. In a healthy cell, positive and negative charges are in balance. The cell membrane has a negative charge, the cytoplasm is neutral, and the nucleus is positively charged (Davis, Rawls, 1979b).

The nucleus of an atom vibrates at 1022 hertz, an atom vibrates at 1015 hertz, molecules oscillate at 109 hertz, and living cells vibrate at approximately 103 hertz (Davis, Rawls, 1993). All matter has a harmonious vibratory frequency and can be made to vibrate at dissonant frequencies. Davis and Rawls found that the negative electrical energies of the body were related to north pole magnetism, whereas positive energy corresponds with the south pole. In 1855 Faraday claimed that man is diamagnetic (1965). The front and right side are positive, whereas the back and left side are negative. As Babbitt observed in 1878, the right foot is a (+) pole, and the right hand is positive (1976).

Stone, a chiropractor, introduced polarity therapy in his book, *Health Building: The Conscious Art of Living.* According to Stone, the polarity of the body is as follows (1985):

Right side of body	Positive
Left side of body	Negative
Front of body	Positive Yin
Back of body	Negative Yang
Right side of palm	Positive
Back of hand	Negative
Right palm	Positive
Back of right hand	Negative
Left palm	Negative
Back of left hand	Positive
Positive energy	Tonifying
Negative energies	Sedating
South Pole	Positive
North Pole	Negative

Through the positive and negative polarities of this field, which appear physically as EM energy, the vital force energy is driven throughout the body, infusing it with life. Obstruction in this flow at the molecular, electromagnetic, and other, more subtle energy levels produces pain. When the polarities are in harmony, health is restored and pain disappears.

Energy Medicine in Veterinary Practice

The most common holistic energy-medicine modalities used in veterinary practice are homeopathy, acupuncture, magnet and magnetic field therapy, low-level laser therapy, and color therapy.

Homeopathy*

Although researchers have not yet documented the exact mechanism of action in homeopathy, they have proposed several theories based on energetic concepts. Nuclear magnetic resonance studies have shown that higher homeopathic potencies dramatically change the structure of water and even when no molecular substance remains, the vehicle has physically changed (Lumry and others, 1983). Infrared spectroscopy analysis of water suggests the following changes:

- The atomic bond angle of the water shifts.
- H-bonding between water molecules decreases.
- Surface tension decreases.

Water can be charged with and store the various subtle energy fields of substances without the molecular structure of the substance. The subtle energy absorption properties of water allow extraction of specific vibrational energy fields. Slawinska and Slawinski (1986) measured ultraweak photon emission from living plant tissues treated with various homeopathic preparations and potencies and found that homeopathically treated water induces measurable changes in plant physiology and growth. Frequency resonance measurements show that homeopathic preparations differ as a function of potency. Clinical results are claimed for homeopathic preparations at higher dilutions such as 100x, 200x, 500c, 1M, and 10M (Reilly and others, 1986). Examining homeopathic preparations in polarized light, Callinan (1985, 1986) showed photographic color changes occurred in potentiation of Pulsatilla 1c, 8c, 200c, and 1M compared with distilled water and rain water (Jayasuriya, 1984).

Thus the physics of magnetoelectric energy, predicted by Einstein's equations, holds the key to deciphering the scientific principles behind the behavior of higher vibrational phenomena. By working on both a physical and an energetic level, homeopathy offers a broad range of benefits in chronic degenerative conditions. Homeopathic remedies have energized EM fields capable of establishing a resonance with the vital force, which can rebalance the energy in the body.

Resonance and Homeopathic Theory

The movement of electrons around the nucleus of an atom is described as a wave when it begins in one direction and then returns to its original location. Each substance has a characteristic wave frequency, or range of frequency, at which it vibrates. A homogeneous elemental substance vibrates at a frequency called its *resonant frequency.* At the resonant frequency, energy is maximized and harmonious. The further a substance deviates from its resonant frequency, the more dissonance occurs (Pauling, Wilson, 1963; Vithoulkas, 1980).

When disease occurs, the first disturbance appears on the EMF of the body, which then challenges the defense system (Royal, Mayfield, 1983). A healthy physical body resonates with a dominant energetic vibration. When the physical body is infected by a bacterium or virus, the frequency of the invader changes the resonance of the physical body (Royal, Mayfield, 1983). Everything has its own EMF, or "energy signature." When the vibrational energy of the body shifts to a disease frequency, a subtle energy of the proper frequency is necessary to reestablish equilibrium through a type of resonance induction (Peterson, 1990).

Homeopathic remedies are "vibrational medicines." If the remedy's frequency matches the patient's illness state, a resonant transfer of energy allows the patient's bioenergetic system to assimilate the needed energy, eliminate dissonant frequencies, and move to a new equilibrium of health. Discussions about the vital energy of a living body are also discussions about resonance. Both subjects concern the interaction of two bodies vibrating at the same

---

*The history and science of homeopathy are discussed in detail in Chapters 25 through 28.

frequency. Homeopathy is the scientific induction of resonance, which alters the arrangement of molecules or electrons, allowing the body's own vital force to take over and reestablish equilibrium (Vithoulkas, 1979).

Acupuncture*

The Chinese believe that *Qi* is the vital force circulating within the meridian channels of energy flow (CEFs) throughout the body. Acupuncture points along the meridians are treated whenever a disease condition blocks the normal flow of energy along these meridians. Each meridian corresponds to an internal organ or system.

The body is endowed at birth with a fixed energy quotient. Daily living depletes this original energy, but it is augmented by energy received from food and air. For an organ to be healthy, the flow of *Qi* must be unobstructed. Mann (1973) explained that the CEF cycle in the body begins with the lungs, where the vital force enters through respiration. The vital force from digestion of food and water in the stomach travels via the spleen to the lungs and throughout the body.

The vital force consists of harmonious forces called *Yin* and *Yang*, which represent opposite polarities of energy. *Yin* is sympathetic, and *Yang* is parasympathetic. Complete balance of *Yin* and *Yang* maintains perfect health. Organ hypofunction or hyperfunction depends on whether *Yin* and *Yang* are balanced. *Yin* indicates deficient or negative, and *Yang* overabundant or positive.

Western technology can now validate the existence of acupuncture meridians and acupuncture points. Pioneering research by Albert Szent-Gyorgyi (1960, 1941) suggests the following:

- Fascia, or connective tissue in the body, forms a continuous network, ensheathing muscles, bones, nerves, and blood vessels and connecting every cell of the body
- All molecules are semiconductors that can conduct energetic electrons
- The collagen that makes up the fascia is a fibrous protein with a crystalline structure that conducts electricity

Becker, a Nobel Prize nominee, identified over 40 meridians (1990). He compared acupuncture meridians to "electrical conductors" that respond to injury by conducting a message to the brain, which responds by sending back the appropriate level of direct current to stimulate healing in the injured area. The conscious mind receives the message from the brain and interprets it as pain. Acupuncture blocks this incoming message and thereby prevents pain. Becker likened acupuncture points to direct current generators, which conduct electricity along the meridians. The acupuncture points are amplifiers; when an acupuncture needle is inserted in a specific acupuncture point, connecting it with nearby tissue fluids, it causes a short-circuit and stops the pain message. Becker found that acupuncture points show specific electrical differences compared with surrounding skin. At the acupuncture point, resistance is less, electrical conductivity is greater, and a DC power source is detectable. Acupuncture points have electrical characteristics; the meridians conduct currents into the central nervous system. Each acupuncture point is positive compared with surrounding skin tissue, and each acupuncture point has a field surrounding it with its own characteristic shape.

Becker established the presence of acupuncture points on the human forearm, showed they had specific, reproducible, electrical parameters, and proved their existence in all subjects he tested. He found that meridians connecting these points had the electrical characteristics of transmission lines, whereas nonmeridian skin did not. Input DC electrical signals at acupuncture points convey the message that an injury has occurred along the acupuncture meridian to the brain, where part of this signal is perceived as pain. The remainder of the signal goes to the more primitive portions of the brain, where it stimulates similar DC signals that cause the cells and chemical mechanisms at the site of injury to begin repair. This process is a complete closed-loop, negative-feedback control system (Becker, Selden, 1985; Reichmanis, 1976).

Direct evidence for the perineural DC system has been accumulating since 1958, when electrical currents were detected in the glial cells of rats' brains. Electron microscopy has shown that the cytoplasm of all Schwann cells is linked, forming a syncytium; other perineural cells (such as ependyma and glial cells) also form a syncytium that provides an uninterrupted pathway for a current. Research indicates that the glial cell network is able to transmit information via slow shifts in DC-current potentials (Becker, 1985). The DC-current system of glial cells appears to be involved in self-healing electrical feedback loops. The glial cell network functions as an interface between the meridian and nervous systems. Living bodies of humans and animals are grids of magnetic blueprints tied together by axiatonal lines. Axiatonal grids are formed by intersecting axiatonal lines that interface with the biologic activities of the organism. The biologic interconnection with the higher-frequency energies takes place through the Acupuncture Meridian System, which is interfaced with the Axiatonal Line and Grid Systems. The acupuncture and axiatonal lines are part of a fifth-dimensional circulatory system (Becker, 1985; Tiller, 1972). The indirect energetic link with the nervous system is the reason that neurologic phenomena can be measured in response to acupuncture stimulation (Gerber, 1988). Scientists are exploring the medical uses of energy for treating illness. These include the use of radiation for treating cancer, use

---

*The history and scientific basis of acupuncture are discussed in detail in Chapters 9 through 11.

of electricity to alleviate pain and shrink tumors, EMFs to stimulate fracture repair, and magnetic fields to alleviate the pain and inflammation of arthritis.

In 1986, Darras and Vernejoul examined energy transport along the meridians and succeeded in visualizing them. Researchers injected a radioactive tracer, sodium pertechnetate, at an acupuncture point and found by using a gamma ray camera that the radioactivity traveled along the acupuncture meridian with a velocity of 3 to 5 cm per minute (Vernejoul and others, 1985). This magnitude causes 25 circulations per day or night but is slower in diseased organs. Darras and Vernejoul confirmed that the radioisotope does not diffuse appreciably if injected at a location other than an acupuncture point and that the radioisotope does not enter the lymphatic or circulatory systems. It diffuses only toward the target organ if injected at an acupuncture point part of the way along a meridian. The rate of diffusion along the meridian increases when the acupuncture point is stimulated, whether by needle, electricity, or laser (Vernejoul, 1985).

Insertion of a needle at an acupuncture point creates an electrical potential. Acupuncture points have decreased electrical resistance and increased electrical conductivity compared with surrounding skin. Stimulation lasting only 1 to 2 seconds at an acupuncture point creates an electrical potential (Royal, Mayfield, 1983). Acupuncture points have an increased electrical capacitance and decreased electrical impedance.

By using Kirlian equipment to photograph the back of the leg, Luciani was able to identify AP points along the bladder CEF. He reported that these discharges were bluish white and flamelike in appearance (Luciani, 1978). Shenberger found that the CEFs retained their identity after death—in fact, he was able to measure electrical activity even in the meridians of a cadaver that had been soaking in formaldehyde for 8 months (Shenberger, 1977).

Magnetic Therapy*

Magnetic therapy is the oldest form of physical therapy. Galen and Paracelsus used magnetic therapy to treat gout, spasms, hernias, dropsy, and jaundice. Lodestones are magnetic stones of iron oxide that were ground into powder, mixed with honey, and applied externally to wounds. Gauss is the unit of measure for magnetism. The primary law of magnetism states that opposite poles attract and similar ones repel. Energy from the magnet leaves the south pole of the magnet and travels halfway around to the magnet's center, where it reverses its spin and travels toward the north pole. Magnetic fields pass through glass, lead, and other solids, whereas electricity does not pass through a nonconductor (such as glass) (Davis, Rawls, 1974).

In their research on magnetic therapy in earthworms and rodents, Davis and Rawls discovered that the north and south poles of a magnet have distinct effects. The north pole slows down the processes of life, controls pain, decreases blood pressure and the growth rate of cancer cells, causes retardation of maturation and growth, and increases sensitivities such as intelligence, reflexes, and environmental reaction.

When the north pole is applied to the forehead, extrasensory perception increases, the rational mind relaxes, and the body becomes more alkaline. The energy produced is negative, with a counterclockwise, centripetal, cohering electron spin (Davis, Rawls, 1993). The south pole strengthens and promotes growth; increases life span, vigor, and vitality; and increases acidity and hyperactivity in the body. It has a clockwise, centrifugal, and electron-expanding spin (Davis, Rawls, 1974). (Box 16-1 compares the poles of a magnet.)

Magnets create polarization of substances. If the plasma is removed from a blood sample, the red blood cells placed on a slide, and a magnet placed under the slide, the red blood cells spin around and point in one direction. This activity demonstrates the polarization of iron and ions in the blood (Cardin, 1933). Magnetic acupuncture uses 800 gauss gold- or ferrite-plated, self-adhesive, north pole magnets, which are placed over specific acupuncture points. The magnets create a healing EMF in the area and eliminate pain (Leviton, 1986).

Magnetic Field Therapy*

Magnetic field therapy was first described by Fichtner, who invented the Vitapulse and the Magnetotron. Magnetic field therapy is based on the law of electricity, which states that electrical currents trigger a series of electrical and magnetic waves that can be measured by frequency. A magnetic field is produced by flowing current or changing electrical fields. Magnetic field lines are continuous and have neither beginning nor end. Pulsating electromagnetic waves are produced by electrical charges undergoing acceleration. These waves can be generated with different frequencies.

Magnetic field lines completely penetrate the body. They hit the ions of the tissues in the frequency rhythm of the pulsed electromagnetic wave. The concentration of ions at the cell membrane increases, causing hyperpolarization and allowing a faster exchange of ions, which increases oxygen use and cell function (Warnke, 1979, 1980). The partial pressure of oxygen in the tissues increases. The ATP level and the metabolic rate of the cell are increased because of membrane polarization. A generalized vasodilation results. These field lines penetrate all organs and bones and affect the body on two levels: cellular and that of the body's EMF.

---

*A comprehensive review of magnetic therapy appears in Chapter 18.

*Magnetic field therapy is discussed in detail in Chapter 18.

BOX 16-1

Poles of a Magnet

N-POLE OF MAGNET	S-POLE OF MAGNET
Alkaline—decreased H^+ ions	Acid—increased H^+ ions
Suppresses cell mitosis	Stimulates cell multiplication
($-$) Energy pole	($+$) Energy pole
Decreases bacteria, viruses	Increases growth of bacteria, viruses
Stops bleeding	Vasodilation
Energy moving counterclockwise	Energy moving clockwise
Shrinks tumors	Increases growth of tumors
Decreases K^+ ion	Increases Na^+ ion
Faster bone healing	Slower bone healing
Dissolves fatty calcium deposits in veins	
Decreases edema and ascites	Increases ascites and edema
Decreases inflammation	Increases inflammation

Data from Davis and Rawls, 1979, 1983.

Pulsating magnetic fields create the following changes in tissues*:

- Increased blood flow to treated area
- Increased oxygen-carrying ability in blood
- Increased enzyme activity
- Increased cell division
- Altered acid-base balance in tissues
- Altered endocrine activity

Low-Level Laser Therapy†

Laser stands for "light amplification by stimulated emission of radiation." This type of electromagnetic radiation was first introduced by Einstein in 1917. In 1953 and 1954 the use of stimulated emission for microwave amplification was suggested by Weber at the University of Maryland, Bosov and Prokhorov in the USSR, and Townes at Columbia University. Townes, Basov, and Prokhorov received the Nobel Prize in physics in 1964 for their original work in quantum electrodynamic theory (Tseung, 1985).

Laser therapy is based on the principle that light consists of oscillating electrical and magnetic fields that carry electromagnetic energy. The EM light waves have both energy and momentum and, when used on specific acupuncture points, can normalize energy flow in the meridians (Goldman, Rockwell, 1971). When laser radiation contacts the surface of the skin, reflection, absorption, and dispersion occur. Of this radiation, 99% is absorbed in the first 3.6 mm of tissue in humans (Goldman, Rockwell, 1971). The resonance of skin tissue absorbs the laser light according to the following equation:

$$E = hv$$

where
E = energy of photon
h = Planck's action quantum
v = oscillating frequency

After absorption, laser radiation is converted by the skin into electrical potential. Laser is used in many medical disciplines, including surgery, internal medicine, dermatology, otorhinolaryngology, obstetrics, and ophthalmology. Laser is also used to reduce pain and edema and treat acupuncture points.

New Energetic Modalities

All biologic processes are electrical, and an electrical change occurs before a biologic or anatomic change appears. Using high-tension transformers, Tesla showed that luminous discharges appear around the body when it is exposed to powerful, high-frequency EMFs. The application of electrographic methods in the examination of living organisms has led to a new scientific discipline called *bioelectrography* (Dumitrescu, Kenyon, 1983). Bioelectrography marked the beginning of advanced techniques in electromagnetic imaging in biology and medicine. Thermography is known to detect energy changes in the body by detecting temperature changes on the skin (Kenyon, 1986). Kirlian photography (high-frequency, high-voltage electrophotography) is excellent for visually recording the energetic change in the body. Kirlian images have shown an acupuncture point to have a central pore with a surrounding halo of photons (Kenyon, 1983).

---

*Delgado (1982); Becker (1969, 1982, 1985); Fahmy (1980); Focke (1983); Lau (1982).

†The energetic basis of low-level laser therapy is discussed in detail in Chapter 17.

Mandel developed a system of medical diagnosis based on Kirlian photographs of the body. Deficiencies in acupuncture meridians are determined by evaluating the control measuring points on the hands and feet and their aura. This new modality is called *Photon Emission Analysis* (Mandel, 1986).

Electrodiagnosis

Research has established that acupuncture points possess electrical conductivity. Voll measured the changes in conductivity at each acupuncture point and discovered that the electrical resistance of the skin decreased at the acupuncture point compared with the surrounding skin (Voll, 1976, 1978a, 1983). Voll, a Nobel nominee, developed a measuring instrument, the Dermatron, that allowed him to measure the electrical resistance at acupuncture points (Voll, 1983). The channels of energy flow (meridians) indicate the general health of each organ or tissue as a whole. Voll determined that higher or lower readings than normal at specific acupuncture points indicate a problem in the corresponding organ. Higher readings suggest inflammation in the organ, and lower readings indicate degeneration.

Voll's extensive research initiated the present era of electrodiagnosis. His pioneering work is called *Electrodiagnosis According to Voll* (Voll, 1983). Dodd pioneered the use of the Dermatron in the treatment of animals, and her observations may prove promising in treating spinal myelopathy and other degenerative conditions (Dodd, 1985).

Today, between 85,000 and 100,000 practitioners in this field exist worldwide (Goldberg, 1993). Peterson invented the Accupath, the first computerized electrodiagnostic computer based on the principles of the Dermatron. Later, Peterson and Curtin invented the Interro Electrodiagnostic Computer (Curtin, 1989; Peterson, 1984).

Tiller made the following statement: "To develop an early warning system concerning the chemical homeostasis of a biological system, a device must be created that monitors the electrical nature of the biological system" (1987a). The Interro Electrodiagnostic Computer contains an experimental and investigational program with the electronic signatures of homeopathic remedies, viruses, bacteria, fungi, pesticides, chemicals, phenolics, and many therapeutic modalities. Diseases can be detected before physical symptoms appear (Madill, 1979, 1984b; Royal, Mayfield, 1983; Werner, Voll, 1983b).

The Interro can find energy imbalances in the body before the body feels adverse effects. The Interro measures the galvanic skin response at each control measuring point (CMP) on the hands and feet to determine organ deficiencies. With the Interro, disease states can be detected at the electromagnetic level before they appear in the physical body. If diseases can be detected on the electromag-

netic level, they can be prevented. When an organism is weak or imbalanced, it oscillates at a different or less harmonic frequency (Voll, 1983a). This abnormal frequency reflects the general state of energetic balance. Imbalances can be corrected by rebalancing the subtle energy with the right frequency. Research indicates that the Interro may be useful in the diagnosis and treatment of animals and the treatment of immunosuppressive diseases such as feline leukemia, peritonitis, and hepatitis (Stefanatos, 1989, 1990). This is a new application of the use of energy medicine in the diagnosis and treatment of animal diseases.

Most of the sophisticated diagnostic systems used today in Western medicine, such as the ECG, EEG, EMG, GSR, PET scanner, computed tomography, Electroacuscope, and MRI, employ the principles of energy medicine. Energy medicine uses diagnostic screening devices to measure the various EM frequencies emitted by the body in order to detect imbalances that may cause current illness or contribute to future disease. These disturbed energy flows can be restored to their normal healthy state through the input of EM signals that specifically counteract the affected frequencies to restore a normal energy balance within the body.

The Electroacuscope

The Electroacuscope 80 is an input/output device that communicates with the body by receiving and transmitting corrective electrical currents based on the existing electrical conductance of the body (Stefanatos, 1984). Stored within it is an integrated circuit chip capable of determining an acupuncture point's exact level of energy graded on a scale of 1% to 100%. If this value is low compared with the normal value, the device transmits a digital signal to bring the energy of the acupuncture point to 100%. The Electroacuscope 80 uses a pulsed square wave form that has been proved most effective in stimulating acupuncture points (Rossen, 1993). The computer senses the existing electrical impedance of the acupuncture point and modifies the next wave form accordingly (Matteson, Eberhardt, 1985; Olsen, 1984).

In veterinary medicine the Electroacuscope has been used with promising results in the treatment of the following conditions: hip dysplasia, arthritis, epilepsy, myelopathy, disk disease, lameness, skin disorders, impaired wound healing, avascular necrosis, colic, and radial nerve paralysis (Stefanatos, 1984).

Biologically Closed Electrical Circuits

In studying the use of electrical currents in cancer treatment, Nordenstrom pioneered the use of platinum needle electrodes in lung tumors. Nordenstrom postulated a mechanism to explain the success of electrotherapy in destroying tumors. He found that white blood cells carry a negative electrical charge. These tumor-fighting lymphocytes are drawn to the cancer site by the positive electrical charge of the platinum electrode, which is placed in the center of the metastatic lesion. A second negative electrode is placed into normal tissue adjacent to the tumor. The resulting electrical field induces ionic tissue changes and acid accumulation in the local environment of the tumor, alterations that are detrimental to the cancer cells. The increased acidity locally destroys red blood cells, depriving the cancer cells of oxygen. The positive electrical field moves water out of the tumor, shrinks it, and causes the surrounding tissue to swell. This swollen tissue puts pressure on local blood vessels and blocks the flow of blood to the tumor. Nordenstrom's research indicates the presence of a "second circulatory system" in the body (Nordenstrom, 1983). Nordenstrom's study of electrical energy in the treatment of cancer and other degenerative diseases suggests intriguing possibilities for veterinary medicine.

Conclusions

Many veterinarians have not been exposed to holistic complementary procedures because established medical journals rarely publish controversial information without references from other established journals. In addition, few double-blind control studies are available in this field. However, energy medicine is of major historical and clinical significance. With its growing importance in complementary modalities using nontoxic medical treatments, energy medicine is an exciting healing paradigm, offering new hope in the treatment of many veterinary medical problems. The future of veterinary medicine includes not only genetic engineering and organ transplants but the examination of bioenergetic and constitutional causes of disease, which can now be diagnosed before physical symptoms appear. The concepts of energy medicine, based on energetic principles involving the mental, physical, emotional, and spiritual dimensions of humans and animals, are rapidly being integrated in traditional veterinary medicine. As information about energy medicine accumulates, a much more effective system of veterinary medicine will emerge.

*R*EFERENCES

Adey WR, Bawin FM, Lawrence AF: Effects of weak amplitude modulated fields on calcium efflux from awake cat cerebral cortex, *Bioelectronics* 3:295, 1982.

Babbitt E: *The principles of light and color: the healing power of color,* Secaucus, NJ, 1976, The Citadel Press.

Baker RR: Signal magnetite and direction finding, *Phys Technol* 15:30, 1984.

Baker RR: Magnetoreception in man and other primates. In Kirschvink JL, Jones DS, McFadden BJ, editors: *Magnetite and biomineralization and magnetoreception in organisms: a new magnetism,* New York, 1985, Plenum.

Barnard GP, Stephenson JH: Fresh evidence for a biofield, *J Am Inst Homeopathy* 562:73, 1969.

Becker RO: Original paper on the electrical factors in regenerating limbs of salamanders, *J Bone Joint Surg* 43-A:643, 1961a.

Becker RO: Proof that the direct electrical currents in the salamander are semiconducting in nature, *Science* 13:101, 1961b.

Becker RO: First paper proposing the primitive DC control system, *NY State J Med* 63:2215, 1963.

Becker RO: The effect of magnetic fields on the CNS. In Barnothy M, editor: *Biological effects of magnetic fields,* vol 2, New York, 1969, Plenum Press.

Becker RO, Murray DG: The electrical control system regulating fracture healing in amphibians, *Clin Orthop Rel Res* 75:169, 1970.

Becker RO: Electrical stimulation of partial limb regeneration in mammals, *Bull NY Acad Med* 48:627, 1972a.

Becker RO: Electromagnetic forces and life processes, *MIT Technol Rev,* pp 32-38, Dec 1972b.

Becker RO: Review of Becker's work on electrical controls of regeneration, *J Bioelectricity* 1:239, 1982.

Becker RO: Theory of relationship of living organisms to ELF fields, *J Bioelectricity* 4:133, 1985,

Becker RO: *Cross currents,* Los Angeles, 1990, Jeremy P Tarcher.

Becker RO, Marino AA: *Electromagnetism and life,* Albany, NY, 1982, State University of New York Press.

Becker RO, Selden G: *The body electric: electromagnetism and the foundation of life,* New York, 1985, William Morrow.

Bohm D: *Wholeness and the implicate order,* London, 1980, Routledge and Kegan Paul.

Bohr N: *The structure of the atom: Nobel lectures, physics 1922-1941,* New York, 1965, Elsevier.

Boyers D, Tiller WA: On corona discharge photography, *J Appl Physics,* p 45, July 1973.

Brown BB: *New mind, new body—biofeedback: new directions for the mind,* New York, 1975, Harper & Row.

Brown F: Biological cycles, *Am Scientist* 60:756, 1972.

Burr HS: *The fields of life, our links with the universe,* New York, 1972, Ballantine.

Callinan P: The mechanism of action of homeopathic remedies, *Compl Med* 3(1):35, 1985.

Callinan P: Vibrational energy in water: a model for homeopathic action, *Compl Med* 2:34, 1986.

Capra F: *The tao of physics,* Berkeley, 1925, Shambhala.

Cardin A: Magnetic sensibility of red blood cells, *Arch di fisiol* 32:295, 1933.

Cohen D: First report on the magnetoencephalogram (magnetic field given off by the brain), *Science* 175:664, 1972.

Conti P and others: A role for Ca^{+2} in the effect of very low frequency electromagnetic fields on the blastogenesis of human lymphocytes, *Fed Eur Biochem Soc* 18(1):28, 1985.

Curtin R: Personal communication, May 10, 1989.

Davidson J: *Subtle energy,* Essex, England, 1987, CW Daniel.

Davis AR, Rawls WC, Jr: *The magnetic effect,* Kansas City, Mo, 1993, Acres.

Davis AR, Rawls WC, Jr: *The magnetic blueprint of life,* Hicksville, NY, 1979, Exposition Press.

Davis AR, Rawls WC, Jr: *Magnetism and its effects on the living system,* Hicksville, NY, 1979, Exposition Press.

De La Warr GW, Baker D: *Biomagnetics,* Oxford, 1967, Delaware Labs.

deBroglie L and others: *Einstein,* New York, 1979, Peebles Press.

Delgado JMR and others: Embryological changes induced by weak extremely low frequency EMFs, *J Anat* 134:533, 1982.

Dumitrescu I, Kenyon JN: *Electromagnetic imaging in medicine and biology,* Suffolk, England, 1983, Neville Spearman.

Dunn JR and others: Magnetic material in the human hippocampus, *Brain Res Bull* 36(2):149, 1995.

Einstein A, Infeld L: *The evolution of physics: the growth of ideas from early concepts to relativity and quanta,* New York, 1938, Simon & Schuster.

Einstein A: *Ideas and opinions,* New York, 1954, Crown Publications.

Eisenberg D: Unconventional medicine in the United States: prevalence, costs, and patterns of use, *N Engl J Med* 328(4):282, 1993.

Fahmy Z: Clinical evaluation of magnetic field therapy in osteoarthritis. Proceedings of the second International Congress of Magnetomedicine, Rome, Nov 8-9, 1980.

Faraday M: *Experimental research in electricity,* New York, 1965, Dover Publications (originally published in 1855).

Focke H: Experiences with the use of magnetic field therapy in equine medicine, *Biophys Med Rep,* Jan 1983.

Gamow G: *The great physicists from Galileo to Einstein,* New York, 1961, Dover Publications.

Ganong WF: *Review of medical physiology,* Los Altos, Calif, 1969, Lange Medical.

Geddes LA, Hoff ME: The discovery of bioelectricity and current electricity: the Galvani-Volta controversy, *IEEE Spectrum* 8(12):38, 1971.

Gerber R: *Vibrational medicine,* Santa Fe, NM, 1988, Bear & Co.

Goldberg B: *Alternative medicine: the definitive guide,* Puyallup, Wash, 1993, Future Medicine.

Goldman L, Rockwell JR: *Laser in medicine,* New York, 1971, Gordon & Breach.

Heisenberg W: *Physics and beyond: encounters and conversations,* New York, 1971, Harper & Row (Translated by Arnold J Pomerans).

Jayasuriya A: *Clinical homeopathy,* Sri Lanka, 1984, Chandrakanthi Press.

Karagulla S: *Breakthrough to creativity,* Santa Monica, Calif, 1967, De Vorss & Co.

Keeton WT: Homing pigeons and their magnetic migration, *Proc National Acad Sci* 68:102, 1971.

Kirschvink JL, Kobayashi-Kirschvink A, Woodford BJ: Magnetite biomineralization in the human brain, *Proc Natl Acad Sci* 89(16):7683, 1992.

Kuhn T: *The essential tension,* Chicago, 1977, University of Chicago Press.

Lakhovsky G: *The secret of life,* London, 1939, Heinemann (Translated by Mark Clement).

Lakhovsky G: *The secret of life: cosmic rays and radiations of living beings,* Mokelumne Hill, Calif, 1970, Health Research (Translated by Mark Clement).

Lau BHS: Effects of low frequency EMF on blood circulation, Unpublished manuscript, 1982.

Levine RL, Bluni TD: Magnetic field effects on spatial discrimination learning in mice, *Physiol Behav* 55(3):465, 1994.

Leviton R: Healing with nature's energy, *East-West,* p 55, June 1986.

Luciani RJ: Direct observations and photography of electroconductive points on human skin, *Am J Acupunct* 6(4):314, 1978.

Lumry J and others: *Structure and stability of biological macromolecules,* Oxford, England, 1983, Oxford University Press.

Madill P: A true and legitimate preventive medicine, *Am J Acupunct* 7(4):279, 1979.

Madill P: The five areas of discovery of German electroacupuncture or electroacupuncture according to Voll, *Am J Acupunct* 12(2):31, 1984a.

Madill P: The uses and limitations of AP point measurement, German EAP or EAV, *Am J Acupunct* 12(1):33, 1984b.

Mandel P: Personal Communication, March 15, 1986.

Matteson JH, Eberhardt T: Pain management and the new generation of intelligence, *Am J Acupunct,* p 5, June 1985.

Miller PE, Murphy CJ: Vision in dogs, *JAVMA* 207(12):1623, 1995.

Miller R: *Methods of detecting and measuring healing energies,* New York, 1977, Future Sci, Doubleday.

Miller R: Paraelectricity, a primal energy, *Hum Dimens* 5(12):23, 1987.

Olsen E: Miracle worker, *The Runner,* p 3, Sept 1984.

Pauling L, Wilson EB: *Quantum mechanics,* New York, 1963, Dover Publications.

Peterson GP: Personal communication, Jan 10, 1984.

Peterson GP: Personal communication, June 12, 1990.

Planck M: *Scientific autobiography and other papers,* Westport, Conn, 1968, Greenwood (Translated by Frank Gaynor).

Popp FA: Photon storage in biological systems. In Popp FA and others: *EM bioinformation,* Munich, 1979, Urban Press.

Popper K: *The logic of scientific discovery,* New York, 1959, Harper Torchbooks.

Preslock JP: Review of function of the pineal gland, *Endocr Rev* 5:282, 1984.

Reichmanis M and others: Acupuncture points show increased DC electrical conductivity, *Am J Chin Med* 4:69, 1976.

Reilly DT and others: Is homeopathy a placebo effect? Controlled trial of homeopathy, *Lancet,* p 881, Oct 18, 1986.

Rossen J: The Electroacuscope, *Humane Innov Altern* 7:508, 1993.

Royal FF, Mayfield CK: *Physician's electrodiagnostic handbook,* Las Vegas, Nev, 1983, Nevada Clinic.

Schrodinger E: *What is life? and mind and matter,* Cambridge, Mass, 1967, Cambridge University Press.

Semm P: First description of magnetic sensitivites of the pineal gland, *Nature* 228:206, 1980.

Slawinska D, Slawinski J: *Biophoton emission from cucumber seedlings perturbed by formaldehyde as a possible indicator of the efficacy of homeopathic drugs,* Berich an Bonn, Essen, Germany, 1986, Verlag fur Ganzheitsmedizin.

Smith CW, Best S: *The electromagnetic man,* New York, 1989, St Martin's Press.

Stefanatos J: Treatment to reduce radial nerve paralysis, *Vet Med,* pp 67-70, Jan 1984.

Stefanatos J: Clinical workshop in bioenergetic veterinary medicine, Bel Air, Md, 1989, AHVMA.

Stefanatos J: Bioenergetic veterinary medicine: homeopathy and acupuncture for animals, Bel Air, Md, 1990, AHVMA.

Szent-Gyorgyi A: A study of energy levels in biochemistry, *Nature* 148:157, 1941.

Tiller W: Some physical network characteristics of AP points and meridians, Los Altos, Calif, 1972, Academy of Parapsychology and Medicine.

Tiller W: Some energy field observations of man and nature in the Kirlian aura, New York, 1974, Aura Press/Doubleday.

Tiller W: *Energy yields and the human body: frontiers of consciousness,* New York, 1974, Avon Books.

Tiller W: Preface. In Gerber R: *Vibrational medicine: new choices for healing ourselves,* Santa Fe, N.M., 1988, Bear & Co.

Tseung ACH: Laser acupuncture in family practice, *Internat J Chin Med* 2(2):42, 1985.

Vernejoul P and others: Etude des meridiens d'acupuncture par les traceurs radio-actifs, *Bull Acad Natl Med* 169:1071, Oct 22, 1985.

Vithoulkas G: *Homeopathy: medicine of the new man,* New York, 1979, Arco Publish Co.

Vithoulkas G: *The science of homeopathy,* New York, 1980, Grove Press.

Voll R: Topographical positions of the measuring points in electroacupuncture, Vols I-III, Velzen, West Germany, 1976, ML-Verlag.

Voll R: Verification of AP points by means of EAV, *Am J Acupunct* 6(1):5, 1978.

Voll R: Foci and fields of disturbance as reasons for short term or insufficient therapeutic success in classical acupuncture, *Am J Acupunct* 6(2):97, 1978.

Voll R: *Electroacupuncture according to Voll: bioenergetic diagnostic and therapy on the basis of acupuncture,* Sri Lanka, 1983, Medicina Alternativa, Institute of Acupuncture.

Voll R: *The 850 EAV measuring points of the meridians and vessels, including the secondary vessels,* Velzen, West Germany, 1983, ML-Verlag.

Walcott C: First ID of a magnetic organ in homing pigeons, *Science* 205:1027, 1979.

Walker M: Associating magnetic organs with function, *Science* 205:1027, 1984.

Warnke U: Infrared emission of the human body as monitor of the influence of a pulsed frequency electromagnetic field. Paper presented at the Symposium Internat des Therapeutiques Ondulatoires 19-20 Mar, 1979, Ubertragsband.

Warnke U: Infrared radiation and O_2 partial pressure of tissue in human beings as indicative of the therapeutic effects of pulsating magnetic fields. Abstracts of the First National Conference of Biophysics and Bioengineering Sciences, Academy of Scientific Research and Technology, Arab Republic of Egypt, Cairo, Dec 22-23, 1980.

Werner F, Voll R: *Electroacupuncture primer,* Velzen, West Germany, 1979, ML-Verlag.

Wolf FA: *Taking the quantum leap: the new physics for nonscientists,* San Francisco, 1981, Harper & Row.

Woolridge DE: *The machinery of the brain,* New York, 1963, McGraw-Hill.

SELECTED READING

Aries ML: *Electromedicine: separating fact from fiction,* New York, 1989, Turning Point.

Bagley L: A new method for locating acupuncture points and body field distortions, *Am J Acupunct* 12(3):219, 1984.

Baker DW: Introduction to theory and practice of German EAV and accompanying medications, *Am J Acupunct* 12(4):327, 1984.

Baker RR: Human magnetoreception for navigation. In O'Conner ME, Loveley RH, editors: *Electromagnetic fields and neurobehavioral function,* New York, 1984, Alan Liss.

Bannerman RH, Burton J, Wen-Chiek C: *Traditional medical and health care coverage,* Geneva, 1983, WHO.

Bansal HL: *Magneto therapy,* New Delhi, 1993, B Jain.

Becker RO: A description of the integrated system of direct currents in the salamander, *IRE Transactions Biomed Electronics* 7:202, 1960.

Becker RO and others: Electrophysiological correlates of acupuncture points and meridians, *Psychoenergetic Systems* 1:105, 1976.

Becker RO: Report that very-low-strength negative electrical currents could cause bone growth and healing, *Clin Orthop Rel Res* 124:75, 1977.

Becker RO: An attempt to "put it all together," *J Bioelectricity* 3:105, 1984.

Bendit L, Bendit P: *The etheric body of man,* Wheaton, Ill, 1977, Theosophical Publishing House.

Bengali NS: *Magnet therapy theory and practice,* New Delhi, 1993, B Jain Publishing.

Benveniste J: Human basophil degranulation triggered by very dilute homeopathic dilutions, *Nature* 334:291, 1988.

Bohm D: Interview with David Bohm, Rupert Sheldrake and Renee Weber, *Revision J* 5(2):97, 1982.

Bohm D: *Quantum theory,* Englewood Cliffs, NJ, 1951, Prentice-Hall.

Bohm D: *The special theory of relativity,* New York, 1965, WA Benjamin.

Bohm D: *Science, order and creativity,* New York, 1980a, Bantam Books.

Bohm D: *Wholeness and the implicate order,* London, 1980b, Routledge and Kegan Paul.

Bohr N: *Atomic theory and the description of nature,* Cambridge, England, 1934, Cambridge University Press.

Bohr N: *Atomic theory and human knowledge,* New York, 1958, John Wiley.

Boiron J, Abecassis J, Belon P: *Aspects of research in homeopathy,* vol 1, Lyon, France, 1983, Boiron.

Boyd WE: *Research on the low potencies of homeopathy,* London, 1936, Heinemann.

Boyd WE: The action of microdoses of mercurius chloride on diastase, *Br J Homeopathy* 32:106, 1942.

Briggs J, Peat F: *David Bohm's looking glass map in looking glass universe: the emerging science of wholeness,* New York, 1984, Simon & Schuster.

Brown ML, Ulett GA, Stern JA: Acupuncture loci: technique for location, *Am J Chin Med* 2:67, 1974.

Brugemann H: *Bioresonance and multiresonance therapy (BRT),* vol 1, Brussels, 1993, Haug International.

Burr HS: *Blueprint for immortality: the electric patterns of life,* London, 1972, Neville Spearman.

Burr HS, Northrup FSC: The electrodynamic theory of life, *Q Rev Biol* 10:322, 1935.

Burr HS, Northrup FSC: Evidence for the existence of an electrodynamic field in living organisms, *Proc Natl Acad Sci* 25(6):284, 1939.

Cheney M: *Tesla: man out of time,* New York, 1981, Doubleday.

Cohen BJ: *Revolution in science,* Cambridge, Mass, 1985, Belknap Press of Harvard University Press.

Collin R: *The theory of celestial influence: Mars, the universe and cosmic mysteries,* Boulder, Colo, 1984, Shambhala.

Constable TJ: *The cosmic pulse of life: borderland sciences,* Garberville, Calif, 1990, Elsevier.

Curtin R: Traditional and emerging methods of electrodiagnosis, *J Soc Ultramolecular Med* 1(1):48, 1986.

Dankin HS, Luciani: *High voltage photography,* San Francisco, 1978, HS Dankin.

Darras JC: Thermography and acupuncture, *J Soc Ultramolecular Med* 1(1):56, 1983.

Davenas E, Poitevin B, Benveniste J: Effect on mouse peritoneal macrophages of orally administered, very high dilutions of silica, *Eur J Pharm* 135:313, 1987.

Davenas E and others: Human basophilic degranulation triggered by very dilute antiserum against IgE, *Nature* 333:816, 1988.

Davis AR, Bhattacharya AK: *Magnet and magnetic fields of healing by firma,* Calcutta, 1986, KLM Private.

Davis AR, Rawls WC: *The magnetic effect,* New York, 1974, Exposition Press.

Delgado JMR: *Physical control of the mind: towards a psychocivilized society, vol 41, World perspectives,* New York, 1969, Harper & Row.

Del Guidice E and others: A quantum field theoretical approach to the collective behavior of biological systems, *Nuclear Physics* B251 FS13: 375, 1985.

Dobrin R, Conaway B, Pierrakos J: *Instrument measure of the human energy field,* New York, 1978, Institute for the New Age.

Dodd G: Electrodiagnosis and veterinary medicine: EAV priciples applied to the dog and cat, *J Soc Ultramolecular Med* 3(2):51, 1985.

Dossey L: *Beyond illness: discovering experience of health,* New Science Library, Boulder, Colo, 1984, Shambhala.

Dubrov AP: *The geomagnetic field and life: geomagnetobiology,* New York, 1978, Plenum Press.

Dumitrescu IFL, Kenyon J: *Electrographic imaging in medicine and biology,* Suffolk, England, 1983, Neville Spearman.

Einstein A, Infeld L: *The evolution of physics,* New York, 1961, Simon & Schuster.

Einstein A, Podolsky B, Rosen N: Can quantum-mechanical description of physical reality be considered complete, *Phys Rev* 47:777, 1935.

Einstein A: On physical reality, *Franklin Institute J* 221:349, 1936.

Einstein A: Autobiographical notes. In Schelpp P, editor: *Albert Einstein, philosopher-scientist,* New York, 1949, Harper & Row.

Foulkes G, Scott-Morley A: *J Altern Med,* July 1984.

Friedman N: *Bridging science and spirit,* St Louis, 1994, Living Lake Books.

Galvani L: Unpublished manuscript, Norwalk, Conn, 1971, Burndy Library.

Gamaleya NF: Laser biomedical research in the USSR. In Wolbarsht ML, editor: *Laser applications in medicine and biology,* vol 3, New York, 1977, Plenum Press.

Gibson R: Homeopathic therapy in rheumatoid arthritis: evaluation by doubleblind clinical trial, *Br J Clin Pharm,* p 453, May 1980.

Goldman L: *Basic reactions in tissue—the biomedical laser: technology and clinical applications,* New York, 1981, Springer Verlag.

Hahnemann S: *Organon of medicine,* Los Angeles, 1982, JP Tarcher (originally published in 1810).

Heisenberg W: *Physics and philosophy,* New York, 1958, Harper Torchbooks, Harper & Row.

Herbert N: *Quantum reality: beyond the new physics,* New York, 1984, Doubleday.

Hiley BJ, Peat FD, editors: *Quantum implications: essays in honor of David Bohm,* New York, 1987, Routledge and Kegan Paul.

Holzapfel E, Crepon P, Phillipe C: *Magnet therapy,* New Delhi, 1989, B Jain Publishing.

Ionescu-Tirgoviste C, Bajenaru O: Electric diagnosis in acupuncture, *Am J Acupunct* 12(3):229, 1984.

Ionescu-Tirgoviste C and others: *The electrophysiology of acupuncture points,* Bucharest, 1965, Communication USSM.

Kaptchuk T: *The web that has no weaver,* New York, 1983, Congdon & Weed.

Keeton WT: Avian orientation and navigation, *Br Birds* 72:451, 1979,

Kenyon JN: *Modern technique of acupuncture,* vol 2, New York, 1983, Thorsons Publishing.

Kenyon JN: Diagnostic techniques using bio-energetic recording methods: the science of bioenergetic regulatory medicine, *J Compl Med,* p 22, Feb 1986.

Kervan CL: *Biological transmutations,* Lockwood, NJ, 1972, Crosby.

Kirlian S, Kirlian V: Photography and visual observations by means of high frequency currents, *J Scientific Appl Photogr* 6:145, 1961.

Kleinkort JA, Foley RA: Laser acupuncture: its use in physical therapy, *Am J Acupunct* 12(1): Jan-Mar 1984.

Kollerstrom J: *Basic scientific research,* Los Angeles, 1982, Brain/Mind Bulletin.

Kreiger D: The relationship of touch with intent to help or to heal, to subjects' in vivo hemoglobin values. Proceedings of the ninth annual research conference of the American Nurses Association, San Antonio, Tex, March 21-23, 1973.

Kreiger D: Therapeutic touch: searching for evidence of physiological change, *Am J Nurs* 79(4):660, 1979.

Kuraisky T: Ultramolecular medicine: a hybridized approach to homeopathy and electrodiagnosis, *J Ultramol Med* 1(1):45, 1983.

Lee R: *Protomorphology: the principles of cell autoregulation,* Fort Collins, Colo, 1946, Selene River Press Archives.

Lerner EJ: Biological effects of electromagnetic fields, *IEEE Spectrum,* p 57, May 1984.

Liberman J: *Light medicine of the future,* Santa Fe, NM, 1991, Bear & Co.

Lucero KM: The Electroacuscope/Myopulse system: impedance-monitoring microamperage electrotherapy for tissue repair, *Rehabilitation Management* 4(3):1, 1991.

Ludwig W: Papers presented at the Seminar of the Brugemann Institute, Gauting, West Germany, 1986, 1988.

MacIvor V, La Forest S: *Vibrations,* York Beach, Maine, 1982, Samuel Weiser.

Mann WE: *Orgone, reich, and eros,* New York, 1973, Simon & Schuster.

Manning CA, Vanrenen LJ: *Bioenergetic medicine E/W acupuncture and homeopathy,* Berkeley, Calif, 1988, North Atlantic Books.

Miller JB: *Food allergy: provocative testing and injection therapy,* Springfield, Ill, 1972, Charles C Thomas.

Miller LA: An explanation of the therapeutic touch, *Nurs Forum* 18(3):278, 1979.

Miller SL: Production of amino acids under primitive earth conditions, *Science* 117:52, 1953.

Neitz J, Geist T, Jacobs GH: Color vision in the dog, *Neuroscience* 3:119, 1989.

Newton I: *Isaac Newton's philosophies naturalis principia mathematica,* ed 3, Cambridge, Mass, 1972, Harvard University Press (originally published in 1726).

Nordenstrom B: Biologically closed electric circuits: clinical, experimental and theoretical evidence for an additional circulation system, Stockholm, 1983, Nordic Medical Public.

Oldfield H, Coghill R: *The dark side of the brain,* 1988, Shaftesbury Elemental Books.

Ott JN: *Health and light,* Greenwich, Conn, 1973, Devin-Adair.

Ott JN: *Light radiation and you,* Greenwich, Conn, 1973, Devin-Adair.

Paracelsus: *The prophecies of Paracelsus,* Washington DC, Smithsonian Archives.

Pierrakos JC: *The energy field of man and nature,* New York, 1975, Institute for the New Age.

Pierrakos JC: *Life function of the energy centers of man,* New York, 1975, Institute for the New Age.

Pierrakos JC: *The core energetic process,* New York, 1977, Institute for the New Age.

Pietri PJ: Good vibrations: the Electroacuscope, *Health and Fitness Los Angeles Weekly,* p 23, Feb 1990.

Planck M: *The origin and development of the quantum theory,* Oxford, England, 1922, Clarendom Press.

Planck M: *The philosophy of physics,* New York, 1936, Norton.

Popp FA and others: *EM bioinformation,* Munich, 1979, Urban & Schwarzenberg.

Prigogine I: *From being to becoming: time and complexity in the physical sciences,* San Francisco, Calif, 1980, WH Freeman.

Ravitz LJ: Applications of the electrodynamic field theory in biology, psychiatry, medicine and hypnosis, *Am J Clin Hypnosis* 1:135, 1959.

Reich W: Discovery of orgone, *Int J Sex Economy and Orgone Research,* vol 1, New York, 1942.

Reichmanis M and others: A direct relationship between electrical measurements and acupuncture points, *IEEE Transactions on Biomedical Electronics* 22:533, 1975.

Reichmanis M and others: Acupuncture meridians have transmission-line characteristics, *IEEE Transactions on Biomedical Electronics* 24:402, 1977.

Rosenblatt S: The electrodermal characteristics of acupuncture points, *Am J Acupunct* 10:131, 1981.

Rosengren A: Experiments in color discrimination in dogs, *Acta Zool Fenn* 121:1, 1969.

Sacks AD: Nuclear magnetic resonance of homeopathic remedies, *J Holistic Med* 5(2):172, 1985.

Schmidt-Morand D: Vision in the animal kingdom, *Vet Inst* 1:3, 1992.

Schrodinger E: *Image of matter in modern physics, with Heisenberg W, Born M, and Auger P,* New York, 1961, Clarkson Palter.

Scofield A: Experimental research in homeopathy: a critical review, *Br Homeop J* 73(3):161 and 73(4):211-226, 1984.

Shadowitz A: *The electromagnetic field,* New York, 1975, Dover.

Shaffer RE: Electrotherapy, *Health Express J of Intern Acad of Nutr Consult,* p 10, July 1981.

Shealy CN and others: Electrical stimulation of the tracts in the spinal cord to treat chronic pain, *Anesth Analg* 45:489, 1967.

Shealy CN: Electrical stimulation of the skin for treatment of chronic pain, *Surg Forum* 23:419, 1973.

Shealy N: Wholistic healing and the relief of pain. In *Dimensions of wholistic healing: new frontiers in the treatment of the whole person,* Chicago, 1979, Nelson-Hill.

Sheldrake R: *A new science of life: the hypothesis of formative causation,* Los Angeles, Calif, 1981, JP Tarcher.

Sheldrake R: Interview, *New Realities* 5(5):8, 1983.

Shenberger RM: Acupuncture meridians retain their identity after death, *Am J Acupunct* 5(4):357, 1977.

Shipley M: Controlled trial of homeopathic treatment of osteoarthritis, *Lancet* 8316:97, 1983.

Sills F: *The polarity process,* Rockport, Mass, 1989, Element Books.

Slawinski J: Electromagnetic radiations and the afterlife, *Near Death Studies* 6(2):79, 1987.

Smith WS, Best S: *Electromagnetic man,* New York, 1989, St Martin's.

Smolan R, Moffitt P, Naythons M: *The power to heal: ancient arts and modern medicine,* New York, 1990, Prentice-Hall.

Stefanatos J: Energy medicine, Part I, *AAHA Trends,* p 28, April 1987.

Stefanatos J: Energy medicine, Part II, *AAHA Trends,* p 31, June 1987.

Stefanatos J: Energy medicine, Part III, *AAHA Trends,* p 36, Aug 1987.

Stefanatos J: Bioenergetic veterinary medicine featuring the IN-TERRO. Proceedings of the AHVMA Conference, Seattle, 1989.

Stefanatos J: A holistic approach to cancer treatment and nutrition for animals. Paper presented at the Bioenergetic Veterinary Medicine Seminar in Nevis, West Indies, 1991.

Stefanatos J: *Animals and man: a state of blessedness,* Minneapolis, 1992, Light and Life Publishing.

Still J: Relationship between electrically active skin points and acupuncture meridian points in the dog, *Am J Acupunct* 16(1):55, 1988.

Stone R: *Health building, the conscious art of living well,* New York, 1985, CRCS.

Szent-Gyorgyi A: *Introduction to submolecular biology,* New York, 1960, Academic Press.

Teller WA: *Some energy field observations of man and nature: galaxies of life,* New York, 1973, Interface.

Teller WA: A technical report on some psychoenergetic devices, *ARE J* 7:81, 1973.

Tiberiu R, Gheorghe G, Popescu I: Do acupuncture meridians exist? a radioactive tracer study of the bladder meridian, *Am J Acupunct* 9(3):251, 1981.

Tiller W: Radionics, radiesthesia and physics. In *Varieties of healing experience: exploring psychic phenomena in healing,* Los Altos, Calif, 1971, Academy of Parapsychology and Medicine.

Tiller W: The positive and negative space/time frame as conjugated systems, New York, 1977, Doubleday.

Tiller W: New fields, new laws. In White JK: *Future science,* Garden City, NY, 1977, Anchor Books-Doubleday.

Tiller W: Present scientific understanding of the Kirlian discharging process, *Psychoenergetic System* 3:1, 1979,

Tiller W: Towards a scientific rationale of homeopthy, *J Holist Med* 6(2): 2S, Fall, 1984.

Tiller W: Foreword. In *Vibrational medicine,* Santa Fe, NM, 1987a, Bear & Co.

Tiller W: What do electrodermal diagnostic AP instruments really measure? *Am J Acupunct* 5(1)55, 1987b.

Tsuei JJ and others: Studies of bioenergy in healthy subjects, *Am J Acupunct* 16(2):125, 1988.

Ullman D: Conceptualizing energy medicine: a beginning, *Am J Acupunct* 9(3):261, 1981.

Voll R: Zhu Zong-Xiang research advances in the electrical specificity of meridians and acupuncture points, *Am J Acupunct* 9(3):203, 1981.

Voll R: Twenty years of EA diagnosis in Germany: a progress report, *Am J Acupunct* 3:5, 1975.

Voll R: Twenty years of EA therapy using low-frequency current pulses, *Am J Acupunct,* p 15, Dec 1975.

Voll R: *Electrodiagnosis according to Voll,* Uelzeng, Germany, 1984, C Beckers Buch druckerei.

Walker M: Associating magnetic organ with function, *Science* 224:751, 1984.

Weaver H: *Divining the primary senses,* New York, 1978, Routledge & Kegan Paul.

Weber R: *Dialogues with scientists and sages: the search for unity,* New York, 1986, Routledge & Kegan Paul.

Wever R: *ELF and VLF electromagnetic field effects,* New York, 1974, Plenum Press.

Wilber K: *The holographic paradigm and other paradoxes,* Boulder, Colo, 1982, Shambhala.

Wolf FA: *Parallel universes: the search for other worlds,* New York, 1988, Simon & Schuster.

Young TM: Nuclear magnetic resonance studies of succussed solutions, *J Am Inst Homeopathy* 68:8, 1975.

Zong-Xiang Z: Research in the electrical specificity of meridians and acupuncture points, *Am J Acupunct* 9(3):203, 1981.

Zukav G: *The dancing Wu Li masters: an overview of the new physics,* New York, 1979, William Morrow & Co.

Chapter 17

*L*ow-Energy Photon Therapy

PEKKA J. PÖNTINEN

Lasers play an important role in medicine today. High-power lasers have partially replaced scalpels in the operating room. Laser beams can reopen an occluded artery. They can also coagulate tumors; repair retinal detachment; evaporate condylomata, warts, and tattoos; explode kidney stones; and perform many other functions.

Applications of low-energy lasers ("soft" or "cold" lasers) include preoperative and postoperative care, pain relief, and biomodulation. Other important indications include soft tissue trauma, wounds, ulcers, tendinitis, and fasciitis. The frequently used names *low-level laser therapy (LLLT), low-intensity laser therapy (LILT)*, and *low-energy laser therapy (LELT)* are no longer entirely accurate for this treatment modality. Coherency, the main specific property of the monochromatic laser light, is almost completely lost when the laser beam passes the skin. Furthermore the wavelength and amount of energy photons conveyed to the target zone are more important than coherency for the tissue effects. Therefore the term *low-energy photon therapy (LEPT)* is more appropriate for this treatment modality. The FDA has a new definition for laser treatment, which was announced in 1994 at the Annual Meeting of the American Society for Laser Medicine and Surgery in Toronto: nonthermal interaction of monochromatic radiation with target site (Felten, 1994). When applied during surgery, the high-power laser is a tool rather than a treatment, whereas low-level laser therapy for wound healing or relief of arthralgia may be considered a treatment (Lanzafame, 1995). At present the FDA has not approved any indications for laser therapy. However, General Motors recently performed a multicenter study on the use of LEPT in carpal tunnel syndrome, which may lead to the approval of LEPT for this application (Guynne, 1994).

Physical medicine uses stimulation therapy to activate the body's natural defense systems. LEPT is but one of many forms of physical medicine, which also includes acupuncture. Although acupuncture is rapidly gaining acceptance, LEPT is still seeking its rightful place in medicine and veterinary science.

The most common laser types in LEPT are the visible red helium-neon (HeNe) lasers, invisible infrared (IR) gallium-arsenide (GaAs) lasers, and gallium-aluminum-arsenide (GaAlAs) lasers. Recently, semiconductor, or diode, lasers have undergone development, and rapid growth is occurring in their manufacture and use. Most commonly used in sports medicine and treatment of myofascial pain and dysfunction, these lasers may emit either visible (orange-red) or invisible (IR) laser light.

To achieve positive results with LEPT, practitioners should understand the main indications for this method of treatment. A correct diagnosis is a prerequisite for successful therapy. Practitioners should understand the principles of LEPT, the basics of laser physics (optoelectronics), and even the construction of laser devices.

Because lasers may induce retinal lesions, all laser devices, irrespective of their purpose, must be classified according to their irradiation properties. Regulations for practitioners of laser treatment vary from country to country. The European Union has established the Committee on Laser Safety in Medicine to provide guidelines for the safe use of lasers in medicine.

In human and veterinary practice, sports medicine, physical or manual medicine, dermatology, and neuroendocrinology are the most important fields for LEPT. Another important use is in human rehabilitation medicine. The antiinflammatory and analgesic properties of LEPT, as well as its effect on collagen formation, make it useful in trauma, surgery, and dentistry.

IR (invisible) LEPT is ideal for use in double-blind studies of human and animal subjects: Researchers can easily eliminate the placebo effect by disconnecting the laser output while maintaining all outward appearances of

LEPT. The placebo effect is less relevant in veterinary medicine, however. Recently, many veterinarians have become interested in LEPT, mainly for its clinical and research applications. The thick and hairy skin common to most animals provides new challenges for LEPT. IR LEPT (mainly GaAs and GaAlAs in class 3B lasers) has many applications in equine medicine (Ambronn, Muxeneder, Warnke, 1995; McKibbin, Paraschak, 1983, 1984; Rogers, 1992).

LEPT may be used to treat internal, systemic, and generalized disorders by irradiating important systemic or reflex points, also called *trigger points (TPs), acupuncture points (APs),* and *tender local points,* or *AHSHI points.* LEPT may also be used as a local therapy over painful joints, muscles, tendons, wounds, ulcers, inflamed areas, and hematomas. In both point treatment and local treatment, LEPT can be applied either with a probe (in direct contact with skin or mucosa) or a laser beam (e.g., HeNe and IR lasers) from a distance of 1 to 50 cm.

A special application is irradiation with LEPT through a rotating and oscillating prism (a scanner device that sends a laser beam to sweep over a larger area). Applying LEPT to points provides a high-power density on a small target area, whereas free-beam scanning gives a lower-power density but a more equal distribution of irradiation over a larger target area.

HeNe (visible red) lasers penetrate the skin poorly and are suitable for treatment of superficial (skin and mucosal) lesions and muscle and connective tissue injuries, whereas IR lasers penetrate more deeply and are suitable for superficial and some deeper lesions.

LEPT has certain advantages over needling or point injection in AP and TP therapy (Rogers, 1992):

- It is aseptic, noninvasive, and painless; if used properly, it has no reported side effects. The probe is held within 0 to 5 cm from the skin, and the light is aimed at the point.
- It is ideal for use on painful (AHSHI) points or in nervous or difficult animals. Children and cats tolerate LEPT well.
- It may be used safely on dangerous points in large animals (such as points below the carpus and tarsus of cattle and horses).
- It is ideal for treatment of superficial APs, such as those on the ear.

History

The word *laser* is an acronym for *Light Amplification by Stimulated Emission of Radiation.* The history of laser use is relatively short, although in 1917 Einstein provided the conceptual foundation for the stimulated emission of electromagnetic radiation. Einstein's theory was verified by R. Landberg in 1928, but at that time no practical means existed to produce a functioning laser device.

In the 1930s and 1940s a better understanding of the energy levels of atoms and molecules and the development of advanced optic material provided a basis for the development of laser. The first known theory on amplification of stimulated emission was found in a patent application from 1951 by the Russian physicist V. Fabrikant and his two assistants; however, this application remained unpublished until 1959 and did not influence research work in the West.

The first apparatus using the principles of stimulated emission was called *maser* and was built by C.H. Townes in 1955. The word *maser* is an acronym for *Microwave Amplification by Stimulated Emission of Radiation.* J. Weber proposed a maser amplification in 1952 and gave a detailed report in his article "Amplification of microwave radiation with substances in thermal equilibrium." N. Bloembergen proposed a solid-based maser in 1956.

A.L. Shawlow and C.H. Townes (1958) furthered the development of maser principles for the age of optic radiation, preparing a draft model by September 1957. In 1958, they reported that the amplified light must be monochromatic and coherent. Townes and Shalow had applied for a maser patent by the summer of 1958. At approximately the same time, G. Gould independently solved the problems preventing the development of a functioning laser and initiated a court trial on patent rights against Townes and Shalow.

Before any of the aforementioned experts were ready to present their lasers, however, an unknown researcher, Theodor Maiman, produced a ruby-laser at the Hughes Aircraft Research Laboratory in Malibu, California. Presented to the press on July 7, 1960, this laser consisted of a 1-cm thick, 10-cm long ruby-probe that produced short but very intensive lighting at 694.3 nm. This was the beginning of a surprisingly rapid development: 1 year later, dozens of lasers were ready to use. Among these were HeNe lasers working in the near-infrared wavelengths (1118, 1153, 1160, 1199, and 1207 nm). The first HeNe laser in a visible wavelength (633 nm) became available in 1962. Today, several thousands of different laser media are available, and new laser types are continually being discovered.

In the former Soviet Union, several scientists worked simultaneously in laser development. N. Basov and A. Prokhorov made great technical advances and shared the Nobel Prize in 1964 with C. Townes. Basov and Prokhorov are still working in laser research today. In 1961, Gould reported important biomedical indications based on the high-energy density of laser light. Laser energy was first applied clinically in ophthalmology, and it was here that the first laser complications were found. Retinal lesions produced by focused laser light and leading to the loss of sharp vision were confirmed in animal studies. In 1962, L. Dulberger published an article describing laser risks titled "How Dangerous Are Lasers?" This article resulted in the first safety regulations for lasers in the mid-1960s.

After the first successful trials to repair retinal detachment, new uses for lasers were found. Surgeons used lasers as instruments for coagulation and evaporation and as simple but extremely accurate scalpels. Results were not always positive, and lasers had other disadvantages: They were unwieldy, expensive, and often overly sensitive.

The first reports of the effects of low-energy laser irradiation were published in the mid-1960s. For example, Y. Laor and his associates (1965) reported that ". . . laser irradiation was found to stimulate the rate of healing of burns and mechanically induced wounds . . .". Dr. E. Mester, professor in surgery at the Semmelweiss Hospital in Budapest, was an influential proponent of laser therapy. He published several studies of the biostimulatory effects of lasers on cell cultures, in experimental animal studies, and in clinical trials before experts in conventional Western medicine were aware of low-energy lasers and their role in medicine (Mester, 1968, 1977; Mester and others, 1968).

In the former Soviet Union the development of lasers for medical use took a slightly different path. N.F. Gamaleya had studied the biologic effects of lasers since 1962. Her first reports dealt with the effects of laser light on cell cultures and animal tissue. After these studies were published, lasers (or *Quantum Opticum*, as Soviets called them at that time) were first applied for biostimulation. V. Inyushin replaced needles with low-power laser beams in acupuncture. At the Central Institute for Experimental Surgery and Anaesthesiology in Moscow, low-power laser is routinely used against postoperative pain and dysfunctions (Tsibulyak, Lee, Alisov, 1988). In Kiev, Zalesskiy used fiber optics to conduct laser light through a cannula directly to the nerve trunks at the target region. This application of lasers was used to alleviate pain associated with cancer (Zalesskiy, 1984; Zalesskiy, Frolov, 1987). More recent applications include extracorporeal irradiation of blood in infectious diseases to enhance the immune response and improve the flowing properties of circulating blood cells (Samoilova and others, 1993).

In veterinary medicine, interest in lasers has been twofold: (1) to accelerate the healing of wounds and soft tissue lesions, and (2) to improve physical performance.

Physical, Biochemical, Biophysical, and Biologic Background for Low-Energy Photon Therapy (LEPT)

Electromagnetic Irradiation

A laser is a device that produces electromagnetic irradiation. Electromagnetic irradiation is a form of energy flux that can be understood in two ways: as a wave movement with all typical properties of waves (e.g., wavelength, polarization, interference, diffraction) and also as a flow formed of particles with their properties (e.g., mass, quantified energy, influenced by gravity). To simplify understanding of these two seemingly unrelated behaviors, we may refer to wave particles or wave packages by the term *photons*. A photon has both the character of a wave and the character of a particle. Photons have a certain amount of energy, which is called *photon energy*. The energy of a photon is inversely related to its wavelength: the bigger the wavelength of a photon, the smaller its energy.

When a photon hits an object, it may deliver its energy. This energy may then be reflected from the surface, transmitted further, or absorbed. In the first two cases the photon retains its energy. In the third case the energy of the photon is delivered to the atoms or molecules of the object. This absorbed energy may be transformed in the following ways:

- It may change to heat oscillations (atom/material becomes hot)
- It may excite an atom or a molecule (electrons change their energy level)
- It may ionize an atom or a molecule (to deliver an electron)
- It may break up chemical bindings (to build up new compounds)

The energy absorbed in LEPT is so low that the temperature increase in the radiated tissues remains below 1° C. Still, enough photons are present to induce changes in cell metabolism.

The Light

Approximately 200 years ago, scientists knew about only a small portion of the electromagnetic radiation known as *light:* the part that is visible. Newton, with other physicists, demonstrated the wave character of the light and proposed that these waves might interfere with each other. The next step was to show that various colors correlated with different wavelengths. Red light has the longest wavelength, whereas violet has the shortest. Orange, green, and blue fall between these extremes.

Scientists discovered later that heat radiation has the same characteristics as light but with longer wavelengths. *Infrared radiation* refers to radiation that occurs beyond the wavelength of red light. Although heat radiation is termed *infrared*, it is completely invisible; not enough photon energy is present to excite the visual cells in the retina. Similarly, invisible radiation that has a shorter wavelength than that of violet light is called *ultraviolet radiation* (Table 17-1).

Some properties of light

Two different systems are used to measure light: photometric and radiometric. The photometric system involves the spectral sensitivity of the eye, whereas the radiometric measurement is absolute and linked to the metric system. The measurements, names, and units in Table 17-2 are in common use.

TABLE 17-1

SOME PROPERTIES OF LIGHT

COLOR	WAVELENGTH	EFFECT ON LIVING TISSUE
Invisible heat radiation	>800 nm	No negative reactions
BOUNDARY TO VISIBILITY		
Red	800-610 nm	No negative reactions (light from this area may
Orange	610-595 nm	induce photoallergy in the presence of certain sub-
Yellow	595-560 nm	stances)
Yellow-green	560-530 nm	
Green	530-495 nm	
Blue	495-430 nm	
Violet	430-400 nm	
BOUNDARY TO INVISIBILITY		
Invisible ultraviolet		
UVA	400-320 nm	May induce photoallergy
UVB	320-290 nm	May induce skin cancer
UVC	290-185 nm	Kills all life forms

TABLE 17-2

SYSTEMS OF MEASURING LIGHT

	RADIOMETRY		PHOTOMETRY	
	NAME	UNIT	NAME	UNIT
Flow	Light flow	W	Light effect	Lumen
Luminous intensity:				
Radiation	Radians	W/Sr	Luminance	Candela
Irradiation	Irradians	W/m²	Illuminance	Lux

Measurements for lasers are always performed with radiometry; that is, their light flow (often incorrectly called *luminous intensity*) is measured in watts or, for low-level lasers, in milliwatts (mW).

A 60-watt light bulb does not deliver a light flow of 60 watts—only about 1 or 2 watts. However, it consumes 60 watts of electricity to produce 1 or 2 watts in light flow. A 60-watt laser delivers a 60-watt pure light effect, but it must consume thousands of watts of electricity to produce it. The light beam from a common light bulb is highly divergent (i.e., it has a wide angle and goes in all directions). The light beam from a searchlight is nearly parallel, or collimated. A convergent light can be produced with lenses and mirrors. *Convergent* means that the light beam becomes narrower toward a focus. Between a burning lens and its focus the radiation is convergent.

Light is a wavelike motion wherein the oscillations of photons occur in a polarizing plane. If all photons oscillate in the same plane (in the same direction), the light is polarized. A polarized light has a certain order: All photons are organized to move in the same plane (e.g., horizontally). This does not depend on the geometry of the radiation.

The light from an incandescent bulb includes photons with all wavelengths inside the visible spectrum and some from the infrared area as well. The undesired wavelengths can be filtered so that they disappear. By using filters in this way, we can obtain more or less monochromatic light. All photons have nearly the same energy. To produce real monochromatic light, the photons must have a certain organization. This organization does not depend on the geometry or polarization of the radiation.

Photons can even be arranged into well-organized lines, where they link to form long, attached swings. This type of light is called *coherent* (organized), and the length the waves are attached together is called *coherence length*.

Many people mistakenly believe that coherent light must be parallel, which is not the case. However, coherent light must be monochromatic. Light from conventional bulbs is almost completely incoherent; coherence length is at best only a few tenths of a millimeter, whereas the light of a laser is always more or less coherent—coherence length may reach several meters.

All waves with the same wavelength (and frequency) that travel in the same direction have a certain phase situation. If the crests and troughs of two waves pass a point simultaneously, these waves are in a phase. If the crest of the first wave passes the point with the trough of the second wave, the waves are in a counterphase.

When radiation is coherent, inducing interference phenomena is easy. Interference helps in elucidating the influence two coherent waves with the same wavelength have on each other if they reach a point simultaneously. If they are in a phase, they strengthen each other (constructive interference); if they are in a counterphase, they weaken or even extinguish each other (destructive interference). Interference phenomenona are always much clearer when a pure light from a laser is used rather than a conventional light bulb.

The origin of light

Photons develop when electrons circulating the atomic nucleus change their course. Normally, this happens when extrinsic energy is brought to the atom. This extra energy can produce the following effects:

- Heat oscillation
- Atom or electron collisions
- Electron-hole recombinations
- Energy from chemical reactions
- Other incoming photons

Energy that is brought to an atom in any of the aforementioned forms can be stored when electrons change from a course near the nucleus to one that is farther away. In most substances, these excited electrons can maintain their new courses for only a short time before reverting to their normal courses.

When an electron jumps from a distant course to one nearer the nucleus, its potential energy becomes lower through the release of a photon with exactly the same energy (i.e., with a wavelength or frequency that corresponds precisely to the energy deficit of the jump). Every jump delivers a photon with an exact wavelength that can be calculated in advance. To produce a great mass of photons with the same wavelength, all excited electrons must have precisely the same course (or energy level) and then jump together to the precisely same (lower-energy) course. When this occurs, a laser is produced.

The same movement of electrons traveling up and down between different energy levels takes place in all natural light or other forms of radiation but in a very disorganized and uncontrolled way. This leads to the whole spectrum of light, heat radiation, and other forms of electromagnetic radiation.

Radiation Sources and Light Sources

Sun

The oldest source of radiation and light, the sun has an enormous spectrum. The sun delivers all forms of electromagnetic radiation (e.g., radio waves, microwaves, x-rays, γ-rays). The ozone layer in the higher atmosphere absorbs most of the dangerous ultraviolet radiation. Some carcinogenic UVB rays and all of the extremely dangerous UVC rays are filtered out. Ultraviolet radiation, with a shorter wavelength and x-ray and γ-ray radiation, is absorbed by oxygen, nitrogen, and other gases in the air. This means that the most dangerous radiation from the sun never reaches us. The most dangerous photons that may reach us have a wavelength of 290 nm. All radiation with shorter wavelengths is filtered by the atmosphere. However, a certain amount of ultraviolet radiation (with a wavelength between 320 and 290 nm) manages to reach the earth and may induce cancer growth.

Neon tube

The first experiments with a gas discharge tube were performed at the beginning of this century. A glass tube containing a minimum amount of gas—almost a vacuum—served as a prototype. After the air was pumped out, neon gas was added and then electrical current, which illuminated the gas in dark red. Light is generated through a process whereby the free electrons of the electrical current rush through the thin gas and collide with the gas atoms (energy process number 2). This collision energy throws the bound electrons of an atom to the outer courses (higher energy levels). When these electrons return to their normal basic condition, they give up the energy difference from this downward jump in the form of photons. Because only one gas exists and it contains easily excitable electrons, light is produced with a wavelength that corresponds to a certain jump between the courses of the electrons in a neon atom.

A gas discharge tube and gas lasers share many characteristics. Other examples of gas discharge tubes are yellow sodium lamps along motorways, mercury lamps (street lighting), and common fluorescent tubes. In all these a flow of free electrons is allowed to rush through a thin mercury vapor. Ultraviolet and visible radiation is generated through collision energy produced when these free electrons collide with mercury atoms and change their energy levels. To increase the portion of visible light, the inner surface of the tube is covered with a fluorescent illuminating powder. When atoms in this illuminating powder collide with ultraviolet photons, electrons are projected to the outer courses (higher energy levels). When they return to their normal courses (normally through several steps), a visible light is generated (energy process number 5).

Light-emitting diode (LED)/superluminous diode (SLD)

Light-emitting diodes (LEDs), or superlumious diodes (SLDs), are recently developed sources of light, only a little older than lasers. They are small and produce red, yellow, or green light. Some newer LEDs produce blue light. Infrared LEDs are found in remote-control devices for television sets. LEDs are inexpensive and frequently used in indicator lamps and calculator displays.

Light is generated through energy process number 3 in a semiconductor. A semiconductor is a crystal (most often silicon) that is mixed with a small amount of a support substance. When electrical current travels through a semiconductor, free electrons are generated, but a "hole" is formed when an atom in the crystal delivers a rather unstable electron. This atom may steal an electron from its neighbor, which in turn may rob an electron from another atom nearby. In this way a "hole" wanders through the crystal. These holes are positive (because a negative charge has been taken away from a neutral atom), and they move through the crystal against the direction of the electrons. If an electron hits a hole, recombination energy is generated, which is directly delivered as a photon (energy process number 3). LED is similar to a laser diode or a semiconductor laser.

Laser: Properties of a Laser Light

Light from a laser differs from light from other sources in at least two ways: (1) It is always monochromatic (i.e., it has a narrow spectrum), and (2) it is always coherent (i.e., it has a long cohererence length). The light from the laser may also have one of the following qualities:

- A small divergence (nearly parallel beam)
- A high output power (many watts)
- Polarization (light waves oscillate in the same plane)

The common belief that laser beams are parallel and have a high power output is mistaken. However, a parallel beam from a laser is easy to produce in comparison with other light sources. Strong light is also easier to produce from a laser than from other sources, especially if small divergence, monochromaticity, and high coherence are also necessary. Light from a laser may or may not be polarized depending on whether it is provided with a polarizing device, or Brewster-window.

Lasers may have more or less specific properties according to the preceding list. Lasers with a long cavity (e.g., HeNe lasers) have a narrow spectrum and greater coherence length, whereas those with a very short cavity (e.g., semiconductor lasers) have a rather broad spectrum and a much shorter coherence length.

Light from a laser, like that from any source, can be conducted through optic fibers. This type of cable can lead light from a large laser tube to a handy probe or "laser pen." However, everything has its price. In this case the coherence length is greatly reduced (from decimeters to millimeters), and a great deal of radiation power is lost (10% to 50%). Polarization is lost simultaneously.

Lasers for Biomodulation

Commonly used low-energy lasers for biomodulation are presented in Table 17-3. HeNe, GaAs, and GaAlAs lasers dominate the field.

Helium-neon lasers (HeNe lasers)

Helium-neon (HeNe) lasers are the oldest and best documented of all lasers with a biostimulating effect. HeNe lasers emit red visible light at 632.8 nm wavelength. Emission is continuous, but it can be switched on and off so that outcoming laser light is pulsed. HeNe lasers have a long coherence length and an output power that can be raised up to 100 mW (although at this level the tube length increases accordingly, and the laser device becomes too large to be practical). HeNe lasers are common and have a great variety of applications beyond medicine. For example, they can be used in surveying and construction work, the production of holograms, and bar code readers and pointers.

The main disadvantages of HeNe lasers are their size and the need for a sensitive laser tube made of glass. HeNe lasers require a high voltage for driving, and the demand for ignition is over 10,000 V. For these reasons the price of an effective medical HeNe laser is relatively high.

Gallium-arsenide lasers (GaAs lasers)

GaAs lasers belong to a newer semiconductor laser family. The first GaAs lasers for biostimulation were produced in the early 1980s. The emission from a GaAs is invisible in the infrared range (904 nm), and it is always pulsed as a flashlight, with a pulse length of 100 to 200 nanoseconds and a pulse peak power up to 100 W. The mean effect is much lower and depends on pulse parameters and pulse repetition frequency. One of the great advantages of GaAs lasers is their small size. Fig. 17-1 shows a typical laser diode mounted in a protective can. The p-n junction laser diode is an excellent light source in optical integrated circuits and fiberoptic signal transmission applications.

Disadvantages relate to the construction of the diode and its mounting. The active region of a laser diode is not only small but also quite asymmetric. Typically the junction of a GaAs laser diode has an effective thickness of only 0.1 micron, but the active region may be 5 microns wide (Fig. 17-2). This leads to a very small and asymmetric beam waist. Consequently the beam divergence is typically between 15 and 30 degrees, although divergences up to 90 degrees are not unusual. Divergence in the plane parallel to the layer is a factor of about 2 degrees less than this.

Optical output power strongly depends on the input pumping current (Fig. 17-3). At low-current levels the

TABLE 17-3

LASERS FOR BIOMODULATION

LASER	WAVELENGTH(S) (nm)
Helium-Neon (HeNe)	632.8
Indium-Gallium-Aluminum-Phosphide (InGaAlP)	635, 670, 780
Gallium-Aluminum-Arsenide (GaAlAs)	820, 830
Gallium-Arsenide (GaAs)	904
Neodymium:Yttrium-Aluminum-Garnet (Nd:YAG)	1064
Carbon dioxide (CO_2)	10600

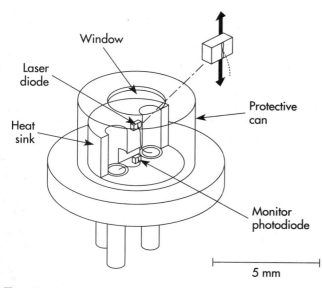

Fig. 17-1 Schematic cross section of a laser diode mounted in a protective can. (From Kolari PJ and others, *Scand J Acup Electrother* 3:96, 1988.)

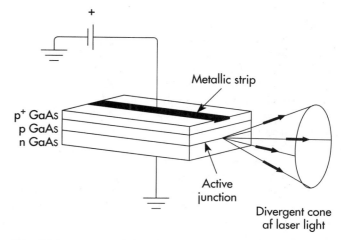

Fig. 17-2 Basic structure of a laser diode. (From Kolari PJ and others: *Scand J Acup Electrother* 3:96, 1988.)

light that is emitted is mostly the result of spontaneous emission, and it has a characteristic spectral line width of dozens of nanometers. It is incoherent light. As the input current exceeds the threshold value, a sharp break can be observed in the slope of the optical output power versus the pump current curve. In addition, the output power markedly decreases with the increasing temperature of a laser diode.

Gallium-aluminum-arsenide laser (GaAlAs laser)

GaAlAs lasers are the latest addition to lasers used for biomodulation. They are solid and small. The composition of the semiconducting, light-emitting crystal may vary considerably. Depending on the percentage of each substance used, the wavelength of outgoing radiation may vary between 660 and 860 nm. The most common measurements in today's commercially available GaAlAs lasers

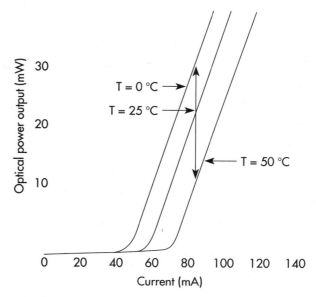

Fig. 17-3 Optic output of a laser diode as a function of input pumping current. (From Kolari PJ and others: *Scand J Acup Electrother* 3:96, 1988.)

are, in descending order, 820, 830 nm (infrared), 635, 670 nm (red), and 760 nm (near IR), a modified Indium-Gallium-Aluminium-Phosphide laser (InGaAlP). These lasers emit either continuously or in the pulsed mode. Their optical output can rise to several hundred mW in a continuous mode or half of that as a mean in a pulsed mode. For biomodulation the output power for single diode lasers is commonly around 30 to 100 mW. For better results in the treatment of bigger joints and deeper-sited lesions in sports medicine, diodes up to 300 mW or multidiode heads (clusters) up to 500 mW (or even higher) are the most recent developments. Multidiode heads (clusters) often combine two laser diodes with multiple SLDs emitting, in some constructions, different wavelengths.

Other laser types for biomodulation

Outside the range of LEPT lasers, biomodulating effects have been reported in connection with treatments with Nd:YAG lasers, argon-laser, ruby lasers, crypton lasers, and CO_2 lasers. Other laser types with biomodulating effects may appear in the future.

Fibers and other extensions/accessories

A common laser accessory is an optic fiber. Optic fiber conducts laser light from an impractically large laser tube to a convenient penlike probe. Two types of optic fibers are available: single fibers (monofibers) and fiber bundles. The challenge is to find light and flexible material with a minimal loss of optic power. Practitioners are advised to allow for a 15% to 40% reduction of optic power per one meter length in present materials.

When light leaves a monofiber or a fiber bundle, it is always more or less divergent. If it was polarized when entering the optic fiber, it is nonpolarized at the outlet. Certain fibers may maintain polarization, but they are expensive and never used in low-power lasers. If the incoming light has a great coherence length, this will get markedly shorter. However, coherence length is still long enough for biomodulation in living tissue.

Scanner devices

With the increased sophistication of laser technique a degree of automation has occurred. The first step toward automation was the so-called laser cannon, which allowed operators to direct radiation from one or several laser diodes or a HeNe tube from a distance of 30 to 80 cm to the target area. The next step was the development of a scanner device that permits the laser beam to sweep over the area under treatment.

A major problem with these laser types is that their beams cannot penetrate as deeply as those of a handheld laser probe. The marked reflection from the skin, due to the wide incident angle, decreases the photon flow and energy density at the target area. The laser probe offers superior optic contact with the skin. The subcutaneous tissue may be pressed lightly to decrease the distance to the peripheral nerves endings and myofascial trigger areas.

Their large size and the difficulty of finding the right angle and distance are other drawbacks of scanner devices, to say nothing of their higher price. For some special applications (e.g., treatment of large areas, including biostimulation for hair growth), specially constructed scanners are practical and reasonably effective.

Important Laser Parameters for Biomodulation

Obviously, practitioners cannot use just any laser to treat patients. Every laser type has its own characteristic properties and different biologic effects. The following are some parameters known to be important in biomodulation, although precise details are not yet available:

- All lasers are not useful in biomodulation. Wavelength should be longer than 600 nm, according to Kana and others (1981).
- Lasers inducing biomodulation may exert different biologic effects (Abergel and others, 1984). For wound and ulcer treatment, HeNe lasers seem to be the best (Mester, Mester, Mester, 1985), for pain relief in the deeper tissues, GaAs lasers are recommended (Schwanitz, 1988), and GaAlAs lasers are reasonably effective in the more superficial complaints (Oshiro, Galderhead, 1988).
- Different laser types may require different energy doses for optimal results (Abergel and others, 1984).
- The effect in the tissues is laser specific (coherent light), whereas the effect in the tissue cultures also includes polarized light (noncoherent) with a narrow waveband (Bihari and others, 1989; Kubota and others, 1989; Mester, Mester, Mester, 1985; Timea and others, 1988).
- In certain cell cultures in which laser light has produced a measurable biomodulatory effect, this effect may diminish or completely disappear in the presence of a noncoherent light with a wide wave band. Therefore another light source (e.g., sun or other strong light, including the LED light from the laser device) may produce a negative or disruptive effect on the biomodulation through the laser light (Karu, 1987).
- A combination of two different laser types may produce a better effect than either of them alone (Bihari and others, 1989; Lonauer, 1987).
- In pulsed lasers, different frequencies seem to produce different biologic effects (Dyson, Young, 1986).
- Energy density is important. An increased dose of irradiation may decrease the biomodulatory effect (Shiroto, Ono, Oshiro, 1989).

With regard to many of these laser parameters, scientists know only that they play an important role in biomodulation (Box 17-1). Although a small number of stud-

BOX 17-1

Laser Parameters for Biomodulation

Wavelength	632.8, 635, 670, 780, 820, 830, 904 nm
Output power/radiant power in CW mode	Average 5-150 mW (300-600 mW in cluster heads)
Peak pulse power (GaAs)	10-100 W corresponding 5-50 mW average radiant power
Waveform	Continuous wave (CW), pulsed (1-10 kHz), frequency modulated (Nogier, von Bahr, etc.)
Power density/irradiance	1-300 J/cm^2
Dosage/site in point treatment	1-4 J (spot size: 1 mm^2 to 1-2 cm^2)

ies demonstrate the importance of pulse frequency, scientists do not know exactly which frequencies are optimal in certain indications. Much work will have to be done before the role of these parameters is clarified.

Should It Be a Laser?

Some people believe that results similar to those produced by lasers can be achieved with cheaper light sources. This argument implies that the narrow wavelength band and coherent light (characteristic of lasers) are probably not necessary to produce effects confirmed in cell cultures, living tissue, experimental animal research, and human experiments. One argument has been that coherence length is markedly reduced when the laser light spreads into the tissue.

Several studies compare the effect of laser light on cell cultures and living tissue with that of light emitted from other sources, with a wider wavelength band. Karu (1987), among others, has investigated the use of a monochromatic light with a wider wavelength band on cell cultures. Her study shows results that are for the most part similar to those produced by laser light. She appears to have used nonpolarized light in her experiments.

Mester (1977) has studied the way lymphocytes in a cell culture react to polarized and nonpolarized red light with a narrow wavelength band. He concluded that polarization plays an important role in the biostimulating effect. Fennyö (1984) has confirmed that even a polarized light with a broad wavelength band has a marked effect on cell membrane; this light produced approximately 80% of the effect of laser light with the same irradiation dose, whereas corresponding experiments with nonpolarized light showed no significant effect.

The aforementioned studies, among others, suggest two different types of phenomena: a phenomenon in which photon energy is the essential parameter and a phenomenon in which the polarization of light plays a major role (i.e., an electric field vector with a specific direction). Research has confirmed, for example, that a linearly polarized light reorganizes floating crystals differently from

the way a nonpolarized light does. Research also shows that certain lipids in the cell membrane behave very much like floating crystals.

However, cell cultures and living tissue have important differences. In a cell culture, polarized light is essential for certain phenomena (e.g., cell metabolism), whereas polarization is not as important when living tissue is irradiated. Open wounds and ulcers may characterize a borderline case. A possible reason for this difference is that a cell culture is commonly a thin and transparent layer of cells that float in a nutrient. When the cell culture is radiated with polarized light, polarization is maintained throughout the cell layer. However, when a living tissue is irradiated, the light beam spreads into the tissue and the polarization is lost after the beam reaches a depth of approximately one half of a millimeter. In a wound secretion, polarization may be maintained to the depth of several millimeters. In other words, all light is nonpolarized beneath the skin, whether it was originally polarized or nonpolarized.

Both coherence and collimation are rapidly lost through scattering and backscattering in the tissues. Laser diodes with a high divergence and poor coherence in time and space can alter cell metabolism and induce clear clinical effects (e.g., in myofascial pain and dysfunction). The same is true with noncoherent but monochromatic radiation from SLDs. For absorption and biologic effects a certain wavelength (monochromaticity) is important (Karu, 1987).

Irradiation Dose

The irradiation dose may be the most important parameter for laser treatment. The irradiation dose is measured in joules (J) per treated point or square centimeter (J/cm^2). The dose should not be so low that no measurable effects are produced, but neither can it be too high. A biomodulating irradiation dose has a lower and higher limit, with an optimum level in the middle. An overly high dose that exceeds the biomodulating level may induce no effect at all or even undesirable effects. For successful therapy, the following should be observed:

- Repeated low doses within a specific time interval produce a stronger effect than the same total dose in a single treatment (Abergel and others, 1984; Laor and others, 1965).
- The biomodulating effect is cumulative. Repeated doses with a suitable, relatively short interval produce an additional response (Mester, Mester, Mester, 1985).
- Doses that are too low produce no demonstrable effect. Doses that are too high either produce no effect or damp the biologic activity (Kana and others, 1981).
- Mester (1968) has found that an optimal weekly irradiation dose for HeNe laser treatment through the skin is about 1 J/cm². Abergel and others (1984) have reported that the dose for a GaAs laser on fibroblasts is clearly lower than that for a HeNe laser.
- Doses for acupuncture points recommended in the literature of the former Soviet Union are about 0.1 J/AP-point.

Calculation of the irradiation dose

The joule is a unit of measurement for energy. One joule is identical to 1 watt-second (i.e., the energy that is generated when 1 watt of power flows for 1 second). The irradiation dose is therefore the amount of energy conducted into the tissue. Because of the importance of conducting this energy through one or several square centimeters, it is better to describe the dose in terms of energy density, or J/cm². Because *joule (J)* is the same as *watt-second (Ws)*, the irradiation dose can be calculated as follows:

$$\frac{\text{Laser power conducted to the tissue in watts} \times \text{time in seconds}}{\text{Treated surface in centimeters}}$$

This can be written as

$$D = \frac{P \times t}{A} \ (J/cm^2) \ (1)$$

For example, if a laser has a 15 mW mean output power, it emits 0.015 joule per second in energy. In 10 seconds, the following equation holds true: $10 \times 0.015 = 0.15$ joule. Table 17-4 shows the way a high dose is emitted in 1 second and 1 minute from different lasers with output power between 6 and 90 mW (mean power). The emission time to reach a total dose of 1 and 2 joules is presented in the same table.

In GaAs lasers working in a fixed pulsed mode, the mean output power becomes very low with low frequencies. Pulse energy for pulsed lasers should be given in a standard approval report. Typical measured values for energy per pulse are from 0.1 μJ to 5 μJ. The mean output power of a single pulsed laser depends only on the frequency, as shown in Table 17-5.

Table 17-5 demonstrates that a fixed pulsed laser is hardly effective when used with frequencies lower than 1000 Hz. For example, a laser with a pulse energy of 1 μJ is driven with 1 kHz (=1000 Hz) frequency. The mean output power for this laser is 0.1 mW. If we want to perform a laser treatment on a 5 × 5 cm area with a dose of 1 J/cm², we may calculate according to the following equation:

Dose: 1 J/cm²
Power: 0.1 mW = 0.0001 W
Target area: 25 cm²

$$D = \frac{P \times t}{A}$$

which is transformed to calculate the time needed for this treatment

$$t = \frac{D \times A}{P} \ (2) \ t = \frac{1 \times 25}{0.0001} = 250,000 \text{ s} = 4000 \text{ min} = 11 \text{ h}$$

The calculation above demonstrates that the laser is useless for this form of therapy. It also demonstrates the need for practitioners to know the output power of the laser or lasers they are using and be able to calculate roughly the

---

TABLE 17-4

CALCULATING THE IRRADIATION DOSE

MEAN OUTPUT POWER (mW)	EMISSION DOSE PER SECOND (mJ/J)	EMISSION DOSE PER MINUTE (mJ/J)	EMISSION TIME PER JOULE (min sec)	EMISSION TIME PER 2 JOULES (min sec)
6	6 mJ = 0.006 J	360 mJ = 0.36 J	2 min 47 sec	5 min 34 sec
8	8 mJ = 0.008 J	480 mJ = 0.48 J	2 min 5 sec	4 min 19 sec
10	10 mJ = 0.010 J	600 mJ = 0.60 J	1 min 40 sec	3 min 20 sec
12	12 mJ = 0.012 J	720 mJ = 0.72 J	1 min 23 sec	2 min 46 sec
15	15 mJ = 0.015 J	900 mJ = 0.90 J	1 min 7 sec	2 min 13 sec
20	20 mJ = 0.020 J	1.2 J	50 sec	1 min 40 sec
30	30 mJ = 0.030 J	1.8 J	33 sec	1 min 7 sec
40	40 mJ = 0.040 J	2.4 J	25 sec	50 sec
60	60 mJ = 0.060 J	3.6 J	17 sec	33 sec
90	90 mJ = 0.090 J	5.4 J	11 sec	22 sec

irradiation dose needed for an effective therapy. Mainly because of widespread ignorance of laser parameters, thousands of laser treatments have been given with irradiation doses far below those that are clinically effective.

These calculations and Table 17-5 demonstrate the advantage of the continuous wave HeNe, GaAlAs, and pulsetrain-modulated GaAs lasers over fixed pulsed lasers. The output power does not depend entirely on the frequency.

The diameter of the laser beam and the irradiation area (spot size) at the target (skin level) are important (Figs. 17-4 to 17-6).

TABLE 17-5

MEAN OUTPUT POWER FOR A FIXED PULSED GaAs-LASER WITH DIFFERENT FREQUENCIES AND INCREASING PULSE ENERGY

PULSE ENERGY FREQUENCY	0.1 μJ	0.3 μJ	1 μJ	3 μJ	5 μJ
10 Hz	0.001 mW	0.003 mW	0.01 mW	0.03 mW	0.05 mW
100 Hz	0.01 mW	0.03 mW	0.1 mW	0.3 mW	0.5 mW
1000 Hz	0.1 mW	0.3 mW	1 mW	3 mW	5 mW
10000 Hz	1 mW	3 mW	10 mW	30 mW	50 mW

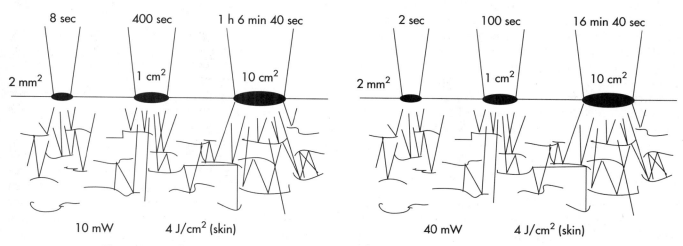

Figs. 17-4 and 17-5 The effect of spot size on the irradiation time needed to reach 4 J/cm² energy density using 10 mW and 40 mW lasers emitting in a continuous wave mode.

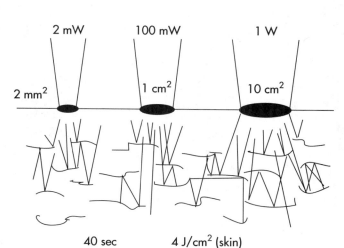

Fig. 17-6' The effect of spot size on the output power to reach 4 J/cm² in 40 seconds.

Three-Dimensional Light Distribution in Biotissue

A light beam from any light source is partially reflected from the surface. The amount of reflection depends on the incident angle of the beam and the quality (color) of the skin. To minimize reflection, a contact treatment is recommended. In noncontact form the beam should hit the skin at a 90-degree angle. Reflection loss is increased in any form of scanner treatment in which the incident angle varies. A longer distance between the skin and laser tip means a greater loss of energy through scattering and greater reflection. The same is true of any noncollimated diode laser in which the divergence angle may easily reach 100 to 150 mrad. The maximum distance for an effective therapy is no more than two centimeters.

Light propagation through biotissue is regulated by scattering, absorption, and backscattering. *Scattering* refers to the change in the direction of light propagation, which depends on relative refractive indices of tissue types (e.g., molecules). Some photons are reflected back toward the surface, which is called *backscattering*. Other photons are absorbed by water and some organic molecules, or chromophores. Every chromophore has a specific absorption coefficient. Absorption is wavelength specific, also. Wavelengths longer than 1200 nm (infrared) and shorter than 200 nm (ultraviolet) are absorbed by water. Typical wavelengths of therapy lasers (633 to 900 nm) are better able to penetrate (optical window) because their photons are not so easily absorbed by living tissue (about 70% water). Moreover, hemoglobin and melanin absorption coefficients are relatively low in near infrared field.

Penetration

Direct penetration of light in biotissue is minimal (Langer, Lange, 1992). Penetration partly relates to the wavelength of radiation, from 0.5 mm for red (HeNe) light to 2 to 3 mm for infrared (820 to 904 nm). Some 2% to 3% of HeNe laser light is measurable at 2 mm depth,

whereas 15% to 17% of IR laser light continues at this level according to studies (Kolari, 1985; Kolari and others, 1988). For a better understanding of light distribution, penetration depth may be conceived as a unit. In a penetration depth of 1, 36% of the irradiation is present at the skin surface. The radiant power, energy density at the surface, and total irradiation dose needed to achieve a therapeutically valid dose at the target zone can all be calculated. Table 17-6 presents the radiant power (power density) for 820 (830) nm single diode lasers of 30, 60, and 150 mW output power at $1\times$ to $5\times$ penetration depths in contact treatment mode (spot size 0.125 cm^2) This theoretical model does not take into account the specific absorption coefficients for different tissues or scattering and backscattering.

Approximately 80 seconds may be necessary for a 30 mW laser to achieve an energy density of 0.1 J/cm^2 at 1.5 to 2.0 cm depth (80 seconds $\times$ 1.3 mW/cm^2); 15 seconds for 150 mW laser or 40 seconds for a 60 mW laser would produce the same energy density at the same target zone.

Laser-Induced Temperature Changes

The degree of temperature elevation in the irradiated tissues is related to the rate of energy absorption at any point in the tissue. The rate of energy absorption in turn depends on the absorption coefficient of the specific tissue type as well as that of every atom and molecule. Because the average water content in the adult human body is about 70%, about 30% is left mainly to organic molecules. An infrared spectrum over 1200 nm and an ultraviolet spectrum shorter than 200 nm predominate in photon absorption by water. Within the commonly used wavelengths in LEPT (630 to 950 nm), absorption may happen either by the amino acids and nucleic acid bases or by chromophores. Typical chromophores, or photoacceptors, are hemoglobin and melanin. Their "antennas" are tuned to specific wavelengths (e.g., oxygenated hemoglobin has absorption peaks at 420 and 577 nm; reduced hemoglobin

TABLE 17-6

CHANGES IN RADIANT POWER OF SINGLE DIODE IR LASER (820 nm) AT 1X-5X PENETRATION DEPTHS IN CONTACT TREATMENT MODE*

TARGET AREA	IR DIODE 30 mW	60 mW	150 mW
Surface	240 mW/cm^2	480 mW/cm^2	1.2 W/cm^2
$1 \times$ PD	87 mW/cm^2	174 mW/cm^2	432 mW/cm^2
$2 \times$ PD	31.2 mW/cm^2	62.4 mW/cm^2	155 mW/cm^2
$3 \times$ PD	10.8 mW/cm^2	21.6 mW/cm^2	54 mW/cm^2
$4 \times$ PD	3.8 mW/cm^2	7.6 mW/cm^2	19 mW/cm^2
$5 \times$ PD	1.3 mW/cm^2	2.6 mW/cm^2	6.5 mW/cm^2

*Spot size at skin surface 0.125 cm^2.
PD, Penetration depth.

at 560 nm). Melanin is responsible for the tanning of human skin by irradiation of near UV light. Both hemoglobin and melanin mediate photothermal effects of light energy photon (LEP) irradiation.

Temperature elevation at the target site during LEPT is minimal, usually 0.5° to 0.75° C with fluences of 1 to 4 J/cm². Temperature elevations of 0.4° to 0.6° C have been measured at the skin level, with fluences of 0.36 to 1.36 J/cm². Anders and others (1993) reported a 0.4° C rise in temperature in the facial nerves of rats after 90 min irradiation with 8.5 mW HeNe laser (total dose 45.9 J, fluence 162.4 J/cm²). Higher-output powers may induce marked elevations in tissue temperature (e.g., 110 mW, 2.45° C; 142 mW, 4.76° C). Gurevich, Filonenko, and Salansky (1994) have calculated temperature distribution curves in laser-irradiated mediums with an external cooled surface; 1 W lasers may induce a 5.8° C increase at the skin level and an approximately 0.9° C increase at the depth of 10 mm. If the surface is cooled, the maximum temperature is transferred deeper in the tissue. For example, 2.7 W irradiation produced a 5.2° C temperature increase at the depth of 3.5 mm. Surface cooling may be applied in acute soft tissue injuries and in sports medicine when higher fluences are necessary. Heat produced by continuously emitting lasers or IR diodes is more stable when excess heat is evenly distributed than during high peak energy pulse irradiation, where a local heat accumulation may take place, especially with high pulse frequencies.

LEPT-Induced Phenomena

Skin and Mucosal Cell Metabolism (e.g., Fibroblast and Keratinocyte Proliferation, Keratinocyte Motility Stimulation, Collagen Synthesis Enhancement)

Mester (1968, 1977) began to study the biologic effects of laser radiation by the early 1960s. He focused on the effect of laser light on wound healing. The irradiation of low-power lasers seemed to accelerate cell division. The number of leukocytes that participate in phagocytosis increased significantly. He also observed increases in the activity of fibroblasts and collagen formation. These changes were maximal in the wound area after the regeneration of lymphatic and blood vessels and with an abundant formation of granulation tissue.

HeNe lasers have a clear effect on mast cells. The number of mast cells is reduced after laser irradiation, and the cells show a marked degranulation. These changes may explain some typical laser effects in tissues (vasodilation, analgesia, antiinflammatory, and edema-reducing effects) corresponding to the release of histamines, prostaglandin, heparin, hyaluronic acid, mucopolysaccharides, and chemotactic factors of eosinophilic and neutrophilic leukocytes as a response to irradiation.

In addition to vasodilation and regeneration of lymph and blood vessels, laser irradiation of cell cultures increases mitochondrial ATP in human lymphocytes and activates RNA synthesis and therefore DNA production. Using similar test conditions, scientists have demonstrated a stimulation of enzyme activity that accelerates maturation of epithelium.

The speed and magnitude of collagen synthesis have been monitored in electron microscope measurements of glycine and proline contents taken simultaneously. On the basis of these studies, the acceleration and increase of collagen formation appear to be the most important factors behind the effect of lasers on wound healing. The laser effect clearly spreads outside the treated area, probably through humoral factors. These findings suggest that it is not necessary to irradiate the whole wound or ulcer area simultaneously to achieve a biostimulation effect. Rodrigo, Zaragoza, and Iturrate (1985) studied the effect of HeNe lasers on osteomyelitic fistulas. According to this study, a contralateral, nontreated fistula healed when only the other leg was treated.

Laser irradiation of leukocytes increases phagocytosis. Lasers can activate enzyme processes on wound edges, an important factor for wound healing. Seen mainly in the deeper layer of the epithelium (stratum basale), this effect leads to an increase in collagen formation in response to the stimulation of fibroblast activity.

Dyson and Young (1986) have clarified the effects of a continuously emitting (cw) HeNe laser and a pulsed IR laser on wound healing. According to their studies, an IR laser irradiation using 700 Hz accelerated scar formation, whereas a treatment using 1200 Hz had no effect if all other parameters remained unchanged. In another study, Steinlechner and Dyson (1993) examined the effects of HeNe and IR laser (904 nm) irradiation on the proliferation of keratinocytes. Energy densities as low as 0.25 J/cm² (HeNe and GaAs) increased keratinocyte proliferation. Energy densities at 4 J/cm² or higher may exert an inhibitory effect.

Abergel and others (1984), Lam and others (1986), and Cisneros (1984) have shown that laser irradiation increases collagen formation and therefore can have an effect on keloid formation, to use one example. A pathologically abundant keloid growth can cease as a result of HeNe laser treatment; the color of the scar can become lighter, and the height of the already formed keloid lower. Similar changes are also produced by acupuncture treatment.

Lubart and others (1993) examined the effect of various wavelengths from noncoherent light sources on fibroblast proliferation. The results were not only dose dependent; they also had a nonlinear dependence on the intensity of the light source. The maximum effect with a noncoherent but monochromatic (540 nm) light was obtained at 4 J/cm², whereas a broad band (600 to 900 nm) irradiation yielded the maximum increase of fibroblast proliferation at 24 J/cm². The corresponding intensities were 9 to 12 mW/cm² for 540 nm irradiation and 150 to

350 mW/cm² for broad band irradiation. An Italian research group (Terribile Wiel Marin and others, 1992) compared the effects of coherent and noncoherent radiation on experimental wound healing, using the same energy density (3.6 J/cm²) and wavelength (633 nm). Both coherent and noncoherent radiation accelerated wound healing over controls, with coherent HeNe laser radiation giving the best result.

Loevschall and Arenholt-Bindslev (1994) studied the effects of different radiant exposures from an 812 nm diode laser on human oral mucosa fibroblasts in vitro. The maximum increase of incorporation on tritiated thymidine followed irradiation with 0.45 J/cm² and suggests an increased DNA synthesis. Gomez-Villamandos and others (1995) examined the effect of a HeNe laser (10 mW, 207 mW/cm², 8 J/cm²) on the cicatrization of superficial wounds in the pharyngeal mucosa of the horse. Irradiated lesions cicatrized after 10.5 days, compared with 18.0 days in nonirradiated controls. Samples from irradiated lesions showed no inflammatory edema, intensive epithelial regeneration, and numerous active fibroblasts, which suggests the beneficial effects of laser irradiation on equine pharyngeal ulcerative lesions (Box 17-2).

LEP Effect on Blood and Blood Cell Physical Properties

Chemiluminescence of peripheral blood reflects changes in cellular oxidative metabolism. LEP irradiation decreased abnormally high chemiluminescence during acute viral respiratory illness. No effect was produced when the blood of a healthy donor was irradiated (Karu, Andreichuk, Ryabykh, 1993). The best response was achieved with a diode emitting at 660 nm, 5000 Hz, 5 to 10 J/cm². Other wavelengths (820, 880, and 950 nm) were nearly as effective. Low frequency (16 Hz) and low dose (0.037 J/cm²) had negligible effect. The chemiluminescence recorded in this experiment originated from the cellular components of blood.

Salansky, Brill, and Filonenko (1994) reported increases in white blood cells (56%) and red blood cells (19%) in human volunteers after a transcutaneous LEP irradiation (660 nm, 6 mW, 15 min, total dose 5.4 J). White rats exposed to red light (630 nm, 5.7 mW/cm²) for 2 minutes reacted under stress with an activation of lipid peroxidation and reduction of hypercoagulation induced by immobilization stress.

Vascular Effects

The antiinflammatory and edema-reducing effects of low-power lasers are caused partly by increased microcirculation and partly by accelerated lymphatic flow. Lievens (1986) has shown that lymphatic flow returns very quickly in mice after laser radiation. The regeneration of lymphatic vessels in the mesenterium of laser-treated mice was complete in 9 days, whereas in the control group the regeneration was still incomplete at the end of the follow-up period (55 days). Moreover the vein network was restored in laser-treated animals in less than half the time needed by the control group. Peritoneal adhesions were rare in laser-treated mice but common in the control group.

BOX 17-2

Summary of Radiant Exposure/Dose-Dependent LEPT Effects at Cellular Level

Proliferation of fibrocytes and keratinocytes
Collagen formation
DNA synthesis
ATP synthesis
Cell growth and differentiation
Cell motility
Phagocytosis
Protein synthesis
Membrane potential and binding affinities

Increase with a radiant exposure over (0.01) 0.25 J/cm² at the target site (coherent and monochromatic irradiation)
Decrease when energy density exceeds 4 J/cm²

Similar cellular effects are possible with the following:
Coherent + monochromatic irradiation (0.26 J/cm²);
Noncoherent + monochromatic irradiation (4 J/cm²);
Noncoherent + broad band (600-900 nm) irradiation (24 J/cm²)

Laser light can increase the consumption of oxygen and glucose in the radiated cells, which reflects the biostimulation effect. If the irradiation dose exceeds a certain threshold (approximately 1 J/mg tissue weight), the response may turn to decreased cell breathing, according to laboratory experiments. The flow of water and electrolytes through the intestinal wall is retarded with a simultaneous increase in intracellular potassium after a laser irradiation of 1 J/cm².

HeNe-laser irradiation has been shown to increase and accelerate vascularization in growing tissue. This effect is clearly seen in a rabbit's ear, for example. The most intensive vascularization takes place at the dermoepidermal junction, where the prominent nuclei of the endothelial cells of the vessels are rich in polysaccharides.

Benedicenti (1982), Lievens (1986), and Miro (1984) have shown that circulation in the nail bed and mesenterial capillary increases after laser irradiation. The increased flow continued 20 minutes after the cessation of laser treatment, even when the target area was cooled. The laser effect on circulation clearly does not depend on the heat produced by light energy. The changes in blood flow in the skin may depend on the intensity and energy density of irradiation. Energy densities between 0.68 and 1.36 J/cm² induced temporary vasoconstriction, whereas vasodilation was seen with fluences between 0.12 and 0.36 J/cm² in a Finnish study with so-called hair lasers (Pöntinen and others, 1995). The first to respond are the sphincters of the end capillaries, and the degree to which they respond depends on the severity of the microcirculation impairment. Mayayo and Trelles (1984) achieved similar results in their study on the anal mucosa of rats. According to Miro and others (1984), both vasodilation and increased microcirculation result from increased tissue metabolism and normalization of homeostasis. Fiszerman and Rozenbom (1995) have demonstrated an increased oxygen partial pressure in lower extremities after laser irradiation.

LEP Effect on Endocrine Function

The effects of laser irradiation on endocrine function have been widely studied. These studies have focused primarily on cell cultures and tissues of small rodents and are therefore not directly transferable to clinical practice. In all these studies, HeNe and IR lasers were shown to stimulate endocrine function and cell division. Both the hypophysis and thyroid glands showed increased activity after laser irradiation (Rodrigo, Lerma, Zaragoza, 1985). Although no evidence suggests that a laser treatment can lead to actual hyperthyroidism, laser radiation over the thyroid should be avoided.

LEP Effect on Nerve Regeneration

Rochkind and his research group in Israel have extensively studied the effects of photobiomodulation on mammalian peripheral and central nervous system (Rochkind, 1992; Rochkind and others, 1987a, 1987b, 1988, 1991). They showed that the HeNe laser has a dose-dependent effect on the nerve tissue. Between 3.5 and 10 J/cm² at the skin level causes a pronounced stimulating effect on the electrophysiologic activity, whereas densities higher than 10 J/cm² exert an inhibitory effect. Daily low-power laser irradiation also accelerated nerve regeneration in rats. A similar effect was demonstrated with a direct irradiation of intact but dissected nerves when the dose was approximately 0.2 J/cm². This amount corresponds with the calculated attenuation of energy density in the living tissue. The same principles have been applied in fetal brain allograft transplantations into adult rat brain and spinal cord allograft transplantations into the spinal cord of dogs. To suppress immune reactivity the irradiation dose was increased to 30 to 70 J/cm². Glial scar formation was minimal, and abundant capillaries developed in the irradiated transplants. The beneficial influence of laser irradiation was evident also when applied to the spinal cord of dogs.

Anders and others (1993) have demonstrated that transcutaneous low-power irradiation increased the rate of regeneration in the facial nerves of rats after a crush injury. The best results were achieved with HeNe and argon-pumped tunable dye lasers with a wavelength of 633 nm, 8.5 mW output power administered for 90 minutes (45.9 J total dose, 162.4 J/cm² energy density at the skin level). The power at the nerve itself was 0.02 mW and the total irradiation dose approximately 0.1 J. Ochi, Osedo, and Ikuta (1995) have developed a superior nerve anastomosis using a low-output CO_2 laser (10,600 nm) on fibrin membrane placed over the site of anastomosis. Before laser irradiation, two stay sutures were applied to hold the nerve stumps in proximity. Three sheets of fibrin films were placed on posterior and anterior aspects of the repair site and irradiated with a 70 mW CO_2 laser beam (total dose 10.5 J) from a distance of about 12 cm. No deleterious effect of the irradiation on nerve regeneration was observed at any time after surgery. The tensile strength was sufficiently strong to connect the dissected nerve. The fibrin film played an important role as a barrier to prevent the escape of nerve fibers and the invasion of excessive scar tissue into the repair site. The number of myelinated axons over 5 μm in diameter was markedly higher in the laser group.

LEP Effect on Muscle and Tendon Regeneration

Bibikova and Oron (1994) have studied the effects of HeNe (6 mW, 31.2 J/cm²) and GaAs (904 nm, 0.005 mW mean, 9 W peak, 2.82 Hz) laser irradiation on muscle regeneration after cold injury to the gastrocnemius muscle of toads. Red noncoherent light (660 nm, 0.4 J/cm²) was used in the control group. Muscle regeneration was promoted equally by single HeNe or GaAs laser irradiation and multiple irradiations by HeNe. HeNe irradiation also promoted the regeneration of skeletal muscle in rats.

Enwemeka and others (1994) examined the biomechanical effects of GaAs (904 nm, 0.5 J/cm²) laser irradiation on tenotomized, repaired, and immobilized calcaneal rabbit tendons. Laser treatment induced a significant increase in tensile strength, tensile stress, energy absorption capacity, and modulus of elasticity, especially when irradiation was given during postoperative days 8 to 14, the phase of fibroblast proliferation and synthesis of collagen fibrils.

LEP-Induced Immunomodulatory Phenomena

Reports on the effect of lasers on viruses and bacteria are extremely controversial. Although laser light effectively prevents infections in vivo, it may stimulate the growth of bacteria in vitro. For example, genital herpes responds well to a HeNe laser, but Gilioli and others (1985) have documented in vitro studies in which laser irradiation increased the virulence of HSV1 and HSV2 viruses.

Further research on the effects of lasers on the immune system is greatly needed. Preliminary experiments have shown that HeNe-irradiated mice with thymus aplasia (2 to 4 J/cm² every other day) survived longer under an experimental sepsis than those without laser treatment (Mayayo, Trelles 1986). GaAs laser (904 nm) has effectively arrested bacterial growth in a petri dish with an irradiation dose of 2 J/dish. A minor effect was produced when the irradiation dose was increased to 10 J/dish. HeNe lasers had no effect with these doses (Hernandez Gonzales and others, 1987). In another study a HeNe laser (0.325 J/cm² and 0.650 J/cm²) had no effect on the growth of *Staphylococcus aureus* in vitro (Carrillo and others, 1987). Wilson and Pratten (1995) have demonstrated that GaAs laser (904 nm, 11 mW mean, 1.2 J/cm²) killed photosensitized (aluminium disulphonated phthalocyanine, AlPcS₂) methicillin-resistant suspension of *Staphylococcus aureus*. Lee, Kim, and Kim (1993) inoculated open wounds in rat gluteal regions with *Staphylococcus mutans*. One side was irradiated with a GaAs laser (904 nm, 27 W peak, 2 mW mean, 1 kHz, 76.4 mJ/cm²), and the other wound was used as a control. The rate of wound closure was significantly increased and swelling (as an indicator of inflammation) significantly decreased in the irradiated group.

Japanese researchers (Amano and others, 1994) studied changes in the synovial membrane in cases of rheumatoid arthritis before surgery. Transcutaneous GaAlAs laser irradiation (790 nm, 10 mW, 0.8 J/point) was given to six points of the external aspect of the knee joint once a day for 6 days. Synovial membrane from the irradiated external aspect and the nonirradiated medial aspect of the knee was taken for histologic examination 1 day after the last irradiation. The difference was significant, suggesting a laser-induced suppression of inflammation in the synovial membrane of RA.

Applications of LEPT

Trauma and Orthopedics

LEPT as a first aid method in minor injuries (wounds, scratches, bruises, burns) and as an adjuvant to fracture treatment (conservative or operative)

LEPT treatment gives better results in acute soft tissue injuries if therapy is given as early as possible after injury. The minimal risk of increased bleeding is not a contraindication for early LEPT. IR LEPT is most suitable for point treatment and first aid applied directly at the site of the injury (e.g., at a football stadium or race track). Because LEPT does not penetrate to the deeper tissues, results are normally better in superficial injuries. Although LEPT may accelerate the healing process, complete relief of pain does not mean that the injury has healed. Resumption of full athletic activity too soon after a partial muscle rupture may lead to a total rupture (this has also been reported after an AP treatment). Walking on a limb that has a hairline fracture (following analgesia and without proper support and immobilization) can exaggerate the injury.

LEPT is applied to the most painful sites or AHSHI points over the injured region (1 to 4 J/point). These points may form a netlike pattern, with 2 to 3 cm between the points. All active and painful passive (latent) TPs in muscles that show increased tension or are in spasm are also treated. LEPT at ipsilateral AP Yanglingquan (GB34) and APs for the affected area can enhance pain relief.

SCRATCHES AND TRAUMATIC AND SURGICAL WOUNDS Conventional care of wounds includes cleansing, minor surgery (debridement, suturing), topical and systemic medication, and tetanus antitoxin. In addition to conventional measures, patients with suppressed immune system (and those whose sratches and small wounds are easily infected) may be given LEPT as a first-aid treatment for any fresh scratch or wound. One session of LEPT (2 to 4 J/cm²) performed on surgical wounds (in the operating theatre) and 1 to 2 sessions over the next 3 days accelerates wound healing, reduces the risk of postoperative infection, and improves the quality of scar tissue (Ghamsari and others, 1995).

FISSURES AND FRACTURES LEPT is useful as a first-aid treatment to provide analgesia, reduce swelling, and permit thorough manual examination. It improves local microcirculation and enhances lymphatic drainage, thus providing optimal conditions for accelerated healing. Near infrared LEPT, especially pulsed 904 nm irradiation (4.0 J/cm²), significantly accelerated callus formation of bone fractures in mice (Glinkowski, Rowinski, 1995).

Acute, Subacute, and Chronic Postsurgical and Posttraumatic Conditions, Repetitive Strain Injuries

Any slowly healing injury or surgical wound may benefit from LEPT. First, the practitioner must carefully check all possible reasons for the delayed recovery and correct them. Table 17-7 shows two common conditions in which LEP-induced phenomena may radically improve chances for full recovery.

A special application for LEPT is immediate postoperative care in aesthetic surgery. The main problems are edema, pain, survival of skin flaps, inflammation, circulatory disturbance, wound healing, and infection—all indications for LEPT. LEPT is best applied either preoperatively or during surgery and then continued 2 to 3 weeks on a daily or every-other-day basis (1 to 4 J/cm^2). For larger areas (over 100 cm^2), multidiode heads or defocused CO_2 lasers are preferable.

LEPT of Musculoskeletal Pain and Dysfunction

Exact localization of points for treatment is essential for successful therapy. Localization can be done with careful palpation, PTH measurement, or electrical skin resistance measurement (Airaksinen and others, 1989).

Adjustment of laser radiation to treatment points

The laser beam should hit the skin in as vertical a direction as possible to minimize the reflection of laser light and maximize the penetration depth of irradiation in the tissues. The light beam can be focused with collimating lenses to give high-energy density to minimal target zones. When the light beam hits the skin, it creates a halo around the point of impact. The distance from its center to the edge corresponds roughly to the penetration of the light beam.

Evaluation of immediate results of LLLT

When point-treatment of APs and TPs is used, responses of the following can be evaluated immediately after irradiation:

- Pressure pain threshold (PTH measurement)
- Muscle force (e.g., hand dynamometer)
- Range of movement (ROM)
- Tissue compliance (TCO measurement)

Checking the patient's response after single-point radiation allows the practitioner to make adjustments for the optimum laser dose and select the most effective points for restoration of normal function (Pöntinen, 1993; Pöntinen, Airaksinen 1989, 1995).

Combination of different point groups for LEPT

In acute cases, laser treatment can be directed first to local AHSHI points. If local therapy creates excessive reactions (e.g., increase of pain for over 24 hours), the practitioner is advised to check for complicating underlying factors. These may include overstimulation (hyperstimulation reaction), osteoarthritis, spondyloarthritic changes, chronic nerve-root irritation in the same spinal nerve segment, and other factors that may induce TP activation. These patients are better treated through regional, segmental, and peripheral APs until the local hypersensitivity ceases (Pöntinen, Pothmann, 1993).

In chronic cases a combination of local treatment with peripheral APs and segmental TPs seems to produce the most effective response. In functional disorders, tender paravertebral segmental (SHU) points are often an important addition to the basic scheme.

When choosing many points for LEPT to be used over a number of sessions, practitioners may select the TPs, tender SHU points, local AHSHI points, and local APs as the primary points and combine them with alternating selections from a secondary list of other AHSHI points, distant points, and special (ear and extra) points.

TABLE 17-7

LOW-ENERGY PHOTONS (LEPS) IN REPETITIVE STRAIN INJURIES

CONDITION	UNDERLYING PATHOLOGY	LEP PHENOMENA
CTS (carpal tunnel syndrome)	Inflamed tendons	Systemic effect
	Swelling	Antiinflammatory
	Median nerve compression	Antiedematous
	Microcirculation (arterial, venous, lymphatic)	Local tissue effect
	Neurogenic factors (cervical spine, TOS)	Lymph flow enhancement
		Microcirculation improvement
		Analgesic effect
Soft tissue injury	Hematoma	Reduction of edema, swelling, pain
	Swelling	Relief of spasm
	Inflammation	
	Muscle spasm	

Lasers can be used immediately after application of ice packs. Lasers do not increase or prolong bleeding. To avoid a complete muscle tear, do not start full activity after a partial muscle rupture despite pain relief. *TOS,* Thoracic outlet syndrome.

LEPT of Wounds, Burns, and Ulcers

LEPT is ideal for the treatment of wounds, burns, and ulcers, even in long-standing and infected cases. Because the lesions usually are superficial, the laser beam's depth of penetration is not as critical as, for example, in treatment of deep-seated TPs or joints. Although the IR laser usually penetrates deeper than the HeNe laser, the latter can be used successfully.

Successful LEPT requires a high energy density. Thus most experts recommend point-treatment, in which points on the wound surface and surrounding healthy tissue are radiated in a netlike pattern, 1 to 2 cm between the points (0.5 to 2 J/point).

Strict sterility should be followed in the application of LEPT, especially to infected wounds, ulcers, and burns. The laser probe can be protected with a thin plastic cover, or HeNe LEPT may be applied from a distance. The session can be completed with a scanner (Fig. 17-7).

Ulcers and pressure sores

The edges of these lesions respond first. Infection is quickly controlled, and the swelling and erythema disappear. Granulation tissue is formed next (from the center and the periphery), followed by epithelial regrowth from the periphery. If epithelial regrowth stops after approximately 2 weeks, arterial circulation must be checked again. Daily TENS (transcutaneous electric nerve stimulation) treatment should be used to support the vasodilatory and antiinflammatory effects of LEPT.

Burns

LEPT of burns is similar to other wound treatments. Its purpose is to provide analgesia, prevent infection, hasten epithelial regrowth, and improve the quality of the scar. According to experimental and clinical work by

Abergel and others (1984), Cisneros (1984), and Trelles (1983), LEPT accelerates epithelial regrowth and prevents keloid formation.

In contrast to other types of wounds, burns should be treated daily to fulfill the high energy demand of the healing tissue. Here, as in other wound treatment, direct contact between the skin and laser probe should be avoided. The basic procedure is to administer 4 to 8 J/cm² in a net-like fashion with 2 to 3 cm between the treated points throughout the burned area and around the edge of the wound on the healthy skin. Scanner treatment over the burned area (0.5 to 1.0 J/cm²) completes the treatment.

Mucosal ulcers, aphthae (herpes simplex)

The biostimulatory effect of LEPT is beneficial in the treatment of mucosal ulcers and aphthae in the mouth. Aphthae can be treated with IR LLLT 1-2 J/aphtha as a contact treatment. Ulcers and mucosal lesions of the vulva react to LEPT, but condylomas and ulcerative vulval lesions induced by human papilloma virus (HPV) should be treated by a combined high- and low-power laser treatment (Rubenstein, 1987). LEPT is also suitable for postoperative treatment of excisions and extirpations of hemorrhoids, polyps, and papillomas.

Scar tissue

By continuous nociceptive discharge from the active TPs in scar tissue, active scars often play an important role in maintaining chronic pain conditions and functional disorders. The activity of TPs in or near scar tissue can be reduced or blocked by administering a microinjection of a local anesthetic (blebbing), needling, or performing LEPT at the TPs and relevant APs.

HeNe and IR LEPT lasers are suitable for treatment of so-called active scars. One treatment is sometimes enough, but treatment should be repeated every other day or week as indicated by the response of the patient. In some cases, LEPT must be continued for many years at monthly or bimonthly intervals.

In addition to relieving pain and eliminating the associated functional disorders, LEPT often causes scar tissue to become lighter in color, softer in consistency, and smaller (or even nonexistent) with time. Similar results can be achieved with needles alone. Patients with the tendency for keloid formation may benefit greatly from early LEPT or needle treatment of the wound, whether surgical or traumatic.

Sumano and his colleagues (1987a, 1987b) have studied the effect of electroacupuncture (EA) on the healing of surgical wounds in rats. The EA-treated wounds healed without infection (per primam intentionem), and their tensile strength was markedly better than in the control group (63% to 88% infected). These rats were treated daily for 10 minutes. Both EA and electrical stimulation to nonacupuncture points (ES) increased the amount of fibroblasts and collagen formation verified in histologic

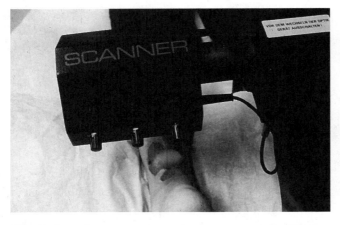

Fig. 17-7 HeNe + IR scanner device: 633 nm 10 mW, 904 nm 72 W (peak), 8 mW (mean at 5 kHz)(Medical Scanlaser, Espoo, Finland). Scanning over the ulcer (1-2 J/cm²) combined with a spotwise treatment around the ulcer on normal, healthy skin (0.5-1.0 J/cm²).

samples, but the effect on the infection rate and tensile strength of the scar was better in the EA group (Sumano, Cosaubon, 1987).

In the treatment of ulcers and poorly healing wounds, electric stimulation (TENS) has been used for years. At the beginning of the 1980s, Kaada reported peripheral vasodilation after a low-frequency (2 Hz), high-intensity TENS (Kaada, 1982, 1983; Kaada, Emru, 1988). This effect spreads over the segments and may last up to 6 to 10 hours after 30 to 45 minutes of stimulation. The main vasodilating mechanism, according to Kaada, is the release of a neuropeptide, VIP (vasoactive intestinal polypeptide) (Kaada, Eielsen, 1983; Kaada, Helle, 1984; Kaada, Olsen, Eielsen, 1984; Kaada, Lygren, 1985). Later, Eriksson, Knutsson, and Skoglund (1986) reported similar results in wound and ulcer treatment with high-frequency (60 to 100 Hz) TENS. They placed the electrodes locally around the wounds and ulcers.

LEPT of Rheumatoid Arthritis and Osteoarthritis

The purpose of LEPT in patients with rheumatoid arthritis (RA) is to relieve pain, reduce local swelling at the joints, and increase joint mobility. The small joints usually respond better than the large joints (e.g., knee and hip joints). Surprisingly, patients with Bekhterev's arthritis (ankylosing spondylitis) also react favorably to LEPT.

LEPT cannot replace conventional medication, surgery, and rehabilitation in patients with RA, but it can reduce their use of analgesic medication and improve their quality of life. Pain relief is achieved both with HeNe and IR LEPT. IR seems to be more effective than HeNe in the reduction of inflammatory signs and the restoration of muscle force and function.

Pain has been the main indication for LEPT in osteoarthritis. Treatment is often given to myofascial TPs, AHSHI points, and APs. The small joints in the hands and feet react especially well to either continuously emitting (cw) or modulated HeNe LEPT.

IR LEPT is effective in the treatment of spondyloarthritis and osteoarthritis of the larger joints, excluding the hip joint (Flöter, 1987; Galante, 1985). LEPT can be started locally at the joint space, and this simple therapy may lead to fast relief of pain. At the first stage of any form of osteoarthritis, patients frequently experience pain-free intervals or only minor symptoms. However, muscle atrophy is an important early sign. Therefore practitioners should add TPs in the affected muscles and relevant APs to the local LEPT and start active mobilization simultaneously. Another approach is to add segmental (often AHSHI) points near the spine. Application of these principles has produced positive results, even in patients with long-lasting, incapacitating pain.

Patients who have been nearly immobilized for a long time (and who often have simultaneous osteoporosis) must be warned against overenthusiasm; they often may experience complete relief of pain after the first sessions of LEPT, and this may cause problems. Overloading may lead to fractures (e.g., in metatarsal bones) when patients with hip and knee osteoarthritis are able to walk freely and without pain after a long interval. With proper medical advice and patient compliance, no signs of abnormal progression of the disease process are apparent in lengthy follow-up studies, despite the increased loading of affected joints and limbs that has become possible through relief of pain. Recent studies on cartilage metabolism support the view that rhythmic loading of joints increases the proteoglycan content of joint cartilage (Helminen and others, 1992). Immobilization decreases the proteoglycans and elasticity of joint cartilage. Therefore careful mobilization of osteoarthritic joints and gradual increases in loading are important.

Neurologic Applications

LEPT produces excellent results in neuralgia caused or maintained by active TPs in scars. It also may give good results in postherpetic and trigeminal neuralgia. The main focus of LEPT in neuralgia is on TPs and AHSHI points in the painful segment and the paravertebral AHSHI points.

Neuralgia caused and/or maintained by active TPs in tender scars

Neuralgia and autonomic dysfunction, which can be severe, are often caused or maintained by active TPs in tender scars. These scars can be postoperative, posttraumatic (including burn scars), and postinfectious (e.g., superficial abscesses). LEPT tends to produce the best results in these types of neuralgia. The scar tissue itself reacts to LEPT and may become softer, smoother, and less discolored. Excellent results have also been obtained in cases that were chronic for several years before LEPT.

Besides TPs and AHSHI points on or near the scar, in the painful segment, and at the paravertebral AHSHI points, one or two distant APs on a meridian passing through or near the scar can also be used. For example, practitioners might add AP GB-34 for an active scar on the lateral thorax, ST-36 or ST-45 for an active scar below the eye, or SP-6 for an appendectomy or cesarean scar.

Postherpetic neuralgia

In cases of postherpetic neuralgia, LEPT should be started as early as possible. Herpes eruptions can be treated with 1 to 2 J per eruption, administered twice a week during the acute phase. In the acute phase, LEPT helps reduce scar formation, and postherpetic pain rarely develops. In the chronic stage, LEPT is less satisfactory, but good results can be expected in 60% of cases. The whole injured area, especially the lesions in the affected dermatomes, can be scanned over with HeNe or IR LEPT

(0.5 to 1.0 J/cm^2). If there are few lesions, point treatment with IR or HeNe LEPT is appropriate.

Trigeminal neuralgia

In trigeminal pain, it is necessary to include muscular TPs from the neck and shoulder muscles with local TPs and AHSHI points from the affected branch in the face. Local APs along the course of the affected nerve are also helpful. Scanning over the affected area completes the treatment.

Nerve injuries

As shown by Rochkind and his group (1987, 1988, 1991), LEPT is an effective additional tool for noninvasive treatment of peripheral nerve and spinal cord injuries in rats and dogs. LEPT also reduces local swelling and enhances and accelerates the functional and morphologic recovery of severely injured nerve tissue in human patients. LEPT can be given preoperatively and postoperatively (neurolysis, nerve graft, neurotization) or as a sole treatment when surgery is not indicated.

Sports Medicine

The most common sports injuries treated with LEPT include soft tissue contusions, partial muscle tears, tendinitis, fasciitis, periostitis, and ankle sprains. In acute injuries, LEPT accelerates the healing process and permits an early return to active training. However, LEPT is by no means a miracle cure, and careful diagnosis and a detailed rehabilitation plan are prerequisites for a fast and full recovery. Selection of an appropriate device to convey the precalculated irradiation dose to the target zone is particularly important. Superficial lesions can be treated with 30 to 60 mW GaAlAs lasers or combined HeNe and IR lasers (Fig. 17-8). Bigger muscles and deep-seated lesions may need higher-output powers (up to 100 to 300 mW) (Fig. 17-9). Defocused CO$_2$ and Nd:YAG lasers (0.5 to 2 W) have been successfully applied in typical deep sports injuries. Galleti (1994) and Parra and others (1993) have confirmed the deep tissue interaction with these laser types. In practice, LEPT should be directed to reactive points (AHSII and trigger points) at a dose of 1 to 8 J per point. Muscles in pain spasm often react favorably to noncoherent but sufficient monochromatic irradiation (880 nm, 300-600 mW, 3-6 J/cm^2) (Box 17-3).

Diagnostics with LEPT

Because LEPT elevates the pressure pain threshold and restores impaired neuromuscular function, it may also be used as a diagnostic tool. To differentiate between nerve root compression (e.g., disk protrusion) and activation of trigger mechanism as in myofascial pain syndromes and musculoskeletal disorders, LEPT may be used for trial treatment of the affected segment. First, to confirm the functional importance of detected reactive (tender) muscle trigger (AHSHI) points or area, a test dose (1 to 2 J/point

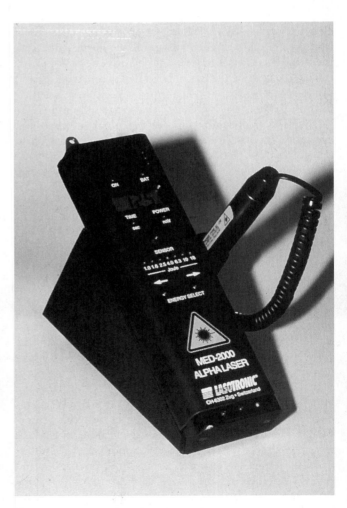

Fig. 17-9 Physiotherapy laser, 3 x 40 mW = 120 mW, 830 nm, cw (Lasotronic AG, P.O. Box 2086, CH-6302 Zug, Switzerland) for deep-sited lesions (see Tables 17-8 and 17-9).

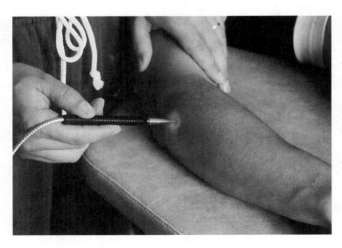

Fig. 17-8 Glassfiber extension for a HeNe-, IR-laser combination therapy.

for large animals; 0.5 to 1 J/point in small animals) may be administered. The immediate restoration of normal range of movement and muscle strength confirms the peripheral (trigger point) level of the disorder. When no change in function occurs, the practitioner should move to the paravertebral area and locate any tender point at the transverse process or over the facet joints. The test dose and functional tests are then repeated. This method allows the practitioner to check the level of the possible nerve root irritation and differentiate between disk disease and peripheral musculoskeletal problems. It also gives the practitioner a better sense of the prognosis.

Limitations, Side Effects, and Complications of LEPT
General

Even today, many people have an irrational fear of laser technology because they do not understand it; sometimes, they confuse it with radioactive radiation. Most accidents with LEPT lasers resulted from direct contact with the electrically active parts. In some LEPT lasers (e.g., HeNe lasers), high voltage is used. When the so-called Q-switch is used, the voltage may increase to 100,000 V.

Risk of Eye Injury with LEPT

Except with collimated IR and HeNe lasers, the risk of eye injury is almost nonexistent with the optical output levels used in LEPT today. Theoretically a light beam from the tube of these lasers, if directed accidentally through the lens, could burn the retina. However, no eye injuries resulting from LEPT have been reported in the literature.

On the other hand, high-energy lasers (as used in surgery and ophthalmology) are extremely dangerous to the eyes. All lasers should be considered as potentially dangerous. To avoid future discussions of possible eye injuries in connection with LEPT, practitioners should always provide patients with protective goggles. However, with LEPT, this precaution is more for psychologic reasons than protection against a genuine risk. In fact, LEPT lasers may elicit positive reactions in certain eye diseases. For example, Meno and others (1989) reported favorable responses in infectious bovine keratoconjunctivitis. Schwartz and others (1987) showed that use of a low-energy HeNe laser greatly affected posttraumatic degeneration of the optic nerve in adult rabbits, whereas the injured optic nerve remained permanently damaged in the untreated control group.

As the cornea and lens focus radiation onto the retina, the power density increases more than 100,000 times higher than the primary energy density on the skin or cornea. The cornea, aqueous humor, lens, and vitreous humor are more conductive of radiation with a wavelength of 450 to 900 nm. The risk of retinal injury is reduced if LEPT is given in a bright light when the pupil size is smallest. In daylight the area of the pupil is only $\frac{1}{16}$ the size it is in a dark room. The amount of energy and the energy density at the retina are correspondingly reduced. IR lasers are more dangerous than visible lasers because the invisible beam does not provoke an eye-blink reflex.

Risk of Radiation Injuries on the Skin with LEPT

Photon energy from all lasers used for biostimulation and pain relief is low (usually 1 to 100 mW) and remains far below the levels needed for ionization. Light from these lasers, even in high doses, does not induce cancer growth.

A laser beam with mean optical power of approximately 200 mW, carefully focused on an area of 1 cm² (power density of 0.2 W/cm²) for approximately 10 minutes, is required to produce first-degree burns. LEPT devices usually have mean optical output values in the range of 5 to 100 mW and are used at power densities of 1 to 100 mW/cm². LEPT cannot produce skin lesions if these power densities and recommended irradiation doses are applied. Even the most powerful diode lasers used in LEPT are safe in that respect.

If a 40 to 100 mW (mean output) diode laser is focused on the skin, nothing more than a slight sensation of heat results. If the tip of a diode laser is in contact with the skin, the subject may feel the tip become hotter over time.

BOX 17-3

Facts About Lasers

- The most commonly used low-energy lasers in pain treatment are helium-neon (HeNe) lasers, gallium-arsenide (GaAs) lasers, gallium-aluminum-arsenide (GaAlAs) lasers, and indium-gallium-aluminum-phosphate (InGaAlP) lasers.
- Skin and mucosal lesions (including body openings) are the main indications for HeNe and InGaAlP lasers. These lasers are also effective in superficial soft tissue injuries and treatment of minor joints.
- GaAs and GaAlAs have their main applications in sports medicine and in the treatment of myofascial pain and dysfunction.
- Recently, high-energy carbon dioxide (CO$_2$) lasers and neodymium:yttrium-aluminum-garnet (Nd:YAG) lasers have been applied in a defocused mode to treat major joints (hip, knee) and deeper soft tissue injuries in sports medicine.

A hot metal tip can induce first-degree burns, but these can be prevented by checking the tip regularly during the session and asking the subject to report any heat sensations. A hot tip can be withdrawn a few millimeters from the skin, which should prevent skin damage.

Contraindications for LEPT

There are no absolute contraindications for LEPT. However, practitioners are advised to be cautious when treating patients in high-risk categories. LEPT should be avoided or administered with special caution in the following cases:

- *Patients with pacemakers:* LEPT should not be applied to the thorax or over the pacemaker itself in patients with pacemakers (especially older models).
- *Patients who are pregnant:* LEPT should not be applied to abdominal or lumbosacral points in pregnant females. The so-called forbidden APs (e.g., LI-4 and SP-6) should be avoided.
- *Patients with cancer:* LEPT should be avoided in cancer patients if recurrence and metastases are possible. Pain relief during the terminal phase is an exception to this rule. Although LEPT has not induced cancer growth in any of the reported studies, the precise reactions of existing tumors to LEPT are unknown.
- *Patients with labile epilepsy:* Labile epilepsy is a relative contraindication of LEPT.
- *Growing children (epiphyseal plates):* LEPT should not be applied to the epiphyseal lines in children.
- *Endocrine glands:* Use of LEPT over the thyroid gland, ovaries, and testicles is not advised.
- Direct contact of laser probes with infected areas or body orifices (e.g., ear canal, nostrils, mouth, vagina, anus) should be avoided unless there is specific reason for it. Disposable laser-light–permeable protective sheaths should be put on the laser probe if local contact–LEPT is needed in those areas.

Although these guidelines are recommended, published reports of any negative effects from LEPT in the aforementioned cases are not available. In contrast, some positive results have been reported (e.g., in the treatment of male infertility through LEPT of the testicles) (Hasan and others, 1989).

LEPT Parameters and Applications Techniques: Implications for Veterinary Practice

Main Differences Between Human and Veterinary LEPT

In human medicine the main indications for LEPT are myofascial pain and dysfunction, other chronic pain problems (e.g., neuralgias, repetitive strain injuries [typical occupational health problems], osteoarthritis), wound and ulcer healing, posttraumatic and postsurgical rehabilitation, rehabilitation of stroke patients, and soft tissue injuries in sports medicine. The following tend to be the most common indications for LEPT in veterinary medicine: tendinitis, fasciitis resulting from overuse or misuse, disk disease and lameness, acute and chronic inflammations with local edema, wounds, scratches, and postoperative wound dehiscences in large animals and joint problems, disk disease, local infections (skin, otitis externa), postsurgical rehabilitation, and alopecia in pets (Ambronn, Muxeneder, Warnke, 1995; Muxeneder 1987, 1990). Improved physical performance is a goal in both human and veterinary medicine.

Large animals present specific application problems. Thick and hairy skin certainly affects the light beam, and a 30% decrease in energy density at the skin level is typical. Higher-power densities and use of the contact mode for treatment are preferred whenever possible. Reflection and scattering in the subject's hair may create the risk of laser radiation reaching the practitioner's retina. Therefore safety goggles are necessary when treatment is given from a distance (e.g., with a scanner). A multidiode head (see Fig. 17-9) with high-power density (200 to 300 mW/cm^2) and an IR diode (noncoherent light) cluster (300 to 600 mW) are other possible choices (Fig. 17-10). A thin plastic cover on the laser tip is recommended when treating wounds and ulcers. The irradiation loss is minimal (3% to 5%). Laser treatment may be administered through an adhesive or wound dressing, but this creates a higher irradiation loss (about 30% to 50%) because of reflection and scattering.

Small animals typically need smaller doses and can be treated with lower-power densities (20 to 90 mW). Animals are often more sensitive than human patients and may sense photon energy. In some cases the practitioner may choose to administer ketamine to quiet the animal. The contact mode is recommended to produce optimal conditions for treatment. Practitioners should comb the hair of dogs and cats aside before administering point treatment. Special extension fibers are available for intraoral and ear-canal therapy and treatment of other orifices.

When local alopecia is treated, a multidiode head or IR cluster sonde is convenient. The most common indications and corresponding LEP sources are presented in Tables 17-8 and 17-9.

Special Applications for Small Animals

Skin and mucosal lesions, scratches, and wounds react favorably to visible (HeNe or 670 nm diode) or IR (820, 830, 904 nm) radiation. A battery-operated pocket-size laser pen (20 to 60 mW) is ideal as a first-aid treatment for on-site injuries (Fig. 17-11). Local infections such as external otitis and gingivitis can be treated effectively with LEPT (Fig. 17-12). In chronic or repeated otitis, local

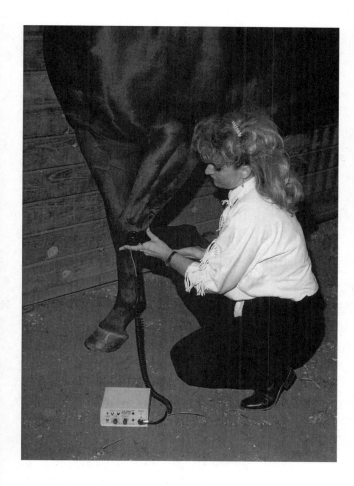

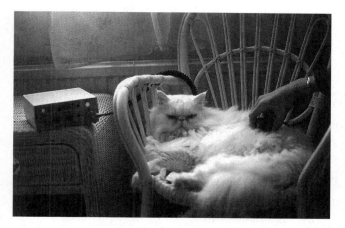

Fig. 17-10 Multidiode (noncoherent) head/cluster probe (880 + 50 nm; 30 × 20 mW = 600 mW/at 50% duty cycle = 300 mW; output area 11.5 cm²; power density 26 mW/cm²) (Cefco Inc, PO Box 429, Inola, Oklahoma 74036) for analgesia, muscle relaxation, antiinflammatory treatment, and reduction of edema.

chemotherapy with no systemic antibiotics in combination with LEPT is recommended.

Antiinflammatory effect and marked reduction of local edema as an immediate response to LEPT are extremely important when treating acute disk disease in dogs. IR (830 or 904 nm) should be applied directly to the tender paravertebral or intervertebral points (4 to 8 J/cm²) in the affected segment. In subacute and chronic cases, treatment should be repeated daily or on alternate days for up to 6 sessions. When osteoarthritic joints are treated, IR laser irradiation should be directed not only to the joint space (2 to 4 J/cm²) concerned but also to the tender (trigger) points (0.5 to 1 J/point) in the muscles moving the joint.

Special Applications for Large Animals

The principles discussed for small animals are also valid for large animals.

When equine muscle pain and lameness are treated, special attention should be given to any tender or trigger points in the whole body quadrant involved. Bilateral irradiation is recommended for better muscle and movement coordination and balance after the treatment. In horses, back muscles may need higher-power densities than are normally applied today in the treatment of myo-

fascial problems. A combination therapy beginning with a multidiode head (30 × 20 mW) over the muscle body (2 to 4 J/cm²) to relieve the spasm and ending with a point-directed contact treatment (90 to 120 mW) to the TPs (6 to 8 J/TP) may restore full function in typical cases of myofascial pain.

Oda and others (1994) investigated the effect of low-level laser acupuncture on subclinical mastitis and reproductive disorders in dairy cattle. They applied a GaAlAs laser (830 nm, 80 mW) in the contact mode, using a probe covered with transparent plastic film. For subclinical mastitis, four acupuncture points were used: *Youmei*, in the depression lateral to the base of each teat; *Nyuzoko*, at the center of each teat; *Nyuki*, at the base of the mammary vein in front of the anterior mammary gland; and *Nyukon*, at the lymph node dorsal to the posterior mammary gland (3 min/day for 5 days). The efficacy of LEPT for subclinical mastitis, measured as a decrease in somatic cell count, was 80.6%. Three AP points were used for reproductive disorders: *Koso*, in the depression between the anus and the ventral tail base; *Einbu*, at the center of the perineum; and *Inkaku*, at the clitoris (3-9 min/day for 3 days). Within a month after LEPT, 37 of the 46 cows (80.4%) exhibited estrus within a month after LEPT. The results suggest that LEPT can be used as an alternative therapy for subclinical mastitis and reproductive disorders, excluding pyometra, in dairy cattle.

Controversial Issues

To date, LEPT usually has been excluded from the range of treatment modalities generally accepted in conventional medicine. Controversal results in in vivo experiments, both animal and human, and even more controversy in clinical trials, along with some negative reports in

TABLE 17-8

PHOTON SOURCE FOR VARIOUS INDICATIONS (SMALL ANIMALS)

INDICATIONS	GINGIVITIS	WOUNDS	MUSCLE TPs	AP (BODY POINTS)	AP (EAR POINTS)	JOINTS	DISK DISEASE	OTITIS EXT. CHRON. INF.	ALOPECIA (ECZEMA)
HeNe 10-30 mW (scanner)	-	+	-	-	-	-	-	-	+
InGaAlP 10-30 mW	++	++	+	++	++	+	-	++	+
InGaAlP 20-40 mW	++	++	++	+	+	++	+	++	++
GaAlAs 10-30 mW	++	++	++	++	+	+	-	++	+
GaAlAs 60-90 mW	++	++	+++	+	-	+++	++	+++	++
GaAlAs 90-150 mW	+	+	++	-	-	+++	+++	+	+
GaAs 70-100 W	+	+	+	-	-	++	++	+	+
Multiple diode 150-300 mW	-	++	++	-	-	++	+	+	++
IR cluster (LED) 300-600 mW	-	++	++	-	-	++	+	+	++

TABLE 17-9

PHOTON SOURCE FOR VARIOUS INDICATIONS (LARGE ANIMALS)

INDICATIONS	GINGIVITIS	WOUNDS	MUSCLE TPs	AP (BODY POINTS)	AP (EAR POINTS)	TENDINITIS BOWED TENDON	FASCIITIS	CHECK. LIGAMENT	PHARYNGEAL HYPERPLASIA
HeNe 10-30 mW (scanner)	-	++	-	-	-	-	-	-	-
InGaAlP 10-30 mW	+	+	-	+	++	-	-	-	-
InGaAlP 20-40 mW	++	+	+	++	+	+	+	+	+
GaAlAs 10-30 mW	+	+	+	++	+	-	-	-	+
GaAlAs 60-90 mW	+++	+	++	+	-	++	++	++	++
GaAlAs 90-150 mW	++	++	+++	-	-	+++	+++	+++	+
GaAs 70-100 W	+	+	++	-	-	++	++	++	+
Multiple diode 150-300 mW	-	+++	+++	-	-	+++	+++	+++	-
IR cluster (LED) 300-600 mW	-	+++	+++	-	-	++	++	++	-

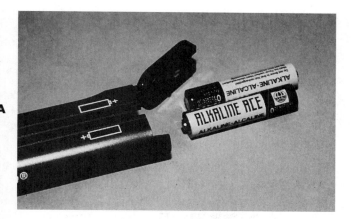

A

B

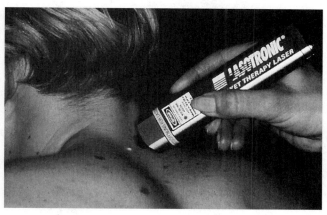

Fig. 17-11 **A** and **B** Laser pen, battery operated 670 nm (visible red) or 830 nm (infrared), 20-40 mW, cw or alpha frequency (Nogier, von Bahr and specific individually set frequencies available in computerized model)(Lasotronic AG, PO Box 2086, CH-6302 Zug, Switzerland). Contact treatment.

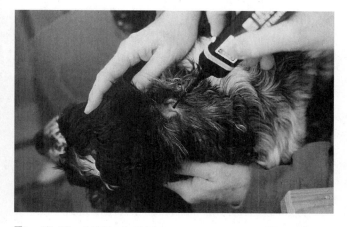

Fig. 17-12 LEPT of otitis externa in cocker spaniel using 30 mW, 670 nm, cw diode laser with an extension tube for local irradiation of ear channel (1-2 J/cm²), combined with local chemotherapy.

respected medical journals, have caused uncertainty and suspicion about the value of low-energy lasers in medicine.* A main argument was the poor penetration of the laser beam through the skin and an almost nonexistent temperature increase at the target site. Today, opinions are changing. We know that laser light (coherent, collimated) is not necessary to induce alterations in cellular function (see Table 17-4.). Highly divergent and noncoherent but monochromatic light can alter biologic processes if the tissue interaction threshold ($0.01 J/cm^2$) is reached. A normal irradiance (dose) of $4 J/cm^2$ at the skin level maintains an effective irradiance to the depth of 0.5 to 2.5 cm (6 penetration depths). When the bigger joints and muscles are treated, the initial irradiance of 100 to $300 J/cm^2$ at the skin level is attenuated to $20 J/cm^2$ at 6 penetration depths, and an effective irradiance can be maintained to the depth of 5 to 10 cm. Therefore it is not surprising that defocused high-power lasers (Nd:YAG and CO_2) have been used successfully in sports medicine and the treatment of hip and knee osteoarthritis. The same irradiance to a wound or ulcer may stop the healing process. No simple linear dose response curve exists for LEPT. For wound healing and biomodulation the minimum irradiance to alter cell function is about $0.01 J/cm^2$. If the irradiance exceeds 4 to $6 J/cm^2$, a suppression effect often results. With the addition of a certain, subject-dependent latency period (as in acupuncture and TENS) that is necessary before tissue reaction can occur, comparison of various clinical reports and standardization of treatments clearly become difficult. Experiments have shown that normal subjects may not react to AP, TENS, or laser therapy to the same extent as patients experiencing pain or peripheral vascular disorders. For example, pressure pain threshold (PTH) reacts to laser, SLD, and TENS if the initial level is lower than normal. Normal PTHs do not react. However, LEPT and TENS may elevate lower-than-normal levels to normal ones. Many of the "correct" double-blind studies have used healthy normal subjects or abnormally low irradiation doses. Often necessary information such as wavelength, radiant power, irradiance, dose, spot size, exposure time, and total dose are missing. The minimal requirement for an acceptable, reliable, and valid treatment is daily checking of the output power of every laser (Fig. 17-13).

Future Trends in LEPT

The following is a short list of topics and fields that have promising preliminary results, although further basic and clinical research is urgently needed.

*Basford (1995); Basford and others (1993); Baxter and others (1991); Bork, Snyder, Mackler (1988); Walker (1985); Walker, Akhanjee (1985); Wu and others (1987).

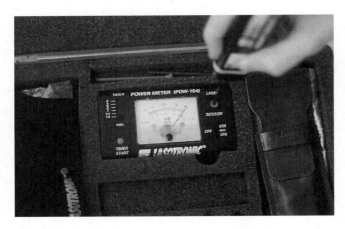

Fig. 17-13 Adjustable power meter for 830 nm and 670 nm laser radiation. Every laser should be measured daily, and battery operation measured before and after every treatment session.

- Immunological aspects of LEPT
  - LEPT to combat immunoreactivity (transplantations, etc.)
  - Blood irradiation, transcutaneous or extracorporeal
- LEPT as a noninvasive method in acupuncture
  - Wavelengths, frequencies
- Photodynamic therapy with LEPT
- LEPT as part of routine operating procedures
  - Smooth scar formation
  - Healing per primam intentionem
  - Accelerated recovery
- LEPT to control recurrent, mixed flora (iatrogenic) superficial skin, mucosal infections
- LEPT as a diagnostic tool in musculoskeletal disorders
- LEPT in trauma surgery and sports medicine
  - Muscle, tendon, nerve repair
  - Postoperative rehabilitation

REFERENCES

Abergel RP and others: Laser treatment of keloids: a clinical trial and an in vitro study with Nd:YAG laser, *Lasers Surg Med* 4:291, 1984.

Airaksinen O and others: Effects of infra-red laser irradiation on the treated and non-treated trigger points, *Acupunct Electrother Res* 14: 9, 1989.

Amano A and others: Histological studies on the rheumatoid synovial membrane irradiated with a low-energy laser, *Lasers Surg Med* 15:290, 1994.

Ambronn G, Muxeneder R, Warnke U: *Laser-und Magnetfeldtherapie in der Tiermedizin,* Jena, Stuttgart, 1995, Gustaf Fischer Verlag.

Anders JJ and others: Low power laser irradiation alters the rate of regeneration of the rat facial nerve, *Lasers Surg Med* 13:72, 1993.

Basford JR: Low intensity laser therapy: still not an established clinical tool, *Lasers Surg Med* 16:331, 1995.

Basford JR and others: Effects of 830 nm continuous wave laser diode irradiation on median nerve function in normal subjects, *Lasers Surg Med* 13:597, 1993.

Baxter GD and others: Effect of laser (830 nm) upon conduction in the median nerve, *Laser Surg Med Suppl* 3:79, 1991 (abstract).

Benedicenti A: La valutazione dell'effetto della luce laser 904 nm nella circolazione ematica in vivo, *Paradontol e Stomatol Nuova* 1:109, 1983.

Bibikova A, Oron U: Attenuation of the process of muscle regeneration in the toad gastrocnemius muscle by low energy laser irradiation, *Lasers Surg Med* 14:355, 1994.

Bihari I and others: The biostimulative effect of low level laser therapy of long-standing crural ulcers, using helium neon laser, helium neon plus infrared lasers, and noncoherent light: preliminary report of a randomized double blind comparative study, *Laser Ther* 1:97, 1989.

Bloembergen N, *Phys Rev* 104:324, 1956.

Bork CE, Snyder Mackler L: Effect of helium-neon laser irradiation on peripheral sensory nerve latency, *J Am Phys Ther Assoc* 68:223, 1988.

Carrillo JS and others: Acción del laser de HeNe sobre el crecimiento de una cepa de stafilococus aureus in vitro, *Laser España 87, Abstracts, Tarragona* Nov 26-28, 1987.

Cisneros JL: Tratamiento de los queloides con laser He/Ne + I.R., *Investigación y Clínica Laser* 1(3):32, 1984.

Dyson M, Young S: Effect of laser therapy on wound contraction and cellularity in mice, *Lasers Med Sci* 1:125, 1986.

Enwemeka CS: Ultrastructural morphometry of membrane-bound intracytoplasmic collagen fibrils in tendon fibroblasts exposed to He:Ne laser beam, *Tissue Cell* 24:511, 1992.

Enwemeka CS and others: Biomechanical effects of three different periods of GaAs laser photostimulation on tenotomized tendons, *Laser Ther* 6:181-188, 1994.

Eriksson A, Knutsson E, Skoglund CR: Smärtlindring och påskyndad läkning av bensår genom transkutan nervstimulering (TNS). XLIII Läkaresällskapets Rikstämma, Stockholm, Dec 3-5, 1986.

Felten RP: FDA status of biostimulation lasers. Abstracts of ASLMS fourteenth annual meeting, Toronto, Ontario, Canada, April 8-10, 1994.

Fennyö M: Theoretical and experimental basis of biostimulation by laser irradiation, *Optics Laser Technol* 8:209, 1984.

Fiszerman R, Rozenbom CY: Low energy therapy effect in low extremity transcutaneous oxygen partial pressure. Abstracts of ASLMS fifteenth annual meeting, San Diego, California, April 2-4, 1995.

Flöter T: Laser in the management of chronic pain, *Scand J Acup Electrother* 2:18, 1987.

Galante O: Tratamiento de artrosis en el geronte con rayo laser, *Investigación y Clínica Laser* 2 (2):78, 1985.

Galleti G: Further elements in favour of low energy-density (LED) CO_2 laser capacity to penetrate tissues, *Laser Ther* 6:9, 1994.

Ghamsari SM and others: Histopatho-logical effects of low level laser therapy on secondary healing of teat wounds in dairy cattle, *Laser Ther* 7:81, 1995.

Gilioli G and others: Effetti sperimentali del laser infrarosso: studi in vitro con l'Herpes virus, *Med Laser Rep* 3:2831, 1985.

Glinkowski W, Rowinski J: Effect of low incident levels of infrared laser energy on the healing of experimental bone fractures, *Laser Ther* 7:67, 1995.

Gomez-Villamandos RJ and others: He-Ne laser therapy by fibroendoscopy of the equine upper airway, *Lasers Surg Med* 16:184, 1995.

Gordon JP, Zeiger HJ, Townes CH: The maser: new type of amplifier, frequency standard and spectrometer, *Phys Rev* 99:1264, 1955.

Gurevich Y, Filonenko N, Salansky N: Analytical method for calculation of temperature distribution in laser-irradiated media with an external cooled surface, *Appl Phys Lett* 64:3216, 1994.

Guynne P: Cold laser uses move beyond carpal tunnel, *Biophotonics* 1:28, 1994.

Hasan P and others: The possible application of low reactive level laser therapy (LLLT) in the treatment of male infertility, *Laser Ther* 1(1):49, 1989.

Helminen HJ and others: Kuormituksen vaikutus nivelrustoon, *Duodecim* 108:1097, 1992.

Hernandez Gonzales LC and others: Comportamiento "in vitro" de las candidas albicans frente a la energia laser (He-Ne/I.R.), *Investigación y Clinica Laser* 4:86, 1987.

Kaada B: Vasodilation induced by transcutaneous nerve stimulation in peripheral ischemia (Raynaud's phenomenon and diabetic neuropathy), *Eur Heart J* 3:303, 1982.

Kaada B: Promoted healing of chronic ulceration by transcutaneous nerve stimulation (TNS), *VASA* 12:262, 1983.

Kaada B, Eielsen O: In search of mediators of skin vasodilation induced by transcutaneous nerve stimulation. I. Failure to block the response by antagonists of endogenous vasodilators, *Gen Pharmacol* 14:623, 1983.

Kaada B, Eielsen O: In search of mediators of skin vasodilation induced by transcutaneous nerve stimulation. II. Serotonin implicated, *Gen Pharmacol* 14:635, 1983.

Kaada B, Emru M: Promoted healing of leprous ulcers by transcutaneous nerve stimulation, *Acupunct Electrother Res* 13:164, 1988.

Kaada B, Helle K: In search of mediators of skin vasodilation induced by transcutaneous nerve stimulation: IV. In vitro bioassey of the vasoinhibitory activity of sera from patients suffering from peripheral ischemia, *Gen Pharmacol* 15:115, 1984.

Kaada B, Lygren I: Lower plasma levels of some gastrointestinal peptides in Raynaud's disease: influence of transcutaneous nerve stimulation, *Gen Pharmacol* 16:153, 1985.

Kaada B, Olsen E, Eielsen O: In search of mediators of skin vasodilation induced by transcutaneous nerve stimulation. III. Increase in plasma VIP in normal subjects and in Raynaud's disease, *Gen Pharmacol* 15:107, 1984.

Kana JS and others: Effect of low power density laser radiation on healing of open skin wounds in rats, *Arch Surg* 116:293, 1981.

Karu TI: Photobiological fundamentals of low-power laser therapy, *IEEE J Quant Elect* 23:1703, 1987.

Karu T, Andreichuk T, Ryabykh T: Suppression of human blood chemoluminescence by diode laser irradiation at wavelengths 660, 820 or 950 nm, *Laser Ther* 5:103, 1993.

Kolari PJ: Penetration of unfocused laser light into the skin, *Arch Dermatol Res* 277:342, 1985.

Kolari PJ and others: Lasers in physical therapy: measurement of optical output power (part I), *Scand J Acupunct Electrother* 3:96, 1988.

Kubota J and others: The effects of diode laser low reactive level laser therapy (LLLT) on flap survival in a rat model, *Laser Ther* 1:127, 1989.

Lam TS and others: Laser stimulation of collagen synthesis in human skin fibroblast cultures, *Lasers Life Sci* 1:61, 1986.

Langer H, Lange W: Vergleichende Untersuchungen zum Transmissions- und Absorptionsverhalten menschlichen Gewebes bei Bestrahlung mit HeNe-Laser, Infrarot-Laser und Infrarot-Emitterdiode, *AKU* 20:19, 1992.

Lanzafame RJ: Treatment or tool, *Lasers Surg Med* 17:302, 1995.

Laor Y and others: The pathology of laser irradiation of the skin and body wall of the mouse, *Am J Pathol* 47:643, 1965.

Lee P, Kim K, Kim K: Effects of low incident energy levels of infrared laser irradiation on healing of infected open skin wounds in rats, *Laser Ther* 5:59, 1993.

Lievens P: The influence of laser irradiation on the motricity of lymphatic system and on the woundhealing process. Proceedings of the

International Congress on Laser in Medicine and Surgery, Monduzzi Ed, Bologna, 1986.

Loevschall H, Arenholt-Bindslev D: Effect of low level diode laser irradiation of human oral mucosa fibroblasts in vitro, *Lasers Surg Med* 14:347, 1994.

Lonauer G: Controlled study of the efficacy of HeNe-laser beams in the therapy of activated osteoarthritis of finger joints, *Clin Exper Rheuma* 2(suppl):39, 1987.

Lubart R and others: Light effect on fibroblast proliferation, *Laser Ther* 5:55, 1993.

Maiman TH: Optical maser action in ruby, *Nature* 187:493, 1960.

Mayayo E, Trelles MA: Irradiación laser experimental de la mucosa anal en el raton de laboratorio, *Investigación y Clinica Laser* 1(4):28, 1984.

Mayayo E, Trelles MA: Laser e inmunidad, *Investigación y Clinica Laser* 3:73-74, 1986.

McKibbin LS, Paraschak D: A study of lasering chronic bowed tendons at Wheatley Hall Farm Limited, *Lasers Surg Med* 3:55, 1983.

McKibbin LS, Paraschak D: Use of laser light to treat certain lesions in standardbreds, *Mod Vet Pract*, March, p 210, 1984.

Meno N and others: Effects of LLLT, using helium-neon laser on infectious bovine keratoconjunctivitis, *Laser Ther* 1(2):79, 1989.

Mester E. Über die Wirkung der Laserstrahlen auf die Bakterienphagozytose der Leukozyten, *Acta Biol Med Germ* 21:317, 1968.

Mester E: Neuere Untersuchungen über die Wirkung der Laserstrahlen auf die Wundheilung—Immunologische Effekte, *Z Exper Chirurg* 10:301, 1977.

Mester E, Mester AE, Mester A. The biomedical effect of laser application, *Lasers Surg Med* 5:31, 1985.

Mester E and others: Untersuchungen über die hemmende bzw. fördernde Wirkung der Laserstrahlen, *Arch Klin Chir* 322:1022, 1968.

Miro L and others: Estudio capilaroscopico de la acción de un laser AsGa sobre la microcirculación, *Investigación y Clinica Laser* 1(2):9, 1984.

Muxeneder R: Soft laser in the conservative treatment of chronic skin lesions in the horse, *Der Prakt Tierarzt* 68(1):12, 1987.

Muxeneder R: Die Behandlung ovarieller Dysfunktionen von Stuten mit Akupunktur und biologischen Heilmitteln. Eine Alternative zur Hormonbehandlung? Der praktische Tierarzt, *Collegium Veterinarium* 21:88, 1990.

Ochi M, Osedo M, Ikuta Y: Superior nerve anastomosis using a low-output CO_2 laser on fibrin membrane, *Lasers Surg Med* 17:64, 1995.

Oda Y and others: Effect of low level laser acupuncture on subclinical mastitis and reproductive disorders in dairy cattle, *Laser Ther* 6:157, 1994.

Oshiro T, Galderhead RG: *Low level laser therapy: a practical introduction*, Chichester, England, 1988, Wiley.

Parra PF and others: Laser ad alta energia tipo Neodimio-YAG defocilizzato: valutazione sperimentale del potere di penetrazione tissutale, *Laser Technol* 3:31, 1993.

Pöntinen PJ: Evaluation and measurement of response to acupuncture and laser therapy. Proceedings of the nineteenth annual International Conference on Veterinary Acupuncture, Tromsø, June 24-27, 1993.

Pöntinen PJ, Airaksinen O: The effect of low power infrared laser on latent myofascial trigger points, first International Symposium on Myofascial Pain and Fibromyalgia, Minneapolis, May 8-10, 1989.

Pöntinen PJ, Airaksinen O: Evaluation of myofascial pain and dysfunction syndromes and their response to low level laser therapy, *J Musculoskel Pain* 3(2):149, 1995.

Pöntinen PJ, Pothmann R: *Laser in der Akupunktur*, Stuttgart, 1993, Hippokrates Verlag.

Pöntinen PJ and others: The effect of hair lasers on skin blood flow. Abstracts of ASLMS, fifteenth annual meeting, San Diego, California, April 2-4, 1995.

Rochkind S: Central nervous system transplantation benefitted by low-power laser irradiation, *Lasers Med Sci* 7:143, 1992.

Rochkind S and others: Response of peripheral nerve to HeNe laser: experimental studies, *Lasers Surg Med* 7:441, 1987.

Rochkind S and others: Stimulatory effect of He-Ne low dose laser on injured sciatic nerves of rats, *Neurosurgery* 20:843, 1987.

Rochkind S and others: The in-vivo nerve response to direct low-energy laser irradiation, *Acta Neurochir* 94:74, 1988.

Rochkind S and others: Intraoperative clinical use of LLLT following surgical treatment of the tethered spinal cord, *Laser Ther* 3:113, 1991.

Rodrigo P, Lerma E, Zaragoza JR: Efectos de la irradiaciÛn laser obre el tiroides: rstudio experimental en la rata blanca, *Investigación y Clinica Laser* 2:7, 1985.

Rodrigo P, Zaragoza JR, Iturrate C: Un caso de osteomielitis tratado con laserterapia. *Investigación y Clinica Laser* 2:94, 1985.

Rogers P: Clinical use of an infra-red diode-laser, *Scand J Acup Electrother* 7:7, 1992.

Rubenstein E: Combined high-power and low-power laser treatment for ulcerative vulval lesions induced by human papillomavirus (HPV), *Laser España*, Tarragona, Nov 26-28, 1987.

Salansky N, Brill G, Filonenko N: Blood indexes changes under low energy photon (LEP) irradiation in vivo experiments. Abstracts of ASLMS, fourteenth annual meeting, Toronto, Ontario, Canada, April 8-10, 1994.

Samoilova KA and others: Photomodification of blood. Therapeutic effects and trigger mechanisms: improvement of the haemorheology, transport and detoxicative functions of blood (Ist pat), *Laser Technol* 3:55, 1993.

Schwanitz R: The position of acupuncture and the importance of its methods in sportsmedicine. Abstracts, Third World Congress of Scientific Acupuncture, ICMART '88, Prague.

Schwartz M and others: Effects of low-energy He-Ne laser irradiation of posttraumatic degeneration of adult rabbit optic nerve, *Lasers Surg Med* 7:51 1987.

Shawlow AL, Townes CH: Intrared and optical masers, *Phys Rev* 112:1940, 1958.

Shiroto C, Ono K, Oshiro T: Retrospective study of diode laser therapy for pain attenuation in 3635 patients: detailed analysis by questionnaire, *Laser Ther* 1:41, 1989.

Steinlechner CWB, Dyson M: The effects of low level laser therapy on the proliferation of keratinocytes, *Laser Ther* 5:65, 1993.

Sumano HL, Cosaubon T: Evaluation of electroacupuncture effects on wound- and burn-healing, *Scand J Acup Electrother* 2:159, 1987 (abstract).

Sumano HL, Cosaubon T, Lopez G: Effect of electrostimulation on second intention wound healing, *Scand J Acup Electrother* 2:154, 1987 (abstract).

Timea Berki M and others: Biological effect of low power helium neon (HeNe) laser irradiation, *Lasers Med Sci* 3:35, 1988.

Terribile Wiel Marin V and others: Experimental wound healing with coherent and non-coherent radiation, *Laser Technol* 2:121, 1992.

Trelles MA: La cicatrización de las heridas en la oreja del conejo bajo la influencia del rayo He/Ne. Estudio histologico, *Antol Dermatol Rev Practica-Medico-Quirurgica de la Med de la Piel y de sus Anexos*, Barcelona 11-15, 1983.

Tsibulyak VN, Lee TS, Alisov AP: Reflexotherapy for analgesia and treatment of infected wounds, *Scand J Acup Electrother* 3:137, 1988.

Walker JB: Temporary suppression of clonus in human by brief photostimulation, *Brain Res* 340:109, 1985.

Walker JB, Akhanjee LK: Laser-induced somatosensory evoked potentials: evidence of photosensitivity in peripheral nerves, *Brain Res* 344:281, 1985.

Weber J: Tran IRE Prof Group on Electron Devices, 3 June, 1953. Presented at tenth International Conference on Electron Tube Research, Ottawa, Canada, June 1952.

Wilson M, Pratten J: Lethal photosensitisation of *Staphylococcus aureus* in vitro: effect of growth phase, serum, and pre-irradiation time, *Lasers Surg Med* 16:272, 1995.

Wu W and others: Failure to confirm report of light-evoked response of peripheral nerve to low power helium-neon laser light stimulus, *Brain Res* 401:407, 1987.

Zalesskiy VN: Use of laser acupuncture for cancer pain relief, *Pain* 2 (suppl):154, 1984.

Zalesskiy VN, Frolov GV: Fiberoptic laser acupuncture for cancer pain relief, *Scand J Acup Electrother* 1:105, 1987.

SELECTED READINGS

Cobo Plana J and others: El laser I.R. en el tratamiento de la osteonecrosis mandibular. A proposito de un caso, *Investigación y Clinica Laser* 3:61, 1986.

Gordon JP, Zeiger HJ, Townes CH, *Phys Rev* 99:1264, 1955.

Karu TI: Molecular mechanism of the therapeutic effect of low-intensity laser radiation. *Lasers Life Sci* 2:53, 1988.

Karu TI and others: Helium-neon laser-induced respiratory burst of phagocytic cells, *Lasers Surg Med* 9:585, 1989.

Mester E, Toth N, Mester A: The biostimulative effect of laser beam, *Laser Basic Biomed Res* 22:4, 1982.

Strassl H, Porteder H, Zetner K: Tierexperimentelle Studie Hüber den Einsatz von Laserstrahlen zur Beeinflussung der Wundheilung, *Acta Chir Austriaca* (2):33, 1983.

Trelles MA, Mester E: Ulceras cronicas en las extremidades inferiores, *Investigación y Clinica Laser* 1(2):32, 1989.

Chapter 18

Magnetic Field Therapy

DONALD E. HUDSON, DOREEN O. HUDSON

For centuries, magnetism has been used as a cure for a variety of illnesses. Magnetic therapy has enjoyed a recent resurgence as a safe, simple, and inexpensive method that produces positive results without harmful side effects. This chapter explores the form and function of different types of magnets and offers a historical perspective on their uses. The literature review gives a scientific view of this modality, and the section on the traditional use of magnets provides background for current veterinary practices. Concerns about the safety of magnetic therapy are thoroughly considered in the context of magnetic field theory. Suggestions are provided to allow for the smooth integration of magnetic therapy into clinical practice. Any additional questions can be answered by consulting the reference list at the end of the chapter.

Magnetism is defined as the alignment of magnetic, or permeable, material so that the molecules face in a uniform direction (i.e., north facing one direction, and south facing the opposite direction). Both the composition and the size of the magnet affect its strength, or intensity. Larger animals require therapies with more magnetic strength than smaller animals simply because of their greater body mass. Magnets are thought to work by means of magnetic lines of force, measured and quantified in units called *gauss*. Gauss, a German mathematician and astronomer, discovered a precise method to measure magnetic field strength. The symbol G is now used to denote the level of magnetic field density. The Earth has a natural magnetic field of 0.5 G, although it is determined to have been much greater earlier in the Earth's history (Smith, Best, 1989).

Classifications of Magnets

The two major classifications of magnets used in therapy are permanent magnets (also called *static magnets*) and pulsed electromagnetic field (PEMF) magnets. In general use, both types are applied to the area of injury. Depending on the strength of the magnetic field, magnetic lines of force permeate the area of injury and stimulate healing.

Magnet Types

A number of magnetic products are now available commercially. The first magnets used in medicine were found in naturally magnetic lodestone, or magnetite. Of all the 92 elements, only iron, cobalt, and nickel are affected by magnetic fields. A number of alloys, or combinations of materials, also have magnetic characteristics (Wheeler, 1978). Magnets have defined north and south poles. If a small piece of magnet is broken off, both pieces of the magnet still contain a north pole and a south pole, so the magnetic alignment of the molecules is "permanently" placed (Wheeler, 1978). Permanent magnets are affixed to the patient and left in place for a period of minutes, hours, or days. A relatively recent addition to the permanent magnet family is the bipolar magnetic strip or pad. Finally, pulsed electromagnetic field therapy systems are devices that generate a pulsating electromagnetic field. Coils that produce the field are placed on the patient, generally for 30 to 60 minutes for each daily therapy session. Magnetic therapy devices come in many different sizes and strengths.

For practical use, static manufactured magnets are preferred over naturally occurring magnetic material because the strength and pole configurations are defined and sometimes marked. Static manufactured magnets are constructed of a variety of materials, usually a combination of neodymium, ceramic, aluminum, nickel, iron, and cobalt. These metals are magnetized to contain a permanent magnetic field. Those made of neodymium, iron, and boron generally have a higher gauss rating. When purchasing magnets from an industrial or scientific supplier, practitioners should note that measurements are indicated in gauss, and lift capability in pounds. A small magnet made of neodymium and boron is very powerful despite its small size. A magnet the same size made of aluminum, nickel, and cobalt (ALNICO) would have a smaller gauss rating. Neodymium, iron, and boron magnets are also the most expensive because they are stronger. Industrial strength magnets up to 35 million gauss are available for heavy industry. Therapeutic permanent magnets usually range from 200 to 3000 gauss, whereas stronger magnets, termed *super magnets*, of 1000 to 3000 gauss are also coming into more frequent clinical use.

> Weight is closely related to depth of penetration, as is strength or intensity. Size is extremely important because the more area covered, the greater the volume of tissue influenced and the more effective the results. Too often it is forgotten that the amount of tissue affected is directly related to the rate of healing (Washnis, Hricak, 1993).

Bar magnets are unipolar (i.e., a north pole on one surface, and a south pole on the opposite surface). Most manufacturers mark the north and south poles for proper application. The term *unipolar* has led some to suppose that the magnet has only a single pole. This is not possible; a magnetic field cannot exist without both poles, one to attract the other. Even if only one side of the magnet is marked, the opposite side must contain the opposite pole, or by definition it could not be a magnet.

Magnetic lines of force are thought to flow from north to south, with the greatest magnetic field near the end points of the magnet. At the center of the magnet, where the two fields are closest, very little magnetic field exists. Assuming two magnets are of the same composition, the smaller magnet has negligible lines of force and a limited gauss field because the distance between the north and south poles is short, whereas the larger magnet has a greater magnetic field because a greater distance exists between the two poles. This phenomenon is best demonstrated by the magnetic field of the earth. Field strength is strongest at the poles and weakest at the equator.

Bar magnets, or magnetic beads, can be applied with tape but are more often applied with super glue or eyelash glue, which hold them in place more effectively.

Bipolar magnets are the most recent addition to the field of magnetics. They are usually manufactured in long rolls or strips (usually 0.06 inches thick) and can be cut in specific shapes. The north and south magnetic materials are laid down parallel to each other or in concentric circles. One manufacturer lays down the field in a checkerboard pattern. This means that when placed on the skin, both north and south poles come in contact with the patient. Magnetic field strengths vary, but in general the magnetized roll and strip materials have fields at the surface of approximately 500 gauss. The materials used in the magnetic strips are the same as those used in promotional items by advertisers, frequently seen as calendar magnets that affix to a file cabinet or a refrigerator. The major differences in the bipolar strips are the thickness and pattern of magnetization. Generally the thicker the strip, the more powerful the field, although the composition of the material also has an effect on its gauss rating. In other words, a 0.125-inch strip would have a greater magnetic field than a 0.06-inch strip, given the same composition. The manufacturers that use concentric circles and the checkerboard pattern claim their pattern of magnetization leads to a greater magnetic effect.

A study conducted by Applied Magnetics Laboratory (Nolan, 1994) documented gauss readings on samples of three commercially available, widely promoted magnetic strips. At the surface the gauss field ranged from approximately 200 to 500 gauss. It also measured the field at short distances from the surface, finding that moving beyond 0.33 inches from the surface of the three pads, the measurable magnetic field was below 20 gauss. Evidently, even though the strength of the magnetic field produced on the surface of the strip is high, the magnetic field strength a short distance away is quite low. This factor is important when considering the penetration of the magnetic field into tissue. Bipolar strips are generally applied with wraps, but smaller pieces may be cut from a larger section and glued on, with the understanding that the size and weight of the magnet are directly related to the depth of penetration of the field. (Different magnetic patterns seen in bar magnets, bipolar, and pulsed electromagnetic field devices are shown in Fig. 18-1.)

Pulsed electromagnetic field therapy (PEMF) is a

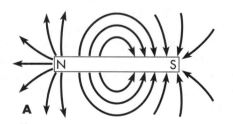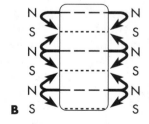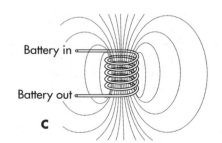

Fig. 18-1 Different magnetic patterns seen in bar magnets, bipolar, and pulsed electromagnetic field devices. **A,** Magnetic field—simple bar magnet. **B,** Bipolar magnetic field—blood vessel is ideally perpendicular to lines of force. **C,** Magnetic field produced by pulsed magnetic field therapy system.

method of creating a pulsating magnetic field by means of pulsing current through a coil of wire. These systems usually contain several coils of wire, a control box with different pulse settings, and a battery-fed direct current power source. A basic principle of physics states that whenever current flows through a wire, a magnetic field develops around the wire. When the current ceases to flow, the magnetic field collapses. Another pulse of current causes the magnetic field to reappear, and turning off the current makes the field collapse again. This action is repeated a number of times per second. The greater the amount of current flow, the greater the magnetic field. A greater number of turns of the wire also increases the strength of the magnetic field.

The coils that generate the magnetic field are placed over the area to be treated; however, coil placement is not crucial because the pulsating magnetic field can extend beyond the coil by more than 15 inches, which greatly increases the amount of tissue affected and positively influences the rate of healing (Washnis, Hricak, 1993). Therapy devices are positioned so that the injury is between two coils, placed in a Helmholz coil pair. This arrangement produces magnetic fields that go in the same direction and therefore enhance each other, increasing the overall magnetic field strength. For example, if treating a leg, the practitioner places one coil laterally and the other medially. This arrangement pulls the magnetic field in on one side of the leg and pushes it out the other side of the leg because the fields aid each other. The rate of pulsing is called the *frequency*, and usually higher frequencies correspond to higher energy levels.

Widespread use of this therapy began in Germany in the early 1970s, where it continues today. Modern systems are battery powered to simplify use in stables and barns and eliminate the risk of using electricity in wet areas. PEMF is applicable to both acute and chronic injury and is frequently used as a maintenance therapy for chronic musculoskeletal conditions. Therapy sessions last from 30 to 60 minutes. Its use in the United States is approved by the U.S. Food and Drug Administration for nonunion fractures.

This brief introduction should demonstrate that the term *magnetic therapy* can represent many things. The method can be varied by using permanent or pulsed magnetic fields. The strength of the magnet may vary depending on the size and composition of the magnet. The length of therapy may range from minutes to days. These variations make quantifying the effects of magnetic therapy difficult. Researchers and clinicians who use a variety of magnetic materials in their studies make replication of results difficult unless the specifications of the magnets used in their studies are made explicit.

History of Magnetics in Medicine

We all have something of magnetic and electric forces in ourselves, and in the same way as the mag-

net itself, we exercise an attracting and a repelling force, depending on whether we are in contact with something similar or dissimilar (Johann Wolfgang von Goethe).

Early medical practitioners used simple magnetic tools, usually natural magnets in the form of lodestone. A number of scrolls from 2800 BC report what appears to be use of healing magnetism to ease pain and suffering (Schiegl, 1987). Cleopatra reportedly wore a lodestone on her forehead to offset the effects of old age. The first direct reference to magnets in medicine occurs in the *Yellow Emperor's Book of Internal Medicine,* attributed to Houang-Ti in about 2000 BC. Lodestones were placed over acupuncture points to assist in balancing the meridians, in addition to using needles and moxa (Becker, 1990).

Hindu scriptures refer to treatment of disease using *siktavati,* or *ashmana,* which have been translated as *instruments of stone* (perhaps lodestone). Tibetan monks used bar magnets in training new monks. In many parts of the world, healing magnetism and magnets were apparently used for thousands of years before the birth of Christ to influence bodily energy systems (Becker, 1990).

Egyptian medicine systems were passed on to the Greeks, as seen in the writings of Hippocrates, who called magnetism "the force which flows from many people's hands." Galen, another important figure in medical history, wrote that "a sick body can gain strength from the unbroken contact with a healthy body" (Becker, 1990). In the mid-1400s, Paracelsus, who wrote and lectured widely about medicine and surgery, added his own theories to the art in his *Great Surgery Book.* He wrote that the earth is a great magnet, and all living beings are affected by the invisible effects of magnetic attractions and repulsions. He studied the application of magnetism, writing about polarities, the attraction of unlike energies, and the repulsion of like energies. He used magnets in the belief that the body could be healed by applying the proper energy forces to the weakened body. Paracelsus is a controversial figure in medical history because he ridiculed many established concepts, yet he occupies a place of importance because of his willingness to explore unusual solutions and embrace the possibilities of forces that could not, at that time, be seen, felt, or measured (Schiegl, 1987).

A contemporary of Mozart, Franz Mesmer wrote his doctoral thesis on the influence of the planets, particularly the influence of the stars on human health. He describes a universal force that permeates the human body and everything on earth (hence the term *mesmerism,* which denotes induction of a hypnotic state). Mesmer became famous and opened a popular clinic in France where he practiced magnetic healing. His theories were collected in his "Report on the Discovery of Animal Magnetism" (Mesmer, 1779). Like most scientists who attempted to question contemporary tenets, he was considered unorthodox and he died in disrepute (Schiegl, 1987).

Magnetic medicine became more scientific and less astral when William Gilbert, the physician to Queen Elizabeth, wrote *De Magnete (The Magnet)* (Gilbert, 1600). Gilbert distinguished magnetism from electricity and described the Earth as a huge magnet. According to Gilbert, the Earth's magnetic quality causes the compass to point north (Hanneman, 1990). A near contemporary of Gilbert, Luigi Galvani concluded from his years of practice as an anatomist and obstetrician that biologic electricity is the vital energy force in all living beings. He developed laboratory experiments that demonstrated muscle contraction when electricity was applied to the spinal cord via metallic wires. His experiments were conducted using the latest equipment available to generate sparks of electricity by means of friction. Galvani demonstrated the flow of direct current (i.e., continuously flowing current, versus alternating current, which flows first in one direction and then back in the other direction). Galvani discovered what is now called the *current of injury,* the electrical current that flows from any injured tissue (Becker, 1990).

By the mid-1800s, Emil DuBois Reymond discovered that nerve impulses could be detected electrically (Becker, 1990). It was Herman von Helmholz who measured the speed of the nerve impulse and determined that it was much slower than an electrical impulse flowing through wire. He concluded that the nerve impulse therefore could not represent the actual passage of electrical particles (Becker, 1990). Julius Bernstein proposed that the conduction of the nerve impulse was actually a chemical reaction. He believed that ions (electrically charged particles) inside the nerve cell contained different electrical charges than the fluid outside the cell. This difference resulted in the electrical potential of the cell membrane (i.e., an electrical difference from the surrounding fluid). Fig. 18-2 demonstrates the difference in potential that Bernstein postulated. The nerve impulse was due to a breakdown in the potential (i.e., the movement of the ions across the cell membrane). This hypothesis is still considered essentially correct for all cells of the body (Becker, 1990).

In the 1920s, physiologist Otto Loewi proved that the transmission of the nerve impulse across the synaptic gap, the space between the nerve and the muscle tissue, is also chemical in nature. This view of medicine, based upon the chemical-mechanistic model, has since dominated medicine, leading to the emphasis on drug-based cures. Otto Loewi's work on nerve impulses and their chemical transmission and his subsequent Nobel Prize led to the established belief that only high-voltage currents can have any effect on the body and that weaker electrical charges can have no impact. Because magnetically sensitive particles were known to exist within the body, magnetic fields were thought to have no effect. The body's inherent electrical nature was ignored as science and medicine focused on chemical reactions (Becker, 1990). In spite of this tendency, an impressive amount of scientific literature has come about in the last 20 years that discredits this singular approach.

Literature Review

A short review of the electrochemical foundation of the cell is helpful to understand the action of the magnetic field on tissue and cellular fluids. Regardless of the action or interaction, all cellular events begin with the organization and behavior of atoms and molecules. All matter contains one or more of approximately 90 different types of elements, materials that cannot be decomposed into a substance with a different property. The special properties of elements such as potassium, calcium, magnesium, phosphorus, and chlorine are the basis of action in pulsed electromagnetic therapy, wherein atoms, which are the smallest identifiable component of the element, take on negative or positive charges, becoming ionized. An isolated atom has a net electrical charge of zero (i.e., an equal number of electrons [negatively charged], and protons [positively charged]). Through various chemical and electrical interactions the element can lose or gain an electron and become an ion, an element with a positive or negative charge. Compounds, a mixture of two or more elements, can also become ionized. For example, a sodium (Na) atom has 11 protons and 11 electrons. If it loses one electron, it becomes a positively charged sodium ion, Na^+. A chlorine atom has 17 protons and 17 electrons. It can gain another electron, becoming a negatively charged chloride ion (Cl^-).

Ionized atoms can be affected by the charged fields of the magnet. A sequence of events must occur for an electrochemical transfer. These events begin with some of the same characteristics that affect any electrical circuit. The movement of electrons governs all cellular reactions, allowing molecules to zip open and closed so that vital tasks can be performed at their surface. (Box 18-1 outlines electrochemical concepts that are relevant to the scientific studies discussed later in the chapter.)

A magnet is a convenient method to produce an electromotive force (EMF). In fact, most of the electric power that serves our homes and businesses is made in this manner. A magnet in motion around a conductor creates a dif-

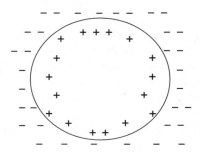

Fig. 18-2 Simplified diagram of a cell with a positive potential in the interior and a negative potential in the exterior.

ference in potential. Conversely a conductor in motion around a magnet also creates a difference in potential. If the conductor (or the magnet) moves back and forth, the flow of electrons reverses or alternates. This type of current is called *alternating current*, or *AC*.

Another convenient method to generate an electromotive force is by means of a battery, a chemical action called *electrochemistry*. A solution called the *electrolyte* interacts with copper and zinc to transfer electrons from the zinc electrode, which gives up positive ions, to the copper electrode, which gives up electrons. This leaves the zinc with a surplus of electrons and a net negative charge. The copper is left with a surplus of protons and a net positive charge. The difference in electron potential always flows from the zinc electrode to the copper electrode in a direct current configuration. This is called *direct current*, or *DC*.

BOX 18-1

$\mathcal{C}$ELLULAR $\mathcal{E}$LECTROCHEMICAL $\mathcal{C}$ONCEPTS

1. Electrons move only if a difference of electrical potential, or voltage, exists. Voltage and electric potential are also known as *electromotive force*. A potential exists to move electrons from one place to another if a difference exists between the two charges. A conductor with a higher voltage at one point and a lower voltage at another point results in the movement of electrons until both points are equal in voltage. The movement of electrons represents the potential to do work, binding atoms or compounds together or breaking them apart.

2. Electrons are thought to flow from a negative charge to a less negative, or positive, charge in the attempt to equalize the difference of potential. Thus a negatively charged chloride ion is attracted to a positively charged sodium ion, forming the compound NaCl with a net neutral electrical charge. (Because no one has actually seen a negative charge move, the question of whether the electron [the negative charge] or the hole [which is considered to be the absence of a negative charge, a positive charge] moves is controversial. The point is, a charge is in motion.)

3. In the cell the flow of the electrical charge is accomplished by ions, and in the electrical circuit the flow is accomplished by electrons. The cellular flow is done by ions because the water and ionic solutions found in the cell are poor electrical conductors. By contrast a good electrical circuit uses a conductor that has a minimum of resistance.

Friction is another common method of developing an electrical potential. Walking across a wool rug in the winter and touching a door knob is a way to demonstrate the effects of friction. The difference in potential between you and the door knob is caused by a buildup of electrons on your body. The electrons move from your hand to the door knob in an effort to neutralize the differences. Light, heat, and pressure can also be used to develop an electric potential.

If the conductor (like a piece of copper wire) is a closed loop, with one end connected to the negative electrode and one end to the positive electrode, the electrons will flow from the most negative end to the most positive end. If a light bulb (or an ionized compound in a cell) is connected in this circuit, the bulb will light, or the compound will be affected according to the aforementioned electrochemical concepts. In the case of static magnets, the magnetic field is stationary and the conductor (the blood flowing in the vessel) is in motion. The magnetic field of the static magnet acts to separate the ionized material (Fig. 18-3), but it lacks the ability to move the ions from one side of the vessel to the other. Pulsing electromagnetic field therapy overcomes this deficiency, affecting the ions continuously as it pulses on and off, affecting any conductor, whether moving, such as blood in motion, or stationary, such as an ionized compound in tissue. Fig. 18-3 depicts how this might appear in the blood vessel.

Static Magnets: Bars, Beads, and Strips

A limited number of articles describe the physics and physiology of applying static magnets to the body and are reviewed here. The studies that are available look not at unipolar magnets but at bipolar magnets. Most revert to Faraday's law as the initiation of effect. This law states that the voltage induced in a conductor is directly proportional to the rate (or speed) at which the conductor cuts the magnetic lines of force. This law is most clearly seen when generating AC. If the conductor alternates back and forth more quickly, the magnetic lines of force are cut faster and more electric current is induced. In the body the electrical conductor is considered to be the blood flowing through the vessel or capillary. If the vessel or capillary is perpendicular to the magnetic lines of force, the magnet forces the separation of charged ions and produces a voltage in the blood. Zablotsky (1989) describes it as follows: "The deflection of these charges is proportional to the field strength (of the magnetic field), the velocity of the charged particles, and the angle between the direction of the charge and the magnetic field vector. It must be emphasized that these principles of physics hold true for steady magnetic fields" (Zablotsky, 1989).

According to Faraday's law and the Hall effect, the stationary magnetic field, if oriented perpendicular to the blood vessel, can affect the flow of blood:

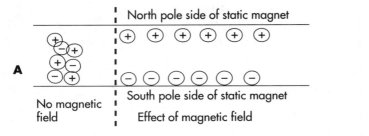

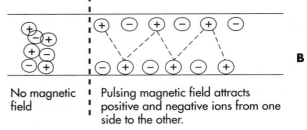

Fig. 18-3   A, Magnetic field of static magnet acts to separate ionized material. **B,** Pulsing electromagnetic field action on blood vessel.

The electrically charged ions in the blood will be deflected by the magnetic pole encountered. For example, NaCl normally circulates through the blood with zero net charge. As the ions encounter a magnetic field, how they react will depend upon the magnetic pole encountered. If a South Pole is first, with its characteristic positive charge, it will deflect the Na$^+$, but attract the Cl$^-$. As the ions separate from each other there is a slight liberation of heat—an electromotive force (EMF). If the next pole encountered is a North Pole with its negative charge, the Cl$^-$ will be repelled while the Na$^+$ will be attracted to it. When a series of alternating North-South poles is established over a blood vessel, the positive and the negative ions will travel a dual sinusoidal path within the vessel (as seen in Fig. 18-3) similar to the action of the pulsing magnetic field. Between the peaks of these waves, small, circulating eddy currents form. Just as one sees at the sides of a river, eddy currents act to "push" the banks outward, effectively widening the river. The combination of (1) the EMF, (2) the altered ionic flow pattern, and (3) the whirling eddy currents acts to dilate the vessels, allowing a greater volume of blood to flow into the area (Zablotsky, 1989).

Baerman (1989) discusses the importance of using circular and radial pole patterns when using static magnetic pads for therapy. When various electromagnetic theories are applied to blood and tissue, some evidence suggests that the blood vessels affected in therapy must be perpendicular, rather than parallel, to the magnetic field. This is a result of Faraday's law, which states that the strength of the EMF is greater if the angle at which the conductor (the electrolyte in the blood vessel) cuts the magnetic field is greater. This law holds true because, as the conductor moves at right angles to the magnetic lines of force, it will cut a maximum number of lines of force per second, producing a maximum EMF.

The practitioner applying bipolar magnetic material or static magnets must know the location of the blood vessels and the direction of the magnetic field on the magnetized pads for maximal action. To avoid static-electric effect (see Fig. 18-3), the blood vessels should cross the alternating magnetic fields at an angle as close to 90 degrees as possible, for maximal action.

The manufacturers of bipolar "liner" pads do not always mark the pads to indicate the direction of the magnetized

fields, making optimal placement difficult. However, practitioners can easily determine the direction of the field by sprinkling iron filings on the pad. The filings will line up according to the direction of the magnetized pattern on the pad. The practitioner may then mark the pad, positioning the blood vessel perpendicular to the magnetic lines of force for optimal effect.

If the manufacturers have marked their materials with the direction of the magnetic field, the placement of the magnetic pad cannot always be certain relative to the direction of blood vessels, because even though the basic placement of major vessels is known, individual variation still occurs. To overcome this difficulty, some manufacturers have devised a radial or checkerboard pattern for the N/S placement so that the blood vessel will always cross the magnetized material at an angle greater than 0 degrees. Fig. 18-4 demonstrates the blood vessel traversing N and S material in an alternating circular pattern.

Although not scientifically proven, the theory is logically consistent: When static magnets are used, the most desirable magnetization pattern for maximal effect and ease of use is bipolar and circular, a pattern that alternates north and south material and places the alternating material in a radial pattern. The blood vessel, with its electrolyte mixture, traverses the alternating north and south poles. This results in moving the blood through an alternating magnetic field. As the electrolyte moves through the alternating north and south field, the ions separate as they are attracted to the opposite charge, then move to the opposite wall and back again.

In an attempt to demonstrate whether static magnets influence the circulation of blood, a 5% solution of NaCl was exposed to a static magnetic field (Pratt, 1989). The 5% saline solution was chosen instead of blood because of the complication of dealing directly with blood products. A statistically significant effect was found ($p < 0.001$) on the flow of the saline solution when the capillary transporting the fluid was exposed to a magnetic pad. A reservoir of distilled water showed no effect from the magnetic pad.

Another study points to clinical results obtained in using a static bipolar magnetic pad. In one study of eight healthy horses, a cross-over trial demonstrated an increase in blood flow of the equine third metacarpus (Kobluk,

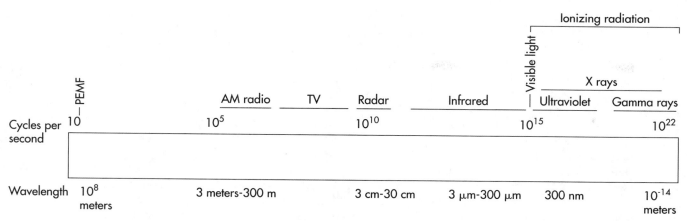

Fig. 18-4 Electromagnetic spectrum.

1994). A linear, bipolar magnetic pad (7.75″ × 4.5″) was applied to the dorsal aspect of 16 clinically normal limbs for 48 hours. A nuclear scintigraphy scan taken in three different phases demonstrated an increased uptake in the limbs that received magnetic therapy, evidenced by the accumulation of ^{99m}Tc-methylene diphosphonate, a bone-seeking pharmaceutical substance injected into the horse. Further studies are indicated on the effect of magnetic therapy in injuries such as soft tissue trauma, inflammation, periostitis, and fracture to duplicate successful studies using pulsing magnetic fields.

A double-blind test compared a magnetized foil versus a sham foil on 100 humans with secondary myotendofasciopathies (Martin, no date). The test population was divided into three groups, one with vertebral local lumbar pain syndrome, one with cervical pain syndrome, and one with periarthritis humeroscapularis. Permanent use of the foil was required. The trial was concluded after 14 days, at which time 43 patients demonstrated unchanged subjective pain sensation, 48 reported reduced pain, and 9 reported increased pain. The study also reported improvement in restricted movement and reduced use of medicines.

A clinical study to determine the relative efficacy of the different static magnet types would be useful (e.g., comparison of bar magnets and bipolar magnets, magnetic strips in the parallel design and strips using the concentric circle and checkerboard designs). Conceivably, one type of magnet might work better on a specific injury, and individual variations among animals are possible as well.

Pulsed Electromagnetic Fields

A number of international societies are devoted to the study of electricity and magnetism in biology and medicine, leading to a growing body of literature concerning the biologic and clinical effects of low frequency, nonionizing forms of energy. Clinical results are reported in nonunion fractures (Bassett, Pawluk, Pilla, 1974), avascu-

lar necrosis of the hip (Aaron, 1989; Bassett, 1989), Perthes' disease (Harrison, Bassett, 1984), lumbar fusions (Mooney, 1990), persistent rotator cuff tendinitis (Binder, 1984), and osteoarthritis (Trock and others, 1993). Three societies investigate and publish results from their studies using pulsed electromagnetic fields (PEMF). PEMF has been used for over a decade in the treatment of delayed union fractures. More than 200,000 human patients have been treated safely over a 17-year period; no toxic effects have been reported.

With such a large number of studies, most questions about PEMF can be addressed. Some studies review very high frequencies and very high depositions of magnetic energy, energy densities much higher than those used in PEMF therapy. For example, microwave therapy is used to produce deep heating of localized areas in the treatment of cancer. This method, termed *diathermy*, has been used as an adjuvant to ionizing radiation therapy and as a primary therapy for relatively heat-sensitive neoplasms (Chou, Luk, 1990). Whole body hyperthermia is used for extensive cancer. The energy output of a diathermy system has vastly different characteristics from that of a PEMF system, which causes no thermal effect in tissue. The common frequencies used in diathermy are 2450, 915, and 433 MHz (millions of cycles per second), whereas PEMF systems range from 1 to 60 Hz (60 cycles per second). The shorter wavelengths used in diathermy allow the energy to be directly focused into the cancer site, because shorter wavelengths are absorbed by the body. The longer wavelengths of 1 to 60 Hz pass through the body. The literature reports a wide range of devices using different frequencies, with a wide range of effect.

Most of the literature reviewed here concentrates on techniques that are in wide veterinary use, the low-frequency devices. The electric and magnetic properties of tissue are outlined, and a review of studies describing the working mechanisms of PEMF forms the basis for an understanding of the results obtained in veterinary therapy.

Many researchers have conducted studies that provide information about the electric and magnetic properties of tissue. These studies are relevant because of the growing use of therapies in which tissue interacts with magnetic fields, such as hyperthermia, impedance pneumography, impedance plethysmography, electrical impedance tomography, and pulsed magnetic therapy to aid tissue and bone healing. Although the electric properties of the cell have been known for decades, the relatively recent discovery of magnetite crystals in the human brain points to the complex relationship between electricity and magnetic energy in the body (Herman, 1992). Magnetite, a microscopic biologic bar magnet, has already been identified in nonhuman subjects such as honey bees, pigeons, whales, and bacteria. Primitive bacteria were thought to have benefited from internal magnets that helped them find nutrient-rich mud. This improved nutrition enabled the bacteria to evolve into more complex life forms, eventually into higher plant, animal, and human forms. A study of dissected brain samples produced crystals one-millionth of an inch wide and ten-millionths of an inch long that could be moved about by magnetic fields only slightly stronger than the Earth's natural field. Researchers found that the average human brain contained approximately one-millionth of an ounce.

Although the discovery of magnetite in the human brain is recent, the electric and electromagnetic qualities of human cells have been analyzed and measured for decades (Fricke, 1925; Hüber, 1910; Oncley, 1943). After Hüber measured the electric impedance of red blood cell suspensions as they were subjected to frequencies of up to 10 MHz, he concluded that red blood cells are surrounded by a poorly conducting membrane and that they contain cytoplasm of low resistivity. He also found that their impedance decreased with increasing frequency (Hüber, 1910). Later studies established values for the ultra-thin membrane at 3.3 nm (Fricke, 1925). In 1954, Linus C. Pauling received the Nobel Prize in chemistry after he discovered that hemoglobin has magnetic properties. Iron is a good carrier of energy because it can be magnetized, which allows it to perform an important role in the cell (Hanneman, 1990). Charman (1990, 1991) thoroughly summarized research findings and theories regarding the role of endogenous bioelectric currents in tissue growth, adaptive remodeling, and tissue healing and the effects of different forms of externally applied currents and fields on biologic activity. He reviews the theory that cell systems might recognize each other and communicate through a range of specific frequencies, with illness and injury resulting in unresponsiveness.

Efforts are ongoing to explain electric and magnetic field cellular effects. These theories attempt to model functions at the cellular and subcellular level. Living systems are surrounded by relatively high levels of random thermal energy, and the challenge for any theory is to explain the way these systems can detect weak fields, which deposit tiny amounts of energy. Investigators focus on finding the site where electrical energy can be transformed into a biochemical reaction. Cell physiologists believe that the cell membrane or its surrounding biologic structure provides the needed tools for this conversion. Each individual cell has an electric charge at its nucleus, various charged particles within the cell, and electric potentials at the inside and outside layer of the cell membrane. The dielectric and electric conduction properties of biologic materials vary, depending on the relative permittivity (the ease with which a magnetic field penetrates), conductivity (the ease with which an electrical charge is passed) of the material, and frequency (the pulse rate). Except for magnetite, which is known to be associated with navigation and orientation abilities of some bacteria, insects, and mammals (including humans), most biologic tissues have a permittivity level close to that of air.

Mammals have a total water content of approximately 70%, and the majority of this water is influenced by dissolved ionic salts (Pilla, 1988). The influence of the ion in the regulation of cell structure and function has widespread acceptance. The action of the ion at the cell surface, which is electrically charged, demonstrates the cell's use of a voltage-dependent process. In his excellent review of the literature, Pilla (1988) reviews the role of electrochemistry in the electromagnetic modulation of tissue. In 1974 he proposed a theory that explained the electric effects on tissues and cells based on charges at the interfaces of the cell membrane, the intracellular fluid, and the extracellular fluid. Electric fields at these sites can be altered by a few millivolts, resulting in changes in adsorbed or bound species, culminating in an electrochemical information transfer. Pilla demonstrated that DC field changes of 0.01 to 100 μV/cm resulted in changes in red blood cell morphology and pointed to the potential action of calcium ions in this change. This theory was confirmed when the addition of calcium alone to these cells caused similar changes.

Blank (1988) reviews the ability of an ionic flux to proceed in a direction opposite to that predicted on the basis of electrochemical potentials, the primary attribute of the ion pump. The ionic channel opens in response to a stimulus that results in a shifting of charge from a high–charge density region to a low–charge density region. The changes result in a reversed local concentration gradient driving ions through the open channel and a reduced gradient across the channel. These types of processes could create the local gradients needed to lead to ion pumping. The steady state ionic concentrations of sodium and potassium normally control the activity of the ion pump. Enhanced ion transport can be seen as these concentrations increase at specific frequencies.

This model is fully developed by the Surface Compartment Model (SCM) theory, which considers the many membrane processes involved in ion transport and accounts for the observed effects of oscillating electric fields on biologic tissue (Blank, Findl, 1987). In the SCM the cell interior, inside surface, membrane, outside surface, and exterior are each defined as compartments with specific properties. Channel functions are modeled as a voltage-dependent permeability, and a set of independent differential equations is then derived to describe the system. Gating, or opening, of the channel can result from any event that leads to changes in surface charge. Gating may result from binding of ligands or enzymatic reactions. This depolarization shifts negative charges to the inside of the cell membrane. An effect of the charge shift is that concentrations of bound counter ions in the channel can be changed in such a way that a reversed local concentration gradient is produced, promoting ion transport in the opposite direction (i.e., ion pumping). Rapid electric changes result in temporary electrochemical imbalances and transient fluxes. If a charged surface is changed by an imposed electromagnetic field or the binding of charged species, the ions reequilibrate. In a membrane system the two charged surfaces can be equilibrated by the opening of an ion channel that connects the two surfaces. Much more is now known about the electrostatic potentials and ion adsorption at membrane-solution interfaces (Zon, Tien, 1988).

After a review of published data in 40 studies, Cadossi and others (1988) concluded that PEMF acts by interfering with membrane processes that govern an active substance and its receptor. They suggested that the cell membrane is a likely target. PEMF appears capable of triggering an increase in the Ca^{2+} across the cell membrane and to increase the amount of free intracellular Ca^{2+}. An increase in intracellular Ca^{2+} seems to be a metabolic signal for the cell to progress to the DNA synthesis phase of the cell cycle (Poenie, 1985). The Genova group investigators studied the effect of PEMF on normal human lymphocytes. The computerized model they developed predicted that PEMF exposure increased the availability of free Ca^{2+} near the membrane and the Ca^{2+} influx via existing channels. A study conducted by Cadossi and others (1988) found that a PEMF-exposed culture of activated lymphocytes significantly increased in activity compared with controls. The increase was observed in both DNA synthesis and mitotic index. It not only suggested an increased number of activated lymphocytes but also favored the entry into the S phase, where DNA synthesis takes place. In another study of PEMF stimulation, brain slices demonstrated an optimal release of calcium ions when stimulated by PEMF at 16 Hz (Adey, 1981).

This calcium release is thought to induce cellular field effects on the biochemistry and activity of immune cells and the immune system (Walleczek, 1992). Walleczek's review argues that considerable evidence supports the existence of PEMF effects in immune system cells, suggesting that the immune system can be influenced by PEMFs too weak in intensity to act through any thermal mechanism. This responsiveness is similar to that documented

for cells and tissues of the neuroendocrine and musculoskeletal system, indicating that PEMF sensitivity might be a general property of biologic systems.

Teneforde (1991) also concludes that changes in the inner membrane surface in response to electrochemical events at the surface of the cell can influence the calcium ions and cyclic nucleotides that regulate DNA synthesis and control cellular metabolism. Once again, the details of these events remain to be specified by careful experimentation, but the cell membrane is strongly implicated as the site of field transduction and signal amplification. Experimental evidence with in vitro cell and organ cultures indicates that extremely-low-frequency (ELF*) currents lead to structural and functional alterations in the cell membrane (Teneforde, 1991). Teneforde's study reports on ELF effects such as altered Ca^{2+} binding at the outer membrane surface and suppression of T-lymphocyte cytotoxicity. Certain combinations of static magnets, comparable in strength to the earth's geomagnetic field, and a pulsing EMF can produce resonance interactions that influence ion movements through membrane channels. This combination has produced alterations in (1) the rate of calcium ion release from the surfaces of cells in brain tissue, (2) calcium-dependent diatom mobility, and (3) calcium ion uptake by human lymphocytes (Blackman, Benane, Rabinowitz, 1985; Liboff and others, 1987; Smith, McLeod, Liboff, 1987).

Gradients across the cell wall are stimulated by PEMF, increasing the channel pumping action. This increase in activity results in cells working together when an injury occurs to reestablish normal cellular function. Becker (1961) measured current over injured salamander limbs, which normally measured − 10 mV, over a period of 20 days as the limb was regenerating (Becker, 1961). When amputated, the stump measured +20 mV, after 15 days it peaked at − 30 mV, and after approximately 20 days, it returned to its normal potential of − 10 mV. He concluded that the neuroepidermal junction is the source of the negative DC current that stimulates regeneration. A study conducted by G. Marsh and H. Beam (cited by Becker, 1961) used the planarium (flatworm) to demonstrate that various levels of current could cause a head to regenerate at the rear and a tail to regenerate at the head. These researchers were convinced that the gradation of electrical charge from front to back controlled the growth. The existence of DC currents is revealed in another study by Barker, Jaffe, and Vanable (1982), which measured voltages across glabrous regions of cavy skin from 30 to 100 mV, inside positive. When an incision is made through the glabrous epidermis at a bald spot of the guinea pig, a microampere flows through each millimeter of the cut's edge. The wound currents generate voltages of about 100 to 200 mV/mm near the cut. This paper references stud-

---

*ELF denotes pulse rates between 0 and 100 cycles per second.

ies that report the active electric properties of adult mammalian skin. Illingworth and Barker (1980) found that 10 to 30 $\mu A/cm^2$ leaks out of the stumps of amputated human finger tips when the finger tips are immersed in saline.

DC currents in the body produce magnetic fields that have been measured by a sensitive magnetic detector called the SQUID (super conducting quantum interference device). The body's fields are produced by either naturally occurring electric currents in the body or ferromagnetic particles. A common example of these naturally occurring currents is seen in the EEG (electroencephalogram) and the ECG (electrocardiogram). The same currents that produce the ECG and the EEG also produce varying magnetic fields. DC magnetic fields are also found in other parts of the body, including the abdomen, upper arm, chest, and eyes. These fields were measured by Cohen and others (1980) with a SQUID detector, which documented a field of 0.1 $\mu G/cm$ over the head and limbs. The field over the head is produced mainly by hair follicles of the scalp; the field over the limbs is associated with electrical sources of the muscles. The field over the forearm appeared spontaneously; when absent, it could be evoked by mild twisting or rubbing. A number of experiments and observations were conducted, including manipulation of the human body and injections of electrolyte solution into muscle tissue, to assess the role of polarized membranes in producing DC magnetic fields. The results suggest that the generation of this steady current is caused by a non-closed, polarized layer across an elongated semipermeable membrane such as a muscle fiber, with the polarization caused by a gradient of extracellular K^+ along the membrane (Cohen and others, 1980). Bassett (1989) summarized PEMF mechanisms of action in a table depicting first order (cell and tissue), second order (subcellular), and third order (biophysical) mechanisms, supported by applicable citations. He stressed the importance of specifying the multiple physical attributes that contribute to the effectiveness of PEMF, including amplitude, frequency, uniformity, timing, and length of exposure. This approach requires an integrated, interdisciplinary approach that includes physics, biology, engineering, and biochemistry in study designs, execution, and analysis.

The aforementioned studies aid in an understanding of the mechanisms at work in these clinical studies of animals and humans. Bassett (1978) studied the use of PEMF in surgically resistant pseudarthroses and nonunion fractures in children and adults. He reported a success rate of 85% in more than 100 patients. Many of the patients in his study were candidates for amputation. Preliminary applications in fresh fractures in humans indicate a 50% reduction in disability time. Bassett's clinical results with human subjects were matched in veterinary populations. For example, with PEMF therapy, defects in rat femurs were repaired more rapidly, with highly organized, mechanically sound osseous tissue. Secondly, the profound disuse osteoporosis that usually follows myec-

tomy, tenotomy, and cast immobilization of the rat hind limb is completely or largely ameliorated. Third, radial osteomies in mature rats heal at a faster rate and reach the mechanical values of 4-week controls in 2 weeks. Fourth, after extraction of canine premolars, the extraction sockets fill with bone more rapidly. Fifth, race horses with traumatic periostitis (bucked shin) are symptom free after 3 weeks of treatment and exhibit healing of fractures of the coffin bone. These results occurred in bone only in the presence of fields with highly specific pulse characteristics, including narrow amplitudes and pulse widths (Bassett, 1978).

A later study by Bassett, Valdes, and Hernandez (1982) assayed different PEMFs and their effects on the mechanical and histologic repair properties of an osteotomy of the radius of the rat. A magnetic pulse that produced an increase (above the control level) in initial load by a factor of 2.4 was characterized by more extensive calcification of fibrocartilage and its replacement by fibrous bone at this early stage in fracture healing. The primary action of the PEMF is to increase early mechanical stability by improving the tempo of maturation, not the volume of callus. This study set the standard for pulse characteristics used in most human PEMF systems.

Sisken (1988) summarizes much of the work that examines the effects of PEMF on nerve regeneration. This study is comprehensive, covering both in vitro and in vivo studies. She supports the findings of Bray, Thomas, and Shaw (1978), who found that low extracellular calcium induced the formation of growth cones along the length of cultured sensory neurons. Work in the area of neural regeneration compares values of the electric field, energy density, and time of stimulation with varying results. Sisken was able to draw parallels between the work done on DC current stimulation and PEMFs because both modalities are in the same effective dosage levels (3 to 10 coulombs) on a time-exposure basis.

PEMFs affected the rate and quality of neural regeneration in a study of 60 rats undergoing high bilateral transection of the sciatic nerve (Ito, Bassett, 1983). After 2 weeks of PEMF or control conditions, the rats were euthanized and examined. Regenerating axons had penetrated the distal stump nearly twice as far in the PEMF-exposed rats as in the controls. Motor function returned earlier in the PEMF subjects and to significantly higher load levels than in controls. Both histologic and functional data indicated that PEMFs improve the rate and quality of peripheral nerve regeneration in the severed rat sciatic nerve by a factor of approximately 2.

Warnke (1980) investigated the physiologic effects of PEMFs having a specific pulse form, pulse frequency, and amplitude on humans. He experimented with 50 Hz at a magnetic field range of 6 to 30 gauss. Results were measured via thermography and showed dilation of large and small blood vessels. The blood vessels of the hands and arms dilated in many cases even when the magnetic field was applied only to the back of the head, with a measurable increase taking place within 3 minutes. Warnke reported increased circulation in the body originating at the blood vessels. About 30% of his subjects showed no thermographic effect from PEMF. He repeated the experiments with chicken embryos, concluding the effect is not limited to humans.

Warnke also documented increased oxygen partial pressure in the tissue. The highest measured and reproducible oxygen value for a given subject (a 25-year-old athlete in good health) after a 10-minute exposure to the PEMF (compared with a value recorded without the PEMF) was more than 1000%. Using the Clark electrode, which measures through the skin of the subject, the average value increase for 58 experiments was about 200%. No effect was found in about 20% of the subjects. The effect remained for an individually specific time after the field was turned off. Warnke found the most effective pulse rate for increase in O_2 to be 21 Hz. Warnke's results were supported by a research report that demonstrated increased blood flow of 200% to 400% when stimulated with PEMF at a frequency between 12 and 20 Hz, with no statistically significant increase in heart rate or blood pressure (Lau, no date). Warnke also studied treatment of 21 patients with diabetic neuropathy, including results of nerve conduction studies at the end of treatment and 2 months later. Patients rated their symptoms before and after the treatment series and at the follow-up session 2 months later. The study showed significant changes of all symptoms in patients receiving magnetic field treatment, whereas members of the control group that did not receive the treatment reported no significant changes in pain.

An analysis of the biophysical, physiologic, and clinical data pertaining to the use of electricity and electromagnetic fields to control wound healing minimizes much of the prevailing confusion (Lee, Canady, Doong, 1993). This study places special emphasis on the role of cells in wound repair. The paper concludes that when the healing process is delayed or arrested, therapeutic intervention can be successful in accelerating the healing process.

A large number of studies have been published demonstrating the effectiveness of PEMF. Those cited here are particularly helpful because many contain excellent summaries of work that has already been done. They provide a starting point for a study of PEMF.

Traditional Medical Theory

Permanent magnets have been used medically for thousands of years in many cultures. Egyptian documents in hieroglyphic and cuneiform script demonstrate that magnets were a valuable and respected method for treating patients. Drawings on walls and sculptures in temples attest to its use, and ancient writers and poets refer to this type of therapy. Magnets were placed directly on the area of injury to eliminate symptoms. In addition, magnet therapy was thought to influence the magnetic current in the system, as when Cleopatra placed a magnet on her forehead to preserve her beauty. Mesmer used magnets to treat malaise, depression, and anxiety. The earliest known use of magnetic therapy occurred in China, where use of magnets was combined with acupuncture medicine. Magnets served as another method of stimulating acupuncture points. Perhaps the first use was in attaching the magnets to ferrous needles already inserted in the point (Schoen, 1994).

More recent theories recommend the placement of specific poles (north or south) on the injury. Proponents believe that the north pole corresponds to the Earth's north pole, negative ionization, and the negative pole (cathode) of a DC circuit. Conversely the south pole corresponds to the Earth's south pole, positive ionization, and the positive pole (anode) of a DC circuit (Philpott, 1990). Many magnet therapists now recommend using the north pole to heal injuries and normalize and calm the system.

Many studies demonstrate differences in the way tissue reacts to DC current. Patel and Poo (1981) report that extracellularly applied steady electric fields of 0.1 to 10 V/cm were found to have marked effects on neurite growth. Neurites facing the cathode showed accelerated growth, whereas those facing the anode showed reduced growth. Neurites growing perpendicular to the field axis were prompted to curve toward the cathode. Some practitioners report that the south pole encourages strength and life in all living systems, including bacteria and viruses, with the conclusion that the south pole should never be used (Hannemann, 1990). However, manufacturers of bipolar magnetic strips and pads place layers of north and south material side by side, with apparent disregard for this caution. There is a lack of widespread agreement regarding this matter.

A number of books espouse static magnetic therapy for a variety of illnesses. The human protocols offered represent years of clinical experimentation by individual practitioners, which accounts for variations in placement, gauss strength, and duration of exposure needed for individual relief. Because no risk has been associated with use of magnets and the cost of purchasing the materials is small, many practitioners have been willing to try this modality. Several authors fail to suggest gauss rates, which could result in a wide range of outcomes. Most experts suggest leaving the magnet in place until the condition resolves or moving the magnet to another area if it fails in one spot.

Use of magnets in acupuncture therapy has become more popular. Use of magnetic ceramic beads to stimulate acupuncture points instead of needles offers several benefits. Many patients cannot tolerate needles, and when the bead is glued or taped to the point, the point can be stimulated over a longer period for sustained action. The beads vary in strength from 500 to 1500 gauss and are used to treat either *ah shi* points or traditional acupuncture points (Schoen, 1994).

Although regularly used in equine therapy since the 1970s, pulsed electromagnetic devices are a recent addition in veterinary therapy. European and Australian manufacturers marketed the first commercial devices, which were used on show horses and racehorses. Compared with newer models, the old equipment was bulky and complicated to use. It required an electrical outlet to operate the pulse generator. The pulse generator would be placed on the floor and was connected to pads by long cables. The pads housed coils that were placed over the area of injury or soreness. The coils generated the magnetic field as they were pulsed with current. Wide acceptance among trainers and owners of performance-horse owners ensued as they realized the benefits of using this type of therapy for 30 to 60 minutes each day. The cost of the early devices limited their use to facilities with large numbers of horses or those with expensive horses. PEMF was not widely used on other veterinary patients because of the cost and the fact that the equipment had been designed primarily for equine patients.

Changes in technology have produced lighter, less expensive versions of this equipment, making this therapy more practical for a wider range of patients. Modern versions are battery powered and have coils that cover the majority of areas requiring therapy. A therapy session can be completed in 30 minutes. In addition, packages have been developed to make the equipment available for use on dogs and other small animals. These improvements, coupled with increasing clinical studies of PEMF, have encouraged veterinarians to apply this therapy to a wider range of conditions on a more diverse group of patients.

Controversial Issues

Magnetic therapy has been controversial since the discovery of natural magnets. Magnetic lines of force cannot be seen, so their effects have been both refuted and inflated. Paracelsus called the force *Mumia.* Mesmer called it *animal magnetism.* The German scholar Burdach termed the process *neurogomy,* meaning "union of nerves." Reichenbach called it the *Od force* (Schiegl, 1987). Although magnetic therapy enjoyed the support of Egyptian pharaohs, its reputation suffered in Western medicine during the 1800s and 1900s, when medicine began to look to science to answer all questions about the body and the healing process. The magnet's wide availability and low cost meant that it was readily available to all socioeconomic groups, without medical supervision. The controversy was fueled by an absence of approval from the medical establishment and the wild claims of some proponents. The dearth of scientific studies slowed the growth of magnetic therapy for many years, and the confusion between static magnets and PEMF has exacerbated this situation. Another closely related concern involves possible negative effects from the south pole of static magnets and electromagnetic fields.

The lack of scientific studies continues to influence use of static magnets. Although static magnets are widely used by millions of people, no double blind studies demonstrate the effectiveness of magnets in the treatment of injury or illness. A handful of studies, however, demonstrate that magnets produce biologic effects. Although a large double blind study using magnets is unlikely to be funded without a commercial interest, a national organization such as the National Institutes for Health would perform a valuable service in providing funds to study simple magnets.

Pulsing magnetic fields have received more interest and attention by researchers. A large body of literature exists on this subject and includes both in vivo and in vitro research. To assist others who wish to reproduce the studies, researchers are now more careful to specify the parameters of the pulsing field, including hertz rate, gauss field, and pulse characteristics. Current research continues to elucidate the mechanism of action and the effects of dosimetry. Biologic interaction appears to be an all-or-nothing response that occurs by way of a threshold mechanism (O'Connor, Bentall, Monahan, 1990). When researchers begin to understand the level of the threshold, dosimetry will become much more specific and precise than the gross blueprints given today. Clinicians, both medical and veterinary, are most interested in physiologic results from PEMF that can be monitored, such as a reduction in edema.

Many clinicians and patients are concerned with the general safety of magnetic fields. The Earth has a natural magnetic field, which varies. It is now measured at approximately 0.5 gauss, but it is popularly thought to be higher in places where inexplicable cures have taken place, such as Sedona, Arizona, and Lourdes, France. The Earth has had a greater gauss field in the past, measured by drilling into ancient volcanoes and analyzing the materials extricated. In addition, some evidence suggests that the magnetic poles have switched place more than once over the many millions of years of Earth's existence. Washnis and Hricak (1993) claimed that the Earth has a negative charge at the surface, a positive charge below the crust, and a positive atmosphere above its surface. The weakened natural magnetic field of the Earth is further reduced by barriers such as steel buildings, cars, and many complex and interacting manmade electrical fields. According to these authors, this phenomenon has led to a barrage of insults to the body's chemical and immune balances. The interaction of magnets and pulsing magnetic therapy systems may stimulate the body to return to its natural state of health (Washnis, Hricak, 1993).

Public concern about the effects of magnetic fields focuses on high-voltage power lines and the electromagnetic energy that can emanate from simple electric wiring and home appliances. The majority of the public has little understanding of the electromagnetic spectrum and the wide range of frequencies that continually bombard the Earth. This energy is transmitted in the form of waves and is systematically depicted in the electromagnetic frequency spectrum (see Fig. 18-4).

As the frequency of the energy wave increases, the wavelength decreases. The shorter wavelengths inherent in high frequencies increase the likelihood of energy being deposited in the body. The greater the frequency, the greater the energy content and the greater its ability to deliver biologic effects. Energy at very high frequencies is termed *ionizing* (i.e., the energy has the capability to break electrons away from their atoms, creating highly reactive ions). Lower frequencies, at approximately 500 nm and greater, do not have the energy required to make these atomic changes and are termed *nonionizing*. Gamma rays and x-rays are known by most people to cause radiation damage. Lower frequencies can be seen as light (in the 10-4 to 10-7) wavelengths. Wavelengths even lower carry radio and television signals to nearly 100% of homes in the United States and many countries around the world.

Significant differences exist between electromagnetic fields produced by PEMF systems, which have been demonstrated to produce therapeutic results, and electromagnetic energies, which have given rise to public concern. Bassett described apparent windows and thresholds influencing the beneficial effects of PEMF (Bassett, 1992). The windows and thresholds result from variances in the pulse that develops the electromagnetic field. Pulses are distinguished by voltage levels (size or amplitude), wave form characteristics (shape), voltage sources (origin), and frequency of pulsing (speed). Voltages produced by electric transmission lines average 345,000 volts, whereas battery-powered PEMF systems operate at only 24 volts, a difference of greater than 10,000 to 1 (Becker, 1990). Standard household electric service operates at 110 to 120 volts, more than a fivefold difference. Another factor is the wave form developed by PEMF systems. Most state-of-the-art PEMF systems generate a specific wave form that produces superior results compared with three other wave forms (Bassett, Valdes, Hernandez, 1982). This wave form is a square shape, and at 15 pulses per second is 20 msec wide. Each "on" pulse is further divided by minute pulses that are on for 250 μsec and off for 33 μsec (Bassett, Valdes, Hernandez, 1982). A third major difference is that newer PEMF systems use direct current, a battery system, as the power source, compared with alternating current, which is found in all aspects of our commercial power grid. Finally the frequencies used by PEMF therapy systems are very low. Higher frequencies, such as those emitted by radar, and microwaves, consisting of short wavelengths that result in energy being deposited into the body, have been a source of concern. The characteristics of these wavelengths vary greatly from those used in PEMF for therapeutic purposes. PEMF therapy generally uses pulse rates of 5 to 30 Hz, resulting in very long wavelengths that pass through the body. A 1-Hz frequency has a wavelength of millions of miles. Human organs and the earth have natural pulsing frequencies that are tuned from 0 to 30 Hz (Becker, 1990; Washnis, Hricak, 1993). PEMF therapies normally occur within these naturally occurring frequencies, which may account for their beneficial effect.

If environmental electromagnetic fields pose a risk to public health, many experts believe it is the chronic nature of these stressors that makes them determinants of human disease; the persistence of these fields in the environment might stress the body, thus reducing the effectiveness of the immune system (Marino, 1988). Conducting studies of exposed versus control subjects has proved difficult. All potential candidates for study have been exposed to a number of energy sources with varying levels of energy density, simply by existing in an environment where communications and electricity are ubiquitous. Selection of control subjects (i.e., subjects who have not been exposed) is therefore problematic.

Many studies have been conducted to determine the potential risks associated with this energy explosion. It is important when reviewing these studies to determine the pulse wave form, frequency, and power source because they often differ from those used in therapeutic PEMF (O'-Connor, Bentall, Monahan, 1990). For example, a study that reported calcium efflux from neonatal chick brains used 50 megahertz (1 megahertz equals one million pulses per second) radio frequency fields, compared with the 15- to 30-Hz field used in therapeutic PEMF. Another study cited changes in central nervous system amines in rats subjected to 60-Hz AC fields (O'Connor, Bentall, Monahan, 1990). Once again, these pulse characteristics are not the same as those used in therapeutic PEMF. Whole body animal studies were conducted that used the microwave frequency of the electromagnetic spectrum; safety levels specified by the American National Standards Institute (ANSI) were derived from studies that reviewed exposure at a range of 300 kHz (thousand hertz) and 300 GHz (billion hertz). The wide variances in pulse frequency, wave forms, and power source used in these studies make it difficult for most veterinary practitioners to evaluate studies of PEMF. Adding to the difficulty is the general lack of training in biophysics among veterinary practitioners.

Media reports of epidemiologic studies based primarily on the exposure of the whole body over extended periods have heightened public concern about the safety of living near or working with electric power lines. These studies have focused on chronic exposure of power line workers and people living near power lines to determine their effect on cancer incidence. A recent statement by the council of the American Physical Society addressed this issue. The American Physical Society is a nonprofit scientific and educational organization devoted to the advancement and diffusion of the knowledge of physics. It is the principal membership organization of physicists in the United States, with over 43,000 members in academia, industry, and government. It concluded, after reviewing over 1000 papers, epidemiologic data, and interviews with experts, that "no consistent, significant link between cancer and power-line fields exists" (Council of the American Physical Society, 1995). Furthermore, the expensive mitigation efforts, lengthy and divisive court proceedings, and general concern caused by these fears has resulted in significant costs—already billions of dollars. According to the Society, "the diversion of these resources to eliminate a threat which has no persuasive scientific basis is disturbing to us. More serious environmental problems are neglected for a lack of funding and public attention, and the burden of cost placed on the American public is incommensurate with the risk, if any" (1995).

Researchers involved with therapeutic PEMF continue to search out the beneficial aspects of this therapy. One study sought to determine the potential benefit of pulsing magnetic fields to cure cancer or ameliorate the clinical situation of patients with tumors. In 1988, 75 patients with tumors were treated with low-frequency (8 Hz and 20 Hz) pulsing magnetic fields (Sauerwein, 1992). Biologic investigations were carried out concomitantly to determine the effect on the tumor mass itself. In addition, when melanoma and squamous cell carcinoma were cultured and treated with pulsing magnetic field, no alterations in cell adherence, spreading, or structure were evident. Permanent cell cultures that remained several months in the magnetic fields showed no effect when compared with controls. These cell lines were also implanted in rats and subsequently treated with pulsing magnetic fields. These preliminary investigations did not show any significant changes. Although no effects on tumor growth, proliferation, or metabolism could be shown, nor were side effects apparent, some patients experienced significant pain relief.

Kraus (1992) also reports that no accelerated growth of a tumor or metastasis has been observed under the influence of PEMF therapy applied according to his method. Instead, he reports examples in which cancerous growth has been inhibited (Kraus, 1992). He surmises that the increased blood supply caused by vascularization of the chronically injured, PEMF-treated tissue leads to an increased absorption of oxygen, which allows the neoplastic cell to differentiate. However, a fatal concentration of hydrogen peroxide and death of the cell result from its incomplete reduction of oxygen.

Controversy regarding the potentially negative effects of magnets and pulsing magnetic therapy may continue until the wide variety of energy associated with environmental magnetic fields is fully understood. At this juncture, little evidence suggests that the energy associated with PEMF therapy either initiates or promotes cancer, but similar conclusions cannot extend to other areas of the electromagnetic spectrum. For example, Adey (1988) concludes that microwave fields may "act synergistically with chemical cancer promoters to disrupt normal intercellular communication through gap junctions, leading to autonomous growth." Additional environmental electromagnetic radiation studies could help clarify the effects of different wave forms, amplitudes, and pulse frequencies and deserve continued support. Long-term follow-up of patients treated continuously for up to 12 years has failed to reveal problems, both in adults treated for femoral head osteonecrosis and in children with congenital pseudarthrosis requiring chronic episodic use of PEMF (Bassett, Schink-Asconi, Lewis, 1989).

New studies elucidate certain aspects of PEMF, but they also stimulate more questions. Most helpful for the veterinarian would be an increased number of in vivo studies investigating a number of different disease conditions. However, the work done to date provides a basis for introducing aspects of this therapy into the practice.

Practical Theory and Applications

Magnetic therapy can be used alone or in conjunction with other modes of therapy, both traditional and alternative. In practice, static magnets and pulsing magnetic fields have usually been used in different ways and for different conditions. Their noninvasive nature and lack of side effects make this simple remedy attractive for a number of conditions.

Anecdotal results provide limited guidance to the veterinarian in using static magnets to treat injuries. Magnets are sometimes used in conjunction with acupuncture, in which the magnet becomes the focal point for extended stimulation when applied directly to the acupuncture point (Schoen, 1994). Schoen (1994) describes use of disk magnets less than 1 cm in diameter applied to the point with sticking plaster. For extended application, the most common dosage is 500 gauss. The Japanese Health and Welfare Ministry presides over the wide use of static magnet therapy in Japan, where a large magnet manufacturer grosses over 1 million dollars annually. Over 10 million magnetic beds and over 30 million magnetic devices are purportedly in use. Considering the extended life expectancy of the Japanese, one might consider that the wide use of magnets plays a part in their health and wellness. The ministry will not approve magnetic devices unless they measure at least 500 gauss because they believe anything less is simply not effective. Experts disagree about the field strength required to cause adaptation, which occurs as a result of the body compensating for the prolonged exposure to static magnetic energy. Static magnets are typically worn for days or weeks. At some point, the magnet ceases to assist in the healing process. To obviate the concern about adaptation, some practitioners recommend applying the magnet for 10- or 20-minute periods at daily intervals until the ache or swelling disappears.

Because of the wide variation in the size of animals treated with magnetic therapy, magnet strength is relevant. The Japanese Ministry of Health makes recommendations for human subjects, as do Philpott (1990) and Davis and Rawls (1993). Magnetic effect in tissue is determined by the size, strength, and composition of the magnet, as described earlier. The larger and heavier the magnet, the deeper the magnetic field penetrates into tissue. If the therapy involves direct application of the magnet to the injured area, large animals such as horses and cows require greater magnetic fields compared with small animals such as cats and dogs. Bipolar magnets and magnetic wraps are not as powerful as simple north/south bar magnets because checkerboard and other bipolar configurations place small concentrations of north and south material next to each other, with one field canceling the other and leading to an overall reduced magnetic effect (Washnis, Hricak, 1993). High-strength applications (up to 12,000 gauss) are discussed by Washnis and Hricak, and super magnets of 1000 to 3000 gauss are reportedly used with success on birds, dogs, cats, rabbits, lions, raptorial birds, goats, elephants, and cattle.

The debate concerning the relative safety and effectiveness of north versus south poles developed because of the negative current of injury that develops soon after an injury occurs. Although initially measuring positive, the site of a broken bone measures negative within 3 hours. Washnis and Hricak (1993) believe that the negative polarity is a more appropriate field to use because it adds to the negative energy produced by the system in an effort to heal the injury. They believe the application of a negative pole mimics the action of the brain when it feeds signals for negative energy to the site of injury. Philpott (1990) supports the use of negative poles when treating injuries and disease conditions. He considers negative energy to be antistressful at all levels and the use of south pole energy to be stressful. Some veterinary practitioners recommend using only the north pole when treating cancer because the south pole is thought to stimulate all types of tissue. Manufacturers of bipolar magnetic products ignore the debate and produce materials with both poles side by side. Philpott reports bipolar fields (exposure to both fields simultaneously) can be antistressful for a brief period but stressful after prolonged exposure. Most anecdotal evidence supports the use of north polarity for best results. Philpott's book (1990) provides a compendium of conditions with suggested strategies for human use. It frequently recommends placing a magnet on the afflicted area until the condition subsides; if no improvement is seen in several days, the magnet should be moved to an area nearer the site of injury.

Most manufacturers predict varying results within varying time frames. The magnets are applied with glue or an adhesive material for the duration of the therapy. The major difficulty when placing magnetic wraps or magnets on dogs, cats, and other small animals is keeping them in place. Manufacturers of the bipolar material have integrated the magnetic material into convenient wraps that are used with equine patients, and magnetic beads come with an accompanying sticky material to help keep them stationary.

Pulsing magnetic therapy has been used primarily on equine patients, with recent advances in technology leading to small, battery-powered equipment packages that are offered at significantly reduced prices from those sold in the 1980s. This has made pulsing magnetic therapy systems available to a wider variety of veterinary patients, including bovine and canine. The same technology with different packaging is used in human orthopedics for nonunion fractures, failed arthrodeses, rotator cuff tendinitis, and a number of other conditions. The equipment is available only by prescription.

Pulsing magnetic field therapy devices have been used extensively in equine sports medicine for musculoskeletal and neurologic conditions (Schoen, 1994.) A blanket containing a number of coils is placed on the horse. If indicated, coils are placed on the legs, hocks, and neck. A pulse generator is connected to a battery pack, and treatment commences, generally for a 30- to 60-minute period. Daily treatment is recommended until the condition subsides. Some devices have been developed strictly for the leg because of the number of leg injuries suffered by sport horses. The most extensive clinical work using PEMF was documented by Focke (1982), who used PEMF to treat a wide variety of equine injuries, including tendon and joint conditions, muscle afflictions, and complex conditions such as navicular disease. Focke usually began therapy using 5 Hz and gradually increased the pulse rate after every four or five treatments. He found periodic treatments were helpful in the case of chronic injuries on older horses. He specified an average of 8 to 10 treatments, 15 minutes daily for acute tendon inflammations, and 12 to 20 treatments for chronic tendon and joint affections. Focke demonstrated that PEMF could be used as a replacement for some drugs, and more recent use of PEMF has been associated with a reduction in irritative procedures such as pin firing and blistering. Its use is adjuvant to antibiotic therapies that may be required for infection. PEMF therapies were ineffective when the patient had been treated with cortisone.

Bull stud facilities have employed PEMF to improve chronic degenerative conditions of the lumbrosacral regions. Sessions lasting 30 minutes are easily included in the daily routine and are well tolerated. PEMF is considered a long-term maintenance therapy for these conditions. It improves the quality of life for the bull, which results in a longer period of production. PEMF has been reported to extend the effects of acupuncture, allowing a longer period of time before the next acupuncture session is needed (Lerch, 1994).

Clinical Indications

Contraindications

Many practitioners discourage use of south pole, bipolar magnets and PEMF on cancerous growths and acute viral and bacterial infections. The use of magnetic products is contraindicated in fresh injuries, pregnant females, and patients using pacemakers or artificial cardiac devices. Rest, ice, compression, and elevation are recommended for the first 48 hours.

Small Animal and Avian

Many musculoskeletal conditions benefit from magnet therapy, including degenerative joint disease, hip dysplasia, rheumatoid arthritis, and vertebral disorders. In addition, PEMF therapy was helpful in treating children with tibial pseudarthrosis who faced amputation after repeated failure to achieve union by surgical means; healing was achieved in 50% of the cases, and functional union in an additional 21% (Bassett, Caulo, Kort, 1980). Injuries causing sprains and lameness, as well as conditions brought about by trauma, benefit from magnetic treatment. Magnetic therapy simplifies treatment of trigger points and muscle injuries that occur in deep tissue. When used in conjunction with acupuncture therapy, magnetic pellets stimulate the acupoint.

PEMF has recently been studied in the treatment of osteoarthritis (Trock and others, 1993). A 1993 report demonstrated improvement of symptoms in 70% to 80% of 861 patients in an uncontrolled observation. Based upon these results, a controlled, double blind study of 27 patients with osteoarthritis, primarily of the knee, was undertaken. Treatment consisted of 18 half-hour periods of exposure over approximately 1 month. Observations were made of six clinical variables at four time points. An average improvement of 23% to 61% occurred in the clinical variables observed with active treatment, whereas 2% to 18% improvement was observed in placebo-treated patients in the control group. No toxicity was observed.

The value of PEMF for the treatment of persistent rotator cuff tendinitis was tested in 29 patients whose symptoms were refractory to steroid injection and other typical measures (Binder and others, 1984). The treated group (15 patients) experienced significant benefit compared with the control group (14 patients) during the study. This double blind crossover study demonstrated that PEMF may be useful in the treatment of severe and persistent rotator cuff and possibly other chronic tendon lesions in small and large animals. A study of 45 athletes with tendon injuries found at the end of treatment that 5 subjects were pain free, 25 had some improvement, and 15 were unchanged. In the case of the 15 unchanged patients, all had been treated with one or more cortisone injections and 12 had to undergo surgery. Of those who demonstrated improvement, 20% were reinjured after the first sporting event and 60% experienced improvement for at least 6 months and were able to achieve relief again after a new PEMF therapy treatment (Hess, Rothaar, 1980).

Equine, Bovine

PEMF has been used in the treatment of degenerative diseases of the support and locomotor system, acute and chronic inflammations of the tendons and tendon sheaths, tendinous fiber lacerations, contusions, chronic disease of the joints, delayed wound healing, and diseases of the back and lumbar regions. Pulsing magnetic therapy simplifies treatment of trigger points and muscle injuries that occur in deep tissue. A simple review of this therapy, which uses both pulsing magnetic fields and magnetized foil wraps, is provided by Jones (1983). Auer, Burch, and Hall (1983) reviewed PEMF literature along with suggested application and treatment times for the equine limb. They reported two cases in which PEMF was used in equine fracture treatment. A 2-year-old thoroughbred colt in race training had multiple cortical stress fractures and dorsal metacarpal disease. After 1 month of PEMF therapy, x-ray examination revealed that the fractures had healed. A 4-year-old quarter horse stallion exhibited lameness of the left hind limb and a swollen fetlock. X-ray examination revealed a fracture of the sesamoid bone. Complete healing occurred after 3 months of PEMF treatment.

Bullock and May (1984) reported a wide range of indications for PEMF therapy, including orthopedics, traumatology, rheumatology, fractures, wounds, burns, degenerative diseases of the apparatus of support and locomotion, coronary and circulatory diseases, and disorders of the neurologic system.

Although use of PEMF therapy immediately after cannon bone osteotomy was not found to improve rates of healing (Bramlage, Weisbrode, Spurlock, 1984), Bassett (1978) reported a 50% reduction in disability time in fresh human fractures. Collier and Brighton performed a study using electrostimulation therapy in fresh fractures (Jager, 1985). They found that electrostimulation was helpful in healing delayed union or nonunion fractures but fresh fractures were not improved or healed more slowly. Bassett, Valdes, and Hernandez (1982) proposed that fresh fractures could be treated if optimal pulse characteristics could be identified and used.

After 3 years treating 250 patients, Focke (1982) summarized his own experiences and concluded that in many cases PEMF should be regarded as an alternative to conventional treatment methods such a neurectomy, caustics, steroids, and phenylbutazone. He successfully treated navicular disease, tendon injuries, arthrotic deformations of the joints, skeletal deformations, arthroses, spavins, contusions, delayed wound healing, and diseases in the back and lumbar regions. Focke was able to keep older horses suffering from severe diseases of the joints and tendons free from lameness for up to 6 months after the discontinuation of phenylbutazone. Older horses sometimes needed further treatment after about 6 months. Bromiley (1987) suggests treatment durations of not less than 3 weeks, even if clinical signs have disappeared. She cautions against ending therapy too soon, although painful symptoms may have improved.

Some recent developments using electromagnetic energy have potential future applications, including stimulation and measurement of nerve activity, soft tissue wound healing, osteoarthritis, electroacupuncture, nerve and spinal cord regeneration, immune system therapies, and potential neuroendocrine modulation (Rubik and others, 1992). Hyperthermia has been used to treat cancer since 3000 BC. More recently a combination of heat and radiotherapy or heat and chemotherapy has been reported. Hyperthermia remains an experimental treatment in the United States (Chou, Luk, 1990). This technique involves using heat to produce selective necrosis in the tumor, without damage to normal tissue. Cancerous tissue is heated by whole body heating, infrared radiation, radio frequency fields, microwave, or ultrasound to a range of 41° to 45° C. Effective therapy requires this narrow range of temperature. Because of the difficulty in setting proper frequency, intensity, and polarization, it is unlikely that electromagnetic methods of cancer treatment will be quickly approved for human use. Still more time will elapse before its benefits can be realized in animals. Advanced hyperthermia equipment might hasten its advance.

A potential therapy for patients with multiple sclerosis uses large pulse magnetic fields to stimulate the motor cortex and deep peripheral nerve in humans (Barker and others, 1987). The results of the first clinical study using magnetic stimulation are described and show clear central motor pathway slowing in multiple sclerosis patients.

Incorporating Magnetic Field Therapy into the Practice

Magnetic therapy is a helpful tool that can be easily integrated into veterinary practice (Table 18-1). Many people already know something about magnetic therapy, and some have used magnets on themselves. Some practitioners use magnets not only to treat specific disease conditions but also to purify the body of toxins found in drinking water and counteract the reaction caused by preservatives in vaccines. Preparation consists of placing the vaccines and water in contact with the north pole of a 1000-gauss magnet for 4 hours. Occasionally, magnetic or PEMF therapy can result in a release of toxins in the body that temporarily cause aches, pains, tingling, or itching; therefore very ill or very toxic pets should be treated with caution and for short periods of time at the beginning of the therapy sessions (DeHaan, 1995). In the few patients who have these reactions, symptoms quickly subside as the body adjusts to a new level of functioning.

The products are widely available in a variety of sizes and shapes. Pebble magnets for use in acupuncture therapy can be purchased for less than 25 cents each; magnetic wraps (bipolar or "bio-north") for placement around limbs cost approximately 20 dollars, although some specialty manufacturers charge much more when they are incorporated into wraps (Fig. 18-5).

Securely fixing magnetic wraps on dogs and cats is difficult, and a magnet of any size, if applied to small animals, can disappear quickly. Acupuncture therapy incorporating the use of small pebble magnets is the best method of using static magnets on small animals. Another strategy to keep a permanent magnet in place is to affix it to a harness, positioning the magnet on the area of injury or disease. Many disease and injury conditions benefit from a daily, general application of magnetic field therapy. Permanent magnets are sewn into the pet's bed. A medium-size "Pet Pad" contains 72 magnets, placed so that a magnetic field extends 12 to 14 inches above the pad (DeHaan, 1995).

PEMF therapy is simple to administer. It does not require either physical or electrical contact with the patient, so no special preparation of the skin is needed. Coils are usually in contact with the subject, although they may be up to an inch away from the body, which reduces risks associated in the treatment of open wounds, traumatized regions, and infection. PEMF therapy is available in a bed for use on animals with both acute and chronic conditions. With the pulsing magnetic system, acute conditions are treated 2 or 3 times weekly in the office, and chronic conditions are treated daily in the client's home. Therapy sessions of 30 minutes are generally pleasant and relaxing for the patient, who simply reclines on the bed and receives the pulsing magnetic therapy treatment. Fig. 18-6 shows pulsing magnetic therapy being given to a 14-year-old keeshond suffering from degenerative joint disease. The unit fits into an existing bed or may be placed in a washable bed cover. The coils in the bed need not be in direct contact with the injured area because the magnetic field can be detected with another magnet or a magnetic sensing unit from 12 to 14 inches away from the coils. This means that lumbar, pelvic, and other areas that are not directly touching the bed receive the benefits of the therapy.

A number of magnetic devices are available to large animal practitioners, including leg wraps, hock wraps, knee and foot wraps, and blankets. Specialty bipolar magnet marketers such as BIOflex and Norfields package their products in attractive wraps that contain pieces of bipolar material. The boots and wraps are lined with a nonbreathable foam backing that helps heat the limb, benefiting local circulation. The manufacturers warn that the patient should be monitored, however, if these products are used for extended periods in hot weather.

Magnetic wraps and strips of bipolar magnetic materials are available from Lhasa Medical in a number of sizes and gauss ratings; for example, a 3″ × 7″ piece of bipolar magnetic material can be purchased for approximately 5 dollars. These strips can be applied as a wrap or with adhesives. Practitioners can experiment by devising a magnetic wrap by using two refrigerator magnets. They are usually a 2″ × 3″ pad of bipolar magnetic material, about half the strength of bipolar magnetic strips. Stack one on top of the other, sew into an Ace bandage, and apply.

Pulsing magnetic therapy systems have been available for equine use since the 1970s. The state-of-the-art model is a portable, battery-powered system with coils built into the blanket at strategic areas. These systems are in wide use at race tracks and show barns, where they are used in maintenance therapy for equine athletes. PEMF systems

TABLE 18-1

COMPENDIUM OF DISEASE CONDITIONS*

CONDITION	STATIC MAGNET TREATMENT†	BIPOLAR TREATMENT‡	PEMF TREATMENT§
Hip dysplasia, spinal myelopathy, Legg-Perthes', osteochondritis dissecans, spinal arthritis	N-pole gold-stick on magnets along bladder meridian BL-18 to 25, GB-29, GB-30, GB-34, BL-67		Animal placed on PEMF coil for each treatment; treated once daily, 30 min; acute: 30 min; daily, low; chronic: 30 min daily, high
Immune deficiency with joint pain	Magnet bed: 24 to 100 magnets; N-pole, 2 to 12 hr daily under pet bed		Acute: 30 min daily, low; chronic: 30 min daily, high
Lumbar spondylosis-disk prolapse, arthritis in extremities	Neodymium N-pole, 9 magnet flexible magnetic pad: 20 min to 4 hr daily		Acute: 30 min daily, low; chronic: 30 min daily, high
Chronic heart disease, arrhythmia, congestive heart failure, systolic murmurs.	1000 to 3000 gauss super magnet taped on a harness on the heart chakra; N-pole against body		PEMF 3 times weekly, first day low, second time medium, third time high
Chronic liver, kidney or pancreas disease	Magnets applied to BL-18 to 23 bilaterally		PEMF daily for 5 days: acute-low day 1 and 2 for 1 hr; day 3: med, 1 hr; days 4 and 5: high, 1 hr
Rickets			Day 1 and 2: low, 1 hr; day 3: med, 1 hr
Nonunion fractures, non-healing wounds			3 times per week until healed on high, 1 hour per treatment
Pain relief	N-pole magnet: 4-8 hr; N-pole drinking water (1 gallon of water next to N pole of magnet for 4 hr)	Wrap applied for 8 hr daily	2 hours, low setting
Abscesses	N-pole 9 magnet flexible pad: 20 min to 4 hr daily		Abscess placed on PEMF coil for 1 hour, med setting, daily
Injuries of tendon, ligament, muscles	N-pole 9 magnet flexible pad: 20 min to 4 hr daily	Wrap applied for 8-12 hr daily	Day 1: low, 30 min; day 2-15: med, 30 min
Inflammation	N-pole 9 magnet flexible pad: 20 min to 4 hr daily	Wrap applied for 8-12 hr daily	Low setting, 1 hr
Epilepsy	N-pole 9 magnet flexible pad: 20 min to 4 hr daily; applied by owner at time of seizure (not a cure-all)		
Cancer	N-pole magnet: 3000 gauss to shrink tumor, or N-pole 9 magnet flexible pad: 20 min to 4 hr daily; N-pole drinking water (1 gallon of water next to N pole of magnet for 4 hours)		

*Very ill or toxic patients should be treated with caution for short periods of time when beginning therapy.
†Affix magnets with eyelash glue or tape, or use flexible pad with static magnets sewn in.
‡Owner applied.
§Low: 3-8 Hz (acute); medium: 10-15 Hz; high: 30 Hz (chronic). Owner or doctor applied.

TABLE 18-1

COMPENDIUM OF DISEASE CONDITIONS*—cont'd

CONDITION	STATIC MAGNET TREATMENT†	BIPOLAR TREATMENT‡	PEMF TREATMENT§
Toxicity caused by pesticides, vaccines			PEMF 3 times weekly: first time low, second time med, third time high
Vaccine reactions	Place vaccine on 1000 gauss N pole in the refrigerator for 4 hr		
Ascending paralysis			PEMF med setting: one 30- or 60-min treatment sometimes helpful
Lethargic older animals	S-pole drinking water (1 gallon of water next to S pole of magnet for 4 hr)		PEMF 3 times weekly: first day on low, on med thereafter

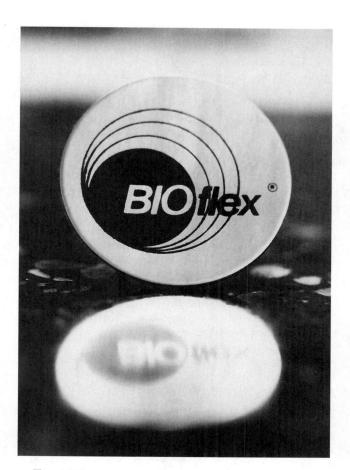

Fig. 18-5   BIOflex magnetic Bi-Polar Magnetic Pad.

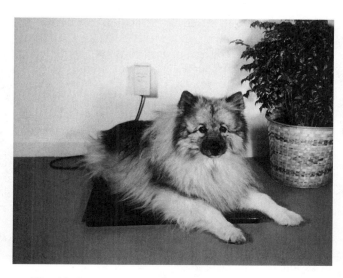

Fig. 18-6   Bio-Pulse 9000 by Respond Systems, Inc.

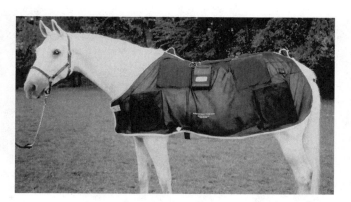

Fig. 18-7   Bio-Pulse 3000 System on a horse.

travel with U.S. equestrian teams to various equine competitions (Fig. 18-7).

PEMF systems have a place in the equine practice for wound healing and nonunion fractures, as well as for bruising and trauma caused by accidents. Artificial insemination centers use PEMF on bulls who suffer from degenerative diseases of the locomotor system. This treatment frequently extends the bull's productive capacity.

Conclusions

Magnetic therapy is used widely in the equine field and with increasing frequency in small animal practices. Many practitioners using magnetic therapy on small animals use it in conjunction with acupuncture therapy. Now that smaller, more cost-effective systems have been developed, PEMF use will probably increase. No single group in the alternative veterinary organizations supports exclusive use of magnetic therapy, although the AHVMA has identified veterinarians who use magnetic therapy with other modalities. For a list of names, contact the AHVMA by writing to them, and include a self-addressed, stamped envelope for a reply.

There is no text written specifically on the subject of magnetic therapy, although the reference section lists good resources to assist in study of the subject. Most of the authors write about pulsing magnetic fields and discuss a wide range of frequencies and energy densities, so the neophyte must read selectively to focus on those therapies that would be useful in the veterinary practice. Their primary value is in documenting scientifically the cellular effects of PEMF and in providing references for further study.

There is no authoritative source with well-documented references on the use of static and bipolar magnets, although Washnis and Hricak (1993) and Philpott (1990) report interesting anecdotes, make intriguing assertions, and are widely quoted. For that reason, they are recommended.

ANNOTATED BIBLIOGRAPHY

Marino AA, editor: *Modern bioelectricity*, New York, 1988, Marcel Dekker. (This is an expensive hard-cover book. However, the references cited in each chapter will save days of on-line searching and will open up the widest possible range of avenues for study.)

O'Connor ME, Bentall RHC, Monahan JC, editor: *Emerging electromagnetic medicine*, New York, 1990, Springer Verlag. (1-800-777-4643) (Covers proceedings from a conference held in 1989 in Tulsa sponsored by the University of Tulsa and the FDA Center for Devices and Radiological Health. 298 pages, soft cover, and very well referenced; contains good sections on cellular mechanisms and covers a wide range of magnetic therapies, from cancer hyperthermia to pulsing electromagnetic fields for bone healing.)

The American Physical Society, Washington Office, Statement by the Council of The American Physical Society, Power Line Fields and Public Health, April 1995. (202-662-8700) (23 pages, a review of epidemiologic data, selected and suggested data, and a report to the public regarding the power line/cancer controversy. The best summary of cogent material contained in one document, and it is free.)

REFERENCES

Adey WR: Tissue interaction with nonionizing electromagnetic fields, *Physiol Rev* 61:435, 1981.

Adey WR: Biological effects of radio-frequency electromagnetic radiation. In Lin JC, editor: *Interaction of electromagnetic waves with biological systems*, New York, 1988, Plenum.

Auer JA, Burch GE, Hall P: Review of pulsing electromagnetic field therapy and its possible application to horses, *Equine Vet J* 15(4):354, 1983.

Baerman H: The influence of multipolar static magnetic fields on the electrolytic system of the living organism with special reference to circular and radial pole patterns. Paper presented at the International Symposium Biomagnetology Magnetotherapy and Postural Activity, Newport, R.I., 1989.

Barker AT and others: Magnetic stimulation of the human brain and peripheral nervous system: an introduction and the results of an initial clinical evaluation, *Neurosurgery* 20:109, 1987.

Bassett CA: Skeletal effects of pulsing electromagnetic fields, AAMI annual meeting, Washington, DC, 1978.

Bassett CA: Fundamental and practical aspects of therapeutic uses of pulsed electromagnetic fields (PEMFs), *Critical Reviews in Biomedical Engineering* 17(5):451, 1989.

Bassett CA: Medical applications and beneficial effects of electric and magnetic fields, The First World Congress for Electricity and Magnetism in Biology and Medicine, Lake Buena Vista, Fla, 1992.

Bassett CA, Caulo N, Kort J: Congenital "pseudarthroses" of the tibia: treatment with pulsing electromagnetic fields, *Clin Orthop* 154:136, 1980.

Bassett CA, Pawluk RJ, Pilla AA: Augmentation of bone repair by inductively coupled electromagnetic fields, *Science* 184:575, 1974.

Bassett CA, Valdes M, Hernandez E: Modification of fracture repair with selected pulsing electromagnetic fields, *J Bone Joint Surg* 64A:888, 1982.

Becker RO: The bioelectric factors in amphibian limb regeneration, *J Bone Joint Surg* 43A:643, 1961.

Becker RO: *Cross currents*, Los Angeles, 1990, Jeremy P Tarcher.

Binder A and others: Pulsed electromagnetic field therapy of persistent rotator cuff tendinitis, *Lancet*, p 695, March 31, 1984.

Blank M: Recent developments in the theory of ion flow across membranes under imposed electric fields. In Marino AA, editor: *Modern bioelectricity*, New York, 1988, Marcel Dekker.

Bramlage LR, Weisbrode SM, Spurlock GE: The effect of a pulsating electromagnetic field on the acute healing of equine cortical bone. Proceedings of the thirtieth annual convention of the American Association of Equine Practitioners, vol 30, 1984.

Bray D, Thomas C, Shaw G: Growth cone formation in cultures of sensory neurons, *Proc Nat Acad Sci* 75:5226, 1978.

Bromiley M: *Equine injury and therapy*, New York, 1987, Howell Book House.

Bullock JE, May KJ: Explaining magnetic field therapy, *The Thoroughbred of California*, 242, Jan 1984.

Cadossi R and others: Lymphocytes and pulsing magnetic fields. In Marino AA, editor: *Modern bioelectricity*, New York, 1988, Marcel Dekker.

Chou C-K, Luk KH: Recent technical developments in cancer hyperthermia. In O'Connor ME, Bentall RHC, Monahan JC, editors: *Emerging electromagnetic medicine*, New York, 1990, Springer Verlag.

Cohen D and others: Magnetic fields produced by steady currents in the body, *Proc Natl Acad Sci USA* 77:1447, 1980.

Council of The American Physical Society: Power line fields and public health, Washington, DC, 1995.

Davis AR, Rawls WC: *The magnetic effect,* Kansas City, MO, 1993, Acres USA.

DeHaan R: Personal correspondence, 1995.

Focke H: Experiences with the use of magnetic field therapy in equine medicine, Mainz, Germany, 1982, Der Praktische Tierarzt.

Fricke H: The electric capacity of suspensions with special reference to blood, *J Gen Physiol* 9:137, 1925.

Gilbert W: *De magnete,* London, 1600, Petrus Short.

Hannemann H: *Magnet therapy: balancing your body's energy flow for self healing,* New York, 1990, Sterling.

Harrison MHM, Basset CA: Use of pulsed electromagnetic fields in Perthes' disease: report of a pilot study, *J Pediatr Orthop* 4:579, 1984.

Hess H, Rothaar J: Experience with magnetic field therapy in affections of the tendon insertions. Lecture at the second International Congress for Magnetomedicine, Rome, Nov 1980.

Herman R: Magnetite found in human brain, *Washington Post,* May 12, 1992.

Hüber R: Eine methode die elektrische leitfahigkeit im innern von zellen zu messen, *Arch Gesamt Physiol Mensch* 133:237, 1910.

Illingworth WM, Barker AT: Measurement of electrical currents emerging during the regeneration of amputated finger tips in children, *Clin Phys Physiol Meas* I:87, 1980.

Ito H, Bassett C: Effect of weak, pulsing electromagnetic fields on neural regeneration in the rat, *Clin Orthop Rel Res* 181:283, 1983.

Jager N: Electrostimulation of fracture repair: shortcut or short circuit, *Quarter Horse J,* p 760, Nov 1985.

Kobluck C: A scintigraphic investigation of magnetic field therapy on the equine third metacarpus, *Vet Comparative Orthop Traumatol* 7:9, 1994.

Kraus W: The treatment of pathological bone lesion with non-thermal, extremely low frequency electromagnetic fields, *Bioelectrochemistry and Bioenergetics* 27:321, 1992.

Lau BHS: AC magnetic field therapy. Unpublished Paper, Department of Microbiology, School of Medicine, Loma Linda University, Loma Linda, Calif.

Lee RC, Canady DJ, Doong HA: Review of the biophysical basis for the clinical application of electric fields in soft tissue repair, *J Burn Care Rehab* 14(3):319, 1993.

Lerch J: Personal correspondence, 1994.

Marino AA, editor: *Modern bioelectricity,* New York, 1988, Marcel Dekker.

Martin J: Double blind study of the therapeutic effectiveness of permanently magnetized foils on secondary myotendofasciopathies at selected different locations. Unpublished test report.

Mesmer FA: *Memoire sur la decouverte du magnetisme animal,* Geneva, 1779, PF Didot le jeune.

Mooney VA: Randomized double blind prospective study of the efficacy of pulsed electromagnetic fields for interbody lumbar fusions, *Spine* 15:708, 1990.

Nolan L: Personal correspondence to Mr. Zablotsky, 1994.

O'Connor ME, Bentall RHC, Monahan JC, editors: Emerging electromagnetic medicine, New York, 1990, Springer Verlag.

Oncley JL: The electrical moments and relaxation times of proteins as measured from their influence on the dielectric constant of solutions. In Cohen EJ, Edsall JT, editors: *Proteins, amino acids and peptides,* New York, 1943, Reinhold.

Patel N, Poo M: Orientation of neurite growth by extracellular electric fields, *J Neurosci* 2(4):483, 1982.

Philpott WH: *Biomagnetic handbook,* Choctaw, Okla, 1990, Enviro-Tech Products.

Pilla AA: An electrochemical consideration of electromagnetic bioeffects. In Marino AA, editor: *Modern bioelectricity,* New York, 1988, Marcel Dekker.

Poenie M: Changes of free calcium levels with stages of the cell division cycle, *Nature* 315:147, 1985.

Pratt G: The effect of the BIOflex magnetic pad on the flow rate of 5% aqueous saline solution. Paper presented at the International Symposium Biomagnetology, Magnetotherapy, and Postural Activity, Newport, R.I., 1989.

Rubik B (Chair) and others: Bioelectromagnetics applications in medicine, alternative medicine: expanding medical horizons. A Report to the National Institutes of Health on Alternative Medical Systems and Practices in the United States, Workshop on Alternative Medicine, Chantilly, Virginia, Sept 14-16, 1992 (U.S. Government Printing Office).

Sauerwein W: Can low frequency, low intensity magnetic fields be used in cancer treatment? *Bioelectrochemistry Bioenergetics* 27:347, 1992.

Schiegl H: *Healing magnetism, the transference of vital force,* York Beach, ME, 1987, Weisner.

Schoen A: *Veterinary acupuncture,* St Louis, 1994, Mosby.

Sisken BF: Effects of electromagnetic fields on nerve regeneration. In Marino AA, editor: *Modern bioelectricity,* New York, 1988, Marcel Dekker.

Smith CW, Best S: *Electromagnetic man,* New York, 1989, St Martin's.

Teneforde TS: Biological interactions of extremely low frequency electric and magnetic fields, *Bioelectrochemistry Bioenergetics* 25:1, 1991.

Trock DH and others: A double blind trial of the clinical effects of pulsed electromagnetic fields in osteoarthritis, *J Rheumatol* 20(3):456, 1993.

Walleczek J: Electromagnetic field effects on cells of the immune system: the role of calcium signaling, *FASEB J* 6:3177, 1992.

Warnke U: Effect of pulsating magnetic fields on biological systems, *Therapiewoche* 30:4609, 1980.

Washnis G, Hricak R: *Discovery of magnetic health,* Rockville, Md, 1993, NOVA.

Wheeler P, editor: *DC electronics,* New York, 1978, Heath.

Zablotsky T: The application of permanent magnets in musculoskeletal injuries. Unpublished paper, 1989.

Zon JR, Tien HT: Electronic properties of natural and modeled bilayer membranes. In Marino AA, editor: *Modern bioelectricity,* New York, 1988, Marcel Dekker.

SELECTED READING

Aaron RK and others: The conservative treatment of osteonecrosis of the femoral head: a comparison of core decompression and pulsing electromagnetic fields, *Clin Orthop* 249:209, 1989.

Barker AT, Jaffe LF, Vanable JW, Jr: The glabrous epidermis of cavies contains a powerful battery, *The American Physiological Society* 242:R358, 1982.

Bassett CA, Schink-Ascani M, Lewis M: Effects of EMF on Steinberg ratings of femoral head osteonecrosis, *Clin Orthop* 246:172, 1989.

Blackman CF, Benane SG, Rabinowitz JR: A role for the magnetic field in the radiation-induced efflux of calcium ions from brain tissue in vitro, *Bioelectromagnetics* 6:327, 1985.

Blank M, Findl E: *Mechanistic approaches to interactions of electric and electromagnetic fields with living systems,* New York, 1987, Plenum.

Charman RA: Bioelectricity and electrotherapy: towards a new paradigm? *J Chartered Soc Physiother,* Sept to Dec 1990, Jan to March 1991.

Jones W: Magnetic field therapy, *Equine Vet Data,* p 337, Nov 20, 1983.

Liboff AR and others: Ca++ -45 cyclotron resonance in human lymphocytes, *J Bioelectr* 6:13, 1987.

Smith SD, McLeod BR, Liboff AR: Calcium cyclotron resonance and diatom mobility, *Bioelectromagnetics* 8:215, 1987.

ACKNOWLEDGMENT

The authors would like to acknowledge and thank the following individuals for contributing their prescriptions to the disease compendium: Dr. Roger DeHaan, Haverhill, Mass., Dr. Joanne Stefanatos, Las Vegas, Nev.

Botanical Medicine

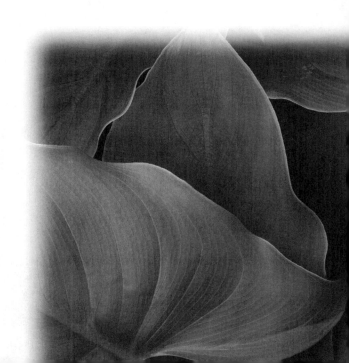

Chapter 19

Western Herbal Medicine: Traditional Materia Medica

JAMES A. DUKE, JUDI duCELLIER, STEPHEN BECKSTROM-STERNBERG

This chapter lists some of the safest and most efficacious herbal medicines. Many of these will likely also prove useful in veterinary medicine. One common argument against the use of experimental data for herbal prescriptions is the difficulty in extrapolating from animal data to humans and the numerous experimental differences between rats and mice and humans. This pharmacopoeial list of potential veterinary applications was prepared by extrapolating data from a list of substances used with promising results in humans.

The following lists were compiled from several reliable sources of information about the most important herbs, leaning especially heavily for modern usages on Varro Tyler's *Herbs of Choice* (1994) and Williamson and Evans' remarkably improved *Potter's New Cyclopaedia of Botanical Drugs and Preparations* (1989). Also included are all herbs recently featured in a brochure of the American Botanical Council, *Herbs and Health. An Introductory Guide to Herbal Healthcare* (1995). The ethnobotanical data are based on a U.S. Department of Agriculture data base of folk uses of medicinal plants, with the information transcribed for this veterinary compendium. These data are frequently updated in the EthnobotDB data base (Duke, Beckstrom-Sternberg, Wain, 1995), an updated version of the former *Medicinal Plants of the World* (Duke, Wain, 1981). Currently the data base has some 80,000 entries, an entry consisting of scientific name, common name (complete), folk use, location of use, and source of data. The common names, as well as the authority for the scientific name, are gradually being completed. This data base is now available on the Internet (URL: http://www.ars-grin.gov/~ngrlsb/).

Some caveats must be noted with regard to the ethnobotanical data. Some relatively toxic herbs are mentioned. All medicines are toxic; the dosage is the determinant. It is probable that therapeutic and lethal doses exist for every phytomedicinal and synthetic compound. The ethnobotanical data are derived from the folklore. Published figures indicate an approximate 25% "hit rate" in several Amerindian compendia compared with nearly 50% in the National Academy of Sciences (NAS) (National Academy of Sciences, 1975) evaluation of Chinese folk medicinal plants. That NAS study counted the folk medicine rationale if the plant contained one or more chemicals that had a biologic activity corresponding to one of the folk uses of the plant. As data bases improve, a 100% rationale figure should be approximated, because almost all plants contain thousands of chemicals with thousands of biologic activities. One can hardly miss in seeking a single chemical, even at levels as small as parts per billion, that would contribute to a resolution of one or more of the diseases being treated folklorically. This approach may seem naive, but now more than ever, practitioners are aware of the many biologically active compounds in herbal medicines. We believe that our bodies, like those of pets and domesticated animals, can "reach" into this herbal potpourri and find at least traces of a compound, with which we coevolved, that will help resolve a medical problem. Conversely, if the veterinary doctor or the physician prescribes a single "magic bullet" for an ailment, there will be only one chemical present. This strategy is fine, *if* the diagnosis and prescription are correct. However, if the diagnosis is incorrect, as sometimes happens, the herb has a better chance of offering a useful biologic activity than the magic bullet. If, as is almost always the case, unidentified comorbid conditions exist, the herb has a better chance of offering something useful than the magic bullet.

Some of the herbs mentioned here, if standardized to their major synergic active ingredients, could be as safe and efficacious as their synthetic counterparts. The herbal shotgun may be better than the magic silver bullet. Until unbiased, head-on comparative trials are pursued, the answer remains unknown. Americans should (but do not) know the best alterative because the alternatives have not yet had fair trials in the scientific courtroom. We believe that humans and animals will be well served by careful investigations of the herbs mentioned herein; however, almost none of the herbal indications have been subjected to rigorous scientific scrutiny.

"In 1993, it cost $231 million to prove a new drug safe and effective according to pharmaceutical industry estimates" (Duke, 1993). Who will invest that much money to prove (or disprove) that horsetail, for instance, can improve arthritis, bursitis, or tendinitis, if horsetail is available for free (nature permitting)? We know more about the drawbacks of horsetail (thiaminase problems) than its brighter medicinal side. The establishment is quick to accept *any* negative report about an herb as proven fact, more readily than it is to believe an upbeat report of 10 anecdotal "cures." In their opinion, the poisoning remains a proven "fact" while the "cure" remains an anecdote.

Practitioners want the best, most affordable medicines for humans, pets, and domestic animals. Until scientific trials of the empirically acceptable herbal medicines and unbiased comparisons with their synthetic counterparts are available, the "best" medicines will not always be known. Americans deserve the best. Are they getting the best?

Adonis, False Hellebore, *Adonis vernalis* L. (Ranunculaceae)

Diuretic and cardiotonic, adonis contains glycosides, which, with digitalis-like action, stimulate the vagus and increase heart contractility and work output. For these reasons, this herb is useful in congestive heart failure. This dangerous plant should be used only under the advice of a physician (Tyler, 1994; Williamson, Evans, 1989).

Ethnobotanical uses: Cancer, cardiac, cardiotonic, diuretic, emmenagogue, poison, sedative, stimulant, vermifuge (Duke, Beckstrom-Sternberg, Wain, 1995).

Alfalfa, *Medicago sativa* L. ssp. *sativa* (Fabaceae)

Alfalfa has been deemed an aperitif, bactericide, cardiotonic, diuretic, estrogenic, stomachic, and tonic. It clearly contains estrogenic isoflavones such as genistein. Sprouts of germinating alfalfa augment the genistein content when infected by fungus. Genistein is reported to have the following activities: antiaggregant, antiangiogenic, anticarcinomic, antifertility, antihemolytic, antiimplantation, antiinflammatory, antiischemic, antileukotrienic, antileukemic, antimelanomic, antimitogenic, antimutagenic, antioxidant, antiprostatadenomic, antispasmodic, antiulcer, apoptotic, cancer-preventive, and estrogenic. It is also reported to be a fungicide and an inhibitor of catechol O-methyltransferase, histidine kinase, lipase, monoamine oxidase, peroxidase, topoisomerase II,

trypanosoma, and tyrosine kinase. However, seeds and sprouts may contain 13,000 ppm canavanine, which may be implicated in hypocomplementenemia, lupus, and pancytopenia. Stachydrine and l-homostachydrine in the seeds may account for its use as an emmenagogue and lactogenic agent (Duke, 1992a, 1992b, 1997; Kaufman and others, 1997).

Ethnobotanical uses: Anodyne, arthritis, bactericide, boil, cancer, cardiotonic, cyanogenetic, depurative, dysuria, emetic, emmenagogue, fever, gravel, intellect, lactagogue, scurvy (Duke, Beckstrom-Sternberg, Wain, 1995).

Aloe, *Aloe vera* (L.) Burman f. (Aloaceae)

Topically, aloe is used as a vulnerary for abrasions, burns, dermatoses, frostbite, skin infections, sores, sunburn, and wounds. Internally, it is used as a laxative for colonic irrigation. The concentrated resin is a strong laxative, containing the anthraquinone glycosides aloin A and B. Aloin reportedly also has antiherpetic, antispermatogenic, cholagogic, hypothermic, peristaltic, uricosuric, and viricidal activities. Extracts enhance phagocytosis. With antibacterial and antifungal properties, the gel is widely used in beverages and cosmetics. It may prove useful in asthma and bronchitis—possibly even cancer and HIV. Acemannan, derived from aloe, reportedly has antiherpetic, anti-HIV, antirhinitic, antitracheitis, and fungicidal properties (American Botanical Council, 1995; Duke, 1992a, 1992b; Tyler, 1994; Williamson, Evans, 1989).

Ethnobotanical uses: Alopecia, aperient, asthma, burn, cancer (stomach), chest, congestion, convulsion, cough, eczema, excrescence, fever, gonorrhea, headache, laxative, pregnancy, purgative, skin, stomachic, swelling, tuberculosis, vermifuge (Duke, Beckstrom-Sternberg, Wain, 1995).

Anise, *Pimpinella anisum* L. (Apiaceae)

A carminative, digestive, and expectorant, anise is an aromatic herb and spice used in cough mixtures and lozenges. Aniseed increases mucociliary transport in vitro (supporting its use as an expectorant). It significantly increases liver regeneration in rats. The plant has mild estrogenic activity, presumably due to dianethole and photoanethole, which explains its use to increase milk secretion, facilitate birth, and increase libido. Anethole (to 5.4% in the seed) has antihepatotic, antiseptic, bactericidal, cancer-preventive, carminative, estrogenic, expectorant, fungicidal, gastrostimulant, immunostimulant, lactogogic, secretogogic, and spasmolytic activities (Duke, 1992a, 1992b; Tyler, 1994; Williamson, Evans, 1989).

Ethnobotanical uses: Abortifacient, anodyne, asthma, balsamic, cancer, carminative, cholera, colic, cough, diaphoretic, diuretic, expectorant, fumitory, fungicide, galactogogue, gonorrhea, kidney, lactogogue, spasm, spice, stimulant, stomachache, stomachic, sudorific (Duke, Beckstrom-Sternberg, Wain, 1995).

Apocynum, Black Indian Hemp, Canadian Hemp, Dogbane, *Apocynum cannabinum* L. (Apocynaceae)

A diaphoretic, diuretic, emetic, and expectorant, apocynum is sometimes used for cardiac dropsy, with dangerous results. Its actions are similar to those of strophanthus. The cardioactive glycosides have been used for congestive heart failure (Tyler, 1994; Williamson, Evans, 1989).

Ethnobotanical uses: Alopecia, asthma, cardiac, cardiotonic, cathartic, condyloma, diaphoretic, diuretic, dropsy, dysentery, dyspepsia, emetic, expectorant, fever, inflammation, intestine, laxative, malaria, masticatory, pneumonia, poison, purgative, sudorific, tonic, vermifuge, wart (Duke, Beckstrom-Sternberg, Wain, 1995).

Arnica, *Arnica montana* L. (Asteraceae)

A stimulant and vulnerary, especially for bruises and muscle pain, arnica is only recommended for topical use; it is considered toxic internally and irritating to the mucous membranes. The dried flower heads, approved by Commission E as antiinflammatory, analgesic, and antiseptic, are used for acne, bruises, myalgia, and sprains and as a general topical counterirritant. Very popular in sport medicine, arnica has shown immunostimulant activity (both helenalin and the polysaccharide fraction stimulate phagocytosis in vitro). Sesquiterpene lactones, especially those with an alpha-methylene-gamma-lactone structure, have antiinflammatory activity. Helenalin, reportedly analgesic, antiaggregant, antiarthritic, antibacterial, antibiotic, antiedemic, antifeedant, antihyperlipidemic, antiinflammatory, antirheumatic, antiseptic, antitumor, antiulcer, fungicide, immunostimulant, and inotropic, is one of the most active compounds. The herb should not be taken internally (Tyler, 1994; Williamson, Evans, 1989).

Ethnobotanical uses: Anodyne, cancer, cancer (intestine), cardiotonic, discutient, diuretic, expectorant, fever, hemostat, irritant, nervine, poison, sternutatory, tonic, vulnerary (Duke, Beckstrom-Sternberg, Wain, 1995).

Ashwagandha, *Withania somnifera* (L.) Dunal (Solanaceae)

The dried root is extensively used as a tonic in Ayurvedic medicine, where it is traditionally used for many conditions (e.g., coughs, debility, fevers, nausea, senility, tumors, and wounds), including enhancing physical and sexual fortitude and improving the complexion. In In-

dia, it is revered for its adaptogenic antistress, antiinflammatory, antitumor, and hypotensive activity. The neurotransmitter acetylcholine affects learning, memory, and sex. Choline dissolves cholesterol and fat and has been used to treat atherosclerosis, cirrhosis, glaucoma, hepatosis, nephrosis (nephritis, nephrorrhagia). Withanolide E, however, may be immunosuppressive to human B and T lymphocytes but also has antitumor activities. The alkaloids (38% withanine) show bradycardic, cerebrodepressant, hypotensive, and respirostimulant activities (Duke, 1992a, 1992b; Linder, 1996; Tyler, 1994).

Ethnobotanical uses: Abortifacient, adenopathy, anodyne, arthritis, asthma, bactericide, bronchitis, cancer, candida, cold, contraceptive, cough, debility, diuretic, dropsy, dyspepsia, enema, eye, fever, fungicide, gynecopathy, hiccup, hypertension, inflammation, intestine, lumbago, marasmus, narcotic, pediculicide, poison, psoriasis, rectitis, rectum, rennet, rheumatism, ringworms, scabies, sedative, senility, sore, spasmolytic, syphilis, tonic, tubercle, tumor, tumor (abdomen), uterus, viricide, witchcraft, wound (Duke, Beckstrom-Sternberg, Wain, 1995).

Astragalus, *Astragalus membranaceus* (Fischer ex Link) Bunge (Fabaceae)

Viewed as the Chinese counterpart to *Echinacea*, astragalus is used in traditional Chinese and East Indian medicine for its immune-boosting and tonic properties. It is useful for several chronic immune problems (American Botanical Council, 1995).

Ethnobotanical uses: Anorexia, anhydrotic, arthritis, bactericide, cardiotonic, cold, debility, diuretic, edema, hyperglycemia, numbness, oliguria, prolapse, rectocele, tonic, tumor (lung), uterus (Duke, Beckstrom-Sternberg, Wain, 1995).

Barberry Bark, *Berberis vulgaris* L. (Berberidaceae)

Weedy species of barberry should be carefully studied as inexpensive alternatives to goldenseal and goldthread, endangered medicinal species used for a wide array of indications. In the Far East, berberine-containing plants are specifically used for bacillary dysentery and diarrhea. Berberine has well-documented antiseptic activities, and the mechanism of its antidiarrheal activity has also been investigated. Berberine enters the cytosol or binds to the cell membrane and inhibits the catalytic unit of adenylate cyclase. It is active in vitro and in animals against cholera. Berberine reportedly also has the following activities: amebicidal, analgesic, antiadrenergic, antiaggregant, antiarrhythmic, antibacterial, anticirrhotic, anticonjunctivitic, anticonvulsant, antidiarrheic, antidysenteric, antigiardial, antiinflammatory, antileishmanic, antimalarial, antineoplastic, antinephritic, antipharyngitic, antipneumonic, antisalmonella, antitumor, antiulcer, cardiotonic, carminative, choleretic, emetic, febrifugal, fungicidal, hemostatic, hypocholesterolemic, hypoglycemic, hypotensive, immunostimulant, sedative, spasmolytic, stomachic, trichomonicide, trypanocidal, uterotonic, vasoconstricting, and viricidal. Berbamine is strongly active against some strains of *Escherichia coli*, *Pseudomonas aeruginosa*, *Salmonella typhi*, *Staphylococcus aureus*, and *Streptococcus viridans*. It increases white blood cell and platelet counts in animals with iatrogenic leukocytopenia. Chinese practitioners use it successfully for leukopenia caused by chemotherapy and radiotherapy. Berbamine is reported to have the following properties: analgesic, antiaggregant, antialopecic, antiarrhythmic, antiarthritic, antidandruff, antiflu, antihistaminic, antihypertensive, antiinflammatory, antioxidant, antipyretic, antiseptic, antispasmodic, antitubercular, antitumor, antiviral, bactericidal, cardioprotective, choleretic, hypotensive, immunostimulant, plasmodicidal, protisticidal, and vasodilating. Palmatine has analgesic, antiarrhythmic, anticholinesterase, antiinflammatory, antileukemic, antimalarial, antipyretic, antiviral, bactericidal, central nervous system (CNS)-depressant, hypotensive, inotropic, plasmodicidal, and uterotonic activities. Its complex effects on the adrenal glands in animals are not fully understood. Jatrorrhizine has antiinflammatory, antimalarial, CNS-active, fungicidal, hypotensive, and sedative effects. Isotetrandrine has analgesic, antialopecic, antiarthritic, anticarcinomic, antiinflammatory, antimalarial, antipyretic, antitubercular, and hypotensive activities. Oxycanthine and magnoflorine are hypotensive. Many of the alkaloids are antineoplastic in a variety of in vitro systems, particularly berberine. No toxicity problems have yet been observed. Alkaloid fractions should be avoided during pregnancy, when uterine-stimulant activity is undesirable (Duke, 1992a; 1992b; Williamson, Evans, 1989).

Ethnobotanical uses: Ache (stomach), alterative, antiseptic, cancer (stomach), cholagogue, diuretic, dysentery, dyspepsia, expectorant, fever, hemorrhage, jaundice, laxative, medicine, purgative, tonic, uterotonic (Duke, Beckstrom-Sternberg, Wain, 1995).

Barley, *Hordeum vulgare* L. (Poaceae)

Barley grass is used as a demulcent nutritive during convalescence and for colitis, diarrhea, and related conditions. Barley water is prepared from the grains, as is malted barley, which is used in making malt extracts, beers, confections, and whiskeys (Williamson, Evans, 1989).

Ethnobotanical uses: Abortifacient, antilactogogue, bladder, bronchitis, burn, cancer, cancer (stomach), catarrh, chest, chilblain, coffee, cough, debility, demulcent, diarrhea, digestive, diuretic, dyspepsia, emollient, expectorant, febrifuge, fever, inflammation, intoxicant, measles, phthisis, poultice, preventive (gray hair), preventive (fever),

puerperium, sore, stomachic, tumor (abdomen), urogenital (Duke, Beckstrom-Sternberg, Wain, 1995).

Bearberry, *Arctostaphylos uva-ursi* (L.) Sprengel (Ericaceae)

An astringent, diuretic, and urinary antiseptic, bearberry has been used for cystitis, pyelitis, urethritis, and other urinary tract infections (UTIs). Both the extracts and arbutin, an active ingredient also found in the related cranberry, have bacteriostatic activities in vitro. Arbutin also reportedly has antiseptic, antitussive, bactericidal, candidicidal, diuretic, and insulin-sparing activities. Arbutin hydrolyzes to antiseptic hydroquinone, which is more effective as a urinary antiseptic. Large doses should be avoided, especially by patients with hepatitis, nausea, nephrosis, stomachache, or vomiting (Duke, 1992a, 1992b; Duke, 1997; Tyler, 1994; Williamson, Evans, 1989).

Ethnobotanical uses: Ache (ear), ache (stomach), antidote (rhus), antiseptic, astringent, cold, cough, cystitis, demulcent, depurative, diuretic, fumitory, inflammation, narcotic, tonic (Duke, Beckstrom-Sternberg, Wain, 1995).

Bilberry, *Vaccinium myrtillus* L. (Ericaceae)

Astringent, diuretic, and refrigerant, bilberries are another food pharmaceutical with many indications. Bilberry extract is rich in purple-blue pigments; in Europe, bilberry extracts are used as an antioxidant to strengthen the cardiovascular system and visual acuity (may help prevent cataracts, glaucoma, macular degeneration) and to increase microcirculation by stimulating new capillary formation, strengthening capillary walls, and increasing overall circulatory health. Dried bilberries are used for diarrhea. Their anthocyanosides inhibit barium-induced contractions in isolated thoracic vein and coronary artery smooth muscle in vitro, possibly via stimulation of vasodilatory prostaglandin production. Anthocyanosides, from this and many other red and blue berries, reportedly have antiaggregant, anticataract, antidiabetic, antiedemic, antiinflammatory, antimenorrhagic, antiretinopathic, antisecretory, antispasmodic, antiulcer, myorelaxant, vasodilating, and vasoprotective activities—several good reasons to eat more fruit (American Botanical Council, 1995; Duke, 1992a, 1992b; Tyler, 1994; Williamson, Evans, 1989).

Ethnobotanical uses: Antidote, antiseptic, astringent, catarrh, diabetes, diuretic, dysentery, hemostat, inflammation, intestine, refrigerant, scurvy, tonic, typhoid (Duke, Beckstrom-Sternberg, Wain, 1995).

Birch, *Betula pubescens* Ehrh. (Betulaceae)

Aquaretic, astringent, and diuretic, birch leaves are used in mouthwash and teas for nephrosis and urethrosis. Birch tar oil is used in ointments for eczema and psoriasis (Tyler, 1994; Williamson, Evans, 1989). Pisha and others (1995) discovered antimelanomic activity in betulinic acid, a melanoma-specific cytotoxic agent. In athymic mice carrying human melanomas, tumor growth was completely inhibited without toxicity. The antitumor activity was mediated by inducing apoptosis. No toxicity was noted at levels of 500 mg/kg. (White birch can yield up to 22% betulin, easily converted to betulinic acid.) Betulinic acid also shows anti-HIV, antiinflammatory, antitumor, and antiviral activities.

Ethnobotanical uses: Antiseptic, diuretic, irritant, ointment, skin (Duke, Beckstrom-Sternberg, Wain, 1995).

Birch, Sweet, *Betula lenta* L. (Betulaceae)

Sweet birch oil, rich in methyl salicylate, is applied topically as a counterirritant analgesic. Methyl salicylate has analgesic, antiinflammatory, antipyretic, antiradicular, antirheumatalgic, antiseptic, cancer-preventive, carminative, and counterirritant activities, often exploited in over-the-counter preparations. Heat and physical activity may increase dermal absorption of methyl salicylate, which can be toxic in large doses (Tyler, 1994). Salicylate-containing herbs should be used with great caution in cats.

Ethnobotanical uses: Anodyne, burn, chafe, dandruff, depurative, diuretic, gout, medicine, parasiticide, rheumatism, scald, sciatica, skin, sugar, tea, wound (Duke, Beckstrom-Sternberg, Wain, 1995).

Bitterroot, Dogbane, *Apocynum androsaemifolium* L. (Apocynaceae)

Cardiotonic, cathartic, diuretic, and emetic, the rather toxic bitterroot has little more than folklore to support it. An alcoholic extract, bitterroot damages transplanted tumors in mice at a subtoxic dose (Williamson, Evans, 1989).

Ethnobotanical uses: Ache (head), cardiotonic, cathartic, diaphoretic, diuretic, emetic, heart, kidney, laxative, narcotic, poison, pregnancy, purgative, sterility, sudorific, tonic (Duke, Beckstrom-Sternberg, Wain, 1995).

Black Cohosh, *Cimicifuga racemosa* Nutt. (Ranunculaceae)

Antiinflammatory, antitussive, and diuretic, black cohosh is used for bronchitis, cough, dysmenorrhea, pertussis, rheumatism, and sciatica. It may also be used as a sedative and emmenagogue. The dried rhizome, sometimes called *black snakeroot,* has long been used for dysmenorrhea and was one ingredient, along with estrogenic fenugreek, in Lydia E. Pinkham's Vegetable Compound. In a clinical study

comparing various estrogens and extracts, the beneficial effects of black cohosh extracts were slow to appear (up to 4 weeks). The alcoholic extract suppressed hot flashes in menopausal women by reducing luteinizing hormone (LH) secretion. LH production in ovariectomized rats was also suppressed. German Commission E has found black cohosh effective for dysmenorrhea, premenstrual syndrome (PMS), and nervous conditions associated with menopause. The methanol extract binds to estrogen receptors in vitro and in rat uteruses, possibly because of formononetin, which black cohosh shares with red clover and many other legumes. The extracts also have antiinflammatory, antispasmodic, CNS-depressant, hypoglycemic, hypotensive, and peripheral vasodilatory activity. Formononetin has abortifacient, anticephalalgic, antiulcer, cancer-preventive, estrogenic, fungicidal, hypocholesterolemic, and hypolipidemic activities. Racemoside has antiulcer activity in mice, and isoferulic acid has antiedemic, antiinflammatory, and hypothermic activities. Nausea may be a side effect. In Chinese medicine a number of other *Cimicifuga* species are used, including *C. heracleifolia* Kom., *C. dahurica* Turcz., and *C. foetida* L. These, called *Shengma,* are used for headache, gingivitis, measles, rectal prolapse (caused by chronic diarrhea), and uterine prolapse. *Shengma* have analgesic, anticonvulsant, and bactericidal action and depress heart rate and blood pressure (Duke, 1992a, 1992b; Tyler, 1994; Williamson, Evans, 1989).

Ethnobotanical uses: Alterative, bite (snake), bronchitis, cancer (tongue), chorea, dysmenorrhea, emmenagogue, female itch, kidney, malaise, malaria, medicine, nerve, parturition, rheumatism, sedative, sore (throat), stomachic, sudorific, tonic, tumor, uterus, yellow fever (Duke, Beckstrom-Sternberg, Wain, 1995).

Blackberry, *Rubus plicatus* Weihe and Nees (Rosaceae)

With astringent, tonic leaves containing 8% to 14% tannin, blackberry is used in teas for diarrhea and in mouthwashes and gargles for sore mouth and throat. Root bark is effective against diarrhea (Tyler, 1994; Williamson, Evans, 1989).

Ethnobotanical uses: Astringent, cough, depurative, diarrhea, diuretic, dysentery, fever, intoxicant, liqueur, resolvent, tea, tonic, tumor, wound (Duke, Beckstrom-Sternberg, Wain, 1995).

Black Currant, *Ribes nigrum* L. (Grossulariaceae)

Reportedly diuretic, hypotensive, and refrigerant, black currant leaves are used for hoarseness, inflammation, and sore throat. Fruits, useful for diarrhea, are a source of vitamin C. The anthocyanosides reportedly have antiinflammatory, bacteriostatic, and vasoprotective (so-called vitamin P) activity. Mildly spasmolytic, black currants are antisecretory against cholera toxin–induced intestinal fluid secretion in vitro. Black currants are widely used as food and flavoring. Seeds, a byproduct of juice and jam production, yield a fixed oil containing 14% to 19% gammalinolenic acid (GLA), useful in the treatment of atopic eczema, PMS, and associated mastalgia (Tyler, 1994; Williamson, Evans, 1989).

Ethnobotanical uses: Cough, cyanogenetic, depurative, detergent, digestive, diuretic, liqueur, refrigerant, scurvy, sudorific, tea, tumor (Duke, Beckstrom-Sternberg, Wain, 1995).

Black Hellebore, *Helleborus niger* L. (Ranunculaceae)

This dangerous diuretic and cardiotonic herb has digitalic glycosides that stimulate the vagus and increase cardiac contractility and work output. It should be used only under medical supervision (Tyler, 1994; Williamson, Evans, 1989).

Ethnobotanical uses: Cancer, cardiac, cardiostimulant, cardiotonic, cathartic, diuretic, emmenagogue, hydragogue, mydriatic, narcotic, nervine, poison, rodenticide (Duke, Beckstrom-Sternberg, Wain, 1995).

Black Mustard, *Brassica nigra* (L.) W.D.J.Koch (Brassiacaceae)

Black mustard is a counterirritant, diuretic, emetic, refrigerant, and stimulant bitter herb, used externally for bronchitis, colds, rheumatic pains, and similar conditions. Ground seeds, macerated in water, are applied in plasters. Isothiocyanates have bactericidal, hypotensive, and respiratory-depressant activity. Skin may blister from the continued release of volatile mustard oil if plasters are left on too long. Mustards are used as condiments and flavorings (Tyler, 1994; Williamson, Evans, 1989).

Ethnobotanical uses: Ache (foot), anodyne, aperitif, arthritis, carminative, counterirritant, dandruff, diuretic, emetic, herpes, laxative, lumbago, lymphoma (neck), mustard plaster, neuralgia, pleurisy, pneumonia, poultice, rheumatism, rubefacient, sciatica, sclerosis (spleen), scurvy, stimulant, stomachic, tumor (viscera), vesicant (Duke, Beckstrom-Sternberg, Wain, 1995).

Blessed Thistle, *Cnicus benedictus* L. (Asteraceae)

Antihemorrhagic, antiseptic, expectorant, stomachic, and vulnerary, this bitter herb is used internally for anorexia, catarrh, and dyspepsia and externally for wounds and ulcers. Cnicin has proven antibiotic, antifeedant, antiinflammatory, antileukemic, antitumor, antiyeast, bactericidal, and emetic activities (Duke, 1992a; Duke, 1992b; Williamson, Evans, 1989).

Ethnobotanical uses: Aperitif, cancer, catarrh, cholagogue, contraceptive, depurative, diaphoretic, diuretic, dyspepsia, emetic, emmenagogue, fever, hemostat, homeopathy, hysteria, inflammation, intestine, intoxicant, liver, lung, medicine, respiratory, scrofula, stomach, stomachic, sudorific, tonic, tumor (spleen), vermifuge (Duke, Beckstrom-Sternberg, Wain, 1995).

Bloodroot, *Sanguinaria canadensis* L. (Papaveraceae)

Bloodroot occurs in many cough, fever, and tonic preparations and has recently been added to antiplaque toothpastes and mouthwashes. *Sanguinaria* extract has been shown to be safe and efficacious for the prevention of plaque and subsequent periodontal disease. Bloodroot has been used externally for burns, dermatoses, skin infections, and tumors. The bloodroot rhizome contains a mixture of isoquinoline alkaloids, including sanguinarine. Both sanguinarine and chelerythrine uncouple oxidative phosphorylation and intercalate with DNA, possibly explaining their bactericidal activities. Sanguinarine has anesthetic, antiinflammatory, antiplaque, antiseptic, antitumor, antiviral, bactericidal, candidicidal, cardiotonic, expectorant, fungicidal, hypertensive, oculotensive, sialogogic, and viricidal properties (Duke, 1992a, 1992b; Tyler, 1994; Williamson, Evans, 1989).

Ethnobotanical uses: Alterative, anemia, aphrodisiac, burn, cancer, cosmetic, cough, divination, emetic, emmenagogue, expectorant, fever, laxative, medicine, narcotic, poison, polyp (nose), preventive, rheumatism, sedative, sore (throat), sternutatory, stimulant, tea, tonic, vermifuge (Duke, Beckstrom-Sternberg, Wain, 1995).

Bogbean, Buckbean, *Menyanthes trifoliata* L. (Menyanthaceae)

Bogbean is often used for hepatosis and rheumatism. It is a bitter, deobstruent tonic and laxative in large doses. Caffeic and ferulic acids have choleretic and antiinflammatory activities, among others. They may be synergistic with iridoids (Duke, 1992a, 1992b; Williamson, Evans, 1989). Pish and others (1995) discovered the promising antimelanomic activity of betulinic acid. In athymic mice carrying human melanomas, tumor growth was completely inhibited without toxicity. Betulinic acid also shows anti-HIV, antiinflammatory, antitumor, and antiviral activities.

Ethnobotanical uses: Aperitif, bitter-principle, cancer, cancer (skin), cathartic, cholagogue, deobstruent, depurative, diaphoretic, diuretic, dropsy, dyspepsia, emetic, eruption, fever, flu, gout, hemoptysis, hypnotic, intoxicant, jaundice, laxative, narcotic, nervine, rheumatism, scurvy, sedative, skin, stomach, stomachic, tea, tonic, vermifuge (Duke, Beckstrom-Sternberg, Wain, 1995).

Boldo, *Peumus boldus* Mol. (Monimiaceae)

Analgesic, antiinflammatory, carminative, cholagogic, choleretic, diuretic, laxative, spasmolytic, and uricosuric, boldo is used for cramps, cystitis, dyspepsia, enterosis, gallstones, gastroses, and obesity. It is also a hepatostimulant. In animal studies, total alkaloidal extract has a greater choleretic activity than boldine alone. Because of its ascaridole content, boldo is contraindicated in patients with serious liver problems and obstruction of the bile duct (Duke, 1997; Tyler, 1994; Williamson, Evans, 1989).

Ethnobotanical uses: Anodyne, antiseptic, diuretic, hepatotonic, liver, rheumatism, sedative, stimulant, stomach, stomachic, tonic, vermifuge (Duke, Beckstrom-Sternberg, Wain, 1995).

Boneset, *Eupatorium perfoliatum* L. (Asteraceae)

Diaphoretic, expectorant, febrifugal, laxative, and tonic, boneset is used for bronchitis, catarrh, and dermatoses. Polysaccharides and sesquiterpene lactones are immunostimulatory at low levels, enhancing phagocytosis in vitro. Extracts are weakly antiinflammatory in rats. Some sesquiterpene lactones and eupatorin exhibit cytotoxic activity in vitro and are being studied for antineoplastic activity. Some *Eupatorium* spp. contain pyrrolizidine alkaloids (Duke, 1992a, 1992b; Williamson, Evans, 1989).

Ethnobotanical uses: Ague, anodyne, cathartic, chest, cold, cough, dengue, diaphoretic, emetic, expectorant, fever, fracture, hemostat, laxative, malaria, medicine, nervine, steam bath, stimulant, stomachic, sudorific, tea, tonic tumor, vermifuge (Duke, Beckstrom-Sternberg, Wain, 1995).

Borage, *Borago officinalis* L. (Boraginaceae)

Demulcent, diuretic, emollient, and refrigerant, borage is taken internally for fevers and pulmonary disease. It is used externally as a poultice. Because commercial samples of the plant contain pyrrolizidine alkaloids (PAs), internal consumption is discouraged, especially when the plant is fresh. The oil, with no PAs, does contain 20% to 26% GLA, useful in treating atopic eczema, mastalgia, and PMS (Tyler, 1994; Williamson, Evans, 1989).

Ethnobotanical uses: Corn, cyanogenetic, depurative, diaphoretic, diuretic, emollient, febrifuge, fever, laxative, nervine, pectoral, spasm, sudorific, tumor, urogenital (Duke, Beckstrom-Sternberg, Wain, 1995).

Buchu, *Agathosma betulina* (P. Bergius) Pill. (Rutaceae)

Diaphoretic, diuretic, and stimulant, buchu is used as a urinary antiseptic for bladder inflammation. However, in vivo effects against urinary pathogens have not yet been proved. Diuresis is due to diosphenol, which also has antiseptic and bactericidal activities. Its LD_{50} is only 212 mg/kg when administered orally to rats, making it slightly less toxic than caffeine. Dipentene, myrcene, pinene, quercetin, and rutin are also bactericidal (Duke, 1992a, 1992b; Williamson, Evans, 1989).

Ethnobotanical uses: Antiseptic, bladder, carminative, catarrh, diuretic, emollient, stimulant, stomachic, sudorific, tonic (Duke, Beckstrom-Sternberg, Wain, 1995).

Buckthorn, *Rhamnus cathartica* L. (Rhamnaceae)

So-called syrup of blackthorn, made from buckthorn berries, is a veterinary laxative. Its laxative properties result from anthraquinone derivatives, particularly glucofrangulin A and B and frangulin A and B. A berry extract produces tumor necrosis in mice. Buckthorn bark should age for 1 year before use to allow the harsh reduced glycosides to convert to milder oxidized forms. Properly aged buckthorn bark is a relatively gentle laxative. The bark may adulterate other *Rhamnus* species (Tyler, 1994; Williamson, Evans, 1989).

Ethnobotanical uses: Aperient, cancer, cyanogenetic, purgative (Duke, Beckstrom-Sternberg, Wain, 1995).

Bugleweed, *Lycopus virginicus* L. (Lamiaceae)

An antitussive, astringent, and sedative, bugleweed is used for hyperthyroidism (thyrotoxicosis or Graves' disease in human medicine). A thyroid-stimulating antibody in the blood binds to and is inhibited by extracts. Recent research shows antihormonal, particularly antithyrotropic, activity. Freeze-dried extracts induce pituitary thyroid stimulating hormone (TSH) repletion in hypothyroid rats and reduction of TSH levels in euthyroid rats. Extracts prevent bovine TSH from binding to and stimulating adenyl cyclase in human thyroid membranes. Antigonadotrophic activity has been demonstrated in rats. Oxidative adducts of caffeic, chlorogenic, ellagic, lithospermic, and rosmarinic acids may be the active ingredients. Lithospermic acid, first discovered in an Amerindian contraceptive, produces anestrus when fed to mice. Reportedly, it possesses antigonadotrophic, antihormonal, antinephritic, antipituitary, antiprolactin, antithyroid, antiuremic, cardiotonic, hypotensive, and vasodilator activities (Duke, 1992a, 1992b; Tyler, 1994; Williamson, Evans, 1989).

Ethnobotanical uses: Aperitif, astringent, cough, diabetes, diarrhea, digestive, hemorrhage, lung, medicine, narcotic, sedative, tuberculosis (Duke, Beckstrom-Sternberg, Wain, 1995).

Burdock, *Arctium lappa* L. (Asteraceae)

Exhibiting alterative, antirheumatic, antiseptic, diaphoretic, and orexigenic activities, burdock has shown promise in the treatment of dermatoses, eczema, lymphoma, psoriasis, tumors, and similar conditions. Arctigenin has antileukemic, antilymphomic, antitumor, and antiviral activities. Trachelogenin has antihypertensive, antilymphomic, and calcium-antagonistic properties. Antiseptic properties accrue to the polyacetylenes and caffeic, chlorogenic, and isochlorogenic acids. One uncharacterized desmutagenic factor counteracts many mutagens. Caffeic acid, chlorogenic acid, and dehydrocostus lactone also have antimutagenic properties. Extracts of the fruit are hypoglycemic in rats (Duke, 1992a, 1992b; Williamson, Evans, 1989).

Ethnobotanical uses: Abscess, acne, alexiteric, alterative, antidote, antiphlogistic, aperient, aperitif, aphrodisiac, bactericide, boil, burn, cancer, carminative, catarrh, cold, corn, cough, depurative, diaphoretic, diuretic, edema, estrogenic, eye, fever, flu, food, fungicide, gonorrhea, gout, hair tonic, hoarseness, hyperglycemia, impetigo, infection, insecticide, laxative, measles, parotitis, pertussis, piles, pneumonia, poultice, prurigo, psoriasis, refrigerant, rheumatism, scarlet fever, scrofula, skin, smallpox, sore, sore (throat), stomachic, sty, sudorific, swelling, syphilis, throat, tonsillitis, tumor, tumor (glands), tumor (spleen) (Duke, Beckstrom-Sternberg, Wain, 1995).

Butcher's Broom, *Ruscus aculeatus* L. (Liliaceae)

Antiinflammatory, aperient, demulcent (with up to 15% mucilage), and diaphoretic, butcher's broom is used for varicose vein syndrome (venous insufficiency). Alcoholic extracts and the steroidal saponins (ruscogenins) have antiinflammatory activity and diminish vascular permeability. The hydroethanolic extract produces alpha-adrenergic effects on isolated cutaneous veins, causing contraction. Extracts are taken internally, applied topically as ointments, or inserted as suppositories for hemorrhoids (Duke, 1992a, 1992b; Tyler, 1994; Williamson, Evans, 1989).

Ethnobotanical uses: Aperient, aperitif, deobstruent, diaphoretic, diuretic, emmenagogue, female complaints,

fever, gravel, jaundice, laxative, lung, sudorific, tumor (prostate) (Duke, Beckstrom-Sternberg, Wain, 1995).

Camphor, *Cinnamomum camphora* (L.) J.S.Presl. (Lauraceae)

Camphor, obtained from natural or synthetic sources, is used as a topical counterirritant. Camphor is both a species and a chemical; the latter is more often used today as an analgesic rubefacient in balms, liniments, and lotions for many ailments (e.g., fibrositis, muscle stiffness). Small doses can be taken internally for colds, diarrhea, and other complaints. Reportedly, camphor has the following activities: analgesic, anesthetic, antiacne, antiemetic, antifeedant, antineuralgic, antipruritic, antiseptic, cancer-preventive, carminative, CNS stimulant, decongestant, ecbolic, expectorant, fungicidal, spasmolytic, and verrucolytic. Large quantities should not be applied externally because camphor is absorbed through the skin and may cause systemic toxicity; overdoses may cause convulsions, nausea, palpitations, and even death. Doses as low as 1 g have killed children (Duke, 1992a, 1992b; Tyler, 1994; Williamson, Evans, 1989).

Ethnobotanical uses: Abdomen, ache (stomach), ache (tooth), analeptic, anodyne, anthelmintic, antiperspirant, antiseptic, antispasmodic, arthritis, beri-beri, calmative, cancer (nose), carminative, circulation, convulsion, dermatophytosis, diarrhea, energy, favus, fumigant, hysteria, inflammation, insecticide, insect repellant, itch, myalgia, myocarditis, nerve, neuralgia, rheumatism, rubefacient, sedative, spasm, stimulant, trauma, tumor, vermifuge, vulnerary, wound (Duke, Beckstrom-Sternberg, Wain, 1995).

Caraway, *Carum carvi* L. (Apiaceae)

Antispasmodic, carminative, and expectorant, caraway is used in both adults and children as a stimulant and for bloating, borborygmus, colic, gas, gastritis, and rugitus. Confirmed antispasmodic effects may accrue to carvacrol, limonene, linalol, myrcene, myristicin, quercetin, and thujone. Carminative effects result from carvacrol and carvone (Duke, 1992a, 1992b; Tyler, 1994; Williamson, Evans, 1989).

Ethnobotanical uses: Ache (head), ache (stomach), anus, bactericide, balsamic, cancer, carminative, cholera, diaphoretic, digestive, diuretic, emmenagogue, fistula, fungicide, lactogogue, laxative, prolapse, scabies, sore, spasm, stimulant, stomachic, syphilis, tonic, venereal, vermifuge (Duke, Beckstrom-Sternberg, Wain, 1995).

Cascara sagrada, *Rhamnus purshiana* DC. (Rhamnaceae)

Laxative and tonic, cascara sagrada is used for constipation, dyspepsia, digestive complaints, and hemorrhoids. The peristaltic cascarosides act on the large intestine and are more effective than hydrolyzed aloins. Cascara and cascara extracts are found in many over-the-counter laxative preparations in the United States. Probably the mildest of the anthraquinone-stimulant laxatives, cascara produces only minor effects on the small intestine. It is considered less likely than some other natural laxatives to produce griping or dependence. Active principles are excreted in mother's milk, so nursing and pregnant women should avoid taking anthraquinone-containing herbs (American Botanical Council, 1995; Tyler, 1994; Williamson, Evans, 1989).

Ethnobotanical uses: Aperient, bilious, cancer, laxative, purgative, tonic (Duke, Beckstrom-Sternberg, Wain, 1995).

Catnip, *Nepeta cataria* L. (Lamiaceae)

Antidiarrheal, calmative, diaphoretic, febrifugal, refrigerant, sedative, and spasmolytic, catnip teas may help colds and colic. Its folklore reputation as a hallucinogen seems undeserved. Minor behavioral effects, similar to those caused by valerian, occur in young chicks, rodents, and cats (Tyler, 1994; Williamson, Evans, 1989). According to de Vincenzi, Mancini, and Dessi (1996), LD_{50} in mice of catnip oil is 1300 mg/kg; nepeta-lactone enriched fraction is 1550; and nepetalic acid is 1050. Catnip oil is less toxic and less sedative than nepetalic acid. At 500 mg/kg, catnip oil, like nepetalic acid at one-seventh the dose, increases hexobarbital sleeping time in mice.

Ethnobotanical uses: Ache (head), ache (stomach), cancer, carminative, catarrh, cold, colic, debility, diaphoretic, emmenagogue, fear, fever, fumitory, hives, hysteria, medicine, nerve, nervine, neurasthenia, pectoral, pneumonia, poultice, refrigerant, respiratory, sclerosis, sedative, spasm, stimulant, stomach, stomachic, sudorific, swelling, tea, tonic (Duke, Beckstrom-Sternberg, Wain, 1995).

Cayenne, *Capsicum frutescens* L. (Solanaceae)

Analgesic, antiseptic, carminative, counterirritant, diaphoretic, rubefacient, spasmolytic, stimulant, and tonic, cayenne is one of the most widely used food pharmaceuticals, used for colic, dyspepsia, gas, and laryngitis. Cayenne is used to improve peripheral circulation. Topically, it is used for chilblains, lumbago, myalgia, and stiffness. Capsaicin is a vasodilator and calcium antagonist that also prevents cancer and inhibits lipoxygenase and cyclooxygenase. Capsaicin has many pharmacologic actions: anesthetic, antiaggregant, antiarrhythmic, antiinflammatory, antiischemic, antimastalgic, antineuralgic, antinociceptive, antioxidant, antipsoriatic, antiseptic, antiulcer, cardiotonic, catabolic, digestive, hypothermic, rubefacient, sialogogic, and spasmolytic. Capsaicin desensitizes the sensory nerve endings to pain stimulation by depleting substance P. Capsicidin has antibiotic activity in some microorganisms. Several external over-the-counter products (usually containing 0.025% to 0.075% capsaicin) are used for arthritic and rheumatoid conditions and pain associated with cluster headache, diabetic neuropathy, herpes zoster, and postmastectomy and postamputation neuralgia (phantom pain syndrome) (American Botanical Council, 1995; Duke, 1992a, 1992b; Tyler, 1994; Williamson, Evans, 1989).

Ethnobotanical uses: Ache (tooth), cancer, dysmenorrhea, impotence, migraine, poison (arrow) (Duke, Beckstrom-Sternberg, Wain, 1995).

Celery, *Apium graveolens* var. *dulce* (Miller) Pers. (Apiaceae)

Reportedly antiinflammatory (and containing over 20 such chemicals), antipodriac, antirheumatic, aphrodisiac, carminative, diuretic, sedative, and tonic, celery is a promising food pharmaceutical. It contains at least six antiarrhythmics (adenosine, apigenin, apiin, magnesium, potassium, and protocatechuic acid), five calcium blockers (apigenin, bergapten, isopimpinellin, psoralen, and xanthotoxin [some photodermatotic]), a dozen diuretics (adenine, apigenin, apiole, asparagine, caffeic acid, chlorogenic acid, glycolic acid, isopimpinellin, isoquercitrin, mannitol, myristicin, terpinen-4-ol), and nine hypotensives (apigenin, bergapten, 3-n-butyl-phthalide, isoquercitrin, myristicin, psoralen, rutin, scopoletin, and valeric acid). It appears to offer equally promising results in arthritis and gout, with apigenin, ascorbic acid, bergapten, butylidene phthalide, caffeic acid, chlorogenic acid, cnidilide, copper, coumarin, eugenol, ferulic acid, gentisic acid, isopimpinellin, linoleic acid, luteolin, magnesium, mannitol, myristicin, alpha-pinene, protocatechuic acid, quercetin-3-galactoside, rutin, scopoletin, thymol, umbelliferone, and xanthotoxin as antiinflammatories; and with caffeic acid, chlorogenic acid, p-cymene, eugenol, falcarindiol, ferulic acid, gentisic acid, menthone, myrcene, and scopoletin as analgesics (Duke, 1992a, 1992b, 1997).

Ethnobotanical uses: Alterative, anasarca, anodyne, antigalactogogue, antiseptic, aperitif, aphrodisiac, arthritis, baldness, bruise, calmative, carminative, colic, deobstruent, depurative, digestive, diuretic, dropsy, dysmenorrhea, dyspepsia, emmenagogue, flux, gout, hoarseness, melancholy, metrorrhagia, nervine, poultice, refrigerant, resolvent, rheumatism, scurvy, sedative, sore, stimulant, stomachic, tonic, tumor, tumor (breast), wen (Duke, Beckstrom-Sternberg, Wain, 1995).

Centaury, *Centaurium erythraea* Rafn. (Gentianaceae)

Aromatic, bitter, stomachic, and tonic, centaury is widely used for disorders of the upper digestive tract, dyspepsia, liver and gallbladder complaints, and inappetence.

Its antipyretic activity may be due to the phenolic acids, and its antiinflammatory activity to caffeic acid, ferulic acid, gentianidine, gentianine, oleanolic acid, protocatechuic acid, sitosterol, and vanillic acid (Duke, 1992a; 1992b; Tyler, 1994; Williamson, Evans, 1989).

Chamomile, Roman, *Chamaemelum nobile* L. All. (Asteraceae)

When taken internally, Roman chamomile is an analgesic, antiemetic, antiinflammatory, antispasmodic, carminative, sedative, and stomachic. Roman chamomile has many of the same uses as German chamomile. As a lotion, it is applied to the skin as a treatment for dermatitis (e.g., diaper rash, sore nipples) and wounds; as a mouthwash, it is used to treat gingivitis and stomatitis. The sesquiterpene lactones have antitumor activity in vitro. Chamomile is an ingredient of shampoos and hair rinses for blond hair (Tyler 1994; Williamson, Evans, 1989).

Ethnobotanical uses: Ache (tooth), carminative, colic, debility, dyspepsia, emetic, hysteria, nervine, stimulant, tonic (Duke, Beckstrom-Sternberg, Wain, 1995).

Chaparral, *Larrea tridentata* (Sesse & Mocino ex DC.) Cov. (Zygophyllaceae)

Brinker (1994) suggests that the combined effects of constituents imply a synergism that enhances the effect of nordihydroguaiaretic acid (NDGA) and indicates the advantage of using whole extracts instead of isolated ingredients. NDGA reportedly has the following activities: analgesic, antiaggregant, anticarcinogenic, anticonjunctivitic, antigalactagogic, antiinflammatory, antimutagenic, antioxidant, antiseptic, antithyroid, antitumor, antiulcer, bactericidal, and fungicidal. It also inhibits lipoxygenase, lyase, and phospholipase. (Brinker, 1994; Duke, 1992a; Duke, 1992b).

Ethnobotanical uses: Antiseptic, arthritis, bruise, cancer (stomach), chafe, diarrhea, diuretic, dysuria, emetic, gastritis, hematochezia, intestine, knee, rheumatism, sore, tuberculosis, venereal, wound (Duke, Beckstrom-Sternberg, Wain, 1995).

Chasteberry, Chaste Tree, *Vitex agnus-castus* L. (Verbenaceae)

The small fruits of the chaste tree have been used for millenia to treat dysmenorrhea. Extracts appear to adjust the monthly menstruation cycle, alleviating premenstrual discomforts. An extract of vitex is approved in Germany for dysmenorrhea, mastalgia, and PMS. The aromatic fruit may have dopaminergic properties; it inhibits the secretion of prolactin by the pituitary gland. (Amenorrhea can be associated with elevated blood levels of prolactin, and

drugs that reduce prolactin concentrations can normalize the menstrual cycle.) The average dose is 20 mg daily of a concentrated alcoholic extract of the fruit. Sensitive animals may develop a rash (American Botanical Council, 1995; Tyler, 1994).

Ethnobotanical uses: Ache (stomach), alterative, anaphrodisiac, anodyne, aperitif, aphrodisiac, carminative, chill, cold, colic, diaphoretic, diuretic, emmenagogue, eye, lactogogue, psychosis, purgative, sclerosis (liver), sedative, soporific, spasm, spice, stimulant, stupefacient (Duke, Beckstrom-Sternberg, Wain, 1995).

Chickweed, *Stellaria media* (L.) Vill. (Caryophyllaceae)

Antipruritic, antirheumatic, emollient, and vulnerary, chickweed is used externally as an ointment or poultice for boils, eczema, psoriasis, and ulcers. It is taken internally for rheumatism. Once used as a source of vitamin C, chickweed reportedly contains gamma-linolenic acid, genistein, rutin, and saponins (Duke, 1992a, 1992b; Williamson, Evans, 1989).

Ethnobotanical uses: Cancer, debility, demulcent, diuretic, eczema, erysipelas, expectorant, eye, fever, fracture, inflammation, mucus, piles, poison, refrigerant, skin, sore, spasm, swelling, urogenital (Duke, Beckstrom-Sternberg, Wain, 1995).

Chicory, *Cichorium intybus* L. (Asteraceae)

Diuretic, laxative and tonic, chicory root decoction is used for gout, hepatosis, and rheumatism. Alcoholic extracts have antiinflammatory effects and depress heart rate and amplitude in vitro. Recently, cichoric acid has been reported to have antiflu, anti-HIV, antiintegrase, antioxidant, antiradicular, antistomatitic, antisunburn, immunostimulant, phagocytotic, and viricidal activities. Roasted roots are used in coffee mixtures and substitutes (Duke, 1992a, 1992b; Williamson, Evans, 1989).

Ethnobotanical uses: Aperient, cancer, cholagogue, coffee, consumption, depurative, diuretic, fever, gall, inflammation, laxative, liver, lung, refrigerant, sclerosis (spleen), sedative, stomachic, sudorific, tonic, typhoid (Duke, Beckstrom-Sternberg, Wain, 1995).

Chiretta, Bitterstick, *Swertia chirata* Buch.-Ham. (Gentianaceae)

Bitter, antimalarial, febrifugal, orexigenic, and tonic, chiretta contains several constituents (e.g., amarogentin) that protect the liver from carbon tetrachloride toxicity. Swertianin and other xanthones are reputedly antituberculous, and swerchirin has in vivo antimalarial activity.

Swertia japonica, used in Oriental medicine, has similar constituents (Tyler, 1994; Williamson, Evans, 1989).

Ethnobotanical uses: Alterative, asthma, atrophy, bronchitis, cachexia, consumption, cough, depurative, fever, gonorrhea, gravel, hypnotic, laxative, liqueur, phthisis, puerperium, stomachic, tonic, vermifuge (Duke, Beckstrom-Sternberg, Wain, 1995).

Cleavers, *Galium aparine* L. (Rubiaceae)

Alterative, aperient, astringent, diuretic, and tonic, the herb cleavers is used in cystitis, lymphedema, and psoriasis. Asperuloside, like other iridoids, is mildly laxative and also reportedly antiinflammatory (probably via prostanoid activities), antineoplastic, cathartic, and herbicidal. Extracts lower arterial blood pressure in dogs without slowing the heart rate or showing any toxicity (Duke, 1992a; 1992b; Williamson, Evans, 1989).

Ethnobotanical uses: Alterative, aperient, astringent, cancer, depurative, diuretic, febrifuge, fever, hemostat, hepatoma, hypertension, intestine, jaundice, leukemia, obesity, parasite, refrigerant, rennet, scurvy, sudorific, tonic, tumor (breast) (Duke, Beckstrom-Sternberg, Wain, 1995).

Clove, *Syzygium aromaticum* (L.) Merr. & Perry (Myrtaceae)

Clove oil is the best-known herbal product used for toothache relief. The volatile oil has local analgesic and antiseptic properties as a result of several phenolic substances, eugenol foremost among them. Used as a local analgesic, eugenol acts on contact to depress sensory receptors involved in pain perception. The undiluted oil is swabbed on the surface of the aching tooth and surrounding tissue or inserted directly into the cavity. The oil is also used in mouthwashes (Tyler, 1994).

Ethnobotanical uses: Abdomen, ache (tooth), analgesic, anesthetic, anodyne, antidote (scorpion), antioxidant, antiperspirant, antiseptic, bactericide, callus, caries, carminative, cholera, dentifrice, deodorant, diarrhea, digestive, dyspepsia, flux, fumitory, gargle, gastritis, gestation, hairblack, halitosis, heart, hernia, hiccup, insect repellant, intestine, nausea, nipple, parturition, polypus, rubefacient, sore, spasm, sterility, stimulant, stomachic, tonic, uterus, vermifuge, wart (Duke, Beckstrom-Sternberg, Wain, 1995).

Coffee, *Coffea arabica* L. (Rubiaceae)

Caffeine, the major xanthine in coffee, reportedly has the following activities: antiapneic, antiapoptotic, antiasthmatic, anticarcinogenic, anticariogenic, antidermatitic, antiemetic, antifeedant, antiflu, antiherpetic, antihypotensive, antinarcotic, antiobesity, antioxidant, antirhinitic, antiserotonergic, antitumor, antiviral, cancer preventive, cardiotonic, catabolic, choleretic, CNS stimulant, diuretic, hypertensive, hypoglycemic, and virucidal. It also inhibits phosphodiesterase and function as a vasodilator. Excess dosages may induce unpleasant side effects such as anxiety, tachycardia, and wakefulness. Caffeine is found in many analgesic preparations (often with salicylates, which it potentiates, as it does paracetamol) (Duke, 1992a, 1992b; Tyler, 1994; Williamson, Evans, 1989).

Ethnobotanical uses: Ache (head), analgesic, anaphrodisiac, anorexic, antidote, antidote (atropine), antidote (narcotic), antidote (opium), asthma, cardiotonic, CNS stimulant, counterirritant, diuretic, fever, flu, hypnotic, intellect, jaundice, kidney, malaria, nausea, nervine, poison, scorpion, sore, stimulant, vertigo (Duke, Beckstrom-Sternberg, 1995).

Colchicum, *Colchicum autumnale* L. (Liliaceae)

Steeped in port wine, the bulb of the autumn crocus, a poisonous ornamental herb, was once used to arrest gout in European royalty, or so the story goes. (Today, red wine is contraindicated in gout.) The corm has been used for more than half a millennium; the seeds for about 150 years. The active principle, colchicine, was first isolated in 1820 and has replaced the herb as the dosage form of choice. Colchicine has also been used in antirheumatic preparations but must be used with extreme caution because it is highly toxic. As a mitotic poison that inhibits microtubule formation during cell division, it has been used experimentally in leukemia but with little success. Although most scientists attribute the hepatoprotective activity to colchicine, Ulrichova and others (1995) suggest that phenolics, especially luteolin, may be responsible for the cytoprotective effects on peroxide-induced injury to isolated rat hepatocytes. Side effects include severe diarrhea, gastrointestinal distress, nausea, and with larger doses, hair loss and nephropathy. Colchicine reportedly has antiarthritic, anticirrhotic, antidermatitic, antierythemic, antiherpetic, anti-HIV, antiinflammatory, antimalarial, antimelanomic, antimeningitic, antipericarditic, antipsoriac, antitumor, bactericidal, carcinogenic, cardioactive, emetic, febrifugal, hepatoprotective, hypertensive, purgative, and uricosuric activities. It may cause fetal abnormalities, and the lethal dose for adults is as low as 7 mg (Duke, 1992a, 1992b; Tyler, 1994; Williamson, Evans, 1989).

Ethnobotanical uses: Alterative, cancer, corn, diuretic, gout, homeopathy, laxative, leukemia, poison, rheumatism, sedative, sudorific (Duke, Beckstrom-Sternberg, Wain, 1995).

Coltsfoot, *Tussilago farfara* (Asteraceae)

Anticatarrhal, antitussive, demulcent, and expectorant, coltsfoot is used for asthma, bronchitis, cough, laryngitis, and pertussis. Herbalists have long smoked coltsfoot for asthma and prepared coltsfoot candy for cough. Its polysaccharides are antiinflammatory, demulcent, and immunostimulant. The flavonoids are antiinflammatory and antispasmodic. The total extract and a lipophilic fraction stimulate phagocytosis in mice inoculated with *E. coli*. In high doses, the PAs are hepatotoxic in rats; use of the herb is therefore discouraged in the United States. PAs do not damage human chromosomes in vitro (Tyler, 1994; Williamson, Evans, 1989).

Ethnobotanical uses: Antihistamine, antitussive, apoplexy, asthma, bactericide, bronchitis, catarrh, cold, cough, demulcent, diarrhea, diuretic, dyspepsia, emollient, expectorant, eye, fumitory, gargle, nerve, pectoral, phthisis, rheumatism, scrofula, styptic, sudorific, tea, tumor (Duke, Beckstrom-Sternberg, Wain, 1995).

Comfrey, *Symphytum officinale* L. (Boraginaceae)

Long used as a vegetable, comfrey has astringent, antiinflammatory, antimutagenic, antipsoriatic, demulcent, and vulnerary properties. For centuries, it has been used for gastric, joint, and pulmonary complaints. However, comfrey has recently received negative attention from the FDA because of carcinogenic PAs present at levels that are not particularly alarming (comfrey leaf tea is less carcinogenic than beer, according to one study). The PAs are hepatotoxic in animals. Comfrey has been implicated in one case of hepatic veno-occlusive disease after chronic use. Not all *Symphytum* species contain the same amounts of dangerous echimidine. About one fourth of the samples of *Symphytum officinalis* studied contained very small amounts of echimidine; the others had none. Species identification is difficult but important. Comfrey roots, which contain about 10 times the concentration of PAs found in the leaves, should not be used for any therapeutic application (Tyler, 1994). The PAs seem to be poorly absorbed through the skin. Hence comfrey is still used as an ointment, oil, and poultice to treat eczema, psoriasis, and ulcers and promote wound healing. The demonstrable antiinflammatory activity may be due in part to rosmarinic acid, which reportedly also inhibits deiodinase and has antianaphylactic, anticomplementary, antiedemic, antigonadotropic, antihemolytic, antihepatotoxic, antiherpetic, antioxidant, antithyreotropic, antithyroid, antiviral, bactericidal, cancer-preventive, thyrotropic, and viricidal activities. An aqueous extract stimulates release of a prostaglandin-like material from the gastric mucosa of rats, which may explain the use of comfrey as a gastric sedative. The soothing and wound-healing properties accrue to allantoin, with reported antidandruff, antiin-

flammatory, antipeptic, antipsoriac, antiulcer, immunostimulant, keratolytic, sunscreen, suppurative, and vulnerary activities. Aqueous extracts of comfrey leaves increase survival of mice bearing spontaneous tumors and decrease tumor growth. In one test, these extracts demonstrated antimutagenic activity. Tyler (1994) states that internal use of comfrey should be avoided. Williamson and Evans (1989) discourage the use of fresh comfrey leaves in salads (Duke, 1992a, 1992b; Williamson, Evans, 1989; Tyler, 1994).

Ethnobotanical uses: Analgesic, antidiarrheic, astringent, cancer, cicatrizant, circulation, demulcent, diarrhea, diuretic, expectorant, hemoptysis, hemostat, inflammation, lung, pectoral, sedative, sore, stimulant, sudorific, swelling (Duke, Beckstrom-Sternberg, Wain, 1995).

Coriander, *Coriandrum sativum* L. (Apiaceae)

Aromatic, antispasmodic, carminative, and digestive, the spice coriander has shown antiinflammatory and hypoglycemic activities. Coriander is a well-known source of linalol, which reportedly has antiallergic, antianaphylactic, anticariogenic, anticonvulsant, antihistaminic, antiseptic, bactericidal, bronchorelaxant, cancer-preventive, candidicidal, expectorant, fungicidal, hypothermic, sedative, and spasmolytic activities. Coriander is the second-best source of alpha-pinene, with its reported antiseptic, bactericidal, expectorant, fungicidal, and spasmolytic activities. The essential oil is reportedly bactericidal and larvicidal. Coriander seeds and fresh leaves are used widely in cooking, and the oil is frequently used in carminatives and flavorings (Duke, 1992a, 1992b; Tyler, 1994; Williamson, Evans, 1989).

Ethnobotanical uses: Ache (head), ache (stomach), ache (tooth), alexiteric, antidote, aperitif, aphrodisiac, aromatic, bilious, carminative, condyloma, cough, digestive, diuretic, dysentery, emmenagogue, fever, flux, halitosis, hernia, hysteria, intoxication, measles, nausea, nerve, ophthalmia, pectoral, piles, ptomaine, refrigerant, rheumatism, sclerosis (limb), sedative, soap, sore, spasm, splenitis, stimulant, stomachic, syphilis, tonic, tumor (abdomen), venereal (Duke, Beckstrom-Sternberg, Wain, 1995).

Corn, *Zea mays* L. (Poaceae)

Corn silk, clearly choleretic, demulcent, diuretic, and hypotensive, is used mainly for cystitis, prostatitis, and urethritis. The diuretic activity has been demonstrated in animals and clinically. Chinese practitioners use cornsilk for edema and hepatobiliary disease. Bisset (1994) mentions the use of cornsilk by Peruvian Indians as an intoxicant. Inhalation apparently induces psychotropic stimulation and finally colic, diarrhea, and vomiting (Bisset, 1994; Williamson, Evans, 1989).

Ethnobotanical uses: Alexiteric, alterative, amenorrhea, analgesic, anodyne, antidote (bromine), antidote (iodine), antiseptic, astringent, Bright's disease, cardiac, corn, cyanogenetic, cystitis, demulcent, diabetes, diuretic, dropsy, dysentery, dysmenorrhea, excipient, flu, gout, gravel, gum, hepatitis, hypertension, inflammation, intoxicant, liqueur, litholytic, lithotriptic, menorrhagia, metritis, nephritis, oliguria, panacea, pneumonia, prostatitis, renitis, rheumatism, shampoo, soap, stimulant, stomachache, stomachic, stone, strangury, tumor, urogenital, wart (Duke, Beckstrom-Sternberg, Wain, 1995).

Cranberry, *Vaccinium macrocarpon* Ait. (Ericaceae)

Cranberry helps prevent urinary tract infections caused by *E. coli* bacteria, particularly in people with recurrent infections. It prevents microorganisms from adhering to the epithelial cells that line the urinary tract. Antiseptic compounds include arbutin, benzaldehyde, benzoic acid, benzyl alcohol, chlorogenic acid, eugenol, oxalic acid, and alpha-terpineol (American Botanical Council, 1995; Duke, 1992a, 1992b; Tyler, 1994).

Ethnobotanical uses: Cancer, scurvy (Duke, Beckstrom-Sternberg, Wain, 1995).

Damiana, *Turnera diffusa* Willd. ex Schultes (Turneraceae)

Damiana has recently been promoted as the long-sought female aphrodisiac. However, this claim should be treated with skepticism. No aphrodisiac activity has been proved, and the herb was once dismissed as a hoax. The leaves are reportedly antidepressant. Duke has enumerated the phytochemicals (Duke, 1992a, 1992b; Williamson, Evans, 1989).

Ethnobotanical uses: Ache (head), ache (stomach), amaurosis, aphrodisiac, astringent, catarrh, cold, diabetes, diuretic, dysentery, dysmenorrhea, dyspepsia, enuresis, expectorant, infection, intestine, kidney, laxative, liqueur, malaria, nerve, nervine, panacea, paralysis, renitis, stimulant, syphilis, tea, tonic, venereal (Duke, Beckstrom-Sternberg, Wain, 1995).

Dandelion, *Taraxacum officinale* Wigg. (Asteraceae)

Regarded as antiinflammatory, antirheumatic, aperient, aperitif, aquaretic, choleretic, diuretic, and tonic, dandelion is used chiefly for kidney and liver disorders, for rheumatism, and as a general tonic. The polysaccharides and aqueous extracts have antitumor activity in animals. When roasted, the root is used as a coffee substitute or flavor additive, and the fresh young leaves are widely used as salad greens. The flowers, used to make wine, are an excellent source of carotenoids and lecithins (American Botanical Council, 1995; Duke, 1992a, 1992b; Tyler, 1994; Williamson, Evans, 1989).

Ethnobotanical uses: Abscess, alterative, aperient, aperitif, bactericide, bilious, bite (snake), bitter-principle, bruise, cancer, cancer (esophagus), cancer (breast), caries, catarrh, cholagogue, coffee, depurative, diuretic, dyspepsia, galactogogue, heart, heartburn, hepatitis, inappetence, intoxicant, jaundice, kidney, laxative, liver, sclerosis (spleen), skin, spleen, stomachic, swelling, tea, tonic, tumor, tumor (breast), wart (Duke, Beckstrom-Sternberg, Wain, 1995).

Digitalis, *Digitalis purpurea* L. (Scrophulariaceae)

The cardiotonic digitalis glycosides, used to treat congestive heart failure, increase the force of contraction of the heart without increasing oxygen consumption, slowing the heart rate when atrial fibrillation is present. Digitalis leaf, even in the standardized form, is rarely used. Use of isolated glycosides may be safer, and even then, close medical supervision is necessary. The lethal dose is only twice the therapeutic dose—a very narrow therapeutic window. Digoxin is the preferred glycoside because it is least cumulative and most rapidly excreted. The cumulative effects of glycosides can easily cause toxic symptoms such as anorexia, nausea, and vomiting (Tyler, 1994; Williamson, Evans, 1989).

Ethnobotanical uses: Asthma, bactericide, cardiotonic, diuretic, dropsy, edema, fever, heart, insanity, neuralgia, palpitation, poison, renitis, sedative, stimulant, stimulant (cardio), tonic, tumor (abdomen) (Duke, Beckstrom-Sternberg, Wain, 1995).

Dill, *Anethum graveolens* L. (Apiaceae)

Dill is a carminative and stomachic annual herb used for pediatric colic and gas. Like caraway, dillseed is a good source of carvone (3.8%), which reportedly has antiacetylcholinesterase, antiseptic, cancer-preventive, carminative, and sedative activities. (Duke, 1992a, 1992b; Williamson, Evans, 1989).

Ethobotanical uses: Useful as a treatment for ache (stomach), balsamic, bruise, carminative, cough, detersive, digestive, diuretic, dropsy, jaundice, lactogogue, laxative, narcotic, psychedelic, resolvent, sclerosis, scurvy, sedative, sore, stimulant, stomachic, tumor, tumor (abdomen) (Duke, Beckstrom-Sternberg, Wain, 1995).

Dong quai *(Tang kwei, Danggui), Angelica sinesis* (Oliv.) Diels (Apiaceae)

One of the most widely used herbs in traditional Chinese medicine, dong quai is primarily used for dysmenorrhea, hot flashes, menstrual pain, muscular cramps, and PMS. Among its analgesic compounds are cymene, falcarindiol, falcarinol, ferulic acid, and scopoletin. Described as analgesic, antiallergic, antiinflammatory, antiseptic, antispasmodic, and hypotensive, dong quai should not be used during pregnancy (American Botanical Council, 1995; Duke, 1997).

Ethnobotanical uses: Amenorrhea, anemia, cancer (esophagus), cancer (cervix), constipation, dysmenorrhea, menoxenia, thrombosis (venous), tranquilizer, tumor (lung), tumor (nose), uterotonic, virucide (Duke, Beckstrom-Sternberg, Wain, 1995).

Echinacea, Coneflower, *Echinacea angustifolia* (DC.), *Echinacea purpurea* (L.) Moensch. (Asteraceae)

Alterative, antibacterial, antiviral, immunostimulant, and vulnerary, echinacea has outstripped garlic as the leading herbal product in sales in the United States, with about 10% of a $3 billion market. It is sold mostly as an immune booster. A decade ago, some researchers claimed that no plant could boost the immune system. However, in vitro and in vivo tests show that total extracts and the polysaccharide fraction stimulate the immune system, promoting lymphocyte activities, increasing release of tumor necrosis factor, inhibiting hyaluronidase, inducing production of interferon and properdin, and stimulating the adrenal cortex and phagocytosis. The polysaccharides activate macrophages and increase secretion of free radicals and interleukin I. German research has confirmed the usefulness of *Echinacea purpurea* in strengthening the body's immune system and preventing colds and flu. It is also used for arthritis, boils, cancer, carbuncles, dermatoses, septicemia, side effects of radiation therapy, wounds, and infections such as bronchitis, candidiasis, colds, flu, laryngitis, pharyngitis, tonsillitis, and urethritis. Echinacin inhibits bacterial formation of hyaluronidase, helping to localize the infection. Echinacea flowers are the best known source of cichoric acid, which is considered potentially useful against HIV because of its antiintegrase activity. Extracts of *E. angustifolia* inhibit *Trichomonas vaginalis* growth in vitro (American Botanical Council, 1995; Duke, 1992a, 1992b; Duke, 1997; Tyler, 1994; Williamson, Evans, 1989).

Ethnobotanical uses: Alterative, antiseptic, aperient, aperitif, aphrodisiac, bite (snake), cancer (breast), cough, depurative, digestive, fever, rabies, sialogogue, skin, sore (throat), sudorific, syphilis (Duke, Beckstrom-Sternberg, Wain, 1995).

Elderberry, *Sambucus nigra* L. (Caprifoliaceae)

Reportedly alterative, antiinflammatory, and antiinfluenzic, elderberry is being intensively studied in Israel as an antiviral agent. Flowers used in teas have demonstrable antiinflammatory activity, perhaps as a result of ursolic acid, which also has reported analgesic, antiarthritic, antidiabetic, antiedemic, antihepatotoxic, antihistaminic, anti-HIV, antileukemic, antimutagenic, antioxidant, and antitumor activities. The flowers are baked in pancakes, and the berries are used in jellies and wines. Warm elderberry wine is used for colds. A mixture of elderberry flowers and peppermint is an old remedy for influenza. Scientists have recently shown antiviral activity, identifying three new nontoxic antiviral compounds, nigrin b, nigrin f, and ebulin f (Citores and others, 1996; Duke, 1992a, 1992b; Williamson, Evans, 1989).

Ethnobotanical uses: Alterative, aperient, asthma, bronchitis, catarrh, cathartic, cold, cyanogenetic, depurative, diaphoretic, diuretic, dropsy, emetic, emollient, epilepsy, epistaxis, excitant, expectorant, fever, gargle, gout, homeopathy, hydragogue, inappetence, lactogogue, laxative, mouthwash, neuralgia, poison, psoriasis, purgative, repellant (mole), rheumatism, scalp, sclerosis (breast), sore (throat), stimulant, stomachic, sudorific, syphilis, wen (Duke, Beckstrom-Sternberg, Wain, 1995).

Eleuthero (Siberian Ginseng), *Eleutherococcus senticosus* Maxim (Araliaceae)

This distant relative of true ginseng, native to Siberia, Manchuria, China, and Northern Japan, has been used by astronauts and Olympic athletes as a tonic to reduce physical and mental stress. In Germany, Siberian ginseng is approved to invigorate and fortify the body during fatigue or weakness, increase work and concentration, and aid in patient rehabilitation. The active ingredients, eleutherosides, resemble ginsensosides and show many of the same activities enumerated by Duke (1989, 1992a, 1992b). Some eleutherosides reportedly have androgenic, antistress, gonadotropic, and hemolytic properties and function as immunomodulators. Eleuthero is used by some athletes, who believe it stabilizes blood sugar levels during exercise and helps the body adapt to increased levels of stress. The only documented effect of eleuthero is that of an immunomodulator (Tyler, 1994). The word *immunomodulator* might be viewed with suspicion; many vitamins modulate the immune system, and all plants contain vitamins (American Botanical Council, 1995; Duke, 1989, 1992a, 1992b; Tyler, 1994).

Ephedra, *Ephedra sinica* Stapf., *E. equisetina* Bunge (Ephedraceae)

Used for at least 5000 years in China, perhaps 60,000 in Iran, ephedra is now a commercial source of some antiasthmatic, antiedemic, bronchodilator, cardiotonic, CNS-stimulant, hypertensive, sympathomimetic, and vasoconstrictor alkaloids. Folklorically, it is used for asthma and hay fever; today, it is also used for allergies, enuresis, narcolepsy, and other disorders. Ephedrine and pseudoephedrine are widely used as decongestants in the form of nasal drops, tablets, and elixirs. Ephedrine reportedly has adrenergic, anesthetic, antiallergic, antianaphylactic, antiappetent, antiasthmatic, antibronchitic, anticholinesterase, antiedemic, antiemphysemic, antienuretic, antiepileptic, antiherpetic, antihiccup, antihistaminic, antiinflammatory, antimyasthenic, antinarcoleptic, antirhinitic, antisinusitic, antisyncopic, and antitussive, and many other activities. Combined with caffeine, ephedrine appears in several weight-control formulations. Patients with high blood pressure should avoid these products. Both natural and synthetic alkaloids have been abused. Large doses may cause dizziness, headache, insomnia, nervousness, palpitations, skin flushing, tingling, and vomiting (Duke, 1992a, 1992b; Tyler, 1994; Williamson, Evans, 1989).

Ethnobotanical uses: Anodyne, antitussive, arthritis, asthma, bronchitis, cold, cough, diaphoretic, dyspnea, edema, febrifuge, fever, flu, hay fever, lung, night sweat, oliguria, poison, sweating, swelling, trachitis, typhoid (Duke, Beckstrom-Sternberg, Wain, 1995).

Eucalyptus, *Eucalyptus globulus* Labill. and Other *Eucalyptus* Species (Myrtaceae)

Eucalyptus oil is an antiseptic, antispasmodic, expectorant, febrifuge, and stimulant. It can be taken internally in small doses and added to cough mixtures, inhalators, sweets, and pastilles. Externally, it is used as an antiseptic, decongestant, rubefacient liniment, and ointment. It is also used in cosmetics, dentifrices, mouthwashes, and pharmaceuticals. Eucalyptus leaves have expectorant activity. Eucalyptus is useful as a cough remedy. When ingested, inhaled, or topically applied, cineole, a prominent constituent, is said to improve a rat's ability to get through a maze. Relatively nontoxic, cineole is reportedly anthelminthic, antibronchitic, antihalitosic, antilaryngitic, antiseptic, and choleretic. It hastens transdermal delivery of other topical medicines (Duke, 1992a, 1992b; Tyler, 1994; Williamson, Evans, 1989).

Ethnobotanical uses: Anodyne, antimalaria, antiperiodic, antiseptic, arthritis, asthma, astringent, bitter-principle, boil, bronchitis, burn, cancer, catarrh, cold, cough, deodorant, diabetes, diaphoretic, diphtheria, dysentery, expectorant, febrifuge, fever, flu, hemostat, inflammation, inhalant, insect repellant, laryngitis, malaria, miasma, phthisis, purgative, respiratory, rhinitis, sore, spasm stimulant, suppurative, throat, tuberculosis, tumor (breast), vermifuge, wound (Duke, Beckstrom-Sternberg, Wain, 1995).

Evening Primrose, *Oenothera biennis* L. (Onagraceae)

Evening primrose has gained in popularity as an American herbal medicine and is used for ailments not predicted by the folklore, including alcoholism, arthritis, atopic eczema, and mastalgia. Evening primrose oil (EPO) has been marketed for only about 30 years. Its gamma linolenic acid (GLA) is considered to be most active. EPO is often taken with vitamin E to prevent oxidation. Clearly, deficiencies of essential fatty acids can lead to arthritis, cardiovascular ailments, hyperactivity, and menstrual irregularities. GLA appears to lower blood pressure and inhibit platelet aggregation. It corrects some defects, such as restoring the motility of red cells in the blood of patients with multiple sclerosis (MS). GLA reportedly has antiacne, antiaggregant, antialcoholic, antiarthritic, antiatherosclerotic, antieczemic, antihypercholesterolemic, antimenorrhagic, anti-MS, anti-PMS, antiprostatitic, anti-Raynaud's, antitumor, and hypotensive activities. Proof of efficacy for hyperactivity and schizophrenia is still unavailable. Antiobesity claims have been challenged. Seeds are one of the richest sources of tryptophan, recently banned as a supplement by the FDA. Tryptophan is reportedly analgesic, antianxiety, antidementic, antidepressant, antidyskinetic, antihypertensive, antiinsomniac, antimigraine, antioxidant, antiparkinsonian, antipsychotic, antirheumatic, hypoglycemic, hypotensive, insulinase-inhibiting, prolactinogenic, sedative, and serotoninergic (American Botanical Council, 1995; Duke, 1992a, 1992b; Tyler, 1994; Williamson, Evans, 1989).

Ethnobotanical uses: Astringent, cyanogenetic, depurative, pectoral, sedative, spasm, tumor (Duke, Beckstrom-Sternberg, Wain, 1995).

Eyebright, *Euphrasia rostkoviana* Hayne (Scrophulariaceae)

Perhaps overrated as an herbal remedy, eyebright is used mainly for the eyes (e.g., as a collyrium in conjunctivitis). Aucubin, which stimulates the secretion of uric acid by the kidneys, might be useful in gout. It is also reportedly antidotal (Amanitin), antiinflammatory, antioxidant, bactericidal, cathartic, and diuretic (Williamson, Evans, 1989).

Ethnobotanical uses: Astringent, cancer, conjunctivitis, jaundice, laxative, ophthalmia, tonic (Duke, Beckstrom-Sternberg, Wain, 1995).

Fennel, *Foeniculum vulgare* Mill. (Apiaceae)

Antiinflammatory, carminative, estrogenic, expectorant, orexigenic, and stomachic, the culinary herb fennel is used particularly to treat colic, dyspepsia, and gas. The carminative and spasmolytic essential oil increases liver regeneration in partially hepatectomized rats. Fennel is antiinflammatory in rats. The popular herb is one of the richest sources of anethole, with antihepatotic, antiseptic, bactericidal, cancer-preventive, carminative, estrogenic, expectorant, fungicidal, gastrostimulant, immunostimulant, lactogogic, secretogogic, and spasmolytic activities (Duke, 1992a, 1992b; Tyler, 1994; Williamson, Evans, 1989).

Ethnobotanical uses: Abdomen, abortifacient, ache (back), ache (stomach), ache (tooth), aerophagia, amenorrhea, anodyne, aphrodisiac, balsamic, bite (snake), cancer, cancer (uterus), cardiotonic, carminative, chest, cholera, colic, dermatosis, diaphoretic, digestive, diuretic, dysmenorrhea, dyspepsia, emmenagogue, energy, enteritis, enuresis, expectorant, flux, gas, gastralgia, gastritis, gonorrhea, hepatosis, hernia, kidney, lactagogue, nausea, nerve, parasiticide, parturition, pectoral, respiratory, restorative, rheumatism, sore, spasm, spice, spleen, stimulant, stomachic, strangury, tenesmus, tonic, tumor, vermicide, virility, vision (Duke, Beckstrom-Sternberg, Wain, 1995).

Fenugreek, *Trigonella foenum-graecum* L. (Fabaceae)

Demulcent, expectorant, febrifugal, lactagogic, laxative, and nutritive, phytoestrogenic fenugreek was one ingredient of Lydia Pinkham's famous compound for women. Saponin-rich extracts of fenugreek exhibit antidiabetic and hypocholesterolemic activities. Fenugreek contains several hypoglycemic or antidiabetic compounds: coumarin, fenugreekine, nicotinic acid, phytic acid, scopoletin, and trigonelline. The fibrous fraction is lipolytic. The aqueous extract is useful in gastric ulcers and exhibits a mild myorelaxant effect in rabbits. Trigonelline significantly inhibits liver carcinoma in mice and is reportedly used as a pessary for cervical cancer in China. It is also reported to have antihyperglycemic, antimigraine, antiseptic, hypocholesterolemic, and hypoglycemic activities. Diosgenin (present at up to 1.9%) has antiinflammatory, antistress, estrogenic, hypocholesterolemic, and mastogenic activities. Fenugreek is also a useful source of other sapogenins. It is an ingredient of curry powders, artificial maple syrups, and other flavorings. Aqueous and alcoholic extracts have been reported to be oxytocic in animals (Duke, 1992a, 1992b, 1997; Williamson, Evans, 1989).

Ethnobotanical uses: Abdomen, anodyne, aphrodisiac, arthritis, astringent, baldness, beriberi, bladder, boil, cancer, carminative, chancre, coffee, cosmetic, cystitis, demulcent, deobstruent, diabetes, diarrhea, diuretic, dysentery, dyspepsia, edema, ejaculation, emmenagogue, emollient, frigidity, gastritis, gonorrhea, hairblack, hernia, hydrocoele, impotence, insect repellant, kidney, lactogogue, piles, renitis, smallpox, sore, spice stimulant, syphilis, tonic, tumor (abdomen), uterus, wound (Duke, Beckstrom-Sternberg, Wain, 1995).

Feverfew, *Tanacetum parthenium* (L.) Schultz Bip. (Asteraceae)

There is much renewed interest in febrifugal feverfew, regarded as analgesic, anthelminthic, antimigraine, antirheumatic, and stomachic, with both preventive and curative effects against migraine and rheumatism. Three clinical studies in England in the 1980s confirmed the efficacy of feverfew in migraine. Fresh leaves or standardized extracts taken daily seem to prevent migraine in about two thirds of patients. Extracts also inhibit secretion of serotonin from platelet granules, implicated in migraine, and proteins from polymorphonuclear leukocytes, implicated in rheumatoid arthritis. The active ingredients, a whole series of parthenolides, inhibit prostaglandin production and arachidonic acid release, which explains at least partly the antiplatelet and antifebrile actions. Parthenolides exhibit anticancer, antimicrobial, and antisecretory activity as well. Parthenolide proper reduces calcium secretion in animals; it is also reportedly antiaggregant, antiarthritic, anticancer, antiinflammatory, antineuralgic, antisecretory, antiseptic, antitumor, bactericidal, fungicidal, and spasmolytic. The stomachic effect of feverfew may be due to spasmolytic spirochetal ethers. Like most good medicines, feverfew has side effects, including dermatitis, sore mouth, and mild tranquility (American Botanical Council, 1995; Duke, 1992a, 1992b; Tyler, 1994; Williamson, Evans, 1989).

Ethnobotanical uses: Abortifacient, ache (ear), anemia, aperient, cancer, carminative, cold, colic, depurative, diarrhea, digestion, diuretic, dyspepsia, emmenagogue, fever, insecticide, laxative, resolvent, spasm, stomachic, tonic, vermifuge (Duke, Beckstrom-Sternberg, Wain, 1995).

Flaxseed, Linseed, *Linum usitatissimum* L. (Linaceae)

Antitussive, demulcent, emollient, laxative, and pectoral, flaxseed is useful in bronchitis, colitis, constipation, coughs, diverticulitis, and gastritis. Externally, flaxseed is applied by poultice to boils, burns, and scalds. The oil is used in the art, health food, and paint industries. Whole books have been devoted to flax and the alpha-linolenic acid (ALA) in its health-giving oil. Tollund man, well preserved in a Danish bog for about 2000 years, had flaxseed in his stomach (Cunnane, Thompson, 1995; Duke, 1997; Williamson, Evans, 1989).

Ethnobotanical uses: Anodyne, astringent, boil, bronchitis, burn, cancer, cancer (skin), carbuncle, cold, conjunctivitis, corn, cough, cyanogenetic, demulcent, diarrhea, diuretic, emollient, expectorant, gonorrhea, gout, inflammation, intoxication, labor, laxative, ointment, ointment base, osmotic, poison, posthume, rheumatism, scald, sclerosis (limb), sore, spasm, suppurative, swelling, tumor, urogenital, vulnerary (Duke, Beckstrom-Sternberg, Wain, 1995).

Garlic, *Allium sativum* L. (Liliaceae)

Antiaggregant, antibiotic, antidiabetic, antithrombotic, bactericidal, expectorant, diaphoretic, fungicidal, hypolipidemic, hypotensive, lipolytic, and sudorific, the food, spice, and medicine known as garlic is used extensively for asthma, bronchitis, colds, and flu. According to folklore, it can be used for almost every ailment that exists. Allicin is active in vitro against *Candida albicans, Escherichia coli, Salmonella typhi, S. paratyphi, Shigella dysenteriae, Staphylococcus aureus, Trichomonas* spp., and *Vibrio cholerae.* Allicin and allylpropyldisulfide are hypoglycemic, but hyperglycemic compounds are also reported. The active hypoglycemic compounds have an insulin-sparing effect, perhaps because of thiol groups competing for insulin. Garlic contains various antihistaminic compounds: caffeic acid, citral, kaempferol, linalol, quercetin, and rutin; the antiinflammatory compounds: caffeic acid, chlorogenic acid, ferulic acid, kaempferol, oleanolic acid, quercetin, and rutin; and the lipoxygenase inhibitors: ajoene, allicin, caffeic acid, chlorogenic acid, p-coumaric acid, kaempferol, and rutin. Ajoene, a potent antithrombotic agent, is also a broad-spectrum antibiotic and has antiinflammatory, hypocholesterolemic, and lipolytic activities. 2-Vinyl-4H-1,3-dithiin is a weaker antithrombotic. Chinese practitioners use garlic for abscesses, dermatoses, diarrhea, dyspepsia, edema, and pertussis. In clinical tests for amebic and bacillary dysentery, garlic had success rates of 88% and 67% respectively. It has also proved useful for appendicitis. Garlic is approved in Europe for cardiovascular conditions, especially high cholesterol and triglyceride levels associated with risk of atherosclerosis. It is also generally regarded as a safe preventive for colds, flu, and other infectious diseases. Garlic can cause heartburn, flatulence, and related gastrointestinal problems in sensitive individuals. Some are allergic to garlic (American Botanical Council, 1995; Duke, 1992a, 1992b, 1997; Tyler, 1994; Williamson, Evans, 1989).

Ethnobotanical uses: Ache (ear), ache (stomach), ache (tooth), alopecia, ameba, antidote, antidote (scorpion), antiseptic, antispasmodic, arteriosclerosis, arthritis, ascaricide, asthma, bactericide, bite (bug), bite (snake), bladder, bronchiectasis, bronchitis, cancer, carminative, cold, colic, corn, cough, dandruff, deafness, demulcent, diaphoretic, diarrhea, diphtheria, diuretic, dysentery, dysmenorrhea, dyspepsia, emmenagogue, expectorant, fever, flatulence, gangrene, hematuria, hepatitis, hypertension, hypertensive, hypotensive, hysteria, internal ulcer, kidney, leukemia, lung, lupus, malaria, malignancy, nerve, oliguria, parasiticide, parturition, pertussis, phthisis, plague, preventive, preventive (cancer), preventive (goiter), preventive (pestilence), repellant (snake), rheumatism, ringworm, rubefacient, scabies, sclerosis, sedative, senescence, skin, sore, spice, spleen, stimulant, sting (bee), stomach, stomachic, thirst, throat, tonic, trachoma, trichomoniasis, tuberculosis, tumor, tumor (abdomen), typhoid, ulcer, vaginitis, vasodilator, vermifuge, wart, wen, whitlow, witchcraft, wound (Duke, Beckstrom-Sternberg, Wain, 1995).

Gentian, *Gentiana lutea* L. (Gentianaceae)

The best known gastric stimulant, the bitter tonic gentian is widely used to improve digestion and stimulate the appetite. It is frequently used to treat diarrhea, dyspepsia, gastritis, heartburn, nausea, and ulcers. Gentian extract is reported to be an aperitif, cholagogue, and choleretic agent and may contain five hepatoprotective compounds—amarogenin, caffeic acid, mangiferin, protocatechuic acid, and sinapic acid. Gentiopicroside stimulates gastric secretion in animals and reportedly has antiinflammatory and choleretic activities. Other choleretic compounds include caffeic acid, mangiferin, nicotinic acid, and swertiamarin. Chinese practitioners use other species of *Gentiana* for conjunctivitis, eczema, hepatitis, jaundice, pruritus, and urinary tract infections. According to some reports, gentian may induce headache (Duke, 1992a, 1992b, 1997; Tyler, 1994; Williamson, Evans, 1989).

Ethnobotanical uses: Aperitif, blood, cancer, gastric juice, stimulant, stomachic, tonic (Duke, Beckstrom-Sternberg, Wain, 1995).

German Chamomile, *Matricaria recutita* L. (Asteraceae)

German chamomile has analgesic, antiinflammatory, antiseptic, antispasmodic, carminative, and sedative activities. Often administered as a tea, German chamomile is used internally for bronchitis, colic, cramps, dentition, diarrhea, dyspepsia, gas, gastritis, gout, insomnia, and sciatica. It can be applied topically for dermatitis, gingivitis, proctosis, stomatitis, and vaginitis. (-)-Alpha-bisabolol and matricine have significant antiinflammatory and analgesic activity; chamazulene, guiazulene and oxides of alpha-bisabolol have less. Natural (-)-alpha-bisabolol is more effective than synthetic racemic bisabolol for burns; it decreases skin temperatures after exposure to ultraviolet light. Bisabolol also has an ulceroprotective effect; it prevents the formation of ulcers induced by indomethacin and alcohol and also produces the healing antispasmodic effect caused by a number of constituents. (-)-Alpha-bisabolol has spasmolytic effects comparable to papaverine; the oxides are about half as potent; spiroethers, particularly the *cis*-isomer, are about 10 times as potent as papaverine; and the flavonoids, especially apigenin, are about three times as potent. Other spasmolytic compounds include borneol, caffeic acid, chrysosplenol, geraniol, isorhamnetin, jaceidin, kaempferol, patuletin, quercetin, rutin, and thujone. The flavonoids also have antiedemic activity. Chamazulene and alpha-bisabolol have antimicrobial properties, umbelliferone is fungistatic, and an extract demonstrates inhibition of poliovirus replication in vitro. German chamomile is considered nontoxic, and tests done on alpha-bisabolol show no teratogenicity or toxicity. The polysaccharides, as with many composites, are immunostimulating; they activate macrophages and B lymphocytes. Chamomiles are used in shampoos and hair rinses for blonds (American Botanical Council, 1995; Duke, 1992a, 1992b; Tyler, 1994; Williamson, Evans, 1989).

Ginger, *Zingiber officinale* Rose. (Zingiberaceae)

Antiemetic, antiflatulent, antispasmodic, antitussive, and carminative, ginger is a splendid example of "food pharmacy." In one recent study, capsules containing the dried rhizome proved superior to dimenhydrinate in the prevention of gastrointestinal consequences of motion sickness. Fresh ginger extracts inhibit gastric secretion and stress-induced lesions in small animals. Both fresh and dried rhizomes suppress gastric secretion and reduce vomiting. The shogaols and the gingerols, pungent components in ginger, have analgesic, antiaggregant, anticancer, antihepatotoxic, antiinflammatory, antipyretic, antitussive, antiulcer, cardiotonic, hypotensive (transient), and sedative activities. Their hepatoprotective activity depends on chain length, with the gingerols being more active than the homologous shogaols. (6)-Gingerol and (6)-shogaol have been shown to suppress gastric contractions. Ginger also contains the proteolytic enzyme zingibain. In Oriental medicine, ginger, like licorice, is so highly regarded that it occurs in about half of the polyherbal prescriptions. According to Williamson and Evans (1989), fresh rhizomes are used for abdominal distention, cough, pyrexia, and vomiting, whereas processed rhizomes are used for diarrhea, enteralgia, and lumbago. Chinese clinical and animal studies suggest the use of injected ginger preparations for lumbago and rheumatic pain. Ginger is a digestive aid and treatment for motion sickness, nausea, and vertigo. It has also been used to treat burns, convulsions, depression, headache, hepatotoxicity, high cholesterol, impotence, migraine, peptic ulcers, rheumatism, and age-related penile vascular changes. According to Fulder and Tenne (1996), ginger "has been shown to be as effective as conventional drugs in the prevention of motion sickness in trials at sea and also in careful clinical studies. . . . Ginger, which acts locally on the digestive system, is undoubtedly much safer than the current drugs for motion sickness" (American Botanical Council, 1995; Duke, 1992a, 1992b, 1997; Tyler, 1994; Williamson, Evans, 1989).

Ethnobotanical uses: Abortive, ache (stomach), ache (tooth), ague, alopecia, amenorrhea, anodyne, antidote

(Brassica), antidote (mushroom), antidote (scorpion), antihistamine, antioxidant, antiseptic, anus, aperitif, aphrodisiac, asthma, astringent, backache, balsamic, bite (dog), bite (snake), bronchitis, cancer, cancer (breast), cancer (stomach), carminative, cataplasm, chill, cholera, colic, congestion, cosmetic, cough, depression, diarrhea, digestive, diuretic, dysentery, dyspepsia, ecbolic, ecchymosis, expectorant, fatigue, fever, fistula, flatulence, flu, gas, gingivosis, gout, gynecology, head cold, headache, helminthiasis, hemorrhage, hemostat, hepatosis, indigestion, infection, intestine, laryngitis, laxative, liqueur, lochia, malaria, marasmus, narcosis, nausea, opacity, panacea, paralysis, parturition, pediculicide, perfume, phthisis, poison, proteolytic, puerperium, rabies, rheumatism, rhinosis, roundworms, rubefacient, sialogogue, sore, spice, spleen, sternutatory, stimulant, stomach, stomachache, stomachic, sudorific, swelling, syphilis, tetanus, tonic, tumor (abdomen), tumor (hand), ulcer, urogenital, vermifuge, wen (Duke, Beckstrom-Sternberg, Wain, 1995).

Ginkgo, *Ginkgo biloba* L. (Ginkgoaceae)

The living fossil, ginkgo, has only recently emerged as a billion-dollar European phytomedicinal, selling as much as a half billion dollars a year. Numerous European studies confirm the use of standardized ginkgo leaf extracts for many geriatric conditions, including cold extremities, intermittent claudication, memory loss, peripheral vascular disease, poor circulation, tinnitus, and vertigo. Ginkgo is reportedly an antiaggregant (platelet-activating factor [PAF] antagonist), antiasthmatic, antioxidant, bronchodilator, and circulatory stimulant. PAF is involved in allergic inflammation, anaphylactic shock, and asthma. The ginkgolides, particularly ginkgolide B, known commercially as BN 52021, are PAF antagonists. BN 52021 also inhibits the other pharmacologic effects produced by PAF, such as platelet aggregation and the wheal-and-flare response. Ginkgo extracts have complex vasoactive effects on isolated blood vessels. The flavonoid extract is used to improve circulation in the brain and treat hemorrhoids. One study showed that extracts protect normal healthy males against cerebral hypoxia. Extracts improve mental performance in elderly subjects with impairments but may have little or no effect on normal subjects. Kleijnen and Knipschild (1992) list the main symptoms of cerebral insufficiency as follows: (1) Difficulties of concentration, (2) difficulties with memory, (3) absentmindedness, (4) confusion, (5) lack of energy, (6) tiredness, (7) decreased physical performance, (8) depressive mood, (9) anxiety, (10) dizziness, (11) tinnitus, (12) headache. Ginkgo has been reported to cause coagulation deficits, dermatitis, diarrhea, irritability, restlessness, and vomiting (American Botanical Council, 1995; Duke, 1997; Tyler, 1994; Williamson, Evans, 1989).

Ethnobotanical uses: Antitussive, asthma, astringent, bactericide, bladder, blennorrhea, bronchitis, cancer, corn, cosmetic, cough, detergent, digestive, dyspepsia, dysuria, expectorant, flux, gonorrhea, intoxicant, leucorrhea, lung, metrorrhagia, quackery, sedative, tranquilizer, tuberculosis, uterus, vasodilator, vermifuge, vesicant, wet dream, wound (Duke, Beckstrom-Sternberg, Wain, 1995).

Ginseng, *Panax ginseng* C.A.Meyer; *Panax quinquefolius* L.; *Panax schinseng* Nees. (Araliaceae)

With fewer than a dozen authentic species, the genus *Panax* is still not well understood. Although Williamson and Evans considered them the same pharmacologically (as do many American scholars), Asian practitioners attributed different properties to the major Oriental species. Oriental ginseng is used for aging, debility, diabetes, fatigue, impotence, insomnia, inability to concentrate, sexual inadequacy, and stress. Sponsored studies have shown that the ginsenosides (panaxosides) have immunomodulatory activity, stimulating protein synthesis (in rat liver and kidney) and raising plasma levels of adrenocorticotropin and corticosterone. Ginsenosides also show antiaggregant activity (reducing conversion of fibrinogen to fibrin and preventing platelet aggregation) and maintain homeostasis by endocrine activity. The often conflicting activities of various ginsenosides may account for the homeostatic reputation of ginseng. (For detailed enumeration of the biologic activities, see Duke, 1989, 1992a, 1992b). In animals an extract increases the capacity of skeletal muscle to oxidize free fatty acids in preference to glucose in production of cellular energy, which would help explain the antifatigue activity seen in conventional exhaustion tests. The hypoglycemic glycans, panaxans A-E, are probably responsible for ginseng's modulation of carbohydrate metabolism. Minor side effects include estrogenism, hypertension, irritability, and related symptoms (Williamson, Evans, 1989). Ginseng is classed as an adaptogen, an herb that increases overall resistance to stress. Other herbal adaptogens, according to the American Botanical Council (1995), include astragalus, Siberian ginseng, and schizandra. In animal studies, ginseng increases activity of the immune system, prevents platelet aggregation, prevents stress-induced ulcers, prolongs swimming time, stimulates hepatic ribosome production, and stimulates protein biosynthesis. All these factors conceivably contribute to the tonic or adaptogenic effects of ginger (American Botanical Council, 1995; Duke, 1989, 1992a, 1992b; Tyler, 1994, Williamson, Evans, 1989).

Ethnobotanical uses: Anemia, anodyne, aperitif, aphrodisiac, asthma, cachexia, cancer (breast), cancer (stomach), cardiotonic, cough, debility, diabetes, divination, dyspepsia, emetic, evil eye, expectorant, fear, fever, forgetfulness, heart, hemorrhage, hyperglycemia, impotence, intestine, longevity, magic, malaria, menorrhagia, nausea, neurasthenia, palpitation, polyuria, rectocele, respiratory, restorative, short-windedness, sialogogue, sore,

spermatorrhea, spleen, stimulant, stomachic, sweating, swelling, thirst, tonic, tranquilizer, weakness (Duke, Beckstrom-Sternberg, Wain, 1995).

Goldenrod, *Solidago virgaurea* L., *S. gigantea* Ait., *S. canadensis* L. (Asteraceae)

Although few taxonomists are able to identify the many species of goldenrod, its many activities have been reported: analgesic, antifungal, antiinflammatory, antiseptic, antitumor, antispasmodic, bacteriostatic, carminative, diaphoretic, and diuretic. Leicarposide has analgesic, antiinflammatory, antilithic, and diuretic effects in animals. The saponins are active against *Candida* species. Extracts show transient hypotensive effects in experimental animals. Aerial shoots are used to treat kidney stones and urinary tract infections (Duke, 1992a, 1992b; Tyler, 1994; Williamson, Evans, 1989).

Ethnobotanical uses: Hemostat, poison, wound (Duke, Beckstrom-Sternberg, Wain, 1995).

Goldenseal, *Hydrastis canadensis* L. (Ranunculaceae)

Among the top ten best-selling herbs sold in the United States, goldenseal is considered alterative, antiinflammatory, hemostatic, and laxative. It is used internally for colitis, dysmenorrhea, dyspepsia, gastritis, menorrhagia, and peptic ulceration. Topically, it is used for canker sores, conjunctivitis, eczema, otitis, and stomatitis. The herb is popular for colds and flu in the United States (American Botanical Council, 1995), although proof of its effectiveness is scanty. Berberine and hydrastine have similar actions, including stimulating bile in humans and producing hypotensive and sedative effects in animals. Herbalists recently challenged the belief that internal antisepsis is likely to result from normal dosages of goldenseal or that goldenseal can mask illegal drugs in urinalyses. Berberine is reportedly amebicidal, analgesic, antiadrenergic, antiaggregant, antiarrhythmic, antibacterial, anticholeric, anticirrhotic, anticonjunctivitic, anticonvulsant, antidiarrheic, antidysenteric, antigiardial, antiinflammatory, antileishmanic, antimalarial, antineoplastic, antinephritic, antipharyngitic, antipneumonic, antisalmonella, antitumor, and antiulcer. Despite its longstanding popularity, the herb has undergone increasing criticism regarding its efficacy and safety (Duke, 1992a, 1992b, 1997; Tyler, 1994; Williamson, Evans, 1989).

Ethnobotanical uses: Alterative, antiperiodic, antiseptic, aperient, aperitif, astringent, cancer, catarrh, cicatrizant, detergent, diuretic, enterorrhagia, eye, hemorrhoids, hemostat, hemostatic, insect repellant, liver, malaria, medicine, metrorrhagia, mucous membrane, poison, sore, stomach, stomatitis, tonic, uterotonic, wound (Duke, Beckstrom-Sternberg, Wain, 1995).

Gotu Kola, Fo-ti, Hydrocotyle, *Centella asiatica* (L.) Urban. (Apiaceae)

Regarded as antidermatitic, antiedemic, antiinflammatory, antileprotic, diuretic, immunostimulant, sedative, tonic, and vulnerary, gotu-kola is used for burns, edema, failing memory, keloids, phlebitis, psoriasis, scars, ulcers, varicose veins, and wounds. It improves venous disorders of the lower limbs and helps prevent and treat scarring caused by burns and surgical procedures. It inhibits the growth of human fibroblasts in vitro. The extract stimulated phagocytosis in mice. The plant contains 0.1% betulinic acid, recently touted as a promising antimelanomic phytochemical, and has reported anticarcinomic, anti-HIV, antiinflammatory, antitumor, and antiviral activities as well. Clinicians proved healing properties of the tincture on wounds. It is taken orally, often as a tea, and administered topically (Duke, 1992a, 1992b, 1997; Williamson, Evans, 1989).

Ethnobotanical uses: Ache (head), ache (rib), alexiteric, alterative, anodyne, aphrodisiac, astringent, boil, brain, cancer, cataract, cholera, circulation, convulsion, dermatosis, diuretic, dysentery, eye, fever, hypertension, infection, insanity, insecticide, lactogogue (veterinary), leprosy, longevity, lung, medicine, narcotic, nervine, pleuritis, poultice, refrigerant, respiratory, spasm, stimulant, tonic, tuberculosis, tumor (abdomen), venereal, wound (Duke, Beckstrom-Sternberg, Wain, 1995).

Guarana, *Paullinia cupana* Kunth (Sapindacaea)

Guarana is one of several caffeine-containing Amazonian CNS stimulants. The active ingredient caffeine is mainly used to counteract drowsiness but also used therapeutically in combination with salicylates for the treatment of headache. Caffeine also has antiasthmatic, anticarcinogenic, anticariogenic, antidermatitic, antiemetic, antiherpetic, antiobesity, antioxidant, and antiviral activities, among many others (Duke, 1992a, 1992b; Tyler, 1994; Williamson, Evans, 1989).

Ethnobotanical uses: Astringent, coffee, diarrhea, intoxicant, migraine, nervine, neuralgia, stimulant, tonic (Duke, Beckstrom-Sternberg, Wain, 1995).

Hawthorn, *Crataegus laevigata* (Poiret) DC., *C. rhipidophylla* Gand., *C. monogyna* Jacq. (Rosaceae)

Widely respected in Europe as a gentle cardiac tonic with antianginal, antiatherosclerotic, antiarrhythmic, and hypotensive properties, hawthorn is an excellent food pharmaceutical. Animal studies have indicated improvements in blood pressure, coronary blood flow, and heart rate. Williamson and Evans (1989) attribute some of these properties to amines. Clinical studies show significant improvement in cardiac function, dyspnea, and edema in pa-

tients treated with a hawthorn preparation. In Europe, hawthorn preparations are widely used for angina. Hawthorn is safe to use for extended periods of time, according to European studies. Hawthorn induces dilation of the smooth muscles of the coronary vessels, thereby lowering their resistance and increasing blood flow, which reduces anginal tendencies. Hawthorn has positive inotropic effects. It accelerates heart rate and increases nerve conductivity and heart muscle irritability (American Botanical Council, 1995; Tyler, 1994; Williamson, Evans, 1989).

Ethnobotanical uses: Arteriosclerosis, cardiotonic, cyanogenetic, depurative, discutient, diuretic, dyspnea, fumitory, hypertension, hypotensive, intestinal tonic, spasm, stomachic, tea (Duke, Beckstrom-Sternberg, Wain, 1995).

Hop, *Humulus lupulus* L. (Cannabaceae)

An anodyne and aromatic bitter with diuretic, hypnotic, sedative, and tonic effects, hops are well known for their tranquilizing activity, caused in part by methylbutenol. Taken orally, hop resin has no CNS-depressant effect, but when stored, bitter principles such as humulone and lupulone undergo autooxidation to produce methylbutenol (Tyler, 1994). Methylbutenol does produce CNS-depressant effects when inhaled, although a single effective dose would require all of the compound in 150 g of hops. Hop pillows are popular with insomniacs. Hops also have antiseptic and spasmolytic activity; the extracts are strongly spasmolytic on isolated smooth muscle tissues. Most hops are grown for the brewery industry. Whether useful pharmacologic effects survive the brewing process is debatable. Recently, beer has been reported to have estrogenic activity (Duke, 1997; Tyler, 1994; Williamson, Evans, 1989).

Ethnobotanical uses: Anaphrodisiac, anodyne, antiseptic, astringent, bitter principle, boil, cancer, cystitis, debility, diuretic, dyspepsia, fever, hypnotic, inflammation, nerve, nervine, poultice, rheumatism, sedative, shampoo, soporific, stomachic, sudorific, tea, tonic, tuberculosis, tumor (liver), vermifuge (Duke, Beckstrom-Sternberg, Wain, 1995).

Horehound, *Marrubium vulgare* L. (Lamiaceae)

Horehound is an antiseptic, cholagogic, expectorant, and bitter tonic herb used for asthma, bronchitis, colds, and coughs (the latter for more than 400 years). By stimulating secretions of the bronchial mucosa, it helps bronchial catarrh, dyspepsia, and inappetence. Marrubiin is considered expectorant. It has also been shown to normalize extrasystolic arrhythmias. When the lactone ring is open, the corresponding acid is strongly choleretic. Marrubiin is also reportedly choleretic and secretogogic. The antiseptic essential oil is reportedly hypotensive and vasodilatory. Extracts of horehound are antiedemic and antiinflammatory and exhibit antiserotonin activity. An ingredient of some tonics, horehound has been added to candies and lozenges and brewed into ales. It may also be consumed as a tea (Tyler, 1994; Williamson, Evans, 1989).

Ethnobotanical uses: Alterative, antiseptic, asthma, astringent, bilious, bronchitis, carminative, catarrh, cholagogue, cholera, cold, cough, debility, diarrhea, diuretic, dysmenorrhea, emmenagogue, expectorant, extrasystole, fever, heart, hepatitis, hypertension, kidney, larvicide, laxative, liqueur, lung, obesity, palpitation, pertussis, sore (throat), spasm, stimulant, stomachic, sudorific, tea, tonic, tumor, vermifuge, witchcraft (Duke, Beckstrom-Sternberg, Wain, 1995).

Horsechestnut, *Aesculus hippocastanum* L. (Hippocastanaceae)

More popular in Europe than the United States, horsechestnut is considered antiinflammatory, astringent, and febrifugal. Extracts of horsechestnut preparations of aescin are used for hemorrhoids, rheumatism, varicosities, and other venous congestion. Aescin has been shown to eliminate edema and reduce exudation. It antagonizes the effects of bradykinin, although it is not a direct bradykinin antagonist. It has antiinflammatory activity and causes an increase in plasma levels of ACTH, corticosterone, and glucose in rats. Aescin is also active against the influenza virus in vitro (Williamson, Evans, 1989). Hippocaesculin and barringtogenol-C-21-angelate have antitumor activity in vitro (Williamson, Evans, 1989). Germany's Commission E has approved the use of horsechestnut seeds for the treatment of chronic venous insufficiency, a feeling of heaviness in the legs, varicose veins, and postthrombotic syndrome. Horsechestnut is antiexudative and acts to increase tonus of the veins. It may cause gastrointestinal irritation, renal and hepatic toxicity (rare), and anaphylactic reaction following intravenous administration (Tyler, 1994).

Ethnobotanical uses: Alterative, analgesic, anodyne, astringent, back, cancer, fever, hemostatic, malaria, narcotic, neuralgia, pertussis, piles, poison, preventive (rheumatism), rectitis, rectum, rheumatism, sclerosis (breast), sore, sternutatory, tonic, vasoconstrictor, vulnerary (Duke, Beckstrom-Sternberg, Wain, 1995).

Horsetail, *Equisetum arvense* L. (Equisetaceae)

Regarded as astringent and hemostatic, horsetail is used for cystitis, enuresis, prostatitis, and urethritis. It is used internally as an antihemorrhagic and externally as a styptic and vulnerary. The hemostatic substance is active orally. It has no effect on blood pressure and vasoconstriction. Because of its high natural silica content, it is marketed in the United States as a treatment for arthritis, poor bone development, and poor hair and skin (Duke, 1997; Williamson, Evans, 1989).

Ethnobotanical uses: Albuminuria, anodyne, antiseptic, astringent, bladder, calculus, cancer, cancer (bones), carminative, consumption, diabetes, diarrhea, diuretic, dropsy, dyspepsia, gout, gravel, hematuria, hemopoietic, hemoptysis, hemostat, kidney, lung, pile, poison, sore, tuberculosis, tumor, wound (Duke, Beckstrom-Sternberg, Wain, 1995).

Hyssop, *Hyssopus officinalis* L. (Lamiaceae)

Regarded as carminative, pectoral, sedative, and stimulant, hyssop is used for bronchitis, colds, and coughs. Marrubiin is reportedly antiarrhythmic, choleretic, expectorant, and secretogogic. Another component, ursolic acid, has analgesic, antiarthritic, antidiabetic, antiedemic, antihepatotoxic, antihistaminic, anti-HIV, antiinflammatory, antileukemic, antimutagenic, antioxidant, and antitumor activities. The extracted oil is nontoxic and nonphotosensitizing to the skin. Hyssop may be taken as an herbal tea. Some researchers have recently speculated that hyssop may help in AIDS. Crude extracts showed strong anti-HIV activity as measured by inhibition of syncytia formation, HIV reverse transcriptase, and antigen expression (Duke, 1992a, 1992b, 1997; Kreis and others, 1990; Williamson, Evans, 1989).

Ethnobotanical uses: Ache (tooth), asthma, bronchitis, carminative, catarrh, cold, cough, diuretic, dyspepsia, emmenagogue, expectorant, gall, hoarseness, kidney, lung, nerve, night sweat, ophthalmia, pectoral, resolvent, sclerosis (liver), stimulant, stomachic, sudorific, tonic, tonsillitis, tumor, tumor (abdomen), urogenital, vermifuge (Duke, Beckstrom-Sternberg, Wain, 1995).

Iceland Moss, *Cetraria islandica* (L.) Ach. (Parmeliaceae)

The antiemetic, demulcent, expectorant, and nutritive properties of Iceland moss (actually a lichen) are mostly due to polysaccharides. Some lichen acids have antibiotic properties. The decoction is reportedly effective for dry coughs and sore mouth and throat (Tyler, 1994; Williamson, Evans, 1989).

Ethnobotanical uses: Demulcent, laxative (Duke, Beckstrom-Sternberg, Wain, 1995).

Ipecac, *Phychotria ipecacuanha* (Brot.) Stokes (Rubiaceae)

The root of this small rainforest shrub is regarded as an amebicidal, diaphoretic, emetic, and expectorant stimulant. In large doses, it is poisonous. Ipecac extract is used in many cough syrups because of its expectorant activity. In larger doses, ipecac is emetic and used to induce vomiting in children who have ingested poisons or adults who have overdosed on certain drugs. Emetine and cephaeline have proven antiamebic activities. They also show some antitumor activity in vitro but have not proved useful in leukemia (Duke, 1992a; Duke, 1992b; Tyler, 1994; Williamson, Evans, 1989).

Ethnobotanical uses: Ameba, amebiasis, amebicide, aperitif, astringent, cancer, cholagogue, diaphoretic, dysentery, emetic, epithelioma, expectorant, hemostat, insect repellant, poison, spasm, sternutatory, sudorific (Duke, Beckstrom-Sternberg, Wain, 1995).

Irish Moss, *Chondrus crispus* (L.) Stackh. (Gigartinaceae)

This antitussive, demulcent, nutritive alga is used for bladder problems, bronchitis, coughs, and nephritis. The carrageenins of low molecular weight (around 20,000 kilodalton), including degraded forms, have been reported to be toxic in animals when injected and ingested. No toxicity has been observed in humans. Food grades of high molecular weight are not normally absorbed through the gut and are considered to be nontoxic. Irish moss is used extensively in processed foods (Williamson, Evans, 1989).

Jewelweed, *Impatiens capensis* Meerb. (Balsaminaceae)

The American species is one of the most widely known folk remedies for poison ivy and urticaria. Fresh crushed leaves are rubbed onto the body immediately after contact with poison ivy to prevent fixation of the urushiol. The juice, perhaps because of the lawsone it contains, seems to have antihistaminic activity with nettle stings. (One acquaintance of the senior author found it prevented an unusual black and blue contusion that otherwise followed the sting.) Elsewhere, fresh plants are poulticed or made into unguents for hemorrhoids. The juice is reputed to remove warts and corns and alleviate ringworm (Tyler, 1994; Williamson, Evans, 1989).

Ethnobotanical uses: Anodyne, antidote (rhus), antidote *(Urtica),* bruise, poison ivy, wart (Duke, Beckstrom-Sternberg, Wain, 1995).

Juniper, *Juniperus communis* L. (Cupressaceae)

With berries that are considered antiinflammatory, antiseptic, carminative, and diuretic, juniper is used for cystitis, rheumatism, and urethritis. The antiinflammatory effects have been demonstrated in vivo. It is normally avoided during pregnancy because it is potentially toxic. Juniper is a main flavor ingredient in gin. Among the an-

tiseptic compounds in juniper are borneol, camphor, citronellal, formic acid, limonene, linalol menthol, alpha-terpineol, and umbelliferone (Duke, 1992a, 1992b; Tyler, 1994; Williamson, Evans, 1989).

Ethnobotanical uses: Arteriosclerosis, bite (snake), bronchitis, carminative, cephalic, colic, deobstruent, depurative, diaphoretic, digestive, diuretic, dropsy, dysentery, emmenagogue, empyreumatic, fumigant, gleet, gonorrhea, gout, hysteria, incense, kidney, leucorrhea, liniment, liqueur, lung, medicine, medicine (veterinary), rheumatism, short-windedness, skin, stimulant, stomachic, sudorific, tenesmus, tumor, urogenital, venereal, vermifuge, wart, wound (Duke, Beckstrom-Sternberg, Wain, 1995).

Kola, *Cola acuminata* (Beauv.) Schott & Endl. (Sterculiaceae)

Like most caffeine-containing plants, kola yields an antidepressant, astringent, cardiotonic, diuretic, and stimulant beverage. Its extracts are used in many tonics and soft drinks for depression, lack of appetite, and fatigue. It is therapeutically combined with salicylates for headache. The main active ingredient is caffeine, which has antiasthmatic, anticarcinogenic, anticariogenic, antidermatitic, antiemetic, antiherpetic, antiobesity, antioxidant, and antiviral activities, among many others. As an astringent, kola is also effective in diarrhea (Duke, 1992a, 1992b; Tyler, 1994; Williamson, Evans, 1989).

Ethnobotanical uses: Aphrodisiac, cancer, cardiotonic, CNS-stimulant, digestive, diuretic, hunger, nerve, stimulant, tonic, tumor (Duke, Beckstrom-Sternberg, Wain, 1995).

Lavender, *Laveandula angustifolia* Mill. (Lamiaceae)

Aromatherapy may originate with lavender, the oil of which was used to treat the burns of an early proponent of aromatherapy. Volatile compounds from lavender oil, applied topically, can be detected in the exhaled breath within minutes, demonstrating a little-known fact: Many volatile aromatic compounds are absorbed through the skin. Cineole, one active CNS stimulant, actually speeds up transdermal absorption of other compounds, sometimes 100-fold. Antidepressant, carminative, spasmolytic, and tonic, the antiseptic oil of low toxicity reportedly has CNS-depressant activity in mice. Lavender is widely used in lotions and perfumes. Spike lavender serves as an insect repellant (Duke, 1997; Williamson, Evans, 1989).

Ethnobotanical uses: Carminative, cholagogue, diuretic, nervine, perfume, repellant (insect), spasm, stimulant, stomachic, sudorific, vermifuge (Duke, Beckstrom-Sternberg, Wain, 1995).

Lemon, *Citrus limon* (L.) Burm. f. (Rutaceae)

The citroflavonoids from lemon (and other citrus fruits) are used in vascular disorders such as hemorrhoids and other varicosities related to venous insufficiency. Citroflavonoids control vascular permeability of liquids and proteins by decreasing porosity. They are also reportedly antiinflammatory, antihistaminic, and diuretic. A modest source of vitamin C, lemons are used in beverages, essences, foods, and flavorings (Duke, 1997; Williamson, Evans, 1989).

Ethnobotanical uses: Aperitif, arteriosclerosis, carminative, cold, corn, diaphoretic, diarrhea, digestive, diuretic, dysentery, epilepsy, fever, inflammation, pneumonia, rheumatism, rubefacient, scurvy, sedative, shampoo, spleen, stimulant, stomach, stomachic, tonic, tumor (glands), wart (Duke, Beckstrom-Sternberg, Wain, 1995).

Lemongrass, *Cymbopogon citratus* (DC. ex Nees) Stapf; *C. flexuosus* (Nees ex Steudel) J.F.Watson (Poaceae)

Closely related to citronella, the lemon grasses are widely used in folk medicine, herbal teas, and perfumery. Most share many of the same insect repellant compounds.

Ethnobotanical uses: *C. citratus:* Abdomen, ache (head), ache (stomach), ache (tooth), anodyne, antiseptic, antispasmodic, carminative, cold, consumption, cough, cyanogenetic, dentifrice, depurative, diaphoretic, diuretic, dyspepsia, elephantiasis, emmenagogue, expectorant, eye, fever, flu, gingivitis, hypertension, insecticide, intestine, leprosy, malaria, mouthwash, neuritis, pectoral, perfume, pneumonia, preventive (cold), pyorrhea, rheumatism, spasm, sprain, stimulant, sudorific, tea, tonic.

Ethnobotanical uses: *C. flexuosus*: Cholera, insect repellant, rheumatic (Duke, Beckstrom-Sternberg, Wain, 1995).

Licorice, *Glycyrrhiza glabra* L. (Fabaceae)

With proven antiinflammatory, antitussive, antiulcer, demulcent, expectorant, and spasmolytic activities, licorice, commonly used in European, Arabian, and Asian traditional medicine, is frequently used for gastric and duodenal ulcers and adrenocortical insufficiency. Licorice extract stimulates the adrenal glands and is therefore used for fatigue caused by adrenal exhaustion. The major active ingredient is glycyrrhizin, which is 50 times sweeter than sugar. Some derivatives are comparable to codeine in antitussive activity. Both glycyrrhizin and glycyrrhetinic acid have antiinflammatory and antiallergic activities, making them useful for asthma. As antioxidants, they are also hepatoprotective. Chinese practitioners use licorice for liver diseases because it improves liver function tests in hepatitis, clears jaundice, and alleviates abdominal distension, nausea, and vomiting. These effects may also be due in part to the ability of glycyrrhizin to induce interferon. A derivative of glycyrrhetinic acid, carbenoxolone, is used in Great Britain for ulcers. Deglycyrrhizinized licorice extracts still protect against experimentally induced ulcers, but this effect has not yet been clinically proved. Possibly by inhibiting bacterial growth and plaque formation, glycyrrhizin has anticarcinogenic activity. The polysaccharide fraction has immunostimulating activity. Licorice has estrogenic activity in animals, perhaps because of its isoflavonoids. Licorice contains nearly a dozen in vitro MAO-inhibitors that may counteract depression: isoliquiritigenin, licocoumarone, licopyranocoumarin, licofuranone, genistein, glycyrrhisoflavone, glicoricone, glycyrrhizin, glycoumarin, licochalcone-A and B, and medicarpin. Liquiritin also has significant antiinflammatory activity. Licorice extracts have antihistamine activity in rats. They appear to have muscle relaxant activity and aid in detoxification of certain drugs such as cocaine, mercurous chloride, picrotoxin, strychnine, and urethane in animals. Licorice is also said to be antianemic, anticariogenic, antihepatotoxic, antimicrobial, antiviral, immunosuppressive, and lipolytic. It has potential in local application as a hydrocortisone potentiator in dermatologic preparations. Duke (1992a, 1992b) reports hundreds of biologically active compounds in licorice; in fact, dozens of activities are reported for glycyrrhizin alone. Unfortunately, glycyrrhizin and glycyrrhetinic acid have mineralocorticoid activity, which may result in edema, hypertension, and hypokalemia when large doses are taken over time (American Botanical Council, 1995; Duke, 1992a, 1992b; Tyler, 1994; Williamson, Evans, 1989).

Ethnobotanical uses: Addison's disease, alexiteric, alterative, anodyne, antidote, antispasmodic, antitussive, bactericide, boil, burn, cancer, cancer (esophagus), cancer (uterus), candida, catarrh, cough, demulcent, deodorant, depurative, diuretic, dyspnea, emollient, expectorant, fever, fungicide, internal ulcer, laxative, masticatory, pectoral, pill, rejuvenation, scald, sore, thirst, tonic, tumor, tumor (abdomen), urogenital, wound (Duke, Beckstrom-Sternberg, Wain, 1995).

Lily of the Valley, *Convallaria majalis* L. (Convallariaceae)

The cardiotonic convallaria has actions similar to digitalis but is less cumulative; it is therefore used in Europe to treat congestive heart failure. The isolated glycoside convallatoxin is the major active compound. Convallamaroside has antifungal and antibiotic activity but tends to form a complex with cholesterol in the body. Lily of the valley flowers are used in perfumery (Tyler, 1994; Williamson, Evans, 1989).

Ethnobotanical uses: Cardiotonic, diuretic, emetic, nervine, poison (Duke, Beckstrom-Sternberg, Wain, 1995).

Lime, *Citrus aurantifolia* (Christm.) Swingle (Rutaceae)

Limes are used more for flavoring than medicine, although the antiscorbutic lime juice, once used for the prevention of scurvy, allegedly gave rise to the term "limey" for British sailors. The expressed oil is used in perfumery. Experimentally, at levels of 0.1 µl/ml, lime oil inhibits acetylcholinesterase. Coumarins, like bergapten, have synergistic antifeedant and insect-repelling properties and may cause photosensitivity, although they are used in some suntan formulas. Related coumarins are used in PUVA (psoralen + ultraviolet-A) treatments for psoriasis. They may cause allergies in sensitive individuals (Duke, 1997; Williamson, Evans, 1989).

Ethnobotanical uses: Ache (tooth), antidote (manihot), antiseptic, aperitif, bactericide, bilious, catarrh, cold, cough, cystitis, depurative, dermatosis, diarrhea, dropsy, dysentery, dysmenorrhea, dyspepsia, emetic, empacho, epistaxis, erysipelas, fever, flu, gonorrhea, hair, headache, insomnia, liver, neuralgia, newborn, ophthalmia, pneumonia, purgative, refrigerant, rheumatism, scorpion, scurvy, soap, sore, sore (throat), stomachache, stomachic, thrush, urogenital, venereal, vermifuge, witchcraft, yaws, yellow fever (Duke, Beckstrom-Sternberg, Wain, 1995).

Lobelia, Indian Tobacco, *Lobelia inflata* L. (Campanulaceae)

Regarded as a diaphoretic, emetic, expectorant, and respiratory stimulant, lobelia is highly regarded for the treatment of asthma and bronchitis. Although the U.S. Food and Drug Administration (FDA) has not approved its use in smoking cessation programs, it is a major ingredient in some antismoking mixtures. With activities that are similar to but weaker than those of nicotine, lobeline may help alleviate nicotine withdrawal symptoms (Duke, 1997). Like nicotine, lobeline can be absorbed transdermally. Lobeline stimulates respiration in animals by stimulating the respiratory center; at high doses, it stimulates the vomiting center. The herb is sometimes used as a poultice on boils and ulcers. In Chinese medicine, *L. radicans* Thunb. (*L. chinensis* Louv.) is used for these purposes and also snake bite (when respiratory depression is involved) and jaundice (Tyler, 1994; Williamson, Evans, 1989).

Ethnobotanical uses: Antidote, antismoking, asthma, bronchitis, cancer, cancer (breast), convulsion, emetic, expectorant, eye, fumitory, narcotic, nervine, nicotinism, poison, sialogogue, spasm, sudorific, urticaria (Duke, Beckstrom-Sternberg, Wain, 1995).

Longleaf pine, *Pinus palustris* Mill. (Pinaceae)

The counterirritant and rubefacient turpentine, composed of resin from any of several pine species, is used externally in rheumatism and stiff muscles. Turpentine has been also taken internally but is relatively toxic. Turpentine is also used in the fragrance, music, and solvent industries. Volatile oil distilled from the oleoresin obtained from long-leaf pine has a long history of use in counterirritant preparations. It should not be applied more than 3 or 4 times daily (Tyler, 1994; Williamson, Evans, 1989).

Ethnobotanical uses: Antiseptic, arthritis, bronchitis, carminative, colic, cystitis, dandruff, diarrhea, diuretic, emmenagogue, expectorant, gonorrhea, hemostat, hiccup, inhalant, kidney, laxative, odontorrhagia, rheumatism, rubefacient, skin, skin stimulant, taenifuge, tapeworms, tuberculosis, tumor, tumor (abdomen), vermifuge (Duke, Beckstrom-Sternberg, Wain, 1995).

Lovage, *Levisticum officinale* W.D.J.Koch (Apiaceae)

Regarded as antiseptic, aquaretic, carminative, diaphoretic, diuretic, expectorant, sedative, and spasmolytic, the culinary herb lovage is used for colic, cystitis, dyspepsia, dysmenorrhea, kidney stones, and urethritis and as a gargle or mouthwash for sore throat, stomatitis, and tonsillitis. Phthalides, found in celery, lovage, and other umbellifers, have proven sedative and spasmolytic activity in animals. Extracts and essential oil are reportedly strongly diuretic in mice and rabbits. Lovage is used as a flavoring in food products and alcoholic beverages (Tyler, 1994; Williamson, Evans, 1989).

Ethnobotanical uses: Abortifacient, antiseptic, cancer, cancer (mouth), carminative, cordial, diaphoretic, diuretic, emmenagogue, expectorant, fever, nervine, stimulant, stomachic, sudorific, tonic (Duke, Beckstrom-Sternberg, Wain, 1995).

Marshmallow, *Althaea officinalis* L. (Malvaceae)

Antitussive, demulcent, emollient, and expectorant, the leaves and roots of the marshmallow are used for bronchitis, coughs, cystitis, enteritis, gastritis, peptic ulcers, and urethritis. They are used externally as soothing vulnerary ointments and poultices for abscesses, boils, and ulcers. The mucilages stimulate phagocytosis in vitro and produce hypoglycemic activity in mice. Extracts of marshmallow root are used in confectionery. Caffeic, chlorogenic, and ferulic acids share many important biologic activities, including analgesic, antihepatotoxic, antiinflammatory, antimutagenic, antitumor, and antiviral ones (Duke, 1992a, 1992b; Tyler, 1994; Williamson, Evans, 1989).

Ethnobotanical uses: Cancer, catarrh, cough, demulcent, emollient, expectorant, inflammation, intestine, lubricative, mucus, pectoral, piles, poultice, respiratory, sclerosis, sore (throat), tumor (Duke, Beckstrom-Sternberg, Wain, 1995).

Melissa, Balm, *Melissa officinalis* L. (Lamiaceae)

Lemon-scented lemon balm, widely known as melissa, is considered carminative, diaphoretic, febrifugal, and sedative. The weedy herb is frequently used in herbal teas, which have antiviral properties mainly because of rosmarinic acid and other polyphenolics. Creams with melissa extracts alleviate cutaneous lesions of herpes simplex. Aqueous extracts inhibit tumor cell division, and tannin-free extracts inhibit protein biosynthesis in cell-free systems of rat liver. The sedative effects, useful in psychiatric disorders such as dystonia, excitability, headache, palpitations, and restlessness, may result from synergistic interactions of several mild sedatives, including benzaldehyde, caryophyllene, citral, citronellal, citronellol, eugenol, geraniol, limonene, and linalol. Antihormonal and antithyroid effects of melissa are well documented. Freeze-dried aqueous extracts can inhibit many effects of exogenous and endogenous thyroid stimulating hormone (TSH) on bovine thyroid gland by interfering with the binding of TSH to plasma membranes and by inhibiting the enzyme iodothyronine deiodinase in vitro. These extracts also inhibit the receptor-binding and biologic activities of immunoglobulins in the blood of patients with Graves' disease, a condition that results in hyperthyroidism. Rosmarinic acid, one thyrotropic agent in lemon balm, reportedly also has the following activities: antianaphylactic, anticomplementary, antiedemic, antigonadotropic, antihemolytic, antihepatotoxic, antiherpetic, antiinflammatory, antioxidant, antithyreotropic, antithyroid, antiviral, bactericidal, and viricidal. It may also inhibit deiodinase and prevent cancer. The reputed spasmolytic effect has not been thoroughly substantiated (Duke, 1992a, 1992b; Williamson, Evans, 1989). Melissa shows some promise in the treatment of cold sores. Aqueous extracts have antiviral activity. A strong tea prepared from 2 or 3 teaspoonsful of finely cut leaves and about ½ cup of water applied to lesions several times daily inhibits herpes simplex virus types 1 and 2. Commission E found melissa an effective and safe calmative and carminative (Duke, 1992a, 1992b; Tyler, 1994; Williamson, Evans, 1989).

Ethnobotanical uses: Ache (head), ache (tooth), anodyne, antiseptic, calmative, carminative, cordial, cosmetic, digestive, emmenagogue, fever, lactogogue, nervine, perfume, sclerosis (liver), sedative, spasm, sternutatory, stimulant, stomachic, sudorific, tonic, tumor, virucide (Duke, Beckstrom-Sternberg, Wain, 1995).

Milk Thistle, *Silybum marianum* (L.) Gaertn. (Asteraceae)

Milk thistle was used in biblical times by nursing mothers (if not the Virgin Mary) and is regarded as antidepressant, choleretic, hepatoprotective, and tonic. German studies verify its effectiveness in liver diseases and jaundice, its most important uses today. Silymarin exerts an antihepatotoxic effect in animals against several toxins, notably those of the death cap mushroom, *Amanita phalloides,* which is occasionally ingested by mistake. The potent liver toxins are amatoxins and phallotoxins, which cause hemorrhagic liver necrosis. Pretreatment with silymarin and silybin affords 100% protection. Silybin given intravenously to humans up to 48 hours after ingestion of *Amanita* can prevent death. Silymarin, used for cirrhosis and chronic hepatitis, also has antierythemic, antiinflammatory, antileukotriene, antioxidant, antiulcer, antiviral, hypolipidemic, laxative, lipolytic, and sunscreen activities. It is active against hepatitis B virus and lowers fat deposits in the liver in animals. It protects against alcohol and many types of chemical toxins. The extract improves liver function, protects against liver damage, and enhances regeneration of damaged liver cells. Protein synthesis is stimulated, accelerating the regeneration process and the production of liver parenchyma cells. Silymarin functions as a free-radical scavenger and antioxidant. At least five lignans—silybin, silychristin, silydianin, silymarin and silymonin—seem to work together in protecting the liver (American Botanical Council, 1995; Duke, 1992a, 1992b; Tyler, 1994; Williamson, Evans, 1989).

Ethnobotanical uses: Alterative, asthma, calculus, cancer, chest, cholagogue, coffee, depurative, diabetes, dropsy, emmenagogue, fever, galactogogue, gallbladder, hemostat, hepatitis, jaundice, leukorrhea, poison, purgative, spleen, stimulant, sudorific, tonic (Duke, Beckstrom-Sternberg, Wain, 1995).

Mistletoe, *Viscum album* L. (Loranthaceae)

Somewhat poisonous but considered antineoplastic, antispasmodic, cardiotonic, hypotensive, immunostimulant, and sedative, mistletoe is used for high blood pressure and tachycardia, as a nervine, and for certain cancers. The cardiotonic activity is thought to be due to the lignans, which show significant cAMP-phosphodiesterase inhibitory activity. The polysaccharides stimulate the murine immune response. A commercial preparation increases antibody production in rats stimulated with antigen after irradiation. Antineoplastic activity has been documented. Viscotoxins bind to DNA, and viscumin inhibits protein synthesis. Alkaloids, where present, have antileukemic activity. A commercial preparation has been used for several types of cancer. In a study of 50 patients with malignant pleural effusions, the exudation disappeared in a remarkable 92% of patients after three or four treatments. In another study on the prophylactic postoperative treatment of carcinoma of the bronchial tree, patients showed better survival time. When treated with a mistletoe preparation, women with advanced ovarian carcinoma showed much better survival times than those in a group treated with conventional therapy, despite the less favorable prognosis of the group treated with mistletoe. Unproven and controversial, its antineoplastic effects when administered by injection are the subject of serious study. When mistletoe is properly administered, its side effects are said not to be serious (Tyler, 1994; Williamson, Evans, 1989).

Ethnobotanical uses: Antiseptic, arteriosclerosis, arthrosis, asthma, astringent, cancer, cardiac, cardiotonic, chorea, diuretic, emetic, epilepsy, galactogogue, hemorrhage, hepatomegaly, hypertension, hysteria, lumbago, malaria, metrorrhagia, narcotic, nervine, otitis, piles, poison, purgative, sedative, spasm, splenomegaly, styptic, tonic, tumor, uterus (Duke, Beckstrom-Sternberg, Wain, 1995).

Mullein, *Verbascum thapsus* L., *V. thapsiforme* Schrad., *V. densiflorum* Bertol., *V. phlomoides* Bertol. (Scrophulariaceae)

Regarded as demulcent, diuretic, emollient, expectorant, and vulnerary, mullein is used internally for bronchitis and catarrh and externally for inflammation and sores. Older herbal texts recommended steeping the yellow flowers for piles (Williamson, Evans, 1989). Teas are used for cough, respiratory catarrh, and sore throat. Aucubin, hesperidin, rotenone, and verbascoside are antiseptic (Duke, 1992a, 1992b; Tyler, 1994).

Ethnobotanical uses: Ache (ear), alterative, anodyne, antiseptic, aphrodisiac, asthma, astringent, baldness, bronchitis, bruise, cardiotonic, catarrh, chest, cold, congestion, cough, cramp, croup, dandruff, demulcent, diarrhea (veterinary), diuretic, dysentery, ear, emollient, expectorant, fever, frostbite, fumitory, hairblack, inflammation, lung, lung (veterinary), malaria, medicine, migraine, mucous, narcotic, pectoral, piles, piscicide, poultice, ringworm, shampoo, sore (throat), spasm, sudorific, sunburn, tumor, vulnerary (Duke, Beckstrom-Sternberg, Wain, 1995).

Myrrh, *Commiphora myrrha* (Nees) Engl., *C. habessinica* (O. Berg) Engl., and Possibly Other *Commiphora* spp. (Burseraceae)

Biblical myrrh, regarded as antiinflammatory, antiseptic, antispasmodic, carminative, and expectorant, is used internally for gastroses, gingivitis, pharyngitis, and tonsillitis. Externally, it is used for boils, ulcers, and wounds. Myrrh, the oleoresin that exudes from bark incisions, has been used for mild inflammations of the mucous membranes of the mouth and throat. The tincture is applied locally to canker sores 2 or 3 times daily. Five to ten drops of tincture is mixed in a glass of water as a gargle for sore throat. Reportedly antiseptic in vitro, extracts of *C. abyssinica* stimulate phagocytosis in mice inoculated with *E. coli*. India's gugul resin is hypolipidemic and hypocholesterolemic in both humans and animals and may lower triglycerides; it increases catecholamine biosynthesis and

activity in cholesterol-fed rabbits and has antiaggregant, antiinflammatory, and possibly thyrotropic effects in rats and chickens (Tyler, 1994; Williamson, Evans, 1989).

Ethnobotanical uses: Alterative, antiseptic, astringent, embalming, emmenagogue, expectorant, hysteria, lochia, mania, sedative, sore, spasm, stimulant, stomachic, uterus, wound (Duke, Beckstrom-Sternberg, Wain, 1995).

Nettle, *Urtica dioica* L., *U. urens* L. (Urticaceae)

The astringent hemostatic tonic, stinging nettle, has moved from folklore to the phytomedicinal arena, at least in Europe, where it is now recommended for allergy, benign prostatic hyperplasia, and hay fever. According to folklore, it was once popular for bleeding and dermatoses such as eczema and skin eruptions. Extracts are said to be mildly aquaretic and hypoglycemic. Nettles were a classical source of chlorophyll. The stinging hairs deliver microinjections of acetylcholine, choline, histamine, and serotonin. Massive exposure to nettle plants has caused severe symptoms of shock in animals. (Duke, 1992a, 1992b, 1997; Tyler, 1994; Williamson, Evans, 1989).

Ethnobotanical uses: Ache, ache (back), alopecia, anodyne, asthma, astringent, ataxia (locomotor), bactericide, blood, bronchitis, bruise, burn, cancer, catarrh, chest, cholecystitis, cholangitis, constipation, cosmetic, cough, counterirritant, dandruff, depurative, diuretic, dropsy, dyspnea, emmenagogue, epilepsy, epistaxis, evil eye, fit, gout, hair tonic, hematemesis, hematoptysis, hemorrhage, hemostat, homeopathy, insanity, massage, menorrhagia, metrorrhagia, paralysis, parturition, purgative, rheumatism, shampoo, shigellosis, sore, sprain, stimulant, stomachic, suppository, swelling, tantrum, tea, tonic, tumor, urticaria, vasoconstrictor, vermifuge, wound (Duke, Beckstrom-Sternberg, Wain, 1995).

Night-Blooming Cereus, *Hylocereus undatus*, (Haw.) Britton and Rose (Cactaceae)

With a reputation as a cardiotonic and diuretic, this epiphytic cactus has been used for angina, arrhythmia, and other cardiopathies. The effects of night-blooming cereus may be due to cactine, and its steroidal structures and physiologic functions are similar to those of digitalis (Tyler, 1994; Williamson, Evans, 1989).

Ethnobotanical uses: Dropsy, fungoid, rheumatism (Duke, Beckstrom-Sternberg, Wain, 1995).

Oak, *Quercus* sp. (Fagaceae)

Oak bark, usually antiseptic, astringent, and hemostatic, is used for diarrhea, hemorrhoids, and sore throat (Williamson, Evans, 1989). In the United States, practitioners originally used the dried inner bark of white oak, *Quercus alba* L.; many different oaks are now used medicinally. Various tannins, including quercitannic acid, underlie the activity. A decoction (1 pint water and 2 teaspoonsful coarsely powdered bark) applied directly to the skin is used for dermatitis. It is also used as a mouthwash for inflammations of the oral cavity (Tyler, 1994).

Ethnobotanical uses: Adenopathy, anodyne, astringent, cancer, coffee, congestion, diarrhea, diuretic, dysentery, epilepsy, erythema, flux, fungicide, gum, intestine, piles, poison, puerperium, sore, spasm, stomach, styptic, tea, thirst, tubercle, tumor, vermifuge, vertigo (Duke, Beckstrom-Sternberg, Wain, 1995).

Oats, *Avena sativa* L. (Poaceae)

Oat straw, equivocally reported to be antidepressant, cardiotonic, and thymoleptic, is used for debility, depression, dysmenorrhea, and impotence. Reports that extracts counteract morphinism and nicotinism have been contested. Externally emollient, oat extracts and the colloidal fraction are used in baths for dry skin and eczema (Duke, 1997; Williamson, Evans, 1989).

Ethnobotanical uses: Demulcent, diuretic, nervine, poison, spasm, stimulant, tonic, tumor, tumor (abdomen), vulnerary (Duke, Beckstrom-Sternberg, Wain, 1995).

Oleander, *Nerium oleander* L. (Apocynaceae)

Oleander plants contain cardioactive glycosides with steroidal structures and physiologic functions similar to those of digitalis (Tyler, 1994). Oleander is too dangerous for folk use.

Ethnobotanical uses: Aposteme, atheroma, carcinoma, cardiac, cardiotonic, corn, cyanogenetic, diuretic, emetic, epithelioma, eruption, homicide, insecticide, insect repellant, parasiticide, poison, psoriasis, purgative, repellant (insect), rodenticide, scabies, skin, sore, sternutatory, stimulant, tonic, tumor, wart, weakness (Duke, Beckstrom-Sternberg, Wain, 1995).

Orange: Bitter Orange, Sweet Orange, *Citrus aurantium* L., *C. sinensis* (L.) Osbeck (Rutaceae)

Leaves, oils, and peels of oranges and many other citrus species are regarded as carminative and stomachic. The flavonoids are antiinflammatory, bacteriostatic, and fungistatic. Limonene has been widely promoted as a breast cancer preventive and an insecticide. Orange peel and oils are used to flavor beverages, candies, foods, and medicine. The juice is a mediocre source of vitamin C (Duke, 1992a, 1992b; Williamson, Evans, 1989). Whether the startling ability of

grapefruit juice to potentiate calcium channel blockers and certain anti-AIDS drugs is due to phytochemicals shared with other citrus species remains unknown.

Ethnobotanical uses: Abdomen, ache (head), ache (stomach), anodyne, antidote (fish), antidote (lobster), antidote (shrimp), antifertility, antiseptic, aperitif, bactericide, bubo, cancer, cancer (breast), cancer (stomach), carminative, chest, congestion, deobstruent, depurative, diarrhea, dysmenorrhea, dyspepsia, dyspnea, emmenagogue, expectorant, fever, freckle, fungicide, gallbladder, heart, hemostat, hypertension, laxative, liver, marasmus, menorrhagia, mouthwash, narcotic, nausea, nerve, nervine, oliguria, panacea, pectoral, pimple, prolapse, purgative, rectocele, refrigerant, rib, scurvy, sedative, shampoo, sore, spasm, splenitis, splenomegaly, stimulant, stomach, stomachic, styptic, sudorific, tea, thirst, thrush, tonic, tranquilizer, urogenital, uterus, vermifuge, wine-nose (Duke, Beckstrom-Sternberg, Wain, 1995).

Papaya, *Carica papaya* L. (Caricaceae)

The papaya is the source of two medicinal proteolytic enzymes, chymopapain and papain. These and other enzymes hydrolyze polypeptides, amides, and esters, particularly in alkaline media, to aid digestion and counteract digestive disorders. Papain is being strongly promoted for arthritis because it may break up circulating immune complexes. These enzymes are also used for healing wounds and ameliorating scarring. Enzymes are used for ocular disorders and slipped disks. Inhalation of the enzyme powder can induce allergies; it is otherwise nontoxic orally. Papain is used to tenderize meat. The leaves and seeds of the papaya are used in native medicine as an anthelmintic, the latex to remove warts, and the roots and leaves as a diuretic (Duke, 1992a, 1992b, 1997; Williamson, Evans, 1989).

Ethnobotanical uses: Abortifacient, ache (head), ache (tooth), amebicide, anodyne, antibiotic, antiphlogistic, arthritis, asthma, bactericide, boil, cancer, cardiac, cardiotonic, cholagogue, colic, constipation, corn, decoagulant, diarrhea, digestive, diphtheria, diuretic, dysentery, dyspepsia, dysuria, ecbolic, elephantiasis, emmenagogue, enteritis, epithelioma, expectorant, fever, flu, freckle, fumitory, fungicide, gravel, hemoptysis, hypertension, infection, itch, laxative, leukoderma, liver, longevity, madness, oliguria, pectoral, pediculicide, psoriasis, rheumatism, ringworm, scorpion, soap, sore, splenitis, stomachic, suppurative, tea, tenderizer, tuberculosis, tumor, tumor (uterus), ulcer, venereal, vermifuge, wart, wound (Duke, Beckstrom-Sternberg, Wain, 1995).

Parsley, *Petroselinum crispum* (Mill.) Nym. ex A.W. Hill (Apiaceae)

The culinary herb parsley is credited with aperient, antirheumatic, antiseptic, carminative, diuretic, expectorant, sedative, and spasmolytic activities. The flavonoids, particularly apigenin, have antihistaminic, antiinflammatory, and antiradicular activity to inhibit histamine release and act as free radical scavengers. Apiole is reportedly antipyretic, diuretic, emmenagogic, hepatotoxic, secretolytic, spasmolytic, and uterotonic. It may also function as a vasodilator. Phthalides are sedative in mice (Duke, 1992a, 1992b; Williamson, Evans, 1989). Data above, like those of Tyler (1994), seem to imply that overdoses of parsley could be abortifacient, phototoxic, and uterotonic. Despite these drawbacks, it is used to reduce urethritis and eliminate kidney stones (Tyler, 1994).

Ethnobotanical uses: Abortifacient, antibiotic, antifertility, aperient, aperitif, bite (bug), bruise, cancer, carminative, depurative, diuretic, ecbolic, emmenagogue, fever, kidney, parasiticide, pediculicide, poison, spice, stimulant, stomachic, sudorific, uteritis (Duke, Beckstrom-Sternberg, Wain, 1995).

Passionflower, *Passiflora incarnata* L. (Passifloraceae)

The beautiful North American maypop, or passionflower, is considered to have anodyne, antispasmodic, hypnotic, hypotensive, sedative, and tranquilizing activities. *Passiflora* extracts have CNS-depressant and hypotensive activities; they are used for their antitachycardic, anxiolytic, hypotensive, sedative, and soothing properties. The harmaline alkaloids and the flavonoids are sedative, as is the 8-pyrone derivative. Apigenin is well known for its antiaggregant, antiinflammatory, antiplatelet, and spasmolytic activities. It was only recently proved to be the sedative ingredient in chamomile. Harmaline has anthelminthic, antileishmanial, antimalarial, antiparkinsonian, aphrodisiac (5 mg per mouse), bactericidal, bradycardic, desmutagenic, and hallucinogenic (4 mg/kg orally in man) activities. It may also be a CNS stimulant and an MAO inhibitor. (Duke, 1992a, 1992b; Duke, 1997; Williamson, Evans, 1989). Germany's Commission E has authorized its use in the treatment of nervous unrest (American Botanical Council, 1995; Tyler, 1994).

Ethnobotanical uses: Aphrodisiac, burn, cyanogenetic, diarrhea, dysmenorrhea, epilepsy, eruption, eye, insomnia, morphinism, narcotic, neuralgia, neurosis, perfume, pile, sedative, skin, soporific, spasm (Duke, Beckstrom-Sternberg, Wain, 1995).

Pau d'Arco, *Tabebuia impetiginosa* (C. Martius ex DC.) Standley (Bignoniaceae)

This bark, sold under the names *ipe roxo, lapacho, pau d'arco,* and *taheebo,* is used as a tea to treat cancers, fungal infections, and yeast infections. Some researchers suggest that it is effective in cancer because of its content of lapachol derivatives, but this effectiveness remains unproven.

The National Cancer Institute was unable to obtain blood levels of lapachol that were high enough to be effective. Antibacterial, antiinflammatory, antifungal, antitumor, and candidicidal activities are reported for some of the phytochemicals. Pau d'arco is being promoted for immune dysfunction, mycoses, and yeast infections (Duke, 1997; Tyler, 1994).

Peppermint, *Mentha piperita* (Lamiaceae)

Grown around the world, peppermint is esteemed as an antiemetic, antiseptic, antispasmodic, bactericide, carminative, cholagogue, diaphoretic, refrigerant, and stimulant. It is used in herbal teas for colic and dyspepsia and is an ingredient in some cough and cold remedies. Menthol, similarly ingested or inhaled, has dozens of reported activities (e.g., analgesic, anesthetic, antiacetylcholinesterase, antiaggregant, antiallergic, antibronchitic, antidandruff, antihalitosic, antihistaminic, antiinflammatory, antineuralgic, antiodontalgic, antipruritic, antipyretic, antirheumatic, antiseptic (4 × phenol), antisinusitic). The spasmolytic and carminative effects have been demonstrated in vivo and in vitro. Like many mints, peppermint extracts also have antiviral effects. Peppermint is still popular as a flavoring for candies, gums, ice cream, liqueurs, sauces, gargles, medicines, mouthwashes, and toothpastes. Menthol is still used in cigarettes. Internally, peppermint has an antispasmodic action, with a calming effect on the stomach and intestinal tract that is often exploited by proctologists. Peppermint is used for biliary problems, dyspepsia, gastritis, gingivitis, irritable bowel syndrome, and nausea (American Botanical Council, 1995; Duke, 1992a; Duke, 1992b; Tyler, 1994; Williamson, Evans, 1989).

Ethnobotanical uses: Ache (head), ache (stomach), anesthetic, anodyne, antidote, antiseptic, aphrodisiac, astringent, bronchitis, cancer, carminative, cholagogue, cold, colic, dyspepsia, liqueur, massage, migraine, myalgia, nausea, navel, nervine, preventative (dyspepsia), rheumatism, sclerosis (limb), spasm, stimulant, stomach, stomachic, tea, tooth whitener, tumor, vermifuge (Duke, Beckstrom-Sternberg, Wain, 1995).

Plantain, *Plantago major* L., *P. lanceolata* L. (Plantaginaceae)

Picturesquely known as the white man's footprint, plantain leaves are considered antihistaminic, antiinflammatory, astringent, and diuretic. Plantain is a common folkloric remedy for bee and nettle stings. Aucubin, which stimulates the secretion of uric acid by the kidneys, might be useful in gout. Aucubin is also reportedly antidotal (Amanitin), antiinflammatory, antioxidant, bactericidal, cathartic, and diuretic. Apigenin, an antiinflammatory, antiplatelet, and spasmolytic compound, has recently proved to have sedative activity also. Baicalein exhibits antiallergic, antiinflammatory, choleretic, diuretic, febrifugal, fungicidal, hypocholesterolemic, lipoxygenase-inhibiting, and triglycerolytic activities. Chinese practitioners use plantain for bacillary dysentery, hepatitis, tuberculous ulcers, urinary diseases, and other conditions. The antiseptic extracts have complex effects on the cardiovascular system. Plantain is a soothing cough suppressant when prepared as a tea and can also be used for dermatitis and stomatitis (Duke, 1992a, 1992b; Tyler, 1994; Williamson, Evans, 1989).

Ethnobotanical uses: Ache (ear), ache (head), ache (tooth), alexiteric, alterative, amebiasis, anodyne, antidiarrheic, antidote (bee sting), antiphlogistic, antitussive, aperitif, aphrodisiac, astringent, bacteriostat, bite (bug), bite (snake), bladder, bladder stone, blepharitis, blisters, boil, bruise, burn, cachexia, cancer, cancer (mouth), cancer (uterus), catarrh, chest, cold, collyrium, conjunctivitis, cough, debility, demulcent, deobstruent, depurative, diabetes, diarrhea, diuretic, dysentery, dysuria, ecthyma, edema, emission, epistaxis, expectorant, fever, gargle, gonorrhea, gravel, hematuria, hemostat, homeopathy, hypertension, impetigo, infection, inflammation, kidney, labor, laxative, liver, lung, nephritis, neuroblastoma, onychosis, ophthalmia, piles, poultice, prostatitis, protisticide, refrigerant, renitis, rheumatism, sedative, skin, sore, spermatorrhea, sterility (male), stimulant, sting, stomatitis, stone, suppurative, thrush, tonic, tumor, tumor (feet), ulcer, urethritis, urogenital, vermifuge, vulnerary, wart, wound (Duke, Beckstrom-Sternberg, Wain, 1995).

Pleurisy Root, *Asclepias tuberosa* L. (Asclepiadaceae)

The pleurisy root is believed to be antispasmodic, aperient, carminative, diaphoretic, expectorant, and tonic. As its name suggests, its main use is to ease pain and facilitate breathing in pleurisy. It is also used for uterine disorders. Estrogenic activity has been demonstrated in rats (Williamson, Evans, 1989).

Ethnobotanical uses: Aperient, bronchitis, carminative, cathartic, colic, debility, diaphoretic, diuretic, emetic, expectorant, fungoid, hemorrhage, hysteria, medicine, panacea, pleurisy, poultice, sore, spasm, sudorific, tonic (Duke, Beckstrom-Sternberg, Wain, 1995).

Pot Marigold, Calendula, *Calendula officinalis* L. (Asteraceae)

Nearly a panacea, the carotenoid-rich calendula flowers reportedly have antihemorrhagic, antiinflammatory, antiseptic, antispasmodic, styptic, and vulnerary activities. Internally, marigold tea is taken for dysmenorrhea, gastroses, and gastric and duodenal ulcers; externally, it is applied to bruises, burns, cuts, diaper rash, sore nipples, and scalds. Alcoholic extracts show in vitro antitrichomonal activity. The orange petals (more properly ligulate florets) alleviate various skin ailments and facilitate wound healing. Tea can be used as a gargle or mouthwash for sores in the mouth, poulticed onto skin ailments, and occasionally swallowed for its antispasmodic and other putative effects. Wounds treated with calendula flower extract showed increases in hyaluronan and the number of microscopic blood vessels. Hyaluronan is associated with the development of new blood vessels. Flavonoids, major components of the aqueous extract, may also promote healing. For this reason the extract is approved in Europe for slow-healing wounds (Patrick and others, 1996). An excellent source of lycopene (to 3600 ppms), marigold flowers are now believed to help prevent cancers, especially prostate cancer. Calendula extracts are used in cosmetic creams, ointments, soaps, and sprays (Duke, 1992a, 1992b; Tyler, 1994; Williamson, Evans, 1989).

Ethnobotanical uses: Ache (stomach), ache (tooth), amenorrhea, analgesic, astringent, bactericide, bruise, cancer, carminative, cholagogue, choleretic, corn, depurative, diaphoretic, diuretic, emmenagogue, fever, flu, hemorrhage, internal ulcer, intestine, kidney, lung, mouthwash, piles, scrofula, sprain, stimulant, stomach, styptic, sudorific, syphilis, tonic, tuberculosis, vermifuge, wart (Duke, Beckstrom-Sternberg, Wain, 1995).

Prickly Ash, *Zanthoxylum americanum* **Mill.** and *Z. clava-herculis* L. (**Rutaceae**)

Regarded as analgesic, antirheumatic, astringent, carminative, diaphoretic, and febrifugal, both American species of prickly ash are used internally and externally for arthritis, fever, poor circulation, rheumatism, and toothache. Chelerythrine, one of the active alkaloids, is reportedly analgesic, antiacetylcholinesterase, antiaggregant, antiinflammatory, antimitotic, antineoplastic, antiseptic, antitumor, and antitussive. The West African species, *Z. zanthoxyloides* (Lam.) Watson, is used similarly. It has related but different constituents, including fagaramide, a potent prostaglandin inhibitor with antiinflammatory and molluscicidal activities. Chewing the bark produces an anesthetic tingling sensation in the mouth, which relieves toothache. American Indians chewed the bark and then packed it around an aching tooth to relieve the pain. Other species seem to hold promise for sickle cell anemia (Duke, 1992a, 1992b; Tyler, 1994; Williamson, Evans, 1989).

Ethnobotanical uses: Ache (tooth), cancer, colic, cough, expectorant, gonorrhea, poultice, rheumatism, sialogogue, sore, spasm, stimulant, stomatitis, sudorific, suppurative, tonic, wound (Duke, Beckstrom-Sternberg, Wain, 1995).

Psyllium, *Plantago ovata* Forsk., *P. scabra* Moench (Plantaginaceae)

When hydrated, seeds and husks of the bulk laxative psyllium swell into a gelatinous mass, promoting peristalsis and hydrating the feces. Such bulk is beneficial in diarrhea. Seeds of *P. ovata* absorb some food additives, including cyclamate, preventing harmful effects in rats. Alcoholic anticholinergic extracts seem to lower blood pressure, slow heart rate, and stimulate peristalsis in animals. The mucilage of *P. asiatica* is hypoglycemic in mice. Seeds appear to protect against carbon tetrachloride-induced hepatotoxicity in mice as a result of aucubin, which is also reportedly antidotal (Amanitin), antiinflammatory, antioxidant, bactericidal, cathartic, and diuretic. Chinese practitioners use the fresh plant for hepatitis with success. A major source of fiber, psyllium seeds and husks are used in over-the-counter bulk laxatives and are especially useful in cases of chronic constipation. Like other high-fiber products, psyllium has been shown to lower blood cholesterol levels. Increasingly, physicians are developing allergies to the dust generated by psyllium powders (American Botanical Council, 1995; Duke, 1992a, 1992b; Tyler, 1994; Williamson, Evans, 1989).

Ethnobotanical uses: Ameba, amebiasis, anodyne, bladder, bronchitis, cold, cough, demulcent, diarrhea, dysentery, emollient, gastritis, kidney, laxative, poultice, rheumatism, styptic, swelling, urethritis (Duke, Beckstrom-Sternberg, Wain, 1995).

Red Raspberry, *Rubus idaeus* L. (Rosaceae)

Properly regarded as antiinflammatory, astringent, spasmolytic, and sudorific, raspberry leaves are taken in teas to relieve dysmenorrhea, sore throat, and thrush and facilitate childbirth. It is drunk freely before and during pregnancy for maximal benefit. Uterine-relaxant effects have been demonstrated in animals. The extract appears to affect only the pregnant uterus of both rats and humans, with no activity on the nonpregnant uterus. Polypeptides, possibly the active constituents, are extremely difficult to isolate. Dried leaves contain appreciable amounts of procyanidins and complex tannins. The tea can also be used for diabetes, diarrhea, morning sickness, and stomatitis (Tyler, 1994; Williamson, Evans, 1989).

Ethnobotanical uses: Astringent, bilious, bowel, cancer, depurative, diabetes, diarrhea, dysmenorrhea, eye, fever, gastritis, gout, inflammation, liqueur, paralysis, parturition, rheumatism, scurvy, sore (throat), spasmolytic, stimulant, sudorific, tea, urogenital (Duke, Beckstrom-Sternberg, Wain, 1995).

Red Clover, *Trifolium pratense* L. (Fabaceae)

Regarded as alterative, antidermatitic, antispasmodic, estrogenic, expectorant, and sedative, clover has been used for bronchoses, cancer, coughs, dermatoses, eczema, and psoriasis. Clover may contain four fungicidal isoflavones (biochanin, daidzein, formononetin, and genistein) that are estrogenic in animals ingesting large quantities as forage. Kaufman and others (1997) showed that clover contained more genistein, a substance now believed to prevent cancer and metastasis, than the highly touted soybean. Interestingly, red clover is an ingredient in many "quack" cancer remedies. Red clover is also reported to have antispasmodic and expectorant properties (Duke, 1992a, 1992b; Williamson, Evans, 1989).

Ethnobotanical uses: Alterative, asthma, bronchitis, burn, cancer, cancer (bowel), catarrh, corn, cough, depurative, diuretic, dyspepsia, expectorant, eye, pertussis, scrofula, sedative, skin, sore, spasm, tonic, tumor, whitlow (Duke, Beckstrom-Sternberg, Wain, 1995).

Rhatany, *Krameria lappacea* (Dombey) Burdett and B.B. Simpson (Krameriaceae)

The astringent tanniniferous root of rhatany is antidiarrheal, antihemorrhagic, antiviral, styptic, and vulnerary. It has been administered internally for diarrhea, dysentery, dysmenorrhea, hemorrhage, and menorrhagia and topically for chilblains, gingivitis, hemorrhoids, pharyngitis, and wounds. The tincture of rhatany root, which contains more than 20% tannin, is used for mouth sores and lesions. It may be used alone or with an equal amount of myrrh tincture and applied locally 3 or 4 times daily. The tincture is also effective as a mouthwash (Tyler, 1994; Williamson, Evans, 1989).

Ethnobotanical uses: Astringent, cough, dentifrice, diarrhea, dysentery, expectorant, hemorrhage, hemostat, incontinence, leukorrhea, ophthalmia, piles, prolapse, sore (throat), stomatitis, styptic, tonic, tooth preservative, tumor (Duke, Beckstrom-Sternberg, Wain, 1995).

Rhubarb, *Rheum officinale* Baill. (Polygonaceae)

Medicinal rhubarb is aperient, astringent, laxative, stomachic, and tonic. English rhubarb is similar but milder in action and has amphoteric (i.e., astringent and cathartic) properties; the anthraquinones are laxative, and the tannins astringent. Chinese practitioners use rhubarb for amenorrhea, burns, carbuncles, dyspepsia, enteralgia, jaundice, and scalds. Rhubarb shows cholinergic action in rodents, enhancing peristalsis and increasing the water content of stools. In low doses, rhubarb increases gastric secretion (and thereby stimulates the appetite) and increases bile secretion. Emodin, one active anthraquinone, reportedly has antiaggregant, antifeedant, antiinflammatory, antileukemic, antimutagenic, antiseptic, antispasmodic, antitumor, and antiulcer activities, in addition to its conventional laxative activity. As a stimulant laxative, it is more potent than cascara or senna and often causes intestinal griping or colic. Nonetheless, it is used in the tonic preparation Swedish bitters, along with senna and aloe (Duke, 1992a, 1992b; Tyler, 1994; Williamson, Evans, 1989).

Ethnobotanical uses: Aperient, astringent, bactericide, boil, burn, cancer, cancer (cervix), cancer (stomach), congestion, cosmetic, decoagulant, depurative, diarrhea, dysentery, dyspareunia, dysuria, fever, freckles, fumitory, gynecopathy, jaundice, laxative, malaria, poison, purgative, sore, stomachic, tonic, vermifuge (Duke, Beckstrom-Sternberg, Wain, 1995).

Rose, *Rosa* sp. (Rosaceae)

Syrups made from the vitamin-rich rosehips (the fruits of the rose) are regarded as antidiarrheic and astringent and are reportedly suitable for infants (Williamson, Evans, 1989).

Ethnobotanical uses: Calmative, cancer, collyrium, diarrhea, fumitory, gargle, mouth, sclerosis, soporific, stomachic, tumor (Duke, Beckstrom-Sternberg, Wain, 1995).

Rosemary, *Rosmarinus officinalis* L. (Lamiaceae)

Rosemary and its namesake, rosmarinic acid, possess anticomplementary, antioxidant, and antiinflammatory activities that, coupled with as many as 10 choline-sparing compounds (carvacrol, carvone, cineole, p-cymene, fenchone, isopulegol, limonene, alpha-terpinene, gamma-terpinene, terpinen-4-ol), should lead to its study as a potential treatment for Alzheimer's. The well-known culinary herb is also viewed as anodyne, antiseptic, astringent, diaphoretic, nervine, and stomachic. Rosmarinic acid has also been suggested as a possible treatment for septic shock because it suppresses the endotoxin-induced activation of complement, the formation of prostacyclin, both hypotensive phases, thrombocytopenia, and the concomitant release of thromboxane A_2. Diosmin at 600 mg/day and hesperidin are reported to decrease capillary fragility (diosmin more than rutin). Long popular in hair preparations, shampoos, and tonics, rosemary leaves and volatile oil are recommended as circulatory tonics. Taken internally or applied externally (often in the form of a bath), rosemary oil has been said to improve chronic circulatory weakness, including hypotension. Whether ingested, inhaled, or applied topically, cineole, a prominent constituent, is said to improve a rat's ability to get through a maze. Rosemary has some carminative properties and may be useful for indigestion (Duke, 1992a, 1992b; Tyler, 1994; Williamson, Evans, 1989).

Ethnobotanical uses: Abortifacient, ache (head), ache (stomach), alopecia, amenorrhea, antiseptic, aperient, asthma, astringent, bactericide, bilious, calmative, cancer, cancer (liver), cardiotonic, carminative, catarrh, chill, chol-

agogue, cold, colic, contraceptive, diaphoretic, disinfectant, diuretic, douche, dysmenorrhea, dyspepsia, emmenagogue, evil eye, fumigant, fumitory, head cold, intellect, liniment, lung, metrorrhagia, nerve, nervine, paralysis, protisticide, repellant (witch), rheumatism, rubefacient, sinusitis, sore (throat), spasm, stimulant, stomach, stomachic, stress, sudorific, tea, tonic, tranquilizer, tumor, vermifuge, vulnerary, wart, wen (Duke, Beckstrom-Sternberg, Wain, 1995).

Sage, *Salvia officinalis* L. (Lamiaceae)

Antidiaphoretic, antiseptic, aromatic, astringent, and spasmolytic, sage tea can be used as a gargle or mouthwash for gingivitis, pharyngitis, stomatitis, tonsillitis, and related disorders. Rosmarinic acid is anticomplementary, antiinflammatory, antioxidant, and choline-sparing, all of which have led English researchers to consider it a potential treatment for Alzheimer's disease. Sage oil has more than a dozen antiseptic compounds and several nontoxic spasmolytic compounds. Sage infusion is used internally for dyspepsia and excessive perspiration. Although widely used as a spice, sage does contain thujone, and frequent internal use is not recommended. Other culinary sages may not contain thujone (Duke, 1992a, 1992b; Tyler, 1994; Williamson, Evans, 1989).

Ethnobotanical uses: Antioxidant, antiseptic, anhydrotic, astringent, baldness, cancer (mouth), carminative, cold, cordial, cough, dandruff, dentifrice, deodorant, diaphoretic, digestive, diuretic, dysmenorrhea, dyspepsia, emmenagogue, estrogenic, fever, fumitory, gargle, gingivitis, hair oil, hemostat, immortality, insecticide, mouthwash, nausea, nervine, night sweat, perspiration, resolvent, sore, sore (throat), spasm, spice, stimulant, stomachic, thrush, tonic, vermifuge, vulnerary, wart, weaning, wen, wound (Duke, Beckstrom-Sternberg, Wain, 1995).

Saint-John's-Wort, *Hypericum perforatum* L. (Clusiaceae)

With proven antidepressant, antiinflammatory, anxiolytic, astringent, and sedative active compounds, Saint-John's-wort is used for colds, coughs, depression, dysmenorrhea, insomnia, and rheumatism and can be used topically for arthritis, bruises, and similar problems. The hypericins have an anxiolytic effect by MAO inhibition in vitro, but apparently do not in vivo. In clinical trials of the standardized extract, anxiety improved significantly in women after 4 to 6 weeks. Fresh flowers, crushed and macerated in olive oil and left to stand several weeks in the sun, may be taken internally or applied locally to relieve inflammation and promote healing. Antidepressive effects are attributed to its content of hypericin, pseudohypericin, and related naphthodianthrones. Several activities seem synergistically involved in antidepressive activity: (1) COMT (catechol-O-methyl-transferase) inhibition (COMT may deplete "feel-good amines"); (2) suppression of interleukin-6-release, affecting mood through neurohormonal pathways; (3) MAO inhibition; (4) regulation of serotonin uptake. Hypericum extracts (but not hypericin) increase dopamine. Hypericin and pseudohypericin exhibit antiretroviral and antileukemic effects in mice with two leukemia retroviruses, and Saint-John's-wort is being studied for patients infected with HIV and AIDS. Hypericin is phototoxic in grazing animals, resulting in dermatitis of the skin and inflammation of the mucous membranes on exposure to direct sunlight (Duke, 1992a, 1992b, 1997; Tyler, 1994; Williamson, Evans, 1989).

Ethnobotanical uses: Abortifacient, alopecia, anodyne, antibiotic, antiseptic, astringent, bactericide, cancer (stomach), catarrh, cholagogue, depression, diarrhea, digestive, diuretic, emmenagogue, expectorant, gastrointestinal, kidney, lumbago, lung, nervine, phototoxic, poison, resolvent, rheumatism, sore, stimulant, sunburn, swelling, tumor, urogenital, uterotonic, vermicide, vermifuge, vulnerary, wound (Duke, Beckstrom-Sternberg, Wain, 1995).

Sarsaparilla, *Smilax aristolochiaefolia* Mill., *S. regelii* Killip and C. Morton, *S. febrifuga* Kunth, *S. officinalis* Kunth (Smilacaceae)

Introduced by the Spanish in 1563 as a treatment for syphilis, sarsaparilla has been regarded as alterative, antiinflammatory, antipruritic, and antiseptic. It has been used for skin diseases, including psoriasis, and has received unwarranted attention as a treatment for impotence because it is a reputed source of testosterone. When patients with psoriasis were treated for 2 years with tablets prepared from sarsaparilla, approximately 62% improved. Diosgenin, present in the roots, can be converted in the laboratory to testosterone. Parillin has antibiotic activity. Chinese species of *Smilax* have been successfully used for dermatoses, dysentery, rheumatism, and even syphilis. Sarsaparilla still appears in some root beers and other soft drinks. Although recently advertised as a natural source of testosterone and a legal replacement for illegal androgenic steroids, it does not contain testosterone nor does it increase testosterone levels in the body. In fact, Tyler (1994) regards this claim for sarsaparilla as a hoax. Steroids, including sarsapogenin and smilagenin, as well as their glycosides, do occur in the plant but do not function as anabolic steroids, nor are they converted to anabolic steroids in the body (Duke, 1992a, 1992b, 1997; Tyler, 1994; Williamson, Evans, 1989).

Ethnobotanical uses: Tumor (Duke, Beckstrom-Sternberg, Wain, 1995).

Sassafras, *Sassafras albidum* (Nutt.) Nees. (Lauraceae)

Once respected but now feared in the United States, sassafras is regarded as antiodontalgic, antirheumatic, antiseptic, carminative, diaphoretic, and diuretic. The fear is generated by safrole, which is carcinogenic in animals at doses much higher than those normally consumed by humans. Safrole-free sassafras extracts lack the pleasant aroma and flavor. Tyler (1994) considers it unsafe and ineffective and therefore does not recommend it. However, it is widely used by laypersons as a tonic and performance enhancer. Safrole is also reportedly anesthetic, antiaggregant, anticonvulsant, antiseptic, bactericidal, and carminative. The root bark was originally recommended for syphilis. Safrole, a phenolic ether in the aromatic oil, was shown to be carcinogenic in 1960. The FDA has prohibited the use of sassafras volatile oil and safrole as food additives or flavors (Duke, 1992a; Duke, 1992b; Tyler, 1994; Williamson, Evans, 1989).

Ethnobotanical uses: Ache (tooth), alterative, analgesic, anodyne, antiseptic, astringent, bronchitis, cancer, carcinogenic, carminative, catarrh, cold, demulcent, dentifrice, dentistry, depurative, diaphoretic, diuretic, dysentery, emmenagogue, eye, fungicide, gout, hypertension, insect repellant, kidney, massage, mouthwash, pediculicide, perfume, repellant (ant), respiratory, rheumatism, rubefacient, scurvy, skin, sore, stimulant, sudorific, swelling, syphilis, tea, tonic, virucide, weaning (Duke, Beckstrom-Sternberg, Wain, 1995).

Saw Palmetto, *Serenoa repens* (Bartr.) Small (Arecaceae)

The saw palmetto is regarded as an anabolic, diuretic, sedative, and mildly androgenic and estrogenic endocrine agent. It is used primarily for benign prostatic hypertrophy, cachexia, cystitis, debility, and wasting diseases. Enlarged prostate is common in men over 50 years of age. Saw palmetto should be used only after a physician's diagnosis. Clinical studies indicate that the extract can increase urine flow and reduce frequency of nighttime urination. Generously endowed with phytosterols and amino acids, the saw palmetto seems to inhibit alpha-reductase, thereby inhibiting aromatase, conversion of testosterone to dihydrotestosterone, the activity of estrogenic receptors in the prostate, phospholipase A2, and 5-lipoxygenase enzymes. These effects inhibit the arachidonic acid cascade and reduce inflammation (American Botanical Council, 1995; Duke, 1997; Tyler, 1994; Williamson, Evans, 1989).

Ethnobotanical uses: Aphrodisiac, diuretic, sedative, stimulant, tumor (Duke, Beckstrom-Sternberg, Wain, 1995).

Schizandra, *Schisandra chinensis* (Turcz.) Baill. (Schisandraceae)

Several of the many (more than 30) lignans found in Chinese schizandra appear to protect the liver from toxic substances (Tyler, 1994). Rats given intragastric schisandra containing 13% lignans (approximately 200 mg lignans/kg) were protected from aflatoxin liver damage and showed lower levels of malondialdehyde in the liver. Additionally, the herb seems to increase excretion of the toxins (Ip and others, 1996).

Ethnobotanical uses: Antitussive, asthma, bactericide, cough, dysentery, ejaculation, hyperglycemia, hypertension, insomnia, night sweat, tonic, tumor (lung), vasodilator (Duke, Beckstrom-Sternberg, Wain, 1995).

Senega Snakeroot, *Polygala senega* L. (Polygalaceae)

Regarded as diaphoretic, diuretic, emetic, and expectorant, senega root is often used as a tea, for asthma, bronchitis, catarrh, colds, croup, and pertussis. The decoction is used as an expectorant for upper respiratory catarrh (Tyler, 1994; Williamson, Evans, 1989).

Ethnobotanical uses: Alterative, asthma, bite (snake), bronchitis, cancer, diuretic, emetic, expectorant, gout, hives, medicine, pleurisy, poison, rheumatism, sudorific, tonic (Duke, Beckstrom-Sternberg, Wain, 1995).

Senna, *Cassia alexandrina* Miller (Fabaceae)

Pods of several senna species containing anthraquinones and glycosides are widely used as over-the-counter cathartics and laxatives. The glycosides are absorbed in the gastrointestinal tract with the active anthraquinones excreted into the colon, where they stimulate the laxative effect. Fruits can be prepared as an infusion. Today, senna is recognized as one of the most popular and reliable stimulant laxatives. Although generally regarded as safe, long-term dependence can develop for anthraquinones; hence, long-term use is discouraged. Senna is more popular and less expensive than cascara but not as mild in its action. Senna produces more smooth muscle contractions with attendant cramping. The active sennosides are synergistic in their laxative activities. Increasingly, German practitioners suggest that prolonged use may be detrimental (American Botanical Council, 1995; Duke, 1997; Tyler, 1994; Williamson, Evans, 1989).

Ethnobotanical uses: Cancer, cathartic, dyspepsia, laxative, purgative (Duke, Beckstrom-Sternberg, Wain, 1995).

Skullcap, *Scutellaria lateriflora* L. (Lamiaceae)

Anticonvulsant, nervine, and sedative, the American skullcap *S. lateriflora* is used for cramps, hysteria, and nervous tension but has not been as extensively studied as the Asian variety, *S. baicalensis*. Activities of its component baicalin include antiaggregant, antiallergic, antianaphylactic, antiarthritic, antiasthmatic, anticholinergic, antiedemic, antiinflammatory, and antileukotrienic properties.

Baicalin inhibits calcium ionophore–induced leukotriene synthesis in human lymphocytes and also inhibits lipoxygenase and cyclooxygenase products in leukocytes, rendering baicalin useful in arthritis. The closely related compound baicelein exhibits many of these activities and is also choleretic, diuretic, febrifugal, fungicidal, hypocholesterolemic, and triglycerolytic. The herb inhibits lipid peroxidation in rat liver. It has been clinically tested in China on patients with hepatitis and improved symptoms in over 70% of the subjects, alleviating abdominal distention, increasing appetite, and improving liver function tests (Duke, 1992a, 1992b; Williamson, Evans, 1989).

Ethnobotanical uses: Afterbirth, astringent, cancer, convulsion, diarrhea, emmenagogue, heart, hysteria, nervine, rabies, rickets, sedative, spasm, sudorific, tonic (Duke, Beckstrom-Sternberg, Wain, 1995).

Slippery Elm Bark, *Ulmus rubra* Muhl. (Ulmaceae)

Antioxidant, antitussive, demulcent, emollient, and nutrient, slippery elm bark is used in porridges for convalescents and ulcer patients by adding boiling water to the powdered bark and flavoring. The mucilage is made by steeping the powder in water, heating gently for about an hour, and straining the solution. Powdered bark is poulticed onto boils, burns, and dermatoses, where it soothes and draws out the infection (Williamson, Evans, 1989). In the United States the inner bark is used as a constituent in Essiac tea and medicines of the Ojibwa peoples (Duke, 1997) and added to commercial throat lozenges (Duke, 1997; Tyler, 1994; Williamson, Evans, 1989).

Ethnobotanical uses: Burn, demulcent, diarrhea, fever, gunshot, laxative, parturition, preventive (chafe), respiratory, skin, tumor, wound (Duke, Beckstrom-Sternberg, Wain, 1995).

Spearmint, *Mentha spicata* L. (Lamiaceae)

Spearmint is a pleasant, antispasmodic, carminative, stimulant, widely used culinary herb and flavoring (Williamson, Evans, 1989).

Ethnobotanical uses: Antidote, astringent, bronchitis, cancer, cancer (stomach), carminative, diarrhea, fever, hysteria, nausea, nervine, neuralgia, parturition, sore, spasm, stimulant, stomach, stomachic, tea, tooth whitener (Duke, Beckstrom-Sternberg, Wain, 1995).

Squill, *Urginea maritima* (L.) Baker (Liliaceae)

Squill contains cardioactive glycosides with steroidal structures and physiologic functions and hazards similar to those associated with digitalis glycosides (Tyler, 1994).

Ethnobotanical uses: Bronchitis, cancer, cardiac, cardiotonic, catarrh, cathartic, diuretic, dropsy, ecbolic, edema, emetic, emmenagogue, expectorant, gout, insecticide, insect repellant, pneumonia, poison, preventative, raticide, restorative, rheumatism, rubefacient, stimulant, suppurative, tumor, vermifuge, vesicant, wart, wound (Duke, Beckstrom-Sternberg, Wain, 1995).

Strawberry, *Fragaria vesca* L. (Rosaceae)

Chemistry suggests that strawberry leaves, rich in ellagic acid and other polyphenolics, may be used as a mild astringent and diuretic instead of tea leaves and raspberry leaves. Fruits have been used to remove dental tartar (Duke, 1992a, 1992b, 1997).

Ethnobotanical uses: Alterative, astringent, bladder, blennorrhagia, blood, calculus, cancer, coffee, depurative, diabetes, diarrhea, discutient, diuretic, gravel, hypertension, laxative, refrigerant, renitis, sore (throat), stone, tea, tuberculosis, tumor, urogenital (Duke, Beckstrom-Sternberg, Wain, 1995).

Strophanthus, *Strophantus kombe* Oliv. or *S. hispidus* DC. (Apocynaceae)

Like digitalis, strophanthus contains useful but dangerous cardiac glycosides, but it is poorly absorbed from the gastrointestinal tract and therefore not used orally. Ouabain can be used in cardiac arrest and acts rapidly when injected. Seeds have been used in making African arrow and dart poisons. Extracts of the leaves and roots inhibited pathogenic bacteria, including multiple drug resistant strains *(Escherichia coli, Klebsiella pneumoniae, Neisseria gonorrhoeae, Proteus mirabilis, Pseudomonas aeruginosa, Staphylococcus aureus, Streptococcus pyogenes)* (Ebana and others, 1993; Tyler, 1994; Williamson, Evans, 1989).

Ethnobotanical uses: Cardiotonic, diuretic, heart, poison, poison (arrow), stimulant (Duke, Beckstrom-Sternberg, Wain, 1995).

Tea, *Camellia sinensis* (L.) O. Kuntze (Theaceae)

An antioxidant, astringent, CNS stimulant, diuretic, nervine, and tonic, tea is now receiving attention as a cancer and cardiopathy preventive, in addition to older folk uses for diarrhea, dysentery, and dyspepsia. The antiasthmatic, diuretic, and stimulant properties are due to caffeine and theophylline, and the antiviral and astringent properties to the tannins. Tea tannins also show antioxidant and antitumor-promoting ability. Tea polyphenols are known to be antioxidant, anticarcinogenic, and antimutagenic and may protect against many diseases. This CNS stimulant is used to counteract drowsiness, and the caffeine is therapeutically combined with salicylates for headache. Several tea chemicals (cadinene, fluorine, geraniol, linalol, nerolidol) may help prevent caries and dental plaque (Duke, 1992a, 1992b; Tyler, 1994; Williamson, Evans, 1989).

Ethnobotanical uses: Ache (head), analgesic, antidote, antidote (wine), astringent, bite (dog), cancer, carminative, CNS stimulant, cold, conjunctivitis, debility, demulcent, deobstruent, digestive, diuretic, dropsy, dysentery, epilepsy, eruption, expectorant, fever, hemoptysis, hemorrhage, intellect, lactogogue, lung, malaria, narcotic, nervine, poison, refrigerant, smallpox, soap, stimulant, stomachic, stomatitis, sudorific, toxemia, tumor (head) (Duke, Beckstrom-Sternberg, Wain, 1995).

Tea Tree, *Melaleuca alternifolia* (Maiden and Betche) Cheel (Myrtaceae)

Verghese and others (1996) state the following: "Of the hundreds of species of tea tree, *Melaleuca alternifolia* Cheel (Myrtaceae) is the source of an exceptionally valuable essential oil." This oil is famous for strong bacteriostatic and fungistatic properties and is used in contraception and dental, health care, surgical, and veterinary practice. Antiseptic, antispasmodic, diaphoretic, expectorant, and stimulant, tea tree oil is used externally for arthritis, myalgia, and rheumatism. Internally, it is used for colds, headaches, and toothaches. Cineole, one main active ingredient, is relatively nontoxic and reportedly anthelminthic, antibronchitic, antihalitosic, antilaryngitic, antiseptic, and choleretic. It is a component of many essential oils used as perfumes and flavorings. Australian aborigines, who have inhabited Australia for at least 40,000 years, used the oil as a local antiseptic; early colonial settlers used it for abrasions, bites, burns, cuts, fungal infections, and other skin problems. Tyler attributes the germicidal activity to terpinen-4-ol, which reportedly has antiasthmatic, antiseptic, antitussive, bactericidal, diuretic, fungicidal, herbicidal, nematicidal, and even spermicidal activities. Tea tree oil has proved useful in various vaginal and skin infections (e.g., acne vulgaris) (Duke, 1992a, 1992b; Tyler, 1994; Williamson, Evans, 1989).

Ethnobotanical uses: Ache (ear), ache (head), ache (tooth), acne, astringent, bronchitis, bruise, carminative, cholera, cold, colic, cough, diarrhea, eczema, emollient, expectorant, gout, hiccup, infection, inflammation, insect repellant, laryngitis, malaria, neuralgia, paralysis, parasiticide, pediculicide, pharyngitis (veterinary), pityriasis, pleuritis, pneumonia, psoriasis, pulicide, rheumatism, rhinitis, rubefacient, scabies, scurvy, sedative, skin, sore (throat), spasm, sprain, stimulant, tea, tumor, vermifuge, wound (Duke, Beckstrom-Sternberg, Wain, 1995).

Thyme, *Thymus vulgaris* L., *T. thracius* Velen., and Other *Thymus* species (Lamiaceae)

The culinary herb thyme, regarded as antiseptic, antispasmodic, antitussive, carminative, and expectorant, is used for backache, bronchitis, cold, cough, pertussis, and related ailments. Thymol and carvacrol, major active ingredients, are anesthetic, anthelminthic, antibronchitic, antiinflammatory, antioxidant, and antispasmodic; the flavonoid fraction has potent activities on the smooth muscle of guinea pig trachea and ileum. Other spasmolytic components include anethole, apigenin, borneol, bornyl acetate, caffeic acid, camphor, cinnamic acid, cirselineol, eugenol, ferulic acid, geraniol, kaempferol, limonene, linalol, linalyl acetate, luteolin, menthone, myrcene, naringenin, and thymonin. Thymol and carvacrol both appear in over-the-counter mouthwashes and toothpastes. Like all phytochemicals, these can be toxic in overdose. Thyme tea, when sweetened with honey, acts as an effective demulcent, effective for symptoms of bronchitis, catarrh, and whooping cough (Duke, 1992a, 1992b; Tyler, 1994; Williamson, Evans, 1989).

Ethnobotanical uses: Ache (tooth), antiseptic, astringent, carminative, catarrh, convulsion, cordial, depurative, emmenagogue, epilepsy, eruption, expectorant, hair, lung, nervine, pertussis, radiculalgia, sedative, skin, spasm, stomachic, tonic, tumor, vermifuge (Duke, Beckstrom-Sternberg, Wain, 1995).

Turmeric, *Curcuma longa* L. (Zingiberaceae)

Recently, turmeric is moving from the spice rack to the medicine chest, with impressive reports of antiarthritic, antiinflammatory, antihepatotoxic, and antilymphomic activities. Curcumin has recently been patented as an antiinflammatory (Duke, 1997). Comparable to phenylbutazone, it inhibits carrageenin-induced inflammation in rats, partly via cyclooxygenase inhibition. Several activities may synergistically alleviate arthritic conditions: analgesic (borneol, curcumin, p-cymene, eugenol); antiedemic (borneol, caryophyllene, curcuminoids [tetrahydrocurcumin > curcumin > triethylcurcumin], eugenol); antiinflammatory (azulene, bis-[4-hydroxycinnamoyl]-methane, borneol, caryophyllene, cinnamic acid, curcumin, eugenol, feruloyl-4-hydroxycinnamoylmethane, alpha-pinene, protocatechucic acid, beta-sitosterol, vanillic acid); cyclooxygenase inhibitor (curcumin, galangin); interleukin-1-inhibitor (curcumin). These combined with the antidermatic and antieczemic activities of curcumin and guaiacol suggest that turmeric might be useful in dermatitis as well. Curcuminoids are considered hepatoprotective, and some of them cleave to caffeic acid, which is also hepatoprotective. Turmeric has antifertility effects in rats and is antiseptic in vitro. Tyler (1994) considers turmeric antiinflammatory, choleretic, cholekinetic, digestive, and hepatoprotective. Turmeric remains important as a natural yellow food colorant and an ingredient in curry powders (Duke, 1992a, 1992b; Tyler, 1994; Williamson, Evans, 1989).

Ethnobotanical uses: Abscess, amenorrhea, antibilious, balsamic, bite (leech), bruise, catarrh, chickenpox, cholagogue, cold, colic, congestion, conjunctivitis, cosmetic, depurative, dermatosis, diarrhea, diuretic, dysentery, escharotic, fumitory, gonorrhea, gravel, hemostat, hepatosis, jaundice, lactagogue, parturition, pyuria, scabies, smallpox, sore, stomachic, swelling, tonic, urogenital, vulnerary, wound (Duke, Beckstom-Sternberg, Wain, 1995).

Valerian Root, *Valeriana officinalis* L. (Valerianaceae)

Regarded as anxiolytic, hypnotic, hypotensive, and nervine, valerian is widely used in Europe for insomnia and stress. The sedative activity is generally believed to be caused, at least in part, by valepotriates and some of their degradation products and valerenic acid, valerenone, and other components of the essential oil, all of which have in vivo activity. Synergistic reactions may occur among these various components, a few of which have demonstrable CNS-depressant activity. Valerian, valerenic acid, and the eugenyl and isoeugenyl esters tend to relieve cramps and spasms. Valepotriate degradation products may be more effective than didrovaltrate. Valerenic acid and related compounds can inhibit gamma-amino-butyric acid (GABA), an activity that could prove useful in anxiety and related depression. Valepotriates show antitumor activity in some in vitro experiments. They reportedly inhibit the synthesis of DNA and proteins by covalent bonding. Few or no adverse reactions have been reported in humans; animal tests indicate very low toxicity. Valerian improves the quality of sleep (as measured subjectively by patients) and speeds the onset of sleep in patients who have not responded to other measures. Valerian extracts are occasionally used for dermatitis and eczema. According to Tyler (1994), valerian is an effective and reliable sedative sleep aid, useful in anxiety, insomnia, and nervous irritability. It does not induce addiction or hangover, like some prescription and over-the-counter medications. The German Commission E has approved valerian as a calmative and sleep-promoting agent useful in treating unrest and anxiety-produced sleep disturbances. Valerian may be administered several times a day as a tea, tincture, or extract. Sometimes, it is used externally in the form of a calmative bath (American Botanical Council, 1995; Duke, 1992a, 1992b; Tyler, 1994).

Ethnobotanical uses: Ache (back), anodyne, antispasmodic, apprehension, bactericide, bruise, carminative, catarrh, CNS depressant, cold, convulsion, epilepsy, fever, flu, hypnotic, hypochondria, hysteria, insomnia, intestine, menoxenia, narcotic, nerve, nervine, neurasthenia, numbness, perfume, polyp (nose), rheumatism, sedative, sore, spasm, spice, stimulant, stomachic, sudorific, tonic, tranquilizer, trauma, vermifuge, wound (Duke, Beckstrom-Sternberg, Wain, 1995).

Violet, *Viola odorata* L. (Violaceae)

Regarded as antiseptic, antitussive, and expectorant, violet syrups have long been used for bronchitis, catarrh, colds, and coughs. According to folklore, violets are used for cancerous conditions and some show anticancer activity in mice (Williamson, Evans, 1989). Flowers are a good source of rutin, which is famous for preventing capillary fragility. Chinese species show immunostimulant activity (Duke, 1992a, 1992b; Williamson, Evans, 1989).

Ethnobotanical uses: Antiseptic, antitussive, aperient, bactericide, bilious, cancer, catarrh, cathartic, cough, depurative, diaphoretic, diuretic, eczema, emetic, emollient, expectorant, eye, fever, fungicide, laxative, liqueur, lung, nervine, pectoral, perfume, poison, purgative, sedative, sudorific, tea, tumor (Duke, Beckstrom-Sternberg, Wain, 1995).

Walnut, black, *Juglans nigra* L. (Juglandaceae)

Sharing juglcone and serotonin with English walnut, black walnut is used in a similar fashion.

Ethnobotanical uses: Diphtheria, gargle, hair dye, insecticide, leukemia, medicine, sore, syphilis, tapeworms, vermifuge (Duke, Beckstrom-Sternberg, Wain, 1995).

Walnut, English, *Juglans regia* L. (Juglandaceae)

Alterative, antiseptic, laxative, and antiseptic, walnut infusions have been used for dermatitis, eczema, eruptions, ringworm, and sores. The essential oil is fungicidal; juglone has antineoplastic, antiseptic, and herbicidal activity. According to the Doctrine of Signatures, it was considered useful in epilepsy and headaches because of its resemblance to the brain. It is one of the best food sources of serotonin. A dye made from walnut shells can darken the hair. Containing about 10% of ellagic acid–derived tannin, the leaves serve well as a local astringent. A decoction is applied to the affected skin 3 or 4 times a day, as with witch hazel (Duke, 1992a, 1992b; Tyler, 1994; Williamson, Evans, 1989).

Ethnobotanical uses: Ache (back), alterative, anodyne, anthelmintic, anthrax, antiscrophulosum, aphthae, astringent, bactericide, caligo, cancer (breast), cancer (cervix), chancre, cholagogue, colic, conjunctivitis, cough, dentifrice, depurative, detergent, digestive, diuretic, dysentery, eczema, ejaculation, favus, hairblack, heart-

burn, hemostat, impotence, inflammation, insecticide, intellect, intestine, intoxication, kidney, laxative, leg, leukorrhea, lithotriptic, lung, rejuvenation, rheumatism, scrofula, semen, skin, sore, stimulant, syphilis, toe, tonic, vermicide, vermifuge (Duke, Beckstrom-Sternberg, Wain, 1995).

White Willow, *Salix alba* L. (Salicaceae)

Based on its proven analgesic, antiinflammatory, and febrifugal activities, willow has been a traditional treatment for arthritis, fever, gout, rheumatism, and pain such as toothache. Willow bark is still used in America and Germany, usually with other herbs or drugs. Synthetic salicylates are used more often now because they are more potent and reliable (Tyler, 1994; Williamson, Evans, 1989).

Ethnobotanical uses: Antiseptic, astringent, callus, convalescence, diarrhea, dysentery, dysmenorrhea, fever, gout, hemoptysis, malaria, medicine, rheumatism, tea, tonic, wart (Duke, Beckstrom-Sternberg, Wain, 1995).

Wild Cherry, *Prunus serotina* Ehrh. (Rosaceae)

Regarded as antitussive, astringent, and sedative, wild cherry has long been used in cough elixirs for irritable and persistent coughs such as those that accompany bronchitis and pertussis. The bark is most commonly used. Wild cherry is also used for diarrhea, dyspepsia, and gastritis (Williamson, Evans, 1989).

Ethnobotanical uses: Anodyne, astringent, bronchitis, calmative, cancer, cold, cough, cyanogenetic, diarrhea, dyspepsia, expectorant, fever, liqueur, measles, metrorrhagia, myalgia, nervine, parturition, pectoral, phthisis, poison, scrofula, sedative, syphilis, tonic, tuberculosis, vermifuge (Duke, Beckstrom-Sternberg, Wain, 1995).

Witch Hazel, *Hamamelis virginiana* L. (Hamamelidaceae)

Extracts of astringent, hemostatic witch hazel are highly regarded for their use in bleeding, hemorrhoids, and varicose veins. The distilled extract, "witch hazel water," is used for bruises, dermatoses, and sprains. It is also used in aftershave lotions, collyriums, and other cosmetics; for example, it may be mixed with equal parts of rose water and used as a skin bracer. Although reportedly tannin-free, distilled witch hazel is still astringent, which makes it popular for the various conditions mentioned. It is approved for use in hemorrhoids. Widely used for various skin ailments, witch hazel leaves contain 8% to 10% tannins. The hydroalcoholic extracts are effective styptics and used to alleviate inflamed skin and mucous membranes

(American Botanical Council, 1995; Tyler, 1994; Williamson, Evans, 1989).

Ethnobotanical uses: Ache (back), alterative, anodyne, antidiarrheic, antiseptic, astringent, bruise, cancer, chew stick, cosmetic, eye, hemorrhage, hemorrhoids, hemostatic, inflammation, lameness, myalgia, piles, poultice, refrigerant, scalp, sedative, skin, sprain, steam bath, tea, tonic, tumor, varicose veins, wound (Duke, Beckstom-Sternberg, Wain, 1995).

Wormwood, *Artemisia absinthium* L. (Asteraceae)

Wormwood is regarded as anthelmintic, anodyne, antiinflammatory, antiseptic, cardiotonic, carminative, choleretic, emmenagogic, spasmolytic, and stomachic. It has long been used for arthritis, cardiopathy, colds, cramps, and rheumatism. Azulene has antiallergic, antiinflammatory, antiulcer, and febrifugal activities; thujone is hallucinogenic and toxic and may interact with a common CNS receptor for tetrahydrocannabinol (the active constituent in marijuana). Wormwood was the major ingredient in the liqueur absinthe, which was declared dangerous and banned. In large doses, thujone and absinthe cause convulsions, cramps, insomnia, nightmares, and vomiting. The anthelmintic properties probably stem from sesquiterpene lactones (Duke, 1992a, 1992b; Williamson, Evans, 1989).

Ethnobotanical uses: Abortifacient, anthelmintic, antifertility, antiseptic, aperitif, balsamic, cancer (liver), deobstruent, depurative, digestive, diuretic, emmenagogue, febrifuge, fever, leukemia, liqueur, narcotic, sclerosis, stimulant, stomachic, sudorific, tonic, tumor (breast), vermifuge, wen (Duke, Beckstrom-Sternberg, Wain, 1995).

Yarrow, *Achillea millefolium* L. (Asteraceae)

Regarded as antiinflammatory, diuretic, febrifugal, hemostatic, hypotensive, spasmolytic, and sudorific, yarrow is widely used for amenorrhea, catarrh, colds, dysmenorrhea, fever, and high blood pressure. It is often used for rheumatism, catarrh, and amenorrhea. Yarrow, usually considered innocuous, is also used as a collyrium and for diarrhea, dyspepsia, itch, and ulcers. Apigenin, an antiinflammatory, antiplatelet, and spasmolytic compound, has recently proved to produce sedative effects also. Azulenes, like salicylic acid, also have antiinflammatory activity. Betonicine is hemostatic. Eugenol has dozens of activities but is best known as an analgesic and anesthetic (Duke, 1992a, 1992b; Williamson, Evans, 1989).

Ethnobotanical uses: Abscess, ache (back), ache (ear), ache (head), ache (leg), ache (tooth), antiseptic, aperitif, astringent, atony, bite (snake), bladder, bruise, cancer, carminative, cathartic, cold, colic, condyloma, consumption, cough, cyanogenetic, deodorant, depurative, diaphoretic, dyspepsia, emmenagogue, enteritis, enterorrhagia, epistaxis, expectorant, eye, febrifuge, felon, fever, gastritis, hematemesis, hematochezia, hematuria, hemorrhage, hemostat, hypochondria, kidney, litholytic, nervine, piles, poultice, puerperium, rash, rheumatism, scurvy, skin, sore, sore (throat), spasm, stimulant, stomach, sudorific, swelling, tonic, tuberculosis, vulnerary, wound (Duke, Beckstrom-Sternberg, Wain, 1995).

Yellow Dock, *Rumex crispus* L. (Polyegonaceae)

Yellow dock, an alterative, cholagogic, and laxative herb, is used for chronic dermatitis, constipation, jaundice, nettle stings, and ringworm. Consumers should be warned that those plants are sometimes high in anthraquinones and oxalic acids (Duke, 1992a, 1992b; Williamson, Evans, 1989).

Ethnobotanical uses: Alterative, antiseptic, astringent, boil, cancer, cathartic, constipation, depurative, diuretic, dysentery, emollient, fever, hives, homeopathy, itch, laxative, nerve, parasiticide, poison, purgative, refrigerant, ringworm, scurvy, sedative, skin, suppurative, tea, tinea, tonic, tumor (Duke, Beckstrom-Sternberg, Wain, 1995).

Yohimbe, *Pausinystalia johimbe* (K. Schum.) Pierre ex Beille (Rubiaceae)

The major alkaloid of yohimbe, yohimbine, is an alpha-adrenergic blocker with a deserved reputation as a sexual stimulant. Animal studies confirm its effectiveness, despite earlier equivocal results. Excess quantities of yohimbine may be depressant. Yohimbine also has anesthetic, antiacetylcholinesterase, antianginal, antiatherosclerotic, antidepressant, antidiuretic, antihypertensive, anxiogenic, aphrodisiac, cardiotonic, cholinergic, emetic, hypertensive, hypothermic, mydriatic, and sialogogic activities. It is also known as a calcium channel blocker and MAO inhibitor. Clinical studies confirm the value of yohimbine in treating male impotence. Side effects of yohimbine include agitation, anxiety, hypertension, insomnia, nausea, tachycardia, tremors, and vomiting (Duke, 1992a, 1992b; Tyler, 1994).

Ethnobotanical uses: Aphrodisiac, fever (Duke, Beckstrom-Sternberg, Wain, 1995).

Yucca, *Yucca* sp. (Agavaceae)

Yucca, viewed as antiinflammatory, is sometimes used as a source of compounds, such as diosgenin, that can be converted into steroids in the laboratory (but not necessarily in the body).

Ethnobotanical uses: Dysentery (Duke, Beckstrom-Sternberg, Wain, 1995).

References

American Botanical Council: Herbs and health: an introductory guide to herbal healthcare [brochure], Austin, Tex, 1995, The Council.

Bisset NG, editor: *Herbal drugs and phytopharmaceuticals*, Boca Raton, Fla, 1994, CRC Press (*English translation of* Wichtl, 1984, 1989).

Brinker F: *Larrea tridentata* (DC.) Coville (Chaparral or Creosote Bush), *Brit J Phytotherapy* 3(1):10, 1994.

Citores L and others: Isolation and characterization of a new non-toxic two-chain ribosome-inactivating protein from fruits of elder *(Sambucus nigra* L.), J Exp Bot 47(303):1577, 1996.

Cunnane SC, Thompson LU, editors: *Flaxseed in human nutrition,* Champaign, Ill, 1995, AOCS Press.

de Vincenzi M, Mancini E, Dessi MR: Monograph on botanical flavoring substances used in foods. Part V, *Fitoterapia* 67(3):241, 1996.

Duke JA: *Ginseng: a concise handbook,* Algonac, Mich, 1989, Reference Publications.

Duke JA: *CRC handbook of biologically active phytochemicals and their activities,* Boca Raton, Fla, 1992a, CRC Press (Published both as hardcopy book and as WordPerfect Database).

Duke JA: *CRC handbook of phytochemical constituents of GRAS herbs and other economic plants,* Boca Raton, Fla, 1992b, CRC Press (Published both as hardcopy book and as WordPerfect Database).

Duke JA: The botanical alternative, *Herbalgram* 28:48, 1993.

Duke JA: Herbalist's desk reference: module 5 in online *Medical Botany* database, http://www.inform/umd.edu:8080/EdRes/Colleges/LFSC/life_sciences/.plant_biology/.WWW/duke.html

Duke JA, Beckstrom-Sternberg SM, Wain K: EthnobotDB, an updated database version of medicinal plants of the world, 1995. (Duke and Wain, 1981). (Internet URL: http://www.ars-grin.gov/~ngrlsb/)

Duke JA, Wain KK: *Medicinal plants of the world,* Unpublished USDA database, USDA-ARS, 1981, Beltsville, Md, 20705; available online at http://www.ars-grin.gov/~ngrlsb

Ebana RUB, Madunagu VE, Etok CA: Antimicrobial effect of *Strophanthus hispidus* and *Secamone afzeli* on some pathogenic bacteria and their drug-resistant strains, *Nigerian J Bot* 6:27, 1993.

Fulder S, Tenne M: Ginger as an anti-nausea remedy in pregnancy—the issue of safety, *Herbalgram* 38:47, 1996.

Ip SP and others: Effect of a lignan-enriched extract of *Schisandra chinensis* on aflatoxin B1 and cadmium chloride–induced hepatotoxicity in rats, *Pharmacol Toxicol* 78:413, 1996.

Kaufman PB and others: A comparative survey of leguminous plants as sources of the isoflavones genistein and daidzein: implications for human nutrition and health, *J Altern Compl Med* 3(1):7, 1997.

Kleijnen J, Knipschild P: *Ginkgo biloba, Lancet* 340:1136, 1992.

Kreis W and others: Inhibition of HIV replication by *Hyssopus officinalis* extracts, *Antiviral Res* 14:323, 1990.

Linder S: *Withania somnifera* winter cherry, Indian ginseng, ashwagandha, *Austr J Med Herbalism* 8(3):78, 1996.

National Academy of Sciences: Herbal pharmacology in the People's Republic of China: a trip report of the American Pharmacology Delegation, Washington, DC, 1975, The Academy.

Patrick KF and others: Induction of vascularization by an aqueous extract of the flowers of *Calendula officinalis* L., the European marigold, *Phytomedicine* 3(1):11, 1996.

Pish E and others: Discovery of betulinic-acid as a selective inhibitor of human melanoma that functions by induction of apoptosis, *Nature Med* 1(10):1046, 1995.

Tyler VE: *Herbs of choice—the therapeutic use of phytomedicinals,* New York, 1994, Pharmaceutical Products.

Ulrichova J and others: Cytoprotective effect of phenolics from Colchicum on rat hepatocytes, *Fitoterapia* 66(5):399, 1995.

Verghese J and others: Indian tea tree (*Melaleuca alternifolia* Cheel) essential oil, *Flav Frag J* 11:219, 1996.

Williamson EM, Evans FJ: Potter's new cyclopaedia of botanical drugs and preparations, rev ed, Saffron Walden, Essex, UK, 1989, CW Daniel.

Chapter 20

Western Herbal Medicine: Clinical Applications

ENRIQUETA DE GUZMAN

We live in a time of renewed interest in herbology and its application to human medicine. In this chapter, these applications are extended to veterinary medicine. Current scientific research on common herbs and their applications is presented. In the first half of the chapter, history, controversial issues, quality control, common forms, and dosages are reviewed. Also included is a basic materia medica with scientific references. Western herbs are defined as botanicals found to have therapeutic properties that are commonly available in the United States and Europe.

History

Recorded use of plants to treat physical ailments dates back to the Bronze Age. More than 5000 years ago, the Sumerians described uses for laurel, caraway, and thyme. The oldest surviving herbal medicine book dates to 2700 BC China. Even the Old Testament refers to herbs such as vetch and mandrake (Lust, 1987).

Major contributions to herbal medicine were made by three prominent Greek physicians: Hippocrates, Dioscorides, and Galen. Hippocrates, who lived circa 300 BC, is considered the father of modern medicine. He believed health could be maintained with the use of a few simple herbs, proper rest and diet, and letting the body's own natural life force deal with illness (Lust, 1987). Dioscorides lived circa 50 AD; he wrote the first European treatise on the medical use of plants, *De Materia Medica* (Tierra, 1992). *De Materia Medica* was a popular medical reference in Europe through the fifteenth century. Galen, who lived circa 130 AD, was the founder of experimental physiology and wrote the famous herbal text *De Simplicibus*. Galen was a promoter of direct intervention in illnesses with large dosages of plant mixtures (Tierra, 1992).

During the Middle Ages, few advances were made in Western herbalism. Monasteries preserved the few written references, and primitive folk medicine was passed verbally from generation to generation among the peasants (Lust, 1987).

The invention of the printing press in the mid-1400s gave renewed vigor to the study of Western herbalism by popularizing the few existing herbals. This popularization was accomplished through the translation of Greek and Latin manuscripts into the common languages of Europe (Lust, 1987). Over the next 300 years, several still-popular herbals were written, including Nicholas Culpepper's seventeenth-century classic *Pharmacopoeia* (renamed *A Physicall Directory*). Culpepper was ostracized by his physician peers for his decision to translate the most exclusive herbal texts of time from Latin into common English (Tierra, 1992).

Some researchers believe that the split between herbal and orthodox medicine occurred in 1785. William Withering discovered that, by using precise amounts of the foxglove leaf, he could treat heart failure. He then proceeded to isolate and purify foxglove's active ingredients: digitoxin and dioxin. From that point forward, conventional medical and pharmaceutical researchers have believed that the active principle of plants should be extracted, purified, and given in specific dosages to ensure its safety (Mabey, 1988).

Western herbal medicine moved to North America with the European and Scandinavian colonists. In America, European herbalism was combined with existing Native American traditions to yield such groups of herbalists as the "White Indian doctors." The most famous of these was Samuel Thomson. The thomsonian school preached that life and health were positive virtues that were to be improved by the natural gifts of God. Thomsonism heavily influenced the eclectic and physiomedical herbal movements of the late nineteenth century in the United States and Europe (Mills, 1991). These herbal traditions and many newly discovered useful plants, such as goldenseal and American ginseng, were exported widely to Europe and Asia from the 1600s until about 1920. This sharing of ideas and material has led to the survival of American herbal traditions. At the turn of the twentieth century, the main American colleges of physiomedicalism, eclecticism, and homeopathy were brought under the umbrella of mainstream medical training as specified by the American Medical Association. Those independent institutions have largely disappeared (Mills, 1991). Many proponents of thomsonism and physiomedicalism returned to Europe and incorporated much of their diagnostic tools and materia medica into existing Western herbal practice. The herbalists of Europe have formed effective organizations such as the National Institute of Medical Herbalists (in Britain). These organizations have promoted scientific research into the efficacy of herbal remedies and have been largely successful in keeping a place in most European medical communities for Western herbalism.

Western herbalism has a prominent and resurgent position in modern medicine. As of 1988, 30% to 40% of all medical doctors in France and Germany relied on herbal preparations as their main medicines (Herbalgram, 1988). In the past 25 years, about 25% of all prescribed drugs in the United States have contained an active constituent from plants (i.e., nonsynthetic) (Werbach, Murray, 1988). Much of the increased interest in herbalism is the result of the desire to find more alternatives for treatment of many chronic illnesses such as arthritis, AIDS, and cancer. Furthermore, herbal medicine is regaining popularity because of the ever-escalating cost of health care and the desire by patients to treat the cause as well as the symptoms of disease.

The history of veterinary herbalism follows a path similar to that of its human counterpart. The first verbal records are from the Shang dynasty in China (1766-1027 BC), and the first formal veterinary manuals are from the Tang dynasty (618-907 AD). The ancient Asians put a strong emphasis on equine and bovine health. They practiced rudimentary herbology, physiology, pathology, and acupuncture (Dunlop, Williams, 1995; OIE, 1994).

Similar developments occurred in India. The ancient Indians were documented to have used garlic as a panacea, Indian snakeroot *(Rauwolfia serpentina)* for its calming effects, hemp for anesthesia, and *Berberis aristata* (similar to goldenseal) for diarrhea (Dunlop, Williams, 1995).

Much of this herbal knowledge influenced the Greeks, Arabs, and, later, the western Europeans. Veterinary herbology (and veterinary medicine in general) made slower progress in the West than it did in China and India (Dunlop, Williams, 1995). As the popularity of veterinary medicine increased in the seventeenth and eighteenth centuries, the popularity of herbalism also grew. It was not until the late nineteenth century that veterinary medicine made the transition from herbal to conventional pharmaceuticals.

Today, human and veterinary herbalism share similar concerns and challenges. Both depend largely on the work of European and Asian researchers to determine the application and efficacy of herbal therapies. Also, the literature is particularly thin with regard to the specific veterinary applications of these therapies. Veterinarians must conduct more research and publish their results in the scientific media.

Controversial Issues

Regulatory Issues

The main role of the U.S. Food and Drug Administration (FDA) is to ensure that all products marketed as medicines are safe and effective. Herbs pose a difficult dilemma. They have been used for thousands of years in many different human cultures. During those thousands of years, they have been well tested through self-experimentation to determine what works and how these herbs are best applied. Yet the pharmacology of the active ingredients of some of the most popular herbs is still unclear. This leaves the FDA in a difficult situation.

The FDA has classified herbal products as food supplements, and they can be only marketed as such. Herbal companies are not allowed to make health claims about their herbal products because the FDA requires the same standards of proof as for any other drug. Furthermore, pharmaceutical companies are not interested in investing millions of scarce research dollars in herbal products that cannot be patented.

So where does this leave us? Medical professionals and the general public are kept uneducated about the proper usage, standards of purity, and quality of the herbal products available. They instead rely on herbal industry literature, word of mouth, and personal experimentation. Also, the American pharmaceutical industry is rapidly falling behind European, Japanese, and Chinese competitors in knowledge of herbal modalities and their commercial application.

How is this dilemma to be handled? At the Workshop on Alternative Medicine at Chantilly, Virginia, in September 1992, the Panel on Herbal Medicine made the following recommendations to the National Institutes of Health (Workshop on Alternative Medicine, 1992):

1. A research organizational conference should be held to help organize herbal medical research. The conference would target pertinent ethnomedical issues.
2. The training and funding of ethnobotanists and their research should become a priority of governmental agencies such as the National Science Foun-

dation and National Institutes of Health. Training of researchers in the field of ethnomedicine would help preserve our native herbal traditions and encourage the identification of other medicinal plants before they become scarce or extinct.

3. Reform the FDA "proof of efficacy" requirements for herbal remedies to focus on safety and product quality. A model such as the German Commission E monographs could be used as a guide.

4. Restructure FDA guidelines to help clarify its mission with regard to herbal medicines. Congress could focus the FDA on verifying the potency and safety of remedies. Producers could participate with the FDA in a voluntary certification system similar to those used in other developed countries. This three-tiered system would reward ethical producers who consistently maintain strict quality standards and help educate the public on the uses, safety, and quality of herbal products. Under this system, manufacturers could apply for a specific health condition label indications based on FDA-approved standards.

Most American ethnobotanists and herbalists agree that the role of the FDA must change. Congress should allow the FDA to perform the important functions of verifying the safety, potency, and quality of herbal remedies. The FDA should be encouraged to provide information about effective herbal remedies to medical professionals and the general public.

Use of Whole Herb versus Active Ingredient

Many herbalists prefer using whole herbal extracts as opposed to the isolated active constituent of the herb (Mills, 1991; Murray, 1995; Tierra, 1990). These herbalists believe that, by using only the isolated active ingredient, some of the other constituents that may act synergistically are lost, thereby decreasing the efficacy of the product. Murray (1995) notes that evidence indicates that crude extracts have greater therapeutic effects than does the active constituent alone.

Other herbalists believe it is best to use the purified active ingredient. Many herbs contain toxins and other principles that may divert or decrease the activity of the desired ingredient or produced undesirable side effects. Tyler, Brady, and Roberts (1988) present the example of cinchona bark, which contains 25 related alkaloids. Of these, only quinine is effective as a treatment for malaria. Yet cinchona bark also contains quinodine, a cardiac depressant, and cinchotannic acid, the astringent qualities of which can induce constipation.

The answer lies beween the two positions. For some herbs, it may be best to use only the isolated active ingredient, whereas others lose effectiveness if the whole herb is not used.

Quality Control, Common Forms, and Dosages

Herbal remedies are sold commercially in various forms such as bulk herbs (usually dried), oils, tinctures (hydroalcohol, glycerin), capsules, tablets, ointments, and creams. The value of these herbal products is variable and is determined by many factors. The best way to ensure consistent performance is to buy high-quality products from a large, established, reputable supplier. Such suppliers attempt to mitigate the many circumstances that can affect the quality of herbal medicines, including the following:

1. Environment in which the plant grows. Is the plant a commercial crop, or wild-harvested? What is the fertility of the soil, the climate? What types of fertilizers were used?

2. Part of plant used. For example, only the ligulate florets of the calendula, *Calendula officinalis* L., have any medicinal use.

3. Age of the plant at harvest is important for some herbs such as ginseng, *Panax ginseng* C.A., and goldenseal, *Hydrastis canadensis* L.

4. Handling after harvest. Each plant must be prepared appropriately (dried at proper temperatures, kept out of sunlight, tinctured in a medium in which the active ingredients are soluble). Because most herbal products are sensitive to light, heat, and the material of the container, it is preferable to store herbal medicines in opaque glass containers in cool, dark areas. Some products such as glycerin-based tinctures must be refrigerated after the container is opened.

High-quality manufacturers also label their products well.

1. Know exactly what you are purchasing. Ideally, the product label should include genus and species. Because of the duplication of common names, it is possible to mistakenly prescribe the wrong herb, resulting in limited or no medicinal effect or even poisoning. It is estimated that because of supplier error and improper identification, up to 50% of the *Echinacea* sp. sold in the United States between 1908 and 1991 was actually *Parthenium inthegrifolium,* which is referred to as Missouri snakeroot (Awang, Kindack, 1991).

2. Product labels should also include an expiration or harvest date. Herbal products typically have a short shelf life. For example, a finely chopped or powdered herb bought in bulk or in capsule form will likely have lost a significant amount of its potency after a year. Herbs preserved in tinctures, oils, or other media typically remain viable for 2 or 3 years.

3. Last, the label should have the part(s) of herb used, the amount of active constituents, and any other ingredients such as fillers.

Many regulators and herbalists are searching for a method of ensuring the identity, quantity, and quality of active constituents in herbal remedies. One approach is a formulary of standardized extracts. These standardized extracts would contain laboratory-verified quantities of certain active ingredients of a given herb or herbs. The primary advantages of this proposal are assured quality and greater safety. The primary disadvantage is the tendency to focus on individual chemical constituents, and away from the synergistic advantages of using the whole herb. Also, herbs can have many active ingredients; as a result, standardization is difficult.

Common Forms

Herbs are administered to patients in several forms: as tea (infusion and decoction), capsules or tablets, extracts, poultices or ointments, and in bulk. What follows is a brief description of each.

Teas

Teas are probably the best known forms of herbal treatments because of their popularity at the local health food store and because most active constituents of herbal medicines are water soluble (making this a valuable method of application). Unfortunately, the forms and dosages of the most common commercial teas are rarely sufficient to elicit the desired medicinal effect.

Teas are divided into two main types: infusions and decoctions. The method used is largely determined by the part of the herb being extracted. Leaves, young stems, flower petals, and finely chopped or powdered herb can all easily and quickly be processed with a hot water infusion. Decoctions are usually reserved for woody stems, barks, berries, rhizomes, and root material. Decoction is performed with hot or cold water; the process typically takes much longer than infusion.

To make an infusion, place two teaspoonfuls of dried herb in a strainer and the strainer in a ceramic cup. Pour about 8 ounces of freshly boiled water over the herbs. Cover the cup and let stand about 10 minutes. After the lid and strainer are removed, the infusion is ready. Infusions can typically be stored in a cool place for up to 48 hours.

To make a decoction, place sliced or chopped herb in a saucepan, then pour cold water over the herb and heat. Bring the mixture to a boil and simmer slowly for 20 to 40 minutes. During this time the total volume should be reduced by one third to one half. Remove the saucepan from heat and pour its contents through a strainer into a storage container. Decoctions can also be stored in cool places for up to 48 hours.

A cold water infusion/decoction is also called a *maceration*. Macerations are necessary for certain herbs for which the release of certain less desirable components must be limited or when the desired active ingredient is particularly sensitive to heat (e.g., senna, valerian, parsley). To prepare a maceration, place the herb and cold water, in a 1:6 ratio, in a container. Let the mixture stand in a cool place for approximately 12 hours and then strain it. Like infusions and decoctions, macerations will keep for up to 48 hours.

Capsules and tablets

Many herbs are found commercially in capsule or tablet form. These forms can be a particularly effective way of administering herbs to small animals. Capsules can include herbs in powdered or tincture form and come in a variety of sizes. Some companies are beginning to sell herbal products with a guaranteed amount of active ingredients, or "guaranteed potency," typically listed in milligrams.

Extracts

Herbal extracts offer a wide variety of opportunities for use. Extracts come in glycerin, water, and alcohol tinctures; powder in capsules and in pills. Because of commercial standardization to a certain number of milligrams of active ingredient per dose, they also offer the advantage of more consistent efficacy. Liquid extracts can then be applied in a variety of forms (teas, poultices, vaporizers).

Poultices and compresses

The poultice is a common and ancient way of applying herbs topically. When using poultices and compresses, remember that animals will lick any medicine applied to the skin. Avoid topical application of toxic herbs. First boil the fresh or dried herb for about 5 minutes, then squeeze out the excess liquid and let the boiled herb cool. Apply the herb to the skin and wrap with cotton gauze to hold the poultice in place. It may be necessary to rub oil on the skin to prevent the herb from sticking. Depending on the intent, the poultice is left in place for only a few minutes or as long as several hours.

Compresses are similar to poultices except that an herbal extract and not the plant itself is applied to the skin. Soak a cloth or cotton wrapped in gauze in warm or cool herbal extract. The extract can be in the form of a diluted tincture, decoction, or infusion.

Ointments

Commercial ointments are available for a variety of purposes, and combinations of herbs are often used. Some herbal ointments should be applied only to unbroken skin.

Bulk herbs

Bulk herb is defined as herb purchased in a loose form (generally chopped, fresh, or powdered). In the case of some good-tasting herbs and for some cooperative patients, direct administration of herbs as a food supplement works well. Typically the amount of whole herb that would have to be consumed to yield an effective dosage of the active ingredients makes this method difficult.

Administration of herbs to some patients may be difficult. Creativity is necessary. Some patients will accept pills, capsules, and teas readily. Others will accept the medicine mixed in food. It is also possible to crush or powder medicine and mix it with bouillon, honey, and other liquids the animal will accept. Liquids can also be given with a syringe.

Common Dosages

The dosage of herbs to apply in a given situation depends on several factors, including the weight of the patient, the concentration of active ingredients in the form chosen, and the absorption of active elements.

No standard, scientifically validated method of dosing animals exists. Veterinarians have been using trial and error to find correct dosages. Typically the veterinarian starts with conservative dosages and carefully gauges the animal's reaction before increasing medication. Also, herbal medication typically takes longer to achieve the desired

effect. It is common for practitioners and owners to become discouraged and not give the medication enough time to achieve its full effect.

In most modern herbal textbooks and herbal product packaging, dosages are given for 150-pound human males. Many veterinary practitioners determine dosages by determining the ratio of the weight of the patient to that of a 150-pound human being. For example, a 50-pound dog would receive one third to one half the human dosage.

Dr. Ihor John Basko presented the following protocol for small and large animals at the 1995 American Holistic Veterinary Medical Association Annual Conference in Snowmass, Colorado (Tables 20-1 and 20-2). I have included it because of its completeness, simplicity, and similarity to my own practices (Basko, 1995).

Materia Medica

The herbs included in this section are those that have been investigated thoroughly and for which significant evidence of efficacy exists. I have not discussed other common uses for these herbs here because of lack of evidence. Other herbs are not mentioned because of questions of toxicity or lack of scientific evidence to support the various

TABLE 20-1

CARNIVORES*

PREPARATION	CATS (10 LB)	DOGS (25 LB)
Decoction	0.5 oz	1.0 oz
Extract powder capsule (100 mg)	1	1
Extract tablet (250 mg)	0.5	1
Freeze-dried granules, 100 mg capsules	1	1 to 1.5
Loose granules	0.25 tsp	0.25 to 0.5 tsp
Syrups (crush extract tablet, or use granules mixed with hot honey)	0.25 tsp	0.25 to 0.5 tsp
Tinctures (remove alcohol by heating first)	5 to 10 drops	5 to 10 drops
Chinese patent medicines (pills)	20% of human dose	25% of human dose

*Carnivores require more per pound on the basis of human dosage. These doses are given two to three times daily depending on the severity of the condition.

TABLE 20-2

HERBIVORES*

PREPARATION	GOAT (250 LB)	COW (1500 LB)	HORSE (1000 LB)
Decoction	4.0 oz	12 oz	8 oz
Extract powder	1 tsp	2 T	2 T
Extract tablet	3 to 5	10 to 15	10 to 15
Freeze-dried granules	1 tsp	2 T	2 T
Tincture	1 tsp	2 T	2 to 3 T

*Herbivores require less per pound on the basis of human or carnivore dosage. These doses are given two to three times daily depending on severity of the condition.

claims about their effects (e.g., yucca, sassafras, blue cohosh, comfrey, chaparral).

The following section is organized roughly by body system or application. These categories include the following:

- Antibacterial
- Antiparasitic
- Cardiovascular system
- Gastrointestinal and hepatic systems
- Immune system
- Nervous system
- Musculoskeletal system and musculoskeletal pain
- Genitourinary system
- Respiratory system
- Skin and mucous membranes

Many of the listed herbs are useful in several body systems. Such herbs are included in the section in which they are mostly commonly applied. Those with multiple primary uses are described fully in one section and noted in others. I have listed as active ingredients those items that researchers have isolated or have hypothesized to be causative agents of the herb's medicinal properties. In some cases the mechanism of action of the active ingredient does not fully explain the clinical findings attributed to the herb. For this reason, many herbalists believe it is important to administer the "whole herb" and not just an isolated constituent of the herb (Mowrey, 1993; Weiss, 1988; Mills, 1991).

Three common ways of prescribing herbs are symptomatic treatments, detoxification treatments, and tonic treatments.

Symptomatic treatments are used to treat the symptoms in the same fashion as allopathic medicines. For example, goldenseal, *H. canadensis* L., is used for bacterial infections.

Detoxification treatments are used to cleanse various organs and systems of the body. For example, milk thistle, *Silybum marianum*, is used to clean and protect the liver.

Tonic treatments are unique to herbal medicine. In small amounts and over long periods, tonics invigorate, strengthen, and protect some or all systems of the body. In other words, they bring into homeostasis the different biochemical and physiologic functions of specific body systems (Mowrey, 1993). When the whole herb is used, tonics provide a balancing effect. For example, research has shown that ginseng, *Panax ginseng*, increases blood pressure in some situations and decreases it in others (active constituents: Rb ginsenosides and Rg ginsenosides) (Bissett, Wichtl, 1994; Chen and others, 1994; Mowrey, 1993). Even though scientists know how the individual constituents act on the body, they have yet to provide a good explanation about how the body recognizes which of the seemingly opposing actions the herb needs to promote.

Antibacterial

Herbs listed include garlic, goldenseal, and tea tree.

Garlic

Latin name:	*Allium sativum* L.
Family:	Liliaceae
Common names:	Garlic

Active ingredients:
1. Garlic contains 0.1% to 0.3% volatile sulfur compounds: allicin (diallyldisulfide-*S*-oxide) and methyl allyl trisulfide.
2. Ajoene (a self-condensation product of allicin) is also found in garlic.
3. Garlic has high levels of vitamins C and A, thiamin, and protein; trace amounts of copper, zinc, iron, tin, calcium, potassium, aluminum, sulfur, germanium, and selenium (Mowrey, 1986).

Major uses:
1. Garlic is an excellent antibiotic. One milligram of the primary active ingredient, allicin, is equal in potency to 15 standard units of penicillin (Cavallito, Bailey, 1945; Mowrey, 1986). Sensitive bacteria include *Staphylococcus, Streptococcus, Brucella, Bacillus, Vibrio, Klebsiella, Proteus, Escherichia, Salmonella, Hafnia, Aeromonas, Citrobacter,* and *Providencia* (Mowrey, 1986).
2. Garlic is an excellent herb for the cardiovascular system. It reduces serum cholesterol and blood lipid and is used as a tonic to help prevent atherosclerosis (Bordia, Bansal, 1973). Garlic reduces blood pressure (Korotkov, 1966). Ajoene helps prevent platelet aggregation (Srivastava, 1984). Werbach and Murray (1994) list 24 studies on the effects of garlic and other members of the lily family on atherosclerosis.

Minor and anecdotal uses:
1. Garlic is effective against roundworms, pinworms, tapeworms, and hookworms (Rao, Rao, Venkatoraman, 1946).
2. Garlic has been shown experimentally to be effective against *Capillaria* sp. worms in the intestinal tract of cichlids (Fairfield, 1995). Also found to be an antinematodal agent in the digestive tract of *Pterophylum scalare* (Fairfield, 1995).
3. Garlic has proven antifungal properties (including against ringworm and *Candida albicans*) (Mowrey, 1986; Tansey, Appleton, 1975; Werbach, Murray, 1994).
4. Small dosages improve the tone of smooth intestinal muscle and therefore increase peristaltic activity. Large dosages reverse the effect (Foster, 1991).

5. Garlic has been shown effective in reducing or preventing various cancers of the skin and gastric system (Werbach, Murray, 1994).
6. Garlic is used in Eastern medicine as a geriatric tonic herb (Weiss, 1988).
7. Garlic may be effective in the treatment of diabetes by increasing the amount of free insulin, resulting in decrease of blood sugar.

Forms:
1. The fresh pulped bulb (pulpy juice) is used.
2. For internal use, garlic is administered, dried, in enteric-coated capsules or as a tincture.

Toxicity and cautions:
1. Large dosages should be avoided in patients with clotting problems.
2. Large dosages (five or more cloves per day for an adult human subject) can cause heartburn, flatulence, and other gastrointestinal disorders (Tyler, 1993).
3. Long-term usage of garlic has caused Heinz body anemia (Poppenga, 1995).

Interesting notes:
1. Albert Schweitzer reportedly used garlic effectively against typhus, cholera, and typhoid (Mowrey, 1986).
2. Antibacterial effectiveness decreases quickly with extended storage of bulbs (Weiss, 1988).
3. When making garlic tea, infuse the herb in hot water. Do not boil.

Goldenseal

Latin name:	*Hydrastis canadenis* L.
Family:	Ranunculaceae
Common names:	Goldenseal, yellow root, yellow puccoon

Active ingredients:
1. Goldenseal contains isoquinoline alkaloids, including 1% to 3% hydrastine, 3% to 4% berberine, and tetrahydroberberine (Tyler, 1994).
2. The plant also contains traces of candine, resin, albumin, starch, fats, sugar, lignin, and a volatile oil (Spoerke, 1990).

Major uses: Goldenseal has antibacterial and amoebicidal properties (Wren, 1988). Sources are mixed as to the value of goldenseal when taken internally. It is used in tincture and in powdered form (internally) as an antibiotic of last resort, only because it is overharvested and becoming scarce in the wild. A promising substitute is Oregon grape *(Berberis aquifolium).*

Minor and anecdotal uses: Berberine and the other alkaloids of goldenseal have very diverse and powerful uses. Their efficacy, in acceptable herbal doses, is unclear.

1. Goldenseal is used to treat gastroenteritis and diarrhea (Kamat, 1967; Lahiri, Dutta, 1967; Werbach, Murray, 1994).
2. The berberine constituent of goldenseal is effective against giardiasis (Gupte, 1975; Werbach, Murray, 1994).
3. Goldenseal has a very bitter taste. Goldenseal has been used to treat dyspepsia, especially with hepatic symptoms (Spoerke, 1990).
4. Goldenseal historically has been used to treat urinary tract infections and internal hemorrhages.
5. The plant is commonly used to treat mouth sores (Tyler, 1994).
6. Goldenseal has traditionally been used to treat inflammation of the eyes (Ellingwood, 1983).
7. Goldenseal is considered a valuable part of herbal formulas for inflammation and infection in lungs, kidneys, and reproductive tract (Mills, 1991).
8. The plant has been used in China for two decades to treat a variety of cancers (Werbach, Murray, 1994).
9. Berberine has been shown effective in treating ventricular dysrhythmia caused by ischemia (Werbach, Murray, 1994).

Forms:
1. The dried rhizome and roots are used.
2. For external use, goldenseal is administered as a strong tea.
3. For internal use, tincture or capsules are used.

Toxicity and cautions:
1. Large doses can cause diarrhea.
2. In toxic doses, goldenseal can cause convulsions and other severe central nervous system effects. Deaths have resulted from large overdoses (Spoerke, 1990).
3. Do not give goldenseal to pregnant animals. It is a uterine stimulant, and large doses can cause abortion (Hobbs, 1992).

Interesting notes:
1. Goldenseal is one of the most popular herbs among eclectics, a cure-all in every sense of the word, at least traditionally. The plant is used as a tonic and in acute cases.
2. It is believed erroneously by some that goldenseal blocks the detection of morphine and other narcotics.

Tea Tree

Latin name:	*Melaleuca alternifolia*
Family:	Myrtaceae
Common names:	Tea tree, melaleuca

Active ingredients: Tea tree leaves distill into 2% volatile oil. Oil comprises one part of terpene hydrocarbons (pinene, terpinene, cymene) and two parts oxygenated terpenes (terpinen-4-ol). Tea tree oil also contains small amounts of sesquiterpene hydrocarbons and oxygenated sesquiterpenes (List et al, 1976).

Major uses:
1. Tea tree oil is widely used as a topical antibiotic and fungicide. The terpinen-4 oil (up to 60% of the volatile oil) is particularly effective (List et al, 1976).
2. Tea tree oil has been found to be an effective treatment for vaginal candidiasis (Pena, 1962).
3. Tea tree oil is incorporated into some pet shampoos to repel fleas (Tyler, 1993).

Minor and anecdotal uses: Tea tree oil is reportedly used to treat acne, aphthous stomatitis, athlete's foot, boils, burns, carbuncles, corns, empyema, gingivitis, herpes, impetigo, infections of the nail bed, insect bites, lice, mouth ulcers, psoriasis, sinus infections, sore throat, skin and vaginal infections, tinea, thrush, and tonsillitis (Altman, 1988).

Forms: For external use, a volatile oil is administered.

Toxicity and cautions:
1. Do not use the tree oil internally.
2. Tea tree oil can cause minor reactions (rash) in allergic individuals.
3. High external dosages can also cause weakness, incoordination, tremors, and depression in animals (Villar and others, 1992).

Interesting notes: Melaleuca was introduced into the Florida Everglades several decades ago. Its invasive nature and a lack of natural predators have allowed it to spread uncontrollably. This unchecked spread has the potential to damage the Everglades ecosystem.

Antiparasitic

The current generation of conventional anthelmintic drugs are quick acting and relatively safe, with proven efficacy. Many herbal anthelmintics can take weeks to act properly and are of questionable toxicity, with variable efficacy. In most cases, conventional anthelmintics are still administered. If a client insists on an herbal anthelmintic, formulas including black walnut, garlic (fully described in antibiotic section), pennyroyal, and wormwood may be used.

Black Walnut

Latin name:	*Juglans nigra*
Family:	Juglandaceae
Common names:	Black walnut

Active ingredients:
1. Black walnut has a high tannin content.
2. Juglandin, juglone, and julandic acid are found in black walnut.
3. Ellagic acid is also a component of black walnut.

Major uses:
1. Black walnut is an anthelmintic, effective against tapeworms (Leung, 1984). Used in Asian and Native American cultures against a variety of worms (Mowrey, 1986).

Minor and anecdotal uses:
1. A University of Missouri research team has reported some anticancer effects of black walnut (Bhargava, Wesfall, 1968).
2. Black walnut is used topically to treat skin disorders, ringworm, and psoriasis (Crellin, Philpott, 1990), largely because of its astringent effect (Spoerke, 1990).
3. Black walnut's close relative, butternut *(Juglans cinerea)*, is well known for its mild laxative properties (Crellin, Philpott, 1990).
4. Alcohol tincture of black walnut has been investigated as a treatment against *Giardia* (Crellin, Philpott, 1990).
5. White walnut leaves *(Juglans regia)* are used in Europe to treat chronic eczema, scrofula, inflammation of the eyelids, and other skin complaints (Weiss, 1988).

Forms:
1. The husks, inner bark, root, leaves, kernel, and shell of the black walnut are used.
2. For internal and external use, black walnut is administered as a decoction.

Toxicity and cautions: Toxicity is low (internal and external).

Interesting notes: The hull of black walnut yields a wonderful dark brown dye.

Pennyroyal

Latin name:	(1) *Mentha pulegeum* L., (2) *Hedeoma pulegiodes* L.
Family:	Lamiaceae
Common names:	Pennyroyal, dittany, (1) European pennyroyal, (2) American pennyroyal

Active ingredients: Pennyroyal contains a pungent volatile oil of not less than 85% ketone and pulegone. This oil accounts for as much as 2% of the plant (Tyler, 1993).

Major uses: An infusion of dried pennyroyal leaves has been used as a stimulant, carminative, and diaphoretic (Coon, 1979), but its toxicity may overshadow any therapeutic use.

Minor and anecdotal uses:
1. Pennyroyal is also traditionally believed to be an effective insecticide. Some claim that its essential oil, rubbed on the skin or hair coat, repels ticks, fleas, and flies (Crellin, Philpott, 1990; Wittmann, 1990).
2. Pennyroyal has the reputation of being a strong but inconsistent abortifacient (Crellin, Philpott, 1990). Abortifacient effects are reliable only in near-lethal dosages (Tyler, 1993).

Forms:
1. The dried leaves of pennyroyal are used.
2. For internal use, an infusion is administered.
3. For external use, a tincture of essential oil, which can be quite toxic, is administered.

Toxicity and cautions:
1. Pennyroyal can be toxic to cats.
2. Pennyroyal is toxic to dogs at high dosages (Sudekum and others, 1992).
3. Because of its abortifacient properties, pennyroyal should not be administered to pregnant animals (Spoerke, 1990).
4. Pennyroyal should not be used in subjects with existing kidney disease.
5. As little as 4 ml of oil has caused convulsions in adult human subjects. Larger dosages can cause even greater problems (Spoerke, 1990).

Interesting notes: Because of its toxic nature and the availability of other, milder bitter tonics, many herbalists recommend that pennyroyal be used only topically, with great caution.

Wormwood

Latin name:	*Artemisia absinthium*
Family:	Asteraceae
Common names:	Wormwood, absinthe, Wurmkraut (German), herbe d'absinthe (French)

Active ingredients:
1. Wormwood comprises 0.15% to 0.4% bitter substances, sesquiterpene lactones with dimeric guianolide absinthin (0.2% to 0.28%; the main component), artabsin, matricin, and anabsinthin. Other bitter substances include pelenolides (hydroxypelenolide) (Hartke and others, 1991).
2. Wormwood contains 0.2% to 1.5% volatile oil containing mainly terpenes. As much as 40% of the oil contains the following chemicals: β or α-thujone (see below) (Chialva, Liddle, Doglia, 1983; Sacco, Chialva, 1988; Vostrowsky and others, 1981), *trans*-sabinyl acetate (Chialva, Liddle, Doglia, and others, 1983; Sacco, Chialva, 1988), *cis*-epoxyocimene (Vostrowsky and others, 1981), or chrysanthenyl acetate (Schneider and others, 1979). The oil may contain as many as 50 other mono- and sesquiterpenes. *Absinthium* is a common name for the oil.
3. Wormwood oil contains 3% to 12% thujone, which is a toxic agent (Hoppe, 1975). It is banned in many countries because of its side effects (Tyler, 1994).
4. Other components of wormwood oil include flavonoids (Hoffman, Herrmann, 1982), caffeine and other phenolic carboxylic acids (Swiatek, Kurosawa, Rotkiewiez, 1984), traces of two diastereoisomeric homoditerpene peroxides (which have in vitro antimalarial activity) (Rucker, Mannas, Wilbert, 1992), and minor amounts of 24-ethylcholesta-7,22-kien-3b-ol (antipyretic activity) (Ikram and others, 1987).

Major uses:
1. As an aromatic bitter, wormwood has strong carminative and choleretic properties (*Bundesanzeiger*, 1984; Kreitmair, 1951). Give the infusion before meals (Weiss, 1988).
2. Wormwood stimulates the gallbladder. For this purpose, give the infusion after meals (Weiss, 1988).

Minor and anecdotal uses:
1. Wormwood infusion is used as a bitter tonic for patients with peptic ulcers or chronic dyspepsia (Weiss, 1988).
2. Wormwood strengthens the body against colds and influenza (Weiss, 1988).
3. The volatile oil is somewhat effective against worms (especially threadworms) (Weiss, 1988).

Forms and dosages:
1. The leaves and young tops are used.
2. For internal use, volatile oil in tincture (known as wormwood drops) and infusion are employed.

Toxicity and cautions:
1. The essential oil is toxic, and as little as 15 ml can cause serious nervous disorders or coma. However, Weiss claims that normal doses have relatively small amounts of the dangerous (−)thujone and (+)isothujone (Spoerke, 1990; Weiss, 1988).
2. Wormwood may have some abortifacient effects and therefore should not be administered during pregnancy (Mills, 1991).

Interesting notes:
1. According to Weiss, "*Artemisia cina*, the Levant wormwood, is the real worm remedy, used not only against threadworms...but also against roundworms."

2. Wormwood is a flavoring used in vermouth.
3. Wormwood oil was used in absinthe, a strong French liquor renowned for its narcotic and hallucinogenic effects. Some say Vincent Van Gogh was under its influence when he cut off his ear (Mills, 1991; Tyler, 1993).

Cardiovascular System

These herbs include alfalfa, garlic (described fully in the section on antibacterial agents), gingko, hawthorn, and motherwort.

Alfalfa

Latin name:	*Medicago sativa* L.
Family:	Fabaceae (Leguminosae)
Common names:	Alfalfa, buffalo grass, lucerne

Active ingredients:
1. Alfalfa comprises up to 50% protein.
2. Other ingredients include β-carotene, chlorophyll, octascanol, saponins, sterols (β-sitoseterol, stigasterol, and α-spinasterol), flavonoids, coumarins, alkaloids, acids, vitamins (A, B_1, B_6, B_{12}, C, D, E, K, niacin, pantothenic acid, biotin, folic acid), amino acids, sugars, minerals (calcium, phosphorus, potassium, magnesium, iron, zinc, and copper), and other nutrients (Duke, 1985; Pedersen, 1987).
3. Alfalfa contains large amount of dietary fiber.

Major uses: Mowrey notes that alfalfa's reputation is that of an excellent food, appetite stimulant, and general vitality tonic. He states that modern herbalists have prescribed alfalfa in a wide variety of applications, mainly on the basis of its wide array of nutrients. Most of these applications are tonic in nature and are meant to affect entire organ systems (e.g., urologic, hepatic, digestive, reproductive, musculoskeletal, glandular) (Mowrey, 1993). Other authors agree, especially with regard to its value as a nutritious food (Crellin, Philpott, 1990; Spoerke, 1990; Tyler, 1993).

Minor and anecdotal uses:
1. Alfalfa is one of the best herbal sources of chlorophyll. Chlorophyll may be useful topically as an antiinfectious agent (Smith, Livingston, 1943). The benefit of chlorophyll to the hemoglobin is a matter of considerable speculation among researchers (Mowrey, 1993).
2. Alfalfa is believed to reduce blood cholesterol by blocking its absorption in the intestines (Bricklin, 1976; Cookson, Fedoroff, 1968; Malinow and others, 1978).
3. Alfalfa may aid in the treatment of diabetes (Adams, Murray, 1975).

4. Alfalfa is used in the long-term treatment of arthritis (despite a lack of scientific evidence of its efficacy) (Mowrey, 1993; Spoerke, 1990).
5. Alfalfa has some estrogenic effects in ruminants (Bickoff, Livingston, Booth, 1964; Keeler, 1975; Schaible, 1970).

Forms:
1. The fresh or dried tops (flowers, stems, and leaves) are used.
2. For internal use, dried herb is ground and pressed into pills, used to fill capsules, or infused.

Toxicity and cautions:
1. Alfalfa can cause allergic reactions in those sensitive to pollens.
2. Large dosages can cause flatulence and diarrhea, blood disorders, and other dangerous side effects (Tyler, 1993).
3. Alfalfa seeds are sometimes recommended as a food additive. Unfortunately, the seeds contain canavanine, which is toxic to mice. Therefore use only the tops (Crellin, Philpott, 1990).

Gingko

Latin name:	*Gingko biloba*
Family:	Ginkgoaceae
Common names:	Gingko, maidenhair tree

Active ingredients: Gingko contains an oil extract with 24% flavoglycosides, 10% quercetin, and terpene derivatives (ginkgolides and bilobalides) (Mowrey, 1993).

Major uses:
1. Gingko has proved to be an excellent tonic for geriatric patients (Mowrey, 1993). One double-blind crossover study of commercial gingko preparations showed increased alpha activity and decreased slow-wave activity similar to that seen in the presence of cognitive activating drugs (Itil, Martorano, 1995). The extract has demonstrated a positive effect on the cerebrovascular system. It is believed to increase the energy level of the brain by increasing levels of glucose and ATP and helps reduce the likelihood and severity of cerebral edema (Borzeix, Lavos, Hartl, 1980).
2. The herb has a revitalizing effect on the brain. It is specifically helpful in reducing the impact of aging on the nervous system. Gingko stimulates the release of a variety of neurotransmitters that affect communication throughout the noradrenergic nervous system. Gingko has also been shown to have a positive effect on dementia (Auguet and others, 1982; Le Poncin-Lafitte and others, 1982; Racagni, Brunello, Paoletti, 1986; Taylor, 1986).

3. Gingko has hypotensive qualities without the typical complications of reduced cerebral circulation (Mowrey, 1993).

Minor and anecdotal uses:

1. Gingko's anticoagulant properties led to its use in patients recovering from heart attacks and strokes and in the prevention of coronary thrombosis (Borzeix, Lavos, Hartl, 1980). It has also been shown to increase microcirculation in patients with vascular dementia (Koltringer, Langsteger, Eber, 1995).
2. It is believed that gingko is an effective neutralizer of free radicals affecting the brain, heart, circulatory system, and adrenal and thyroid glands (Brunello and others, 1985).
3. Mowrey (1983) lists eight other studies detailing other applications of gingko's positive effects on the nervous and circulatory system.

Forms:

1. Oil is extracted from leaves. The Chinese also use the fruits and seeds.
2. Gingko is used internally and externally: Filled capsules, tincture, or infusion is employed.

Toxicity and cautions:

1. Gingko has low toxicity and few side effects even in large doses (Mowrey, 1993).
2. Although little research has been conducted on the subject, it is recommended that animals with blood-clotting problems should not be given ginkgo on a long-term basis.

Interesting notes: The species is believed to predate the last ice age. Specimens 1000 years old have been found. The gingko is incredibly hardy and thrives among urban pollution and in a variety of climates.

Hawthorn

Latin name:	*Crataegus oxyacantha, Crataegus monogyna, Craetagus laevigata*
Family:	Roseaceae
Common names:	Hawthorn, mayflower, whitethorn, quickset, maybush, Hagedorn (German), herbe d'aubepine avec fleurs (French)

Active ingredients:

1. Hawthorn contains 1% to 2% flavonoids that vary substantially among species and parts of the plant (Hecker-Niediek, 1983). Flavonoids include quercetin, acetylated and unacetylated vitexin 2-rhamnoside, hyperoside, rutin, spiraeoside, and glavonoglycosylis (Lamaison, Carnart, 1991; Harmon, 1988).

2. Hawthorn contains 1% to 3% oligomeric procyanidines (Schussler, Holzl, 1992).
3. Other components include amines (cardiotonic activity) (Wagner, Grevel, 1982), catechols, phenol-carboxylic acids (especially chlorogenic acid), triterpene acids, sterols, and purines (Harmon, 1988; Hobbs, Foster, 1990).

Major uses:

1. The flowers and leaves of *Crataegus* are a popular long-term heart remedy (*Bundesanzeiger*, March 1984; Weiss, 1988; Mowrey, 1993). It has no digitalis-like components; therefore it is not effective against acute anginal attacks. But according to Weiss, it does have the following tonic indications:
   - Improved coronary circulation (opens vessels, relaxes smooth muscles).
   - Treatment of certain cardiac dysrhythmias: extrasystoles and paroxysmal tachycardia.

   The consensus of multiple researchers is that hawthorn has the following cardiac influences (Echte, 1960; Hammerl and others, 1967; Kandziroa, 1969; Kovach, Foldi, Fedina, 1959; Mann, 1963; Mavers, Hensel, 1974; Mowrey, 1986; Roddewig, Hensel, 1977; Ullsperger, 1951):

   - Peripheral vasodilation
   - Mild dilation of coronary vessels
   - Increased enzyme metabolism in the heart muscle
   - Improved oxygen use by the heart
2. General tonic for the aging heart (O'Conolly and others, 1986).

Minor and anecdotal uses:

1. Helps increase low blood pressure (part of its stabilizing influence on heart) (Mills, 1991).
2. Helps strengthen hearts weakened by the stress of pneumonia, influenza, diphtheria, and other infectious diseases (Weiss, 1988).

Forms:

1. The dried flowers and leaves of hawthorn are used.
2. For internal use, tinctures and infusions are used.

Toxicity and cautions: Hawthorn is safe in normal dosages for long-term use. No evidence of habituation or negative side effects has been reported (Bissett, Wichtl, 1994; Tyler, 1993; Weiss, 1988).

Interesting notes:

1. Hawthorn and digitalis appear to sensitize the heart to each other. It has been reported that when a patient had been treated previously with one herb, only half the normal dosage of the other was required for the desired effect (Bersin, Mueller, Schwarz, 1955).

2. Instant results cannot be expected. The effects of hawthorn are cumulative and long term. The patient should be given the tonic for months.
3. Hawthorn was clinically tested for more than 4 years at the request of the German Federal Ministry of Health, with positive results (Ammon, Handel, 1981).
4. A 125-page book, *The Hawthorn Berry*, is devoted to the medicinal effects of this herb (Rodale, 1971).

Motherwort

Latin name:	*Leonurus cardiaca, Leonurus sibiricus*
Family:	Labiatae
Common names:	Mother herb, mother weed, heartwort, (1) motherwort, (2) East Asian motherwort.

Active ingredients:
1. Motherwort contains various alkaloids (leonurinine) and glycosides (Mowrey, 1986).
2. Tannic acid is a component of motherwort.
3. A bitter principle (leonurine) is also contained in the herb.

Major uses: Motherwort has been shown to be a mild general heart tonic. It must be used for many weeks or months for maximum effect (Weiss, 1988). Mowrey (1993) states that it has an effect similar to that of valerian root. Cardiac effects include (Arustanmova, 1963; Erspamer, 1948; Isaev, Bojadzieva 1960; Kubota, Nakashima 1930; Polyakov, 1964; Schramm, 1958):

• Hypotensive
• Sedative
• Antispasmodic

Minor and anecdotal uses: Motherwort has been reported anecdotally used to treat bronchitis, diarrhea, asthma, and rheumatism (Stuart, 1987).

Forms:
1. The dried leaves and flowers of motherwort are used.
2. For internal administration, infusion or capsules are used.

Toxicity and cautions: Motherwort has caused contact dermatitis in some cases.

Interesting notes:
1. Research into the action of motherwort on the heart has yielded conflicting results. This discrepancy should not be taken as a "negative." Rather, this is usually the sign of good results for most tonic herbs.
2. Motherwort has been used for centuries for "female" support, especially during pregnancy.

Gastrointestinal and Hepatic Systems

Herbs in this category include cascara, chamomile (fully described in the section on nervous system agents), dandelion, ginger, licorice, milk thistle, peppermint, plantago, senna, and slippery elm.

Cascara

Latin name:	*Rhamnus purshiana* D.C.
Family:	Rhamnaceae
Common names:	Cascara sagrada ("sacred bark"), western buckthorn, Californian buckthorn, Americani Faulbaumrinde (German), ecorce de cascara (French)

Active ingredients:
1. Cascara contains a 10% hydroxyanthracene glycoside mixture (Hobbs, 1992). These glycosides include C(10)-glucosylanthrone type (cf. aloes) (70% to 90%) and 11-desoxyaloins A and B (10% to 30%). This mixture also contains O-glucosides and cascarosides A, B, C, and D (*Deutsches Arzneiburch*, 1993).
2. Minor ingredients include tri- and dihydrooxyanthraquinones (emodin, frangulin, isoemodin, aloeemodin, physcion, and chrysophanol), rhein, iso- and heterodianthrones, and aloins (Mowrey, 1986; Hager, 1979).

Major uses:
1. Cascara is a medium-strength laxative affecting the large intestine (Bissett, Wichtl, 1994; Mabey, 1988). Expect results 6 to 8 hours after ingestion.
2. Cascara restores bowel tone and muscle activity without astringent effects or cramping (Mowrey, 1993). Cascara does not affect the small intestine (except with excessive dosages).

Minor and anecdotal uses: Cascara has minor constituents that have proved useful against leukemia, in expelling worms, in preventing formation of calcium-containing urinary stones, and in curing liver disease. It also has strong antibiotic properties (Mowrey, 1986).

Forms:
1. The powdered bark of cascara is used.
2. For internal use, tincture and capsules are used.

Toxicity and cautions:
1. Cascara use should be avoided in subjects with frequent, watery stools or ulcers (Hobbs, 1992).
2. Cascara is not as habituating as senna, but large dosages given for more than 1 week should be avoided (Hobbs, 1992).

3. Cascara may be used in small quantities as a daily tonic (Mowrey, 1993).
4. Cascara can be passed to the fetus and through mother's milk. Therefore its use should be avoided in pregnant and nursing subjects (as with all anthraquinone-containing herbs) (Tyler, 1994).

Interesting notes:

1. Cascara gained popularity in 1870s and 1880s because of promotion by Parke-Davis (Crellin, Philpott, 1990).
2. Cascara is officially recognized by *The United States Pharmacopoeia XXII* (Tyler, 1993).
3. Cascara should be stored for at least a year or heated in a warm air stream to reduce its bitter taste (and the amount of strong anthrones) (*Bundesanzeiger,* 1984). Storage for up to 4 years is reputed to increase potency (Trease, Evans, 1983).
4. Cascara is best used in combination with aromatic herbs such as ginger or fennel (Hobbs, 1992).

Dandelion

Latin name:	*Taraxacum officinale*
Family:	Asteraceae
Common names:	Dandelion, lion's tooth, fairy clock, Lowenzahnkraut or Lowaenzahnwurzel (German), racine et herbe de dent de lion or racine et herbe de pissenlit (French)

Active ingredients:

1. Dandelion is rich in vitamins C and A, niacin, and other nutrients (proteins, fats, and iron).
2. Dandelion is a digestive bitter known previously as *taraxacin.* It contains eudesmanolides (tetrahydroridentin-β and taraxacolide β-D-glucopyranoside) and germacranolides (taraxic β-D-glucopyranoside, 11,13-dihydrotarzix acid β-D-glucopyranoside, and p-hydroxyphenylacetic acid derivative taraxacoside) (Rauwald, Huang, 1985).
3. Dandelion contains triterpenes: taraxasterol and isolactucerol, their acetates and 16-hydroxyl derivatives (arnidiol and faradiol), and b-amyrin (Bissett, Wichtl, 1994).
4. Dandelion contains sterols (sitosterol, stigmasterol), carotenoids (xanthophylls), flavonoids (apigenin and luteoli 7-glucosides), caffeic acid, and carbohydrates (1.1% mucilage) (Bissett, Wichtl, 1994).
5. Dandelion contains gluten, gum, and potash (up to 4.5%) (Bissett, Wichtl, 1994).
6. Dandelion contains inulin (2% to 40%) (Bissett, Wichtl, 1994).

Major uses:

1. Dandelion is a highly nutritious food.

2. The plant stimulates liver secretions, particularly bile (cholagogue) (Bohm, 1959; Bonsmann, 1942; Bussemaker, 1937; Bussemaker, 1936).
3. Dandelion improves the secretion of bile in the gallbladder. Lessens the chances of developing gallstones and reduces their resulting impact (Chabrot, Charonnat, 1935; Leclerc, 1935).
4. Dandelion is an effective digestion and appetite stimulating bitter (*Bundesanzeiger,* 1992).

Minor and anecdotal uses:

1. Dandelion is a remedy for a variety of liver problems, including chronic liver congestion, hepatitis, swelling of the liver, jaundice, and dyspepsia with deficient bile secretion (Kroeber, 1950; Leclerc, 1935).
2. Dandelion is believed to be an effective diuretic and stimulant for the kidney (Mowrey, 1986; Racz-Kotilla, Racz, Solomon, 1974; Weiss, 1988).
3. In long-term tonic therapies, dandelion is used to improve cell metabolism (Weiss, 1988).
4. Some suggest that dandelion has a hypoglycemic effect and is therefore helpful to diabetic patients (Mowrey, 1986).
5. Other reputed uses for dandelion include anticancer and laxative applications (Baba, Abe, Mizuno, 1981; Tyler, 1993).
6. The milk of dandelion leaves may be applied to a wart daily for several weeks to eliminate it (Crellin, Philpott, 1990).

Forms:

1. Fresh, young leaves or dried root is used.
2. For internal use fresh leaves are eaten; the root is chopped and decocted or used in capsules; fresh juice may also be used.

Toxicity and cautions: Dandelion has no known toxicity.

Interesting notes:

1. The Germans made ersatz coffee from roasted dandelion root during World War II.
2. Dandelion is native to Tibet. Hundreds of varieties populate the world.

Ginger

Latin name:	*Zingiber officinale Roscoe*
Family:	Zingigeraceae
Common names:	Ginger, Ingberwurzel (German), fingembre (French)

Active ingredients:

1. Ginger contains pungent phenolic compounds: phenylalkanones or phenylalkanonols (gingerol, zingerone, shogaol) (Kikuzaki, Tsai, Nakatani, 1992)

and diarylhepatnois (including gingerenones A-C, isogingerenone B, and gingerdione) (Endo, Kanno, Oshima, 1990; Kikuzaki, Kobayashi, Nakatani, 1991).
2. Ginger contains 2.5% to 3% volatile oil, which typically includes sesquiterpenes (zingiverene, arcurcumene, beta-bisabolone, and epsilon-alpha-farnesene. The exact components vary with area of cultivation. Australian ginger contains mainly monoterpenes (Elrer and others, 1988; Harvey, 1981). Vietnamese ginger is two thirds monoterpenes. Japanese ginger contains mainly acyclic oxygenated monoterpenes.

Major uses:

1. Ginger's major use is as a digestive tonic. It gently stimulates the entire digestion process (Mowrey, 1993).
2. Other major uses for ginger include reduction of motion sickness, flatulence, heartburn, diarrhea, vertigo, nausea, and dizziness resulting from gastrointestinal causes. It does not affect central nervous system activity (*Bundesanzeiger,* 1988; Kawai and others, 1994; Mowrey, Clayson, 1982).
3. Ginger is used in several commercially available gastrointestinal formulas, including cleansing enemas and liver flushes (Hobbs, 1992).

Minor and anecdotal uses:

1. The antiinflammatory properties of ginger reduce frequency and severity of some symptoms of arthritis (Mowrey, 1986; Srivastava, 1984; Srivastava, Mustafa, 1992).
2. Ginger has some energizing cardiotonic (Shoji and others, 1982), antipyretic, analgesic, antitussive, and sedative properties in small lab animals (*Lawrence Review of Natural Products,* 1986).
3. Hypocholesterolemic properties for ginger have been demonstrated in rats (Gujral, Bhumra, Swaroop, 1978).

Forms:

1. The ginger rhizome is used.
2. For internal administration, powdered and capsulated ginger is used; it is also found in teas, tablets, and candied form.

Toxicity and cautions:

1. Large overdoses can cause depression of the central nervous system and cardiac dysrhythmia (Mowrey, 1986).
2. Ginger inhibits thromboxane synthetase and acts as a prostacyclin agonist. Therefore it is not recommended for postoperative nausea (Backon, 1991).
3. Use smaller doses during pregnancy. Ginger is not dangerous in tonic or culinary doses.
4. Ginger use should be avoided in subjects with ulcers (Weiss, 1988).

Interesting notes:

1. Ginger is generally considered safe by the FDA (Mowrey, 1986).
2. Ginger is used in all major medicinal systems, including traditional Western herbalism, traditional Chinese medicine, and Ayurvedic medicine (Hobbs, 1992).

Licorice

Latin name:	*Glycyrrhiza glabra* L., *G. glandulifera*
Family:	(1) Leguminosae, (2) Fabaceae
Common names:	Glycyrrhiza, *Gan Cao,* (1) Spanish licorice, (2) Russian licorice, licorice root, liquorice.

Active ingredients:

1. Licorice contains glycyrrhizin (the calcium and potassium salts of glycyrrhizic acid) (also known as GL).
2. Hydrolysis of GL in the gut yields glycyrrhetinic acid (a triterpene glycoside) (also known as GLA), 2% to 14%. GLA reduces the metabolism of prostaglandins E and $F_{2\alpha}$, therefore encouraging the healing of peptic ulcers. GLA also inhibits 11b-hydroxysteroid dehydrogenase. This action increases the glucocorticoid concentration in mineralocorticoid-responsive tissues, which in turn increases sodium retention, potassium excretion, and blood pressure (Mills, 1991; Tyler, 1994).
3. Licorice also contains triterpenoid saponons, flavonoids, bitter principle, estrogenic substances, asparagin (2% to 4%), volatile oil, coumarins, and trace amounts of tannins (Mills, 1991).

Major uses:

1. Licorice has been shown to have significant antitussive and expectorant properties. It is especially useful in formulas for treating coughs and the common cold (Chandler, 1985).
2. The combination of GLA and hydrocortisone seems to be effective in the treatment of several skin conditions, including atopic, subacute, and chronic eczematous conditions; itching dermatoses; pruritus; seborrheic, infective, sensitization, contact, neurofoliative, and exfoliative dermatitis; pustular psoriasis (Sommerville, 1957).
3. GLA is 50 times sweeter than sucrose (by weight). Therefore it is helpful in making an otherwise unsavory herbal tea more palatable to the patient (Mills, 1991).

Minor and anecdotal uses:

1. Licorice is considered by many practitioners to be one of the two or three most important herbs available. It

has also been researched for the following uses (Mowrey, 1993; Tyler, 1993):

- Hypolipidemic (cholesterol- and triglyceride-lowering) (Donomae, 1960; Nakamura, Ishiara, 1966).
- Anticariogenic (antiplaque and anti–tooth decay).
- Antimicrobial (Tomoda and others, 1990).
- Antiviral (GL) (Pompei and others, 1980).
- Mildly immunosuppressive (Takagi, Watanabe, Ishi, 1965).
- Invigoration of the reticuloendothelial system (Tomoda and others, 1990).
- Antihepatotoxic (Fujisawam and others, 1980; Mowrey, 1993).
- Antiarthritic and antiinflammatory (Anderson, Smith, 1961; Gujral and others, 1961; Ichioka, 1968; Nasyrov, Lazareva, 1980; Parmar and others, 1964; Sommerville, 1957; Zhao and others, 1983).
- Anticancer (Shvarev and others, 1966).
- Laxative (Mills, 1991).
- Antiasthmatic (Mills, 1991).
- Posttuberculosis healing (effect similar to that of hydrocortisone) (Mills, 1991).
- Transitional treatment for patients ending a long-term steroid regimen (Mills, 1991).
- Combined with small amount of cortisone to treat adrenal exhaustion and Addison's disease (Borst and others, 1953; Groen and others, 1951).
- Eye wash for conjunctivitis and other inflammatory conditions (Mills, 1991).
- Antipyretic results similar to those of sodium salicylate (Aleshenshaya, Aleshkina, 1967; Saxen, Ghalla, 1968).

2. Licorice is useful for treating peptic and duodenal ulcers (Anderson, Smith, 1961; Brogden, Speight, Avery, 1974; Cliff, Milton-Thompson, 1970; Takagi, Watanabe, Ishi, 1965). The German Commission E recommends that it be used for only 4 weeks at a time (*Bundesanzeiger*, 1986; Tyler, 1994).

Forms:
1. The dried rhizome and roots are used.
2. For internal administration, the powdered herb infusion, decoction, ointment, or tincture is used.

Toxicity and cautions: Long-term, excessive usage of licorice can lead to edema, lethargy, high blood pressure, and even more serious aldosteronal side effects. Consumption should be limited to 4 to 6 weeks. Licorice should be used with particular caution in older subjects, as well as in those with cardiovascular, liver, and kidney problems (Tyler, 1994). The most common side effects occur when isolated GLA is used. When possible, use a preparation of the whole plant (Mills, 1991).

Interesting notes:
1. Licorice has been a favorite agent in candies and tobacco products, but, according to Tyler (1993), "most

licorice candy manufactured in this country [the United States] is simply flavored with anise oil."
2. Licorice is found in more traditional Chinese medicine formulas than any other single herb (Hobbs, 1992).
3. Werbach and others (1994), and Mowrey (1986) suggest that all side effects of licorice can be avoided by supplementing the patient's diet with potassium and restricting sodium intake.
4. A major effect of GLA seems to be prevention of the breakdown and prolongation of the half-life of endogenous cortisol (Werbach, Murray, 1994).

Milk Thistle

Latin name:	*Silybum marianum*
Family:	Asteraceae
Common names:	Milk thistle, Marian, St. Mary's, Our Lady's thistle

Active ingredients: The milk thistle fruit has 1% to 4% silymarin comprising a variety of flavonolignans: silybin, isosilybin, dehydrosilybin, silydianin, silychristin, and others (Seligmann, 1985).

Major uses:
1. Silymarin has been found to be protective of and restorative to the liver. Applications include use against phallotoxins of the deadly *Amanita* mushrooms, chronic hepatitis, and cirrhosis. Silymarin also helps combat inflammation of the bile ducts and fatty infiltration of the liver (chemical- and alcohol-induced fatty liver) and reduces impact of leukotrienes.*
2. Milk thistle is an effective antioxidant, many times more potent than vitamin E (Deak and others, 1990; Rauen, Schriewer, 1971; Werbach, Murray, 1994).
3. Milk thistle has been shown to increase the glutathione (GSH) content of the liver by as much as 35%. More GSH, in turn, helps the liver more successfully process environmental toxins such as heavy metals and pesticides (Szilard, Szentgyorgyi, Demeter, 1988; Werbach, Murray, 1994). It also improves protection against carbon tetrachloride, *Amanita* toxin, galactosamine, and praseodymium nitrate (Hikino and others, 1984; Vogel and others, 1975; Wagner, 1986; Wagner, 1981).

Minor and anecdotal uses:
1. Milk thistle helps the liver regenerate healthy cells and repair old damage (Homann and others, 1982).

---

*Boari and others (1985); Canini and others (1985); Ferenci and others (1989); Foster (1991); Hikino and others (1984); Magliulo, Gagliardi, Fiori (1978); Salami, Sarna (1982); Sarre (1971); Scheiber, Wohlzogen (1978); Vogel and others (1975); Wagner (1981); Wagner (1986).

2. It appears to be helpful in the treatment of psoriasis because of its positive impact on liver health (Weber, Galle, 1983).
3. Milk thistle stimulates bile flow (Westphal, 1931).

Forms:
1. Mainly the fruit, but also the shells, seeds, and leaves of milk thistle are used.
2. For internal administration, liquid extract is given in capsule form or injected.

Toxicity and cautions:
1. Milk thistle has no known toxicity.
2. Extremely large doses can cause loose stools as a result of excessive bile production (Werbach, Murray, 1994).

Interesting notes: Milk thistle is also known to some as *Carduus marianus* L. (Mowrey, 1993).

Peppermint

Latin name:	*Mentha x piperita*
Family:	Lamiaceae
Common names:	Peppermint, pfefferminzblatter or Katzenkraut (German), menthe poivree or feuilles de menthe (French)

Active ingredients:
1. Peppermint contains 0.5% to 4.0% volatile oil that is composed of 50% to 78% free menthol and 5% to 20% menthol with various esters such as acetate and isovalerate (Bissett, Wichtl, 1994; Tyler, Brady, Robbers, 1988).
2. Peppermint also contains (+)-and (−)-menthone, (+)-isomenthone, (+)-neomenthane, (=)-menthofuran, and eucalyptol, plus other monoterpenes. It also contains minimal amount of sesquiterpenes (Bissett, Wichtl, 1994; Tyler, Brady, Robbers, 1988).
3. Peppermint contains flavonoids including lipophilic aglycones with o-methylation patterns that vary with age (Voirin, Bayet, 1992).
4. 6% to 12% to tannins, triterpenes, and bitter substances (Bissett, 1994).

Major uses:
1. Peppermint is a tonic for the digestive tract. It has been shown to reduce gas and vomiting, to increase the flow of bile, and to aid in digestion (*Bundesanzeiger,* November 1985; Dinckler, 1936; Mowrey, 1993; Pasechnick, 1967; Steinmetzer, 1926; Tyler, 1993).
2. Peppermint is an appetite stimulant. It temporarily inhibits hunger pangs, which subsequently return with increased vigor (Sollmann, 1948).

3. Peppermint is a flavoring agent in many herbal formulae (Spoerke, 1990).
4. Peppermint relieves symptoms of irritable-bowel syndrome (Werbach, Murray, 1994).

Minor and anecdotal uses:
1. Peppermint has topical antibacterial properties (*Bundesanzeiger*, 1985).
2. It has been shown to inhibit or kill 30 different harmful microorganisms (Mowrey, 1986).
3. Peppermint oil is used as a topical antiinflammatory agent in arthritis, chronic skin disease, and pleurisy (Mills, 1991).
4. Peppermint is used in an alcohol solution to treat ringworm (Mills, 1991).
5. Peppermint is used to cleanse and treat disorders of the liver, pancreas, and gallbladder diseases (Giachetti, Taddei, Taddei, 1988; Mowrey, 1993; Weiss, 1988).

Forms:
1. The leaves are used.
2. For internal administration, volatile oil tincture, infusion of dried leaves, or capsules are used.
3. For external administration, compress of infusion or poultice of leaves is used.

Toxicity and cautions: Peppermint is not useful in treating ulcers (Weiss, 1988).

Interesting notes: Peppermint must be transplanted every 2 years for its properties to be maintained (Weiss, 1988).

Psyllium

Latin name:	*Plantago psyllium, Plantago indica, Plantago ovata Forskal*
Family:	Plantaginaceae
Common names:	Psyllium, (1) Spanish psyllium, (2) French psyllium, (3) blonde psyllium, Indian psyllium, flea seed, isapughula, Spogel seed, indische Flohsamen or indisches Psyllium (German), ispagul (French)

Active ingredients:
1. Psyllium contains oil, protein, and small amounts of iridoids (such as aucubin) (Bissett, Wichtl, 1994).
2. Mucilage (20% to 30%) comprising weakly acidic arabinoxylans (xylose, arabinose, galactose) (Stuart, 1987), rhamnose, and galacturonic acid (Kennedy, Singh, Southgate, 1979).

Major uses: Varieties are used interchangeably.

1. Grain (seed and seed coats) are used as a bulk laxative. Mucilage-filled cells are not absorbed or digested by the gut. Psyllium swells to about eight to 14 times its original mass in gut. It must be taken with large quantities of fluids (*Bundesanzeiger,* 1990; Bissett, Wichtl, 1994; Spoerke, 1990).
2. Psyllium is particularly effective when used in combination with senna (63% psyllium, 37% senna) (Marlett and others, 1987).
3. Psyllium is effective in treating irritable-bowel syndrome (Werbach, Murray, 1994).

Minor and anecdotal uses:
1. Mucilaginous gum is used as emulsifying agent for oil-in-water emulsions (Mills, 1991).
2. Psyllium is effective in the treatment of Crohn's disease (Weiss, 1988).
3. Some evidence suggests that it may slightly lower cholesterol levels in human subjects (*Bundesanzeiger,* 1990; Howard, Marks, 1984).

Forms: (150 ml of liquids required per 5 g of herb) (*Bundesanzeiger,* 1990).
1. The whole or powdered seeds and seed husks are used.
2. For internal administration, psyllium in capsules or mixed in liquid is used.

Toxicity and cautions:
1. Psyllium not recommended for subjects with obstructed bowels.
2. Some may be allergic to psyllium (Berton, 1970).

Interesting notes:
1. Because of its gentle nature, it may take 2 or 3 days of psyllium use to show results.
2. The U.S. FDA will not allow psyllium in "commercial" food products because they consider it a drug.
3. Psyllium is listed in *The United States Pharmacopoeia XXII* (Tyler, 1994).

Senna

Latin name:	*Cassia acutifolia delile, Cassia augustifolia vahl, Cassia marilandica*
Family:	Caesalpinaceae
Common names:	Khartoum or Alexandria senna, Tinnevelly senna, American senna

Active ingredients:
1. Senna contains agents with laxative effects: anthraquinone derivatives, 1.5% to 3.0% dianthrone glycosides (sennosides A, B, C, D, and G) (Jaket, Winterhoff, Kemper, 1990).

2. Senna is an inhibitor of fluid absorption in gut, containing 10% mucilage and tartrates (Weiss, 1988).

Major uses:
1. Dried senna leaves are a strong laxative (Tyler, 1994). Dried pods are gentle (Weiss, 1988). Senna is frequently combined with potassium tartrate and aromatics in laxative formulas (Anton, Haag-Berrurier 1980).
2. Used as part of an overall digestive stimulant with laxative properties; see formulas below.

Minor and anecdotal uses: Senna may be of use in some skin conditions such as psoriasis (Anton, Haag-Berrurier, 1980).

Forms:
1. The leaves of senna are used.
2. For internal administration, cold water infusion, fluid extracts, and tablets are used.

Toxicity and cautions:
1. Two to 4 g of senna can cause liquid stools or pain. Eight to 12 g can cause severe colic, nausea, and vomiting.
2. Do not use senna as a tonic. Senna is habituating and requires larger and larger doses to remain effective (Mowrey, 1993).
3. Excessive senna use can irritate the colon (Pahlow, 1979).
4. Do not use senna during pregnancy; it may stimulate the uterus (Weiss, 1988).

Interesting notes:
1. The laxative properties of senna have led the FDA to categorize it as an over-the-counter class 1 drug.
2. American senna is an effective substitute for Asian varieties (Crellin, Philpott, 1990).
3. Weiss's digestive aid/laxative formula (1988):
   • Components in equal parts: caraway seed, fennel seed, peppermint leaves, senna leaves.
   • One tablespoon of herbs to 0.25 L boiling water, infuse for 15 minutes and let cool to room temperature.
   • One cup morning and night. The infusion may be stored in refrigerator for 2 or 3 days.

Slippery Elm

Latin name:	*Ulmus rubra,* formerly *Ulmus fulva*
Family:	Ulmaceae
Common names:	Slippery elm tree, red elm

Active ingredients:
1. The slippery elm's inner bark contains large amounts of the viscid mucilage polysaccharide.

2. Small amount of starch, tannins, calcium oxalate, and calcium are also found in slippery elm (Spoerke, 1990).

Major uses: Slippery elm is an effective demulcent and antitussive (*Lawrence Review of Natural Products,* 1991).

Minor and anecdotal uses:
1. Slippery elm is used in laxative formulae as an adjunct to soothe the mucous membranes of the gut (Mowrey, 1993).
2. Used internally in Native American medicine to treat diarrhea, urinary and bowel complaints, and dysentery (Mowrey, 1986).
3. Used externally in Native American medicine to treat wounds, ulcers, and burns (Mowrey, 1986).
4. The root tea of slippery elm is used to assist in childbirth or as an abortifacient (Stuart, 1987).

Forms:
1. The dried inner bark or root is used.
2. For internal administration, infusion, commercial "natural" throat lozenges, and capsules are used.
3. For external administration, compresses and poultices are used.

Toxicity and cautions:
1. Slippery elm may cause an allergic rash (Spoerke, 1990).

Interesting notes: According to Tyler (1994), slippery elm was listed in the official compendia in the United States (United States Pharmacopeia [USP] and National Formulary [NF]) from 1820 through 1960.

Immune System

These herbs tone the immune system and improve its overall response. They include echinacea and ginseng.

Echinacea

Latin name:	*Echinacea angustifolia* D.C., *Echinacea pallida, Echinacea purpurea* L.
Family:	Asteraceae
Common names:	Echinacea, coneflower, black Sampson, Sonnenhutwurzel or Igelkopfwurzel (German), racine d'echinacea (French), purple coneflower

Active ingredients:
1. The most important ingredients are the variety of polysaccharides found in each genus. The most heavily researched are from *E. purpurea:* PS I (a-4-O-methylglucuronoarabinoxylan, M, 35 kD) and PS II (an acid rhamnoarabinogalactan, M, 450 kD) (Bauer, Wagner, 1990; Bauer, Wagner, 1991).
2. Echinacea contains 0.3% to 1.3% caffeic acid ester echinacoside (Bauer, Wagner, 1990; Bauer, Wagner, 1991).
3. Cynarin, 1,5-di-O-caffeoylquinic acid, is a component of echinacea (Bauer, Wagner, 1990; Bauer, Wagner, 1991).
4. Echinacea contains a large variety of alkylamides (mainly isobutylamides), including isomeric dodeca-2E,4E,8Z,10E/Z-tetraenoic acid (Bauer, Wagner, 1990; Bauer, Wagner, 1991).
5. Essential oils are found throughout the plant, especially in the tops (Bissett, Wichtl, 1994).
6. Echinacea contains 0.006% pyrrolizidine alkaloids tussilagine and isotussilagine (Roder and others, 1984).

Major uses:
1. Echinacea has been demonstrated to be a nonspecific immunostimulant. It is particularly effective on colds, influenza, and other infectious processes (Steinmuller and others, 1993; *Bundesanzeiger,* 1992; Bauer, Wagner, 1991; Bauer, Wagner, 1990). This effect is achieved by the activation of phagocytosis and stimulation of fibroblasts (Roesler and others, 1991; Bauer, Wagner, 1991; Gaisbauer and others, 1990; Wagner, Proksch, 1981; Korting, Born, 1954; Kuhn, 1953).
2. Echinacea is used topically to reduce inflammation and stimulate wound healing (*Bundesanzeiger,* 1992; Bonadeo, Botaxxi, Lavazza, 1971).

Minor and anecdotal uses:
1. The isobutylamides found in echinacea have demonstrated insecticidal properties (Bohlmann, Genz 1966; Jacobson, 1954).
2. Some ingredients of echinacea may have oncolytic properties (Bauer, Wagner, 1991; Bauer, Wagner, 1990; Luettig and others, 1989).

Forms:
1. The dried rhizome and roots are used.
2. For internal administration, infusion, decoction, tincture, or capsules are used.
3. For external administration, compresses or poultices are used.

Toxicity and cautions: Echinacea has no known toxicity.

Interesting notes: Echinacea herbal products have been subjected to widespread adulteration and used to perpetrate fraud, so much so that in 1990 the German Pharmacopoeial Commission deleted the *Echinacea* monograph from its reference guide. In 1992, Commission E published two new monographs discussing *Echinacea angustifolia* and *Echinacea pallida* separately (Bissett, Wichtl, 1994). Echinacea products are among the most common to be of low quality or to be adulterated. Echinacea products must be purchased from reputable vendors or with known and specific concentration of active ingredients.

Ginseng

Latin name:	(1) *Panax ginseng* C.A. *Meyer*, (2) *Panax quinquefolius*, (3) *Eleutherococcus senticosus*
Family:	Araliaceae
Common names:	(1) Ginseng, Asian ginseng, Korean ginseng, Chinese ginseng, Ginsengwurzel or Kraftwurzel (German), racine de ginseng (French), (2) American ginseng, (3) Siberian ginseng

Active ingredients: Most scientific research has been conducted with Korean ginseng, but all the types of ginseng have similar active ingredients. Korean ginseng is considered superior in quality to American and Siberian ginseng.

1. 2% to 3% triterpene saponins. It is largely made up of ginsenosides Rg1, Rc, Rd, Rb1, Rb2, and Rbo (also known as panaxosides A–F) (Bissett, Wichtl, 1994; Hirakura and others, 1992; Hirakura and others, 1991)
2. Ginseng is about 0.05% essential oil, including limonene, terpineol, citral, and polyacetylenes (Bissett, Wichtl, 1994; Hirakura and others, 1992; Hirakura and others, 1991).
3. A series of ginsenoynes, A–K—of which some are acetylated—is found in ginseng (Bissett, Wichtl, 1994; Hirakura and others, 1992; Hirakura and others, 1991).

Major uses:

1. Researchers are just beginning to investigate the actions of ginseng using the Western scientific method. Until this research is completed, the best way to describe ginseng is as a tonic herb whose long-term use helps the patient adapt to the various environmental stresses that lead to illness (an "adaptogen"). Simply said, ginseng helps the patient avoid disease (Merson, 1984; Sonnenborn, 1987).
2. Animal experiments have demonstrated that ginseng is an immunostimulant (Jie, Cammisuli, Baggiolini, 1984; Singh, Agarwal, Gupta, 1984; Singh and others, 1983).
3. The adaptogenic action of ginseng may be caused in part by seemingly opposing actions of the main active ingredients, the ginsenosides. Some have been found to increase blood pressure and to act as central stimu-

lants. Others have been found to decrease blood pressure and to act as CNS depressants (Chen and others, 1994; Bissett, Wichtl, 1994).
4. Ginseng has also been found to enhance the biosynthesis of RNA and protein (Lu, Dice, 1985; Iijima, Higashi, 1979). Ginseng enhances carbohydrate and lipid metabolism (Avakia, Evonuk, 1979; Qureshi and others, 1985; Yamamoto, Kumagai, 1982).
5. Ginseng revitalizes, reduces fatigue, and increases energy levels (Brekhman, Dardymov, 1969; *Bundesanzeiger*, 1991; D'Angelo and others, 1986; Hallstrom, Fulder, Carruthers, 1982; Saito, Yoshida, Takagi, 1974; Sterner, Kirchdorfer, 1970).
6. Ginseng has been shown to improve mood and reduce fasting blood glucose and body weight but did not affect the lipid values of patients with non–insulin-dependent diabetes (Sotaniemi, Haapakoski, Rautio, 1995).
7. Chinese researchers found that ginseng and digoxin exhibited synergism in the treatment of congestive heart failure. Ginseng also proved to be an effective and safe adjutant without side effects (Ding, Shen, Cui, 1995).

Forms:
1. The dried rhizome and roots are used.
2. For internal administration, infusion, decoction, tincture, or capsules are used.

Toxicity and cautions: Ginseng toxicity is rare. High dosages or long periods of use may cause diarrhea and nervousness (Roder, 1983).

Interesting notes: Ginseng is one of the most popular herbs of the Chinese, Korean, Russian, and Japanese medicinal traditions. It is heavily cultivated throughout eastern Asia. It is difficult to determine the type and quality of ginseng roots. Often one species is mistaken for another. Many commercial products are adulterated with poor-quality ginseng or contain none at all (Liberti, Der Marderosian, 1978). For these reasons, high-quality roots have sold for as much as several thousand dollars (Tyler, 1994).

Nervous System

Herbs of this variety include chamomile, gingko (described fully in the cardiovascular section), oats, St. John's wort, and valerian.

Chamomile

Latin name:	(1) *Anthemis nobilis* L., (2) *Matricaria recutita* L.
Family:	Asteraceae/Asteraceae
Common names:	(1) Roman chamomile, *Chamaemelum nobile* L., double

chamomile, Romische Kamille or Grobe Kamille (German), fleur de camomille romaine (French), and (2) German chamomile, *Matricaria chamomilla,* matricaria, Hungarian chamomile, wild chamomile, Kamillenbluten or Kleine Kamille or Feldkamille (German), fleur de camomile (French)

Active ingredients:
1. *Anthemis nobilis* contains the following agents:
   - 0.6% to 2.4% volatile oil containing angeloyl, methacryl, tigloyl, and isobutyryl ester of aliphatic C4- to C6-alcohols.
   - 0.6% germacranolide-type sesquiterpene lactones (bitter substances) (Holub, Xamek, 1977): nobil, 3-epinobilin (3α-OH), sesquiterpene peroxides such as 1β-hydroperoxyisonobilin (Mayer, Rucker, 1987).
   - Flavonoids including apigenin and luteolin 7-O-glucosides, quercitrin, apiin (apigenin 7-apiosylglucoside) (Bissett, Wichtl, 1994).
   - Small amounts of *trans*-caffeic and ferulic acids, triterpenes (Bissett, Wichtl, 1994), resin, anthesterol, antheme, chamazulene, acetylenic salicylic derivative, cyanogenic glycoside, coumarins (scopolin), valerianic acid, and apigenin (7-D-glycoside) (Mills, 1991; Spoerke, 1990).
2. *Matricaria chamomilla* contains the following agents:
   - 0.3% to 1.5% volatile oil containing bisabolol and its oxides, chamazulene, bisabolone oxide, chamaviolim, spathelenol, and *cis*- and *trans*-enyne dicyclo ethers (spiroether, poilyacetylenes) (Becker, Forster, 1984), farnesine, and terpenes, including tiglic acids, anelic, pinene, and anthemal (Mills, 1991).
   - Flavonoids such as flavones and flavonols (Becker, Forster, 1981), apigenin (7-D-glycoside) (Bauer, Wagner, 1991), luteoli, quercitrin, 7-mono- and 7-diglycosides and 7-monoglycosides acetylated in the sugar moiety.
   - Sesquiterpene lactones: matricin, matricarin, desacetylmatricarin.
   - Coumarins: umbelliferone and heriarin, mucilage.

For further reading on ingredients, see Becker, Reichling, 1981; Carle, Isaac, 1985; Flaskamp, Nonnenmacher, Isaac, 1981; Luppold, 1984; Schilcher, 1987).

Major uses: The two types of chamomile have similar clinical indications.

1. Chamomile is used to reduce anxiety, nervous tension, spasms, colicky pain, and convulsions. The volatile oil, apigenin, and chamazulene are strong antispasmodic agents (Achterrath-Tuckermann and others, 1980; Becker, Reichling, 1981; Breinlich, Scharmagel, 1968; Breinlich, 1966; Carle, Isaac, 1985; Spoerke, 1990).

2. Chamomile is a digestive aid. It is a bitter (gastric) stimulant but does include constituents that slow and regulate gut activity. Therefore chamomile seems to be a balanced remedy for digestive problems caused by nervous tension. It also positively affects the liver (*Bundesanzeiger,* 1984; Lind, Bruh, 1984; Mills, 1991; Pasechnick, 1969).

3. Chamomile has strong internal and external antiinflammatory and fungicidal effects (*Bundesanzeiger,* 1984; Della Loggia and others, 1986; Della Loggia, 1985; Tubaro and others, 1985; Yakolev, von Schictegroll, 1969). Chamomile has been used since ancient times to treat wounds, tooth ache, skin inflammation, and abscesses (Glowania, Raulin, Swoboda, 1987; Mills, 1991; Spoerke, 1990; Thiemer, Stadler, Forsch, 1973).

4. Chamomile has mild sedative properties (Loggia and others, 1982).

5. Chamomile is an antibacterial (including *Staphylococcus* and *Streptococcus*) (Rucker, Mayer, Lee, 1989; Shipochliev, 1981) and antiphlogistic agent (Breinlich, Scharmagel, 1968; Jakovlev, Osaac, Flaskamp, 1983; Jakovlev, Schlichtegroll, 1969; Kienholz, 1963, Kienholz, 1962).

6. Other sources for clinical evaluations for these indications include Carle and Isaac (1987), Detter (1981), Isaac (1980), and Nasemann (1975).

Minor and anecdotal uses:
1. Chamomile is an antiulcer and antiseptic agent (Isaac, 1975; Szelenyi, Isaac, Thiemer, 1979).
2. Constituents have been investigated as possible anticancer and antitumor agents (Kraul, Schmidt, 1957). Historically chamomile has been used against benign/malignant tumors and carcinomas of the liver, stomach, mouth, skin, and brain (Hartwell, 1968).

Forms:
1. The dried flower heads are used.
2. For internal administration, infusions, tincture, capsules, and volatile oil are used.
3. For external administration, compresses and poultices are used.

Toxicity and cautions:
1. Chamomile may cause a skin rash or other allergic reactions in patients sensitive to ragweed-type pollens (Spoerke, 1990).
2. Excessive dosage of infusion may also cause irritation of the stomach and gut (Spoerke, 1990).
3. Ingestion of excessive quantities (gallons) can inhibit motor function (Mowrey, 1993).

Interesting notes:
1. Chamomile is one of the most popular European tonics and "cure-alls" (Mowrey, 1986).

2. Boiling destroys the volatile oil.
3. The volatile oil is not soluble in water. Steeping in water for 10 minutes only extracts about 10% to 15% of the desired oil (Tyler, Brady, Robbers, 1988).
4. Chamomile is so popular in Germany that it was selected medicinal plant of the year for 1987 (Carle, Isaac, 1987).
5. *Matricaria recutita* L. is the form of chamomile most commonly used on the European continent and in the United States. *Anthemis nobilis* L. is the most popular form in England (Tyler, 1994).
6. Clinical research suggests that the whole chamomile herb is more effective than its isolated constituents (Mowrey, 1993).

Oats

Latin name: *Avena sativa* L.
Family: Graminaceae
Common names: Oats, oats beards, groats, Gruner Hafer (German), herbe d'avoine (French)

Active ingredients:
1. The oat seed contains starch, gluten, albumin, sugar, and gum oil (Spoerke, 1990).
2. Other active ingredients include triterpenoid saponins of the furostanol type (including avenacosides A and B) (Wolters, 1966).
3. Alkaloids (including indole alkaloid, gramine, trigonelline, and avenine), sterol (avenasterol), flavonoids, and silica (SiO_2) (Becker, Forster, 1984) may be found in Oats.
4. The oat is rich in minerals, especially calcium, iron, manganese, and zinc (Schneider, 1985).

Major uses:
1. As a nutritious food and a nourishing tonic, the oat truly straddles the fence between food and medicine. Overall, it is an excellent food for those recovering from exhaustion or other debilitating conditions (Mills, 1991; Spoerke, 1990).
2. Its nutrients seem to be specific to the recovery of the nervous system. The oat has a long-term tonic effect (stabilizing the highs and lows). It is considered the remedy of choice in convalescent programs for the nervous system (*Bundesanzeiger*, 1987; Mills, 1991).
3. Because of its demulcent attributes, the oat has been used topically in soothing poultices to treat wounds and burns (Mills, 1991).

Minor and anecdotal uses:
1. The oat has been used for long-term treatment of herpes, including the genital variety (Mills, 1991).
2. Spoerke (1990) claims the oat has been used as an antidepressant.

Forms:
1. The dried flowering plant and seed are used.
2. Internal: decoction; alcohol tincture; oatmeal.
3. External: compresses, poultices; baths.

Toxicity and cautions:
1. The oat has no known toxicity.

Interesting notes:
1. The oat is gaining popularity as an ingredient in animal shampoos.

St. John's Wort

Latin name: *Hypericum perforatum*
Common names: Saint John's wort, Walpurgiskraut or Hexenkraut (German), herbe de millepertuis (French)

Active ingredients:
1. St. John's wort contains 1% volatile oil (pseudohypericin and related naphthodianthrones) (Holzl, Munker, 1985).
2. The plant contains 10% tannins and a small amount of procyanidins (Holzl, Ostrowski, 1987).
3. St. John's wort contains 0.05% to 0.3% hypericin, a reddish dianthrone pigment that causes photosensitization (Holzl, Ostrowski, 1987).
4. Flavonoids, including rutin and hyperoside, are found in St. John's wort (Berghofer, Holzl, 1987).
5. As much as 3% hyperforin, a phloroglucinol derivative, is found in St. John's wort (Holzl, Ostrowski, 1987; Maisenbacher, Kovar, 1992).

Major uses:
1. The tea is used mainly as a mild, calming nerve tonic. It is prescribed in cases of depression, anxiety, and disturbed sleep (*Bundesanzeiger*, 1984; Holzl, 1990; Muldner, Zoller, 1984; Schmidt, Sommer, 1993).

Minor and anecdotal uses:
1. The essential oil is used on wounds, inflammation, and hemorrhoids (*Bundesanzeiger*, 1984; Pahlow, Mihailescu, 1979).
2. St. John's wort is believed to be an effective diuretic (Schmidsberger, 1980).

Forms:
1. The dried leaves and flowering tops are used.
2. For internal administration, tincture or infusion is used.
3. For external administration, the essential oil of leaves and flowers is used.

Toxicity and cautions: Photosensitization has been recorded in cattle fed hypericum (Spoerke, 1990). This ef-

fect is most likely to occur after prolonged use or extremely large dosages (Tyler, 1993).

Interesting notes:
1. St. John's wort was one of the most popular herbs from the time of Dioscorides and Hippocrates through the Middle Ages. It has recently regained popularity.
2. The plant is called St. John's wort because of likelihood that it will be in full bloom on June 24, St. John's Day in medieval Europe (Tyler, 1993).
3. Preliminary tests suggest that hypericin may be helpful in treating AIDS and Epstein-Barr virus infection (Werbach, Murray, 1994).

Valerian

Latin name:	*Valeriana officinalis, Valeriana wallichii*
Family:	Valerianaceae
Common names:	Valerian, garden heliotrope, all-heal, fragrant valerian, Baldrianwurzel or Katzenwurzel or Balderbrackenwurzel (German), racine de valeriane (French)

Active ingredients: Researchers have had mixed results in determining which constituents cause the observed properties of valerian. What is clear is that the highest-quality herbs are those that are fresh or have been dried carefully at temperatures less than 40° C (Bos and others, 1986; Tyler, 1993).

1. Valerian contains 0.3% to 0.7% volatile oil (including valerianic acid, isovalerianic acid, borneol, pinene, camphene, methyl-2-pyrrole ketone, assorted sesquiterpenes).
2. Epoxy iridoid esters (valepotriates) are found in valerian.
3. Volatile alkaloids, including valerianine and chatarinine, are components of valerian.
4. Valerian contains resin and gum (Mills, 1991; Titz and others, 1983).

Major uses:
Valerian is used as a natural, nonaddictive "tranquilizer," as opposed to a sedative (Becker, Reichling, 1981; Houghton, 1988; Nahrstedt, 1984; Riedel, Hansel, Ehrke, 1982; Veith and others, 1986).

Minor and anecdotal uses:
1. Historically, valerian has also been used for its antispasmodic, diuretic, and expectorant properties (Hendriks and others, 1981; Mills, 1991).
2. Valerian has minor hypotensive properties (Mowrey, 1986; Spoerke, 1990).

3. Valerian may have some antitumor properties (Spoerke, 1990).

Forms
1. The fresh or dried root is used.
2. For internal administration, glycerin and hydroalcohol-based tinctures are used.

Toxicity and cautions: No toxicity has been observed. Valerian is regarded as safe for food use by the FDA (Werbach, Murray, 1994).

Interesting notes:
1. Supposedly valerian oil attracts rats; reportedly the Pied Piper used it to rid the town of Hamelin of the rodents (Hylton, 1974). Weiss (1988) claims that valerian has an effect on cats similar to that of catnip (*Nepeta cataria*).
2. Diazepam (Valium) is not a derivative of valerian (Klotz, 1990).

Musculoskeletal System and Musculoskeletal Pain

Many of these herbs are tonics that can be used as long-term dietary supplements. This list includes alfalfa (described fully in the cardiovascular section), cayenne, cloves, and white willow bark.

Cayenne

Latin name:	*Capsicum minimum, Capsicum frutescens, Capsicum annuum*
Family:	Solanaceae
Common names:	Cayenne, capsicum, chili, red pepper, bird pepper

Active ingredients:
1. Cayenne has been found to contain alkaloids (capsaicin) 0.02%.
2. Carotenoid pigments (including capsanthin, capsorubin) are found in cayenne.
3. Flavonoids, ascorbic acid, and volatile oils (capsico) are also components of cayenne (Mills, 1991; Spoerke, 1990).

Major uses:
1. When capsaicin (the active ingredient in capsicum) ointment is applied topically, it can reduce the pain of diabetic neuropathy, rheumatoid arthritis, trigeminal neuralgia, osteoarthritis, and peripheral neuropathy (Werbach, Murray, 1994).
2. Capsaicin cream was found to be effective against psoriasis (Bernstein and others, 1986; Ellis and others, 1993).

Minor and anecdotal uses:
1. Cayenne may be an effective reliever of postamputation stump pain (Rayner and others, 1989).
2. Cayenne is used internally as a carminative and a gastrointestinal stimulant (Locock, 1985).
3. Historically, cayenne's primary use has been as a stimulant (Crellin, Philpott, 1990).

Forms:
1. The dried and powdered fruit is used.
2. For internal administration, tincture or infusion or capsules of powder are used.
3. For external administration, tincture, ointment, poultices, or compresses are used.

Toxicity and cautions:
1. Avoid capsicum if hyperacidity, hypertension, or peptic ulcers are present (Mills, 1991).
2. Excessive amounts can irritate the mucous membranes (especially of the stomach) (Spoerke, 1990).

Interesting notes:
1. Cayenne is most frequently used in herbal formulas to stimulate various digestive and circulatory functions of the body. It is used as an "activator" in formulas.
2. Several 0.075% capsaicin creams have been approved by the FDA for over-the-counter sales (Tyler, 1994).
3. Cayenne is a good source of vitamin C (Tyler, 1993).

Cloves

Latin name:	*Syzgium aromaticum* L.
Family:	Myrtaceae
Common names:	Clove oil

Active ingredients: The clove contains a volatile oil (eugenol).

Major uses:
1. When clove oil is applied directly to the gums or tooth, it blocks the pain of toothache (Tyler, 1994).
2. Clove oil is added in 1% to 5% concentrations to mouthwashes to provide antiseptic effects (Tyler, 1994).

Minor and anecdotal uses:
1. Clove oil is used externally as a rubefacient and counterirritant (Mills, 1991).
2. Internally, clove oil increases the flow of saliva and gastric juices (Mills, 1991).

Forms:
1. The dried flower buds are used.
2. For internal administration, volatile oil in tinctures, capsules, or infusions is used.

Toxicity and cautions: Prolonged contact of clove oil with the gums can be extremely irritating.

Interesting notes:
1. In many older herbals, the botanical name of this plant is given as *Eugenia caryophyllata* T. or *Caryophyllus aromaticus* L. (Tyler, 1994).
2. Clove oil is accepted by the FDA and American Dental Association for over-the-counter use in dental products. In Germany, it has also been approved for use as a local anesthetic and antiseptic.
3. Clove oil is used as a preservative for pickles.

White Willow Bark

Latin name:	*Salix alba* L., *Salix purpureau* L., *Salix fragilis* L.
Family:	Salicaceae
Common names:	White willow bark

Active ingredients: Most commercial willow bark products contain 1% total of salicin and phenolic glycosides. *S. alba* typically contains about 1% of these active ingredients, *S. purpurea* about 7%, and *S. fragilis* about 10% (Tyler, 1994).
1. White willow bark contains salicin (salicyl alcohol glycoside).
2. Phenolic glycosides (including salicortin, fragilin, tremulacin, and others) are found in white willow bark. When the bark is dried, these are converted to salicin (Meier, Sticher, Bettschart, 1985).
3. White willow bark contains tannins (10%-20%) (Tyler, 1994).

Major uses: White willow bark has analgesic, antiinflammatory, antipyretic, and disinfectant properties. It is used to treat muscle pain, arthritis, headaches, rheumatism, and fevers (Mowrey, 1986; Tyler, 1994).

Forms:
1. The powdered, dried inner bark is used.
2. For internal use, capsules or infusions are used.

Toxicity and cautions: The primary concern about using willow bark in the same fashion as synthetic salicylate (aspirin) is the sheer volume of herb required for a similar dosage of active ingredient. To get just one dose, 14 g of herb would have to be prepared in 2.4 L of water. Moreover, if ordinary 1% white willow bark is used, this volume would have to be multiplied by seven (Tyler, 1994).

Interesting notes:
1. White willow bark is the well-known parent plant of the now-famous drug aspirin.

2. Because of slow absorption of salicin in the intestine and liver, willow bark's effects are slower to appear but longer lasting than an application of salicylate alone (Schneider, 1987).

Genitourinary System

A short list includes black cohosh, cranberry, goldenrod, parsley, raspberry, saw palmetto, and uva ursi.

Black Cohosh

Latin name:	*Cimicifuga racemosa* L., *Actaea racemosa*
Family:	Ranunculaceae
Common names:	Squaw root, bugbane, black snakeroot, cimifuga, rattleweed, rattleroot, bugwort. It should not be confused with blue or white cohosh.

Active ingredients:
1. Black cohosh contains a water-insoluble resin, which in turn contains acteina (15%–20%).
2. Triterpenoid glycosides are found in black cohosh.
3. Other ingredients include isoferulic, palmitic and oleic acids, tannins, and racemosin.

Major uses:
1. Black cohosh is a tonic herb that relaxes the nervous system and smooth muscles of the intestines and uterus (Mowrey, 1993).
2. The plant has proven hypotensive and vasodilatory effect in rabbits and cats (Genazzani, Sorrentino 1962; Salerno, 1955) but not in dogs (Tyler, 1993).

Minor and anecdotal uses:
1. Traditionally, black cohosh has been used to treat the female reproductive tract (Mowrey, 1993). It is given to pregnant patients in the days immediately preceding labor to promote quick, easy, and uncomplicated birth.
2. Black cohosh has some hypoglycemic effects, but more research is needed to quantify them (Farnsworth, Segelman, 1971; Mowrey, 1993).
3. Black cohosh has some antiinflammatory effects (Benoit and others, 1976).
4. Other reputed uses include as an aid in dyspepsia, as a cough suppressant, and as an antidiarrheal agent (Spoerke, 1990). It also has been found to have astringent, diuretic, alterative, and diaphoretic actions (Wren, Wren, 1975).

Forms:
1. The dried rhizomes and roots are used.

2. For internal administration, tinctures and decoctions are used.

Toxicity and cautions:
1. Black cohosh can cause the premature onset of uterine contractions. Pregnant patients should not receive the herb until the week before the due date.
2. The herb has occasionally caused stomach upset and vomiting (Spoerke, 1990; Tyler, 1994).

Interesting notes:
1. Black cohosh was used extensively by Native Americans and eclectic physicians.
2. The herb is found in many commercial herbal formulas, including the famous Lydia E. Pinkham's Vegetable Compound (Burton, 1949).

Cranberry

Latin name:	*Vaccinium macrocarpon*
Family:	Ericaceae
Common names:	Cranberry, American cranberry, trailing swamp cranberry

Active ingredients:
1. Fructose and an unidentified polymeric compound are responsible for the cranberry's effectiveness against urinary tract infections (Tyler, 1994).
2. The cranberry also contains various carbohydrates, fiber, and plant acids (including benzoic, citric, malic, and quinic acids) (Ofek and others, 1991).

Major uses: The cranberry is used to prevent and treat urinary tract infections (Avorn and others, 1994; Moen, 1962; Papas, Brusch, Ceresia, 1966; Tyler, 1994).

Minor and anecdotal uses: In patients with chronic kidney stones, cranberry juice reduced the urinary ionized calcium by an average of 50% (Light and others, 1973).

Forms:
1. The berries are used.
2. For internal administration, juice or capsules of dried powder are used.

Toxicity and cautions: The cranberry has no known toxicity.

Interesting notes: The acidity of cranberry juice was once believed the cause of its effectiveness against urinary tract infections. Recently, research has shown that constituents of cranberry act by preventing microorganisms such as *Escherichia coli* from adhering to the epithelial cells (Schmidt, Sobota, 1984, 1989; Soloway, Smith, 1988; Zafriri and others, 1989).

Goldenrod

Latin name:	*Solidago virgaurea, Solidago serotina, Solidago canadensis, Solidago odora;* many hybrids.
Family:	Asteraceae
Common names:	Goldenrod, European goldenrod, goldenrod, Riesengoldrutenkraut (German)

Active ingredients:

1. Goldenrod contains flavonoids: kaempferol, rhamnetin, isorhamnetin, quercetin, and their 3-O-rutinosides (Batyuk, Kovalera, 1985); isoquercitrin; astragalin; and afzetin.
2. Goldenrod contains saponins: bisdesmoside mixture (Reznicek and others, 1991).
3. Goldenrod contains diterpenes: one diterpene acid and three diterpenes of the labdane type (Bohlmann and others, 1980).
4. Goldenrod contains essential oil: 85% hydrocarbons and 15% oxygenated compounds, including caryophyllene oxid, cyclocolorenone, α-curcumene, γ-salinene, and β-caryophyllene (Bohlmann and others, 1980).
5. Other components include phenolic glycosides such as leiocarposide, tannins, and polysaccharides (Wren, 1988).

Major uses:

1. Goldenrod is widely used in Europe to treat urinary tract infections and to prevent the formation, or promote elimination, of kidney stones (Bissett, Wichtl, 1994; Tyler, 1994).
2. Goldenrod has significant antiinflammatory and analgesic properties (Metzner, Hirshelmann, Hiller, 1984).
3. Goldenrod is an effective diuretic (Chodera and others, 1985).

Minor and anecdotal uses:

Goldenrod is reported to have antitumor (Kraus, Schneider, Franz, 1986), antifungal (Bader and others, 1987), and antispasmodic (Tyler, 1994) properties.

Forms:

1. The dried leaves, roots, and flowers of the goldenrod plant are used.
2. For internal administration, a decoction or capsules are used.

Toxicity and cautions:

Goldenrod has no known toxicity.

Interesting notes:

1. Goldenrod is quite invasive and hybridizes easily.

Botanists have found 27 species in Indiana alone (Deam, 1940).
2. Parke-Davis marketed a fluid extract of goldenrod in the 1890s (Parke-Davis, 1890).
3. Goldenrod is a common ingredient in commercial herbal kidney-support formulas (Weiss, 1988).

Parsley

Latin name:	*Petroselium crispum, Petroselium sativum*
Family:	Apiaceae
Common names:	Parsley, Petersilienfruchte (German), persil (French)

Active ingredients:

1. Parsley contains volatile oil (0.1% in root, 0.3% in leaf, 2%-7% in seeds) that includes myristicin, apiol, and 1-allyl-2,3,4,5-tetramethoxybenzene (Stahl, Jork, 1964).
2. Vitamins A, B_1 B_2, K, and C are found in parsley. The herb also contains protein, iron, and other minerals (Murphy, March, Willis, 1978; Watt, Merrill, 1963).
3. Parsley also contains terpenes (Formacek, Kubeczka, 1982), flavonoids (including apiin), and furanocoumarins (Horhammer, List, 1977).

Major uses:

1. A tea of the leaves and roots of parsley is recommended as a treatment for urinary tract infection and to facilitate the passage of kidney stones (Braun, Frohne, 1987; *Bundesanzeiger*, 1989; Weiss, 1988). Some believe that parsley works best in these situations when combined with other herbs such as buchu and cornsilk (Mowrey, 1986).
2. Parsley is a digestive aid that helps expel gas (*Bundesanzeiger*, 1989; Tyler, 1994).
3. The fresh leaves are a nutritious food.

Minor and anecdotal uses:

1. The volatile oil is a uterine and menstrual flow stimulant (Tyler, 1988).
2. Parlsey is mildly hypotensive (Petkov, 1979) and antibacterial (Abdullin, 1962).
3. Parsley has been used clinically to treat jaundice and other liver ailments for more than 100 years. No experimental data are available, however (Mowrey, 1986).

Forms:

1. The dried leaves, seeds, and roots are used.
2. For internal administration, cold-water infusion of leaves or cold-water decoction of roots or seeds is used.

Toxicity and cautions:

1. Because of the uterine-stimulant properties of the volatile oil, it should be avoided by pregnant patients.
2. The volatile oil also increases the photosensitivity of the patient (Tyler, 1994).
3. Because it irritates the epithelial tissues of the kidney, parsley should be avoided by those with impaired kidney function (Tyler, 1994).

Raspberry

Latin name:	Various varieties of *Rubus idaeus* L. and *Rubus strigosus Michx*
Family:	Rosaceae
Common names:	Raspberry, red raspberry, Himbeerblatter (German), feuille de framboisier (French)

Active ingredients: The raspberry contains 8% to 14% hydrolyzable tannins (containing gallic and ellagic acids) and 1.5% vitamin C (Horhammer, List, 1979).

Major uses:

1. Raspberry is considered the herb of choice for expectant mothers. Reynolds (1982) recommends it as a traditional remedy for uterine pain and profuse bleeding during pregnancy. Evidence suggests that raspberry is a uterine and intestinal smooth muscle relaxant (Burn, Withell, 1941; Noble, 1959).
2. Taken internally as a tea, raspberry is a fast-acting and effective remedy for diarrhea (Tyler, 1993).

Minor and anecdotal uses:

1. Raspberry has astringent and stimulant properties (Grieve, 1971). It is applied as a poultice to wounds and burns and used as a mouthwash to reduce mouth and throat inflammation (Tyler, 1993).
2. The astringent qualities of raspberry also make it useful for treating dysentery, internal bleeding, ulcers, and chronic skin disease (List and others, 1968-1979; Martindale, 1977).

Forms:

1. The dried leaves or powdered root bark is used.
2. For internal administration, strong infusions or decoctions of root bark are used.
3. Externally, tincture is used in mouthwash; poultices, compresses used elsewhere.

Toxicity and cautions: Raspberry has no known toxicity; however, because of its tannin content, excessive use could lead to bowel or kidney irritation.

Interesting notes:

1. Some commercially available "raspberry" teas are nothing more than black tea with an applied volatile oil that smells like raspberries. Be careful to read the list of ingredients (Tyler, 1993).
2. Many traditional herbalists use red and black raspberry leaves and root barks interchangeably. No serious research has been conducted to determine the medicinal difference among the many *Rubus* species. In American eclectic medicine red and black raspberry are highly prized for their astringent effects. Red raspberry seems to be more popular today for its reputed uterine effects.

Saw Palmetto

Latin name:	*Serenoa repens*
Family:	Arecaceae
Common names:	Saw palmetto, sabal

Active ingredients:

1. Saw palmetto contains volatile and fatty (β-sitosterol-3-D-glucoside) oils. The exact active component and its mechanism are not clear.
2. Various acids (including anthranilic, caffeic, and cholorgenic), tannins, sugars, and polysaccharides are also found in saw palmetto (Hansel, Haas, 1984).

Major uses:

1. The antiandrogenic and antiinflammatory effects of saw palmetto seem to be effective in the treatment of benign prostatic hyperplasia (Boccafoschi, Annoschia, 1983; Breu and others, 1992; Champault and others, 1984; Mattei and others, 1988) and chronic cystitis (Spoerke, 1991).

Minor and anecdotal uses:

1. Saw palmetto may stimulate appetite (Mowrey, 1986).
2. The herb is mildly diuretic (Tyler, 1993).

Forms:

1. The berries are used.
2. For internal administration, fluid extract in capsules or infusion is used.

Toxicity and cautions: Saw palmetto has no known toxicity. Extremely large amounts of saw palmetto may cause diarrhea.

Interesting notes:

1. Because of the considerable amount of water-insoluble active ingredients, do not prepare infusions or decoctions of the raw or dried berries of the saw palmetto (Tyler, 1994).
2. Although saw palmetto is popular in Europe and was popular in the United States before 1950, it is not recognized as a remedy for benign prostatic hyperplasia by the FDA (Anonymous, 1990).

Uva Ursi

Latin name:	*Arctostaphylos uva-ursi,*
	Arctostaphylos coactylis,
	Arctostaphylos adenotricha
Family:	Ericaceae
Common names:	Uva ursi, bearberry, bear's grape, mountain box, Barentraubenblatter or Wolfsbeere or Wilderbuchs (German), feuille de busserole or feuille de raisin d'ours (French)

Active ingredients:

1. Uva ursi contains phenolic glycoside arbutin (5%–12%), which hydrolyzes in the gut and releases hydroquinone. It is largely responsible for uva ursi's antiseptic and astringent properties (Bissett, Wichtl, 1994; Tyler, 1993).
2. Other components include iridoid glycoside montrepein (Johada, Leifertova, Lisa, 1978), the flavonoid hyperoside, gallo tannin, and catechol types of arbutrin gallic acid ester (Britton, Haslam, 1965; Herrmann, 1953; Wahner, Schonert, Friedrich, 1974).
3. Ursolic acid and isoquercitrin contribute to diuretic action (Spoerke, 1990).

Major uses:

1. In general, uva ursi soothes inflammations of the lower urinary tract (*Bundesanzeiger,* 1984; Frohne, 1970; Kedzia and others, 1975). It is helpful in the treatment of inflammatory diseases such as urethritis, nephritis, cystitis (Grieve, 1971), and prostatitis (Mills, 1991).
2. Arbutin is an excellent urinary antiseptic, especially if the urine is alkaline (List and others, 1969-1976; Pahlow, 1979; Trease, Evans, 1978).

Minor and anecdotal uses:

1. Uva ursi is used as a mild CNS depressant (Spoerke, 1990).
2. Uva ursi has some anticancer properties (Hartwell, 1960).
3. The herb has been shown to have good antibiotic properties (Benigni, 1948; Danilowski, 1895; Johadar, Leifertova, Lisa, 1990).
4. Uva ursi helps relieve the pain of kidney stones (Mowrey, 1986).
5. Uva ursi is a mild diuretic (Mowrey, 1986; Tyler, 1993). This finding is disputed by Weiss (1988).
6. The tannin content of uva ursi should offer some assistance in managing diarrhea and intestinal irritation (Mills, 1991).

Forms:

1. The dried leaves are used.
2. For internal administration, cold-water infusion or tincture is used.

Toxicity and cautions:

1. Although hydroquinone can be dangerous, doses of uva ursi as large as 20 g have shown no side effects in human subjects (Tyler, 1993).
2. The high tannin content of uva ursi can cause stomach upset, especially with extended use (Weiss, 1988).
3. Uva ursi may stimulate the uterus and therefore should be avoided in pregnant patients (Weiss, 1988).

Interesting notes:

1. The decoction process Weiss recommends likely causes uva ursi to lose its mild diuretic properties, and cold-water infusion or capsules of powdered herb are favored.
2. Uva ursi is found in many commercial kidney and bladder teas (Tyler, 1993).

Respiratory System

These herbs support the respiratory tract in similar but different ways. They include colt's foot, ephedra, marshmallow, mullein, and plantain.

Colt's Foot

Latin name:	*Tussilago farfara* L.
Family:	Asteraceae
Common names:	Colt's foot, coughwort, horsehoof, foal's foot

Active ingredients:

1. Colt's foot contains mucilage.
2. Other constituents include bitter glycosides, tannin (up to 17% in leaves, none in flowers), saponins, volatile oil, a resin, zinc, and pectin (Crellin, Philpott, 1990; Mills, 1991; Spoerke, 1990).

Major uses: Colt's foot is useful as a demulcent antitussive (Tyler, 1994). Weiss (1988) prescribes it for chronic coughs.

Minor and anecdotal uses:

1. Traditionally colt's foot has been prescribed for all types of respiratory and chest problems, including coughs, colds, asthma, and general bronchial congestion (Crellin, Philpott, 1990).
2. The herb is also used topically in poultices for wounds and ulcers (Mills, 1991).

Forms:

1. The dried leaves and flowers are used.
2. For internal administration, tincture or infusion is used.
3. For external administration, compresses or poultices are used.

Toxicity and cautions: Colt's foot contains pyrrol-izidine alkaloid (senkirkine), which was found to cause cancer of the liver in rats when fed in 4% concentration (Spoerke, 1990; Tyler, 1994). This toxin is found in such small amounts in the dried herb, 0.000% to 0.015%, that it should not be a concern in proper dosages (Weiss, 1990).

Ephedra

Latin name:	*Ephedra sinica* (Chinese ephedra) and *Ephedra equisetina*
Family:	Ephedraceae
Common names:	Ephedra, *Ma Huang*

Active ingredients: Ephedra contains various alkaloids, including ephedrine, pseudoephedrine, norephedrine, and norpseudoephedrine (1% to 3%). These ingredients seem to have similar effects on the patient and are active in the treatment of bronchial asthma. Not all varieties of ephedra contain alkaloids. North and Central American species do not contain alkaloids and are therefore not used medicinally (Hegnauer, 1962).

Major uses:
1. Ephedra is a fast-acting treatment for bronchial asthma (Kreig, 1964; Tinkelman, Avner, 1977; Weiss, 1988).
2. Ephedra is a strong nasal decongestant (Kreig, 1964). Often it is combined with an expectorant to manage bronchitis and other upper respiratory tract ailments (Weiss, 1988).
3. Ephedra is a CNS stimulant (Kreig, 1964). It increases systolic and diastolic blood pressure, as well as heart rate (Tyler, 1994).

Forms:
1. The young stems are used.
2. For internal administration, decoctions and commercial liquid preparations are used.

Toxicity and cautions: The FDA warns that large dosages can be extremely dangerous, especially in those with heart conditions, high blood pressure, enlarged prostate, diabetes, or thyroid disease (Tyler, 1994; Werbach, Murray, 1994).

Interesting notes: Because ephedrine is a precursor in the synthesis of methamphetamine, its use is now strictly controlled (Tyler, 1994).

Marshmallow

Latin name:	*Althaea officinalis*
Family:	Malvaceae
Common names:	Marshmallow, Eibischblatter or Altheeblatter (German), guimauva (French)

Active ingredients:
1. Marshmallow contains 5% to 10% mucilage, consisting primarily of arabinogalactans and galacturonorhamans (Karawya, Balbaa, Afifi, 1971).
2. Marshmallow also includes 37% to 38% starch, 10% to 11% pectin, 2% asparagine, 1.25% fat, and 10% to 11% sugars (Spoerke, 1990; Weiss, 1988).
3. Flavonoids found in marshmallow 8-hydroxyluteolin 8-β-gentiobioside and the corresponding 8-glucoside (Gudej, 1987).

Major uses: Marshmallow is an antiinflammatory and demulcent used to treat sore throats and coughs (Bissett, Wichtl, 1994; Spoerke, 1990; Weiss, 1988).

Minor and anecdotal uses:
1. Marshmallow is also used topically as a poultice, especially in wound healing (Bissett, Wichtl, 1994; Mowrey, 1986).
2. Other traditional uses include treatment of inflammation and mucosal disorders of the genitourinary and gastrointestinal tracts (cystitis, incontinence, painful urination, gonorrhea, enteritis, diarrhea, dysentery, and cholera) (Mowrey, 1986).

Forms:
1. The chopped, dried roots (except for the brown outer corky layer) and the dried leaves are used.
2. For internal administration, syrup or cold-water decoction is used.
3. For external use, cold-water decoction (gargle), poultices, or compresses are used.

Toxicity and cautions: Marshmallow has no known toxicity, and its administration should not pose a problem unless the patient has a bowel obstruction (Spoerke, 1990).

Interesting notes: At one time, the marshmallow root was the main ingredient of the spongy white confection that bears its name (Mowrey, 1986).

Mullein

Latin name:	*Verbascum thapsiforme, Verbascum phlomoides, Verbascum thapus*
Family:	Scrophulariaceae
Common names:	Mullein, Wollblumen or Konigskerzenblumen or Windblumen (German), fleurs de molene (French)

Active ingredients:
1. Mullein contains 3% mucilage, which yields after hydrolysis 47% D-galactose, 25% arabinose, 14% D-glucose, 6% D-xylose, 4% L-rhamnose, 2% D-mannose, 1% L-fucose, and 12.5% uronic acids (Kraus, Franz, 1987).

2. Mullein also contains iridoids, including aucubin, 6β-alosylaucubin, datalpol, 6β-xylosylcatalpol, methylcatalpol, and isocactapol (Seifert and others, 1985).
3. Other components include saponins (verbascosaponin) (Tschesche, Delhri, Sepulveda, 1979), flavonoids (apigenin and luteolin and their 7-O-glycosides) (Papav and others, 1980), phenol-carboxylic acids (caffeic and ferulic) (Swiatek and others, 1984), sterols, digiprolactone, and 11% invert sugar (fructose + glucose) (Bissett, Wichtl, 1994).

Major uses:

1. Because of its demulcent and expectorant properties, mullein is often used in antitussive teas (*Bundesanzeiger*, 1990; Kraus, Franz, 1987; Weiss, 1988).
2. Mullein is used topically as a demulcent and astringent to treat skin disorders and irritation (Spoerke, 1990; Tyler, 1993).

Minor and anecdotal uses:

1. Mullein has been reported anecdotally as a treatment for a variety of chest pains (Spoerke, 1990) and rheumatism and as a diuretic (Tschesche, Delhri, Sepulveda, 1980).
2. Mullein is also used in tea form to activate lymph circulation in neck and chest (Hobbs, 1992).
3. Mullein may also have antibiotic effects (Fitzpatrick, 1954).
4. Mullein has been used in combination with garlic or goldenseal in eardrops to treat inflammation and infection of the ear.

Forms:

1. The leaves and flowers are used.
2. For internal administration, infusion or capsules are used.
3. For external administration, poultices of fresh leaves and oil for eardrops are used.

Toxicity and cautions: Mullein has no known toxicity.

Plantain

Latin name:	*Plantago lanceolata* L.
Family:	Plantaginaceae
Common names:	Plantain, English plantain, ribwort plantain, jackstraw, ribgrass, snake plantain, Wundwegerich or Spitzwegerich (German), psyllium blond d'allemagne (French)

Active ingredients:

1. Approximately 6.5% of plantain is mucilage, including four polysaccharides (Brautigam, Franz, 1985a).
2. Plantain contains three iridoid glycosides: aucubin, asperuloside, and catapol (Bianco and others, 1984).

3. The herb also has tannins, phenolic carboxylic acids (r-hydroxybenzoic, protocatechuic, and gentisic acids), chlorogenic and neochloroenic acids, minerals (silica, zinc, and potassium), flavonoids (apigenin, luteolin, scutellarein), and saponin (Tarle, Petricic, Kupinic, 1981).

Major uses:

1. Plantain is well known as a soothing antitussive (*Bundesanzeiger*, 1985; Tyler, 1994).
2. The sap from crushed leaves is antibacterial and astringent (Bissett, Wichtl, 1994; Ehlich, 1960; Felklowa, 1958). It is used topically for the treatment of skin inflammations and wounds (*Bundesanzeiger*, 1985). Other mucous membrane irritations can be treated with plantain, including middle-ear infections, oral cavity inflammations, bronchitis, and sinusitis (Mills, 1991).

Minor and anecdotal uses:

1. The tea is mildly diuretic (Mills, 1991).
2. Aucubin has been found to have hepatoprotective properties (chloroform, α-amanitin) (Chang, Yun, Yan, 1984).

Forms:

1. The dried leaves and fresh juice are used.
2. For internal administration, infusion or tincture is used.
3. For external administration, fresh juice is spread liberally on the wound or inflammation.

Toxicity and cautions: Plantain has no known toxicity.

Interesting notes:

1. Plantain's relative *Plantago major* is the more commonly found broadleaf variety. *P. major* appears to be an excellent herb for wounds and inflammations but less effective as an antitussive (Weiss, 1988).
2. The tea is not antibacterial. The boiling water inactivates the hydrolytic enzyme (Wichtl, 1985).

Skin and Mucous Membranes

These herbs are specific to the various needs and repair of the skin and mucous membranes not related to the respiratory system. They include aloe vera, calendula, evening primrose, tea tree (described fully in the antibacterial section), and witch hazel.

Aloe

Latin name:	*Aloe vera, aloe bardadensis, aloe ferox, aloe africana, aloe spicata*
Family:	Aloaceae or Asphodelaceae

Common names: Aloe vera, Curacao aloe or Cape aloe (German), aloes (French)

Active ingredients:
1. Aloe contains hydroxyanthracene derivatives (25%–40%) (anthraquinone laxative properties) (Rauwald, Voetig, 1982).
2. Aloe also contains acemannan: one liter of juice yields about 1600 mg (Werbach, Murray, 1994).

Major uses:
1. Aloe gel is helpful in the topical treatment of wounds, burns, and skin irritations (especially in diabetic patients) (Davis and others, 1988).
2. The gel is used as a stimulating laxative (Bissett and others, 1984; *Bundesanzeiger,* 1985; Werbach, Murray, 1994).
3. Acemannan is a powerful immunostimulant. It has been administered to cats with feline leukemia, with positive results (Sheets and others, 1991).

Minor and anecdotal uses:
1. Dried aloe gel is used to moderate blood sugar levels in diabetic patients (Ajabnoor, 1990; Beppu, Nagamua, Fujita, 1993; Ghannam, 1986).
2. Acemannan may also be helpful in treating cancer (Harris and others, 1991; Peng and others, 1991).

Forms:
1. For topical use, the gel can be squeezed from the raw stem of the plant or purchased commercially. For internal use, the yellow gel found in the pericyclic tubules just under the epidermis of the leaves is dried into a reddish-black, glistening mass.
2. For internal administration, capsules, tinctures, infusions are used.
3. For external administration, gel is liberally applied.

Toxicity and cautions:
1. Excessive ingested amounts of aloe can cause abdominal cramping, diarrhea, and other more serious side effects (Werbach, Murray, 1994).
2. Aloe can be passed in mother's milk to a nursing infant (Werbach, Murray, 1994).
3. If being used as a laxative, aloe should only be administered for a short period of time. It is habituating.

Interesting note: Aloe is used as an ingredient in commercially available aquarium water conditioners.

Calendula

Latin name:	*Calendula officinalis* L.
Family:	Asteraceae
Common names:	Calendula, marigold flowers, garden marigold, pot marigold, mary bud,

Ringelblumen or Goldblume (German), fleur de souci officinal or fleur de tous les mois or fleur de Calendule (French)

Active ingredients:
1. Essential oil (up to 0.12%) contains menthone, isomenthone, γ-terpinene, α-muurolene, γ- and δ-cadinene, caryophyllene, pedunculatine, α- and β-ionone 5,6-epoxide, dihydro-actinidiolide, geranylacetone, carvone, and caryophyllene ketone (Gracza, 1987).
2. Sesquiterpene, alloaromadendrol, epicubebol, and glycosides are found in calendula (Tommasi and others, 1990).
3. Calendula contains flavonol glycosides and corresponding quercetin derivatives (Vidall-Ollivier and others, 1989).
4. A mixture of hemolytically active bisdesmosidic saponins, with oleanolic acid as the basic unit, is found in calendula (Vidall-Ollivier and others, 1989).
5. Other constituents include triterpene alcohols (Wilkomirski, 1985); free, esterified, and glucosidic sterols; carotenes and xanthophylls; polyacetylenes; phenol-carboxylic acids; and bitter substances (Willuhn, Westhaus, 1987).
6. It is not clear which of these principles is responsible for calendula's medicinal action (Scheffer, 1979).

Major uses: Calendula is an antiinflammatory, antiseptic, antibiotic, fungicide, and nontannin astringent. It is commonly used on wounds and skin inflammations (*Bundesanzeiger,* 1986).

Minor and anecdotal uses: Calendula is a mild antispasmodic and antipyretic (Wichtl, 1984).

Forms:
1. The dried flowers, specifically the ligulate florets, are used.
2. For internal administration, hydroalcohol tincture or infusion is used.
3. For external administration, compresses, poultices, and creams are used.

Toxicity and cautions: Use of calendula should be avoided during pregnancy.

Interesting notes: Calendula is used to produce yellow and orange colors in cosmetics.

Evening Primrose

Latin name:	*Oenothera biennis* L.
Family:	Onagraceae
Common names:	Evening primrose, primrose oil

Active ingredients: The oil of primrose seeds contains *cis*-linolenic acid (70%) and *cis*-γ linolenic acid (9%) (GLA). GLA is a precursor to prostaglandin E_1 (Tyler, 1994).

Major uses: Primrose oil is used to treat atopic eczema (Barber, 1988; Wright, Burton, 1982).

Minor and anecdotal uses:
1. It has been reported anecdotally that primrose may be used to treat a variety of conditions including asthmatic cough, bruises, and gastrointestinal disorders (Briggs, 1986).
2. Some claim that the GLA in evening primrose oil can decrease blood cholesterol and blood pressure and cure rheumatoid arthritis (Passwater, 1981).

Forms:
1. The extracted oil is used.
2. For internal use, 500-mg capsules are given.
3. For external administration, compresses or creams are used.

Toxicity and caution: The use of primrose should be avoided in subjects with blood-clotting disorders.

Interesting notes:
1. In 1992 the FDA took the position that evening primrose oil is an unproven food additive and that it is not generally safe for consumption. It is not readily available in the United States (*Health Food Business*, 1992).
2. Less expensive GLA alternatives include the seeds of the European black currant, *Ribes nigrum* L. (Traitler and others, 1984).
3. Because of the recent surge in popularity of evening primrose, the incredible number of claims made about this herb, and the general lack of substantiating evidence, significant further scientific study is necessary.

Witch Hazel

Latin name: *Hamamelis virginiana* L.
Family: Hamamelidaceae
Common names: Witch hazel, hamamelis leaves and bark, Hamamelisrinde or Virginische Zaubernubrinde (German), ecorce d'hamamelis de virginie or ecorce de noisetier de la sorciere (French)

Active ingredients:
1. Witch hazel contains a 10% mixture of tannins (digalloylhamamelose and catechols) and free gallic acid and monogalloylhamamelose (Friedrich, Kruger, 1974; Freudenberg, Blumel, 1924; Ganday, 1946; Gruttner, 1898; Loebich, 1964).

2. Other components include soft fats and waxes (Gruttner, 1898), essential oil (eugenol and sesquiterpene) (Jowett, Pyman, 1913), and, perhaps, saponins (Horhammer, List, vol 5, 12, 1976, and vol 5, 372, 1993).

Major uses: Witch hazel is an excellent astringent for skin and mucous membranes. It is used to treat wounds, local inflammations, and hemorrhoids (*Bundesanzeiger*, 1985; List, Hoerhammer, 1978; Mowrey, 1986; Trease, 1978). It is effective against chronic atopic dermatitis (Pfister, 1981).

Forms:
1. The dried leaves and bark are used.
2. For external administration, nondistilled hydroalcoholic extract, applied directly or in ointment or suppository form, is used.

Toxicity and cautions: Witch hazel should only be used topically.

Interesting notes: Several distilled witch hazel extracts are commercially available. Because the tannins are not transferred in the distillation process, the resulting astringent effect is largely caused by the alcohol or other constituents (Tyler, 1994).

Conclusions

Western veterinary herbal medicine is still in its infancy, and its practitioners are pioneers. Herbs can be used independently or in conjunction with other types of therapy. Veterinarians must cooperate and communicate their experiences with different herbal remedies and therapies.

Practitioners must work with the FDA to reform its policies on herbal medicine. Practitioners can better help their patients by keeping directly involved in high-quality research, monitoring popular periodicals for misinformation about herbal pet products, and publishing the results of our experience.

To achieve the most consistent and best results, practitioners must remember to use herbs of the correct genus and species, obtain high-quality products from reputable manufacturers, and follow other guidelines stated earlier.

Unlike the situation with conventional pharmaceuticals, no formularies exist for veterinary herbal remedies to provide exact dosage guidelines or 50% lethal doses. When using herbs, veterinarians also must consider the differences between species and between herbivores and carnivores, along with other factors (e.g., size, sex) (Table 20-3).

The incorporation of herbs into everyday veterinary practice may seem overwhelming to many readers, with too many variables and uncertainties. Veterinarians are advised to start by learning the use of 20 or fewer herbs. After studying them thoroughly, veterinarians should begin with conservative dosages. Later, they may add five more

TABLE 20-3

HERBS

COMMON NAME	LATIN NAME	CATEGORY
Alfalfa	*Medicago sativa* L.	Cardiovascular, musculoskeletal
Aloe vera (Curacao, Cape)	*Aloe vera, A. bardandensis, A. ferox, A. africana, A. spicata*	Skin and mucous membranes
Black cohosh	*Cimicifuga racemosa* L., *Actaea racemosa*	Genitourinary
Black walnut	*Juglans nigra*	Antiparasitic
Calendula	*Calendula officinalis* L.	Skin and mucous membranes
Cascara	*Rhamnus purshiana* D.C.	Gastrointestinal
Cayenne	*Capsicum minimum, C. frutescens, C. annuum*	Musculoskeletal
Chamomile (Roman, German)	*Anthemis nobilis* L., *Matricaria recutita* L.	Nervous, gastrointestinal
Cloves	*Syzgium aromaticum* L.	Musculoskeletal
Colt's foot	*Tussilago farfara* L.	Respiratory
Cranberry	*Vaccinium macrocarpon*	Genitourinary
Dandelion	*Taraxacum officinale*	Gastrointestinal and hepatic
Echinacea	*Echinacea angustifolia* D.C., *E. pallida, E. purpurea* L.	Immune
Ephedra	*Ephedra sinica, E. equisetina*	Respiratory, nervous
Evening primrose	*Oenothera biennis* L.	Skin and mucous membranes
Garlic	*Allium sativum* L.	Antibacterial, cardiovascular, antiparasitic
Ginger	*Zingiber officinale*	Gastrointestinal
Gingko	*Gingko biloba*	Cardiovascular; nervous
Ginseng	*Panax ginseng* C.A. Meyer, *P. quinqefolia, Eleutherococcus senticosus*	Immune
Goldenrod	*Solidago virgaurea, S. serotina, S. canadensis, S. odora,* and other hybrids	Genitourinary
Goldenseal	*Hydrastis canadensis* L.	Antibacterial
Hawthorn	*Crataegus oxyacantha, C. monogyna, C. laevigata*	Cardiovascular
Licorice (Spanish and Russian)	*Glycyrrhiza glabra* L., *G. glandulifera*	Gastrointestinal, skin

APPLICATIONS	CONTRAINDICATIONS	PART USED AND FORM
General tonic	Allergic reaction in some; seeds	Fresh or dried tops; infusion, pills, capsules
Wounds, burns, and skin inflammations; laxative; immunostimulant	Nursing mothers; habituating laxative	Gel (two types); capsule, tincture, infusion, spread topically
Relaxant of uterus, intestines, and nerves	Pregnancy; sensitive stomach	Dried rhizome and roots; decoction, tincture
Anthelmintic	None	Decoction of inner bark
Antiinflammatory, antiseptic, antibiotic, fungicide, nontannin astringent; wounds	Pregnancy	Dried flowers; tincture, infusion, compress, poultice, ointment
Medium-strength laxative	Pregnant and nursing mothers; ulcers	Powdered bark in tincture or capsules
Pain reduction in joints and muscles; warming	Hyperacidity, hypertension, or peptic ulcers	Powdered fruit; capsules, tincture, poultice ointment
Antiinflammatory; calming; mild sedative; digestive aid	Allergic reaction in some	Dried flower head; used in poultices, tincture, capsules
Antiseptic; blocks pain of toothache	Prolonged contact with gums	Volatile oil of flower buds; tinctures, capsules; infusion
Demulcent antitussive	None in small dosages	Dried flowers and leaves; tincture, infusion, poultice
Prevents and treats urinary tract infections	None	Berries; juices, capsules of dried powder
Nutritious food; stimulates bile production in liver and gallbladder	None	Fresh young tops; dried root decocted or in capsules
Nonspecific immunostimulant, wound healing	None	Root and rhizome; decoction, tinctures, capsules, compress
Bronchial asthma; strong nasal decongestant; central nervous stimulant	Large doses extremely dangerous; heart and thyroid disease; high blood pressure; diabetes	Young stem; decoction, tincture
Atopic eczema	Blood-clotting problems	Extracted oil; compresses, creams
Antibiotic; heart and circulatory tonic; anthelmintic	Blood-clotting problems	Fresh pulp; enteric coated capsules
Digestive tonic; reduces symptoms of gastrointestinal illnesses	Ulcers; postoperative nausea; smaller doses in pregnant subjects	Dried rhizome; capsules, tablets, infusions, and candies
Geriatric tonic; brain vitalizing; hypotensive	Blood-clotting problems	Oil from leaves, fruit, seed; tincture; infusions; capsules
Immunostimulant, adaptagenic, lowers fatigue	Diarrhea or nervousness possible with excessive long-term usage	Rhizomes and roots; decoction, tincture
Urinary tract infections; kidney stones; diuretic; antiinflammatory; analgesic	None	Dried leaves, roots, and flowers; decoction, capsules
Antibiotic; amoebicidal	Pregnancy	Dried roots and rhizome; tea, tincture, capsules
Heart tonic	None	Dried flowers and leaves in tincture or infusion
Antitussive and expectorant; various skin conditions; complementary	Long-term or excessive use; geriatric and weak patients	Dried rhizome and roots; infusion of powder; decoction; tincture; ointment

Continued

TABLE 20-3

HERBS—cont'd

COMMON NAME	LATIN NAME	CATEGORY
Marshmallow	*Althaea officinalis*	Respiratory
Milk thistle	*Silybum marianum*	Hepatic
Motherwort	*Leonurus cardiaca; L. sibiricus*	Cardiovascular
Mullein	*Verbascum thapsiforme, V. phlomoides, V. thapus*	Respiratory, skin
Oats	*Avena sativa* L.	Nervous, skin
Parsley	*Petroselium crispum, P. sativum*	Genitourinary
Pennyroyal (European and American)	*Mentha pulegeum* L., *Hedeoma pulegiodes* L.	Antiparasitic
Peppermint	*Mentha* × *piperita*	Gastrointestinal
Plantain	*Plantago lanceolata* L.	Respiratory, skin
Psyllium (Spanish, French, blonde)	*Plantago psyllium, P. indica, P. ovata Forskal*	Gastrointestinal
Raspberry	*Rubus idaeus* L., *R. strigosus* Michx., and numerous hybrids	Genitourinary
Saw Palmetto	*Serenoa repens*	Genitourinary
Senna (Alexandria, Tinnevelly, American)	*Cassia acutifolia delile, C. augustifolia vahl, C. marilandica*	Gastrointestinal
Slippery elm	*Ulmus rubra*	Gastrointestinal
St. John's wort	*Hypericum perforatum*	Nervous
Tea tree	*Melaleuca alternifolia*	Antibacterial
Uva ursi	*Arctostaphylos uva-ursi, A. coactylis, A. adenotricha*	Genitourinary
Valerian	*Valeriana officinalis, V. wallichii*	Nervous
White willow bark	*Salix alba* L., *S. purpurea* L., *S. fragilis* L.	Nervous
Witch hazel	*Hamamelis virginiana* L.	Skin and mucous membranes
Wormwood	*Artemisia absinthium*	Antiparasitic, gastrointestinal

APPLICATIONS	CONTRAINDICATIONS	PART USED AND FORM
Antiinflammatory and demulcent for throats	Bowel problems	Dried roots; cold water decoction, syrup, poultice
Protectant of liver; antioxidant	None	Fruit, shell, leaves; liquid extract in capsules
Heart tonic	Allergic reaction in some	Dried flowers and leaves tincture or infusion
Antitussive, demulcent and astringent for skin irritations	None	Leaves or flowers; infusion, capsule, compress, poultice
Nutritious food; nervous tonic; demulcent	None	Dried flower, seeds; baths, decoction, tincture, oatmeal
Urinary tract infection; kidney stones; digestive aid; nutritious food	Pregnancy; increases photosensitivity; impaired kidney function	Dried leaves, seeds, roots; cold water infusion or decoction
Topical insect repellent	Pregnancy; dangerous for internal use	Tincture of essential oil
Digestive tonic; appetite stimulant; flavoring agent	Ulcers	Leaves; infusions, tincture of volatile oil, capsules
Antitussive; antibiotic and astringent for mucous membranes	None	Dried leaves, fresh juice; infusion, tincture, juice spread topically
Nonhabituating, bulk laxative	Obstructed bowels; bowel disease; allergic reaction	Powdered seed and seed hulks; capsules
Uterine pain and menstruation during pregnancy; diarrhea	High tannin content sometimes leading to bowel irritation	Dried leaves, powdered root bark; infusion or decoction, tincture, poultice
Benign prostatic hyperplasia	None	Berries; infusion of extract
Strong, habituating laxative	Pregnancy; severe cramping and intestinal discomfort possible with overdosage	Leaves; cold water infusion; fluid extract; tablets
Antitussive and demulcent	Allergic reaction in some	Dried inner bark and root; infusion; lozenges; poultices
Calming nerve tonic	Extreme doses sometimes leading to photosensitivity	Dried leaves and flowering tops; tincture; infusion; oil
Antibiotic; fungicide; vaginal candidiasis; repel fleas	Allergic reaction in some	Volatile oil; used topically
Urinary antiseptic and antiinflammatory	Pregnancy; high tannin content sometimes leading to upset stomach	Dried leaves; cold water infusion, tincture
Mild tranquilizer (does not greatly impair function)	None	Fresh or dried root; tincture
Antiinflammatory; antipyretic; analgesic; disinfectant	Large quantity of herb necessary for effective dosage	Inner bark; capsules; infusion
Astringent; inflammations; chronic atopic dermatitis	Topical use only	Dried leaves, bark; nondistilled hydroalcoholic extract
Anthelmintic; aromatic bitter; gallbladder	Pregnancy; essential oil toxic	Infusion or volatile oil of leaves and young tops

herbs to their repertoires. Practitioners should experiment and build their knowledge base, then share this knowledge with others.

REFERENCES

Abdullin KK: Bactericidal effect of essential oils, *Uch Zap Kazansk Vet Inst* 84:75, 1962.

Achterrath-Tuckermann U and others: *Plant Med* 39:38, 1980.

Adams R, Murray F: *Health foods*, New York, 1975, Larchmont Books.

Ajabnoor MA: Effect of aloes on blood glucose levels in normal and alloxan diabetic mice, *J Ethnopharm* 28:215, 1990.

Aleshenshaya EE and others: Pharmacology of glycyrrhiza glabra (licorice) preparations, *Farmikol I Toksikol* 27(2):217, 1964.

Altman PM: Australian tea tree oil, *Aust J Pharm* 69:276, 1988.

Ammon HTT, Handel M: *Planta Medica* 43/2/3/4:105, 1981.

Anderson DM, Smith WG: The antitussive activity of glycyrrhetic acid and its derivatives, *J Pharm Pharmacol* 13:396, 1961.

Anonymous: *Am Pharm* NS30(6):17, 1990.

Anonymous: *Health Food Business* 38(8):13, 1992.

Anton R, Haag-Berrurier M: Therapeutic use of natural anthraquinone for other than laxative actions, *Pharmacology* 20(suppl)1:104, 1980.

Arustanmova FA: Hypotensive effect of leonaurus caridaca on animals in experimental chronic hypertension, *Izvestiya Akademii Nauk Armyanski SSR, Biologicheski Nauki* 16(7):47, 1963.

Auguet M and others: Effects of an extract of ginkgo biloba on rabbit isolated aorta, *Gen Pharmacol* 13:225, 1982.

Avakia EV, Evonuk E: Effects of *Panax ginseng* extract on tissue glycogen and adrenal cholesterol depletion during prolonged exercise, *Planta Med* 36:43, 1979.

Avorn J and others: Reduction of bacteriuria and pyuria after ingestion of cranberry juice, *JAMA* 271:751, 1994.

Awang DVC, Kindack DG: Echinacea, *Can Pharmacol J* 124:512-516, 1991.

Backon J: *Anaesthesia* 46:705-706, 1991.

Basko IJ: Over the counter herbal pet supplements: fact or fiction? Proceedings of the 1995 American Holistic Veterinary Medical Association Annual Conference, P139, 1995.

Batyuk VS, Kovalera SN: *Khim Prir Soedin* 1985, 566; CA 104:165306, 1985.

Bauer R, Wagner H: Echinacea species as potential immunostimulatory drugs. In Wagner H, Farnsworth NR, editors: *Economic and medicinal plants research*, vol 5, London, 1991, Academic Press.

Bauer R, Wagner H: *Echinacea: Handbuch fur Apotherker und andere naturwissenschaftlicher*, Stuttgart, 1990, Wissenschaftliche Verlagsgesellschaft.

Becker H, Forster W: Biologie, Chemie und Pharmakologie pfanzlicher Sedativa, *Zeitschrift fur Phytotherapie* (Stuttgart) 5:817, 1984.

Becker H, Reichling J: *Dtsch Apoth Ztg* 121:1185, 1981.

Benigni R: The presence of antibiotic substances in the higher plants, *Fitoterapia* 19(3):1, 1948.

Benoit PS and others: Biological and phytochemical evaluation of plants. XIC. Anti-inflammatory evaluation of 163 species, *Lloydia* 39(2-3):160, 1976.

Beppu H, Nagamua Y, Fujita K: Hypoglycaemic and anti-diabetic effects in mice of aloe arborescens Miller var natalensis Berger, *Phytother Res* 7:S37, 1993.

Berghofer R, Holzl J: *Planta Med* 53:216, 1987.

Bernstein JE and others: Effects of topically applied capsaicin on moderate and severe psoriasis vulgaris, *J Am Acad Dermatol* 15(3):504, 1986.

Bersin T, Mueller A, Schwarz H: Substances contained in crataegus oxyacantha. III. A heptahydroxyflavan glycoside, *Arzneimittel-Forschungen* 5:490, 1955.

Bhargava UC, Westfall BA: Anti-tumor activity of juglans nigra (black walnut) extractives, *J Pharm Sci* 57(10):1674, 1968.

Bianco A and others: *J Nat Prod* 47:901, 1984.

Bickoff EM, Livingston AL, Booth AN: Tricin from alfalfa—isolation and physiological activity, *J Pharm Sci* 53(11):1411, 1964.

Bissett NG, Wichtl M, editor: *Herbal drugs and phytopharmaceuticals*, Boca Raton, Fla, 1994, CRC.

Boari C and others: Occupational toxic liver diseases: therapeutic effects of silymarin, *Min Med* 72:2679, 1985.

Boccafoschi S, Annoscia S: Comparison of *Serenoa repens* extract with placebo by controlled clinical trial in patients with prostatic adenomatosis, *Urologia* 50:1257, 1983.

Bohlmann R and others: *Phytochemistry* 19:2655, 1980.

Bohlmann F, Genz M: *Chem Ber* 99:3197, 1966.

Bohm K: *Arzneimit-Forsch* 9:376, 1959.

Bonsmann MR: *Arch Exp Pathol Pharmacol* 199:376, 1942.

Bordia A, Bansal HC: Essential oil of garlic in prevention of atherosclerosis, *Lancet* II:1491, 1973.

Borst JGC and others: Synergistic action of liquorice and cortisone in Addison's and Simmond's disease, *Lancet* 1:657, 1953.

Borzeix MG, Lavos M, Hartl C: Recherches sur l'action antiagregant de l'extrait de ginkgo biloba: activité au niveau des artères et des veines de la pie-mère chez le lapin, *Arch Int Pharmacodyn* 243:236, 1980.

Bos R and others: *Phytochemistry* 25:133, 1986.

Braun H, Frohne D: *Heilpflanzenlexikon fur Artze und Apotheker*, Stuttgart, 1987, Gustoav Fischer Verlag.

Brautigam M, Franz G: *Planta Med* 51:293, 1985a.

Brautigam M, Franz G: *Deutsch Apoth Ztg* 125:58, 1985b.

Breinlich J, Scharmagel K: *Arzneim-Forsch* 18:429, 1968.

Breinlich J: *Dtsch Apoth Ztg* 106:698, 1966.

Brekhman II, Dardymov IV: Pharmacological investigation of glycosides from ginseng and *Eleuterococcus*, *Lloydia* 32:46, 1969.

Breu W and others: *Zeitschrift fur Phytotherapie* 13:107, 1992.

Britton G, Haslam E: *J Chem Soc* 7312, 1965.

Brogden RN, Speight TM, Avery GS: Deglycyrrhizinised liquorice: A report of its pharmacological properties and therapeutic efficacy in peptic ulcer, *Drugs* 8(5):330, 1974.

Bundesanzeiger (Cologne, Germany): German Commission E monograph on Cascara, May 12, 1984.

Bundesanzeiger (Cologne, Germany): German Commission E monograph on Matricaria flowers, May 12, 1984.

Bundesanzeiger (Cologne, Germany): German Commission E monograph on St John's wort, May 12, 1984.

Bundesanzeiger (Cologne, Germany): German Commission E monograph on Uva ursi, May 12, 1984.

Bundesanzeiger (Cologne, Germany) German Commission E monograph on wormwood, May 12, 1984.

Bundesanzeiger (Cologne, Germany) German Commission E monograph on aloe, August 21, 1985.

Bundesanzeiger (Cologne, Germany) German Commission E monograph on witch hazel, August 21, 1985.

Bundesanzeiger (Cologne, Germany) German Commission E monograph on peppermint, November 11, 1985.

Bundesanzeiger (Cologne, Germany) German Commission E monograph on plantain leaf, November 30, 1985.

Bundesanzeiger (Cologne, Germany) German Commission E monograph on peppermint leaf, November 30, 1985.

Bundesanzeiger (Colonge, Germany) German Commission E monograph on marigold, March 13, 1986.

Bundesanzeiger (Cologne, Germany) May 15, 1986.

Bundesanzeiger (Cologne, Germany) German Commission E monograph on oats, October 15, 1987.

Bundesanzeiger (Cologne, Germany) German Commission E monograph on ginger, May 5, 1988.

Bundesanzeiger (Cologne, Germany) German Commission E monograph on parsley, February 3, 1989.

Bundesanzeiger (Cologne, Germany) German Commission E monograph on plantago seed, January 2, 1990.

Bundesanzeiger (Cologne, Germany) German Commission E monograph on mullein, January 2, 1990.

Bundesanzeiger (Cologne, Germany) German Commission E monograph on ginseng, January 17, 1991.

Bundesanzeiger (Cologne, Germany) German Commission E monograph on dandelion, August 29, 1992.

Bundesanzeiger (Cologne, Germany) German Commission E monograph on *Echinaceae augustifoliae*, August 29, 1992.

Bundesanzeiger (Cologne, Germany) German Commission E monograph on hawthorn leaf/flower, March 1, 1984.

Burn JH, Withell ER: A principle in raspberry leaves which relaxes uterine muscles, *Lancet* 6149:1, 1941.

Burton J: *Lydia Pinkham is her name,* New York, 1949, Farrar, Straus.

Bussemaker J: *Pharm Ztg* 82:851, 1937.

Bussemaker J: Concerning the choleretic activity of Dandelion, *Naunyn-Schmiederbergs Archiv fuer Experimentelle Pharmakology und Pathologie* 181:512, 1936.

Canini F and others: Use of silymarin in the treatment of alcoholic hepatic stenosis, *Clin Ther* 114:307, 1985.

Carle R, Isaac O: *Zeitschrift fur Phytotherapie* 8:67, 1987.

Carle R, Isaac O: *Dtsch Apoth Ztg* 125(suppl I):3, 1985.

Cavallito CJ, Bailey JH: Allicin, the antibacterial principle of allium sativum. I. Isolation, physical properties and antibacterial action, *J Am Chem Soc* 66:1950, 1945.

Chabrot E, Charonnat R: Therapeutic agents in bile secretion, *Ann Med* 37:131, 1935.

Champault G and others: A double-blind trial of an extract of the plant *Serenoa repens* in benign prostatic hyperplasia, *Br J Clin Pharmacol* 18:461, 1984.

Chandler RF: Licorice, more than just a flavor, *Can Pharm J* 118:420, 1985.

Chen X and others: The effects of *Panax quinquefolium* saponin (PQS) and its monomer ginsenoside on heart, *China Journal of Chinese Materia Medica* 19(10):617, 640, 1994.

Chialva F, Liddle PAP, Doglia G: *Z Lebensm Unters Forsch* 176:363, 1983.

Chodera A and others: *Acto Poloniae Pharmaceutica* 42:199, 1985.

Cliff JM, Milton-Thompson GJ: A double blind trial of carbenoxolone capsules in the treatment of duodenal ulcer, *Gut* 11:167–70, 1970.

Crellin JK, Philpott J: *Herbal medicine past and present. Vol II. A reference guide to medicinal plants,* Durham, NC, 1990, Duke University Press.

Danilowski U: *Arch Exp Path Pharmacol* 35:105, 1895.

Davis RH and others: Aloe vera: A natural approach for treating wounds, edema, and pain in diabetes, *J Am Pod Med Assoc* 78:60-68, 1988.

Deak G and others: Immuno-modulator effect of silymarin therapy in chronic alcoholic liver disease, *Ory Hetil* 131(24):1291-1292, 1295-1296, 1990 (in Hungarian).

Deam CC: *Flora of Indiana,* Indianapolis, 1940, State of Indiana Department of Conservation, Division of Forestry.

Della Loggia R: *Dtsch Apoth Ztg* 125(suppl I):9, 1985.

Della Loggia R and others: *Prog Clin Biol Res* 213:481, 1986.

Detter A: *Pharm Ztg* 126:1140, 1981.

Deutsches Arzneiburch (German Pharmacopoeia), ed 10, 1991; first supplement 1992; second supplement 1993.

Dinckler K: *Pharm Zentralhalle* 77:281, 1936.

Ding DZ, Shen TK, Cui YZ: Effects of red ginseng on the congestive heart failure and its mechanism, *Chung Kuo Chung His I Chieh Ho Tsa Chih* 15(6):325-327, 1995.

Donomae I: Gycyrhizzin acid, *Nippon Rinsho* 19:1369-1372, 1960.

Duke HA: *CRC Handbook of medicinal herbs,* Boca Raton, FL, 1985, CRC Press.

Dunlop RH, Williams DJ: *Veterinary medicine: an illustrated history,* St Louis, 1995, Mosby.

D'Angelo L and others: A double-blind, placebo controlled clinical study on the effect of a standardized ginseng extract on psychomotor performance in healthy volunteers, *J Ethnopharmacol* 15:15, 1986.

Echte W: Die Einwirkung von Weissdorn-extrakten auf die dynamik des menschlichen herzens (The effect of Hawthorn extracts on the dynamics of the human heart), *Aerztliche Forshung* 14(11):1560, 1960.

Ehlich J: *Dtsch Apoth Ztg* 106:428, 1960.

Ellingwood F: *American materia medica, therapeutics and pharmacognosy,* Portland, Ore, 1983, Eclectic Medical Publications.

Ellis CN and others: A double-blind evaluations of topical capsaicin in pruritic psoriasis, *J Am Acad Dermatol* 29(3):438, 1993.

Elrer J and others: *Z Lenensmitt-Unters-Forsch* 186:231, 1988.

Endo K, Kanno E, Oshima Y: *Phytochemistry* 29:797, 1990.

Erspamer LV: Pharmacology of leonurus cardiaca and leonurus marrubiastrum L, *Arch Int Pharmacodyn Ther* 76:132, 1948.

Farnsworth NR, Segelman AB: Hypoglycemic plants, *Till and Tile* 57(3):52, 1971.

Felklowa M: *Pharm Zentralhalle* 97:61, 1958.

Ferenci P and others: *Hepatology* 4:1093, 1984.

Fitzpatrick FK: Plant substances active against *Mycobacterium tuberculosis, Antibiotics and Chemotherapy* 4(5):528, 1954.

Flaskamp E, Nonnenmacher G, Isaac O: *Z Naturforsch* 36b:114, 1981.

Formacek V, Kubeczka KH: *Essential oil analysis by capillary gas chromatography and carbon-13 NMR spectroscopy,* Somerset, NJ, 1982, John Wiley & Sons.

Foster H: Garlic, *Allium sativum, Botanical Series No 311,* Austin, TX, 1991, American Botanical Council.

Freudenberg K, Blumel F: *Liebigs Ann Chem* 440:45, 1924.

Friedrich H, Kruger N: *Planta Med* 25:138, 1974.

Frohne D: *Planta Med* 18:1, 1970.

Gaisbauer M and others: The effect of *Echinacea purpurea* Moench on phagocytosis in granulocytes measured by chemiluminescence, *Arzneim Forsch* 40(5):594, 1990 (in German).

Ganday R: *Pharm J* 156:73, 1946.

Genazzani E, Sorrentino L: Vascular action of acteina: active constituent of actaea racemosa L, *Nature* 194(5):544, 1962.

Ghannam N: The anti-diabetic activity of aloes: preliminary clinical and experimental observations, *Hormone Res* 24:288, 1986.

Giachetti D, Taddei E, Taddei I: Pharmacological activity of essential oil on Oddis' sphincter, *Planta Med* 54:389, 1988.

Glowania HJ, Raulin C, Swoboda M: Effect of chamomile on wound healing—a clinical double-blind study, *Z Hautkr* 62(17):1262, 1987.

Gracza L: *Planta Med* 53:227, 1987.

Grieve M: *A modern herbal,* vol 2, New York, 1971, Dover Publications.

Groen J and others: Extract of licorice for the treatment of Addison's disease *N Engl J Med* 244:474, 1951.

Gruttner F: *Arch Pharm* 236:278, 1898.

Gudej J: *Acta Pol Pharm* 44:369, 1987.

Gujral ML and others: Anti-arthritic activity of glycyrrhizin in adrenalectomized rats, *Ind J Med Sci* 15(8):625, 1961.

Hallstrom C, Fulder S, Carruthers M: Effect of ginseng on the performance of nurses on night duty, *Comp Med East West* 6:277, 1982.

Hammerl H and others: Klinisch experimentelle stoffwechseluntersuchungen mit einem crataegus extrakt (Clinical and experimental investigations on metabolism with an extract of Crataegus), *Aerztliche Forschung* 21(7):261, 1967.

Hansel R, Haas H: *Therapie mit Phytopharmaka,* Berlin, 1984, Springer-Verlag.

Harmon NW: Hawthornes, the genus *Crataegus, Can Pharm J* 121:708, 1988.

Harris C and others: Efficacy of acemannan in treatment of canine and feline spontaneous neoplasms, *Mol Biother* 3(4):207, 1991.

Hartwell JL: Plants used against cancer: a survey, *Lloydia* 31:71, 1968.

Hartwell JL: Plant remedies for cancer, *Cancer Chemotherapy Rep* 19:24, July 1960.

Harvey DJ: *Chromatography* 212:75, 1981.

Health Food Business 38(8):13, 1992.

Hecker-Niediek A: Thesis, University of Marburg, 1983.

Hegnauer R: *Chemotaxonomie der Pflanzen,* vol 1, Basel, 1962, Birkhauser Verlag.

Hendriks H and others: *Plant Med* 42:62, 1981.

Herbalgram interview: An interview with Prof. H. Wagner, *Herbalgram* 17:16-17, 1988.

Herrmann K: *Arch Pharm* (Weinheim) 286:515, 1953.

Hikino H and others: Antihepatotoxic actions of flavonolignans from *Silybum marianum* fruits, *Planta Medica* 50:248, 1984.

Hirakura K and others: *Phytochemistry* 30:3327, 1991.

Hirakura K and others: *Phytochemistry* 31:899, 1992.

Hobbs C: *Foundations of health: The liver and digestive herbal,* Santa Cruz, Calif, 1992, Botanica Press.

Holub M, Xamek Z: *Collect Chem Commun* 42:1053, 1977.

Holzl J: *Dtsch Apotheker Zeitung* 130:367, 1990.

Holzl J, Munker H: *Acta Agron* 34(suppl):52, 1985.

Holzl J, Ostrowski E: *Dtsch Apotheker Zeitung* 127:1227, 1987.

Homann J and others: Theragpie der akuten Knollenblaetterpilzvergiftungen, *Hepatology* 12:1522-1523, 1982.

Hoppe HA: *Drogenkunde,* ed 8, vol 1, Berlin, 1975, Walter de Gruyter.

Horhammer L, List PH, eds: *Hager's Handbuch der Pharmazeutischen Praxis,* ed 4, vols 1-8, vol 6b, Berlin, 1979, Springer-Verlag.

Houghton PJ: *J Ethnopharmacol* 22:121, 1988.

Hylton WH ed: *The Rodale herb book,* Emmaus, Pa, 1974, Rodale Press Book Division.

Ichioka H: The pharmacological action of glycyrrhizin. I. The effect on the blood bilirubin level in rabbits with ligated common bile duct, *Gifu Daigaku Igakubu Kiyo* Gifu University School of Medicine 115(3):792, 1968.

Iijima M, Higashi T: *Chem Pharm Bull* 27:2130, 1979.

Ikram M and others: *Planta Med* 53:389, 1987.

Isaac O: *Dtsch Apoth Ztg* 120:567, 1980.

Isaac O, Thiemer K: *Arzneim-Forsch* 25:1352, 1975.

Isaev I, Bojadzieva M: Obtaining galenic and neogalenic preparations and experiments for the isolation of an active substance from leonuraus cardiaca, *Nauchnye Trudy Visshiia Meditsinski Institut (Sofia)* 37(5):145, 1960.

Itil T, Martorano D: Natural substances in psychiatry (*Gingko biloba* in dementia, *Psycholpharmacol Bull* 31:147, 1995.

Jacobson M: *Science* 120:1028, 1954.

Jaket FW, Winterhoff H, Kemper FH: *Zeitschrift fur Phytotherapie* 11:177, 1990.

Jakovlev V, Osaac O, Flaskamp E: *Plant Med* 49:67, 1983.

Jakovlev V, Schlichtegroll A: *Arzneim Frosch* 19:625, 1969.

Jie Y H, Cammisuli S, Baggiolini M: *Agents Actions* 15:386, 1984.

Johadar L, Leifertova I, Lisa M: *Pharmazie* 33:536, 1978.

Jowett HAD, Pyman FL: *Pharmacol J* 91:129, 1913.

Kamat SA: *J Association of Physicians of India* 15:525, 1967.

Kandziora J: Crataegutt-wirkung bei koronaren durchblutung-sstoerungen, *Muenchener Medizinische Wochenschrift* 6:295, 1969.

Karawya MS, Balbaa SI, Afifi MSA: *Planta Med* 20:14, 1971.

Kawai T and others: *Planta Med* 60:17, 1994.

Kedzia B and others: *Med Dosw Mikrobiol* 27:305, 1975.

Keeler RF: Toxins and teratogens of higher plants, *Lloydia* 38(1):56, 1975.

Kennedy JF, Singh J, Southgate DAT: *Carbohydrate Res* 75:265, 1979; CA 91: 135932, 1979.

Kienholz M: *Dtsch Apth Ztg* 102:1076, 1962.

Kienholz M: *Arzneim-Forsch* 13:980, 1963.

Kikuzaki H, Kobayashi M, Nakatani N: *Phytochemistry* 30:3647, 1991.

Kikuzaki H, Tsai SM, Nakatani N: *Phytochemistry* 31:1783, 1992.

Klotz U: *Lancet* 335:922, 1990.

Koltringer P, Langsteger W, Eber O: Dose-dependent hemorrheological effects of microcirculatory modifications following intravenous administration of gingko special extract Egb761, *Clin Hemorrheol* 15(4):649, 1995.

Korotkov VM: The action of garlic juice on blood pressure, *Vrachebnoe Delo* 6:123, 1966.

Korting GW, Born W: *Arzneim Forsch* 4:424, 1954.

Kovach AGB, Foldi M, Fedina L: Die Wirkung eines extraktes aus *Crataegus oxyacantha* auf die durchstromung der coronarien von hunden (the effect of extracts from *C. oxyacantha* on the coronary circulation of dogs), *Arzneimittelforschung* 9(6):1959.

Kraul MA, Schmidt F: The growth-inhibiting effect of certain extracts from flores chamomilae and of a synthetic azulene derivative on experimental mice tumors, *Archive der Pharmazie (Wienheim)* 290:66, 1957.

Kraus J, Franz G: *Dtsch Apotheker Zeitung* 127:665, 1987.

Kraus J, Schneider M, Franz G: *Dtsch Apotheker Zeitung* 126:2045, 1986.

Kreig MB: *Green medicine,* Chicago, 1964, Rand McNally.

Kreitmair K: *Pharmazie* 6:27, 1951.

Kroeber L: Pharmacology of inulin drugs and their therapeutic use. II. Cichorium intybus; taraxacum officinale, *Pharmazie* 5:122, 1950.

Kubota S, Nakashima S: The study of *Leonurus sibericus* L. II. Pharmacological study of the alkaloid "leonurin" isolated from *Leonurus sibericus* L, *Folia Pharmacologica Japonica* 11(2):159, 1930.

Kuhn D: Echinacin and its reaction with phagocytes, *Arzneim Forsch* 3:194, 1953.

Lahiri SC, Dutta NK: Berberine and choloramphenicol in the treatment of cholera and severe diarrhea, *J Ind Med Assoc* 48(1):1, 1967.

Lamaison JL, Carnart A: *Plantes Med Phytotherap* 25:12, 1991.

Lawrence Review of Natural Products, Collegeville, Pa, April 1986, Pharmaceutical Information Associates.

Lawrence Review of Natural Products, Collegeville, Pa, March 1991, Pharmaceutical Information Associates.

Le Pocin-Lafitte M and others: Ischemie cérébrale après ligature non simultanée des artères carotides chez le rat: effet de l'extrait de ginkgo biloba, *Semin Hop Paris* 58:403, 1982.

Leclerc H: *Phytotherapie (Paris),* 1927 cited by Ripperger, W Pflanzliche laxantien und cholagogue wirkungen, *Medizinische Welt* 9:1463, 1935.

Leung AY: *Chinese herbal remedies,* New York, 1984, Universe Books.

Liberti LE, Der Marderosian A: *J Pharm Sci* 67:1487, 1978.

Light I and others: Urinary ionized calcium in urolithiasis, *Urology* 1(1):67, 1973.

List PH, Hoerhammer LH: *Hagers Handbuch der Pharmazeutischen Praxis,* six vols, Berlin, 1968-1979, Springer-Verlag.

Locock RA: Capsicum, *Can Pharm J* 118:516, 1985.

Loebich F: Thesis, University of Heidelberg, 1964.

Lu ZQ, Dice JF: *Biochem Biophys Res Commun* 126:636, 1985.

Luettig B and others: Macrophage activation by the polysaccharide arabinogalactan isolated from plant cell cultures of *Echinacea purpurea, J Natl Cancer Inst* 81(9):669, 1989.

Luppold E: *Pharmazie in unserer Aeit* 13:65, 1984.

Lust J: *The herb book,* New York, 1987, Bantam Books.

Magliulo E, Gagliardi B, Fiori GP: Results of a double blind study on the effect of silymarin in the treatment of acute viral hepatitis, carried out at two medical centres, *Med Klin* 73(28-29):1060, 1978.

Maisenbacher P, Kovar KA: *Planta Med* 58:351, 1992.

Mann D: Appropriate cardiovascular therapy: clinical and experimental study of the action of an injectable preparations of *Crataegus, Zeitschrift fuer die Gesamte Innere Medizin und ihre Grenzgebiete* 18(4):145, 1963.

Marlett JA and others: Comparative laxation of psyllium with and without senna in an ambulatory constipated population, *Am J Gastroenterol* 82(4):333, 1987.

Mattei FM and others: *Serenoea repens* extract in the medical treatment of benign prostatic hypertrophy, *Urologia* 55:547, 1988.

Meier B, Sticher O, Bettschart A: *Deutsche Apotheker Zeitung* 125:341, 1985.

Merson FZ: *Adaptionation, stress and prophylaxis,* Berlin, 1984, Springer-Verlag.

Mihailescu G, Mihailescu A: *Planzen helfen heil,* Munich, 1979, Biblio Verlagsgesellschaft MbH.

Mills SY: *The essential book of herbal medicine,* London, 1991, Arkana.

Moen DV: *Wisconsin Med J* 61:282, 1962.

Mowrey DB: *Herbal tonic therapies,* New Canaan, Conn, 1993, Keats.

Mowrey DB: *The scientific validation of herbal medicine,* New Canaan, Conn, 1986, Keats.

Mowrey DB, Clayson DE: Motion sickness ginger and psychophysics, *Lancet* I:655, 1982.

Muldner H, Zoller M: Anti-depressive effect of a hypericum extract standardized to the active hypericine complex, *Arzneim Forsch* 34:918, 1984 (in German).

Murphy EW, March AC, Willis BW: Nutrient content of spices and herbs, *J Am Dietetic Association* 72:174, 1978.

Murray MT: *The healing power of herbs,* Rocklin, Calif, 1995, Prima.

Nahrstedt A: *Schriftenr. Bundesapotheskenkammer,* Wiss Fortbild Gelbe Reihe, 1984.

Nasyrov KM, Lazareva DN: Study of the anti-inflammatory activity of glycyrrhizin acid derivatives, *Farmak-k Toksikol* 43(4):399, 1980.

Noble RL: The report of the proceedings of the Sixth International Conference on Planned Parenthood, 14-21 February, 1959, 243-250, Vigyon Bharan, New Delhi, India.

OIE (International Office of Epizootics): Early methods of animal disease control, Revue, *Scientific et Technique* 13(2): 1994.

O'Conolly VM and others: Treatment of cardiac performance (NYHA stages I to II) in advanced age with standardized *Crataegus* extract, *Fortschr Med* 104:805, 1986 (in German).

Pahlow M: *Heilpflanzen heute,* Munich, Grafe und Unzer GmbH.

Pahlow M: *Das grosse Buch der Heilpflanzen,* Munich, 1979, Grafe und Unzer GmbH.

Pahlow M: *Das grosse Buch der Heilpflanzen,* Munich, 1985, Grafe und Unzer GmbH.

Papas PN, Brusch CA, Ceresia GC: Cranberry juice in the treatment of urinary tract infections, *Southwest Med* 47(1):17, 1966.

Papav V and others: *Pharmazie* 35:334, 1980.

Parke-Davis: 1890, p 87.

Parmar SS and others: Biochemical basis for anti-inflammatory effects of glycyrrhetic acid and its derivatives, *Int Cong Biochem* 6(5):410, 1964.

Pasechnick IK: Choleric action of *Matricaria officinalis, Farmakilogiia I Toksikologiia* 468, 1969.

Pasechnick IK: *Farmakilogiia I Toksikologiia* 29:735, 1966; CA 66:54111 Cf, 36450, 1967.

Pena EO: *Melalaeuca alternifolia* oil: uses for trichomonal vaginitis and other vaginal infections, *Obstet Gynecol* 19:793, 1962.

Peng SY and others: Decreased mortality of Norman murine sarcoma in mice treated with the immuno-modulator acemannan, *Mol Biother* 3(2):79, 1991.

Petkov V: Plants with hypotensive, anti-atheromatous, and coronarodilatating action, *Am J Chinese Med* 7(3):197, 1979.

Pfister R: Problems in the treatment and after care of chronic dermatoses: a clinical study on hanetum ointment, *Forschr Med* 99(31-32): 1264-1268, 1981 (in German).

Polyakov NG: A study of the biological activity of infusions of valerian and motherwort and their mixtures, *Information of the First All Russian Session of Pharmacists,* Moscow, 319, 1964.

Pompei R and others: Anti-viral activity of glycyrrhizic acid, *Experientia* 36:304, 1980.

Poppenga RH: Risks associated with herbal remedies. In Bonagura JD, editor: *Current veterinary therapy,* Philadelphia, Pa, 1995, WB Saunders.

Qureshi AA and others: *Lipids* 20:817, 1985.

Racagni G, Brunello N, Paoletti R: Neuromediator changes during cerebral aging: the effect ginkgo biloba extract, *Presse Med* 15(31):1488, 1986.

Racz-Kottila E, Racz G, Solomon A: *Planta Medica* 26:212, 1974.

Rao RR, Rao SS, Venkatoraman PR: *J Sci Ind Res* 5:31, 1946.

Rauen HM, Schriewer H: Enzymaktivitaetskorrelationen im serum nach experimentellen lebershaiedigungen der ratte, *Arzeimittel-Forschung* 21:1206, 1971.

Rauwald HW, Voetig R: *Arch Pharm (Weinheim)* 315:477, 1982.

Rauwald HW, Huang JT: *Phytochemistry* 24:1557, 1985.

Rayner HC and others: Relief of local stump pain by capsaicin cream (letter) *Lancet* II:1276, 1989.

Reynolds JEF, editor: *Martindale: the extra pharmacopoeia,* ed 29, London, 1982, The Pharmaceutical Press.

Riedel E, Hansel R, Ehrke G: *Plant Med* 46:219, 1982.

Rodale JI: *The hawthorn berry for the heart,* Emmaus, Pa, 1971, Rodale.

Roddewig VC, Hensel H: Reaction of local myocardial blood flow in non-anesthetized dogs and anesthetized cats to oral and parenteral application of a crataegus fraction (oligomere procyanidins), *Arzneim Forsch* 27:1407, 1977 (in German).

Roder E: *Dtsch Apoth Ztg* 122:2083, 1983.

Rucker G, Mayer R, Lee KR: *Arch Pharm (Weinheim)* 322:821, 1989.

Sobota AE: Inhibition of bacterial adherence by cranberry juice: a potential use for treatment of urinary tract infection, *J Urol* 131:1013, 1984.

Saito H, Yoshida Y, Takagi K: Effect of *Panax* ginseng root on exhaustive exercise in mice, *Jap J Pharmacol* 24:119, 1974.

Salmi HA, Sarna S: Effect of silymarin on chemical, functional, and morphological alteration of the liver: a double-blind controlled study, *Scand J Gastroenterol* 17:417-421, 1982.

Salerno: *Minerva Otorinolaringologica* 5:12, 1955.

Sarre H: Experience in the treatment of chronic hepatopathies with silymarin, *Arzneim-Forsch* 21:1209, 1971.

Saxen RC, Ghalla TN: Anti-pyretic effect of glycyrrhetic acid and imipramine, *Jap J Pharmacology* 18(3):353, 1968.

Schaible PJ: *Poultry, feeds and nutrition,* Westport, Conn, 1970, AVI.

Scheffer JJC: *Pharm Weekly* 114:1149, 1979.

Scheiber V, Wohlzogen FX: Analysis of a certain type of 2 × 3 tables, exemplified by biopsy findings in a controlled clinical trial, *Int J Clin Pharmacol* 16:533, 1978.

Schilcher H: *Die Kamille,* Stuttgart, 1987, Wissenschaftliche Verlagsgesellschaft.

Schmidsberger P: *Knaurs Buch der Heilpflanzen,* Munich, 1980, Droemer Knaur.

Schmidt D, Sobota A: An examination of the anti-adherence activity of cranberry juice on urinary and non-urinary bacterial isolates, *Microbios* 55:173, 1988.

Schmidt U, Sommer H: St. John's wort extract in the ambulatory therapy of depression: attention and reaction ability are preserved, *Fortschr Med* 111(19):339-342, 1993 (in German).

Schneider E: *Zeitschrift fur Phytotherapie* 6:165, 1985.

Schneider E: *Zeitschrift fur Phytotherapie* 8:35-37, 1987.

Schussler M, Holzl J: *Dtsch Apoth Ztg* 132:1327, 1992.

Seifert K and others: *Planta Med* 51:409, 1985.

Sheets MA and others: Studies of the effect of acemannan on retrovirus infections: clinical stabilization of feline leukemia virus–infected cats, *Mol Biother* 3(1):41, 1991.

Shipochliev T: Extracts from a group of medicinal plants enhancing the uterine tonis, *Veterinary Sciences (Sofia)* 18(4):94, 1981.

Shoji N and others: Pharmacological studies on Zingiber mioga Roscoe (2), *Folia Pharmacological Japonica* 75(7):731, 1979.

Shoji N and others: *J Pharm Sci* 71:1174, 1982.

Shvarev IF and others: Effect of triterpeniod compounds from glycyrrhiza glabra on experimental tumors, *Voproisy Izuch Ispol'z Solodki SSR, Akad Nauk SSR* 167-170, 1966.

Singh VK, Agarwal SS, Gupta BM: *Plant Med* 50:462, 1984.

Singh VK and others: *Planta Med* 47:234, 1983.

Soloway MS, Smith RA: Cranberry juice as a urine acidifier, *JAMA* 260:1465, 1988.

Sommer H: Improvement of psychovegetative complaints by hypericum, Fourth International Congress on Phytotherapy, Munich, Germany, September 10-13, 1992 (abstract SL55).

Sommerville J: Glycyrrhetinic acid, *BMJP,* Feb 2, 1957.

Sonnenborn U: *Dtsch Apoth Ztg* 127:433, 1987.

Sotaniemi EA, Haapakoski E, Rautio A: Ginseng therapy in non–insulin dependent diabetic patients, *Diabetes Care* 18:1373, 1995.

Spoerke DG: *Herbal medications,* Santa Barbara, Calif, 1990, Woodbridge.

Srivastava KC: Effect of aqueous extracts of onion, garlic, and ginger on platelet aggregation and metabolism of arachidonic acid in blood vascular system: in vitro study, *Prostaglandins Leukot Med* 13:227, 1984.

Srivastava KC, Mustafa T: Ginger (Zingiber officinale) and rheumatism and musculoskeletal disorders, *Med Hypothesis* 39:342, 1992.

Stahl E, Jork H: *Arch Pharm (Weinheim)* 297:273, 1964.

Steinmetzer K: *Wierner Klin Wochenschr* 39:1418, 1926.

Steinmuller C and others: Polysaccharides isolated from plant cell cultures of *Echinacea purpurea* enhance the resistance of immunosuppressed mice against systemic infections with *Candida albicans* and *Listeria monocytogenes, Int J Immunopharmacol* 15(5):605, 1993.

Sterner W, Kirchdorfer AM: Comparative work load tests on mice with standardized ginseng extract and a ginseng containing pharmaceutical preparation, *Z Gerontol* 3:307, 1970 (in German).

Stuart M: *Encyclopedia of herbs and herbalism,* London, 1987, Macdonald & Co.

Sudekum M and others: Pennyroyal oil toxicosis in a dog, *JAVMA* 200(6):817, 1992.

Szelenyi I, Isaac O, Thiemer K: Pharmacological experiments with compounds of chamomile. III. Experimental studies of the ulcerprotective effect of chamomile, *Plant Medica* 35(3):218, 1979.

Szilard S, Szentgyorgyi D, Demeter I: Protective effect of Legalon in workers exposed to organic solvents, *Acta Med Hung* 45(2):249, 1988.

Takagi K, Watanabe K, Ishi Y: Peptic ulcer inhibiting activity of licorice root, *Proc Int Pharmacol Meeting* 7(2):1, 1965.

Tansey MR, Appleton JA: Inhibition of fungal growth by garlic extract, *Mycologia* 67(2):409, 1975.

Taylor JE: Liasons des neuromédiateurs à leurs récepteurs dans le cerveau de rats: effet de l'administration chronique de l'extrait de ginkgo biloba, *Presse Med* 15(31):1491, 1986.

Thiemer K, Stadler R, Isaac O: *Arzneim-Forsch* 23:756, 1973.

Tierra M, ed: *American herbalism: Essays on herbs and herbalism by members of the American Herbalists Guild,* Freedom, Calif, 1992, The Crossing Press.

Tommasi ND and others: *J Nat Prod* 53:830, 1990.

Tomoda M and others: Characterization of two polysaccharides having activity on the reticuloendothelial system from the root of *Glycyrrhiza uralensis, Chem Pharm Bull* 38(6):1667, 1990.

Traitler H and others: *Lipids* 19:923, 1984.

Trease GE, Evans WC: *Pharmacognosy,* ed 11, London, 1978, Baillière Tindal.

Trease GE, Evans WC: *Pharmacognosy,* ed 12, London, 1983, Baillière Tindal.

Tschesche R, Delhri S, Sepulveda S: *Phytochemistry* 18:1248, 1979.

Tyler VE, Brady LR, Robbers JE: *Pharmacognosy,* ed 9, Philadelphia, 1988, Lea & Febiger.

Tyler VE: *Herbs of choice: the therapeutic use of phytomedicinals,* Kent, Wash, 1994, Pharmaceutical Products.

Tyler VE: *The honest herbal: a sensible guide to the use of herbs and related remedies,* Kent, Wash, 1993, Pharmaceutical Products.

Ullsperger R: Vorlaufige Mitteilung ueber den Coronargefaesse Erweiternden Wirkkoerper aus Weissdorn (Preliminary communication concerning a coronary vessel dilating principle from hawthorn), *Pharmazie* 6(4):141, 1951.

Veith J and others: *Plant Med* 52:179, 1986.

Vidall-Ollivier E and others: *Planta Med* 55:73, 1989.

Vidall-Ollivier E and others: *Plantes Med Phytotherap* 22:235, 1989.

Vogel G and others: Studies on pharmacodynamics, site and mechanism of action of silymarin, the anti-hepatotoxic principle from *Silybum marianum* (L) Gaert, *Arzneim-Forsch* 25:179, 1975.

Wagner H: Plant constituents with anti-hepatotoxic activity. In Beal JL, Reinhard E, editors: *Natural products as medicinal agents,* Stuttgart, 1981, Hippokrates-Verlag.

Wagner H, Proksch A: An immunostimulating active principle from *Echinacae purpurea, Z Angew Phytother* 2:166, 1981.

Wagner H: Anti-hepatotoxic flavonoids. In Cody V, Middleton E, Harbourne JB, editors: *Plant flavonoids in biology and medicine: biochemical, pharmacological, and structure-activity relationships*, New York, 1986, Alan R Liss.

Wagner H: Interviewed in *Herbalgram* 17:16, 1988.

Wagner H, Grevel J: Cardiotonic drugs IV, cardiotonic amines from *Crataegus oxyacantha, Planta Medica* 45:98-101, 1982.

Wahner Ch, Schonert J, Friedrich H: *Pharmazie* 29:616, 1974.

Watt BK, Merrill AL: *Compositions of foods—raw, processed, prepared*, Rev, Washington, DC, USDA Agricultural Handbook No 8, 1963.

Weiss RF: *Herbal medicine*, Beaconsfield, 1988, Beaconsfield Publishers.

Werbach M, Murray M: *Botanical influences on illness: a source book of clinical research*, Nijmegen, Netherlands, 1994, Third Line Press.

Westphal K: *Gallenwegsfunktionen und Gallenleider*, Berlin, 1931, Springer-Verlag.

Wichtl M: *Dtsch Apotheker Zeitung (Supplement Videopharm)* 125(38):20, 1985.

Wilkomirski B: *Phytochemistry* 24:3066, 1985.

Willuhn G, Westhaus RG: *Planta Med* 53:304, 1987.

Wolters B: *Dtsch Apoth Ztg* 106:1729, 1966.

Zafriri D and others: Inhibitory activity of cranberry juice on adherence of type I and type P fimbriated *Escherichia coli* to eucaryotic cells, *Antimicrob Agents Chemother* 33(1):92-98, 1989.

Zhao MQ and others: The preventive and therapeutic actions of glycyrrhizin, glycyrrhetic acid and crude saikosides on experimental cirrhosis in rats, *Yao Hsueh Hsueh Pao* 18(5):325-331, 1983.

SELECTED READINGS

Anderson and others: Protective action of deglycyrrhizinated licorice on the occurrence of stomach ulcers in pylorous-ligated rats, *Scand J Gastroenterol* 6:683, 1971.

Baba K, Abe S, Mizuno D: Anti-tumor activity of hot water extract of dandelion, *Taraxacum officinale*—correlation between anti-tumor activity and timing of administration, *Yakugaku Zasshi* 101(6)538, 1981.

Bader G and others: *Pharmazie* 42:140, 1987.

Barber AJ: *Pharmaceutical J* 240:723, 1988.

Berton HS: The allergenicity of psyllium seed, *Medical Annals of the District of Columbia* 39:318, 1970.

Bonadeo J, Botaxxi G, Lavazza M: Perfumi, pianti offici, aromi, saponi, cosmet, aerosol, *Riv Ital Essenze* 53:281, 1971.

Bricklin M: The practical encyclopedia of natural healing, Emmaus, Pa, 1976, Rodale.

Briggs CJ: *Can Pharm J* 119:248, 1986.

Brunello N and others: Effects of an extract of *Ginkgo biloba* on noradrenergic systems or rat cerebral cortex, *Pharm Res Commun* 17:1063, 1985.

Chang IM, Yun HS, Yan KN: *Yakhak Hoechi* 28:35, 1984.

Cookson FB, Fedoroff S: Quantitative relationships between administered cholesterol and alfalfa required to prevent hypercholesterolemia in rabbits, *Br J Exp Pathol* 49:348, 1968.

Coon N: *Using plants for healing*, ed 2, Emmaus, Pa, 1979, Rodale.

Danilowski U: *Arch Exp Path Pharmacol* 35:105, 1895.

Della Loggia R and others: Depressive effects of chamomilla recutiat (1) rausch, tubular flowers, on central nervous system in mice, *Pharmacol Res Commun* 14(2):153, 1982.

Dew MJ, Evans BK, Rhodes J: Peppermint oil for the irritable bowel syndrome: a multi-centre trial, *Br J Clin Pract* 40(7):292, 1986.

Fairfield T: Garlic as an antinematodal agent in the genus: *Symphysodon, Diskus Brief* 2(4):30, 1995.

Fairfield T: Garlic as an anti-nematodal agent, *Aquarium Fish*, Nov 1995.

Forster H: Apasmolytische wirkung pfanzlicher carminativa, *Zeitschrift der Allgemein Medizin* 59:1327, 1983.

Foster HB, Nilkas H, Lutz S: *Planta Med* 40:309, 1980.

Foster S: *Peppermint, Mentha x piperita, Botanical Series No 306*, Austin, Tex, 1991, American Botanical Council.

Friedman CA: Structure-activity relationships of anthraquinone in some pathological conditions, *Pharmacology* 20(suppl)1:113, 1980.

Fujisawam J and others: Therapeutic approach to chronic active hepatitis with glycyrrhizin, *Asian Med J* 23:745, 1980.

Glowania HJ, Raulin C, Swoboda M: Effect of chamomile on wound healing—a clinical double-blind study, *Z Hautkr* 62(17):1262, 1987.

Greenbaum DS: Psyllium and irritable bowel syndrome, *Ann Intern Med* 95:660, 1981.

Griffith HW: Complete guide to vitamins, minerals, and supplements, Tucson, Ariz, 1988, Fisher Books.

Griggs B: *Green pharmacy: the history and evolution of western herbal medicine*, Rochester, Vt, 1991, Healing Arts.

Gujral S, Bhumra H, Swaroop M: Effect of ginger *(Zingiber officinale roscoe)* oleoresin on serum and hepatic cholesterol levels in cholesterol-fed rats, *Nutr Rep Int* 17(2):183, 1978.

Gupte S: Use of berberine in the treatment of giardiasis, *Am J Dis Child* 129:866, 1975.

Hartke K and others, editors: DAB 10—Kommentar. Wisenschaftliche Erlauterungen zum Deutschen Arzneibuch, 10. Ausgabe. (German Pharmacopoeia, ed 2—Commentary), 6 vol. Wissenschaftliche Verlagsgesellschaft mbH, Stuttgart, and Govi-Ver-lag, Frankfurt/M, 1991.

Hobbs C, Foster S. *Herbal Gram* 22:21, 1990.

Hoffman B, Herrmann K: *Z Lebensm Unters Forsch* 174:211, 1982.

Howard AN, Marks J: *Arterioscler Brain Dis* 1983:203, 1984.

Johadar L, Leifertova I, Lisa M: *Pharmazie* 45:446, 1990.

Khmetova BK: The electrocardiographic changes in patients with chronic pulmonary and pulmonary-cardiac insufficiency treated with European wild ginger, *Sbornick Nauchnykh Trudov Bashkirskii Meditsninskii Institut* 17:113, 1968.

Klonz U: Natural benzodiazepines in man, *Lancet* 335:922, 1990.

Lind PO, Bruh JG: Biologiska effekter av kamomill, *Lakartidningen* 81(51)4846, 1984.

Loggia RD and others: Evaluation of the anti-inflammatory activity of chamomile preparations, *Planta Med* 56:657, 1990.

Mabey R: *The new age herbalist*, New York, 1988, Macmillan.

Magliulo E and others: Studies on the regenerative capacity of the liver in rats suspected to partial hepatectomy and treated with silymarin, *Arzneimitte-Forschung* 23(suppl):161, 1973.

Malinow MR and others: Effect of alfalfa meal on shrinkage (regression of atherosclerotic plaques during cholesterol feeding in monkeys), *Atherosclerosis* 30(1):27, 1978.

Martindale W: *The extra pharmacopoeia*, London, 1977, The Pharmaceutical Press.

Mavers VWH, Hensel H: Changes in local myocardial blood flow following oral administration to a crataegus extract to non-anesthesized dogs, *Arzniem Forsch* 24:783, 1974.

Mayer R, Rucker G: *Arch Pharm* (Weinheim) 320:318, 1987.

Merfor I, Willuhn G: *Deutsche Apotheker Zeitung* 125:695, 1985.

Metzner J, Hirshelmann R, Hiller K: Antiphlogistische und Anagestic Wirkongen von Leiocarposid, eimem phenolischem Bisglucosid aus Solidago virgaureale L, *Pharmazie* 39:869, 1984.

Nakamura MY, Ishiara: Effects of dietary magnesium and glycyrhizzin on experimental atheromatosis of rats, *Jap Heart J* 7(5):474 1966.

Nasemann T: *Z Allgemein Med* 51:1105, 1975.

The National Formulary, ed 6, Washington, DC, 1935, American Pharmaceutical Association.

Pahlow M: *Das Grosse Buch der Heilpflanzen*, Munich, 1985, Grafe und Unzer GmbH.

Passwater RA: *Evening primrose oil*, New Canaan, Conn, 1981, Kent.

Pedersen M: *Nutritional herbology*, Boutiful, Utah, 1987, Pedersen.

Reznicek G and others: *Phytochemistry* 30:1629, 1991.

Roder E and others: *Dtsch Apoth Ztg* 124:2316, 1984.

Roesler J and others: Application of purified polysaccharides from cell cultures of the plant *Echinacea purpurea* to test subjects mediates activation of the phagocyte system, *Int J Immunopharmacol* 13(7):931, 1991.

Rucker G, Manns D, Wilbert S: *Phytochemistry* 31:340, 1992.

Sacco T, Chialva F: *Planta Med* 54:93, 1988.

Schneider E: *Zeitschrift fur Phytotherapie* 11:50, 1990.

Schneider G, Mielke B: *Dtsch Apoth Ztg* 118:469, 1978.

Schramm G: Uber Den Gegenwartigen Stand Der Arzneipflanzenforschung in China, *Planta Medica (Stuttgart)* 6:39, 1958.

Smith LW, Livingston AE: Chlorophyll: an experimental study of its water-soluble derivatives in wound healing, *Am J Surg New Series* LXIII(3):358, 1943.

Sollmann T: *A manual of pharmacology*, ed 7, Philadelphia, 1948, WB Saunders.

Swiatek L, Dombrowicz E: *Farm Pol* 40:729, 1984.

Swiatek L, Kurosawa A, Rotkiewicz D: *Herba Pol* 30:173, 1984.

Tarle D, Petricic J, Kupinic M: *Farm Glas* 37:351, 1981.

Tinkelman DG, Avner SE: Ephedrine therapy in asthmatic children, *JAMA* 237:553-557, 1977.

Titz W and others: *Sci Pharm* 51:63, 1983.

Tubaro A and others: *Plant Med* 51:359, 1985.

Verzarne PG, Szegi J, Marczal G: Effect of certain chamomile compounds, *Acta Pharmaceutica Hungarica* 49(1):13, 1979.

Villar D and others: Toxicity of melaleuca oil and related essential oils applied topically on dogs and cats, *Vet Hum Toxicol* 36(2):139, 1994.

Voirin B, Bayet C: *Phytochemistry* 31:2299, 1992.

Vostrowsky O and others: *Z Naturforsch* 36c:369, 1981.

Wagner H, Seligmann O: In Chang HM and others, editors: *Advances in Chinese medicinal materials research*, Singapore, 1985, World Scientific Publishing.

Wagner H: Anti-hepatotoxic flavonoids. In Cody V, Middleton E, Harbourne JB, editors: *Plant flavonoids in biology and medicine: biochemical, pharmacological and structure-activity relationships*, New York, 1986, Alan R Liss.

Weber G, Galle K: The liver: a therapeutic target in dermatoses, *Med Welt* 34:108, 1983 (in German).

Weiss RF: *Herbal medicine*, Beaconsfield, 1988, Arcanum, Gothenburg and Beaconsfield Publishers.

Wichtl M, editor: Teedrogen, Stuttgart, 1984, Wissenschaftliche Verlagsgesellschaft.

Wittmann C: *Herb Quarterly* 48:12, 1990.

Wren RC, Wren RW: *Potter's new cyclopaedia of botanical drugs and preparations*, Hengiscote, England, 1975, Health Science.

Wren RC: *Potter's new cyclopaedia of botanical drugs and preparations*, Saffron Walden, England, 1988, CW Daniel.

Wright S, Burton J: *Lancet*, vol 20, November 1982.

Yakolev V, von Schlichtegroll A: Anti-inflammatory activity of (-)alpha-bisabolol, an essential component of chamomile oil, *Arzneimittel-Forschung* 19(4):615, 1969.

Yamamoto M, Kumagai A: *Planta Med* 45:149, 1982.

Chapter 21

Chinese Herbal Medicine: Pharmacologic Basis

JEN-HSOU LIN, PHILIP A.M. ROGERS, HARUKI YAMADA

Herbal medicine, or phytotherapy, has a well-studied pharmacologic basis. Herbology, the study of herbs, derives from the Chinese term *Ben Cao,* from which the term *bencaology (herbology)* derives. Traditional Chinese medicine (TCM) uses Chinese herbal medicine (CHM), acupuncture (AP), moxibustion, and other methods. The World Health Organization (WHO, 1993), which supports the use of effective and safe remedies, accepts traditional medicine as a valuable and readily available resource for primary health care.

For thousands of years, herbal medicine has been used as a therapy to maintain human and animal health in China. The philosophy and logic of TCM trace back to the Three Mythical Emperors, Fusi (8000-3000 BC?), Huangdi (2852-2737 BC?), and Shen Nong (2838-2698 BC?). *Huangdi Nei Jing* (Huangdi's Internal Medical Classic) and *Shen Nong Ben Cao Jing* (Shen Nong's Herbal Classic) were attributed to the latter two authors. In fact, they were written much later by others. The *Nan Jing* and other classics up to medieval times expanded on those works, which remain the foundation of TCM. Chapters 22 and 23 discuss the early history of TCM.

African, American, Arabian, Egyptian, European, Indian, Japanese, Korean, Lapp, Polynesian, Samoan, Sumerian, Tibetan, and other cultures developed their own forms of herbal medicines over centuries. Today, 75% to 80% of the world's population still relies on herbal medicine (plants and plant extracts) and other tools of traditional medicine in basic health care.*

In Asia, especially in China, Japan, Korea, Taiwan, and Vietnam, medical practitioners are trained to prescribe traditional medicines (TMs) together with Western medicines (Chan and others, 1993). Western medicines often are expensive, and their use may cause the development of drug resistance and iatrogenic disease. To research, develop, register, and market a new pharmaceutical drug in the United States takes approximately 10 years and costs about $200 million (Abelson, 1990; Cox, Balick, 1994). Moreover, Western medicines produce sometimes limited results in many chronic conditions.

Because of these factors, demand for TMs, especially CHM, is increasing and traditional herbal medicine therapy is used widely in the United States and European countries (Otsuka, 1988; Yamada, 1994a). In contrast to Western medicines, appropriately prescribed Chinese herbal medicines can be used for relatively long periods with minimal or no adverse effects.* However, most traditional medicine systems (including herbal medicine and acupuncture) require additional scientific research on aspects of safety and efficacy (Chaudhury, 1995; Dharmananda, 1991; Lin, Yamada, Rogers, 1995).

CHM uses a complex combination of medicinal plants and other natural products (Luo, Shi, 1986; Ou, 1989). Plant products include specifically selected parts (leaves, branches, stems, roots, tubers, and bark) harvested from herbs, flowers, and trees. Other natural products include parts of living or dead tissue (e.g., animals, insects, reptiles, venoms, shell, and coral) and minerals (e.g., mineral salts, certain types of pulverized rocks, and soils). The remedies are carefully balanced mixtures of many ingredients. They are taken as decoctions, extracts in water or alcohol, or dried extracts (e.g., as pills). Some are used externally. Other forms of herbal medicines are being developed such as pills, tablets, powders, capsules, tinctures, syrups, suppositories, ointments, and injections.

---

*Abelson, 1990; Chan and others, 1993; Chaudhury, 1995; Cox, Balick, 1994; Schwartz, 1994; Yamada, 1994a.

*Chan and others (1993); Dharmananda (1991); Hosoya, Yamamura (1988); Hsu (1982); Schwartz (1994); Yamada (1994a).

CHM uses TCM theory and a TCM diagnosis of the patient's pathologic condition. When the TCM syndrome is established, suitable herbal medicines are prescribed. (In TCM, the syndrome is classified by the Eight Principles [*Yang-Yin,* External-Internal, Hot-Cold, Excess-Deficiency], the Six Levels, the External Causes, the Internal Emotions, the Channel(s) involved, the energies affected [*Qi,* Blood, or Fluid], and in other ways. These concepts are discussed elsewhere.) Treatment aims mainly to maintain harmony of body function (homeostasis) and to expel pathogens. Many ingredients are designed to enhance the effects or act as antidotes to unwanted effects of other ingredients.

History of Scientific Research in CHM

The ancient history of TCM and CHM is documented by Xie and others (1994) and Ou (1989) and is summarized in Chapters 22 and 23.

From the nineteenth century to the beginning of this century, the influx of Western ideas adversely affected traditional Chinese culture and science. TCM nearly became extinct. In the past 40 years, renewed interest in the techniques of TCM has occurred in China. In 1990, Hong-Cheng Fong published two books on veterinary herbology that contain more than 10,000 formulas and probably comprise the biggest collection of traditional Chinese veterinary medicine (TCVM) since antiquity. Today a worldwide TCVM society is based in China, with thousands of members who practice TCVM daily. Foreign (non-Chinese) graduates may attend courses on TCVM and veterinary acupuncture in China (Lin, Panzer, 1994). Development and research in TCM for humans and animals have become popular again throughout China, Japan, Korea, and Taiwan (Hosoya, Yamamura, 1988; Hsu, 1982; Lin, Yamada, Rogers, 1995a; Yamada, 1994a). Traditional Oriental medicine (TOM) and Kampo Medicine (KM) are forms of traditional medicine from east Asia and Japan, respectively. Both were derived primarily from CHM or were strongly influenced by it.

Kampo literally means "Han's formulas." Most formulas of KM are from the *Shang Han Lun* (Treatise on Cold-induced [Febrile] Disorders) and the *Jin Kui Yao Lue Fang Lun* (Essentials of the Golden Cabinet), both written by Zhang Zhong-jing (Zhang Ji) in approximately 210 AD and arranged some years later by Wang Shu-He (Wang Xi) (Hsu, 1982; Otsuka, 1988; Xie and others, 1994). Since 1976 the Ministry of Health and Welfare of Japan has approved 146 KM formulations. National health insurance in Japan covers the use of the herb components of such approved KMs.

WHO has issued guidelines for evaluating the safety and efficacy of herbal medicines. International and national conferences, such as those run by the World Veterinary Association, the Japanese Pharmaceutical Society, and the Medical and Pharmaceutical Society for Wakan-Yaku (Japan), also discuss these topics. Journals that publish research on the chemistry and pharmacology of herbal medicines and phytotherapy are listed in Box 21-1.

Pharmacologic Research in Herbal Medicine

Pharmacognosy is the study of compounds ingested or otherwise used by humans and animals as supposed medicines; zoopharmacognosy is the study of the actions of these materials in animals (Robles and others, 1995). Phytotherapeutics is the therapeutic use of these compounds. These disciplines have led to the identification of many useful medicines.

In 1985, worldwide, 3500 new chemical structures were discovered, 2619 of which were isolated from higher plants. In 1987, Japan held 56% of patented natural products summarized in *Phytotherapy Research.* Germany also has been more active than the United States in this field (Abelson, 1990).

Research in phytotherapy can be classified under many different headings. Research on pharmacologic effects of herbal medicines will be discussed under three headings: individual herbs or extracts, individual active compounds of individual herbs, and complex herbal medicine formulas. The boundaries between these headings are not easy to maintain; thus some overlap occurs between them.

Research on Individual Herbs Or Extracts

Documentation of TCM is more than 3000 years old. Thus extensive data and cumulative experience on the use of CHM are available, including recent textbooks.*

Bensky and others (1986) summarize the actions of some potent herbal ingredients. *Ginseng radix* (*ren shen* means "Man Root," or "Man Essence") is sometimes manshaped (like mandrake). The medicinal use of ginseng in China dates from before 100 BC. Many varieties exist, including Appalachian, Korean, Japanese, and Chinese ginseng. Great therapeutic and mystical potency is attributed to ginseng. Much sought-after, it is very expensive and among the most frequently cited herbs in TCM. Experimentally, it has potent effects on the CNS and peripheral nerves. Centrally, it improves nervous responses in a homeostatic way, enhancing both stimulatory and inhibitory processes depending on their initial state of receptivity. In this way, it resembles acupuncture, in which stimulation of the same acupuncture points can have diametrically opposed effects depending on the state of the subject. In normal use, ginseng is a central stimulant like caffeine, but in large doses, it is a sedative. It counteracts the stimulating effects of other stimulants and the in-

---

*Bensky and others (1986); Chaudhury (1995); Dharmananda (1991); Hosoya, Yamamura (1988); Hsu (1982); Luo, Shi (1986); Ou (1989); Xie and others (1994).

JOURNALS THAT PUBLISH RESEARCH ON THE CHEMISTRY AND PHARMACOLOGY OF HERBAL MEDICINES AND PHYTOTHERAPY

Agric Biol Chem	J Ethnopharmacol
Am J Chin Med	J Infect Dis
Am J Dis Child	J Nat Prod
Am J Trop Med Hyg	J Natural Toxins
Ann Trop Med Parasitol	J Ortho Med
Antimicrob Agents Chemother	J Pharm Pharmacol
Antiviral Res	J Pharma Soc Jap
Arch Int Pharmacodyn Ther	J Pharmacobio-Dynamics
Asia Pac J Pharmacol	J Trad Chin Med
Biochem Biophys Res Commun	Jap J of Inflammation
Biochem Pharmacol	Jap J of Oriental Medicine
Biol Pharm Bull	Lancet
C and EN	Life Sci
Can J Microbiol	Med Hypotheses
Cancer Biother	Natural Med
Carbohydr Polymers	Nature
Carbohydr Res	Pharmacol Res
Chem Pharm Bull	Phytochemistry
Chin J Chin Materia Medica	Phytomedicine
Curr Opin Biotechnology	Phytother Res
Excerpta Medica (Amsterdam)	Plant Mol Biol
Exp Hematol	Planta Med
Folia Pharmacol Jap	Pure Appl Chem
Indian J Med Res	Rev sci tech Off int Epiz
Indian Pediatr	Science
Int J Immunopharmacol	Tokai J Exp Clin Med
Int J Immunother	Vet Bull
J Alternative and Complementary Med	Vet Rec
J Chin Med (Taiwan)	Vet Res

hibitory effect of opiates. It enhances the acute hypnotic effect of pentobarbital. Small doses of ginseng have muscarinic effects on peripheral nerves; large doses have nicotinic effects. It shortens the latency of nerve reflexes, accelerates nerve transmission, and strengthens conditioned reflexes. Over long periods, it tends to the middle (i.e., neither stimulatory nor inhibitory). Experimentally, it has cardiotonic effects, similar to cardiac glycosides; it is clinically useful in cardiac dysrhythmia.

Huang (1993) devotes a full chapter to the medicinal uses and pharmacology of the ginseng root. In summary, ginseng root contains volatile oils, saponins (glycosides, panaxosides, ginsenosides), antioxidants, peptides, polysaccharides, fatty acids, vitamins, and other active ingredients, many of whose chemical structures are known. It is known as the "elixir of life" because it has potent antiaging effects and antiirradiation effects, probably from its antioxidants and immunostimulating properties. Experimentally, ginseng increases endurance in animals and has potent antistress effects against many environmental stressors (Huang, 1993). It has antidiabetic and hypoglycemic effects and alpha-2-adrenergic and antihypertensive effects (blocked by yohimibine). It has beta-adrenergic blocker effects in oxygen starvation. It has antiinflammatory effects and activates the reticuloendothelial system, dilates cerebral and coronary vessels, stimulates hematopoiesis in the bone marrow, lowers serum cholesterol levels, and produces antiatherosclerotic effects, which protect against cardiac ischemia. It has potent CNS effects, increasing concentration, awareness, and night adaptation of the eyes, and also functions as a sedative. It has antipyretic effects and increases the release of corticotropin releasing factor (CRF) from the hypothalamus. Because it activates the thyroid, testis, and ovary, it has clinical uses in male and female infertility and male potency via the hypothalamic-gonadal axis. Ginseng also activates the posterior pituitary, exerting an antidiuretic action. An important component of ginseng is its ability to activate the immune system in clinical and experimental cancer, experimental radiation sickness, and after exposure to cytotoxic agents. Symptomatically, it stimulates appetite, promotes a sense of well-being, and increases the will to live during convalescence from chronic diseases. Ginseng is nontoxic at normal dosage but may be toxic at high doses; the LD50 in mice was 5 g ginseng powder/kg LW. Clinically, ginseng is used in a myriad of conditions, such as shock and emergencies (e.g., cardiac, hemorrhagic, septic, and toxic), heart failure, acute myocarditis, angina, arteriosclerosis, cough, fevers, hormonal disorders (e.g., infertility, diabetes mellitus, diabetes insipidus, and thyroid disorders), hypotension, hypertension, stress, insomnia, headaches, anemia, neurasthenia, muscle atrophy, chronic debility, impotence, poor concentration, gastrointestinal disorders (e.g., inappetance, indigestion), cancer therapy, immunosuppression, and senility (Huang, 1993).

Huang (1993) categorized herbs under the following headings in a systematic study of the pharmacology of CHM: those acting on the cardiovascular system (multiple action, cardiac, antiarrhythmic, antihypertensive, antianginal, antihypercholesterolemic, and antishock herbs); nervous system (anesthetic and muscle-relaxing herbs; sedative-hypnotic herbs; anticonvulsive, analgesic, antipyretic, antirheumatic, and central stimulating herbs); alimentary system (stomachic and "wind"-dispelling herbs; herbs promoting digestion, antacid and antiulcer, laxative, antidiarrheal, emetic, antiemetic, choleretic, antihepatitis, tonic, and supporting herbs); respiratory system (antitussive, expectorant, and antiasthmatic herbs); genitourinary system (diuretic and uterine-active herbs); hematopoietic system (promoters of blood formation; hemostatic and antistatic herbs); endocrine system (herbs affecting the thyroid, adrenal cortex, and pancreas); and chemotherapeutics (antibacterial, antiviral, antifungal, antitubercular, antiseptic, disinfectant, anthelmintic, antiamebic, antitrichomonial, antimalarial, and anticancer herbs).

This study and other modern texts and reviews show that medical compounds in herbal medicines include immunomodulators such as antiallergic, antiasthmatic, antiinflammatory, antiinfectious, antihepatotoxic, antineoplastic, antioxidant, and antitoxic compounds. Herbal medicines also include antistress compounds (hypotensives, muscle relaxants, sedatives, and vasodilators), hypoglycemics, and insect repellents (antifeedants).

The roles of individual herbs and formulas (herb combinations) in therapy are discussed under two headings: allergies and the immune system (including antiviral effects). Most of the data for these sections are from the review by Dharmananda (1991).

Antiallergic herbs*

Important antiallergic herbs include achyranthes, alisma, alpinia, apricot seed, arctium, asarum, astragalus, atractylodes, bezoar, bupleurum, cardamom, ching pi, cinnamon, citrus, cluster, cornus, ephedra (*ma huang*), galanga, ganoderma, gentian, ginger, ginseng, hoelen, licorice, magnolia, moutan, pinnelia, polyporus, pueraria, rehmannia, scute, stephania, *tang-kuei*, zedoaria, and zizyphus (jujube).

Type 1 allergies (IgE and chemically mediated *immediate* disorders) are caused by circulating IgE attached to mast cells, which releases chemical mediators (including histamine). They include drug allergies, hay fever, hives, and allergic asthma. Herbs that suppress IgE activity in stage 1 allergic response are alisma, apricot seed, bupleurum, cardamom, gentian, ginseng (Japanese), licorice, *tang-kuei*, and zizyphi fructus (jujube). Herbs that suppress release of chemical mediators (such as histamine) after IgE binding to mast cells in stage 2 allergic response are achyranthes, asarum, bezoar, *ching pi,* cinnamon bark, ephedra (*ma huang*), ganoderma, magnolia flowers, moutan, scute, and sinomenium. These herbs have antiinflammatory and antimediator-release action. Some of them have beta-adrenergic or antihistaminic effects: they suppress the reaction of the target organs (e.g., capillary permeability; smooth muscle contraction in nasal membranes, lungs, gut, and skin; hypothyroidism) after release of chemical mediators in stage 3 allergic response. Asarum (which contains methyleugenol and higenamine), atractylodes, and sinomenium also have antihistaminic activity (Box 21-2).

*Summarized from Tsung (1987).

BOX 21-2

FORMULAS IN TYPE 1 ALLERGY

Antiallergic (Stage 1): Bupleurum and Hoelen Formula, Minor Bupleurum Formula

Antiallergic (Stage 2): Minor Bupleurum Formula, Minor Blue Dragon Formula, Ma Huang and Apricot Seed Formula

Antiallergic (Stage 3): Minor Blue Dragon Formula, Pueraria and Magnolia Formula, Tang-kuei and Arctium Formula

Antiinflammatory, detoxifying, anti–chest distention: Bupleurum + Scute

Antiemetic, antinausea, digestive: Pinnelia and Ginger

Stomachic and antiheartburn: Ginseng, Jujube, and Licorice

Diuretic, antiascitic, antiedematous: Alisma, Polyporus, Hoelen, and Atractylodes

Type 2 allergies

Type 2 allergies (complement-mediated disorders) are caused by activation of complement by complement-fixing antibodies against cell-surface antigens. They include anaphylactic shock (side effects of incompatible blood), hemolytic anemia in autoimmune or drug reactions, and decreased platelet numbers. Herbs with anticomplement activity include cinnamon bark, ganoderma, and licorice. Formulas for type 2 allergies contain these as major ingredients.

Type 3 allergies

Type 3 allergies (immune-complex disorders) are caused by activation of complement after formation of antigen-antibody complexes. They include bacterial glomerular nephritis, chronic hepatitis B, atopic bronchial asthma, erythromatosus, chronic rheumatoid arthritis, and thyroiditis. Therapy for type 3 allergies uses anticomplement or antiinflammatory drugs.

Herbs used in type 3 allergies include ganoderma, bupleurum, cinnamon, citrus, cornus, ginseng, licorice, *ma huang*, moutan, and *tang-kuei*.

Formulas used in type 3 allergies (and those used in kidney disorders) include Atractylodes Formula, Bupleurum and Hoelen Formula, Bupleurum and Dragon Bone Formula, Ginseng and Astragalus Formula, Stephania and Astragalus Formula, and Rehmannia Eight Formula (Box 21-2). These formulas use various combinations of herbs listed in the previous paragraph; they have antiallergic and antiinflammatory effects and anticomplement activity.

Type 4 allergies

Type 4 allergies (no antibody involvement) are mediated by T-lymphocytes. They include contact dermatitis, tubercular lesions, chronic hepatitis, bacterial glomerular nephritis, erythromatosus, rheumatoid arthritis, Hashimoto's thyroiditis, and intestinal ulcers.

Herbs used in type 4 allergy include ganoderma, ginseng, hoelen, licorice, magnolia bark, pinellia, and zizyphus.

Formulas used in type 4 allergy include Minor Bupleurum Formula, Bupleurum and Hoelen Formula, Bupleurum and Schizonpeta Formula, Cinnamon and Atractylodes Formula, *Tang-kuei* and Gardenia Formula, Minor Blue Dragon Formula, and Pueraria Formula (Box 21-2).

In Western medicine, steroids are widely used in controlling allergies. Combinations of herbal medicines (which often contain plant steroids themselves) with steroids reduce the doses of the latter 33% to 50%. This reduces the risk of steroidal side effects.

Herbs with immunostimulatory, antiinflammatory, antitoxic, antiviral, and antioxidant effects include akebia, albizzia, alisma, astragalus, centella, cimicifuga, cistanche, codonopsis, dianthus, dioscorea, ginseng, lycium fruit, melia, mushrooms (coriolus, ganoderma, hoelen, lentinus, polyporus, and tremella), platycodon, polygala, rehmannia, sambucus, and zizyphus. They have been used for centuries to treat inflammation, fevers, intoxications, and infectious and neoplastic diseases.

Research on Individual Active Compounds

Western medicine uses many drugs extracted from natural products such as aspirin, atropine, cocaine, curare, digitalis, ephedrine, hyoscine (scopolamine), opiates (codeine and morphine), pilocarpine, primrose oil, quinine, reserpine, steroids, taxol, and warfarin. Other Western medicines from natural materials include kaolin, bentonite (in preparations of mineral matter), antibiotics, ergotamine, ergometrine, mescaline (from fungi), allergens for desensitization, antitoxins and antivenoms, heparin, hormones (steroids, HCG, PMSG, and insulin), vaccines, and venoms.

Most of these medicines have been discovered on the basis of information derived from traditional medicine and ethnopharmacognostics (Table 21-1). For instance, ephedrine was isolated from *Ephedra sinica* in 1885. *Ephedra sinica* and *Ephedra distachia* were used medicinally for centuries in Asia to treat asthma, hay fever, nasal congestion, and hypotension. Ephedrine is closely related to epinephrine (adrenaline) and the amphetamines. The first successful product of the modern pharmaceutical industry (Otsuka, 1988), ephedrine is still widely used today to relax the bronchioles in asthma and bronchitis, as a nasal decongestant in some allergies, and as a mydriatic. It stimulates the CNS and is used to treat hypotension, cardiac failure, and narcotic poisoning. *Digitalis purpurea* was used to treat ascites and edema in congestive heart failure and its alkaloids are still used for that purpose. *Cinchona* bark is the source of several alkaloids, especially quinine and quinidine. Both have antimalarial, antifebrile, and analgesic effects. Quinidine also is a cardiotonic and is used in the treatment of cardiac dysrhythmia, fibrillation, and heart block.

Raw ingredients used in herbal medicines contain pharmacologically active compounds of low and/or high molecular weight. Low–molecular weight compounds include primary metabolites (e.g., sugars, fatty acids, and peptides) and secondary metabolites (e.g., alkaloids, terpenoids, saponins, and flavonoids). High–molecular weight compounds include proteins, tannins, and polysaccharides. The therapeutic activity of herbal medicines derives from these compounds (Yamada, 1994a,b). Clarification of the active principles of herbal medicines helps us to understand the modes of action at a molecular level, to evaluate efficacy, and to maintain herbal quality. It also helps us to develop novel drugs by extraction from plants, use of biotechnology, or by synthetic methods. This may provide remedies for diseases incurable or poorly controlled by modern chemotherapeutics.

TABLE 21-1

SOME IMPORTANT DRUGS ISOLATED FROM PLANTS

DRUG	MEDICAL USE	PLANT SOURCE
Aspirin	Analgesic and antiinflammatory, reduces platelet stickiness	*Filipendula ulmaria*
Codeine	Analgesic and antitussive	*Papaver somniferum*
Digoxin and digitoxin	Cardiac stimulant	*Digitalis* spp.
Ephedrine	Bronchodilator	*Ephedra sinica*
Forskolin	Cardiac stimulant	*Coleus forskolii*
Ipecacuanha	Emetic	*Psychotria ipecacuanha*
Pilocarpine	Antiglaucomic	*Pilocarpus jaborandi*
Quinine	Antimalarial	*Cinchona pubescens*
Reserpine	Antihypertensive	*Rauwolfia serpentina*
Scopolamine	Eases motion sickness	*Datura stramonium*
Taxol	Treats ovarian cancer	*Taxus brevifolia*
Theophylline	Bronchodilator	*Camellia sinensis*
Vinblastine and vincristine	Treats Hodgkin's disease	*Catharanthus roseus*

The following material is summarized from the review by Dharmananda (1991). In Western medicine and pharmacognosy, active compounds are classified in many different ways: by their physiologic effects, by their clinical indications, or by their chemical and pharmacologic nature. The latter method groups medicines into eight classes:

1. Carbohydrates (sugars, polysaccharides, gums, mucilages, and pectins)
2. Steroids (steroid hormones, sterols, and bile acids)
3. Glycosides (anthraquinones, flavonoids, lactones, and phenols)
4. Alkaloids (tropanes, quinolines, and indoles)
5. Tannins (catechols and pyrogallols)
6. Lipids (fixed oils, waxes, and fatty acids)
7. Volatile oils (alcohols, aldehydes, ketones, and phenols)
8. Resins (oleoresins, gum-resins, and balsams)

Herbal medicines used to treat various disorders of the immune system, including allergies, inflammations, infections, cancer, and AIDS, contain one or more of these active compounds. Some herbal medicines contain mixtures of these compounds; for example, ginseng and hoelen contain potent polysaccharides *and* steroids.

In this chapter, the following active herbal compounds (Dharmananda, 1991) are briefly summarized: polysaccharides, steroids, flavonoids, and alkaloids.

Polysaccharides

Plants contain many sugar molecules in various combinations, sizes, and chemical sequences. Monosaccharides are simple sugars. Long, straight- and/or branched-chain monosaccharide polymers form polysaccharides. Most are not water-soluble (such as gums), but some are (such as

the pectin polysaccharides). Sugars, gums, and celluloses have relatively little use in Western medicine, except as fillers and binders. However, pectins can soothe the gastrointestinal tract and can be used to treat diarrhea and gastroenteritis. Pueraria, dioscorea, and hoelen are used in this way. Inulin (from *Compositae* spp.) can soothe urinary irritation. Cellulose and gums can have a bulking effect and can help relieve constipation (Dharmananda, 1991).

Some polysaccharides have potent effects on the immune system. The clinical results of herbal medicine in the therapy of cancer, AIDS/ARC, and other disorders of the immune system led to their discovery. These herbal medicines contain mushrooms (coriolus, ganoderma, hoelen, lentinus, polyporus, and tremella), codonopsis, ginseng, and other herbs. Polysaccharides from *Coriolus versicolor (yun zhi)* are registered as PSK in Japan and PSG in China. Krestin, the largest-selling antineoplastic drug in Japan, contains mainly polysaccharides from *Coriolus*. Lentinan is another immunostimulant and antineoplastic polysaccharide. It is a six-branched beta (1-3) glucan chain from *Lentinus edotes* (*xiang ling,* the shiitake mushroom). Polysaccharides from *Ganoderma lucidum* and *japonicum (ling zhi)* are used to treat myasthenia gravis and have similar uses to Krestin and lentinan in AIDS/ARC and cancer (Dharmananda, 1991).

Ganoderma, the most widely used medicinal mushroom, is easy to cultivate. It has tonic and sedative effects and is said to prolong life. The *Shen Nong Ben Cao Jing* discussed medical uses of this mushroom. Different colors of *ganoderma* have different effects: red stimulates heart, internal organ, and brain function; black stimulates water metabolism and kidney function; blue helps liver and eye function and is sedative; white helps lung and spleen function and relieves cough; yellow helps stomach and chest problems and problems related to stress, overwork, or abuse of food or drink. Some varieties can act as antiallergic, antithrombotic, and antihyperlipemic agents.

Polyporus (Grifola) umbellata (zhu ling) is used to treat nephritis. Its polysaccharides are 6-branched beta (1-3) glucans, which promote antibody production, normalize liver function, and are antineoplastic.

Hoelen (Poria cocos) is a dense mushroom that grows near pine tree roots. *Fu ling (Poria* stalk) is the main part. It is one of the most frequently used Chinese herbal medicines; it is mild and helps all the organs. Its major polysaccharide (pachymaran) and triterpenoids are not immunologically active unless treated chemically, but its chemically modified pachymaran, a β (1-3) glucan, shows antineoplastic activity. *Fu shen (Poria* spirit) is the part attached to the roots and has sedative effects.

Tremella (bai mu er, white tree ear) is a tonic and expectorant. Its polysaccharides have antineoplastic effects, stimulate phagocytosis, and counter the adverse effects of cortisone treatment.

Based on a beta-1,3 glucan structure, polysaccharides in *coriolus, ganoderma, lentinus,* and *polyporus* have the highest natural antineoplastic activity. These polysaccharides also enhance the immune response to bacteria, fungi, protozoa, and yeasts and help patients to recover more easily from radiation, chemotherapy, or surgery (for cancer or other reasons). *Coriolus* polysaccharides also are used to treat hepatitis (infectious and toxic).

Steroids

In Western medicine, steroids are used to treat dozens of clinical conditions, including Addison's disease (adrenal insufficiency), inflammation, allergy, male and female reproductive disorders, skin and mental health problems associated with hormonal imbalance, menstrual disorders, impotence or frigidity, and postmenopausal syndromes. They also have a sedative action, and some are used as oral contraceptives.

Steroids are lipid-soluble organic compounds that occur naturally throughout the plant and animal kingdoms. All steroids have a four-ring structure. Steroids are diverse and include the sterols (such as cholesterol) of vertebrates, bile acids from the liver, all sex hormones, and adrenal cortical hormones. Hormonal steroids in the body are synthesized from cholesterol. The biosynthetic mechanisms are similar in all steroid-secreting tissue (testis, ovary, placenta, and adrenal cortex). There are two classes of corticosteroids. Glucocorticoids (e.g., cortisone) primarily affect carbohydrate and protein metabolism. They have limited use in the treatment of many immunologic and allergic diseases, such as arthritis. Mineralocorticoids (e.g., aldosterone) principally regulate salt and water balance. Because of the great therapeutic value of corticosteroids, many synthetic steroids have been produced, some more potent than the natural hormones.

Plant steroidal compounds belong to the general category called *saponins.* In CHM, triterpenes yield the most important steroids. The triterpenes of the herbal medicines most commonly used in immunostimulation and allergies (bupleurum, ganoderma, ginseng, hoelen, licorice) have been studied most.

Sterols are chemically similar steroidal compounds with alcohol (hydroxyl [OH]) groups attached to a series of fused rings. The principal sterol in vertebrates is cholesterol, especially abundant in nerve tissue and gallstones. Ergosterol, a sterol found in yeast, ergot, and molds, gives rise to vitamin D_2 (calciferol) when irradiated with ultraviolet light. Higher plant sterols include stigmasterol (from soybean oil) and several spinasterols (from spinach and cabbage). Natural sterols are poorly absorbed and transferred to the circulation by higher animals. Cholesterol is absorbed readily, but coprostanol and cholestanol, which are structurally similar, are not absorbed. Most animals can synthesize their essential sterols from smaller carbon compounds. Immunostimulatory herbs, such as ganoderma, ginseng, rehmannia, and sophora, also contain sterols. Yams *(Dioscorea)* contain steroids or a steroid precursor, diosgenin, from which several steroids (cortisone, estrogen, and progesterone) are manufactured by chemical alteration. The Mexican yam *(D. floribunda)* is a rich source of steroid precursor.

Plant steroids usually have similar action to that of steroid hormones, but at a lower activity (often 10%). Unlike the action of many plant saponins, herbal medicines do not cause hemolysis and their steroids have a mild action, with minimal side effects (unlike Western medicine steroids, which often cause iatrogenic Cushing's disease). Licorice *(Glycyrrhiza)* steroids have aldosterone-like actions. Excessive ingestion of raw licorice candy can cause excess corticoid levels, which can cause heart irregularities, edema, and death. This does not happen with the amounts of licorice used in CHM.

In herbal medicine, plant steroids can be used for the same indications as Western medicine steroids, but can be used for many other indications also. Chinese and Japanese studies of triterpenes, steroids, and sterols in herbal medicines have shown the following actions: stomachic (prodigestive), emmenagogue, and tonic effects on the liver and lung. Some triterpenes, such as the ginsenosides, are immunostimulatory also. Immunostimulatory, antiinflammatory, antihepatotoxic, antiallergic (antihistaminic), sedative, and antispasmodic effects of plant steroids are discussed later.

STOMACHIC (PRODIGESTIVE) EFFECTS   Herbal medicines with triterpenes (alisma, asparagus root, bupleurum, dioscorea, ganoderma, ginseng, hoelen, licorice, and zizyphus) assist digestion and relieve gastritis, stress ulcers, diarrhea, and colitis. Asparagus root is rich in spirostane saponins and strongly inhibits gastroduodenal ulcers.

TONIC EFFECTS ON THE LUNG   Herbal medicines that protect the lung and assist expectoration include albizzia, arisemia, bupleurum, cinnamon, eleuthero, ganoderma, glehnia, hoelen, licorice, lily family (anemarhena, asparagus, lily, and ophiopogon), platycodon, and polygala. Many of these have steroidal action via their saponins, triterpenes, or spirostane glycosides. They are useful clinically in bronchitis, asthma, cough, lung congestion, and pneumonia.

Many other ingredients used in herbal medicine have steroidal activity. They include animal products, such as deer antler, gecko, pipefish, and seahorse, and extracts of ovary, testis, adrenal, and placenta from many species. Their uses in TCM include strengthening of the *Yin* and Blood and the Kidney *Yang*.

Antiaging formulas aim to boost *Yang*, support *Yin*, and avert shrivelling (for example, drying of membranes, wrinkles, and impotence). They contain many herbal medicines with steroidal action.

Agitation, fidgeting, fatigue, and insomnia often accompany immunosuppression (as in AIDS/ARC, hepatitis, and Epstein-Barr virus) and autoimmune disease (especially when pain is present). A combination of herbal medicines with steroidal, immunostimulatory, and sedative actions is especially useful in those conditions.

Flavones and flavonoids

Flavones and flavonoids are found in the aerial parts of many plants (leaves, flowers, and fruits) but are less common in the underground parts. Most herbal medicine formulas contain herbs with some flavonoids; some formulas have flavonoids as the main active compounds. Herbs with flavonoids include astragalus, bauhinia, capillaris, citrus peel, eclipta, eucommia, forsythia, ginkgo (leaf and fruit), *ho-shou-wu*, ilex, ixeris, licorice, lonicera, millettia, pueraria, qingpi, rose fruit, salvia, scutellaria (scute), sophora, swertia, vitex, and zhishi.

Medicinal effects of flavonoids include increased vascular integrity (antihemorrhagic and antiascitic), antithrombotic, and vasodilatory. Antiviral or antifungal, antiallergic, and antihepatotoxic effects are discussed later.

INCREASED VASCULAR INTEGRITY Agents that can enhance capillary integrity are useful clinically to prevent or treat bruising, hemorrhagic diseases, and ascites. Flavonoids in citrus peel and eclipta have that effect.

ANTITHROMBOTIC EFFECTS Low doses of aspirin are used to reduce platelet aggregation to prevent thrombosis, heart attack, and stroke. However, hemorrhage, possibly cerebral, is a side effect. Flavones and flavonoids in bauhinia, ixeris, millettia, scutellaria, and vitex can have the same antithrombotic effect, but their effect on vascular integrity would prevent hemorrhage.

VASODILATORY EFFECTS Vasoconstriction is a significant clinical sign in many cardiovascular conditions (peripheral vasoconstriction, hypertension, migraine, angina, palpitations, and some forms of cerebrovascular accident). Vasodilators used in Western medicine can help such cases, but sometimes cause the "steal effect" (vasoconstriction elsewhere in the body). Flavonoids in ginkgo leaf and

pueraria have marked vasodilatory effects in the heart and brain, without the "steal effect." Such flavonoids include ginkgetins and rutin. Kaempferol, quercetin, and rhamnetin combined, or an extract of ginkgo, achieved good results in a small study of patients with Parkinson's disease. Flavonoids in ilex and scute are useful in treatment of cardiovascular disease, hypertension, headaches, and sore throat (Dharmananda, 1991).

Flavonex is a formula with eight herbs high in flavonoids (eucommia, ginkgo, ho-shou-wu, ilex, lonicera, pueraria, rose fruit, and salvia) and six other herbs (acorus, cistanche, lycium fruit, morus fruit, schizandra, and tang-kuei). In TCM, the formula is used to promote Blood Circulation, nourish the Essence, and prevent the effects of aging (especially on brain function). Clinical uses include allergies and poor cerebral circulation.

Ginseng, Astragalus, and Pueraria Formula is used to treat tinnitus, Bell's palsy, early cataracts, and senility. To aid circulation, especially cerebral, it contains four herbs (astragalus, licorice, pueraria, and vitex) that are high in flavonoids. The formula also contains ginseng (a general stimulant, an immunostimulant, and antiallergic herb), cimicifuga, phellodendron (antitoxic and antiinflammatory herbs), and peony.

Tang-kuei and Anemarrhena Formula is used to treat dermatitis and arthralgia. It contains five herbs high in flavonoids (capillaris, licorice, pueraria, scute, and sophora) and nine others that are immunostimulatory and antiinflammatory (alisma, anemarrhena, atractylodes, chianghuo, cimicifuga, ginseng, polyporus, siler, and tang-kuei).

SESQUITERPENE LACTONES Recently, several sesquiterpene lactones have been identified in plants consumed by animals for presumed medicinal value. They include agents with antineoplastic (parthenin and eupatoriopicrin), antiulcer (dehydroleucodin), and cardiotonic (helenalin) effects (Robles and others, 1995).

Alkaloids

Alkaloids have at least one nitrogen atom or an amine group. There are more than 200 known, and they have the suffix "-ine." Examples include aconitine, andinine, atropine, berbamine, berberine, berberrubine, brucine, caffeine, cocaine, codeine, colchicine, coumbamine, domesticine, emetine, ephedrine, ergometrine, ergotamine, hyoscine (scopolamine), hyoscyamine, isobolidine, isoquinolines, isotetrandine, jatorrhizine, magnoflorine, matrine, mescaline, morphine, nicotine, palmatine, papaverine, phellodendrine, pilocarpine, protoberberines, quinidine, quinine, quinolizidines, reserpine, ricinine, solamargine, solanine, solasonine, strychnine, tetrandine, theobromine, theophylline, tropanes, veratrine, vinblastine, and vincristine.

Alkaloids are alkaline, are acid-soluble, and can be isolated by acid extraction, followed by ammonia precipitation. Some are simple, monocyclic amines, but many are complex, polycyclic amines. Various family groupings are possible according to basic ring structure, such as pyridine or quinoline alkaloids. Most are poorly soluble in water and taste bitter. Thus herbal medicines that contain alkaloids are often taken as pills, syrups, or vinegar extracts, rather than as decoctions.

Alkaloids usually are absorbed fast, act fast, and are rapidly excreted. They act mainly via the nervous system. Most alkaloids have biphasic action. At low doses, many stimulate the heart and respiratory system. Clinically, they promote circulation, breathing, coughing, and expectoration. At higher doses, many act as sedatives. Clinically, they relax the heart and respiratory center, relax muscles, and promote sleep. These effects are more pronounced as the dose increases. At toxic doses, death may occur from cardiac or respiratory failure.

Many alkaloids induce nausea and vomiting as a side effect. This may be used clinically to induce vomiting, for example, syrup of *ipecacuanha* or vinegar extract of *lobelia*. Some may induce vertigo (dizziness), altered perceptions or hallucinations (cocaine, codeine, mescaline, reserpine, and scopolamine). Those with potent CNS effects have potential for addictive abuse and dosage tolerance.

Some Solanaceae, such as datura, atropa, and hyoscyamus (henbane), contain large amounts of atropine, hyoscyamine, and scopolamine (hyoscine). Henbane was used extensively as an anesthetic and analgesic. *Mandragora officinarum* (mandrake), one of the Solanaceae, also contains hyoscyamine. These plants are toxic when consumed in large quantity but are invaluable medicinal agents when given in proper amounts. Atropine is used in Western medicine as a mydriatic and anticholinergic; it inhibits the secretion of body fluids and is used in nasal decongestants. As a smooth-muscle relaxant, atropine is useful in relieving some gastrointestinal problems. It is also used as an antidote to nerve gas and some insecticides. Overdoses of atropine can cause an accelerated heartbeat and shallow breathing, leading in some cases to death. Scopolamine is used as a hypnotic and as an antispasmodic to reduce gastrointestinal contractions. Hyoscyamine has potent CNS effects; it is used as a sedative, especially to control spasmodic conditions. Hyoscyamine and scopolamine have been used to treat alcohol and morphine addiction.

Differences in alkaloid structure influence the dose range needed to produce pharmacologic effects. Some are relatively nontoxic and may be taken safely; others (such as aconitine) may induce potent sedation and may be very toxic at low doses. Sedative alkaloids (the majority) maintain a sedative effect at moderate doses. Stimulant alkaloids maintain a stimulant action over a very wide dose range.

STIMULANT ALKALOIDS Many societies use indigenous plants containing stimulant alkaloids. The Sudanese chew kola nut (origin of cola drinks) for its stimulant effects from its high caffeine content. South American Indians chew coca leaf, a source of cocaine, to attain in-creased energy, alertness, and euphoria. Cocaine, isolated in 1855, was used in Western medicine as a local anesthetic (especially for the nose, throat, and cornea) and nasal decongestant. Used systemically, cocaine stimulates the CNS, producing feelings of excitation, elation, well-being, enhanced physical strength and mental capacity, and a lessened sense of fatigue. It also causes increased heart rate, blood pressure, and temperature; in large doses, it can cause death. It is strongly addictive and has become a major drug of abuse. Khat leaves contain norpseudoephedrine; they are chewed by Middle Eastern peoples. Betel nut, the seed of the betel palm *Areca catechu*, contains arecoline. Many Asians and South Pacific Islanders chew the nut to obtain a mild narcotic stimulation and sense of well-being. In veterinary medicine, the nut has been used for deworming.

Nicotine, in tobacco and snuff, is an addictive stimulant drug, and other alkaloids have potential for dependency/addiction. Some (such as caffeine and cocaine) stimulate the CNS; others (such as hyoscyamine and morphine) depress the CNS. Via central and peripheral neural action, alkaloids influence muscle (especially smooth muscle), usually relaxing it. For example, ephedrine and codeine cause bronchorelaxation, reduce coughing, and assist expectoration; vasodilatory effects of alkaloids can help reduce fevers and relieve muscle spasm and hypertension.

Alkaloids have potent pharmacologic action, and many are used daily as medications in Western and herbal medicine. They are potentially toxic if misused; most plants containing them are classed as toxic. Curares are of different botanical origin, and each contains extracts of several plants. The toxiferins obtained from *Strychos toxifera* are the most potent curare alkaloids. Species of *Chondrodendron* are sources of tubocurarine. Curare alkaloids are inactive orally; parenterally they act as skeletal muscle relaxants by blocking muscle receptors for acetylcholine. The main clinical use of curare is as an adjuvant in surgical anesthesia to obtain relaxation of skeletal muscle or to facilitate diagnostic procedures, such as laryngoscopy and endoscopy.

Most plant families (85% to 90%) contain no alkaloids, but plants that do are seldom used for food. Exceptions are potatoes and tomatoes (solanine), coffee beans (caffeine), tea leaves (caffeine, theophylline), cocoa (caffeine, theobromine), and kola extract (caffeine), and the levels in the consumed portions are relatively low. However, acute solanine toxicity can arise in animals who ingest excessive amounts of potatoes or tomatoes.

Many alkaloids act as stimulant drugs or analeptics. Stimulants excite the CNS, increasing alertness, decreasing fatigue, and delaying sleep. Some that impair appetite are prescribed to promote weight loss in obese people. Most users of these drugs experience a sense of euphoria, but this reaction depends greatly on the drug taken and the dose. Signs of overstimulation by these drugs, such as muscle tremors or irregular heart rate, are common. Caffeine is the most widely used stimulant drug in the world. In small amounts, it acts as a mild stimulant and is harmless to most people. In large amounts, it may cause insomnia, restlessness, and anxiety. Caffeine increases heart rate and can cause heart irregularities; heavy coffee drinkers are more prone to coronary heart disease. Caffeine decreases blood flow to the brain and has been used in treating migraine headaches. It is also used in treating poisoning by depressants such as alcohol and morphine, and studies suggest that it somewhat increases the effectiveness of common analgesics such as aspirin. By widening bronchial airways, caffeine and theophylline can help relieve asthma attacks. Caffeine can cause chronic (low grade) adverse reactions in humans who consume excessive amounts. With increasing age, caffeine users may experience for the first time insomnia or palpitations of the heart associated with irregular beats. Heavy users often become nervous, irritable, apprehensive, restless, and unable to sleep; such symptoms may be construed as a psychiatric disorder unless the history of caffeine misuse is known. Recognition of the drug effects of these beverages has led to the increased use of decaffeinated coffee.

Alkaloids have potent vasodilatory-hypotensive-sedative, antitussive-expectorant, and antiinflammatory-analgesic-antiarthritic effects. Many have immunostimulatory effects, potent antibacterial action, and stimulate leukocytosis and phagocytosis; some also have antifungal and antiviral action. Some alkaloids inhibit neoplastic cells and stimulate excretion of bile and uric acid. They are used clinically to treat immunomediated disorders (allergies, asthma, immunosuppression, bronchitis, autoimmune diseases, arthritis, gout and allied conditions, infections, gastroenteritis, dysentery, constipation, and neoplasia), hypertension, stress, insomnia, and the effects of chronic disease and senility. The alkaloids used in CHM are relatively safe, usually nonaddictive, and confer multiple therapeutic effects, especially when combined with other herbal medicines.

Alkaloid-containing medicinal herbs include aconite, aristolochia, berberis, chin-chiu, cocculus, coptis, corydalis, erythina, Fangji, gentiana, ipecacuanha, lobelia, lycopodium, mahonia, nandina, phellodendron, rauwolfia, sinomenium, solanum, sophora, stemona, stephania, and veratrum.

Commonly used herbs in which alkaloids are the principal active compounds come from two main families: the *Berberidaceae* and the *Menispermaceae*. Within each family, the alkaloid structures and clinical effects are similar. Both families contain species that contain berbamine and tetrandine.

The *Berberidaceae* have antiinflammatory action, inhibit gastrointestinal bacteria, and relieve irritation of mucous membranes in the eye and digestive and respiratory systems. They are used to treat fever, cough with excessive phlegm, gastroenteritis, dysentery, and inflammation of the eyes, throat, mouth, and joints. They include many species of *Berberis* root (high in berberine, palmatine, berbamine, and jatorrhizine). *Mahonia* contains similar alkaloids and magnoflorine. *Nandina* contains domesticine, andinine, isobolidine, and other alkaloids, similar to those in *mahonia* and *berberis*.

The *Menispermaceae* include *cocculus, stephania,* and *sinomenium*. These have potent clinical effect with minimal side effects and are used interchangeably. They contain alkaloids with antiarthritic, antiallergic, antiedematous, hypotensive, and antimicrobial effects, and are used to treat arthritis, allergies, edema, hypertension, and gastroenteritis.

MISCELLANEOUS ALKALOID-CONTAINING HERBS Antiinflammatory herbs used in arthritis include aconite, aristolochia, chin-chiu, corydalis, erythina, lycopodium, and solanum. Antiinflammatory herbs used in irritation of skin and mucous membranes include coptis, gentiana, phellodendron, solanum, and sophora. Antiinflammatory herbs used in cough and bronchitis include solanum and stemona. The solanum used in CHM *(S. nigra)* contains solasonine and solamargine, but little solanine. (*S. dulcamara* contains high levels of solanine and is dangerous if used internally.) It is contraindicated in pregnancy, but its roots, seeds, and leaves are used extensively in China to treat cancer.

Opiate alkaloids are considered the most effective of all analgesics. *Papaver somniferum* yields 26 alkaloids, of which the most important are morphine, codeine, and papaverine. All opiates can be abused, but heroin, a morphine derivative, is the most notorious. Because of their abuse, opiates are restricted and used less and less in routine Western medicine, except in treatment of terminal illness.

Alkaloid-containing herbs are a relatively small part of most formulas used in CHM. They are used mainly to supplement the effects of other herbs. However, the following formulas contain a high content of alkaloids:

- *Coptis and Scute Formula* (coptis, phellodendron, gardenia, and scute). The first two herbs rely mainly on alkaloids for their action. The formula is used in fever, hemorrhagic diseases, insomnia, gastroenteritis, pruritus, and hypertension.
- *Coptis and Evodia Pills* (berberis, coptis, evodia, phellodendron, licorice, peony, and saussurea). The first four herbs contain alkaloids with sedative, hypotensive, and antiinflammatory effects. The formula is used to treat gastrointestinal disorders associated with stress or agitation, including chronic colitis associated with immunodeficiency.

Dharmananda's review of the effects of polysaccharides, steroids, flavonoids, and alkaloids shows that herbal medicines containing these compounds (and others not discussed) can have potent therapeutic action on inflammation, membrane stability, lipid peroxidation, infections, immunomediated disorders, cancer, and nervous, cardiac, pulmonary, hepatic, and renal disease.

The rest of this section discusses data on other active compounds found in herbal medicines: immunomodulators, antiinflammatories, antioxidants, antimicrobials, antivirals, antineoplastics, sedatives or hypotensives, and insect antifeedants.

Immunomodulators

Immunomodulation is critical to the treatment of immunomediated disorders (infections, inflammations, autoimmune disease, and allergies). Many systemic diseases, such as autoimmune diseases, immunosuppression, AIDS, and cancer, are poorly controlled by Western medicines. Based on TCM, Sino-Japanese concepts of homeostasis suggest that there is a regulatory effect on the immune, endocrine, and cardiovascular systems.

AUTOIMMUNE DISEASE   Several herbal medicines are clinically effective in autoimmune diseases such as chronic hepatitis, rheumatoid arthritis, nephrosis, and systemic lupus erythematosus. These herbal medicines are thought to act by modulating the immune system (Labadie and others, 1989; Wagner, 1990). Active compounds (polysaccharides, steroids, flavones, and alkaloids) in herbal medicines have potent action on immunomediated disorders (Dharmananda, 1991), as discussed earlier.

ANTIALLERGIC EFFECTS   *Bupleurum* contains saikosaponins (steroids with antiinflammatory and antiallergic activity). *Sophora* alkaloids have antiallergic action (Dharmananda, 1991). *Scute* contains baicalin, baicalein, and skullcapflavone II; these inhibit release of chemical mediator from mast cells.

Herbs with antihistaminic effects (caused by beta-eudesmol and nerolidol) are alpinia, cardamom, cluster, galanga, ginger, and zedoaria. *Zizyphi fructus* (jujube) contains a compound that increases cAMP production in the body, a beta-adrenergic compound and ethyl-Ó-D-fructofuranoside. These compounds suppress IgE activity. Hot water–extract of ganoderma suppresses histamine release from mast cells and the passive cutaneous anaphylactic (PCA) reaction (Tsung, 1987). Steroidal activity in ganoderic acids (in ganoderma), ginsenosides (in ginseng), and extracts of bupleurum and licorice have antiallergic and antihistaminic effects. They inhibit or reduce mediator release. Antiallergic effects also include other antiinflammatory mechanisms.

Polymethoxyflavones have high antiallergic and high antithrombotic activity. Nobeletin, tengeretin, and heptamethoxyflavone are the active antiallergic compounds in the Chinese citrus products *zhishi* and *qingpi*. These compounds markedly inhibit PCA reaction in experimental allergic challenge in rats. Nobeletin has a similar structure to koganebananin and skullcapflavones (baicalin, baicalein, and skullcapflavone II) from *scute*. The latter inhibit mediator release from mast cells. Baicalin increases the levels of cAMP and PGE_1, which inhibit mediator release. *Capillaris* and *scute* are used to treat urticaria and dermatitis. *Capillaris* contains cirsimaritin, which has a similar structure to baicalin. Antiasthmatic herbal medicine formulas often contain gingko fruit. Ginkolide, both natural and synthetic, is effective in treating human asthma and allergic inflammation and reduces rejection of transplanted grafts in animals. Daidzein and similar compounds are the active compounds in pueraria and sophora, which are important antiallergic herbs for treatment of urticaria, dermatitis, sinusitis, migraine, and asthma (Dharmananda, 1991).

ANTIHEPATOTOXIC EFFECTS   In Western medicine, as in TCM, many allergic, autoimmune, inflammatory, metabolic, and toxic disorders involve seriously disturbed liver functions. These include food and drug allergies, gastro-duodenal-colonic irritation and ulceration, photosensitization, dermatitis, conjunctivitis, migraine, irritability, gout, rheumatoid arthritis, and hepatitis. Therapy that protects or enhances liver function also helps in liver-mediated disorders. Polysaccharides, steroids, and flavones in herbal medicines with hepatoprotective action are also useful in such conditions (Dharmananda, 1991). Herbal medicines that protect the liver against toxins and are useful clinically in hepatotoxic disorders and hepatitis include andrographis, bupleurum, coriolus, eleuthero, ganoderma, gentiana, ginseng, gynostemma, licorice, paeonia, phyllanthus, picrorrhizia, polyporus, and sophora. The effects are mediated by their polysaccharides, steroids, and saponins. Other important herbal medicines used in hepatitis and liver disease are capillaris and scute; they have potent antihepatotoxic action, mediated by their flavonoids. Flavonoids capillarisin, arcapillin, isorhamnetin, and quercetin are hepatoprotective in carbon tetrachloride cytotoxicity. *Swertia* flavonoids (homoorientin, swertiajaponin, and swertisin) are hepatoprotective in galactosamine cytotoxicity (Dharmananda, 1991).

The bitter taste of most alkaloids, especially berberine alkaloids, stimulates bile secretion. Herbal medicines containing such alkaloids are used as appetite stimulants, mild laxatives, and to treat biliary stasis, cholecystitis, and ascariasis of the bile ducts. Their combination with herbal medicines that stimulate liver function increases their efficacy (Dharmananda, 1991).

In controlled experiments in rats, ginseng had a protective effect on the liver; injections of a water extract of ginseng significantly decreased liver enzyme levels (AST, ALT) induced by injections of dexamethasone (Lin and others, 1995c).

Antiinflammatories

Steroids in akebia, alisma, dianthus, licorice, and poria (hoelen), as in the formula *Ba Zhen Tang*, have antiinflammatory effects and are used to treat nephritis and urinary infections. Steroids are thought to underlie the efficacy of *bupleurum* in allergies, hepatitis, gastroenteritis, and dermatitis. The alkaloids tetrandine and isotetrandine have antiinflammatory, antiallergic, and antianaphylactic action. Alkaloids in Fangji, an herbal medicine based on any one or a combination of aristolochia, cocculus, stephania, or sinomenium, activate the self-defense system in infection and inflammation (Dharmananda, 1991).

Alkaloids from the *Berberidaceae* are used mainly to treat inflammation of the skin and mucous membranes; those from the *Menispermaceae* are used to treat inflammation of the joints (Dharmananda, 1991).

Accumulation of urates in tissue, especially in the tendons and joints, can cause gout and gouty arthritis. Classic signs are irritability and pain, especially in the big toe (the "Liver Toe" in TCM). Berberis, coptis, and phellodendron increase uric acid excretion and are used to treat gout. Their alkaloids are thought to be involved in urate elimination. Colchicine, from *Colchicum autumnale,* is used in Western medicine for the same purpose. Other herbs with antiinflammatory and hepatoprotective effect are also used to treat gout.

Protoberberines and isoquinolines have analgesic effects in hot plate–induced experimental pain. Corydalis, menisperma, and sinomenium are used to treat pain, especially in trauma and arthritis. They contain protoberberines, such as corydalimine, stepholidine, and synactine. Cocculus, menisperma, and stephania are used to treat arthritis pain. They contain isoquinolines, such as berbamine, coclobine, dauricine, and tetrandine.

Ginsenoside Ro, isolated from the roots of *Panax ginseng,* reduces acute paw edema (induced by 40/80 or carrageenin) in rats; it also inhibits the increase in vascular permeability (induced by acetic acid) in mice (Matsuda, Samukawa, Kubo, 1990). An extract of ginseng increases the phagocytotic ability of white cells in bovine blood and milk (Hu and others, 1995).

Ginseng is used in TCM for its tonic and restorative effects on stress, neurasthenia, and convalescence. Ginseng extract restores adrenal and thyroid functions inhibited by dexamethasone treatments; the effects of the extract on adrenal and thyroid function may explain some of its effects as a general tonic and antistress herb (Lin and others, 1995c).

New diastereoisomers and sulphur-containing compounds isolated from onion, *Allium cepa* L., have potent inhibitory effects for collagen-induced aggregation, as well as arachidonate-induced aggregation of human platelets in vitro. The most active compound is a diastereoisomer of cis-3-ethyl-2,4,5-trithia-6-octene 2-S-oxide (Morimitsu, Kawakishi, 1990).

Antioxidants

Many disease processes involve the generation of reactive oxygen species—superoxide anionic radical (O_2-), hydrogen peroxide (H_2O_2), and hydroxyl-radical (OH-). If not neutralized, these oxidative radicals cause cellular oxidative stress, increase lipid peroxidation, and cause instability of cellular membranes. The presence of these radicals also compromises the microbicidal activity of polymorphonuclear leukocytes and other phagocytic cells (macrophages and reticuloendothelial cells).

Prooxidants increase the risk of all disorders associated with reactive oxygen species (free radicals) in the body. In the future, antioxidants in herbal medicines may be an important method of maintaining life in a polluted environment. Anthropogenic pollution is a serious threat to life on earth. We burn organic materials to generate power (electricity, heat, transportation) and to dispose of municipal or domestic waste by incineration. Fires also burn organic material. Unless these emissions are removed and/or recycled by expensive technology, they enter our atmosphere. Particulate (fly-ash) and gaseous emissions return to earth by deposition or precipitation. Emissions from combustion or industrial sources (smelters, refineries, pharmaceutical and chemical plants, and fertilizer factories) contain xenobiotic (inherently toxic to life [human, animal, or plant]) organic compounds such as 2,4,5-trichlorophenol (phenoxyacetic acid), halogenated aromatic hydrocarbons, polycyclic aromatic hydrocarbons, pentachlorophenols, polychlorinated dibenzofurans, polychlorinated biphenyls, polychlorinated dibenzo-p-dioxins, tetrachlorodibenzo-p-dioxins, and related xenobiotics. Some herbicides and pesticides also contain them.

Organic hydrocarbon emissions include dioxins, the most toxic anthropogenic chemicals known. Organic toxins enter the food chain, persist for long periods in the environment, and pose toxic hazards to soil, plant, animal, and human life. Xenobiotic effects of dioxins on humans and animals include increased lipid peroxidation and cellular oxidative stress (exaggerating any environmental deficiencies of copper, selenium, and vitamins, especially vitamin E), immunotoxicity (thus increasing susceptibility to cancer, AIDS, viral and bacterial infections, and inflammatory processes), thyrotoxicity (thus exaggerating environmental deficiencies of iron and selenium and compromising reproduction, neonatal survival, lactation, growth, and general metabolism), and disorders of the liver, kidney, skin, heart, and lungs. Dioxins also adversely influence female and male reproduction; they compromise pregnancy and induce birth defects. Dioxins also reduce growth and they influence and are influenced by vitamin A in serum and tissues (Rogers, 1995).

Animals have an extensive antioxidant defense system to minimize the untoward effects of oxygen. Antioxidants alleviate the oxidative load by directly quenching reactive oxygen species before they damage vital cellular components. Mammalian intracellular antioxidants include the selenium-dependent glutathione peroxidases, the copper-dependent superoxidase dismutases, vitamins E and C, beta-carotene, and uric acid.

Medicinal plants also contain large amounts of antioxidants (ascorbic acid, tocopherol, ubiquinone, glutathione, and phenolics). Therefore it is not surprising that these natural sources are used medicinally in many conditions, including aging, atherosclerosis, and immunomediated diseases (immunosuppression, inflammation, infection, and neoplasia).

Gypenoside saponins of *Gynostemma pentaphyllum* have antioxidant properties that counter oxidative stress in phagocytes, liver microsomes, and vascular endothelial cells. The extensive antioxidant effect of gypenosides may be valuable to prevent and treat various diseases such as atherosclerosis, liver disease, and inflammation (Li, Jiao, Lau, 1993).

Tannins are polyphenols widely present in plants. Since phenolic compounds have antioxidant activities, tannins also could be developed to prevent lipid peroxidation and biologic damage caused by free radicals formed under oxidative stress. Of 25 tannins and related compounds tested, catechin, benzylthioether, and procyanidin beta-2 benzylthioether were the most potent in inhibiting lipid peroxidation, with inhibitory effects stronger than Trolox, a water-soluble analogue of vitamin E. Also, conjugation of tannins with a benzylthioether group did not enhance the free radical scavenger activity of tannins. However, it may increase the inhibitory effect on lipid peroxidation (Hong and others, 1995). Recently, magnolol and honokiol, isolated from *Magnolia officinalis,* were shown to be 1000 times more potent than Trolox (Lo and others, 1994). Antioxidant (free radical–scavenging) effects of bupleurum polysaccharide are discussed later in this chapter.

Antimicrobials

Many plants and herbal medicines contain antimicrobial compounds. Such compounds are of interest because of their relationship to phytoalexin production. Phytoalexins are antimicrobial compounds of low molecular weight. They act as a defense against microbial infection of the plant; plants synthesize and accumulate them after exposure to microorganisms (Dixon, Lamb, 1990). Most herbs have weak antimicrobial activity in comparison with that of synthetic antibiotics or those from microbial or fungal origin, but some have antibacterial and/or antifungal activity of practical value in medical and veterinary therapy (Cousins, 1995a,b).

Oryzalide A (Fig. 21-1, *A*) is a novel C19-kaurane type of diterpene. It was isolated from the healthy leaves of a rice plant that was resistant to *Xanthomonas campestris* pv. *oryzae.* That organism is a cause of leaf blight in susceptible rice plants (Watanabe and others, 1990). At 150 ppm, Oryzalide A inhibited approximately 60% of the colony-forming ability of *X. campestris.* Because similar diterpenes were isolated from rice as phytoalexins, it is thought that the biosynthetic pathway of diterpenes may play an important role in the mechanisms of disease resistance in rice plants. In tropical countries, plants from the *Meliaceae*

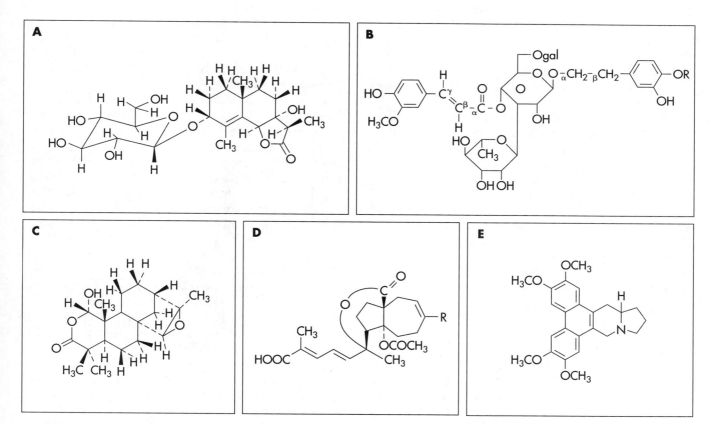

Fig. 21-1 Structures of some natural compounds used medicinally. **A,** Structure of sphaeranthanolide; **B,** structure of Jionoside A₁ (R, H) and Jionoside B₁ (R, CH₃); **C,** structure of Oryzalide; **D,** structure of Pseudolaric acid-A (R, CH₃) and Pseudolaric acid-B₁ (R, COOCH₃); **E,** structure of Tylophorine.

family are used widely in traditional medicine to treat fever. Gedunin, a limonoid recently isolated from *Meliaceae* spp., had moderate antimalarial activity (IC50, 0.72 mg/ml) against *Plasmodium falciparum* (Bay and others, 1990).

Protoberberines (including jatorrhizine, coumbamine, berberine, and phellodendrine) have effective antimicrobial activity. They occur in berberis, coptis, and phellodendron, herbs that are used to treat gastroenteritis, bacillary dysentery, or wound infection. Matrine and other alkaloids in *sophora* are strongly antiseptic and antifungal. Stemona alkaloids are antibacterial and antifungal. Flavonoids have good antifungal activity in the treatment of candidiasis and thrush. Condensed flavonoids form tannins that are useful as astringents and antiseptics. Herbal medicines with flavonoid/tannin effect are useful in gastrointestinal infection (Dharmananda, 1991).

Antivirals

Some herbs have antiviral activity that may have practical value in veterinary therapy (Cousins, 1995a). Several antiviral compounds have been isolated from herbs (Dharmananda, 1991). The Lonicera and Forsythia Formula (*Yinqiao Jiedu San* in TCM) is the world's most commonly used medication for colds and flu. The flavonoid quercetin gave some protection to animals experimentally inoculated with many viruses. It also inactivated herpes simplex, polio, rabies, and some flu viruses. Catechin is more potent than quercetin against herpes virus. Stemona alkaloids are antiviral (Dharmananda, 1991); 5-0-methyl-genistein 7-0-beta-D-glucopyranoside from *Ulex europaeus* inhibited the replication of Herpes simplex virus (HSV) and poliovirus (De Rodriguez and others, 1990). Three proanthocyanidins from *Pavetta owariensis* (Guinean Traditional medicine), proanthocyanidin A2 (dimeric proanthocyanidin), cinnamtannin B1 (trimeric anthocyanidin), and cinnamtannin B2 (tetrameric anthocyanidin), had pronounced antiviral properties against HSV and Coxsackie viruses. It seems that both antiherpetic potency and the cytotoxicity of tannins depend on the molecular weight, as well as the number of polyphenolic groups (Balde and others, 1990; Fukuchi and others, 1989). Recently, 2 of 134 flavonoids isolated from *Scutellaria radix* (scute) were shown to have highly potent antiinfluenza activities in vitro and in vivo (Nagai and others, 1995).

Antineoplastics

Drug resistance is common when single drugs are used to treat a specific cancer. Western medicine usually uses many drugs simultaneously in cancer chemotherapy because tumors are less likely to become resistant to drug therapy by the combination technique. Combination chemotherapy has been most successful in treating cancer, especially leukemia, Hodgkin's disease, testicular cancer, and ovarian carcinoma. Recent cancer therapies combine less radical forms of surgery with radiation, chemotherapy, "preventive" therapy, and support therapy.

Western medicine uses two main types of chemotherapy: cytotoxic chemotherapy and immunotherapy (Dharmananda, 1991; Ogilvie, Moore, 1995).

CYTOTOXIC CHEMOTHERAPY   Cytotoxic chemotherapy aims to kill neoplastic cells by a direct toxic action. The side effects can be severe and may need to be controlled by symptomatic medication. Several types of naturally occurring compounds that react directly with DNA are used. These include steroids, antibiotics, alkaloids, and alkylating agents. Western medicine also uses antimetabolites. These resemble normal metabolites in structure and compete with them for some metabolic function, thus preventing further utilization of normal metabolic pathways.

IMMUNOTHERAPY   Immunotherapy aims to enhance the body's innate ability to recognize, attack, and destroy the neoplastic cells. Active immunotherapy aims to stimulate lymphocytes that are effective in destroying cancer cells. Passive, specific, or nonspecific immunotherapy is conducted by injection of antibodies specific for the neoplasm (such as specific monoclonal antibodies), administration of nonspecific immunoglobulins, interferon, cytokines (such as tumor-necrosis factor [TNF], and interleukin 2 [IL2]). It also includes the use of antioxidants (vitamin E and trace elements—especially selenium) and nonspecific immunostimulants and immunomodulators; the latter act by boosting the body's production of cytokines and other protective agents (Dharmananda, 1991; Ogilvie, Moore, 1995).

Many cytotoxic antineoplastic agents have been isolated from plants, especially the polysaccharide fraction of mushrooms (as in the Japanese formula Krestin) and astragalus (Dharmananda, 1991). Vinblastine and vincristine (alkaloids from *Vinca rosea*, or *Catharanthus roseus*) are used to treat Hodgkin's disease and acute leukemia, respectively. Taxol, from the bark of Pacific yew trees *(Taxus brevifolia)*, gave promising results in advanced ovarian, breast, and other cancers (Borman, 1991). *Mallotus japonicus* husks contain 3-(3,3-di-methylallyl)-5-(3-acetyl-2,4-dihydroxy-5-methyl-6-methoxybenzyl)-phloracetophenone. This compound had excellent cytotoxic activity against target neoplastic cells such as human carcinoma cells (larynx [HEp-2] and lung [PC-13]) and mouse B_{16} melanoma, leukemia P-338 and L5178Y cells. It increased significantly the lifespan of mice bearing L5178Y leukemia (Arisawa and others, 1990).

Novel diterpene acids, pseudolaric acid-A and pseudolaric acid-B (Fig. 21-1, *B*), isolated from *Pseudolarix kaempferi* (*Tu-Jin-Pi* in CHM), are cytotoxic against human cancer cell lines. Pseudolaric acid-A is more effective on leukemia P-388 and melanoma SK-MEL-5, whereas pseudolaric acid-B is more active against leukemia HL-60TB and P-388, CNS cancer TE671, melanoma SK-MEL-5, and ovarian cancer A2780 (Pan and others, 1990). Bryophillin B, a potent cytotoxic bufadienolide, has been isolated from *Bryophyllum pinnatum*. It shows potent cytotoxicity (ED50 <80 ng/ml) against in vitro growth of KB tissue culture cells (Yamagishi and others, 1989).

Cantharidin, isolated from *Mylabris* spp., possesses antihepatoma properties and induces leukocytosis (Wang, 1989). However, it is highly toxic and it decreases synthesis of steroids (Lin and others, 1995b). Because it may be fatal, it seldom is used clinically. Fortunately, several analogues (such as disodium norcantharidate, norcantharidin, dehydronorcantharidin, and methylcantharidimide) have been synthesized. Those analogues may have important uses in antineoplastic therapy (Wang, 1989).

Indirubin, a potent antileukemic agent, was isolated from *Danggui Liuwei Wan* (Six Flavor Tang-kuei Pill). That formula is used to treat cancer in China. Indirubin was the main active compound in an extract of *Qingdai (Baphicacanthus cusia)*, another herb used to treat cancer (Dharmananda, 1991).

Certain glucosides are immunoactive, but only those with immunostimulant effects are indicated in cancer therapy. For example, two new phenylalcohol glucosides, jionosides A1 and B1 (Fig. 21-1, *C*), were isolated from *Rehmannia glutinosa* (Sasaki and others, 1989). They have immunosuppressive effects, as have related glucosides. A new sesquiterpene glucoside, sphaeranthanolide (Fig. 21-1, *D*), from the flowers of *Sphaeranthus indicus*, has immunostimulant activity; it enhances the antibody response to sheep red blood cells (SRBC) (Shekhani and others, 1990).

In immunomediated disorders, alkaloids of the protoberberine, isoquinoline, and quinolizidine groups are of special interest as immunostimulants. Berbamine enhances the antineoplastic effects of cyclophosphamide in chemotherapy of cancer. It also increases white cell counts and counteracts cyclophosphamide-induced leukopenia. Berbamine and isotetrandine activate lymph glands and the cellular reaction of plasmoblasts and plasma cells. Berberrubine is a potent inhibitor of sarcoma 180. Tetrandine and isotetrandine inhibit many forms of cancer, including Erlich ascites tumor and carcinoma of the liver. Sophora alkaloids increase white cell counts and counteract radiation-induced leukopenia. Water extract of sophora inhibits sarcoma 180 and tumor growth of transplanted cervix tumor cells and prolongs survival of animals experimentally inoculated with ascitic and carcinoma cells (Dharmananda, 1991). TJ-48 is a Japanese pharmaceutical preparation used in KM. TJ-48, and its original prescription (JTT), are powerful immunostimulants and have potent effects on cancer patients. These effects are discussed later in this chapter under JTT.

Lien and Li (1985) and Zhang (1989) give much more detailed reviews of the pharmacology of CHMs and their uses in the treatment of cancer.

Sedatives, antispasmodics, and hypotensives

The sedative and hypotensive effects of herbal medicines containing triterpenes and alkaloids and the anticonvulsive effects of saponin-containing herbal medicines are useful in many clinical indications (Dharmananda, 1991).

Polysaccharides in blue ganoderma and poria have sedative effects. Herbal medicines containing saponins, such as arisaemia, bamboo, gleditsia, and typhonium have anticonvulsant effects similar to phenobarbital. These are useful clinically in epilepsy and febrile convulsions. In TCM, insomnia, agitation, and restlessness are caused by disturbed Shen (spirit), often from weak Heart *Yin*. Herbal medicines that calm the Shen by strengthening Heart *Yin* have sedative effects. Herbal medicines with such effect include albizzia, eleuthero, ganoderma, hoelen, lily, ophiopogon, polygala, poria, rehmannia, and zizyphus. The sedative effects are caused by a steroidal action via their saponins and triterpenes. Such herbs prolong the effects of phenobarbital. Herbal medicines with sedative effects not caused by steroids include acorus, biota, lotus seed, and tang kuei. Herbal medicines with sedative action are useful clinically to treat stress, insomnia, and agitation.

The Coptis and Scute Formula is used to treat hypertension. Potent hypotensive agents include the protoberberine alkaloids (at high levels in coptis and phellodendron) and isoquinoline alkaloids (e.g., cyclanoline in stephania). Tetrandine, palmatine, and berberis alkaloids are hypotensive also. Jatorrhizine and related alkaloids, such as palmatine, occur in berberis, coptis, corydalis, and phellodendron. They are sedatives and prolong sleep induced by phenobarbital. Domesticine and andinine, found in the antitussive nandina fruit, have morphinelike effects (Dharmananda, 1991). *Rauwolfia serpentina*, which contains reserpine, was used for centuries as a sedative in snakebite, in mental disease, and insomnia, and for many other purposes. Western medicine also uses reserpine to treat hypertension and as a sedative in psychiatric disorders such as schizophrenia. Its mechanism of action involves the depletion of catecholamines and serotonin.

The pharmacologic activity of the benzodiazepine sedative group is mediated by a specific channel receptor (benzodiazepine-x-gamma-aminobutyric acid$_A$-chloride, BDZ-GABA) complex. Many herbal medicines contain compounds that bind to BDZ receptors in the central nervous system. BDZ-like compounds in plants can be detected by gas chromatography–mass spectroscopy (Unseld, Klotz, 1989), or by their specific interaction with a monoclonal antibody to BDZ (Medina and others, 1989). The clinical significance of these compounds for humans and animals should be explored.

Insect antifeedants

Some plants possess highly active insect antifeedants. These active compounds can be used as novel insecticides.

Under laboratory conditions, tylophorine (Fig. 21-1, *E*), isolated from *Tylophora asthamatica,* completely inhibited feeding by *Spilosama obliqua* under laboratory conditions. The effect persisted in field trials for 2 days, as determined by damage rating scores (Tripathi, Singh, Jain, 1990). Tylophorine may be used as a prototype for the synthesis of safer and more economical molecules to deter insects from feeding. These may have future industrial use.

Four new sesquiterpene alkaloids, 1Ó-nicotinoyloxy-2Ó-acetoxy-6beta-acetoxy-9beta-furoyloxy-11-isobutyryloxy 4beta-hydroxydihydro-beta-agarofuran and related compounds, isolated from the root-bark of *Celastrus angulatus,* showed strong antifeedant action with several different insect species (Liu and others, 1990). Treated insects were paralyzed for many hours after ingesting a small dose of the test sample. They then recovered, fed, and became paralyzed again. As a result, the insects gradually starved to death.

Miscellaneous known medicinal effects of active herbal compounds

The active compounds in herbal medicines can have multiple medicinal effects. Box 21-3 is summarized from Ackerson (1995).

BOX 21-3

MULTIPLE MEDICINAL EFFECTS OF ACTIVE COMPOUNDS IN HMs

Allium sativa (garlic) is used as a spice, a medicine, and a germicide. Its juice contains the antibiotic oil *allicin* (diallyl thiosulphinate). Effects include inhibition of platelet aggregation, enhanced mesenteric circulation, and antimicrobial effects in bacterial, viral, protozoal, and fungal diseases.

Gentiana lutea (gentian glycosides, gentiopicrin, and gentiopicroside): Effects include antiinflammatory, antibacterial, and antimalarial effects; choleretic and digestive effects (useful in hyperchlorhydria and hypochlorhydria); and diuretic and liver-protective effects.

Hydrastis canadensis (isoquinoline alkaloids, berberine, and hydrastine): Effects include antiprotozoal and broad spectrum antibacterial effects, especially against candida and gastrointestinal pathogens. The herb has antispasmodic effects on the gut and is used to treat gastroenteritis, ulcers, and indigestion.

Jugulans nigra (naphthoquinone, juglone): Effects include antifungal, antiviral, antibacterial, and anthelmintic effects, similar to *Hydrastis.*

Quassia amara (quassinoids, gutulactone, and simalikalactone): Effects include antiprotozoal, antineoplastic, and antiviral activity and anthelmintic activity against nematodes (ascaris and pinworms).

Future research on herbal compounds?

Chaudhury (1995) reviewed pharmacologic research, folk medicine, and traditional texts. The herbal medicines in Box 21-4 have good clinical efficacy in the following indications. This justifies the need for detailed research on the identification and clinical potency of the active compounds in the herbal medicines (Chaudhury, 1995).

Pharmacologic Effects of Complex Herbal Medicine Formulas

Because of the number of herbal ingredients in each complex formula, the variety of active compounds, and the probability of interactions between the compounds, research on the effects of traditional formulas is challenging. In spite of the difficulties, research continues. Traditional

---

*The 12 Main Channel-Organ System(s) (COS) of TCM, also called the 12 Main Meridians, are: BL (Bladder); GB (Gallbladder); HT (Heart); KI (Kidney); LI (Large Intestine); LU (Lung); LV (Liver); PC (Pericardium, Circulation-Sex); SI (Small Intestine); SP (Spleen-Pancreas); ST (Stomach); TH (Triple Heater, Respiration-Digestion-Reproduction-Elimination, and Endocrine). The COS sequence (Diurnal Qi Cycle, beginning 0300 h) is: LU → LI → ST → SP → HT → SI → BL → KI → PC → TH → GB → LV (→LU). Each Channel is bilaterally symmetrical and has a superficial and deep path, connects with its respective Organ-Bowel and controls its TCM functions. COSs, with other Channels and Collaterals, form a 3-dimensional network connecting and uniting every cell, organ, and function in the body.

BOX 21-4

CLINICAL INDICATIONS OF SOME HMs

Antiinflammatories, arthritis: *Azadirachta indica, Commiphora wightii,* and *Curcuma longa*
Asthma: *Albizzia laback*
Cardiac disease: *Terminalia arjuna*
Hyperlipemia, atherosclerosis, and obesity: *Commiphora wightii* (gum guggal, steroids, diterpenoids, aliphatic esters, and carbohydrates)
Hyperglycemia, diabetes mellitus: *Gymnema sylvestre, Momordica charantia*
Hypertension: *Moringa oleifera*
Liver disease, hepatitis: *Andrographis paniculata, Glycyrrhiza, Picrorrhizia kurroa,* and *Phyllanthus amarus*
Malaria, antiprotozoals, fever: *Artemisia annua* (sesquiterpene lactones and flavones, artemesinin, artemetin, and casticin), *Dichroa febrifuga, Xanthium strumarum*
Respiratory disease: *Adhala vasica*
To improve quality of life: *Tinosporia cordifolia*
To increase interferon levels: *Glycyrrhiza* (licorice)

From Chaudhury RR: In Munson PL, Mueller RA, Breese GR, eds: *Principles of pharmacology: basic concepts and clinical applications,* New York, 1995, Chapman & Hall International.

formulas in CHM may be evaluated from the perspectives of TCM and Western medicine.* Two examples of traditional formulas, KHHT and JTT, are discussed from Chinese and Western perspectives. They illustrate the historical and scientific background of Chinese herbology.

KHHT from the perspective of TCM

The word *Tang* means decoction. Koken-Huanglien-Huangchin-Tang (KHHT) is discussed in the treatise *Shang Han Lun* (about 210 AD). The formula contains four herbs: pueraria (Koken), coptis (Huanglien), scute (Huangchin), and licorice in a ratio of 20:10:10:3.

Weber (1992) lists the following pharmacologic properties of the individual main ingredients:

- *Pueraria* (Koken, Gegen): Analgesic, anticonvulsant, antidiarrheal, antipyretic, coronary vasodilator, and salivation stimulant
- *Coptis* (Huanglien): anticonvulsive, antidiarrheal, antifungal, anthelmintic, and stomachic
- *Scute* (Huangchin): antiallergic, antiasthmatic, antidermatitic, antiemetic, antihypertensive, antipyretic, cholegogue, sedative, and stomachic
- *Licorice* (Gancao, *Glycerrhiza*): antiallergic, antidiarrheal, antiinflammatory, antipharyngitic, antispasmodic, antitoxic, antitussive, antiulcerative (gastroduodenal), expectorant, harmonizer for all drugs, immunostimulant, stomachic, and tonic

In combination, KHHT is a common formula to treat human gastroenteritis and dysentery. It also controls symptoms of flu, fever, erysipelas, measles, some eye disorders, headache, toothache (Luo, Shi, 1986; Ou, 1989). In TCM, Huanglien (Ministerial drug) clears Damp Heat from the Middle Heater; Huangchin (Assistant drug) clears Damp Heat from the Upper Heater. Together, they help Koken (Principal drug for the digestive system) to stop diarrhea, mainly by releasing Heat and boosting *Yang Qi* of the Earth Channel Organ Systems (ST [Stomach] and SP [Spleen]). Licorice (Guiding drug) enhances the total action of the other drugs and reduces side effects.

KHHT from the perspective of Western medicine

Experimentally, KHHT and gentamycin were highly (and equally) effective (85% and 88%, respectively) in curing piglet scour within 4 days, but only 52% of untreated controls had recovered by then (Lin and others, 1988). However, this does not mean that KHHT works like antibiotics. The mechanism of KHHT is a holistic treatment. The basic principle behind therapy using TCM is to regulate the homeostasis of the whole body through the compound actions of several herbs and to restore the abnormal state to normal. Huanglien and Huangchin (ministerial and assistant drugs) have antiviral and broad-spectrum antibacterial activities in vitro and in vivo (Nagai and others, 1995). Whatever the mechanism, as postulated by Western or Eastern views, KHHT enhances the body defenses, improves gastrointestinal function, and has antibacterial and antiviral action.

JTT from the perspective of TCM

Shiquan Dabu Tang is called *Juzen-Taiho-To (JTT)* in KM. JTT is the Japanese name for Shiquan Dabu Tang (Decoction of Ten Good Herbs), a formula from the Song Dynasty. JTT is another example of a very old formula from CHM that still is used widely today. JTT has a great tonic effect in patients with chronic debilitating diseases. Given to patients after surgery, it promotes rapid postoperative recovery (Xie and others, 1994).

Shiquan Dabu Tang (or JTT) contains 10 herbs to tonify body functions (Table 21-2) (Xie and others, 1994): Ba Zhen Tang (Eight Precious Herb Decoction), cinnamon, and astragalus. Ba Zhen Tang is a combination of Si Wu Tang (Four Material Decoction) and Si Jun Zi Tang (Four Gentleman Decoction). Si Wu Tang and Si Jun Zi Tang are recorded in *Tai Ping Hui Min He Ji Ju Fang* (Prescription of Peaceful Benevolent Dispensary, Song Dynasty). Shiquan Dabu Tang (Decoction of Ten Good Herbs) was described in the same source.

SI WU TANG   Si Wu Tang (Four Material Decoction) is a TCM Formula to treat Blood Deficiency (Xie and others, 1994). It contains angelica, rehmannia, paeonia,

---

TABLE 21-2

THE HERBAL INGREDIENTS OF *SHIQUAN DABU TANG* (OR *JUZEN-TAIHO-TO*, JTT, TJ-48)

FORMULA	CLINICAL USES	HERBS CLASSIFIED BY CHINESE RATIONALE			
		PRINCIPAL	MINISTERIAL	ASSISTANT	GUIDING
Si Wu Tang*	Blood Deficiency	*Angelica*	*Rehmannia*	*Paeonia*	*Cnidium*
Si Jun Zi Tang†	*Qi* Deficiency	*Ginseng*	*Atractylodes*	*Hoelen*	*Licorice*
Shiquan Dabu Tang‡	*Qi*/Blood Deficiency	The above eight herbs plus cinnamon and astragalus, both of which are Assistant and Guiding drugs			

*Four Material Decoction.
†Four Gentleman Decoction.
‡Decoction of Ten Good Herbs.

and cnidium. Its function in TCM is to tonify and regulate Blood. It is used for the Syndrome of Deficiency and Stagnation of Blood, with symptoms such as menstrual disorders, abdominal pain, threatened abortion, and lochia. Other diseases, such as malnutrition, anemia, insomnia, and vertigo, can respond well to this remedy. The Principal drug (angelica) tonifies the Blood (hematopoietic system), relieves stagnation and pain, helps bowel movements, and relieves constipation. The Ministerial drug (rehmannia) tonifies the Blood and *Yin.* The Assistant drug (paeonia) tonifies *Yin,* Blood, Liver, and hemopoietic system. The Guiding drug (cnidium) tonifies the free circulation of *Qi* and Blood and expels Damp. Together, the four ingredients effectively tonify the hematopoetic system (Blood formation) and the circulation.

SI JUN ZI TANG   Si Jun Zi Tang (Four Gentleman Decoction) is a TCM Formula to treat *Qi* Deficiency. It contains ginseng, atractylodes, hoelen, and licorice. Its function in TCM is to tonify *Qi,* the abdominal Organ-Bowels, and digestion. It is used to tonify *Qi* in *Qi* Deficiency, especially in malfunction of abdominal Organ-Bowels, anemia, and fatigue. This remedy is mainly used for dysfunction of Earth COSs (SP, ST). The Principal drug (ginseng) tonifies *Qi, Yang,* and the functions of the abdominal Organ-Bowels, such as Stomach, Spleen, Kidney, and Liver. It also calms the mind. The Ministerial drug (atractylodes) tonifies Spleen to transform Substance into *Qi.* The Assistant drug (hoelen) helps ginseng and atractylodes to tonify Spleen to transform Substance into *Qi;* hoelen tonifies Kidney. It has diuretic effects that can expel Damp. It expels Stagnated Water from the body. The Guiding drug (licorice) regulates the internal organs, via enhancing *Qi* flow through the Channels. Together, the four ingredients tonify digestive function to produce more *Qi* from Substance and to normalize the body defense system.

BA ZHEN TANG   Ba Zhen Tang (Eight Precious Herb Decoction) is a combination of Si Wu Tang and Si Jun Zi Tang. Sometimes, the physician adds ginger and date to increase the Assistant and Guiding effects. See previous discussions for functions.

SHIQUAN DABU TANG   Shiquan Dabu Tang (Decoction of Ten Good Herbs) and Juzen-Taiho-To (JTT) is a combination of Ba Zhen Tang, cinnamon, and astragalus (Table 21-2). In TCM, this formula is a Master Remedy for Syndromes of Deficiency of *Qi* and/or Blood. Indicative symptoms are remittent fever, muscle spasms, coarse skin, nocturnal emissions, pallor, coldness, anemia, weakness, and anxiety. The Principal drugs (angelica and ginseng) tonify the Blood and *Qi,* respectively, and ginseng also tonifies the functions of the abdominal Organ-Bowels and calms the mind. The Ministerial drugs are rehmannia (to tonify *Yin* and Blood) and atractylodes (to tonify Spleen, to transform Substance into *Qi,* and to tonify digestion and decrease Damp Syndrome [edema]).

Its Assistant drugs are paeonia (to tonify *Yin,* Blood, Liver, and the hemopoietic system) and hoelen (to tonify Kidney; it has diuretic effects that can expel Damp). The Guiding drugs are cnidium (to tonify the free circulation of *Qi* and Blood and expel Damp) and licorice (to regulate the internal organs, via enhanced *Qi* flow through the Channels and to adjust and detoxify all the other herbs, making them more effective and safe). Finally, astragalus tonifies *Qi* and *Yang,* to tonify Spleen, Stomach, and digestive function, and cinnamon warms the body and expels Cold, or sensations of chill; it also tonifies the Lung, Heart, and Kidney. It is antifebrile in chills and antierythematous; it coordinates the diuretic effects of other herbs. The combination of the 10 ingredients in JTT is a master tonic; it treats a wide variety of symptoms in patients debilitated after surgery or childbirth and after acute or chronic illness. It is useful in anemia, dysmenorrhea, inappetence, fatigue, and weakness (Xie and others, 1994).

JTT from the perspective of Western medicine

As mentioned, JTT is given to patients recovering from surgery or suffering from chronic diseases to promote improvement of their debilitated general conditions. JTT has been shown to modulate the defense system. It is a powerful immunostimulant. It significantly enhances antibody responses to SRBC (Komatsu and others, 1986), phagocytosis (Maruyama and others, 1988), and mitogenic activities against splenic B cells in mice (Takemoto and others, 1989). Peripheral blood cell counts in patients treated concomitantly with JTT orally and an antineoplastic drug (mitomycin C) were higher than in patients treated with the antineoplastic drug alone (Nabeya, Ri, 1983). Concomitant dosing of JTT with mitomycin C gave significantly longer survival periods in p-388 cancer-bearing mice than those treated with mitomycin C alone (Aburada and others, 1983). JTT facilitated hematopoietic recovery from mitomycin C–induced bone marrow or radiation injuries (Kawamura and others, 1989; Ohnishi and others, 1990; Yamada and others, 1990). These immunostimulating activities may relate closely to the clinical effects of JTT. Thus the efficacy of JTT can be evaluated if immunomodulators are isolated and characterized from the preparation.

TJ-48 is a Japanese spray-dried powder of JTT extract. TJ-48 improved the general condition of cancer patients receiving chemotherapy and/or radiation therapy. Patients who took TJ-48 orally with an antineoplastic drug maintained higher peripheral blood counts than patients not taking TJ-48. It accelerated hemopoietic recovery from bone-marrow injury by mitomycin C (MMC) (Kawamura and others, 1989). It also had many immunostimulating activities, including mitogenic activity against B lymphocytes and anticomplement activity. These effects were the result of pectic polysaccharides in TJ-48. These activities may relate closely to the clinical effects of TJ-48 (Yamada, 1994).

TJ-48 enhanced antibody and interleukin 2 (IL-2) production and promoted granulocyte-macrophage colony forming cells (GM-CFC), and anticomplement and mitogenic activities. To isolate these immunopharmacologically active substances, TJ-48 was fractionated into low– and high–molecular weight fractions. These were F1 (methanol-soluble), F2 (methanol/water-insoluble), F3 (methanol-dialysable), F4 (ethanol-soluble but nondialysable), and F5 (crude polysaccharide). Although F2 had anticomplement activity, F1 and F3 had GM-CFC–enhancing activity. The crude polysaccharide fraction (F5) enhanced antibody and IL-2 production and also showed anticomplement and mitogenic activities (Fig. 21-2) (Ikehara and others, 1992; Kiyohara and others, 1991, 1993; Yamada and others, 1990). Of the TJ-48-derived fractions, F5 displayed anti-SRBC antibody response in vivo when the polysaccharide fraction was given to Balb/c mice, either intraperitoneally or orally (Kiyohara and others, 1995a). Oral dosing of aged mice with F5, or TJ-48 from 6 days before immunization with SRBC, gave a significant increase in anti-RBSC IgG, but at a lower level than that of young mice (Kiyohara and others, 1995a). When the antineoplastic agent cisplatin was given to mice, the anti-SRBC antibody response decreased significantly (Kiyohara and others, 1995a). Both F5 and TJ-48 enhanced the anti-SRBC IgM level similarly to those of their respective oral doses in cisplatin-immunosuppressed mice on post-injection day 7 (Kiyohara and others, 1995a). Oral dosing of the other fractions (F1 and a mixture of F3 and F4) also stimulated the anti-SRBC response (Kiyohara and others, 1995a). Cisplatin inflicted toxic effects on the kidneys. As with the action of TJ-48, high values of blood urea nitrogen (BUN) induced by cisplatin treatment were reduced by dosing with either F1, a mixture of F3 and F4, or F5. Cisplatin-induced toxic effects were markedly relieved by the use of F5 (Kiyohara and others, 1995b). Still, the mechanism of action of this toxicity-attenuating effect remains unknown. The acidic polysaccharide fraction F5-2 showed anticomplement and mitogenic activities, whereas both F5-3 and F5-4 merely showed anticomplement effects. The neutral polysaccharide fraction (F5-5) enhanced both anticomplement activity and IL-2 production (Fig. 21-2). Further fractionation of the individual acidic and neutral polysaccharide fractions (F5-2, F5-5) per se by DEAE-Sephadex gave 22 different polysaccharides with varied immunostimulating activities (Kiyohara and others, 1991, 1993).

Recently, a pectic polysaccharide with free radical–scavenging activities was isolated from *Bupleuri radix* (Matsumoto and others, 1993). This compound may be

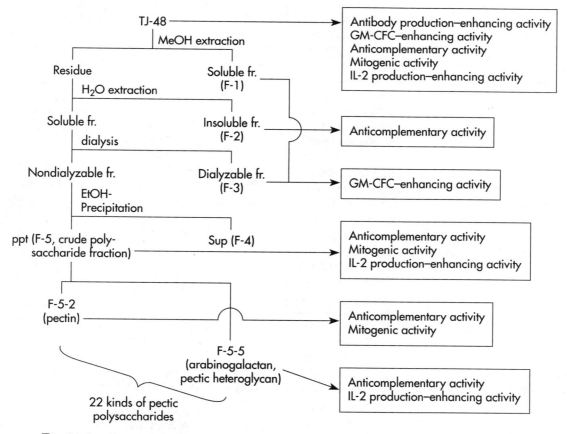

Fig. 21-2 Fractionation and in vitro immunomodulating activities of Juzen-Taiho-To (JTT) extract preparation TJ-48.

related to the antiulcer effect of the medicinal herb. This suggests that the antioxidant (free radical–scavenging) activity in cisplatin-induced toxicity may be involved in the attenuating effect of the polysaccharide fraction.

These results suggest that the immunomodulating activities of JTT are the result of a combination effect of several different pectic polysaccharides that may have different immunomodulating effects, in addition to the effects of compounds of low molecular weight. These activities may contribute to the clinical effects of JTT (Fig. 21-2).

Other aspects of phytopharmacologic research

Although extensive knowledge and cumulative experience of the clinical uses of KM have been acquired from CHM, Japanese workers have made great contributions to the scientific understanding of KM in the last two decades. Every year, hundreds of scientific papers are published. Most support the application of KM. Similarly, many hundreds of CHMs have potent therapeutic effects.

The literature on research into the mode of action of medicinal herbs documents well the low–molecular weight fractions, but the larger molecules, such as polysaccharides, have come under study only recently (Matsumoto, Yamada, 1995; Yamada, 1994b).

The Kitasato team is researching the action of pectic polysaccharides at the cellular and intracellular level. For example, recent work on Bupleurum has given valuable new findings. Bupleurum is a common Chinese herbal medicine, mainly used to treat liver disease. Recently, bupleuran 2IIb, a pectic polysaccharide isolated from *Bupleurum falcatum*, was shown to upregulate the expression of Fc-receptors (FcRs) on macrophages; this action was mediated by enhancing the transcription of both Fc-gamma RI and Fc-gamma RII genes (Matsumoto and others, 1993).

The regulation of intracellular signal transduction pathways can be determined by measuring second messengers in response to the presence of specific inhibitors. Macrophages from the peritoneal cavity of mice were used to study whether protein kinase C and A (PKC and PKA) were involved in FcR upregulation by bupleuran 2IIb. Neither the PKC inhibitor 1-(5-isoquinolinyl-sulphonyl)-2-methylpiperazine dihydrochloride nor the PKA inhibitor N-[2-(methylamino)ethyl]-5-isoquinoliny-sulphonamide dihydrochloride inhibited bupleuran 2IIb–induced upregulation of FcR. However, when macrophages were treated with Ca^{2+}-antagonist 8-(diethylamino)-octyl-3,4,5-trimethoxybenzate hydrochloride, bupleuran 2IIb-induced upregulation of FcR was inhibited in a dose-dependent manner. The two calmodulin antagonists trifluoperazine and N-(6-aminohexyl)-5-chloro-1-naphthalensulphonamide hydrochloride also blocked the action. Also, fluorescence image analysis, using the Ca-sensitive dye Fura-2, showed that bupleuran 2IIb induced a rapid increase in intracellular levels of Ca. These results suggest that bupleuran 2IIb induced the up-regulation of FcR on macrophages by a mechanism dependent on an increase in intracellular Ca^{2+}, followed by activation of the calmodulin, but not by a PKC or PKA pathway (Matsumoto, Yamada, 1995). Fig. 21-3 summarizes this hypothesis.

Herbal Medicine: Controversial Issues and Possible Solutions

Herbal medicine, as with Western medicine, has negative or unresolved as well as positive or resolved aspects, and the status will change (a law of TCM). It is possible to make the changes positive. To do this, leaders and workers in the fields of science, medicine, and national government need to recognize the disadvantages of herbal medicine and work to solve them. Some disadvantages and possible solutions follow.

The Supply of Raw Herbal Ingredients

Some important raw materials used in herbal medicine are found only in a few areas of the world and thus are in limited supply. Some animal-derived ingredients used in the East (such as monkey tissues, tiger bone, rhino or elephant horn, and antler velvet from deer) are banned in the West on grounds of unnecessary cruelty to animals or conservation of endangered species.

Some countries have specific national legislation that bans the use of certain ingredients, such as ruminant brain tissue, because of public fear of bovine spongiform encephalopathy, and tiger bone, because of conservation pol-

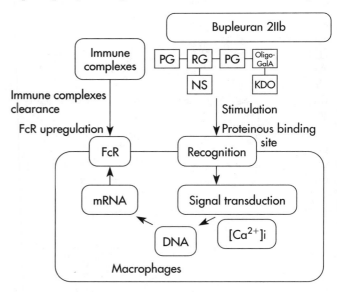

Fig. 21-3 The intracellular action of bupleuran 2IIb, a pectic polysaccharide isolated from *Bupleurum falcatum*. Bupleuran 2IIb upregulates the expression of FcRs on macrophages through an increase in intracellular Ca^{2+} and activation of the calmodulin, but not by a PKC or PKA pathway. *PG*, Polygalacturonan; *RG*, rhamnogalacturon core; *NS*, neutral sugar chain.

icy. Solutions could include guaranteed exclusion of banned ingredients from the marketplace, research into natural propagation of the rarer permitted ingredients, and in vitro production of active ingredients or suitable alternatives. This could include use of biotechnology and genetic engineering to clarify the active components or synthesize similar alternatives (Chaudhury, 1995).

It would also be useful to study substitutes for some rare or special ingredients. It is warranted now to find good substitutes for certain human tissues (for example, human placenta is used in some herbal medicines). Certain animal tissues (bone, horn, penis, testis, and ovary) from domestic animals (buffalo, cattle, deer, and pigs) might be used instead of similar tissues from rare or preserved species (tigers, primates, rhinos, and elephants). Common tissues might be used instead of rare material (for example, bovine bile instead of bovine gallstones). It would also be useful to cultivate medicinal herbs that might have actions similar to much rarer or more expensive herbs (for example, Danhseng [Codonopsis pilosula] instead of ginseng).

Quality Control

Used properly, herbal medicine is safe; if overused, however, the ingredients used in herbal medicine also are toxic. Thus great care is needed in their combinations and dosage. Quality control needs to be improved and increased (Chaudhury, 1995; Dharmananda, 1991).

The levels of active ingredients in the raw materials in herbal medicines vary with time and place of collection, the parts of the plants used, methods of processing, and other factors. For example, although the root is used, ginseng leaves contain more active compounds than the root (Dharmananda, 1991; Sun, Matsumoto, Yamada, 1992). At present, there is little or no quality control on the levels of active ingredients in the final prescriptions of many formulas. This is unacceptable to many professionals in Western medicine.

A solution would be to develop guaranteed methods and standards of quality control. Product labeling and datasheets could be made mandatory. These should state clearly the dosage, clinical indications, contraindications, side effects, emergency procedures, and/or antidotes (if known) in case of severe adverse reaction, as is the case with Western medicines.

Research is needed on the processing and purification of herbal medicines. Decoctions usually are prepared by the patient from the dried crude formulas. Patient errors may occur in the preparation and dosage of decoctions, which are bulky and hard to preserve and transport. They are also tedious to decoct properly and may be unpalatable (Yamada, 1994a). Unit doses of pills or powders, made from the dried extracts, have many advantages over decoctions. Their preparation, purification, and packaging as pill and unit doses are beneficial. Sometimes, however,

decoctions must be used. As a guide to doctors on their relative palatabilities, decocted KMs were submitted to members of a taste panel who assigned a taste-rank score to each decoction for the strength or weakness of its taste. A table of mean taste-ranks with dosage guidelines is available (Kim and others, 1995). Quality control should build on this work and see if flavoring agents or other methods of preparation could offset the more unpalatable tastes.

Registered Versus Unregistered Medicines

Many countries, such as the United States and Europe, make it difficult and expensive to register therapeutic drugs for use in humans or animals. A dossier on each formulation must list details of the type of animal, indications, dosage, contraindications, safety, toxicity studies, antidotes, labeling, levels of active ingredients, quality control procedures, shelf life, residue levels, and withholding time (in meat and milk animals). These statements must be supported by research findings, especially by independent agencies.

Herbal medicines usually are unregistered as therapeutic products in most Western countries. In the United Kingdom, at least 40 herbal medicines are freely available without prescription (Chaudhury, 1995). Use of unregistered products (or adverse interactions between registered and unregistered products) could present professionals with legal problems in the event of untoward (or adverse) effects in their patients. Most herbal medicines used in animals are based on prescriptions for humans. Research is needed on their use in animals. Application of stringent rules to the main remedies or formulas used in herbal medicine would probably make it impossible to register them. Until then, most veterinary associations would not recognize herbal medicine as a valid therapy.

It would be unrealistic to expect Western authorities and insurance companies to give a carte blanche to professionals to use anything they please as a medical therapy. However, there are possible solutions.

The governments could adopt the Japanese medical model: to endorse the use of specific herbal medicines in specific conditions by authorized professionals. It could authorize a list of herbal medicines, mainly complex formulas, whose use has been validated as to their safety and efficacy by centuries of documentation and usage (Chaudhury, 1995). The approved list could be drawn up in association with recognized experts in herbal medicine. Each state also could decide what constitutes minimal competence before licensing the professionals. Use by registered professionals of expert TCM databases (see below) could qualify in that respect.

The state could license the use and dosage of specific approved herbal medicines *in combination* with accepted (conventional) therapies. Contraindications and adverse interactions between Western medicines and the approved herbal medicines would need to be listed formally (Chaudhury, 1995).

The state also could encourage the use of specific herbal medicines as experimental unregistered health products or supplements. In that case, their use would require that the professional obtain from the client a written consent for their experimental use and an indemnity against claims for negligence or malpractice in the event of untoward reactions (Schwartz, 1994).

How to Develop Herbal Medicine Further

Western medicine is highly developed today. The prevalence of acute infectious diseases of humans and animals has fallen significantly since the discovery, development, and use of antibiotics and vaccines, and the use of improved auxiliary techniques (intensive care, fluid therapy, dialysis, and blood filtration). Also essential to this success are improved diagnostic screening techniques and overall improvement of personal and food hygiene, improved overall nutrition, housing, and control of the environment.

However, drug-resistant "superbugs," especially *Staphylococcus aureus,* are becoming prevalent. These and some chronic infectious diseases, such as AIDS, viral hepatitis, and bovine tuberculosis, are especially difficult to eradicate. Also, the prevalence of other chronic diseases, especially those related to stress, environmental pollution, and immunosuppression, seems to be increasing.

TCM is underdeveloped, mainly through lack of adequate funding for basic and clinical research and also because of lack of good information for education and training of practitioners. Even so, complementary therapies using herbal medicines are widely used in the United States and Europe and their use is growing (Micozzi, 1995; Otsuka, 1988; Yamada, 1994a). Although some regard the scientific nature of TCM as inferior to Western medicine, each system has its validity, strengths, and weaknesses. Herbal medicine will continue to grow in popularity and use as an adjunct to Western medicine. TCM has great potential to prevent and cure many chronic diseases (Dharmananda, 1991), but one cannot expect TCM to make a great impact in Western medicine without a proactive approach from both sides and greatly increased international inputs in funding for research, education, and training in TCM.

Personal effort, group effort, the activities of interested organizations, teaching and training at university level, and financial support from governments and industries are the main factors in the development of all sciences. Recent development in biotechnology has proved that. Although modern veterinary medicine in China is underdeveloped, all of these factors are present. However, most other countries lack these factors. Fortunately, the developed countries may use their modern facilities in veterinary science and their educational systems to study and develop herbal medicine. Some suggestions to help such developments are presented elsewhere (Lin, Panzer, 1994).

Easy Access to Expert Information on Herbal Medicine Is Essential

Why do practitioners prescribe the drugs that they use daily? Apart from the constraints of the availability of the products and the ability of the client to pay for them, most practitioners prescribe the best drugs or other therapies that they know for the diagnosed problems. In other words, the key factors in prescribing the "best drugs" are knowledge (especially of diagnostics and therapeutics) and belief (that the prescription will give satisfactory results). In any medical system (Western or TCM) the *knowledge* and *belief* of the practitioner are conditioned by his or her culture and limited by his or her education and by ongoing access to credible information.

With some exceptions, expert use of herbal medicine requires fast, easy access to Oriental medical theory and the ways to select the most appropriate ingredients or formulas (Otsuka, 1988). Busy Western medicine professionals who wish to learn herbal medicine must face this problem. Most are unable or unwilling to take 1 to 3 years or more out of their practice or research to study the huge amount of novel information that must be learned and assimilated. Unless professionals in Western medicine can access the data rapidly and reliably, they are unlikely to use herbal medicine, even on an experimental basis.

If it can be developed, expert TCM software could offer solutions to the knowledge problem. User-friendly, expert, interactive PC-based databases could incorporate all the key aspects of TCM, herbal medicine, the relevant herbal medicine remedies and formulas, TCM syndromes, and diagnosis. All of these could be cross-referenced to the equivalent Western medicine syndromes and medications. Novice (but professional) users could enter the clinical findings into the computer. The software could prompt the user to add other relevant data. A preliminary cross-matching of the input data with the database could activate prompts for further relevant input. The database could then display the TCM diagnosis and the indicated (and contraindicated) herbal medicines. In this way, inexperienced professionals could use herbal medicine quickly and effectively, and alter the herbal medicines by inputting changes in the syndrome or Sho. Further refinements could allow users to browse the various files for study purposes, and to enter hypothetical clinical data for self-testing purposes.

Such databases could be efficient learning aids for inexperienced professionals, as demonstrated some years ago by an expert database in Western medicine developed at Harvard Medical School. Such technology is available to professionals interested in homeopathy and certain aspects of AP, both complementary therapies that MSM professionals find difficult to master.

Chinese Herbal Medicine (Green Medicine, Version 1.1.) is a database for Apple MacIntosh and Windows PCs (Weber, 1992). This seems to be the first attempt to put TCM at the fingertips of PC users. It contains a wealth of data on clinical signs and symptoms, TCM syndromes, herbal actions, indications, CHM formulas, and dosages. However, it needs major revision to make it faster, more user-friendly, and more "intuitive."

Computers can store and recall information faster and more accurately than many humans. However, for best results, skilled humans must interpret the data; one should not rely on computers for basic medical knowledge any more than one should rely blindly on fixed herbal formulations as a cure for all ills. However, computers and formulations have one thing in common: both can help the doctor to help patients cure themselves. Also, computers can help doctors to better manage and reinforce their medical knowledge and can stimulate them to master that knowledge. However, no matter how good they are, computers cannot replace adequate medical knowledge and skill, nor can they replace compassion for and desire to heal the patient. Compassion, love, and service are at the core of healing.

Additional Research

Further pharmacologic experiments are needed to evaluate plant compounds as clinically useful medicines. Plant cell culture, chemical synthesis, or biotechnologic production methods of the compounds may be needed to obtain sufficient amounts for sampling purposes. In the chemical synthesis of medicinal compounds, structure-activity relationships should be considered to prepare compounds that are more active and safe, and that exhibit bioavailability. The search for new drugs from herbal medicines is justified because of the long-term clinical evidence of their clinical value in humans and animals. Such research proves the experimental applications of herbal medicines to be true and helps to explain their clinical effects (Dharmananda, 1991). As with Western medicines, some herbal medicines are toxic. It may be necessary to check for undesirable residues or metabolites in food products from herbal medicine-treated animals (for example, the level of plant alkaloids in milk, cheese, meat).

Future Prospects

The main aim of all good medicine is to improve the quality of human or animal life. TCM and Western medicine have this aim. Advantages of TCM are the lower costs and the absence of side effects relative to those of Western medicines. Also, most herbal medicines come from natural biologically renewable sources. Cultivation and processing of herbal medicines could be a valuable source of income for developing countries.

Development of TCM on the Internet

Western professionals who wish to learn or use complementary therapies often feel isolated. They may have few colleagues nearby with whom to exchange information. Internet bulletin boards on TCM could be developed on all aspects, including herbal medicine. The Internet, also called the electronic information superhighway, is an electronic, computer-based worldwide communication web. Via the Internet, those with sufficient money and computer-based technology can communicate almost instantly with colleagues anywhere in the world.

Herbal medicine abstracts

Occidental researchers have great difficulty accessing information written in Oriental languages and vice versa. Advances in optical scanning devices allow printed data to be scanned in ASCII text into computer files. Advances in computer software now allow articles digitized in one language to be translated into another. Via the application of existing scanning, translation, and communications technology, the Internet could radically enhance the exchange of research and clinical data on herbal medicine. Development of specialist areas on the Internet for herbal medicine research abstracts and herbal medicine clinical abstracts would accelerate its development.

Register of drug reactions

Though most states have a formal reporting system to record adverse effects of medication (or their suspicions of them), professionals may have difficulty accessing the data. Also, they may not be able to check if data that they submitted were actually recorded. Requests to commercial companies for data on adverse reactions may be futile; because of vested interest, companies may deny or play down reported iatrogenic disease. The Internet could help to solve this problem. A password-protected Register of Drug Toxicity/Iatrogenic Disease would allow validated professionals to record (against their name) adverse reactions to specified drugs (Western medicines and/or herbal medicines). The data could be read anywhere in the world by other professionals with authorized access to the Internet register.

Conclusions

Widespread research, development, and use of herbal medicine could save billions of dollars annually on the international cost of conventional drugs, hospitalization, and lost time at work.* This would force major changes in the modern (Western-oriented) pharmaceutical industry and

---

*The AIDS epidemic profoundly impacts many aspects of medicine and health care. The Public Health Service estimates that the annual cumulative lifetime cost of treating all persons with AIDS in the United States in 1991 was $5.3 billion; this was expected to reach $7.8 billion by 1993.

in agricultural production. Initially at least, this could have serious effects on investment and employment. If the major pharmaceutical industries can be persuaded to diversify slowly into herbal medicine, they could save many jobs and create new ones. New areas of work would include biologic research, breeding, refining, tending, processing, and replenishing the herbs, researching the active principles, upgrading quality control, and refining the combinations of medicines to eliminate any risk of toxicity or adverse side effects. Also, governments could reinvest their savings on drug bills into improved systems of health care for all.

TCM and herbal medicine have been used empirically over thousands of years in billions of human and animal patients, and their use is increasing. These factors are strong evidence of their overall safety and efficacy and recent research, both clinical and basic, has confirmed these claims.

In contrast to Western medicines, properly used Chinese herbal medicines can be given for long periods with minimal or no adverse effects.* Thus OM/TCM/herbal medicine shows great promise, especially for sustainable use of medicinal resources (Lin, Yamada, Rogers, 1995a).

The problems of TCM are primarily the result of lack of easily accessible information and lack of funding. Their solution needs greatly increased inputs from researchers, clinicians, relevant industries, and governments. These problems must be resolved if the advantages of both medical systems (TCM and Western medicine) are to be put to better use internationally. Resolution of the problems would lead to the dawn of a new age of medicine. That medicine, based on a combination of the best aspects of Western medicine and TCM, would be safer, less expensive, and more sustainable than is the case today.

Summary

Research, conducted worldwide, has confirmed the great potential benefits of herbal medicine, especially in chronic disorders that respond poorly, if at all, to Western medicine. Parallels and differences between these two are discussed.

TCM has well-documented laws and theories. Its laws have been proved by constant use in humans and animals over millennia; its theories have been tested in-vivo and proved or amended by constant criticism and dynamic discussion by its practitioners. TCM uses mainly Chinese herbal medicine (CHM), physical medicine (acupuncture, thermotherapy [moxibustion], and mental therapy [Qigong, meditation]). CHM is the oldest, best-documented system of medicine known. To understand CHM, one must understand the essential concepts of TCM. Its methods of diagnosis are complex and holistic. By a detailed process of pattern recognition, practitioners determine the TCM Syndrome, and the nature and location of energy *(Qi)* disorder in the subject.

Once a diagnosis is made, CHM uses formulations of 4 to 10 herbal ingredients to apply a complex theory of holistic treatment. Treatment aims mainly to obtain and maintain harmony of body function (homeostasis) and to expel pathogens. Many ingredients are used to enhance the effects of or to act as antidotes to the unwanted effects of other ingredients. The formulation may be changed as the subject's *Qi* patterns change. The history of TCM, its fundamental concepts, syndrome diagnosis, and selection and alteration of remedies are beyond the scope of this chapter. They are discussed elsewhere, primarily in Chapters 22 and 23.

A new look at herbal medicine may stimulate readers to study the subject and to apply it in routine practice. Herbal medicine is a valid science, with great potential for integration with Western medicine to the benefit of human and animal health and welfare. As the pharmacologic basis becomes better understood, it will be easier to integrate herbal medicine into conventional Western medicine. However, herbal medicine needs more research, development, goodwill, and education before it can reach its full potential. Problems of supply of raw ingredients, quality control, registration of proven formulations, and access to expert information need to be addressed urgently.

Acknowledgments

We thank Ms. A. Yamasaki for excellent clerical assistance. We thank all the cited authors, especially Drs. A. Ackerson, D. Bensky, R.R. Chaudhury, S. Dharmananda, and P.K. Tsung, whose material was reproduced in summary form. Finally, we thank the National Science Council, Republic of China, for financial support to Professor J.H. Lin (32056F), without which this article could not have been finished.

References

Abelson PH: Medicine from plants, *Science* 247:513, 1990.

Aburada M and others: Protective effects of Juzen-Taiho-To (JTT), dried decoctum of 10 Chinese herbs mixture, upon the adverse effects of mitomycin C in mice, *J Pharmacobio-Dynamics* 6:1000, 1983.

Ackerson A: Botanical antiparasitic and antimicrobial agents: traditional uses and recent research, 1995. Reprint undocumented.

Arisawa M and others: Cytotoxic and antitumour constituents in pericarps of *Mallotus japonicus, Planta Med* 56:377, 1990.

Balde AM and others: Plant antiviral agents. VII. Antiviral and antibacterial pronathocyanidins from the bark of *Pavetta owriensis, Phytother Res* 4:182, 1990.

Bay DH and others: Plants as sources of antimalarial drugs. Part 7. Activity of some species of *Meliaceae* plants and their constituent limonoids, *Phytother Res* 4:29, 1990.

Bensky D and others: *Chinese herbal medicine: materia medica,* Seattle, 1986, Eastland Press.

---

*Chan and others, 1993; Dharmananda, 1991; Hosoya, Yamamura, 1988; Hsu, 1982; Schwartz, 1994; Yamada, 1994a.

Borman S: Scientists mobilize to increase supply of anticancer drug taxol, *C and EN* Sept. 11-18, 1991.

Chan KL and others, editors: Trends in traditional medicine research, Penang, Malaysia, 1993, The School of Pharmaceutical Sciences, University of Science Malaysia.

Chaudhury RR: In Munson PL, Mueller RA, Breese GR, eds: *Principles of pharmacology: basic concepts and clinical applications*, New York, 1995, Chapman & Hall International, p 1530.

Cousins DJ: Plants with antimicrobial properties: antiviral and antibacterial properties, Vol 1, Wallingford, UK, 1995a, CAB International. (Also on floppy disk.)

Cousins DJ: Plants with antimicrobial properties: antifungal properties, Vol 2, Wallingford, UK, 1995b, CAB International. (Also on floppy disk.)

Cox PA, Balick MJ: The ethnobotanical approach to drug discovery, *Sci Am* June, 1994, p 60.

De Rodriguez DJ and others: Search for in vitro antiviral activity of a new isoflavonic glycoside from *Urex europaeus, Planta Med* 61:59, 1990.

Dharmananda S: Chinese herbal therapies for immune disorders, Portland, Ore, 1991, Institute for Traditional Medicine.

Dixon RA, Lamb CJ: Molecular communication in interactions between plants and microbial pathogens, *Ann Rev Physiol Plant Mol Biol* 41:339, 1990.

Fukuchi K and others: Inhibition of herpes simplex virus infection by tannins and related compounds, *Antiviral Res* 11:285, 1989.

Hong CY and others: The inhibitory effect of tannins on lipid peroxidation of rat heart mitochondria, *J Pharm Pharmacol* 47:134, 1995.

Hosoya E, Yamamura Y, eds: Recent advances in the pharmacology of kampo (Japanese herb) medicines, Amsterdam, 1988, Excerpta Medica.

Hsu HY, ed: Natural healing with Chinese herbs, Los Angeles, 1982, Oriental Healing Arts Institute.

Hu S and others: Ginseng-enhanced oxidative and phagocytic activities of polymorphonuclear leukocytes from bovine peripheral-blood and stripping milk, *Vet Res* 26(3):155, 1995.

Huang KC: The pharmacology of Chinese herbs, Boca Raton, Fla, 1993, CRC Press, p 388.

Ikehara S and others: Effects of medicinal plants on hemopoietic cells. In Friedman H, Klein TM, Yamaguchi H, eds: Microbial infections: role of biological response modifiers, New York, 1992, Plenum Publishing Corp, p 319.

Kawamura H and others: Accelerating effects of Japanese Kampo Medicine on recovery of murine haematopoietic stem cells after administration of mitomycin C, *Int J Immunotherapy* V:35, 1989.

Kiyohara H and others: Characterization of mitogenic pectic polysaccharides from Kampo (Japanese herbal) medicine Juzen-Taiho-To (JTT), *Planta Med* 57:254, 1991.

Kiyohara H and others: Characterization of in vitro IL-2 production enhancing and anticomplementary pectic polysaccharides from Kampo (Japanese herbal) medicine Juzen-Taiho-To (JTT), *Phytotherapy Res* 7:367, 1993.

Kiyohara H and others: Effect of oral administration of a pectic polysaccharide fraction from a Kampo Medicine "Juzen-Taiho-To" on antibody response of mice, *Planta Med* 61:429, 1995a.

Kiyohara H and others: Protective effect of oral administration of a pectic polysaccharide fraction from a Kampo Medicine "Juzen-Taiho-To" on adverse effects of cis-diaminedichloroplatinum, Abstract of 10th General Meeting of Medical and Pharmaceutical Society for Wakan-Yaku 117, 1995b.

Komatsu Y and others: Effect of Juzen-Taiho-To (JTT) on the anti-SRBC response in mice, *Jap J Inflammation* 6:405, 1986.

Labadie RP and others: An ethnopharmacognostic approach to the search for immunomodulators of plant origin, *Planta Med* 55:339, 1989.

Li L, Jiao L, Lau BH: Protective effect of gypenosides against oxidative stress in phagocytes, vascular endothelial cells and liver microsomes, *Cancer Biother* 8:263, 1993.

Lien EJ, Li WY: Structure-activity relationship analysis of Chinese anticancer drugs and related plants, Taiwan, 1985, Oriental Healing Arts Institute.

Lin JH and others: Control of preweaning diarrhoea in piglets by acupuncture and Chinese medicine, *Am J Chin Med* 16:75, 1988.

Lin JH, Panzer R: Use of Chinese herbal medicine in veterinary science: history and perspectives, *Rev Sci Tech Off Int Epiz* 13(2):425, 1994.

Lin JH, Yamada H, Rogers PAM: A sustainable veterinary medicine for the 21st century: a proposal. In Proceedings of the 25th congress of the World Veterinary Association, Yokohama, p 30 (SY 16.5) and *Jap J Vet History* 33:41, 1995.

Lin JH and others: An inhibitory effect of cantharidin on testosterone production from dispersed rat Leydig cells, *J Natural Toxins* 4:149, 1995b.

Lin JH and others: Effects of ginseng on the blood chemistry profile of dexamethasone-treated male rats, *Am J Chin Med* 23:167, 1995c.

Liu JK and others: Insect antifeeding agents: sesquiterpene alkaloids from *Celastrus angulatus, Phytochemistry* 29:2503, 1990.

Lo and others: Magnolol and honokiol isolated from *Magnolia officinalis* protect rat heart mitochondria against lipid peroxidation, *Biochem Pharmacol* 47:459, 1994.

Luo XW, Shi JZ: A Classic of TCM: English translation of Shang Han Lun, by Zhang Zhong-jing: Treatise on febrile diseases caused by cold (circa 210 AD), Beijing, 1986, New World Press, p 442.

Maruyama H and others: Effect of Juzen-Taiho-To (JTT) on phagocytes, *Jap J Inflammation* 8:461, 1988.

Matsuda H, Samukawa K, Kubo M: Anti-inflammatory activity of Ginsenoside Ro, *Planta Med* 56:19, 1990.

Matsumoto T and others: The pectic polysaccharide from *Bupleurum falcatum L* enhances immune-complexes binding to peritoneal macrophages through the receptor expression, *Int J Immunopharmacol* 16:683, 1993.

Matsumoto T, Yamada H: Regulation of immune complexes binding of macrophages by pectic polysaccharide from *Bupleurum falcatum L:* pharmacologic evidence for the requirement of intracellular calcium/calmodulin on Fc receptor up-regulation by Bupleuran 2IIb, *J Pharm Pharmacol* 47:152, 1995.

Medina JH and others: Benzodiazepine-like molecules, as well as other ligands from the brain benzodiazepine receptors, are relatively common constituents of plants, *Biochem Biophys Res Commun* 165:547, 1989.

Micozzi MS: Alternative and complementary medicine: part of human heritage, *J Alternative and Complementary Med* 1:1, 1995.

Morimitsu Y, Kawakishi S: Inhibitors of platelet aggregation from onion, *Phytochemistry* 29:3435, 1990.

Nabeya K, Ri S: *Effect of oriental medical herbs on the restoration of the human body before and after operation*, Proceedings of Symposium on Wakan-Yaku, 16:201, 1983.

Nagai T and others: Mode of action of the anti-influenza virus activity of plant flavonoid, 5,7,4'-trihydroxy-8-methoxyflavonoid from the roots of *Scutellaria baccalesis, Antiviral Res* 26:11, 1995.

Ogilvie GK, Moore AS: Managing the veterinary cancer patient: a practice manual, Trenton, NJ, 1995, Veterinary Learning Systems.

Ohnishi Y and others: Effect of Juzen-Taiho-To (JTT, TJ-48), a traditional Oriental medicine, on haematopoietic recovery from radiation injury in mice, *Exp Hematol* 18:18, 1990.

Otsuka Y: Pharmacotherapy in Oriental medicine. In Hosoya E, Yamamura Y, eds: Recent advances in the pharmacology of Kampo (Japanese herb) medicines, Amsterdam, 1988, Excerpta Medica, p xvii.

Ou M: Chinese-English manual of common-used prescriptions in TCM, Joint Publishing Co. (Hongkong) and Guangdong Science & Technology Publishing House (China), 1989.

Pan DJ and others: The cytotoxic principles of *Pseudolarix kaempferi* pseudolaric acid-A and -B and related derivatives, *Planta Med* 56:383, 1990.

Robles M and others: Recent studies on the zoopharmacognosy, pharmacology and neurotoxicity of sesquiterpene lactones, *Planta Med* 61:199, 1995.

Rogers PAM: *Xenobiosis from combustion of organic materials*, a draft review to the Veterinary Committee of the Irish Environmental Protection Agency (EPA), Dublin, 1995, p 60.

Sasaki H and others: Immunosuppressive principles of *Rehmannia glutinosa var. hueichingensis*, *Planta Med* 55:458, 1989.

Schwartz C: Chinese herbology in veterinary medicine. In Schoen AM, ed: *Veterinary acupuncture: ancient art to modern medicine*, St Louis, 1994, Mosby, p 691.

Shekhani MS and others: An immunostimulant sesquiterpene glycoside from *Sphaeranthus indicus*, *Phytochemstry* 29:2573, 1990.

Sun XB, Matsumoto T, Yamada H: Purification of anti-ulcer polysaccharide from the leaves of *Panax ginseng*, *Planta Med* 58:445, 1992.

Takemoto N and others: Mitogenic activity of Juzen-Taiho-To (JTT, TJ-48) on murine lymphoid cells, *Jap J Inflammation* 9:137, 1989.

Tripathi AK, Singh D, Jain DC: Persistency of tylophorine as an insect antifeedant against *Spilosoma obliqua walker*, *Phytother Res* 4:144, 1990.

Tsung PK: Allergy and Chinese herbal medicine, Monograph, Long Beach, Calif, 1987, Oriental Healing Arts Institute, p 39.

Unseld E, Klotz U: Benzodiazepines: are they of natural origin? *Pharmacol Res* 6:1, 1989.

Wagner H: Search for plant derived natural products with immunostimulatory activity (recent advances), *Pure Appl Chem* 62:1217, 1990.

Wang GS: Medical uses of *Mylabris* in ancient China and recent studies, *J Ethnopharmacol* 26:147, 1989.

Watanabe M and others: Novel C19-kaurane type of diterpene (Oryzalide A), a new antimicrobial compound isolated from healthy leaves of a bacterial leaf blight-resistant cultivar of rice plant, *Agric Biol Chem* 54:1103, 1990.

Weber D: Chinese herbal medicine (Green medicine, version 1.1). Database for AppleMac and Windows PCs, 1992. Cited in Redwing Reviews (June 1995), Redwing Book Company, Brookline, Mass (Fax: +1-617-738-4620; email: redwing@oa.net).

Wiseman N, Ellis A: Fundamentals of Chinese medicine (English translations and amendments of texts by the Beijing, Nanjing and Shanghai colleges of Chinese medicine), Brookline, Mass, 1995, Paradigm Publications, p 532.

World Health Organization: Research guidelines for evaluating the safety and efficacy of herbal medicines, Manila, 1993, WHO.

Xie ZF and others: Beijing Medical College: Dictionary of traditional Chinese medicine, Hong Kong, 1994, The Commercial Press.

Yamada H: Modern scientific approaches to Kampo Medicine, *Asia Pacific J Pharmacol* 9:209, 1994a.

Yamada H: Pectic polysaccharides from Chinese herbs: structure and biological activity, *Carbohydr Polymers* 25:269, 1994b.

Yamada H and others: Fractionation and characterization of mitogenic and anti-complementary active fraction from Kampo (Japanese herbal) medicine Juzen-Taiho-To (JTT), *Planta Medica* 56:386, 1990.

Yamagishi T and others: Antitumour agents, 110, Bryophillin B: a novel potent cytotoxic bufadienolide from *Bryophyllum pinnatu*, *J Nat Prod* 52:1071, 1989.

Zhang DZ: *The treatment of cancer by integrated Chinese-Western medicine*, Translated by Ting-Ling Zhang and Bob Flaws, Boulder, Colo, 1989, Blue Poppy Press, p 213.

SELECTED READINGS

Connoly D: *Traditional acupuncture: the law of the five elements*, Columbia, Md, Centre for Traditional AP.

Essentials of Chinese acupuncture, Beijing, 1993, Foreign Languages Press.

Fong HC: *Meng Jen Shou Yi Ben Cao (Ethnopharmacognostics of veterinary medicine in China)*, Beijing, 1990, Science and Technology (in Chinese).

Kaptchuk T: *The web that has no weaver*, New York, 1983, Congdon & Weed.

Kim SJ and others: A study of the taste of decocted kampo medicines, *Jap J Oriental Med* 46:21, 1995.

Lin JH, Rogers PAM: Acupuncture effects on the body's defence systems: a veterinary review, *Vet Bull* 50:633, 1980.

Lin JH, Rogers PAM: Five elements and hormone regulation, *Intl J Chin Med* 2:15, 1985.

Matsumoto K, Birch S: *Five elements and ten stems: nan jing theory, diagnostics and practice*, Brookline, Mass, 1983, Paradigm Publications.

Matsumoto T, Moriguchi R, Yamada H: Role of polymorphonuclear leucocytes and oxygen-derived free radicals in the formation of gastric lesions induced by HCl/ethanol, and a possible mechanism of protection by anti-ulcer polysaccharide, *J Pharm Pharmacol* 45:535, 1993.

Porkert M: *The essentials of Chinese diagnostics*, Zurich, 1983, Acta Med Sinensis, Chinese Medical Publications.

Yamada H: Natural products of commercial potential as medicines, *Curr Opin Biotech* 2:203, 1991.

Chapter 22

Veterinary Herbal Therapy in China

HUISHENG XIE, JIANXIN ZHU

Introduction and History of Traditional Chinese Medicine

Origin and Development

The origin of traditional Chinese veterinary medicine (TCVM) can be traced to primitive society (remote antiquity to the twenty-second century BC), when human beings began to domesticate wild animals. At that time, methods to treat or prevent animal diseases were developed. For example, from the Yangshao relics (Neolithic Age) found in Henan, many animal bones, stone knives, bone needles, and pottery were unearthed. The knives and needles may represent the original acupuncture needle, and pottery may have been used as a cupping tool. Some disorders of animals, such as dental disease and internal parasitism, were documented in the inscriptions on bones of the Shang Dynasty (sixteenth to eleventh century BC). From the Gaocheng ruins of the Shang Dynasty, found in Hebei, certain classic Chinese medicines such as bunge, cherry seed, and peach kernel were excavated (Cheng, 1991; Yu, 1987).

In the Western Zhou Dynasty (eleventh century to 476 BC), full-time veterinarians appeared. At that time, certain veterinary medical methods, such as oral administration of medications, surgery, and nursing care, had been used. More than 100 Chinese medications were documented in *Zhou Li (The Rites of the Zhou Dynasty)*. In the period of Warring States (475-221 BC), there were equine specialists known as "doctors of horses." The classic traditional Chinese medicine (TCM) textbook, *Huang Di Nei Jing (The Yellow Emperor's Classic of Internal Medicine)*, which set forth the theoretic knowledge and experiences of the ancient Chinese in their struggle against disease, was published during this period. TCVM basic principles and theories originate from this book.

The earliest herbal book, *Shen Nong Ben Cao Jing (The Shen Nong's Book of Medical Herbs)*, was published during the Han Dynasty (106 BC-220 AD). It describes 365 Chinese medical herbs for human beings and animals. During this time, Zhang Zongjing (ca. 150-219 AD) wrote *Shang Han Za Bing Lun (Treatise on Exogenous Febrile Diseases and Internal Diseases)*. He enriched and developed the accumulated knowledge of his predecessors on the determination of treatment, using the differentiation of syndromes (pattern identification).

Yuan Heng Liao Ma Ji (Yuan-Heng's Therapeutic Treatise of Horses) was published in 1608 AD. This representative work of traditional Chinese veterinary medicine was widely used in China (Yu, Yu, 1963). Li Shizhen (1518-1593 AD) wrote the renowned herbal text *Ben Cao Gang Mu (Compendium of Materia Medica)*, which describes 1,892 Chinese medicines and 11,096 formulas, including some veterinary medicines (Yu, 1987).

Educational Systems in China

Historical perspective
Box 22-1 gives a historical perspective of educational systems in China.

Institutions
Table 22-1 compares institutions of TCVM in China.

TCVM education programs
Table 22-2 outlines 4-year and 3-year TCVM programs in China.

Definitions of TCM and TCVM

TCM and TCVM are the summation of thousands of years of medical experience in the treatment and prevention of disease. TCM and TCVM each comprise five parts: theories, diagnosis, herbal medicines, acupuncture, and clinical application. The two systems are similar with regard to the basic principles of theories, diagnosis, and treatment; however, most acupuncture points and herbal formulas for animals are different from those for humans.

BOX 22-1

HISTORICAL PERSPECTIVE OF EDUCATIONAL SYSTEMS IN CHINA

Antiquity-1946: TCVM knowledge and techniques handed down from generation to generation or learned by apprentices from their masters

1947: Professional TCVM education established at Northern China University College of Agriculture, the first professional TCVM educational program in China

1958: First TCVM school, called the Training School for Traditional Chinese Veterinary Medicine, set up in Ding County, Hebei Province

1960: One-year postgraduate training in TCVM offered by the Department of Veterinary Medicine of the Beijing Agricultural University

1979: Four-year DVM program in TCVM offered at the Sichuan College of Animal Science and Veterinary Medicine

1980: Three-year master's degree program offered by Beijing Agricultural University

The most commonly used herbal medicines and formulas are introduced in this chapter.

Chinese Medicines *(Zhong-Yao)* and Veterinary Herbal Therapy

Chinese medicines, or *Zhong-yao*, are substances used to treat diseases according to the theories of Chinese medicine. Chinese medicines have three sources: plants, minerals, and animal products. For example, plantago *(Che Qian Cao)* is a plant. The Chinese medicine gypsum fibrosum *(Shi Gao)* is a mineral. Pilose antler *(Lu Rong)* is an animal product.

Because most Chinese medicines are made from plants, they are also called herbal medicines *(Cao-yao)* or Chinese herbal medicines *(Zhong-cao-yao)*. About 800 Chinese medicines are commonly used in the treatment of animal disease (Qu, 1991); however, only about 400 are introduced in the 4-year veterinary training program (Xie, 1994; Yu, 1987).

Traditional Chinese Veterinary Formulas and Herbal Formulas

Early in the history of traditional Chinese veterinary medicine, practitioners used individual Chinese medicines *(Zhong-yao)* to treat diseases. As combinations of Chinese medicines were found to be more efficient, the concept of formulas gained popularity. Traditional Chinese veterinary formulas are compositions of different quantities of several Chinese medicines. Most comprise two or more Chinese medicines. Because these formulas are composed mostly of herbs, they are also called herbal formulas. There are about 2000 veterinary herbal formulas (Yu, Zhang,

TABLE 22-1

INSTITUTIONS OF TRADITIONAL CHINESE VETERINARY MEDICINE IN CHINA

INSTITUTIONS	4-YEAR VET PROGRAM MASTER'S DEGREE 3-YEAR PROGRAM SPECIALTY	INTERNATIONAL PROGRAM	TRAINING COURSE
Beijing Agricultural University	Yes	Yes	Yes
Sichuan College of Animal Science and Veterinary Medicine	Yes	Yes	
Zhenzhou Institute of Animal Science and Veterinary Medicine	Yes		
Jilin Agricultural University	Yes		
Southern China Agricultural University	Yes	Yes	
Central China Agricultural University	Yes		
Hebei Agricultural University	Yes	Yes	
Lanzhou Institute of Traditional Chinese Veterinary Medicine	Yes		
Veterinary University of Chinese People's Liberation Army	Yes		

1992). About 200 are commonly used in the veterinary clinic (Li, 1987; Zhang, 1988).

Theory of Chinese Medicines

Effects of Chinese Medicine

The effects of Chinese medicine are described by the four Properties and the Five Tastes.

Four properties

The properties refer to the cold, hot, warm, and cool nature of different drugs. Hot and warm nature belong to *Yang,* whereas cold and cool nature belong to *Yin.*

The Four Properties were defined on the basis of the body's response to Chinese medicines. The Chinese medicines used to cure cold diseases are considered to be hot or warm natured, whereas those used to cure hot diseases are considered to be cold or cool natured (Table 22-3). For instance, a horse with symptoms such as cold ears and nose; shivering; loud peristaltic sounds; abdominal pain; watery feces; green, pale mouth; and deep, slow pulse is said to

demonstrate a Cold pattern. Hot or warm Chinese medicines—such as a aconite root *(Fu Zi),* dry ginger *(Gan Jiang),* cardamom fruit *(Sha Ren),* and magnolia bark *Hou Po)*—should be prescribed.

If a horse has high fever; polydipsia; dry feces; scanty, dark urine; rapid respiration; red tongue; and forceful, rapid pulse, it is said to be afflicted with a Heat pattern. Cold or cool medicines, such as coptis root and rhizome (Huang Lian) and scutellaria root (Huang Qin), should be used.

Five tastes

The Five Tastes are pungent, sweet, sour, bitter, and salty. Chinese medicines with different tastes have different components and therefore different actions (Table 22-4).

PUNGENT TASTE   Chinese medicines with pungent taste have diaphoretic actions related to their volatile oil components, which activate *Qi* and Blood. For instance, ephedra *(Ma Huang)* and mentha *(Bo He),* which can be used to treat an Exterior pattern due to Wind-Cold, have a pungent taste. Saussurea root *(Mu Xiang)* and carthamus *(Hong Hua),* which can be used to treat a Stagnation pattern of *Qi* and blood, also have a pungent taste.

TABLE 22-2

FOUR-YEAR AND 3-YEAR TCVM PROGRAMS AND CONVENTIONAL DVM PROGRAMS IN CHINA

COURSES	CREDIT HOURS	COURSE HOURS
TCVM 4-YEAR VETERINARY PROGRAM*		
Conventional Western veterinary medicine portion†		
TCVM portion		
TCVM Theory and Principles	5	100
Traditional Chinese Veterinary Herbology	5	120
TCVM Diagnosis	6	120
TCVM Classical Literature	3	70
Traditional Chinese Veterinary Formulas	5	100
Chinese Veterinary Acupuncture	5	100
TCVM Internal Medicine	7	140
TCVM Surgical Medicine	3	70
TCVM Clinical Practice	Six months	
THREE-YEAR MASTER'S DEGREE‡		
Advanced TCVM	4	80
Herbology Seminar	4	80
Experimental Acupuncture	3	60
Laser Veterinary Medicine	2	40
Other biologic, biochemistry, medical courses	22	440
Research		
CONVENTIONAL DVM PROGRAM		
Conventional Western veterinary medicine		
TCVM segment	6 credit hours	120 course hours

*Based on the program of the university SCASVM (Deng, 1997).
†Covers about 1200 course hours.
‡Based on Beijing Agricultural University program (Lu, 1997).

TABLE 22-3

FOUR PROPERTIES AND THEIR ACTIONS

HERB PROPERTY	CATEGORY	ACTION	EXAMPLES
Cold	Yin	Eliminates Heat and Fire, cools Blood	Coptis root (Huang Lian) Scutellaria root (Huang Qin)
Cool	Yin	Resolves toxins	Bupleurum root (Chai Hu) Mulberry leaf (Sang Ye)
Warm	Yang	Warms the Interior, disperses Cold	Ledebouriella root (Fang Feng)
Hot	Yang	Tonifies Yang Qi and activates the Channels	Dry ginger (Gan Jiang) Cinnamon bark (Rou Gui)

From Xie HS: Traditional Chinese veterinary medicine, Beijing, 1994, Beijing Agricultural University Press.

TABLE 22-4

FIVE TASTES AND THEIR ACTIONS

TASTE	CATEGORY	ACTIONS	EXAMPLES
Sour	Yin	Astringently consolidating	Schisandra fruit (Wu Wei Zi) Mume (Wu Mei)
Bitter	Yin	Eliminates heat and damp Purges intestines	Coptis root (Huang Lian) Rhubarb root (Da Huang)
Salty	Yin	Softens hardness, purges intestines	Mirabilite (Mang Xiao)
Pungent	Yang	Diaphoresis, activating Qi and Blood	Ephedra (Ma Huang) Saussurea root (Mu Xiang)
Sweet	Yang	Tonification, regulation	Ginseng (Ren Shen) Jujube (Da Zao)

From Xie HS: Traditional Chinese veterinary medicine, Beijing, 1994, Beijing Agricultural University Press.

SWEET TASTE Chinese medicines with sweet taste have tonifying effects, regulating the *Middle Jiao,* or middle burner (including spleen and stomach); and mediating effects, which are related to their sugar components. For instance, the glucose and sucrose contained in licorice may help harmonize the actions of other herbs. They are mainly used to treat Deficiency patterns and to coordinate the actions of other drugs. One example is ginseng *(Ren Shen)* and prepared rehmannia root *(Shu Di Huang),* which can tonify *Qi* and blood; these have a sweet taste. Licorice root *(Gan Cao)* and jujube *(Da Zao),* used to mediate other drugs, also have a sweet taste.

SOUR TASTE Chinese medicines with sour taste have astringent functions related to organic acid or tannic material. They are generally used to treat sweating with weakness, chronic diarrhea, and emission. For example, schisandra fruit *(Wu Wei Zi),* which can astringently consolidate and relieve sweating; and mume *(Wu Mei),* which can astringently consolidate the intestines and stop diarrhea, have a sour taste.

BITTER TASTE Chinese medicines with bitter taste eliminate Heat and Damp and purge accumulation from the intestines. These actions are related to alkaloid or glucoside components. Bitter medicines are used mainly to treat Heat patterns, constipation, and Damp patterns. For instance, rhubarb root and rhizome *(Da Huang),* which purges heat and accumulation from the intestines, and coptis root, which eliminates Heat and Damp, have a bitter taste.

SALTY TASTE Chinese medicines with salty taste have the ability to soften hardness, dispel stagnation, and purge accumulation because of their mineral components. They are mainly used to treat constipation. For example, mirabilite *(Mang Xiao),* which purges accumulation from the intestines, has a salty taste.

Coordination of Chinese Medicines

Coordination of Chinese medicines is the simultaneous application of more than two drugs to treat a disease, according to the effects of drugs and the features of the disease. Multiple Chinese medicines used simultaneously yield several results: increase of effect, decrease of effect, increase of toxin, and decrease or elimination of toxin. These results are called the "Seven Features": single action, potentiation, enhancement, antagonism, suppression, counterdrive, and incompatibility.

Single action

Single action is the use of a single Chinese medicine (not a formula) to treat a disease. For instance, licorice root *(Gan Cao)* is used alone to eliminate a poisonous disease; dandelion *(Pu Gong Ying)* is prescribed for hot swelling of the skin.

Potentiation

Potentiation is the combined use of more than two Chinese medicines, similar in effects or nature and taste, that can potentiate each other. For instance, the combined use of gypsum fibrosum *(Shi Gao)* and anemarrhena rhizome *(Zhi Mu)* can augment the elimination of Heat and Fire; the combined use of rhubarb root *(Da Huang)* and mirabilite *(Mang Xiao)* can enhance the purging of accumulation from the intestines.

Enhancement

Enhancement is the combined use of more than two Chinese medicines, one the major drug and the others adjuvant, to enhance the effect. The combined use of astragalus root *(Huang Zi)*, which tonifies *Qi* and excretes water; and poria *(Fu Ling)*, which excretes water and Dampness, can enhance the effect of tonifying *Qi* and excreting water. Scutellaria root *(Huang Qin)*, combined with rhubarb root and rhizome *(Da Huang)*, with purging—as well as the combination of akebia stem *(Mu Tong)* with diuresis—can enhance the effect of eliminating Heat and Fire.

Counterdrive

The belief that toxic or side effects of one Chinese medicine can be counteracted or eliminated by the other is called *counterdrive*. For instance, the toxic effect of fresh pinellia *(Ban Xia)* and arisaema tuber *(Tian Nan Xing)* can be ameliorated or diluted by fresh ginger *(Sheng Jiang)*. Therefore it is said that fresh pinellia and fresh arisaema tuber are subject to counterdrive by fresh ginger.

Suppression

Suppression means that one Chinese medicine decreases or eliminates the toxic or side effects of the other. Suppression is almost the same as counterdrive, but suppression is active, whereas counterdrive is passive. For instance, ledebouriela root *(Fang Feng)* suppresses the toxic effect of arenic *(Pi Shuang)*, and mung bean *(Lu Dou)* suppresses the toxic effect of croton seed (Ba Dou).

Antagonism

Antagonism refers to antagonistic actions between Chinese medicines in which one drug decreases or eliminates the curative effects of the other. For instance, scutellaria root *(Huang Qin)* can decrease the warming effect of fresh ginger *(Sheng Jiang)*, and radish seed *(Lai Fu Zi)* can decrease ginseng's *(Ren Shen)* effect of tonifying *Qi*. Antag-onism is one contraindication for the combined use of certain herbs.

Incompatibility

When the combined use of two Chinese medicines causes severe toxic or side reactions, the drugs are said to be *incompatible*. For instance, licorice root *(Gan Cao)* combined with kansui root *(Gan Sui)* will cause toxic side reactions; the combined use of Sichuan aconite root *(Wu Tou)* and pinellia *(Ban Xia)* also gives rise to side effects. Like antagonism, incompatibility is a contraindication for the combined use of some Chinese medicines.

Commonly Used Chinese Medicines

Ephedra (Ma Huang)

Source: Ephedra is from the stems and twigs of the following three plants: *Ephedra sinica Stapf.*, *Ephedra equisetina Bge.*, and *Ephedra inermedia Schrenk et Mey.* It is produced in the provinces of Shanxi, Inner Mongolia, and Hebei. Ephedra from Shanxi Province is considered the best.

Property and taste: Ephedra is pungent, mildly bitter, and warm.

Channel-tropism: Lung and bladder meridians.

Action and indication:
1. To induce perspiration and release the Exterior. Ephedra is a strong diaphoretic and is the most important Chinese medicine of pungent-warm diaphoretic nature. It is used for the Excess pattern of common cold, commonly is combination with cinnamon twig *(Gui Zhi)*. The clinical signs include aversion to cold and chill, as well as fever without sweating.
2. To disperse congestion in the lung and stop asthma. Ephedra is a good antiasthmatic. It is used for coughs and asthma, often in combination with apricot seed *(Xing Ren)*.
3. To drain water and eliminate the Excess pattern of swelling in the presence of exterior pattern, often in combination with fresh ginger *(Sheng Jiang)* and white atractylodes *(Bai Zhu)*.

Recommended dosage: Horses and cattle may be given 15 to 30 g, dogs 1.5 to 3 g, and cats 1 g.

Contraindications: Ephedra is contraindicated in patients with spontaneous sweating due to Exterior deficiency, asthma or cough due to Lung Deficiency, or swelling due to Spleen Deficiency.

Siler or Ledebouriella (Fang Feng)

Source: *Fang Feng* is the dry root of the plant *Siler divaricatum Benth. et Hook.* It is produced mainly in the Chinese provinces of Helongjiang, Jilin, Inner Mongolia, and Liaolin.

Property and taste: Siler is pungent, sweet, and mildly warm.

Channel-tropism: Bladder, Liver, and Spleen meridians.

Actions and indications:
1. To dispel Wind and release the Exterior. Siler can release the Exterior on the whole body. Its diaphoretic effect is mild. It is often used to treat Wind-Cold pattern, with a combination of Schizonepeta *(Jing Jie)* and Notopterygium *(Qiang Huo)*.
2. To eliminate Wind-Dampness and relieve pain. Ephedra is used to treat rheumatic pain in any part of the body.

Recommended dosage: Horses and cattle may be given 15 to 45 g, dogs 1.5 to 3 g, and cats 1 g.

Contraindications: Siler should not be used in the presence of a Heat pattern due to *Yin* Deficiency.

Anemarrhena Rhizome (Zhi Mu)

Source: Zhi Mu is the rhizome of the plant *Anemarrhena asphodeloides Bunge.* Its major areas of production are the Chinese provinces of Hebei, Shanxi, and Shandong.

Property and taste: *Zhi Mu* is bitter and cold.

Channel-tropism: Lung, Stomach, and Kidney meridians.

Actions and indications:
1. To eliminate the Heat in *Qi*. Zhi Mu is used for the Excess Heat pattern in acute infectious and febrile diseases.
2. To replenish *Yin* and moisten the lung. It is used for Deficiency Heat patterns, often in combination with Phellodendron bark *(Huang Bai)*.

Recommended dosage: Horses and cattle may be given 20 to 45 g, dogs 2 to 4 g, and cats 1 to 2 g.

Contraindications: *Zhi Mu* should not be used in the presence of diarrhea due to a spleen *Qi* Deficiency pattern.

Coptis root (Huang Lian)

Source: *Huang Lian* is the root and rhizome of the plants *Coptis chinensis Franch, Coptis deltoisea* CY *Cheng et* *Hsiao* and *Coptis teetoides* CY *Cheng.* It is produced in the Sichuan and Yunnan provinces of China, as well as the central and southern parts of China. Coptis root produced in the Sichuan province is considered the best.

Property and taste: Coptis root is bitter and cold.

Channel-tropism: Heart, Liver, Stomach, and Large intestine meridians.

Actions and indications:
1. To eliminate Heat and Dampness. Coptis root is a major Chinese medicine for the treatment of any Dampness-Heat pattern, especially in the intestines and stomach, such as acute enteritis, dysentery, and diarrhea. It is often combined with curcuma root *(Yu Jin)*, scutellaria root *(Huang Qin)*, and phellodendron bark *(Huang Bai)*.
2. To purge Heat and Fire. Coptis root has a strong action of purging Fire from the Heart and is used for Heart Fire Excess pattern, which can manifested as delirium, restlessness, and tongue ulcers. It is often combined with scutellaria root *(Huang Qin)*, phellodendron bark *(Huang Bai)*, and akebia stem *(Mu Tong)*.
3. To detoxify heat toxin. Coptis root is also used for local swellings on the body surface caused by Heat toxin.

Recommended dosage: Horses and cattle may be given 10 to 30 g, dogs 1 to 3 g, and cats 0.5 to 1 g.

Contraindications: Subjects with Cold Deficiency pattern or Heat Deficiency pattern should not be given coptis root.

Scutellaria root (Huang Qin)

Source: *Huang Qin* is the root of the plant *Scutellaria baicalensis Georgi.* Its major areas of production are the Hebei, Shanxi, Inner Mongolia, Henan, and Shaanxi provinces of China.

Property and taste: Scutellaria is bitter and cold.

Channel-tropism: Lung, Gallbladder, and Large Intestine meridians.

Actions and indications:
1. To eliminate Heat and Dampness. Scutellaria has the same action as coptis root.
2. To clear Heat and Fire. Because the scutellaria root has good action in clearing excessive Heat or Fire in the lung, it is used for treatment of cough due to lung Heat in combination with *Anemarrhena* rhizome *(Zhi Mu)*.

3. To comfort the fetus. Scutellaria root is often combined with white atractylodes *(Bai Zhu)* in the treatment of fetal restlessness and the prevention of abortion.

Recommended dosage: Horses and cattle may be given 15 to 45 g, dogs 2 to 4 g, and cats 1 to 2 g.

Contraindications: Scutellaria should not be used in the presence of Heat Deficiency pattern and Spleen Cold Deficiency pattern.

Lonicera flower (Jin Yin Hua)

Source: *Jin Yin Hua* is the flower-bud of the plant *Lonicera japonica Thunb.* Its major areas of production are the Henan and Shandong provinces of China.

Property and taste: Lonicera is sweet and cold.

Channel-tropism: Lung, Stomach, and Large Intestines meridians.

Actions and indications:
1. To clear Heat and resolve Heat toxin resulting from excessive Heat or Fire. When excessive Heat invades the body and accumulates in the muscles, it heats the blood. The blood gradually becomes thicker and flows more slowly, leading to stagnation of blood and then stasis of *Qi*. Stagnation of blood and *Qi* may accumulate and become secondary Heat. Both exogenous Heat and secondary Heat cause the muscles to be rotten, resulting in furuncle, skin ulcers, and pus. Because lonicera flower has strong action in eliminating Heat toxin, it is often used for the Excess pattern of skin ulcers or furuncles, which are red, swollen, hot, and painful.
2. To eliminate Wind-Heat. Lonicera flower is used in the common cold resulting from pathogenic Wind-Heat and the initial stage of febrile diseases, often in combination with forsythia fruit *(Lian Qiao)*.

Recommended dosage: Horses and cattle may be given 30 to 60 g, dogs 3 to 6 g, and cats 2 to 3 g.

Contraindication: Lonicera should not be administered to subjects with Cold Deficiency pattern.

Dioscorea Root (Huang Yao Zi)

Source: *Huang Yao Zi* is the root of the plant *Dioscorea bulbifera* L. It is produced mainly in the Hubei, Hunan, Jiangsu, Jiangxi, Shandong, and Hebei provinces of China.

Property and taste: Dioscorea is bitter and mediate.

Channel-tropism: Heart, Lung, and Spleen.

Actions and indications:
1. To clear Heat and cool blood.
2. To resolve toxin and eliminate swelling.
3. Cough due to Lung Heat, sore and swollen throat, skin ulcers and furuncles, and snakebite. Dioscorea root is a commonly used Chinese herbal medicine, especially for horses.

Recommended dosage: Horses may be given 50 to 60 g.

Stephania Root (Bai Yao Zi)

Source: *Bai Yao Zi* is the root of the plant *Stephania cepharantha Hayata.* Its major areas of production are the Chinese provinces of Jiangxi, Hunan, Hubei, Guangdong, Zhejiang, Shaanxi, and Gansu.

Property and taste: Stephania is bitter and cold.

Channel-tropism: Lung, Heart, and Spleen meridians.

Actions and indications:
1. To clear Heat and resolve toxins.
2. To cool blood and stop bleeding.
3. To dispel stagnation and eliminate swelling.
4. Like dioscorea root, stephania root is commonly administered to horses. It can be used to treat cough due to Lung Heat, sore and swollen throat, and skin ulcers and furuncles.

Recommended dosage: Horses may be given 20 to 60 g.

Rehmannia root (Sheng Di Huang *or* Sheng Di)

Source: *Sheng Di Huang,* or *Sheng Di,* is the root of the plants *Rehmannia glutinosa Libosch.* and *Rehmannia glutinosa Libosch. var. hueichingensis (Chao. et Schih.) Hsiao comb. nov.* Its major areas of production are the Henan and Hebei provinces, Inner Mongolia, and the northeastern part of China.

Property and taste: Rehmannia is sweet, bitter, and cold.

Channel-tropism: Heart, Liver, and Kidney meridians.

Actions and indications:
1. To clear Heat and cool blood. Rehmannia root is often used for the Blood Excess Heat pattern, which

is manifested as prolonged fever, restlessness, and petechial hemorrhages on the skin and mucosa. It is combined with scrophularia root *(Xuan Shen)* and rhinoceros horn *(Xi Jiao)*.
2. To nourish *Yin* and produce body fluid. The body fluid *(Yin)* is easily wasted during the course of febrile diseases (Heat). Rehmannia root is good for this situation in febrile diseases, which is manifested as thirst, dry mouth, and red tongue. It is commonly combined with ophiopogon root *(Mai Men Dong)* and glehnia root *(Sha Shen)*.

Recommended dosage: Horses and cattle may be given 20 to 45 g, dogs 2 to 4 g, and cats 1 to 2 g. Double dosage of fresh rehmannia root should be used.

Contraindications: The Spleen *Qi* Deficiency pattern and diarrhea are contraindications to the use of rehmannia.

Rhubarb root (Da Huang)

Source: *Da Huang* is the root of the plants *Rheum officinale Baill.*, *Rheum palmatum L.* and *Rheum tanguticum Maxim. ex Regel*. Its major areas of production are the Sichuan, Gansu, Qinghai, Hubei, Yunnan, and Guizhou provinces of China. The best material is from Sichuan Province.

Property and taste: Rhubarb is bitter and cold.

Channel-tropism: Spleen, Stomach, Large Intestines, Liver, and Pericardium meridians.

Actions and indications:
1. To clear Heat and purge accumulations from the stomach and intestines. Rhubarb root is a major purgative herbal medicine. It is commonly combined with mirabilite *(Mang Xiao)* and magnolia bark *(Hou Po)* for the treatment of constipation colic due to Excess Heat pattern.
2. To clear Fire and cool Blood. Rhubarb root can be used for hemorrhage due to Blood Heat pattern, often in combination with scutellaria root and coptis root.
3. To activate blood circulation and eliminate stasis. Rhubarb root can be used for Blood Stasis pattern due to falls, trauma, contusions, and strains. It is often combined with carthamus *(Hong Hua)* and persica seed *(Tao Ren)*.
4. To eliminate Dampness-Heat. Rhubarb can be combined with evergreen artemisia *(Yin Chen Hao)* and gardenia fruit *(Zhi Zi)* and used for Dampness-Heat pattern in the Liver, which includes jaundice.
5. To resolve Heat toxin. Rhubarb root can be used for burns.

Recommended dosage: Horses and cattle may be given 20 to 90 g, dogs 2 to 10 g, and cats 1 to 5 g.

Contraindication: Rhubarb should not be used in patients with no Heat pattern or with no Excess pattern or in pregnant animals.

Cinnamon bark (Rou Gui)

Source: *Rou Gui* is the bark of the plant *Cinnamomum cassia Presl.* It is mainly produced in the Guangdong, Guangxi, Yunnan, and Guizhou provinces of China.

Property and taste: Cinnamon is pungent, sweet, and very hot.

Channel-tropism: Spleen, Kidney, and Liver meridians.

Actions and indications:
1. To warm the kidney and tonify *Yang*. Cinnamon bark is often used for kidney Yang Deficiency pattern.
2. To warm the spleen and dispel Cold. Cinnamon bark is used for spleen Cold Deficiency pattern, colic due to Cold, and diarrhea due to Cold.
3. To activate blood and relieve pain. Cinnamon bark is also used in the treatment of rheumatic pain and postparturition pain.

Recommended dosage: Horses and cattle may be given 25 to 30 g, dogs 2 to 3 g, and cats 1 g.

Contraindications: Pregnant animals and patients with Excess Heat pattern should not be given cinnamon.

Atractylodes rhizome (Cang Zhu)

Source: *Cang Zhu* is the rhizome of the plants *Atractylodes lancea (Thunb.)* DC, *Atractylodes chinensis* (DC) *Koidz.*, and *Atractylodes japonica Koidz.* ex *Kitam*. Its major areas of production are the Jiangsu, Anhui, and Zhejiang provinces of China.

Property and taste: Atractylodes rhizome is pungent, bitter, and warm.

Channel-tropism: Spleen and Stomach meridians.

Actions and indications:
1. To eliminate Dampness by drying and strengthening the Spleen. Atractylodes rhizome has a strong, pungent taste, with dry and warm properties. It is commonly used for accumulation of Dampness in the spleen-stomach, manifested by loss of appetite, indigestion, diarrhea, and abdominal pain. It is commonly combined with citrus peel *(Chen Pi)* and magnolia bark *(Hou Po)*.

2. To resolve the Exterior (treat superficial symptoms) and eliminate Wind-Dampness. Atractylodes rhizome is also used for rheumatic pain.

Recommended dosage: Horses may be given 15 to 60 g, dogs 4 to 6 g, and cats 2 to 3 g.

Contraindications: Atractylodes rhizome should not be used in the presence of Heat deficiency pattern.

Citrus Peel (Chen Pi)

Source: *Chen Pi* is the dry mature peel or pericarp of the fruits of the plants *Citrus reticulata Blanco* and *Citrus tangerina Hort. et Tanaka.* It is produced in many countries all over the world.

Property and taste: Citrus peel is pungent, bitter, and warm.

Channel-tropism: Spleen and Lung meridians.

Actions and indications:
1. To regulate *Qi* and strengthen the Spleen. Because citrus peel has good function in regulating the flow of *Qi* in the Middle *Jiao* (or Middle Burner), it is used in the treatment of abdominal fullness, loss of appetite, vomiting, and diarrhea due to disorders of the Middle *Qi.* Under these conditions, citrus peel is combined with fresh ginger *(Sheng Jiang)*, white atractylodes *(Bai Zhu)*, and saussurea root *(Mu Xiang)*.
2. To dispel Dampness and resolve phlegm. Citrus peel can be used to treat coughs with profuse phlegm. It is often combined with pinellia *(Ban Xia)* and poria *(Fu Ling)*.

Recommended dosage: Horses may be given 30 to 60 g, dogs 3 to 6 g, and cats 2 to 4 g.

Contraindications: Citrus peel should not be given to patients with *Yin* Deficiency pattern, including symptoms of red, dry tongue.

Magnolia Bark (Hou Po)

Source: *Hou Po* is the dry bark of the plants *Magnolia officinalis Rehd. et Wils.* and *Magnolia biloba (Rehd. et Wils.) Cheng.* Its major production areas are the Sichuan, Yunnan, Fugian, Guizhou, and Hubei provinces of China. The best magnolia bark comes from the Sichuan province.

Property and taste: Magnolia bark is bitter, pungent, and warm.

Channel-tropism: Spleen, Stomach, and Large Intestine meridians.

Actions and indications:
1. To promote the flow of *Qi* and dry Dampness. Magnolia bark can relieve food or gas stagnation in the stomach by promoting the flow of *Qi* and can strengthen the function of the spleen by drying Dampness. Magnolia bark is therefore commonly used for abdominal distension, abdominal pain, and vomiting due to stagnation of Dampness in the Middle *Jiao* or that due to disorders of *Qi* flow. It is commonly combined with atractylodes rhizome, citrus peel, and licorice.
2. To reverse the upward flow of *Qi* and relieve asthma. Magnolia bark can be used in the treatment of cough and asthma with profuse phlegm. It is commonly combined with pinellia and perilla seed *(Su Zi)*.

Recommended dosage: Horses and cattle may be given 24 to 45 g, dogs 3 to 5 g, and cats 2 to 3 g.

Contraindication: Patients without gas or food stagnation in the stomach and intestines should not be given magnolia bark.

Lindera root (Wu Yao)

Source: *Wu Yao* is the dry root of the plant *Lindera strychnifolia (Sieb.) et Zucc. Vill.* It is produced mostly in the Zhejiang, Anhui, Hubei, Jiangsu, Guangdong, and Guangxi provinces of China. The best lindera root comes from Tian-tai, Zhejiang province, so it is called *Tian-tai Wu* or *Tai Wu.*

Property and taste: Lindera root is pungent and warm.

Channel-tropism: Spleen, Stomach, and Kidney meridians.

Actions and indications:
1. To promote the flow of *Qi* and relieve pain. Because lindera root has carminative and anodyne functions, it can be used in the treatment of cold colic and abdominal distension due to the upward flow of *Qi* and stagnation of Cold.
2. To warm the kidney and dispel Cold, lindera root is commonly used for frequent micturition due to Cold deficiency. It is combined with black cardamom seed *(Yi Zhi Ren)* and Chinese yam *(Shan Yao)*.

Recommended dosage: Horses and cattle may be given 30 to 60 g, dogs 5 to 6 g, and cats 2 to 3 g.

Contraindication: Blood Deficiency pattern and *Qi* Deficiency pattern are contraindications to the use of lindera root.

Salvia Root (Dan Shen)

Source: *Dan Shen* is the dry root and rhizome of the plant *Salvia miltiorrhiza Bunge.* It is produced mostly in the Sichuan, Anhui, and Hubei provinces of China.

Property and taste: Salvia root is bitter and cold.

Channel-tropism: Heart, Pericardium, and Liver meridians.

Actions and indications:
1. To activate blood circulation and eliminate Blood stasis. Salvia root is commonly used for any type of Stagnant Blood pattern, including retention of lochia, abdominal pain after parturition, angina pectoralis, and coronary heart disease. It is commonly combined with persica seed *(Tao Ren)*, carthamus *(Hong Hua)*, and Chinese angelica root *(Dang Gui)*.
2. To cool Blood and eliminate swelling. Salvia root can be used for skin ulcers and carbuncles.
3. To tonify Blood and calm the mind. Salvia root is also used for restlessness due to heat invasion into the Blood stage. (In TCM, a disease is divided into four stages: [1] defense, [2] *Qi*, [3] Nutrient, and [4] Blood. The Blood stage is the last stage of disease development).

Recommended dosage: Horses and cattle may be given 25 to 45 g, dogs 3 to 5 g, and cats 2 to 3 g.

Contraindication: Salvia root should not be used with *Veratrum nigrum (Li Lu)*.

Pseudoginseng (San Qi)

Source: *San Qi* is the dry root of the plant *Panax pseudoginseng Wall. var. otoginseng (Burk.). Hoo. et Tseng.* It is mainly produced in the Yunnan, Guangxi, and Jiangxi provinces of China. The best pseudoginseng comes from Yunnan province.

Property and taste: Pseudoginseng is sweet, mildly bitter, and warm.

Channel-tropism: Liver and Stomach meridians.

Actions and indications:
1. To eliminate blood stasis and stop bleeding. Pseudoginseng dispels stagnation and stops hemorrhage. It is commonly used for the treatment of all kinds of bleeding, such as hematuria, epistaxis, and hematemesis. It is also used for coronary heart disease and angina pectoralis.
2. To eliminate swelling and relieve pain, pseudoginseng is widely used for contused wounds and soft-tissue injuries.

Recommended dosage: Horses and cattle may be given 10 to 30 g, dogs 3 g, and cats 1 g.

Carthamus (Hong Hua)

Source: *Hong Hua* is the flower of the plant *Carthamus tinctorius* L. It is mainly produced in the Chinese provinces of Sichuan, Henan, Yunnan, and Hebei.

Property and taste: Carthamus is pungent and warm.

Channel-tropism: Heart and Liver meridians.

Actions and indications:
1. To activate Blood circulation and eliminate stasis. Carthamus is commonly used for any type of pain due to Blood stagnation. It is combined with persica seed, ligustocum rhizome *(Chaun Xiong)*, and Chinese angelica root.
2. To eliminate swelling and relieve pain. Carthamus can be used for soft-tissue injuries due to falls, beatings, contusions, and strains.

Recommended dosage: Horses and cattle may be given 25 to 30 g, dogs 3 to 5 g, and cats 1 to 2 g.

Contraindication: Carthamus should not be given during pregnancy.

Ginseng (Ren Shen)

Source: *Ren Shen* is the root of the plant *Panax ginseng* CA *Mey.* Its major areas of production are the Chinese provinces of Jilin, Liaoning, and Heilongjiang.

Property and taste: Ginseng is sweet, mildly bitter, and mildly warm.

Channel-tropism: Spleen, Lung, and Heart meridians.

Actions and indications:
1. To tonify *Qi* and resuscitate *Yang* collapse. Ginseng is used for prevention of Collapse pattern, including heart failure, shock, and prostration.
2. To tonify *Qi* and strengthen the spleen. Ginseng is used for Spleen *Qi* Deficiency pattern, including chronic diarrhea, indigestion, loss of appetite, and soft abdominal fullness.
3. To produce body fluid and calm the mind. Used for restlessness due to Heart Blood Deficiency pattern.

Recommended dosage: Horses and cattle may be given 9 to 21 g, dogs 2 to 3 g, and cats 1 g.

Contraindications: Patients with Excess Heat pattern should not be given ginseng, and it cannot be used with *Veratrum nigrum* or *Trogopterus* dung (*Wu Ling Zhi*).

American Ginseng (Xi Yang Shen)

Source: *Xi Yang Shen* is the root of the plant *Panax quinquefolium* L. It was originally produced in United States and Canada. It is also cultivated in China.

Property and taste: American ginseng is sweet, bitter, and cool.

Channel-tropism: Lung and Stomach meridians.

Actions and indications:
1. To replenish the stomach and produce body fluid. American ginseng has strong action in replenishing *Yin* and producing fluids, although its action of tonifing *Qi* is weaker than that of ginseng. It is commonly used for low-grade chronic fever due to *Yin* wasted by Heat in febrile diseases. It is combined with glehnia root (*Sha Shen*), dendrobium (*Shi Hu*), and trichosanthes root (*Tian Hua Fen*).
2. To tonify the Lung. American ginseng is used for treatment of chronic cough, exertional asthma, and heaves. It can be combined with glehnia root, ophiopogon root (*Mai Men Dong*), and anemarrhena rhizome.

Recommended dosage: Horses and cattle may be given 10 to 20 g, dogs 2 g, and cats 1 g.

Contraindication: Presence of the Cold Dampness pattern precludes the use of American ginseng. It cannot be fried and should not be used with *Veratrum nigrum*.

Astragalus Root (Huang Qi)

Source: *Huang Qi* is the root of the plants *Astragalus membranaceus (Fisch.) Bunge* and *Astragalus mongholicus Bunge*. It is mainly produced in the Gansu, Inner Mongolia, Shaanxi, and Hebei provinces and the northeast part of China. The best astragalus root comes from the Gansu province.

Property and taste: Astragalus root is sweet and mildly warm.

Channel-tropism: Spleen and Lung meridians.

Actions and indications:
1. To tonify *Qi* and hoist *Yang*. Astragalus root is a major Chinese medicine for tonifying *Qi*. It is commonly used for Spleen-Lung *Qi* Deficiency pattern, including symptoms of emaciation, weariness, shortness of breath, loss of appetite, diarrhea, and prolapse of the uterus or anus.
2. To consolidate the Exterior and stop perspiration. Astragalus root is commonly used for spontaneous sweating. It is combined with ledebouriella root (*Fang Feng*) and ephedra root (*Ma Huang Gen*).
3. To dispel pus and accelerate the healing of wounds. Astragalus root is used for abscesses and chronic skin ulcers. It is commonly combined with angelica (*Bai Zhi*), Chinese angelica root, and gleditsia spine (*Zhao Jiao Ci*).
4. To regulate water metabolism and reduce edema. Astragalus root is used for chronic edema due to *Qi* Deficiency pattern. It is combined with stephania root (*Fang Ji*) and white atractylodes.

Recommended dosage: Horses and cattle may be given 20 to 60 g, dogs 4 to 6 g, and cats 2 to 3 g.

Contraindication: Excess Heat pattern and Yin Deficiency pattern are contraindications to the use of astralagus root.

Chinese Angelica Root (Dang Gui *or* Tang-Kuei)

Source: *Dang Gui* is the dry root of the plant *Angelica sinensis (Oliv.) Diels*. It is mainly produced in the Chinese provinces of Gansu, Ningxia, Sichuan, Yunnan, and Shaanxi.

Property and taste: Angelica root is sweet, pungent, bitter, and warm.

Channel-tropism: Heart, Spleen, and Liver meridians.

Actions and indications:
1. To replenish and activate Blood. Chinese angelica root is used in the treatment of Blood Deficiency patterns, including anemia. It is commonly combined with prepared rehmannia root and astragalus root.
2. To eliminate stagnation and relieve pain. Chinese angelica root can be used for any type of Stagnant Blood pattern, including soft-tissue injuries due to contusions and strains, and heart disease.
3. To lubricate the intestines and purge the feces. Chinese angelica root can be used for constipation due to *Yin* Deficiency or Blood Deficiency pattern.

Recommended dosage: Horses and cattle may be given 15 to 60 g, dogs 3 to 6 g, and cats 2 to 3 g.

Contraindication: Fever due to *Yin* Deficiency is a contraindication to the use of Chinese angelica.

Black Cardamom (Yi Zhi Ren)

Source: *Yi Zhi Ren* is the fruit of the plant *Alpinia oxyphylla Miq.* It is mainly produced in the Guangdog, Yunnan, Fujian, and Guangxi provinces of China.

Property and taste: Black cardamom is pungent and warm.

Channel-tropism: Spleen and Kidney meridians.

Actions and indications:
1. Black cardamom is used to warm Kidney Yang and consolidate Kidney Essence. Black cardamom is mostly used for Kidney *Yang* Deficiency patterns, including spermatorrhea, seminal emission, and frequent micturition.
2. Black cardamom is used to warm the Spleen and stop diarrhea and salivation. Black cardamom is also used for Spleen Yang Deficiency patterns, including diarrhea, abdominal pain, and excessive salivation.

Recommended dosage: Horses and cattle may be given 15 to 45 g, dogs 3 to 5 g, and cats 1 to 2 g of black cardamom.

Contraindication: Heat Deficiency due to *Yin* Deficiency is a contraindication to the use of black cardamom.

Cornus Fruit (Shan Zhu Yu)

Source: *Shan Zhu Yu* is the seedless fruit of the plant *Cornus officinalis Sieb. et Zucc.* Its most important areas of production are the Chinese provinces of Shanxi, Shaanxi, Shandong, Anhui, Henan, Sichuan, and Guizhou.

Property and taste: Cornus fruit is sour and warm.

Channel-tropisum: Liver and Kidney meridians.

Actions and indications:
1. To tonify the Kidney Essence and Liver *Yin.* Cornus fruit is commonly used for treatment of Kidney-Liver Deficiency patterns, including posterior paresis, impotence, premature ejaculation, and frequent micturition. It is combined with prepared rehmannia root, dodder seed *(Tu Si Zi),* and eucommia bark *(Du Zhong).*
2. To astringently consolidate collapse and stop sweating. (When Kidney *Qi* is very weak, it will become exhausted or collapse, followed by spontaneous sweating.) Cornus fruit is used for spontaneous or nocturnal sweating.

Recommended dosage: Horses may be given 30 to 60 g, dogs 3 to 6 g, and cats 2 to 4 g.

Commonly Used Herbal Formulas

Bu Zhong Yi Qi Tang *(Tonifying Spleen-Stomach Decoction)* (Xie, 1994)

Constituents:

Baked astragalus root	75 g *Astragalus membranaceus (Fisch) Bge*	*Huang Qi*
Ginseng	50 g *Panax ginseng C. A. Mey*	*Ren Shen*
White atractylodes	50 g *Atractylodes macrocephala Koidz*	*Bai Zhu*
Chinese angelica root	50 g *Angelica sinensis (Oliv) Diels*	*Dang Gui*
Baked licorice root	25 g *Glycyrrhiza uralensis Fisch*	*Gan Cao*
Citrus peel	30 g *Citrus reticulata Blanco*	*Chen Pi*
Cimicifuga rhizome	15 g *Cimicifuga foetida L*	*Sheng Ma*
Bupleurum root	15 g *Bupleurum chinense DC*	*Chai Hu*

Action: To tonify the Spleen and Stomach, to uplift the *Yang,* and to replenish the *Qi.*

Indication: Qi Deficiency of the Spleen and Stomach with descending disorders of the *Qi* of Zhong-Jiao (Middle Burner). The symptoms are weariness, mental dullness, emaciation, weakening in the limbs, tendency to lie down, reluctance to move, spontaneous sweating, long-standing diarrhea, and prolapse of anus or rectum or uterus.

Application: Long-standing diarrhea or dysentery, rectal or uterine prolapse, spontaneous sweating, weariness.

Usage: Decoction.

Gui Pi Tang *(Strengthening Spleen Decoction)* (Xie, 1994)

Constituents:

Ginseng	60 g *Panax ginseng CA Mey.*	*Ren Shen*
Astragalus root	60 g *Astragalus membranaceus (Fisch)*	*Bge Huang Qi*
Chinese angelica root	50 g *Angelica sinensis (Oliv.) Diels*	*Dang Gui*
Longan aril	50 g *Euphoria longan (Lour.) Steud*	*Long Yan Rou*
White atractylodes	45 g *Atractylodes macrocephala Kodz*	*Bai Zhu*

Saussurea root	25 g *Saussurea lappa Clarke*	*Mu Xiang*
Poria	50 g *Poria cocos (Schw.) Wolf.*	*Fu Ling*
Polygala root	50 g *Polygala tenuifolia Willd*	*Yuan Zhi*
Baked licorice root	25 g *Glycyrrhiza uralensis Fisch.*	*Zhi Gan Cao*
Jujube	15 dates *Ziziphus jujuba Mill. var. inermis (Bge.) Rehd.*	*Da Zao*
Wild jujube	50 g *Ziziphus jujuba Mill. var. spinosa*	*Hu Suan Zao Ren*
Fresh ginger	30 g *Zingiber officinale Rosc.*	*Sheng Jiang*

Action: To tonify *Qi* and Blood, and to strengthen the Spleen and Heart

Indication: Deficiency of *Qi* and Blood due to deficiency of the Spleen and Heart *Qi*. The symptoms are weariness, loss of appetite, bloody feces, bloody urine, pale tongue, and weak and thready pulse.

Application: Anemia, chronic hemorrhage of gastrointestinal tract or uterus.

Usage: Decoction.

Gui Xing San *(Cinnamon Powder)* (Xie, 1994)

Constituents:

Cinnamon bark	20 g *Cinnamum cassia Presl.*	*Rou Gui*
Dry ginger	25 g *Zingiber officinale Rosc.*	*Gan Jiang*
Black cardamon seed	20 g *Alpinia oxyphulla Miq.*	*Yi Zhi Ren*
Cardamon fruit	20 g *Amomum villosum Lour.*	*Sha Ren*
Nutmeg	20 g *Myristica fragrans Hourr.*	*Rou Dou Kou*
Green tangerine peel	20 g *Citrus reticulata Blanco*	*Qing Pi*
Citrus peel	25 g *Citrus reticulata Blanco*	*Chen Pi*
Magnolia bark	20 g *Magnolia officinalis Rehd et wils*	*Hou Po*
Chinese angelica root	20 g *Angelica sinensis (Oliv.) Diels*	*Dang Gui*
Schisandra fruit	15 g *Schisandra chinensis Baill.*	*Wu Wei Zi*
White atractylodes	25 g *Atractylodes macrocephala Kodz.*	*Bai Zhu*
Licorice root	15 g *Glycyrrhize uralensis Fisch.*	*Gan Cao*

Action: To warm the Spleen and Stomach and eliminate Cold; to regulate the *Qi* and activate the Blood.

Indication: Cold Pattern of Spleen and Stomach. The symptoms are cold nose and chilly ears, profuse watery saliva, loss of appetite, diarrhea, colic, pale red tongue, and deep pulse.

Application: Loss of appetite, diarrhea, or colic due to pathogenic Cold.

Usage: Decoction.

Huang Lian Jie Du Tang *(Coptis Detoxifying Decoction)* (Xie, 1994)

Constituents:

Coptis root	45 g *Coptis chinensis Franch*	*Huang Lian*
Scutellaria root	45 g *Scutellaria baicalensis Georgi*	*Huang Qin*
Philodendron bark	45 g *Phellodedron amurense Rupr.*	*Huang Bai*
Gardenia fruit	60 g *Gardenia jasminoides Ellis.*	*Zhi Zi*

Action: To dispel Heat and Toxin from all three Burners.

Indication:
Excess Heat Pattern in all three Burners. The symptoms are high temperature; delirium; boils, maculae, sores, or swelling on the skin; dry, dark red tongue; yellow coating; forceful and rapid pulse.

Application: Septicemia, dysentery, pneumonia, any kind of inflammatory disease belonging to the Excess Heat pattern.

Contraindication: Yin Deficiency pattern due to excessive Heat.

Usage: Decoction.

Ju Pi San *(Tangerine Peel Powder)* (Xie, 1994)

Constituents:

Citrus peel	30 g *Citrus reticulata blanco*	*Chen Pi*
Green tangerine peel	30 g *Citrus reticulata Blanco*	*Qing Pi*
Magnolia bark	25 g *Magnolia officinalis rehd. et wills*	*Hou Po*
Chinese angelica root	25 g *Angelica sinensis (Oliv.) Diels*	*Dang gui*
Areca seed	25 g *Areca catechu L.*	*Bing Lang*

Cinnamon bark	20 g *Cinnamomum cassia Presl.*	Rou Gui
Asarum herb	15 g *Asarum sieboldi Miq.*	Xi Xin
Fennel fruit	25 g *Poeniculum vulgare Mill*	Hui Xiang
Angelica	20 g *Angelica dahurica (Fisch. ex Hoffm.) Benth. et Hook. f.*	Bai Zhi

Action: To regulate the flow of *Qi* and to eliminate Cold and stop pain.

Indication: Ju Pi San is used to treat enterospasm or colic due to drinking cold water. The symptoms are head-turning to observe the abdomen, alternate standing up and lying down, loud peristaltic sounds, pale blue-green tongue, and deep pulse.

Application: Enterospasm, colic.

Usage: Decoction or powder.

Liu Wei Di Huang Wan (Six-Ingredients-with-Rehmannia Pill) (Xie, 1994)

Constituents:

Rehmannia root	80 g *Rehmannia glutinosa Libosch*	Shu Di Huang
Cornus fruit	40 g *Cornus officinalis Sieb et Zucc*	Shan Zhu Yu
Chinese yam	40 g *Dioscorea opposita Thunb.*	Shan Yao
Alisma tuber	30 g *Alisma plantago-aquatica* L *var. orientala*	Sam Ze Xie
Moutan bark	30 g *Paeonia suffruticosa Andr*	Mu Dan Pi
Poria	30 g *Poria cocos (Schw.) Wolf*	Fu Ling

Action: Liu Wei Di Huang Wan is used to tonify *Yin* of Kidney and Liver.

Indication: Yin Deficiency of the Kidney and Liver. The symptoms are weariness; emaciation; low-grade tidal fever or fever just during afternoon; night sweats; dry feces; reduced urine quantity; red, dry tongue; and thready, rapid pulse.

Application: Chronic nephritis, pulmonary tuberculosis, hyperthyroidism, and other chronic diseases that are manifested as a Deficiency Pattern of the Kidney and Liver.

Usage: Pills or decoction.

Ma Huang Tang (Ephedra Decoction) (Xie, 1994)

Constituents:

Ephedra	45 g *Ephedra sinica stapf*	Ma Huang
Cinnamon twig	45 g *Cinnamomum Cassia Presl*	Gui Zhi
Apricot seed	60 g *Prunus armeniaca* L.	Xing Ren
Baked licorice	20 g *Glycyrrhiza uralensis Fish.*	Gan Cao

Action: To induce perspiration and dispel Wind-Cold, mobilize Lung Qi, and stop asthma.

Indication: Exterior Excess Pattern due to pathogenic Wind and Cold. The symptoms are intolerance of cold, fever, weariness, no perspiration but cough and asthma, thin white coating on tongue, and tight floating pulse.

Contraindication: Common cold due to pathogenic Wind and Heat.

Usage: Decoction or powder mixed with boiling water (infusion).

Qing Fei San (Lung-Clearing Powder) (Xie, 1994)

Constituents:

Isatis root	90 g *Isatis tinctoria* L	Ban Lan Gen
Lepidium seed	60 g *Lepidium apetalum Willd.*	Ting Li Zi
Fritillary bulb	30 g *Fritillary cirrhosa* D.	Bei Mu
Platycodon	30 g *Platycodon grandiflorum (Jacq.)* A DC	Jie Geng
Licorice root	25 g *Glycyrrhiza uralensis Fisch.*	Gan Cao

Action: To eliminate Heat from the Lung, and to stop asthma and cough.

Indication: Cough and asthma due to Heat in the Lung. The symptoms are rapid respiration, dyspnea, asthma, cough, warm gas exhaled from the Lung, red tongue and mouth, and forceful and rapid pulse.

Application: Pneumonia, bronchitis, asthma, cough.

Contraindication: Lung deficiency.

Usage: Decoction or powder.

Qu Mai San (Leaven-Barley powder) (Xie, 1994)

Constituents:

| Medicated leaven | 60 g *Massa fermentata medicinalis* | Shen Qu |

Germinated barley	45 g	*Hordeum vulgare* L	*Mai Ya*
Hawthorn fruit	45 g	*Crataegus pinnatifida Bge. var. Major N.E. Br.*	*Shan Zha*
Green tangerine peel	30 g	*Citrus reticulata Blanco*	*Qing Pi*
Magnolia bark	30 g	*Magnolia officinalis Rehd. et Wils*	*Hou Po*
Bitter orange	30 g	*Citrus aurantium* L	*Zhi Qiao*
Radish seed	20 g	*Raphanus sativus* L	*Lai Fu Zi*
Citrus peel	30 g	*Citrus reticulata Blanco*	*Chen Pi*
Atractykodes rhizome	30 g	*Atractylodes lancea (Thunb) DC*	*Cang Zhu*
Licorice root	15 g	*Glycyrrhiza uralensis Fisch*	*Gan Cao*
Lard	60 g		*Zhu You*

Action: To promote digestion and relieve stasis; to strengthen Spleen and enhance appetite.

Indication: Indigestion due to overfeeding. The symptoms are weariness, semiclosed eyes and lowered head, stiff movement, loss of appetite, red tongue with thick coating, and forceful pulse.

Application: Indigestion due to overfeeding.

Usage: Decoction.

Si Jun Zi Tang *(Four-Gentlemen Decoction)* (Xie, 1994)

Constituents:

Ginseng	60 g	*Panax ginseng* CA Mey.	*Ren Shen*
White atractylodes	45 g	*Atractylodes macrocephala Koidz*	*Bai Zhu*
Poria	45 g	*Poria cocos (Schw.) Wolf*	*Fu Ling*
Licorice root	15 g	*Glycyrrhiza uralensis Fisch*	*Gan Cao*

Action: To tonify the *Qi* and strengthen the Spleen and Stomach.

Indication: *Qi* deficiency pattern of the Spleen and Stomach. The symptoms are weariness, lowered head, dry hair, emaciation, muscle weakness in limbs, tendency to lie down, reluctance to move, loss of appetite, diarrhea, light color of mouth or tongue, thin coating, and weak pulse.

Application: Chronic gastritis or other chronic gastric problems that belong to the *Qi* Deficiency Pattern of the Spleen and Stomach.

Usage: Decoction.

Si Wu Tang *(Four-Ingredient Decoction)* (Xie, 1994)

Constituents:

Prepared rehmannia root	75 g	*Rehmannia glutiosa Libosch*	*Shu Di Huang*
Chinese angelica root	50 g	*Angelica sinensis (Oliv.) Diels*	*Dang Gui*
White peony root	50 g	*Paeonia albiflora Pallas* var. *trichocarpa Bunge*	*Bai Shao Yao*
Ligusticum	30 g	*Ligustucum wallichii Franch.*	*Chuan Xiong*

Action: To tonify or replenish Blood and to regulate the flow of Blood.

Indication: Deficiency or stagnation of Blood. The symptoms are abdominal pain due to stagnation of Blood, especially after parturition, anemia, pale tongue or mouth, and thready weak pulse.

Application: Anemia, various types of Blood loss.

Usage: Decoction.

Wu Shi Wan *(No-Failure Pill)* (Xie, 1994)

Constituents:

Rhubarb root	60 g	*Rheum palmatum* L	*Da Huang*
Mirabilite	120 g	Sodium sulfate	*Mang Xiao*
Pharbitis seed	60 g	*Pharbitis nil* (L) *Choisy*	*Qian Niu Zi*
Areca seed	20 g	*Areca catechu* L	*Bing Lang*
Saussurea root	20 g	*Saussurea lappa Clarke*	*Mu Xiang*
Green tangerine peel	25 g	*Citrus reticulata Blanco.*	*Qing Pi*
Bureed tuber	30 g	*Sparganium stoloniferum Buch-Ham*	*San Leng*
Rush-cherry seed	30 g	*Prumus japonica Thunb.*	*Yu Li Ren*
Akebia stem	15 g	*Akebia trifoliata (Thunb.) Koidz. var. australis (Diels) Kehd.*	*Mu Tong*

Action: To purge Heat and keep bowels open; to regulate *Qi* and eliminate stagnation in the intestines.

Indication: Constipation, intestinal obstruction. The symptoms are dry feces and then inability to discharge feces, constipation, colic, repeated standing up and lying down, abdominal fullness or bloating, deep red tongue and mouth, and deep pulse.

Application: Constipation, obstruction or retention in the gastrointestinal tract.

Usage: (1) Powder: taken with boiled water. (2) Pills: drugs ground into powder and then mixed with honey and made into round masses. When used, a pill is dissolved in 1000 ml warm white wine, and augmented with pounded allium bulb (*Allium fistulosum* L *Cong Bai*).

Xi Xin San *(Heart-Clearing Powder)* (Xie, 1994)

Constituents:

Philodendron bark	30 g *Phellodendron amurense Rupr.*	*Huang Bai*
Scutellaria root	30 g *Scutellaria baicalensis Georgi.*	*Huang Qin*
Gardenia fruit	30 g *Gardenia jasminoides Ellis*	*Zhi Zi*
Coptis root	20 g *Coptis chiensis Franch*	*Huang Lian*
Trichosanthes root	30 g *Trichosanthes kirilowii Maxim*	*Tian Hua Fen*
Forsythia fruit	30 g *Forsythia suspensa (Thunb.) Vahl*	*Lian Qiao*
Arctium fruit	45 g *Arctium lappa* L	*Niu Bang Zi*
Platycodon root	25 g *Platycodon grandiflorum (Jacq.) A DC*	*Jie Geng*
Angelica	15 g *Angelica dahurica (Fisch. ex Hoffm.) Benth. et Hook. f.*	*Bai Zi*
Akebia stem	20 g *Akebia trifoliata (Thunb.) Koidz. var. australis (Diels) Rehd.*	*Mu Tong*
Poria	25 g *Poria cocos (Schw.) Wolf*	*Fu Shen*

Action: To eliminate Heat and Toxin from the Heart; to remove stagnation and eliminate swelling.

Indication: Heat in the Heart. The symptoms are tongue ulcer and swollen, restlessness, rapid respiration, reduced urine quantity, salivation (?), difficulty eating, red tongue and mouth, rapid forceful pulse.

Application: Stomatitis, glossitis, tongue ulcer or sore.

Usage: Powder or decoction.

Xiao Chai Hu Tang *(Minor Bupleurum Decoction)* (Xie, 1994)

Constituents:

Bupleurum root	60 g *Bupleurum chinense* DC	*Chai Hu*
Scutellaria root	45 g *Scutellaria baicalensis Georgi*	*Huang Qin*
Ginseng	45 g *Panax ginseng* CA Mey.	*Ren Shen*
Pinellia	45 g *Pinellia ternata (Thunb.) Breit.*	*Ban Xia*
Jujube	20 dates *Ziziphus jujuba Mill. var. inermis (Bge.) Rehd.*	*Da Zao*
Fresh ginger	45 g *Zingiber officinale Rosc.*	*Sheng Jiang*
Licorice root	30 g *Glycyrrhiza uralensis fisch*	*Gan Cao*

Action: To mediate the Shao-Yang (Minor *Yang*) Channel, to treat febrile diseases neither in the Exterior (superficial) nor in the Interior.

Indication: Shao-Yang Channel pattern, which runs between the Exterior and the Interior of the body. The symptoms are alternating fever and chills, weariness, loss of appetite, thin white tongue coating, wiry pulse.

Application: Indigestion caused by prolonged fever, jaundice, malaria.

Usage: Decoction.

Xue Fu Zhu Yu Tang *(Dispersing-Stagnation-in-Chest Decoction)* (Xie, 1994)

Constituents:

Chinese angelica root	45 g *Angelica sinensis (Oliv) Diels*	*Dang Gui*
Ligusticum rhizome	20 g *Ligusticum wallichii Franch*	*Chuan Xiong*
Red peony root	30 g *Paeonia lactiflor Pall*	*Chi Shao Yao*
Persica seed	60 g *Prunus persica (L) Batsh*	*Tao Ren*
Carthamus	40 g *Carthamus tinctorius* L	*Hong Hua*
Achyranthes root	45 g *Achyranthes bidentata Blume*	*Niu Xi*
Fresh rehmannia root	45 g *Rehmannia glutinosa Libosch*	*Sheng Di Huang*
Bitter orange	30 g *Citrus aurantium* L	*Zhi Qiao*
Platycodon root	20 g *Platycodon grandiflorum (Jacq.)* ADC	*Jie Geng*
Bupleurum root	20 g *Bupleurum Chinese* DC	*Chai Hu*
Licorice root	15 g *Glycyrrhiza uralensis Fisch*	*Gan Cao*

Action: To activate the Blood and disperse stagnation; to promote the flow of *Qi* and stop pain.

Indication: Stagnation of Blood in the chest or head. The symptoms are chronic pain in the chest, lameness, dark red tongue with stagnant spots, irregular and tight pulse.

Application: Heart diseases due to Blood stasis, pleuritis, external injury in the chest.

Usage: Decoction.

Yin Qiao San *(Lonicera-Forsythia Powder)* (Xie, 1994)

Constituents:

Lonicera flower	45 g *Lonicera japonica Thunb.*	*Jin Yin Hua*
Forsythia	45 g *Forsythia suspensa Thunb. vahl.*	*Lian Qiao*
Mentha	30 g *Mentha haplocalvx Briq.*	*Bo He*
Schizonepeta spike	25 g *Schizonepeta tenuifolia Briq.*	*Jing Jie Sui*
Prepared soybean	30 g *Glycine Max (L) Merr.*	*Dan Dou Chi*
Arctium fruit	30 g *Arctium Lappa L*	*Niu Bang Zi*
Platycodon root	25 g *Platycodon grandiflorum (Jacq.) A DC*	*Jie Geng*
Henon bamboo leaf	20 g *Phyllostachys nigra var henonis*	*Dan Zhu Ye*
Phragmites rhizome	60 g *Phragmites communis (L) Trin.*	*Lu Gen Gan Cao*

Action: To relieve the Exterior and dispel Wind-Heat; to eliminate Interior Heat and detoxify.

Indication: Common cold caused by pathogenic Wind-Heat, the initial stage of febrile disease caused by pathogenic Wind-Warm factors. The symptoms are fever, slight intolerance of wind and cold, tendency to drink more water, weariness, cough, slight sweat or no perspiration, thin white or yellow coating, red tongue, floating rapid pulse.

Application: Influenza, acute laryngopharyngitis, acute bronchitis pneumonitis, and the initial stages of other febrile diseases, acute tonsillitis, epidemic encephalitis B.

Contraindication: Common cold due to pathogenic Wind-Cold.

Usage: Decoction.

Yu Jin San *(Curcuma Powder)* (Xie, 1994)

Constituents:

Curcuma root	45 g *Curcuma aromatica Salisb.*	*Yu Jin*
Coptis root	30 g *Coptis chinensis Franch*	*Huang Lian*
Philodendron bark	35 g *Phellodendron amurense Rupr.*	*Huang Bai*
Scutellaria root	30 g *Scutellaria baicalensis Georgi.*	*Huang Qin*
Gardenia fruit	30 g *Gardenia jasminoides Ellis*	*Zhi Zi*
White peony root	30 g *Paeonia lactiflora Pall.*	*Bai Shao Yao*
Rhubarb root	45 g *Rheum palmatum L*	*Da Huang*
Terminalia fruit	30 g *Terminalia chebula Retz.*	*He Zi*

Action: To dispel Heat and Toxin from the intestines; to restrain intestines and stop diarrhea.

Indication: Heat accumulated in the intestines. The symptoms are diarrhea; watery, foul-smelling, bloody feces; thirst; yellow coating; red tongue and mouth; and rapid pulse.

Application: Acute gastroenteritis, acute enteritis, dysentery.

Usage: Decoction.

Clinical Application of Herbal Medicines in Horses

STOMATITIS

Stomatitis refers to generalized inflammation of the mouth, which may include the gums (gingivitis), lips (cheilitis), and tongue (glossitis). In TCVM, stomatitis is divided into three types: Mouth Trauma, Up-Flaring of Heart-Fire, and Suffocating of Stomach-Fire.

Mouth Trauma

Main manifestations: Reluctance to eat, painful mastication, food dropping and profuse salivation, slightly warm oral cavity, redness and swelling, mucosal ulceration, or evidence of sharp foreign bodies in the tongue or mouth. Mouth trauma is an Excess Heat pattern.

Treatment principles: To eliminate Heat and resolve swelling; to extract the foreign body, when appropriate.

Treatment:
1. Thorough cleansing of the oral cavity.
2. External application of herbal formula: *Bing Peng San* (Borneol-Borax powder).

Constituents of *Bing Peng San*:

Borneol	(Bing Pian)	30 g
Borax	(Peng Sha)	500 g
Cinnabar	(Zhu Sha)	60 g
Dehydrated mirabilite	(Xuan Ming Fen)	500 g

Usage: The ingredients are ground into fine powder, mixed, and kept in a bottle. This recipe can cover many dosages for thousands of cases. Blow or smear the powdered medicines on the affected areas.

Up-Flaring of Heart-Heat

Main manifestations: Depression; fever; thirst; swollen or necrotic tongue; oral ulceration; thick, malodorous salivation; rapid respiration; dry feces; scanty, dark urine; deep red mouth or tongue; and surging, rapid pulse. It belongs to the Heart Excess Heat pattern.

Treatment principles: To clear Heart Fire and toxin; to dissipate stagnation and swelling.

Treatment:
1. Thorough cleansing of the oral cavity.
2. External application of herbal formula: *Bing Peng San* (see "Mouth Trauma").
3. Internal therapy: *Xi Xin San* (Heart-Clearing Powder) (see "Commonly Used Herbal Formulas"). It is given orally.

Suffocating of Stomach Heat

Main manifestations: Loss of appetite; thick salivation or foam from the mouth, with foul smell and slight warmth; swollen or rotten gum and hard palate, or lips and medial cheek; tongue ulcer; red mouth and tongue; thick yellow coating; and surging, rapid pulse. It belongs to Stomach Excess Heat pattern.

Treatment principles: To clear Stomach fire; to dissipate swelling.

Treatment:
1. Cleansing of the oral cavity.
2. External application of *Bing Peng San* (see "Mouth Trauma").
3. Internal therapy: *Shi Gao Zhi Mu Tang* (Gypsum-Anemarrhena Decoction).

Constituents:

Gypsum fibrosum	(Shi Gao)	250 g (cook first)
Anemarrhena rhizome	(Zhi Mu)	60 g
Mentha	(Bo He)	30 g
Isatis root	(Ban Lan Gen)	30 g
Gardenia fruit	(Zhi Zi)	30 g
Honeysuckle flower	(Jin Yin Hua)	30 g

Forsythia fruit	(Lian Qiao)	30 g
Rhubarb root	(Da Huang)	30 g
Licorice root	(Gan Cao)	30 g

Usage: The ingredients are cooked together and made into a soup extract. The extract is given orally.

PHARYNGITIS

Pharyngitis is inflammatory lesions of the mucosa and submucosal tissues of the pharynx and tonsils. In TCVM, it belongs to the Excess Heat pattern.

Treatment principles: To eliminate Heat and Toxin; to resolve swelling and clear the pharynx.

Herbal treatment: Internal therapy: *Xiao Huang San* (Dissipating Huang pattern Powder).

Constituents:

Anemarrhena rhizome	(Zhi Mu)	30 g
Fritillary bulb	(Bei Mu)	30 g
Coptis root	(Huang Lian)	30 g
Gardenis fruit	(Zhi Zi)	30 g
Scutellaria root	(Huang Qin)	30 g
Forsythia fruit	(Lian Qiao)	30 g
Rhubarb root	(Da Huang)	30 g
Mirabilite	(Mang Xiao)	90 g
Dioscorea stem	(Huang Yao Zi)	20 g
Stephania root	(Bai Yao Zi)	20 g
Curcuma root	(Yu Jin)	30 g
Licorice root	(Gao Cao)	20 g

Usage: Decoction given orally. External therapy: *Bing Peng San* (Borneol-Borax powder no. 108) (See "Stomatitis"). The powdered medicine is blown into the affected area.

GASTROINTESTINAL CATARRH

Gastrointestinal catarrh denotes inflammation of the gastrointestinal mucosa. In TCVM, it belongs to anorexia or diarrhea. It includes six types: anorexia due to Stomach Cold, anorexia due to Stomach Heat, anorexia due to overfeeding, anorexia due to Spleen Deficiency, diarrhea due to Intestinal Cold, and diarrhea due to Spleen Deficiency.

Anorexia Due to Stomach Cold

Main manifestations: Loss of appetite; cold limbs and trunk; clear salivation; coarse or watery feces; too much fluid in the mouth; pale or greenish-yellow mouth and tongue; thin, white coating of the tongue; deep, slow pulse. Anorexia due to stomach cold belongs to the Stomach Cold pattern.

Treatment principles: To warm the Middle Burner and disperse Cold; to strengthen the Spleen and Stomach.

Herbal treatment: *Gui Xing San* (Cinnamon Powder) (see "Commonly Used Herbal Formulas").

Anorexia Due to Stomach Heat

Main manifestations: Depression; lowered ears or head; partial or complete anorexia; dry feces; scanty, dark urine; bright red tongue and mouth with dryness and bad smell; thick yellow tongue coating; and surging, rapid pulse. It belongs to the Stomach Heat pattern.

Treatment principles: To clear Stomach Fire; to nourish *Yin* and moisten Dryness.

Herbal treatment: *Qin Lian Shi Gao Tang* (Scutellaria-Coptis-Gypsum Decoction).

Constituents:

Scutellaria root	(Huang Qin)	30 g
Coptis root	(Huang Lian)	30 g
Gypsum fibrosum	(Shi Gao)	30 g
Anemarrhena rhizome	(Zhi Mu)	30 g
Trichosanthes root	(Tian Hua Fen)	20 g
Forsythia fruit	(Lian Qiao)	20 g
Rhubarb root	(Da Huang)	20 g
Citrus peel	(Chen Pi)	20 g
Medicated leaven	(Shen Qu)	20 g
Licorice root	(Gan Cao)	15 g
Polygonatum rhizome	(Yu Zhu)	20 g
Scrophularia root	(Xuan Shen)	20 g
Ophiopogon root	(Mai Men Dong)	20 g
Wolfberry bark	(Di Gu Pi)	15 g

Usage: Decoction.

Anorexia Due to Overfeeding

Main manifestations: Partial or complete anorexia; preference for grass over grain; depression; reluctance to move; abdominal fullness; red, dry mouth or tongue with sour smell; thick, greasy coating on tongue; and surging, rapid pulse. It belongs to the Excess Heat pattern.

Treatment principles: To eliminate food stasis and promote digestion.

Herbal treatment: *Xiao Shi Tang* (Eliminating Food Stasis decoction).

Constituents:

Hawthorn fruit	(Shan Zha)	60 g
Medicated leaven	(Shen Qu)	60 g
Germinated barley	(Mai Ya)	60 g
Mirabilite	(Mang Xiao)	90 g
Radish seed	(Lai Fu Zi)	60 g

Usage: Decoction, given orally.

Anorexia Due to Spleen Deficiency

Main manifestations: Depression, loss of appetite, emaciation, coarse hair coat, fluctuating peristaltic sounds, soft feces or small dry feces with undigested food, pale or greenish-yellow tongue, and thready, weak pulse. It belongs to Spleen *Qi* Deficiency pattern.

Treatment principles: To strengthen the Spleen and tonify *Qi*.

Herbal treatment: *Shen Ling Bai Zhu San* (Ginseng-Poria-Atractylodes powder).

Constituents:

Ginseng	(Ren Shen)	45 g
White atractylodes	(Bai Zhu)	45 g
Chinese yam	(Shan Yao)	45 g
Lotus seed	(Lian Zi Rou)	30 g
Baked licorice root	(Gan Cao)	45 g
Coix seed	(Yi Yi Ren)	30 g
Poria	(Fu Ling)	45 g
Dolichos seed	(Bian Dou)	60 g
Glehnia root	(Sha Ren)	30 g
Platycodon root	(Jie Geng)	30 g

Usage: Powder or decoction.

Diarrhea Due to Intestinal Cold

Main manifestations: Sudden diarrhea; watery, nonoffensive feces; loud peristaltic sounds; cold trunk and limbs; cool ears and nose; greenish-yellow or pale tongue and mouth with watery saliva; and deep, slow pulse. It belongs to the Stomach Cold pattern.

Herbal treatment: *Ping Wei San* (Neutralizing Stomach Powder) plus *Wu Ling San* (Five-Porias Powder).

Constituents:

Atractylodes rhizome	(Cang Zhu)	60 g
Magnolia bark	(Hou Po)	45 g
Citrus peel	(Chen Pi)	45 g
Licorice root	(Gan Cao)	20 g
Jujube	(Da Zao)	90 g
Fresh ginger	(Sheng Jiang)	20 g
Polyporus	(Zhu Ling)	45 g
Poria	(Fu Ling)	45 g
Alisma tuber	(Ze Xie)	75 g
White atractylodes	(Bai Zhu)	45 g
Cinnamon twig	(Gui Zhi)	30 g

Usage: Decoction, given orally.

Diarrhea Due to Spleen Deficiency

Main manifestations: Prolonged diarrhea; gradual emaciation; harsh, dry hair coat; cold ears and nose; loud peristaltic sounds; coarse, unformed feces or watery feces with undigested grain; pale mouth and tongue; and deep, thready, weak pulse. In serious cases, there may be edema of the four limbs and persistent diarrhea. It belongs to Spleen *Qi* Deficiency Pattern.

Treatment principles: To strengthen the Spleen and dry Dampness; to remove water and stop diarrhea.

Herbal treatment: *Shen Ling Bai Zhu San* (Ginseng-Poria-Atractylodes powder no. 66) (See "Anorexia Due to Spleen Deficiency"). With serious diarrhea and edema, add cinnamon bark *(Rou Gui)* and dry ginger *(Gan Jiang)*.

GASTROENTERITIS

Gastroenteritis refers to inflammatory lesions of the mucosa and submucosal tissues of gastrointestinal tracts. In TCVM, gastroenteritis is divided into three types: Damp-Heat Pattern, Cold-Damp Pattern, and Blood Heat-Toxin pattern.

Damp-Heat Pattern or Acute Gastroenteritis

Main manifestations: Depression; slight or high fever; anorexia; abdominal pain; restlessness; offensive diarrhea (watery feces with mucosal shreds and blood) or dry feces, initially in the form of small balls, then soft feces with mucosal shreds or blood; thirst for cold water; scanty urine; deep red mouth and tongue with halitosis; yellow, greasy tongue coating; and surging, rapid pulse. It belongs to the Damp-Heat pattern of the Stomach-Intestine.

Treatment principles: To eliminate Heat and Toxin; to dry Dampness and stop diarrhea.

Herbal treatment: *Yu Jin San* (Curcuma Powder no. 19) with modification (see "Commonly Used Herbal Formulas"):
1. If feces with mucosal shreds and blood are present, discard white peony root *(Bai Shao Yao)*; add red peony root *(Chi Shao Yao)*, sophora flower *(Huai Hua)*, sanguisorba root *(Di Yu)*, and pulsatilla root *(Bai Tou Weng)*.
2. With persistent diarrhea, discard rhubarb root *(Da Huang)*.
3. With serious abdominal pain, add resina myrrhae *(Mo Yao)*, mastic *(Ru Xiang)*, lindera root *(Wu Yao)*, and saussurea root *(Mu Xiang)*.

4. With scanty fluid (*Yin* deficiency), add ophiopogon root *(Mai Men Dong)* and schisandra fruit *(Wu Wei Zi)* to the formula.

Cold-Damp Pattern or Chronic Gastroenteritis

Main manifestations: Watery feces, depression, tendency to lie down, cold limbs and trunk, cool ears and nose, thirst for cold water, clear salivation, greenish-purple mouth and tongue, and thready pulse. It belongs to the Cold Damp pattern.

Treatment principles: To dispel Dampness and Cold.

Herbal treatment: *Huo Xiang Zheng Qi San* (Agastache-*Zheng-Qi* Powder).

Constituents:

Agastache	*(Huo Xiang)*	90 g
Pinellia tuber	*(Ban Xia)*	60 g
Magnolia bark	*(Hou Po)*	60 g
Citrus peel	*(Chen Pi)*	60 g
Perilla leaf	*(Zi Su Ye)*	30 g
Angelica	*(Bai Zhi)*	30 g
Areca peel	*(Da Fu Pi)*	30 g
Poria	*(Gu Ling Pi)*	30 g
White atractylodes	*(Bai Zhu)*	60 g
Platycodon root	*(Jie Geng)*	60 g
Licorice root	*(Gan Cao)*	75 g
Fresh ginger	*(Sheng Jiang)*	20 g
Jujube	*(Da Zao)*	20 g

Usage: The ingredients are ground into a powder; 50 to 150 g of the powder is given orally at each treatment session.

Blood Heat-Toxin Pattern

Main manifestations: Diarrhea with blood and mucosal shreds, fetid stools; fever; anorexia; rapid respiration; lassitude; weariness; weakness of the limbs; palpitations; harsh dry hair coat; emaciation. In serious cases, restlessness or coma, sweating of whole body, convulsions, deep red or purple mouth and tongue with dryness, and thready, rapid pulse.

Treatment principles: The goal in treatment of this pattern is to eliminate Heat and Toxin, to cool Blood and stop diarrhea.

Herbal treatment: *Qing Ying Tang* (Dissipating-Ying-Stage Decoction) plus the following herb medicines: schisandra fruit *(Wu Wei Zi)* and moutan bark *(Mu Dan Pi)*.

Constituents of *Qing Ying Tang*:

Rhinoceros horn*	(Xi Jiao)	10 g
Scrophularia root	(Xuan Sheng)	45 g
Rehmannia root	(Sheng Di Huang)	60 g
Ophiopogon root	(Mai Men Dong)	45 g
Coptis root	(Huang Lian)	25 g
Forsythia fruit	(Lian Qiao)	30 g
Honeysuckle flower	(Jin Yin Hua)	45 g
Bamboo leaf	(Zhu Ye)	15 g
Salvia root	(Dan Shen)	30 g

INTESTINAL IMPACTION

Intestinal impaction is the incipient colic symptoms of fecal stasis (impaction) or obstruction in the intestinal tract due to disorders of intestinal movement and secretion. It is a common problem in horses. In TCVM, it is considered part of the Constipation pattern.

Heat Constipation

Main manifestations: Lower position of the lumbar area; attempts to discharge feces but difficulty excreting dry, hard, and dark feces; slight abdominal pain; scanty, yellow urine; red tongue with yellow coating; and deep, rapid pulse. In horses, severe abdominal pain, alternately standing up and lying down. It belongs to the Heat Excess pattern.

Treatment principles: To eliminate Heat and purge stasis from the intestines.

Herbal treatment: *Wu Shi Wan* (No-Failing Pill) with modification (See "Commonly Used Herbal Formulas"):
1. With dry feces, add cannabis seed *(Huo Ma Ren)*, rush-cherry seed *(Yu Li Ren)*, and vegetable oil *(Zhi Wu You)*.
2. With dry mouth, add rehmannia root *(Sheng Di Huang)* and ophiopogon root *(Mai Men Dong)*.

Deficiency Constipation

Main manifestations: Lower position of lumbar area, attempts to discharge feces but inability to defecate, depression, weakness of the limbs, pale tongue, weak pulse.

Treatment principles: To tonify *Qi* and moisten the intestines.

Herbal treatment: *Dang Gui Cong Rong Tang* (Angelica-Cistanche Decoction).

Constituents:

Chinese angelica root	(Dang Gui)	200 g
Cistanche	(Rou Cong Rong)	100 g
Senna leaf	(Fan Xie Ye)	30 g
Magnolia bark	(Hou Po)	20 g
Saussurea root	(Mu Xiang)	15 g
Cyperus tuber	(Xiang Fu)	30 g
Bitter orange	(Zhi Qiao)	30 g
Medicated leaven	(Shen Qu)	60 g
Dianthus	(Qu Mai)	15 g
Tetrapanax	(Tong Cao)	10 g

Usage: Decoction.
1. With weakness and fatigue, add astragalus root *(Huang Qi)* and ginseng *(Ren Shen)*.
2. With hard, dry feces, add scrophularia root *(Xuan Shen)* and ophiopogon root *(Mai Men Dong)*.

Cold Constipation

Main manifestations: Straining to defecate, slight abdominal pain, alternate standing and lying down, cold ears and nose, cool limbs, greenish-white mouth or tongue, and deep, slow pulse. It belongs to the Cold Excess pattern.

Treatment principles: To warm Middle Jiao and purge stasis from the intestines.

Herbal treatment: *Wu Shi Wan* (No-Failing Pill) (See "Commonly Used Herbal Formulas") plus the following Chinese medicines: aconite root *(Fu Zi)*, cinnamon bark *(Rou Gui)*, dry ginger *(Gan Jiang)*, astragalus root *(Huang Qi)*, ginseng *(Ren Shen)*, scrophularia root *(Xuan Shen)*, ophiopogon root *(Mai Men Dong)*, and rehmannia root *(Sheng Di Huang)*.

COLIC

Colic is the symptom complex of rolling on the ground and alternately standing up and lying down (all of which suggest abdominal pain), which are caused by stagnation of *Qi* and Blood in the abdomen. In TCVM, it includes Cold Colic, Damp-Heat Colic, Stagnated Blood Colic, Food Stasis Colic, and Constipation Colic.

Cold Colic

Main manifestations: Intermittent abdominal pain, alternate standing lying and down, pawing the ground, turning of the head to observe the abdomen, rolling, soft or watery feces, loud peristaltic sounds, cold ears and nose, and slow, deep pulse.

Treatment principles: To warm Middle Jiao and disperse Cold; to promote the *Qi* Flow and stop pain.

*If rhinoceros horn is not available, substitute water buffalo horn 100 g.

Herbal treatment: *Ju Pi San* (Tangerine-Peel Powder) (See "Commonly Used Herbal Formulas").
1. With severe Cold Pattern, add evodia fruit *(Wu Zhu Yu)* and dry ginger *(Gan Jiang).*
2. With severe pain, add Lindera root *(Wu Yao),* Saussurea root *(Mu Xiang),* and Corydalis tuber *(Yan Hu Suo).*

Damp-Heat Colic

Main manifestations: Alternate lying and standing; fever; thirst; diarrhea; mucous, malodorous stool; scanty, dark urine; deep red tongue or mouth; yellow, greasy tongue coating; and surging, rapid pulse.

Treatment principles: To eliminate Damp-Heat, to promote the *Qi* flow and relieve stasis.

Herbal treatment: *Yu Jin San* (Curcuma Powder) (See "Commonly Used Herbal Formulas").
1. In early stages of the disease, add mirabilite *(Mang Xiao)* and immature bitter orange *(Zhi Shi);* discard terminalia fruit *(He Zi).*
2. With severe fever, add honeysuckle flower *(Jin Yin Hua)* and forsythia fruit *(Lian Qiao).*

Stagnated Blood Colic—Blood Obstruction Abdominal Pain

Main manifestations: Symptoms include abdominal pain during work, restlessness, alternate standing and lying, pawing the ground, intermittent pain; masses in the mesenteric root.

Treatment principles: To strengthen the Spleen and regulate Qi; to activate Blood and eliminate Stagnation.

Herbal Treatment: *Qi Bu San* (Seven-Tonification Powder) with modifications:

Constituents:

Cinnamon bark	(Rou Gui)	30 g
Fennel fruit	(Hui Xiang)	30 g
Black cardamom seed	(Yi Zhi Ren)	30 g
Citrus peel	(Chen Pi)	25 g
Green tangerine peel	(Qing Pi)	40 g
Mastic	(Ru Xiang)	30 g
Resina myrrhae	(Mo Ya)	30 g
Chinese angelica	(Dang Gui)	30 g
Ligustcum rhizome	(Chuan Xiong)	25 g
White peony root	(Bai Shao Yao)	25 g
Sichuan chinaberry	(Chuan Lian Zi)	20 g
Bureed tuber	(San Leng)	20 g
Zedoary	(E Zhu)	20 g

Usage: Decoction given orally.

Stagnated Blood Colic—Postparturition Abdominal Pain

Main manifestations: Postparturition abdominal pain; turning of the head to observe the abdomen; partial to complete anorexia; dark, bloody vaginal discharge; greenish mouth or tongue; and deep, tight pulse.

Treatment principles: To tonify and activate Blood; to dissolve stagnation and stop pain.

Herbal treatment: *Sheng Hua Tang* (Generating Dispersing Decoction) plus Si Wu Tang (Four-Ingredients Decoction).

Constituents:

Chinese angelica root	(Dang Gui)	120 g
Ligusticum rhizome	(Chaun Xiong)	45 g
Persica seed	(Tao Ren)	45 g
Stir-baked ginger	(Gan Jiang)	10 g
Baked licorice root	(Gan Cao)	10 g
Prepared rehmannia root	(Shu Di Huang)	75 g
White peony root	(Bai Shao Yao)	50 g

Usage: Decoction or powder given orally.

Food Stasis Colic

Main manifestations: Abdominal pain soon after eating large amounts of food; alternate standing and lying; pawing; converse peristalsis of esophageal tract; deep red mouth or tongue; yellow, thick tongue coating; and deep, tight pulse.

Treatment principles: To eliminate food stasis and promote digestion.

Herbal treatment: Mild dosage of *Qu Mai San* (Leaven-Barley Powder) plus 250 to 500 ml vinegar (See "Commonly Used Herbal Formulas").

CONSTIPATION COLIC

See "Intestinal Impaction."

COMMON COLD AND INFLUENZA

Common cold is caused by invasion of Wind-Cold and Wind-Heat through the skin, mouth, or nose. It includes two patterns: Wind-Cold and Wind-Heat. Influenza is a special type of Cold, infectious and serious. It belongs mostly to the Wind-Heat Pattern.

Wind-Cold Pattern

Main manifestations: Depression; anorexia; cool nose and ears; aversion to cold, piloerection; fever; no cough; clear nasal discharge; thin, white coating on tongue; and superficial, tight pulse. It belongs to the Wind-Cold pattern.

Treatment principles: To induce perspiration and dispel Wind-Cold.

Herbal treatment: *Ma Huang Tang* (Ephedra Decoction) (See "Commonly Used Herbal Formulas").

Wind-Heat Pattern

Main manifestations: Depression; anorexia; rapid respiration; fever; sweating; cough; thick nasal discharge; aversion to heat; extreme thirst; dry feces; scanty, dark urine; thin white and yellow tongue coating; and superficial rapid pulse. It belongs to the Wind-Heat pattern.

Treatment principles: To relieve the Exterior with pungent and cool nature; to disperse Wind-Heat.

Herbal treatment: *Yin Qiao San* (Lonicera-Forsythia Powder no. 3) (See "Commonly Used Herbal Formulas"). With influenza, add: isatis root *(Ban Lan Gen)*, belamcanda rhizome *(She Gan)*, and pueraria root *(Ge Gen)*.

LARYNGITIS

Laryngitis is inflammation of the laryngeal mucosa and submucosal tissues. In TCVM, it is called *Larynx Huang*. It belongs to the Excess Heat patterns.

Treatment principles: To eliminate Heat and toxin; to resolve swelling and clear the larynx.

Herbal treatment: *Xiao Huang San* (Dissipating-Huang-Pattern Powder) (See Pharyngitis) plus the following Chinese medicines: arctium fruit *(Niu Bang Zi)*, isatis root *(Ban Lan Gen)*, pigeon peel *(Shan Dou Gen)*, belamcanda rhizome *(She Gan)*, platycodon root *(Jie Geng)*, and trichosanthes root *(Tian Hua Fen)*.

BRONCHITIS

Bronchitis is inflammation of the bronchial mucosa and submucosal tissues. It includes acute and chronic bronchitis. In TCVM, bronchitis belongs to the Cough pattern. Acute bronchitis is divided into Wind-Cold Cough and Wind-Heat Cough, whereas chronic bronchitis falls into the Lung *Qi* Deficiency Cough, Lung *Yin* Deficiency Cough, and Spleen-Lung Deficiency Cough categories.

Acute Bronchitis—Wind-Cold Cough

Main manifestations: Fever, aversion to cold, piloerection, frequent loud cough, clear nasal discharge, pale mouth or tongue, and superficial, tight pulse. It belongs to the Wind-Cold pattern.

Treatment principles: To dispel Wind-Cold; to disperse congestion in the Lung and stop cough.

Herbal treatment: *Zhi Sou San* (Cough-Stopping Powder) plus perilla leaf *(Zi Su Ye)* and ledebouriella root *(Fang Feng)*.

Constituents of *Zhi Sou San*:

Aster root	(Zi Wan)	30 g
Stemona root	(Bai Bu)	30 g
Cynanchum root	(Bai Qian)	30 g
Citrus peel	(Chen Pi)	25 g
Schizonepeta	(Jing Jie)	30 g
Platycodon root	(Jie Geng)	30 g
Licorice root	(Gan Cao)	15 g

Usage: Decoction.

Acute Bronchitis—Wind-Heat Cough

Main manifestations: Aversion to heat; flared nostrils and rapid respiration; warm breath; forceful cough; thick nasal discharge; dry, red mouth or tongue; thin white or yellow coating on tongue; and superficial or surging, and rapid pulse. It belongs to the Wind-Heat pattern.

Treatment principles: To dispel Wind-Heat; to disperse congestion in the Lung and stop cough.

Herbal Treatment: *Bei Mu San* (Fritillary Powder) plus the following herbs: honeysuckle flower *(Jin Yin Hua)*, citrus peel *(Chen Pi)*, colt's foot flower *(Kuan Dong Hua)*, aristolochia fruit *(Ma Dou Ling)*, and eriobotrya leaf *(Pi Pa Ye)*.

Constituents of *Bei Mu San*:

Fritillary bulb	(Bei Mu)	30 g
Gardenia fruit	(Zhi Zi)	30 g
Stemona root	(Bai Bu)	30 g
Apricot seed	(Xing Ren)	30 g
Aster root	(Zi Wan)	30 g
Platycodon root	(Jie Geng)	30 g
Arctium fruit	(Niu Bang Zi)	30 g
Licorice root	(Gan Cao)	30 g

Usage: Decoction. It is given orally.

Chronic Bronchitis—Lung **Qi** Deficiency Cough

Main manifestations: Depression; emaciation; harsh, dry hair coat; soft cough; shortness of breath; exertional asthma and sweating; thick or thin nasal discharge;

pale tongue; and weak, thready pulse. It belongs to the Lung *Qi* Deficiency pattern.

Treatment principles: To tonify the Lung *Qi*; to moisten the Lung and stop cough.

Herbal treatment: Chronic bronchitis is treated with *Er Chen Tang* (Two-Old-Herbs Decoction) plus the following herbs: pilose asiabell root *(Dang Shen)*, white atractylodes *(Bai Zhu)*, aster root *(Zi Wan)*, schisandra fruit *(Wu Wei Zi)*, prepared rehmannia *(Shu Di Huang)*, and astragalus root *(Huang Zi)*.

Constituents of *Er Chen Tang*:

Pinellia tuber	*(Ban Xia)*	45 g
Citrus peel	*(Chen Pi)*	45 g
Poria	*(Fu Ling)*	60 g
Licorice root	*(Gan Cao)*	25 g

Usage: Decoction, given orally.

Chronic Bronchitis—Lung Yin Deficiency Cough

Main manifestations: This form of chronic bronchitis is characterized by weak, unproductive cough; nocturnal cough; red, dry, uncoated tongue; and thready, weak pulse. It belongs to the Lung *Yin* Deficiency pattern.

Treatment principles: To nourish Yin; to moisten the Lung and stop cough.

Herbal treatment: *Bai He Gu Jin Tang* (Consolidating-Lung-with-Lily Decoction).

Constituents:

Lily bulb	*(Bai He)*	45 g
Prepared rehmannia root	*(Shu Di Huang)*	60 g
Raw rehmannia root	*(Sheng Di Huang)*	60 g
Ophiopogon root	*(Mai Men Dong)*	45 g
White peony root	*(Bai Shao Yao)*	30 g
Scrophularia	*(Xuan Shen)*	20 g
Tendrilled fritillary bulb	*(Chuan Bai Mu)*	30 g
Chinese angelica root	*(Dang Gui)*	30 g
Platycodon root	*(Jie Geng)*	20 g
Licorice root	*(Gan Cao)*	30 g

Usage: Decoction, given orally.

Chronic Bronchitis—Spleen-Lung Deficiency Cough

Main manifestations: Productive cough, depression, anorexia, pale tongue with greasy coating, and deep, thready pulse. It belongs to the Spleen-Lung *Qi* Deficiency pattern.

Treatment principles: To strengthen the Spleen and dry Dampness; to dissolve phlegm and stop cough.

Herbal treatment: *Er Chen Tang* (Two-Old-Herbs Decoction) (See "Lung *Qi* Deficiency Cough") plus the following Chinese medicines: pilose asiabell root *(Dang Shen)*, white atractylodes *(Bai Zhu)*, astragalus root *(Huang Qi)*, atractylodes rhizome *(Cang Zhu)*, radish seed *(Lai Fu Zi)*, citrus peel *(Chen Pi)*, cinnamon twig *(Gui Zhi)*, and perilla seed *(Zi Su Zi)*.

PNEUMONIA

Pneumonia is defined as inflammation of the lung. In TCVM, pneumonia is called Lung *Huang*, or Lung Heat and Lung Stasis, which includes five types: Affliction of Wind-Heat in the Lung, Lung Extreme Heat, Collapse of Deficient Zheng *Qi*, Lung *Qi* Deficiency, and Lung *Yin* Deficiency.

Affliction of Wind-Heat in the Lung

Main manifestations: Pneumonia is characterized by sudden fever; mild aversion to cold; severe cough; piloerection; thick nasal discharge; red tongue and mouth; thin, white tongue coating; and superficial and rapid pulse. It belongs to the Wind-Heat pattern.

Treatment principles: To relieve the Exterior with pungent and cool agents; to clear the Lung and dissolve phlegm.

Herbal treatment: *Yin Qiao San* (Lonicera-Forsythia Powder) (See "Commonly Used Herbal Formulas") with modifications:
1. With serious fever, add: scutellaria root *(Huang Zin)*, gardemia fruit *(Zhi Zi)*, gypsum fibrosum *(Shi Gao)*, and trichosanthes root *(Tian Hua Fen)*.
2. With serious cough, add trichosanthes fruit *(Gua Lou)*, cynanchum root *(Bai Qian)*, and aster root *(Zi Wan)*.

Lung Extreme Heat

Main manifestations: High fever; severe asthma; occasional cough; suppurative, grayish-yellow nasal discharge; depression; anorexia; dry feces; dark, concentrated urine; marked thirst; dry, red tongue or mouth; thick yellow tongue coating; and surging, rapid pulse. It belongs to Lung-Heat pattern.

Treatment principles: To eliminate Heat and toxin; to clear the Lung and stop asthma.

Herbal treatment: *Ma Xing Shi Gan Tang* (Ephedra-Apricot-Gypsum-Licorice).

Constituents:

Ephedra	*(Ma Huang)*	30 g
Apricot seed	*(Xing Ren)*	45 g
Gypsum fibrosum	*(Shi Gao)*	120 g
Baked licorice root	*(Gan Cao)*	30 g

Usage: Decoction, given orally.

1. With serious fever, add scutellaria root *(Huang Qin)*, honeysuckle flower *(Jin Yin Hua)*, forsythia fruit *(Lian Qiao)*, and isatis root *(Ban Lan Gen)*.
2. With serious asthma, add cynanchum root *(Bai Qian)*, trichosanthes fruit *(Gua Lou)*, and bitter orange *(Zhi Qiao)*.
3. With dry feces, add rhubarb root *(Da Huang)*, mirabilite *(Mang Xiao)*, and cannabis seed *(Huo Ma Ren)*.
4. With thirst and dry mouth, add anemarrhena rhizome *(Zhi Mu)* and ophiopogon root *(Mai Men Dong)*.
5. With suppurative pneumonia, add Wei Jing Tang *(Reed Decoction)*.

Collapse of Deficient Zheng Qi

Main manifestations: Sudden worsening of symptoms; whole-body shivering; profuse, oily sweating; very cold limbs; shallow breath; greenish-purple tongue; and weak, thready pulse. It belongs to the Collapse pattern of *Yang Qi*.

Treatment principles: To resuscitate collapse by reviving *Yang Qi*.

Herbal treatment: *Shen Fu Tang* (Ginseng-Aconite Decoction) plus the following Chinese medicines: oyster shell *(Mu Li)*, dragon bone (Long Gu), white peony root *(Bai Shao Yao)*, licorice root *(Gan Cao)*, and schisandra fruit *(Wu Wei Zi)*.

Constituents:

Ginseng	*(Ren Shen)*	30 g
Baked aconite root	*(Fu Zi)*	45 g

Usage: Decoction, given orally.

Lung *Qi* deficiency: Same as Lung *Qi* Deficiency Cough in Bronchitis.

Lung *Yin* deficiency: Same as Lung *Yin* Deficiency Cough in Bronchitis.

MENINGITIS AND ENCEPHALITIS

Meningitis and *encephalitis* refer to acute or chronic inflammatory lesions of the central nervous system. In TCVM, they are called Cerebral *Huang*, or Wind Pattern, which include *Yang* Mania, *Yin* Depression, and convulsion patterns.

Yang *Mania Pattern*

Main manifestations: Manic behavior, circling, obliviousness to surroundings, deep red mouth or tongue, and surging, rapid pulse. In serious cases: sudden falling, profuse perspiration, foaming from the mouth, and muscle shivers. It belongs to the *Yang* Mania Pattern.

Treatment principles: To eliminate Heat and dissolve phlegm; to calm the Heart and tranquilize the Mind.

Herbal treatment: *Zhen Xin San* (Calming-Heart Powder) plus the following Chinese medicines: pinellia rhizome *(Ban Xia)*, batryticated silkworm *(Jiang Can)*, arisaema tuber *(Tian Nan Xing)*, and bamboo shavings *(Zhu Ru)*.

Constituents of *Zhen Xin San*:

Coptis root	*(Huang Lian)*	30 g
Scutellaria root	*(Huang Qin)*	30 g
Gardenia fruit	*(Zhi Zi)*	30 g
Curcuma root	*(Yu Jin)*	30 g
Cinnabar	*(Zhu Sha)*	10 g
Poria	*(Fu Lin)*	30 g
Polygala root	*(Yuan Zhi)*	30 g
Ephedra	*(Ma Huang)*	20 g
Ledebouriella root	*(Fang Feng)*	30 g
Pilose asiabell root	*(Dang Shen)*	30 g
Honey	*(Feng Mi)*	120 ml
Licorice root	*(Gan Cao)*	20 g

Usage: Decoction, given orally.

Yin *Depression Pattern*

Main manifestations: Depression, ataxia or sudden falls, coma, blindness, cranial nerve abnormalities including deep red mouth or tongue, and surging, rapid pulse. It belongs to the *Yin* Depression pattern.

Treatment principles: To dissolve phlegm and open the orifice; to calm the heart and tranquilize the Mind.

Herbal treatment: *Zhen Xin San* (Calming-Heart Powder) (See "*Yang* Mania Pattern") plus the following drugs: pinellia rhizome *(Ban Xia)*, arisaema tuber *(Tian Nan Xing)*, poria *(Fu Ling)*, saussurea root *(Mu Xiang)*, batryticated silkworm *(Jiang Can)*, and uncaria stem with hooks *(Gou Teng)*.

Convulsion Pattern—Convulsion Due to Extreme Heat

Main manifestations: Fever; thirst; falling, tonic-clonic seizures; neck rigidity; opisthotonos; foaming at the mouth; deep red eyes; yellow, greasy tongue coating; and surging, rapid pulse. It belongs to the Heat Excess pattern.

Treatment principles: To eliminate Heat and Toxin; to calm Wind and tranquilize convulsions.

Herbal treatment: *Ling Yang Gou Teng Tang* (Antelope-Uncaria Decoction).

Constituents:

Antelope horn	(*Ling Yang Jiao*)	60 g
Uncaria stem with hooks	(*Gou Teng*)	30 g
Mulberry leaf	(*Sang Ye*)	20 g
Chrysanthemum flower	(*Ju Hua*)	30 g
Tendrilled fritillary bulb	(*Chuan Bei Mu*)	30 g
Fresh rehmannia root	(*Sheng Di Huang*)	60 g
White peony root	(*Bai Shao Yao*)	30 g
Licorice root	(*Gan Cao*)	15 g
Bamboo shavings	(*Zhu Ru*)	60 g
Poria	(*Fu Ling*)	30 g

Usage: Decoction, given orally.

Convulsion Pattern—Convulsion Due To Blood Deficiency

Main manifestations: Emaciation; harsh, dry hair coat; weakness of the limbs; tonic-clonic seizures; rigidity of the neck; "lockjaw"; falling with inability to rise; cool ears and nose; pale tongue; and weak, thready pulse. It belongs to the *Qi* Blood Deficiency pattern.

Treatment principles: To tonify both Blood and *Qi*.

Herbal treatment: *Si Jun Zi Tang* (Four-Gentlemen Decoction) plus *Si Wu Tang* (Four-Ingredients Decoction) (See "Commonly Used Herbal Formulas"), plus the following Chinese medicines: uncaria stem with hooks *(Gou Teng)*, batryticated silkworm tuber *(Jiang Can)*, cicada slough *(Chan Tui)* and typhonium *(Bai Fu Zi)*.

CHRONIC HYDROCEPHALUS

Chronic hydrocephalus is characterized by accumulation of excess cerebrospinal fluid in the ventricles of the brain and a general increase in intracranial pressure, with dysfunctions of movement and consciousness. In TCVM, it is considered as Spleen Deficiency Damp Pattern.

Treatment principles: To dry Damp and dissolve Turbidity; to eliminate water and clear the brain.

Herbal treatment: *Jie Yin Tang* (Platycodon-Honeysuckle Decoction)

Constituents:

Platycodon root	(*Jie Geng*)	30 g
Honeysuckle flower	(*Jin Yin Hua*)	30 g
Chrysanthemum flower	(*Ju Hua*)	30 g
Cicada slough	(*Chan Tui*)	30 g
Polyporus	(*Zhu Ling*)	24 g
Poria	(*Fu Ling*)	24 g
Alister tuber	(*Ze Xie*)	24 g
Atractylodes rhizome	(*Cang Zhu*)	24 g
Mentha	(*Bo He*)	15 g
Angelica	(*Bai Zhi*)	15 g
Rush pith	(*Deng Xin Cao*)	12 g
Cimicifuga rhizome	(*Sheng Ma*)	12 g
Pinellia tuber	(*Ban Xia*)	18 g
Pilose asiabell root	(*Dang Shen*)	12 g
Chinese yam	(*Shan Yao*)	12 g
White atractylodes	(*Bai Zhu*)	12 g
Astragalus root	(*Huang Qi*)	12 g

Usage: Decoction, given orally.

DIAPHRAGMATIC CHOREA

Diaphragmatic chorea is the spasmodic contraction of the diaphragm and rhythmic tremor of the trunk.

Treatment principles: To regulate and decrease *Qi* flow.

Herbal treatment: *Ju Pi San* (Tangerine-Peel Powder) (see "Commonly Used Herbal Formulas") plus lindera root *(Wu Yao)*, cyperus tuber *(Xiang Fu)*, and dry ginger *(Gan Jiang)*.

NEPHRITIS

In Chinese medicine, nephritis generally includes glomerulonephritis, interstitial nephritis, and inflammatory lesion of renal tubules. In TCVM, it is divided into two types: Accumulation of Damp-Heat and Spleen-Kidney *Yang* Deficiency. It can also be regarded as Edema.

Accumulation of Damp-Heat

Main manifestations: High body temperature; scanty, dark urine; difficulty urinating; painful lumbar area, sensitive to touch; reluctance to move; stilted gait; red, dry tongue and mouth; and surging, rapid pulse. It belongs to the Damp-Heat pattern.

Treatment principles: To eliminate Heat and Damp; to dissolve swelling and stop pain.

Herbal treatment: *Wu Ling San* (Five-Porias Powder) plus the following Chinese medicines: honeysuckle flower *(Jin Yin Hua)*, dandelion *(Pu Gong Ying)*, rehmannia root *(Sheng Di Huang)*, scrophularia root *(Xuan Shen)*, anemarrhena rhizome *(Zhi Mu)*, philodendron bark *(Huang Bai)*, citrus peel *(Chen Pi)*, and resina myrrhae *(Mo Yao)*.

Constituents of *Wu Ling San:*

Polyporus	*(Zhu Ling)*	45 g
Poria	*(Fu Ling)*	45 g
Alisma tuber	*(Ze Xie)*	75 g
White atractylodes	*(Bai Zhu)*	45 g
Cinnamon twig	*(Gui Zhi)*	30 g

Usage: The decoction is given orally.

Spleen-Kidney Yang Deficiency

Main manifestations: Edema of the eyelids, ventral thorax, ventral abdomen, limbs and perineum; pale mouth and tongue; and deep, thready pulse. It is a Spleen-Kidney *Yang* Deficiency.

Treatment principles: To tonify *Yang* and warm the Spleen and Kidney; to eliminate water and dissolve swelling.

Herbal treatment: *Wu Ling San* (Five-Porias Powder), (see "Accumulation of Damp-Heat") plus the following Chinese medicines: pilose asiabell root *(Dang Shen)*, astragalus root *(Huang Qi)*, morinda root *(Ba Ji Tian)*, psoralea *(Bu Gu Zhi)*, magnolia bark *(Hou Po)*, resina myrrhae *(Mo Yao)*, aconite *(Fu Zi)*, and dry ginger *(Gan Jiang)*.

CYSTITIS

Cystitis refers to inflammation of the mucosal and submucosal tissues of the urinary bladder. In TCVM, it is considered to be in the category of Urinary Dripping, which includes Bladder Damp-Heat and Kidney *Yang* Deficiency.

Bladder Damp-Heat

Main manifestations: Pollakiuria with scanty, deep red urine; urgency and apparent pain on urination; abdominal fullness and pain; pawing the ground; alternate standing and lying, red and yellow tongue and mouth; and rapid pulse. This condition belongs to Bladder Damp Heat pattern.

Treatment principles: To eliminate Heat and Damp.

Herbal treatment: *Ba Zheng San* (Eight-Diuretics Powder).

Constituents:

Akebia stem	*(Mu Tong)*	50 g
Dianthus	*(Qu Mai)*	50 g
Plantago seed	*(Che Qian Zi)*	40 g
Talc	*(Hua Shi)*	50 g
Gardenia fruit	*(Zhi Zi)*	40 g
Rhubarb root	*(Da Huang)*	40 g
Rush Pith	*(Deng Xin Cao)*	40 g
Baked licorice root	*(Gan Cao)*	30 g

Usage: Decoction, given orally.

Kidney Yang Deficiency

Main manifestations: Frequent and difficult micturition; scanty, grayish urine; painful urination with weak stream; emaciation; pale tongue and mouth; and deep, thready pulse. It belongs to the Kidney *Yang* Deficiency Pattern.

Treatment principles: To tonify the Kidney and warm *Yang*.

Herbal treatment: *Shen Qi Wan* (Kidney-*Qi* Pill) plus the following Chinese medicines: achyranthes root *(Niu Xi)* and plantago seed *(Che Qian Zi)*.

Constituents of *Shen Qi Wan:*

Dry rehmannia root	*(Gan Di Huang)*	80 g
Cornus fruit	*(Shan Zhu Yu)*	40 g
Chinese yam	*(Shan Yao)*	40 g
Aconite root	*(Fu Zi)*	30 g
Cinnamon twig	*(Gui Zhi)*	30 g
Alisma tuber	*(Ze Xia)*	30 g
Moutan bark	*(Mu Dan Pi)*	30 g
Poria	*(Fu Ling)*	30 g

Usage: Decoction, given orally.

UROLITHIASIS

Urolithiasis refers to complete or incomplete urethral obstruction by various types of concretions. In TCVM, urolithiasis is considered to be in the category of Stone Dripping.

Treatment principles: To eliminate Heat and drive through urinary dripping and diuresis.

Herbal treatment: *Hua Shi San* (Talc Powder) plus the following Chinese medicines: dianthus *(Qu Mai)*, polygonum *(Bian Xu)*, lygodium spores *(Hai Jin Sha)*, lysimachia *(Jin Qian Cao)*, and pyrosia leaf *(Shi Wei)*.

Constituents of *Hua Shi San:*

Talc	*(Hua Shi)*	60 g
Alisma tuber	*(Ze Xie)*	30 g
Polyporus	*(Zhu Ling)*	30 g
Evergreen artemisia	*(Yin Chen Hao)*	30 g
Rush pith	*(Deng Xin Cao)*	10 g
Anemarrhena rhizome	*(Zhi Mu)*	30 g
Philodendron bark	*(Huang Bai)*	30 g

Usage: Decoction, given orally. *Ba Zheng San* (Eight-Diuretics Powder) (See "Cystitis"), plus the following Chinese medicines: chicken's gizzard skin *(Ji Nei Jin)*, lygodium spores *(Hai Jin Sha)*, lysimachia *(Jin Qian Cao)*, and pyrosia leaf *(Shi Wei)*.

ECZEMA

Eczema, an acute or chronic dermatitis, is a reaction of epidermal cells to allergens. In TCVM, it is considered to be in the category of Damp-Toxin, which includes Wind-Heat pattern and Damp-Heat pattern.

Wind-Heat Pattern

Main manifestations: Warm skin surface, patches of erythema with small vesicles, itching and restlessness, scratching and rubbing of the affected area, and alopecia in the affected area. It belongs to the Wind-Heat pattern.

Treatment principles: To eliminate Heat and disperse Wind.

Herbal treatment: *Xiao-Feng San* (Dispersing-Wind Powder).

Constituents:

Schizonepeta	*(Jing Jie)*	25 g
Ledebouriella root	*(Fang Feng)*	25 g
Arctium fruit	*(Niu Bang Zi)*	25 g
Cicada slough	*(Chan Tui)*	20 g
Sophora root	*(Ku Shen)*	20 g
Rehmannia root	*(Sheng Di Huang)*	25 g
Anemarrhena rhizome	*(Zhi Mu)*	25 g
Gypsum fibrosum	*(Shi Gao)*	25 g
Akebia stem	*(Mu Tong)*	20 g

Usage: Decoction or powder.

Damp-Heat Pattern

Main manifestations: Small vesicles that may rupture; thick, yellow discharge from the surface; scabs or ulcers; itching and restlessness; scratching and rubbing; and alopecia. It belongs to the Damp-Heat pattern.

Treatment principles: To eliminate Heat and Damp.

Herbal treatment: *Qing Shi Re Tang* (Eliminating-Heat-Damp Decoction).

Constituents:

Scutellaria root	*(Huang Qin)*	30 g
Philodendron root	*(Huang Bai)*	25 g
Sophodra root	*(Ku Shen)*	25 g
Rehmannia root	*(Sheng Di Huang)*	25 g
Isatis root	*(Ban Lan Gen)*	30 g
Plantago seed	*(Che Qian Zi)*	25 g
Talc	*(Hua Shi)*	25 g

Usage: Powder or decoction.

URTICARIA

Urticaria is an acute allergic skin lesion characterized by wheals and localized skin edema. In TCVM, it is regarded as a Lung Excess Wind-Heat pattern.

Treatment principles: To eliminate Heat and Toxin; to dispel Wind and stop itching.

Herbal treatment: *Xiao Huanbg San* (Dissipating-Huang-Pattern Powder) (see "Pharyngitis"), plus the following Chinese medicines: schizonepeta *(Jing Jie)*, ledebouriella root *(Fang Feng)*, mentha (Bo He), and sophora root *(Ku Shen)*.

CONJUNCTIVITIS

Conjunctivitis is inflammation of the conjunctiva, probably the most common eye disease. In TCVM, it belongs to Liver Wind-Heat pattern.

Treatment principles: To dissipate Wind and eliminate Heat.

Herbal treatment: *Fang Feng San* (Ledebouriella Powder):

Constituents:

Ledebouriella root	*(Fang Feng)*	16 g
Schizonepeta	*(Jing Jie)*	20 g
Cicada slough	*(Chan Tui)*	20 g
Coptis root	*(Huang Lian)*	15 g
Scutellaria root	*(Huang Qin)*	16 g
Gentiana	*(Long Dan Cao)*	16 g
Sea-ear shell	*(Shi Jue Ming)*	16 g
Celosia seed	*(Qing Xiang Zi)*	16 g
Cassia seed	*(Jue Ming Zi)*	16 g
Resina myrrhae	*(Mo Yao)*	15 g
Licorice root	*(Gan Cao)*	15 g

Usage: Powder or decoction; add 125 ml honey for palatability.

KERATITIS

Keratitis is inflammation of the cornea. In TCVM, it is considered to be the result of Liver Heat transmitted to the Eyes. It belongs to the Liver-Heat pattern.

Treatment principles: To clear Liver and eliminate Fire; to clear eyes and to resolve nebula.

Internal herbal treatment: *Jue Ming San* (Sea-Ear Powder):

Constituents:

Cassia sea-ear shell	*(Shi Jue Ming)*	45 g
Cassia seed	*(Jue Ming Zi)*	45 g
Coptis root	*(Huang Lian)*	20 g
Gardenia fruit	*(Zhi Zi)*	30 g
Scutellaria root	*(Huang Qin)*	20 g
Rhubarb root	*(Da Huang)*	30 g
Resina myrrhae	*(Mo Yao)*	20 g
Astragalus root	*(Huang Qi)*	30 g
Dioscorea stem	*(Huang Yao Zi)*	30 g
Stephania root	*(Bai Yao Zi)*	30 g

Usage: Decoction or powder, given orally.

External herbal treatment: *Bo Yun San* (Dispelling Clouds Powder).

Constituents:

Borneol	*(Bing Pian)*	3.2 g
Borax	*(Peng Sha)*	3.2 g
Calamine	*(Lu Gan Shi)*	1.6 g
Cinnabar	*(Zhu Sha)*	1.6 g

Usage: Mix and grind into very fine powder. Keep in a bottle. Put 0.3 g powdered drug into the affected eye. If the problem is caused by trauma, the drug is contraindicated.

PERIODIC OPHTHALMIA

Periodic ophthalmia is a common infectious disease in the horse characterized clinically by recurrent attacks of conjunctivitis, keratitis, photophobia, and lacrimation. In TCVM, it is considered to have three stages: early, later, and recurrent.

Early Stage

Main manifestations: Sudden occurrence of ocular signs such as swollen red conjunctiva, ocular discharge, and photophobia; swollen eyelids and blepharospasm; painful response to touch; corneal opacity; and miosis. Seven to 10 days later, ocular signs become less pronounced, with clearing corneas and normal pupils. This stage usually lasts 2 to 3 weeks (rarely, as long as 4 weeks). It belongs to the Liver Heat pattern.

Treatment principles: To clear the Liver and eliminate Heat.

Internal herbal treatment: *Long Dan Xie Gan Tang* (Puring-Liver-Fire-with-Gentian Decoction) plus the following Chinese medicines: moutan bark *(Mu Dan Pi)*, red peony root *(Chi Shao Yao)*, chrysanthemum flower *(Ju Hua)*, cicada slough *(Chan Tui)*, calcined sea-ear shell *(Shi Jue Ming)*, cassia seed *(Jue Ming Zi)*, and celosia seed *(Qing Xiang Zi)*.

Constituents of *Long Dan Xie Gan Tang*:

Gentian	*(Long Dan Cao)*	30 g
Scutellaria root	*(Huang Qin)*	45 g
Gardenia fruit	*(Zhi Zi)*	30 g
Alisma tuber	*(Ze Xie)*	60 g
Akebia stem	*(Mu Tong)*	30 g
Plantago seed	*(Che Qian Zi)*	45 g
Chinese angelica root	*(Dang Gui)*	25 g
Rehmannia root	*(Sheng Di Huang)*	45 g
Bupleurum root	*(Chai Hu)*	30 g
Licorice root	*(Gan Cao)*	30 g

Usage: Decoction, given orally.

External herbal treatment: *Bo Yun San* (Dispelling-Clouds Powder; see "Keratitis").

Later and Recurrent Stages

Main manifestations: Variable iris atrophy; thick, mucoid ocular discharge; corneal opacity; yellow or grayish sclera. The later stage usually lasts 1 to 6 months. There may be sudden recurrence of the early stage, iris atrophy, and blindness. It belongs to Liver-Kidney *Yin* Deficiency pattern.

Treatment principles: To nourish the Liver and Kidney; to clear the eye and resolve opacity.

Herbal treatment: *Liu Wei Di Huang Wan* (Six-Ingredients-with-Rehmannia Pill) (see "Commonly Used Herbal Formulas"), plus the following Chinese medicines: Chinese angelica root *(Dang Gui)*, chrysanthemum flower *(Ju Hua)*, white peony root *(Bai Shao Yao)*, calcined sea-ear shell *(Shi Jue Ming)*, and tribulus fruit *(Ci Ji Li)*.

LAMINITIS

Laminitis is an inflammation of the laminae in the hoof. It may affect one foot, or there may be bilateral involvement of thoracic or pelvic limbs or of all four feet. In TCVM, it is divided into Over-Food Founder and Over-Walk Founder.

Over-Walk Founder

Main manifestations: Heat and pain of the affected hooves with increased digital pulses, short gait, great reluctance to move, difficulty bearing weight, rapid respiration, red tongue and mouth, increased body temperature. Forelimb involvement alone: thoracic limbs are advanced forward with the weight on the heel of the foot, head and neck are raised and hind feet carried well up under the body to support weight. Hind feet: thoracic limbs placed backward under the body to bear as much weight as possible, head and neck lowered, and rear feet thrust forward to shift weight to the heels. All four feet: refusal to move, shifting of weight to redistribute body weight to avoid pain. In severe cases, the horse remains recumbent.

Treatment principles: To activate Blood and promote *Qi* flow; to dissolve stagnation and stop pain.

Herbal treatment: *Yin Chen San* (Evergreen-Artemisia Powder).

Constituents:

Evergreen artemisia	(Yin Chen Hao)	25 g
Resina myrrhae	(Mo Yao)	25 g
Carthamus	(Hong Hua)	15 g
Chinese angelica root	(Dang Gui)	30 g
Dioscorea stem	(Huang Yao Zi)	15 g
Stephania root	(Bai Yao Zi)	15 g
Platycodon root	(Jie Geng)	15 g
Bupleurum root	(Chai Hu)	15 g
Citrus peel	(Chen Pi)	15 g
Green tangerine peel	(Qing Pi)	15 g
Licorice root	(Gan Cao)	15 g
Apricot seed	(Xing Ren)	18 g

Usage: Decoction.

Overeating Founder

Main manifestations: Anorexia, preference for grass over grain, watery feces, rapid breath, bright red mouth and tongue, and surging, rapid pulse.

Treatment principles: To improve digestion and disperse food stasis; to activate Blood and promote *Qi* flow.

Herbal treatment: *Hong Hua San* (Carthamus Powder)

Constituents:

Carthamus	(Hong Hua)	20 g
Resina myrrhae	(Mo Yao)	20 g
Chinese angelica root	(Dang Gui)	30 g
Bitter orange	(Zhi Qiao)	20 g
Magnolia bark	(Hou Po)	20 g
Citrus peel	(Chen Pi)	20 g
Medicated leaven	(Shen Qu)	30 g
Hawthorn fruit	(Shan Zha)	30 g
Germinated barley	(Mai Ya)	30 g

Platycodon root	(Jie Geng)	20 g
Dioscorea stem	(Huang Yao Zi)	20 g
Stephania root	(Bai Yao Zi)	20 g
Licorice root	(Gan Cao)	15 g

Usage: Decoction, given orally.

Research Organizations for Traditional Chinese Veterinary Medicine in China

- Lanzhou Institute of Traditional Chinese Veterinary Medicine
- Jiangxi Institute of Traditional Chinese Veterinary Medicine
- China Control Institute of Veterinary Drugs
- Jilin Institute of Specialty

Societies of Traditional Chinese Veterinary Medicine in China

Chinese National Society of Traditional Chinese Veterinary Medicine

Liaison: Yu Chuan, professor
College of Veterinary Medicine
Beijing Agricultural University
Beijing 100094
China
PR China

North-China Society of Traditional Chinese Veterinary Medicine

Liaison: Li Chengming, Professor
Department of Veterinary Medicine
Hebei Agricultural University
Baoding, Hebei Province 071001
China

South-West Society of Traditional Chinese Veterinary Medicine

Liaison: Zheng Dongcai, Professor
Department of Veterinary Medicine
Sichuan College of Animal Sciences and Veterinary Medicine
Rongchang County, Chongqing
Sichuan Province 632460
China

South-North Society of Traditional Chinese Veterinary Medicine

Liaison: Yang Yingfu, Professor

The Animal Science and Veterinary Medicine Bureau
of Guangxi
Nanning
Guanxi Province 53001
China
PR China

East-China Society of Traditional Veterinary Medicine

Liaison: Son Dalu, Professor
College of Veterinary Medicine
Nanjing
Jiangsu Province 210095
China

Periodicals on Traditional Chinese Veterinary Medicine in China

Journal of Traditional Chinese Veterinary Medicine *(Zhong-Shou-Yi-Yi-Yao-Za-Zhi)*

Liaison: The Journal Board
Lanzhou Institute of Traditional Chinese Veterinary
Medicine
Xiaoxihu, Lanzhou
Gansu Province 730000
China

Chinese Journal of Traditional Veterinary Science *(Zhong-Shou-Yi-Xue-Za-Zhi)*

Liaison: The Journal Board
Jiangxi Institute of Traditional Chinese Veterinary
Medicine
#2 Fuzhou Road, Nanchang
Jiangxi Province, 330006
China

Chinese Journal of Veterinary Medicine *(Zhong-Guo-Shou-Yi-Za-Zhi)*

Liaison: Journal Board
College of Veterinary Medicine
Beijing Agricultural University
Beijing 100094
China

Journal of Chinese Veterinary Science and Technology *(Zhong-Guo-Shou-Yi-Ke-Ji-Zia-Zhi)*

Liaison: Journal Board
Lanzhou Institute of Veterinary Medicine
Yanchangbao, Lanzhou
Gansu Province, 730046
China

REFERENCES

Cheng LF: *China agricultural encyclopedia: the volume of traditional Chinese veterinary medicine* (in Chinese), Beijing, 1991, China Agricultural Publishing House.

Deng YG: personal communication, 1997.

Li KS: *Clinical essentials of traditional Chinese veterinary medicine* (in Chinese), Chengdu, China, 1987, Sichuan Science and Technology Press.

Lu G: personal communication, 1997.

Qu ZM, Xu FZ, Jiang XJ: *A complete set of veterinary herbology* (in Chinese), Beijing, 1991, China Agricultural Science and Technology Press.

Xie HS: *Traditional Chinese veterinary medicine,* Beijing, 1994, Beijing Agricultural University Press.

Yu BY, Yu BH: *Yuan-Heng's therapeutic treatise of horses (Yuan-Heng Liao Ma Ji)* (in Chinese), Beijing, 1963, China Agricultural Publishing House. (Originally published in 1608.)

Yu C: *Traditional Chinese veterinary medicine* (in Chinese), ed 2, Beijing, 1987, China Agricultural Publishing House.

Yu C, Zhang LQ: *A complete set of secret recipes of traditional Chinese veterinary medicine* (in Chinese), Shanxi, China, 1992, Shanxi Science and Technology Press.

Zhang KJ: *Traditional Chinese veterinary formulas* (in Chinese), Henan, China, 1988, Henan Science and Technology Press.

Chapter 23

Chinese Herbal Medicine in Small Animal Practice

CHERYL SCHWARTZ

This chapter is an introduction to basic terminology and theory regarding the use of Chinese herbs in small animal practice. Examples of commonly used herbal formulas for digestive, musculoskeletal, and renal disorders are listed with their Western and Chinese applications. Although Chinese herbs can be used according to Western diagnosis, they have a wider range of efficacy if prescribed using traditional Chinese medicine, in which formulas can be specifically designed for the individual patient. Dosages and applications are based on my 14 years of clinical experience.

A suggested reading list, as well as a listing of some herbal distributors, can be found at the end of the chapter.

Chinese herbology is a vital and integral part of traditional Chinese medicine (TCM). As one of the main branches of TCM, herbs can be used alone or to enhance other treatment modalities such as acupuncture, acupressure, and food therapy. If desired, most herbs can be used with Western medications, provided their intentions are complementary. Herbs are especially useful for patients with chronic conditions that require long-term therapy. One main advantage of using herbs is that herbs help improve and restore internal organ function.

Historical Perspective

Herbology developed as part of the study of TCM along with acupuncture. Diagnosis is made according to the classical TCM categories of the Five Elements, or Phases, and the Eight Principles. Treatment principles are designed to relieve symptoms and to restore physiologic balance by means of the TCM system.

The *Nei Ching,* or *Yellow Emperor's Classics of Internal Medicine,* compiled by physicians in the third century BC, states, "A cold disease should be treated with hot herbs; and a hot disease by cold herbs. . . . Pungent and sweet herbs will disperse internal energy and they are *yang* herbs; sour and bitter herbs will cause diarrhea and they are *yin* herbs" (Lu, 1991).

TCM is deeply rooted in nature, and its terminology refers repeatedly to internal and external environments. Cold diseases are characterized, among other things, by chills, sluggishness, and problems that are worsened by cold environments. Hot diseases are those that cause fevers and inflammations, such as infections. The *Yin* and *Yang* characteristics of herbs refer to the underlying concepts of restful fluids and active movement as discussed more fully below. It is interesting that these basic concepts described in the third century BC are still in effect today.

During the third century AD, herbs were categorized in the *Shang Han Lun* by Zhang Zong-Jing, in *The Discussion of Cold Induced Disorders and Miscellaneous Disease.* The *Shang Han Lun* discusses the stages of disease and their prognoses. This text is still taught today as a basis of TCM. The herbs listed in the *Shang Han Lun* were regrouped several decades later by Wang Shu-He into *The Discussion of Cold Induced Disorders and the Essentials from the Golden Cabinet;* 20% of the herbs listed in that classic are still used.

As the nature and understanding of diseases changed and expanded, Chinese herbology met the challenge by developing new interpretations of the classic TCM categories. Herbal formulas were prescribed to meet the changing diagnoses of the new school of thought based on *Warm Febrile Diseases* (Bensky, 1990).

As more information is being shared between the East and West, modern texts are being written by or for Westerners or by Easterners growing up in Western countries. Dan Bensky and Andrew Gamble compiled the *Chinese Herbal Medicine Materia Medica* (Bensky, Gamble, Kaptchuk, 1986). Sabhuti Dharmananda wrote *Your Nature, Your Health: Chinese Herbs in Constitutional Therapy,* as well as developing the Institute for Traditional Medicine (ITM), which conducts research on and imports Chinese herbs (Dharmananda, 1986). Hong-yen Hsu and Chau-Shin Hsu wrote *Commonly Used Chinese Herb Formulas with Illustrations* (Hsu, Hsu, 1980) as part of the Oriental Healing Arts Institute (OHAI) with its research and publishing facilities. Both ITM and OHAI issue regular herbal research and information bulletins for the practitioner. Jake Fratkin and Margaret Naesser wrote books on the use of patent herbal formulas available in Chinese "over-the-counter" pharmacies (Fratkin, 1987, 1990; Naesser, 1991). Ron Teeguarden wrote a book on Chinese Tonic Herbs (Teeguarden, 1985). Wiseman, Ellis, and Zmiewski wrote *Fundamentals of Chinese Medicine* (Wiseman, Ellis, Zmiewski, 1985), which lists TCM diagnosis, acupuncture, and herbal prescriptions. These books use the Eight Principle categories. Giovanni Maciocia wrote *The Foundations of Chinese Medicine: A Comprehensive Text for Acupuncturists and Herbalists* (Maciocia, 1989). More recently, Harriet Beinfield and Efrem Korngold wrote *Between Heaven and Earth,* which developed a line of herbs based on the Five-Element system (Beinfield, Korngold, 1991). As more practitioners gain experience and knowledge in this country with Chinese herbs, the field of academic dissertations in this subject will grow.

Empirical Evidence and Western Scientific Research

A number of concerns surround the use of herbal medicine. One major issue discussed is the lack of "scientific Western research," in which double-blind studies are used to determine efficacy of a substance. Another concern regards the *precise* dosage and quality of active constituent present.

Herbs were used for more than 1000 years before the advent of the Western scientific model. Much of the knowledge acquired by herbalists has been of the empirical and experiential type. Although some in the West may consider this anecdotal, others look at the large numbers of patients and considerable time involved in accumulating these data and concede that they constitute more than mere anecdotes. In fact, some (myself included) may consider it an early form of *meta-analysis,* in which a large number of studies are cross-sectioned and interpreted for their general principles and conclusions.

More recently, as economic dealings with China and Japan have increased, herbs have entered the international market. In light of this, an increasing amount of "Western type research" has been conducted to support the claims of the thousands of years of herbal experience. Modern scientific and clinical journals such as *The International Journal of Oriental Medicine* and *The American Journal of Chinese Medicine* publish studies gleaned from academic institutions and journals in the East. In addition, some of this research is conducted on mice, rats, and rabbits, which show their efficacy on veterinary patients.

For example, a study conducted at Yunyang Medical College and Tonji Medical University in China demonstrated the effects of the herb gastrodia on vascular impedance and tolerance to ischemia and hypoxia in rabbits and rats. Precise dosage of the herb, methods of preparation and administration, and corroborating electrocardiographic changes accompany the study, which shows an increased blood flow perfusion in the brain and coronary arteries along with peripheral vasodilation. Gastrodia has been used in Chinese herbal medicine formulas to aid in treatment of headaches, dizziness, numbness, and hemiplegia after stroke (Ren, Yu, Zhao, 1994).

Studies in the endocrine field show that the herb rehmannia, which is part of a basic herb formula to enhance renal function, was "shown to increase the level of estradiol in serum of female and of testosterone in male rats" (Chen, Zang, Wu, 1993). Ginsenosides obtained from ginseng and pantocrine, obtained from deer antler, increase the production of luteinizing hormone in rats (Ge, Pu, 1986). The basic "hormone" content of these herbs is very low, so most herbal researchers believe that Chinese herbs act to stimulate hormones by altering the hormone receptors (Dharmananda, 1994).

Use of Western scientific methods to verify clinical experience is helpful to convince the Western practitioner of herbal efficacy. In some cases, it can also lead to new uses for old herbs to treat conditions heretofore untreatable. However, if Western research is used as the sole reliable measure of herbal effectiveness and an indication of new uses, knowledge of ways to use herbs may be seriously hampered. Aside from the vast heritage of traditional Chinese herbology, TCM is based on a valid system of checks and balances in which disease is perceived in an entirely different way than in our Western model. Western medicine looks for a single cause and single effect, whereas Chinese medicine encompasses multiple variables in causes and effects, with the understanding that a disease process results from imbalances between organ systems. This model includes the piecing together of symptoms that fit into the traditional "Chinese differentiation." Because of this, TCM can recognize and treat imbalances before they manifest as clinical diseases according to a specific Western diagnosis. In these cases, proving that an imbalance has been treated is difficult, except by the resolution of subjective symptoms. Because individuals may have specific symptoms, researchers may have problems finding a sufficiently large sample of patients who exhibit identical symptoms. As the understanding of veterinary TCM grows in the United States, practitioners will be more apt to develop studies that combine the special patterns of Chinese differentiation with the needs of the Western model.

Another controversy between the Eastern and Western approaches is the amount of "active constituent" contained within an herb to produce its qualities. Western practitioners look for specific amounts of a particular component that give the desired effect. Many herbologists, however, believe that it is the *entire* plant or mineral that gives the herb its particular qualities. Each plant is unique in location of growth and conditions for optimal health. This is how some herbs were discovered. For example, the sour mountain date, shanzhuyu *(Fructus cornus)* is known for its long growing season (the flower first appears in May), but the fruit itself is not harvested until November. This means that the plant can withstand temperatures and environmental conditions of three seasons, including heat and cold, wet and dry. Herbalists reasoned that if the plant could be productive for this length of time, it would be helpful in sustaining the life of an individual. Cornus is known as one of the "longevity" herbs that strengthen and tonify the liver and the kidneys, helping to retard the aging process. This herb is also helpful in the control of diabetes mellitus (Lu, 1991).

When the entire plant is used, the conditions for which the substance is effective have a far greater range than for a specific active constituent. When researchers seek only one active constituent, they may miss other attributes of the plant that can treat other disorders or balance potential toxic qualities of the substance. Various active constituents in a plant may actually be synergistic. This concept is sometimes difficult for the Western practitioner to comprehend.

Another controversy centers on quality control of herbal products. Because herbs are imported in the form of syrups, pills, powders, and freeze-dried preparations, practitioners in the United States do not believe that they can depend on the purity of these products. Some herbalists also worry about environmental pollutants and processing procedures. Quality control is an important factor to consider in the use of Chinese herbs. Herbal pharmacies in China are required to register with the Chinese government and are subject to their control. In addition, Western wholesale herb buyers usually supervise the herbs that they import into this country.

Patent herbs present the greatest risk of poor quality control. These are preformed herbal combinations that are sold over the counter, similar to products sold in our pharmacies. These herbal preparations have been so commonly used by practitioners over the centuries that herb companies began packaging them in advance rather than "weighing out" the herbal components. Chinese herbal pharmacies store the individual dried herbs in small cabinet drawers. When the pharmacist receives a presciption from a doctor, the prescription is filled by measuring or weighing each individual herb that comprises the formula and combining them into a packet. The patient takes the packet home and prepares the herbs by making teas from the ingredients. Some herb combinations became so commonplace that manufacturers produced ready-made, or *patented,* varieties in pill or liquid form so that the patient would not need to brew the mixture at home. Patent herbs are manufactured by specific pharmacies in specific geographic areas or districts in China. Although all the pharmacies are supposed to be regulated by the Chinese government, regulation of each plant is difficult. Once the packaged herbs reach this country, the Food and Drug Administration (FDA) randomly chooses preparations to check for specific ingredients.

During the years that I have been using patent herbs, I have not had any problems with the formulas as far as toxins. A controversy arose over the use of the incorporation of the Western drug cortisone into certain formulas with its identification on the label. This patent was removed by the FDA. Aside from listed ingredients, the main detraction for use of patent herbs is that because they are so inexpensive, the quality of the herbs used appears to be less potent than the freeze-dried extracts that are being imported and overseen by the Western companies who deal in China.

Companies such as *Sun Ten* and *Min Tong* freeze-dried herbs, dried herb importers such as the Institute for Preventive Health and Medicine (ITM) in Portland, Health Concerns in California, and herbal tincture producers such as McZand Herbals in California, to name a few, have special buyers in China who perform quality control checks. Individual herbs are chosen by these companies with regard to time of harvesting, processing, and potency.

Because some patients of TCM practitioners live in the West, some herbalists and environmentalists believe that it would be best for these patients to use Western herbs because these herbs are grown locally. In some cases this is an improvement, because the quality control can be greater. It is interesting that there is great overlap of the use of Western and Chinese herbs. Some herbalists trained in TCM are beginning to use Western herbs according to their Chinese indications, and this may prove to be a future use of herbs.

Legal Aspects

Unlike acupuncture, which the American Veterinary Medical Association (AVMA) has recognized as a valid modality, Chinese herbology is classified as a form of holistic medicine, along with chiropractic, homeopathy, and energy medicine. Accordingly, herbs are considered unconventional medicine and of an experimental nature. Patients should be informed of this if herbs are used in practice. Clinically I have found herbs to be of enormous use and efficacy in small animal practice. A client release form may be appropriate before the use of herbs.

Advantages of Using Herbs

Herbs can be used for their *tonifying,* or strengthening, characteristics. They can be used for short-term tonifying to help rebuild the individual about a bout of illness or after chemotherapy or radiation therapy. Herbs can be used long term for chronic degenerative conditions such as osteoarthritis and immune, renal, and hepatic disorders to help strengthen and rebalance the body and alleviate symptoms. Herbs can be used for TCM patterns that are unrecognizable in Western differentiations. Herbs can be tailored to specific individuals for very particular needs. Herbs also can be used preventively to boost the immune system at the outbreak of disease. Herbs have been shown to have antiviral capabilities. They can also be used in the case of drug sensitivities.

Discussion of the categories for herb use requires definitions of some basic terminology used in Chinese medicine. Definitions are important because practitioners must be able to match a category of disease or imbalance with a category of herb, and these categories encompass TCM.

The TCM classifications are broken down into concepts of the Eight Principles and Five Elements (or Phase) system.

Categories of the Eight Principles are derivatives of Yin and Yang. Other important categories are *excess* and *deficiency*, *cold* and *hot*, and *interior* and *exterior*.

Yin is like water, with a tendency to be cold and heavy. *Yin* moistens the surface and interior of the body, helps internal fluids flow, and controls relaxation and restfulness. When *Yin* is out of balance, it can become *excessive* or *deficient*. In practice, an animal with an excess of *Yin* is overly restful (i.e., lethargic). It may become cold easily. Animals with a *Yin* excess tend to be overweight, thirstless, and sluggish in digestion and attitude. Ascites or edema may be evident. Discharges from eyes, nose, and ears are watery and thin. Animals with a deficiency of *Yin* do not have sufficient calming capacity and are therefore restless or irritable. They pace, howl, and are intolerant of heat. Excessive thirst; constipation; red, dry skin; dry eyes; and an increase in metabolic rate occur. A deficiency of *Yin* may cause symptoms similar to those associated with excess *Yang*.

Yang is like fire with its heating, active, moving, and circulating abilities. If the heat is excessive, it can burn up the internal fluid, creating dryness (as with a deficient *Yin* individual) or frank inflammation. Bleeding tendencies, fevers, tachycardia, hyperthyroid, and hypermotile gastrointestinal tracts are examples of excessive *Yang* or internal heat. If the *Yang* is deficient, the animal will be sluggish and exhibit symptoms similar to those associated with excess *Yin*.

Patients with Cold disorders have difficulties with circulation and temperature regulation. Some cannot hold their urine at night or exhibit polyuria. All their symptoms are worse during cold weather. Osteoarthritis exacerbated by cold temperatures is an example. Individuals with cold tendencies usually have sluggish immune systems and repeatedly get low-grade chronic infections that are difficult to resolve. Part of the traditional Chinese medical examination includes tongue analysis. The patient with a cold disorder has a pale tongue with a white coating.

Patients with Heat disorders have an excess of *Yang* internal heat. These animals are intolerant of heat and tend to pant excessively, preferring the shade, cement floors, and open windows. They have odorous, thick discharges, usually yellow, green, or brown in color. Their stool has a strong odor and often contains mucus or blood. The tongue coating is usually yellow or appears dirty, and the tongue body is dark pink or red.

Patients with deficiencies lack confidence, fluids, muscle mass, and stamina. These patients are timid, shy, clingy, and fearful of noise. For example, a dog with a weak whimper rather than a strong bark or a cat with a silent meow may have a deficiency. Animals with deficiencies usually enjoy petting and touching. They often have thin and lusterless hair coats, thin tongue coatings, and small amounts of discharge. *Deficiency* refers to a lack of one of the vital substances of *Qi*, *Blood*, *Yang*, or *Yin*. Depending on which vital substance is deficient, the signs can be varied.

Animals with *excess* disorders are often aggressive. Dogs with excesses may bark loudly and fiercely at everything. Depending on which vital substance is excessive, the animal may exhibit excessive discharge, strong odors, or excessive appetite. The hair coat is usually oily and odorous, and the tongue coating is thick.

Interior and *Exterior* refer to the duration and depth of illness. Exterior conditions are superficial (e.g., acute flu and upper respiratory tract infections). Interior conditions are of longer duration and affect the internal organ systems (e.g., renal and hepatic failure).

The next classifications that correspond to the Eight Principles are the vital essences: the *Qi*, the Fluid, and the blood.

Qi is the energy circulating through the body and the energy channels (called *meridians*). *Qi* promotes vitality and is responsible for all the movement and activity within the body, as well as the immune system. *Qi* directs the digestive process and respiration. *Qi* disturbances can cause vomiting, bile secretion problems, pasty stools, and diarrhea. *Qi* disturbances affiliated with the Kidney in Chinese medicine can affect the spinal column, creating arthritis, calcification, disk problems, and pain. A deficiency of *Qi* causes fatigue. *Qi* is closely associated with the *Yang* of the body and the Blood.

In Chinese medicine the Blood is more than the physical substance we know in Western medicine. The Chinese ascribe other attributes to the Blood. The Blood is said to be stored by the liver during periods of rest and circulated by the heart and the liver during activity. If the Blood movement is hampered, stagnation occurs. Stagnation results in pain and the potential for tumor formation and stroke. The Spleen is said to keep the blood within the vessels, so that oozing-type hemorrhages, such as those that occur in thrombocytopenia, are under the control of the spleen. The Blood is also helpful for bathing the organs and keeping them functioning. The Fluid refers to the *Yin* fluid of the body, including tears and saliva and joint, tissue, and abdominal fluids.

In addition to Cold and Heat, finally environmental factors should be considered—namely, *Wind, Dampness,* and *Dryness. Wind* refers to characteristics that move from one body place to another, like a gust of wind or polyarthritis. Wind, when it enters the body, can also cause pain in the muscles. It also refers to an infection that comes on suddenly, such as upper respiratory tract flus. *Dampness* refers to the state of moisture held within the tissues. Dampness affects water movement throughout the body and can therefore affect digestion, urination, respiration, and joint movement. Dryness reflects a lack of moisture in the tissues that is exacerbated in dry environments.

In addition to the Eight Principles and vital essences, another system known as the *Five Phases,* or *Five Elements,* is studied. Each element refers to a specific internal organ system and its extended definition in traditional Chinese terms.

The Elements are *Earth, Metal, Water, Wood,* and *Fire.* The Earth element is associated with the spleen and Stomach. The Metal element is associated with the Lungs and Large Intestine. The Water element is associated with the Kidney and Urinary Bladder. The Wood element is associated with the Liver and Gallbladder, and the Fire element is associated with the Heart and Small Intestine, along with two Chinese categories of the Triple Heater and Pericardium. Herbs are also used to tonify certain organ systems, as manifested by certain imbalances. Each of the elements can be affected by any of the Eight Principle qualities listed.

Tonification

Tonification herbs are used to strengthen *Qi, Blood, Yin,* and *Yang,* as well as specific organ systems. For example, if an animal has soft, mushy stools, belches frequently, or has a weight problem (too high or too low), *Qi* tonics are used. An example of a *Qi* tonic is ginseng. If an animal has anemia or dry skin or is extremely timid, blood tonics are used. An example of a Blood tonic is *Tang Kuei.* If an animal has excessive agitation, thirst, or dry hot skin, *Yin* tonics are used. An example is ophiopogan. If an animal has excessive lethargy, weak hind legs, and poor circulation worsened by cold temperatures, *Yang* tonics are used. An example is Eucommiae. After chemotherapy or radiation therapy, when an individual is weakened and the immune system is vulnerable to attack, the *Qi* tonic of *Astragalus* has been shown to increase stamina and enhance immune protection.

Preventive and Antiviral

Some herbs can be used to prevent illness. These herbs are categorized as *Qi* tonics (e.g., *Astragalus* and ganoderma mushrooms). Other herbs used as preventives fall under the categories of Heat or toxin-clearing herbs. The herb *Radix isatidis (Ban Lan Gen)* has been shown to "forestall the epidemic nature of mumps" in a study of over 11,000 people (Bensky, Gamble, 1986).

Chronic Degenerative Conditions

Herbs may be used to treat conditions such as arthritis, chronic renal, lung, and hepatic failure; autoimmune problems; and Addison's and Cushing's diseases. The treatment principle in arthritis is to alleviate pain and strengthen the underlying organs whose imbalances have initially caused the problem—namely the Kidney and the Liver. Recent studies in China have shown that a combination of the herbs ligustrum and eclipta satisfactorily treated IgA nephropathy when hematuria was the chief clinical symptom and when Western medication had proved ineffective (Schwartz, 1993). The herb rhizoma coptidis *(Huang Lian)* helps increase the formation of bile and decrease its viscosity. It is used for chronic cholecystitis (Bensky, Gamble, 1986) and in the treatment of chronic flare-ups of hepatitis and cirrhosis of the liver.

Certain herbs, such as the tree mushroom, *Lentinus edodes,* have been shown to enhance immunity by activating the complement system, influencing macrophages, and helper T cells (Bensky, Gamble, 1986). These herbs contain polysaccharides. The polysaccharide family has also been shown to inhibit tumor growth. In studies in Japan and Korea the ganoderma mushroom polysaccharides inhibited up to 98% of implanted tumor cells in mice. Ginseng and eleuthro ginseng also contain polysaccharides (Dharmananda, 1988).

Unrecognizable Western Patterns

Vague symptoms of digestive disturbances, such as abdominal distention after eating or sluggish digestion, may be treatable with TCM when no Western diagnostic test is conclusive. Symptoms of disharmony between the Liver and Spleen qualify in this regard, and herbs such as bupleurum, pinellia, and citrus peel can be used to enhance the digestive processes while bringing the Liver and Spleen back into balance.

Vague symptoms of excessive yawning or flank-biting can be attributed to a function of the liver known as "Liver *Qi* constraint." Yawning is a symptom of a blockage in the *Qi* flow or circulation of the middle compartment of the body. When blockage exists, pain, itching, numbness or tingling, and tumor formation can occur. Yawning may be the first symptom of this, and if this can be addressed, future problems may be avoided. Herbs such as bupleurum, cnidium, and peony can be used.

Drug Sensitivity

Some individuals are sensitive to antiinflammatory agents such as cortisone, which can create excessive urination or mood swings. Depending on the condition, herbs can mediate the inflammation. For example, the combination of clematis and stephania can be used instead of cortisone for muscle and joint pain worsened by damp and cold weather. Skin problems may be lessened with herbs such as *Tribulus* (to decrease pruritus) and anemarrhena (to decrease inflammation). Scutellaria can be used as an antibiotic substitute, especially in conditions of lung inflammations and immune disorders. Scutellaria has the ability to inhibit the release of enzymes from mast cells, making it helpful in formulas in which asthma is an underlying condition for frequent lung infections (Bensky, Gamble, 1986).

Treatment Principles

After identifying an imbalance according to the Eight Principles of *Yin/Yang*, Cold/Hot, Excess/Deficiency, and Interior/Exterior, the practitioner evaluates the individual's constitution and the resulting symptoms. The practitioner then determines the treatment goal and chooses herbs according to their traditional Chinese qualities and classifications to rebalance the patient. Many variables are considered, and the individual, *not* the disease, is treated.

The herbal treatment principles revolve around restoring balance. If the individual exhibits too much *Yang* or internal heat, herbs with cooling capabilities are chosen. If an individual shows deficiency signs, herbs are chosen to strengthen the weak organ or vital substance. If an individual presents excessive signs, herbs are chosen to eliminate the excess. If an individual exhibits cold signs, herbs are chosen for their warming properties. If an individual is suffering from an acute attack, herbs are chosen to relieve the exterior or body surface and promote vasodilation. In summary, the herbal treatment principles are as follows (Table 23-1):

- Cool the Heat
- Warm the Cold
- Clear or Sedate the Excess
- Tonify the Deficiency
- Relieve the Surface

Classifications of Herbs

Herbs have specific (1) flavors or tastes, (2) energies or characteristics, (3) meridians or organs of influence, (4) directions, (5) categories, and (6) actions.

Flavors

Each flavor has its own purpose: Sweet nourishes organs and *Qi*. Astragalus is an example. Sour dries and strengthens mucous membranes of the gastrointestinal and respiratory tracts, as well as the linings of arteries. Chinese hawthorne *(Crataegus)* is an example. Hot/Spicy/Pungent or Acrid disperses *Qi*, fluids, or blood, inducing perspiration, dilating surface blood vessels, and relieving acute conditions such as upper respiratory tract infections. Thorny ginseng (Acanthopanax) is an example. Bitter detoxifies and is useful in infectious or inflammatory conditions. Bitter apricot kernel (Kuxingren) is an example.

Salty softens masses, which the Chinese believe is the first step toward eliminating a tumor that has formed. Salty herbs are also used for thyroid tumors. *Inula japonica (xuanfuhua)* is an example (Lu, 1991).

Energies and Temperatures

Herbs are described as Hot, Warm, Cold, Cool, and Neutral. Hot herbs such as processed aconite are used to warm the vitality, as required by animals in a state of collapse with blue mucous membranes and circulatory shutdown. Warm herbs such as ginger are used to help aid circulation and remove internal coldness. Cold herbs such as scutellaria are used to detoxify bacterial or viral infections. Cool herbs such as Momordicae fruit *(Luohanguo)* are used to decrease inflammation. Neutral herbs such as lycium fruit *(Gouqizi)* are used to balance the formulas and tonify the *Qi*.

Meridians

Influence of meridians corresponds to the paired internal organ systems of the Five Element/Phase system: Spleen/Stomach, Lung/Large Intestine, Kidney/Urinary Bladder, Liver/Gallbladder, Heart/Pericardium, Small Intestine/Triple Heater.

Directions

When internalized, each herb has the ability to disperse in a certain direction. This ability provides their affiliation with certain organs and allows them to be directed to a certain area of the body. The directions follow:

Ascending, or *Yang*—Garlic and bupleurum are examples.
Descending, or *Yin*—Raw rehmannia is an example.
Sinking, such as diuretics or seizure inhibitors—Oyster shell is an example.
Outward, which disperses energy as needed in eliminating an acute attack—*Ma-huang* twig is an example.

Categories

The categories are described as the Eight Principles; the three vital substances of *Qi*, Blood, and Fluid; the Five Elements of Earth, Metal, Water, Wood, and Fire; and the pathologic environmental Factors and Products. This last category is involved with environmental influences, as discussed above—wind, dampness, dryness, and heat. Heat is pathologic if it enters the body, causing heatstroke, severe fevers, and inflammations creating hemorrhage. Dryness is pathologic if it creates dry skin, dry coughs, constipation, or excessive thirst. Individuals with the propensity for *Yin*-deficient problems or lung deficiencies are most susceptible to dryness. Dampness is a factor that causes problems to worsen in wet or damp environments. Exam-

TABLE 23-1

SUMMARY OF TREATMENT PRINCIPLES

COMMON PATIENT SYNDROMES	TREATMENT PRINCIPLE
YIN EXCESS COLD (CAN MIMIC DEFICIENT *YANG*) • Watery eyes, nose, copious discharge • Tendency to diarrhea, loose, pasty stool • Frequent or dilute urination • Lack of thirst • Lack of vital heat • Lethargic • Bloated abdomen, ascites • Edema, coldness of limbs • Need for constant petting, touch	Use herbs to nurture the *Yang*, warm and circulate dry moisture, and tonify *Qi*
YANG EXCESS HOT (CAN MIMIC DEFICIENT *YIN*) • Inflammations, fevers, infections • Thick, purulent, colored, or scanty discharges • Offensive odors from skin, ears • Constipation • Thirst • Scanty, very concentrated urine • Hyperactivity (pacing, anxiety, panting) • Rage syndromes • Hyperthyroid • Tendency to seek shade, cement floors • Refusal of touch	Use herbs to nurture the *Yin*, cool and sedate, and lubricate
QI DISTURBANCES (DEFICIENCY, STASIS, STAGNATION) • Vomiting • Diarrhea, pasty stool • Poor appetite • Malabsorption • Lethargy • Stone formation • Disk, spinal calcification • Tumor/cyst formation • Weak hind legs	Use herbs to circulate the *Qi*, invigorate the *Yang*, dry the moisture, regulate the *Qi*
WIND SYNDROMES (PAIN) • Musculoskelatal pain • Rheumatoid arthritis, polyarthritis • Headaches, watery eyes, common cold • Twitching, spasms, seizures	Use herbs to treat the surface, relieve the pain, clear the channels

ples are arthritis, which is worse in damp weather; asthma; allergic bronchitis; emphysema, which is worse in humid weather; urinary tract infections, in which straining occurs but no blood or crystals appear; and diarrhea of the pasty, watery, low-odor type, in which food particles remain in the feces. Phlegm is a pathologic product that accumulates when a problem with water distribution occurs in the body. An underlying problem with the liver is usually pres-

ent; which creates stagnation in circulation, allowing accumulation of energy (Qi) or fluid in a certain place and absence of *Qi* or fluid in other places. The stagnation causes fluid to heat up and congeal, creating sticky mucus that can affect the respiratory or gastrointestinal systems. In TCM, phlegm can also create pain and inflammation of the joints and contribute to seizures. Phlegm can also congeal, creating tumors, cysts, and growths.

Actions

In Western terms, actions are the indications for use (Bensky, Gamble, 1986). TCM contains classical actions and modern expansions that encompass almost every condition. The 14 classical categories are as follows:

- *Tonification:* Tonification is used to restore deficient conditions of depleted body fluids and vitality.
- *Heat Clearing:* Heat clearing is used to clear excess conditions such as fevers.
- *Diaphoresing:* Diaphoresing is used to create surface vasodilation and sweating to alleviate acute viral and bacterial infections.
- *Draining dampness:* Draining dampness is used to diurese and produce an astringent effect on conditions such as edema and urinary and gastrointestinal straining.
- *Expelling wind:* Expelling wind is used to alleviate pain in the musculoskeletal and nervous systems.
- *Transforming:* Transforming is used to alter phlegm in the lungs, intestines, and joints and softening of masses.
- *Regulating:* Regulating is used to circulate the blood, lymph, and *Qi.*
- *Harmonizing:* Harmonizing is used to aid digestion among the liver, spleen, and intestines.
- *Invigorating:* Invigorating is used to circulate and warm. This is helpful in alleviating abdominal pain, menstrual irregularities, and abdominal masses.
- *Dispersing:* Dispersing is used to break up stagnation in blood and *Qi,* including breaking up masses.
- *Parasiticides:* Parasiticides are used to expel parasites.
- *Calming the spirit:* Calming the spirit tranquilizes the subject and relieves hyperexcitability.
- *Purging:* Purging is used for laxative purposes.
- *Emetics:* Emetics are used for vomiting and food poisonings.

For example, a practitioner would choose an herb such as *Astragalus* for its tonifying characteristics. *Astragalus* helps enhance the immune system by tonifying *Qi,* Blood, and *Yang. Astragalus* is warm and sweet, with an ascending and descending direction. Affiliated with the spleen and Lung meridians, it strengthens vitality, decreases fatigue, enhances the appetite, and normalizes bowel movement. It also helps drain dampness by promoting urination as part of its ability to strengthen the spleen.

Pinellia is a warm, acrid herb that disperses and transforms cold phlegm. It is affiliated with the spleen and stomach. It is used for vomiting of water and mucus in the treatment of borborygmus, watery diarrhea, and watery coughs.

Herbal Formulas

Most herbalists prescribe herbal formulas that combine single herbs in a complete prescription. Although some herbs can be used alone, formulas usually combine 2 to 15 herbs that address specific symptoms and the underlying imbalance. Herbs are combined and balanced according to their energies, properties, tastes, and actions. More than 2000 herbs are available.

Each formula contains a chief herb, whose main action addresses the prevailing symptom; a ministerial herb, whose action enhances the chief herb or addresses a coexisting pattern; assistant herbs, whose actions are minimize side effects or balance the directions and tastes; and *envoy herbs,* whose actions harmonize the formula (Bensky, Barolet, 1990).

Types of Formulations

Freeze-dried herbs have a very long shelf life if kept dry. They usually come in 100-g packages and can be divided as needed. Storage is best in covered, dark-brown jars of plastic or glass. Dried and powdered herbs have a shorter shelf life. Dried herbs can be administered as tablets or loose powders.

Tinctured herbs contain varying amounts of alcohol, usually ranging from 13% to 40%. Small dogs and cats are sensitive to the alcohol; therefore the alcohol should be removed by boiling the tincture before use. Tinctured herbs also can be diluted for animal use. Herbal tinctures can be diluted by 50% with distilled water (half herb/half water) or in a mixture of one third herb/two thirds water, depending on the sensitivity of the animal and the severity of the problem. The diluted herb prescription can be uncapped and the opened bottle placed in the top part of a double boiler over the steam of boiling water below. Steam from the boiling water should be allowed to surround the herbal liquid for 5 minutes.

Patent herbs are packaged in small, black-brown, pelletlike pills, sugar-coated tablets, tiny pellets in small vials, capsules, liquids, and wax eggs.

A list of herb distributors is provided at the end of the chapter.

Dosage and Time of Administration

Herbs can be given with meals. Practitioners are advised to give the herb with a small amount of food at the beginning of the meal. If a meal is not eaten at time of administration, a snack should be given. Herbs can also be given approximately 30 minutes after mealtime (Box 23-1).

The lower dosage should be used when a range of dosages is available. Overdosage of the herbs listed usually results in digestive disturbances, including diarrhea, depressed appetite, and occasionally vomiting. Other effects of sensitivity or overdosage include fatigue and lethargy. If these symptoms occur, use of the herb should be discontinued for 48 hours. Most animals revert to normal behavior within the first 12 hours. The herb can be given again at half the dosage indicated. If the problem

BOX 23-1

Typical Herb Dosages

FREEZE-DRIED HERBS

Cat/small dog (10 to 15 lb):	⅛ to ¼ tsp or 1 to 2 #2 capsules bid/tid
Medium dog (up to 50 lb):	½ tsp bid/tid
Large dog (50 lb or over):	⅔ to ¾ tsp bid

DRIED HERBS PRESSED INTO CAPLET FORM (E.G., I.T.M. SEVEN FORESTS, HEALTH CONCERNS)

Cat/small dog (10 to 15 lb):	½ caplet bid/tid
Medium dog (up to 50 lb):	1 caplet bid/tid
Large dog (50 lb or over):	1½ to 2 caplets bid/tid

TINCTURES (HERBAL APOTHECARY, MCZAND)

Diluted herb: half herb/half distilled water, or one third herb/two thirds distilled water

Cats/small dog (10 to 15 lb):	1 ml bid/tid
Medium dog (up to 50 lb):	1.5 to 2 ml bid/tid
Large dog (50 lb or over):	2.5 cc bid/tid

PATENT HERBS

Pellets

Cat/small dog (10 to 15 lb):	2 pellets bid/tid
Medium dog (up to 50 lb):	4 to 6 pellets bid/tid
Large dog (50 lb or over):	6 to 8 pellets bid/tid

Coated tablets

Cat/small dog (10 to 15 lb):	1 tablet bid
Medium dog (up to 50 lb):	2 tablets bid/tid
Large dog (50 lb or over):	3 to 4 tablets bid/tid

being treated is severe and acute, herbs should be administered 3 times daily. If the problem is chronic, twice daily usually suffices.

If herbs are being given in addition to Western medication, as with cortisone, furosemide (Lasix), and heart medications, the herb is best administered separately, at least 1 hour after administration of Western medication. When herbs are added to the regimen, sometimes a lower dose of the Western medication is required because part of the purpose of the herb is to strengthen the underlying organ system. An illustration of this phenomenon is the use of stephania and ginseng combination, which is used for congestive heart failure with pulmonary edema. Administration of this herbal combination may require a reduction in the furosemide dosage. Observation of the patient during the first 5 days of herb therapy for symptoms of excess diuresis is a good plan. Any dramatic changes, such as a large increase in water intake, should always be monitored when herbs are added to any treatment regimen.

Herbs can be used for months or even years for chronic deficiency problems. In general, tonic herbs are given daily for 6 to 8 weeks, upon which patient reassessment is essential. A long-term plan of herb administration for 5 of 7 days a week or 3 weeks on and 1 week off can be tried. In some cases, such as in chronic renal failure, kidney tonic

herbs are used continuously for months or years. Patients should be monitored, as with use of any other long-term medication.

In acute situations, herbs are used for 3 to 14 days depending on the severity of the symptoms. Many herbs that clear fever or infection can injure the *Qi* if used for longer than 2 weeks without modification.

Specific Formulations

Although Chinese herbs are best prescribed according to each individual's constitutional makeup, the following herbs have been used for periods from 5 to 14 years. They are listed according to their western and Chinese differentiations.

Individual herbs with TCM functions were taken from Bensky's and Gamble's *Chinese Herbal Medicine Materia Medica* and Dharmananda's course book (Bensky, Gamble, 1986; Dharmananda, 1981).

Herbs for Digestion

The classifications of herbs for digestion are those used in the treatment of (1) weakness or "deficiency" spleen or stomach *Qi*, resulting in poor appetite, fatigue, weight problems, and malabsorption (tonic herbs); (2) a disharmony between the liver and stomach, resulting in gas, burping, and abdominal distention (regulating herbs); (3) painful or violent vomiting of bile, food, or blood from gastroenteritis, ulcers, or both (cooling herbs); and (4) painful colitis from a liver, spleen, and large intestine imbalance, which requires cooling and relief (stagnation herbs).

Qi tonics for deficient spleen or stomach

In TCM, digestion is governed by the spleen and stomach, which regulate the *Qi*. The spleen, which is associated with the pancreas in TCM, transforms the food to be used by the body, helping the stomach to break nutrients down and transporting them to the *Qi* and Blood. In conjunction with the kidneys and lungs, the spleen also regulates the moisture throughout the digestive tract.

The spleen is sensitive to dampness-producing foods (e.g., sugars, cold foods) and damp environments. The stomach transports the food and water downward into the small intestine. Spleen *Qi* and *Yang* are closely related with the *Yang*, including the warming and activating aspects of the *Qi*. Many of the Spleen *Qi*–tonifying formulas contain *Yang* and moving herbs.

When Spleen *Qi* is weak, digestive disorders such as vomiting (known as *rebellious Qi*), borborygmus (water stagnation in the stomach), food accumulation and subsequent slow digestive emptying (as in pyloric malfunctions, flatulence, malabsorption, mild ulcers from stagnation and stomach heat), phlegm formation (when the moisture-moving ability of the spleen is impaired, it stagnates and congeals, forming phlegm), and loose, pasty stools with food particles can occur. Chronic *Qi* problems lead to weight loss and fatigue, flaccid musculature, poor appetite, and an anxious appearance. Two basic formulas can be used.

FOUR-MAJOR-HERB COMBINATION (Brion, Min Tong Freeze Dried) (Hsu, Hsu, 1980) This formula enhances *Qi*, appetite, assimilation, and weight gain and alleviates pasty stool in patients exhibiting *Qi* deficiency. Because this formula is considered one of the building blocks of *Qi* tonics, the single herbs are listed with their flavors, thermal temperatures, directions, meridians, and categories. Ingredients include the following:

- Ginseng (sweet, warm, ascending) tonifies Spleen *Qi* and enhances immunity
- Licorice (sweet, warm) tonifies Spleen *Qi* and harmonizes digestion
- Ginger (acrid, warm, outward, or dispersing) warms the center and disperses and tonifies Spleen *Qi*
- Jujube (sweet, neutral) warms the center and tonifies Spleen *Qi*, producing a steroidal-like action
- Atractylodes (sweet, warm, ascending, and descending) tonifies Spleen *Qi* and drains dampness

- Hoelen (sweet, bland, neutral) drains dampness, produces antitumor activity, and tonifies Spleen *Qi*

SHEN QI DA BU WAN (Naesser, 1991) (Patent herb pellets). This formulation is useful for fatigue, poor appetite, weakness after long-standing illness, and weight loss. It is also useful for boosting *Qi* and immunity in cats with FeLV or FIV between outbreaks or for cats in households with continual exposure to FeLV or FIV. The ingredients are *Astragalus* and codonopsis, both *Qi* tonics of the spleen and lung and appetite stimulants.

Harmonizing and regulating herbs

CENTRAL *QI* TEA (Patent Medicine, pellets) (Fratkin, 1987). This formulation is useful for the maintenance of good digestion, especially in cases of abdominal bloating and flatulence. The ingredients include the following:

- *Astragalus*, which is a Spleen and Lung *Qi* tonic that lowers blood pressure in dogs, cats, and rabbits and decreases proteinuria in glomerulonephritis
- Codonopsis, licorice, jujube, and atractylodes, which warm and tonify Spleen *Qi* and regulate moisture
- *Tang Kuei*, which tonifies spleen and liver blood
- Cimicifuga, which cools inflammation from the lung, spleen, and stomach
- Citrus, which acts as a *Qi* regulator
- Bupleurum, which cools the liver and harmonizes digestion between the liver and the spleen

ZISHENG STOMACHIC PILLS (Patent Medicine, pellets) (Fratkin, 1987). This is for chronic digestive disturbances, including pancreatitis, stomach pain, nausea, poor appetite, malabsorption, and congestion of Liver *Qi* that causes pain and bloating. They are also used after splenectomy to help regulate digestion. Ingredients include the following:

- Codonopsis as a Spleen and Lung *Qi* tonic
- Atractylodes and hoelen, which act as a Spleen *Qi* tonic and aid in moisture distribution
- Coix seed, which warms the Spleen *Yang*, regulates moisture, and decreases fatigue
- Citrus, which regulates *Qi*
- *Crataegus* fruit, which functions as a sour spleen, stomach, and liver tonic, aiding in motility through the intestine and pyloric valve (relieves food stagnation in TCM)
- Euryale seed, which astringes the spleen and kidney and stops diarrhea
- Dioscorea, which tonifies the Spleen, Lung and Kidney *Qi*, and hoelen

PINELLIA COMBINATION (Dharmananda, 1988) (Brion Freeze Dried, Herbal Apothecary tincture). This formula is useful for acute or chronic vomiting that occurs either immediately after eating or several hours after eating; vomiting of water; vomiting from kidney weakness, stomach ulcers; nausea; anorexia; borborygmus; diarrhea caused by spleen deficiency; and nervous vomiting. The tongue is usually moist and has a white and sometimes greasy coating. The ingredients include ginseng, ginger, and jujube from the Four Major herb tonic formula, with scute and coptis added to cool inflammation in the heart, lung, gallbladder, liver, and large intestine, along with Pinellia, which transforms phlegm in the gastrointestinal tract that causes vomiting of water or mucus.

Gastroenteritis, fever, dysentery, ulcers

COPTIS AND SCUTE COMBINATION (Brion Freeze Dried, McZand and Herbal Apothecary tinctures) (Fratkin, 1990). This combination is useful for gastroenteritis with vomiting and fever and vomiting or diarrhea caused by ulcerations with bleeding. The formula should be used for no longer than 2 weeks because prolonged use injures the *Qi*. This combination contains bitter and cold herbs to decrease inflammation, fight infection, stop bleeding tendencies, and clear excess moisture from the digestive tract. The ingredients are scute, affecting the heart, liver, stomach, and large intestine; phellodendron, affecting the kidney and bladder; gardenia, affecting the liver, lung, stomach; and coptis, affecting the heart, liver stomach, and large intestine.

PILL CURING (Fratkin, 1987) (Patent herb, vials, use ½ to 1 vial tid up to 5 days, McZand tincture). This combination is used for vomiting and diarrhea of acute onset. The formula mixes cooling and warming bitter and sweet herbs to address flulike syndromes with chills, low fevers, and body aches. Because it also contains some mild Spleen *Qi* tonics, it can be used longer term than the coptis and scute formula. This combination is safe during pregnancy and can be used in human patients to treat morning sickness. In animals it can be used for prolonged periods at one half vial daily to help regulate sluggish digestion in preulcerative conditions with pyloric valve problems. The ingredients include the following:

- Gastrodia, chrysanthemum, pueraria, mentha, and trichosanthis to expel wind (acute-onset infections), stop headache, and cool digestion
- Angelica to alleviate body aches
- Saussurea to regulate *Qi*
- Atractylodes to tonify Spleen *Qi* and regulate moisture
- Magnolia, which transforms phlegm and sticky moisture in the body that slows digestive motility (food stagnation in TCM)

Painful colitis with blood, mucus, and straining

Painful colitis accompanied by blood, mucus, and straining is a complex condition caused by an imbalance among the liver, spleen, stomach, and large intestine. Although no particular herb combination has been successful in all cases, one combination has been helpful in approximately one third of the cases I have seen.

ISATIS COOLING (Health Concerns, caplets) (Health Concerns, 1995). The ingredients include isatis extract, moutain, and gardenia to clear heat; akebia and alisma to drain dampness; red peony to invigorate blood and decrease pain; oyster shell to calm; bupleurum and smilax to clear the liver; *tang kuei* to nourish the blood; codonopsis to nourish the *Qi*; and cyperus to regulate the *Qi*.

Herbs for Musculoskeletal Disorders

According to TCM, pain is caused by a blockage of *Qi* and blood in the channels and meridians (energy pathways) of the body. Muscle pain, stiffness, osteoarthritis, spondylosis, and rheumatoid arthritis are all considered part of the *Bi* syndrome. *Bi* syndrome encompasses four types of arthritis that all have the component of the pathologic factor wind. Wandering *Bi* is pain that travels from joint to joint (like the wind) with acute onset. Fixed *Bi* is caused by a combination of wind and dampness, and creates swelling in the joints or surrounding tissues. Fixed *Bi* is worse in a damp environment. Painful *Bi* is pain in the joints that worsens in cold weather. Febrile *Bi* occurs with inflammation and infection in the joints (Limehouse, 1989). Osteoarthritis can involve parts of each of these syndromes and is the most long-standing and detrimental to patients.

Certain herb combinations can be helpful in reducing pain according to which syndrome is most basic. *Du Huo Jiseng Wan* (Patent Medicine, pellets, McZand tincture) (Fratkin, 1987) is beneficial for the animal with stiffness and pain in the lower back and hind legs that worsens in cold and damp weather. Calcification may be present. The animal's condition improves with massage and pressure of the limbs and back. The ingredients include the following:

- Eucommia, which strengthens the back and is a kidney yang tonic
- Rehmannia, which nourishes the liver and kidney blood
- *Tang kuei*, which nourishes the blood and helps dispel pain
- *Du huo*, which nourishes the kidney yang and bladder to expel wind, dampness, cold, and pain
- Cinnamon bark, codonopsis, and ginger, which warm the circulation and act as Spleen *Qi* tonics
- Hoelen, which drains dampness and acts as a Spleen Qi tonic
- Licorice as a harmonizer

CLEMATIS AND STEPHANIA COMBINATION (Freeze Dried, McZand tincture) (Hsu, 1994). This formulation is useful for the dog or cat with weak hind legs, stiffness that improves with movement, lumbosacral pain, sciatic pain, knee pain, hip dysplasia, and numbness. It is helpful in painful flare-ups of spondylitis. The ingredients include the following:

- *Tang kuei*, peony, persica, rehmannia, and ligusticum to tonify and invigorate the blood
- Hoelen, stephania, and atractylodes to drain dampness and help the spleen transform dampness
- Clematis for pain caused by wind and dampness
- Notopterygium, siler, ginger, and angelica to dispel wind and coldness pain
- Gentiana to clear dampness and heat
- Achyranthis to tonify Kidney *Yin* and *Yang*

DRYNARIA 12 (ITM dried caplets) (Dharmananda, 1992). This formulation is used to treat chronic osteoarthritis, including aspects of wind, cold, and dampness. The ingredients include the following:

- Drynaria, dipsacus, achyranthes, eucommia, and deer antler to tonify the yang and warm and strengthen the bones
- Rehmannia, millettia, cnidium, and *Tang kuei* to nourish the blood and help the circulation to relieve pain
- Asarum to relieve wind and pain
- Astragalus to tonify the *Qi*

KANG GU ZHENG SHENG PIAN* (Patent, sugar-coated pill) (Combat the Bone Hyperplasia Pill) (Fratkin, 1987). This formula is indicated for spinal inflammation or disk injury and can be used after the disk has calcified, after surgery, or in cases when surgery is not recommended. It can also be used preventively to avoid further disk injuries to surrounding spinal areas in individuals with previous injuries. The ingredients include the following:

- Rehmannia as a blood and *Yin* tonic
- Dioscorea as a Spleen *Qi* tonic
- Epimedium as a liver and kidney tonic and to relieve pain, numbness, and dampness
- Hedera to clear heat and drain dampness
- LiquidAmber and Tokoro to invigorate the circulation and clear dampness
- Cistanches as a kidney yang tonic
- "Tiger bone" (probably ox bone) to strengthen bones

Renal Conditions and Incontinence

In TCM, the Kidney oversees and regulates bone formation and metabolism, especially of the spine and hind limbs, in addition to its renal involvement. The Kidney is also partly responsible for the hormonal system (along with the liver and spleen) and sexual functioning (along with the liver and spleen). These functions are all controlled by Kidney *Yang*. According to TCM, the underlying immune system with which patients are born is guided by the "ancestral *Qi* of the kidney." Therefore autoimmune problems are also under the auspices, at least in part, of the kidney. Finally, the kidney is responsible for the underlying *Yin* of the body. The *Yin* fluids keep an individual cool, calm, and collected throughout the day and restful at night.

TCM is helpful in maximizing renal function in animals with chronic renal failure. Because the herbs used contain high concentrations of potassium, potassium supplementation is not often necessary except in severe cases. Because many of the herbs are *Yin* tonics, they can help to moisten the body, and they clinically decrease polydypsia, constipation, and the need for subcutaneous fluid therapy (Schwartz, 1993). Because *Yang* tonics help strengthen and warm the lower body, they aid in polyuria. Because many of the kidney tonic herbs are also blood tonics, they can be used to prevent and treat anemia. Because some of the herbs within formulas are *Qi* tonics, they act as appetite stimulants. Additionally, herbal formulas can be tailored to individual needs by addition of herbs to decrease vomiting. TCM is also beneficial in strengthening the lower back and legs through the use of acupuncture and kidney tonic herbs.

REHMANNIA SIX (Brion, *Min Tong* Freeze Dried, Herbal Apothecary and McZand herbal tinctures, *Liu Wei Di Huang Wan* Patent Medicine pellets). This combination of herbs is a variation of the basic kidney formula to which other herbs can be added to modify the treatment. Rehmannia Six is a Kidney *Yin* and Blood tonic formula. The indications for use of this formula are thirst, constipation, preference for cool temperatures. fatigue, weak lower back, dry skin, poor appetite, and a red tongue with little coating. The ingredients include the following:

- *Rehmannia* (usually cooked): If the rehmannia is cooked, it is processed with wine and has a warming quality. Raw, unprocessed rehmannia has a cooling quality. Rehmannia tonifies blood, decreases blood pressure and cholesterol, and is high in potassium (Bensky, Gamble, 1986)
- Cornus, an astringent that consolidates the kidney essence and ancestral *Qi*, decreases incontinence, decreases low-back pain, decreases blood pressure, and has an antibiotic affect against *Staphylococcus aureus* infection (Bensky, Gamble, 1986)
- Dioscorea tonifies *Qi* of the spleen, kidney, and lung
- Moutan cools blood heat; decreases inflammation, thirst, and blood pressure; lowers body temperature; and tranquilizes (Bensky, Gamble, 1986)
- Hoelen regulates fluid metabolism, decreases abdominal bloating and the "bearing down, frequent urging sensation," and aids in water circulation. It also improves urination, strengthens the spleen, harmonizes digestion, and decreases palpitation and insomnia; it is high in potassium (Bensky, Gamble, 1986)

---

*A variation of this formula is available from ITM as Liquid Amber 14.

- Alisma regulates fluid metabolism, decreases abdominal bloating, cools kidney inflammation, increases the excretion of urea, lowers blood pressure, and is high in potassium (Bensky, Gamble, 1986)

In some individuals, rehmannia can adversely affect digestion. If vomiting, diarrhea, or depressed appetite occur, adding pinellia combination or central *Qi* tea, both at half dosages, may correct the problem.

ANAMARRHENA PHELLODENDRON AND REHMANNIA (Brion, *Min Tong* Freeze dried, McZand, Herbal Apothecary tincture, *Chih Pai Di Huang Wan* Patent Medicine Pellets) (Hsu, 1993). If thirst or constipation is severe, the Rehmannia 6 combination can be modified by adding anemarrhena and phellodendron, which cool relative inflammation of the kidney. This formula can be used for mouth lesions caused by kidney failure. It can also be used if the urine is scanty and appears to be painful to pass.

REHMANNIA EIGHT (Brion, *Min Tong* Freeze dried, McZand, Herbal Apothecary tincture, Sexoton or golden Book Kidney Pills Patent Medicine pellets) (Dharmananda, 1988). This formula was the original kidney tonification combination, helping restore the Kidney *Yin* and *Yang*. The symptoms are polyuria (especially at night), dilute urine, polydipsia, weak or painful lower back, cold extremities, loose stool that is worse in the morning, diminished visual or auditory acuity, and pale tongue. This formula may be effective in treating nephritis, nephrosis, renal calculus, renal atrophy, pyelitis, and proteinuria (Hsu, 1994).

The ingredients are rehmannia 6 with the addition of cinnamon bark and processed aconite to warm the kidneys.

GE JIE DA BU WAN (Gecko great nourishment pills, patent herb, capsules) (Dharmananda, 1988). This formula is useful for weakness, fatigue, frequent urination, pain in the lower body, anemia, and asthmatic wheezing that results from an imbalance between the Kidney yang and lung in TCM differentiation. Because it contains warming herbs, if the formula is too strong for the patient, symptoms such as increased thirst and eye redness can occur. If these symptoms persist, the dosage should be decreased. The ingredients include the following:

- Gecko lizard and eucommia as Kidney, Lung, and liver *Yang* tonics
- Codonopsis, hoelen, and *Astragalus* as Spleen *Qi* tonics
- Dioscorea as a *Qi* tonic of the Spleen, Lung, and Kidney
- Lycium, tang kuei, and rehmannia as Kidney and Liver Blood tonics
- Ligustrum as a Liver and Kidney *Yin* tonic
- Licorice as a digestive harmonizer
- Chaenomelis to relieve pain and strengthen legs

RESTORATIVE TABLETS (ITM, Seven Forest, dried herb caplets). This herbal combination helps restore all as-pects of the kidney. It is used in weak patients with increased thirst, dry skin, urine dribbling, and severe fatigue. It is helpful in certain patients with Cushing's syndrome. This combination aids the Kidney *Yin* and *Yang* and ancestral *Qi* or jing essence. It is useful for "steaming bone syndromes" in which the bones are inflamed from a deficiency of internal fluids (e.g., symptoms of systemic lupus erythematosus with lameness).

The formula contains human placenta, tortoise shell, rehmannia, tang kuei, stone ear, ligustrum, peony, and melletia to nourish the blood and essence; cuscuta and aquilaria to help correct the urine dribbling; anemarrhena and phellodendron to help clear internal heat; *Astragalus* to nourish the *Qi* and promote immunity; and eucommia to strengthen the back (Dharmananda, 1988).

Conclusion

Herbs can be used to treat almost any internal condition treatable by Western medicine. They can also be used to address conditions that cannot be diagnosed with Western medicine but do have patterns consistent with the concepts of TCM. Herbs can be used to enhance the veterinary pharmacopoeia. The herbs listed in this chapter can be used with any of the Western medications applicable to the disorders discussed.

Herbs can also be used when Western medications are not available or recognized; for example, the tonic qualities of herbs may be used to nurture or restore organ systems, such as in renal failure. Herbs can be used according to Western diagnoses, but a much wider range for use exists if the practitioner applies TCM concepts. Herbs can be used for long periods without the deleterious side effects of some Western drugs.

Herb Distributors*

Brion Freeze Dried Herbs, Sun Ten Products
9250 Jeronimo Road
Irvine, CA 92718

Draline Tong (Patent Herbs)
1003 Webster Street
Oakland, CA 94607

Health Concerns
8001 Capwell Drive
Oakland, CA 94621

Herbal Apothecary
El Cerrito, CA

---

*This is a partial listing only. Check with holistic veterinarians in your geographic area for local herb distributors.

Institute for Traditional Medicine & Preventive Health
  Care (ITM)
2242 SE Sherman
Portland, OR 97214

Mayway Trading Company (Patent Herbs)
780 Broadway
San Francisco, CA 92133

McZand Herbal Inc.
P.O. Box 5312
Santa Monica, CA 90405

Min Tong Herbs
Oakland, CA

References

American Veterinary Medical Association (cited p. 9).

Benfield H, Korngold E: *Between heaven and earth: a guide to Chinese medicine*, New York, 1991, Ballantine Books.

Bensky D, Barolet R: *Chinese herbal formulas and strategies*, Seattle, 1990, Eastland Press.

Bensky D, Gamble A: *Chinese herbal medicine materia medica*, Seattle, 1986, Eastland Press.

Chen J, Zang Y, Wu Q: Effect of jingui shenqi pills on sex hormone in aged rats, *China Journal of Chinese Materia Medica* 18(10):619, 1993.

Dharmananda S: *Traditional Chinese medical herbology professional training, guide,* Portland, Ore, 1981, Institute for Traditional Medicine and Preventive Health Care.

Dharmananda S: *Your nature, your health*, Portland, 1986, Institute for Traditional Medicine and Preventive Health Care.

Dharmananda S: *Chinese herbal therapies for immune disorders*. Portland, Ore, 1988, Institute for Traditional Medicine and Preventive Health Care.

Dharmananda S: *Pearls from the golden cabinet*, Long Beach, Calif, 1988, Oriental Healing Arts Institute.

Dharmananda S: *A bag of pearls*. Portland, Ore, 1992, Institute for Traditional Medicine and Preventive Health Care.

Dharmananda S: The effect of Chinese herbal medicine on endocrine function, *International Journal of Oriental Medicine*, 19:3,121-42, 1994.

Fratkin J: *Chinese classics guide for the practitioner*, Santa Fe, N.M., 1990, Shya Publications.

Fratkin J: *Chinese herbal patent formulas: a practical guide,* Boulder, CO, 1987, Shya Publications.

Ge R, Pu H: Effects of ginsenosides and pantocrine on the reproductive endocrine system in male rats, *JTM* 6:301, 1986.

Health Concerns pocket reference for health practitioners: Oakland, Calif, 1995, Health Concerns.

Hsu H-Y: Application of Chinese herbal formulas and scientific research rehmannia six and rehmannia eight formulas, *International Journal of Oriental Medicine* 18:1, 41-6, 1993.

Hsu H-Y: *International Journal of Oriental Medicine* 19:3, 166, 1994.

Hsu H-Y, Hsu C-S: Commonly used Chinese herb formulas with illustrations, Long Beach, Calif, 1980, Oriental Healing Arts Institute.

Limehouse J: Course notes, 1989, International Veterinary Acupuncture Accreditation Course.

Liu H-W, Yang X-J: The therapeutic effect of ligustrum and eclipta formula on IgA nephropathy, *International Journal of Oriental Medicine* 19:3, 160, 1994.

Lu H: *Legendary Chinese healing herbs*, New York, 1991, Sterling Publishers.

Maciocia G: *The foundations of Chinese medicine: a comprehensive text for acupuncturists and herbalists*, New York, 1989, Churchill Livingstone.

Naesser M: *Outline guide to Chinese herbal patent medicines in pill form*, Boston, 1991, Boston Chinese Medicine.

Ren S-L, Yu L-S, Zhao G-J: Effects of gastrodia on vascular impedance and tolerance to ischemia and hypoxia, *International Journal of Oriental Medicine* 19:4, 187, 1994.

Schwartz C: Chronic renal failure in the cat. Paper presented at International Veterinary Acupuncture Society, Minneapolis, Minn, September 1993 (unpublished).

Teeguarden R: *Chinese tonic herbs*, Tokyo, 1985, Japan Publications.

Wang Shu-He: *The discussion of cold-induced disorders and the essentials from the golden cabinet,*

Wiseman N, Ellis A, Zmiewski P: *Fundamentals of Chinese medicine*, Brookline, Mass, 1985, Paradigm Publications.

Zong-Jing Z: *The discussions of cold induced disorders and miscellaneous disease,*

Chapter 24

*A*yurvedic Veterinary Medicine

ROBERT J. SILVER

The Tradition of Ayurvedic Medicine

Ayurveda, which literally means "the science of Life," is the ancient and traditional holistic healing system of India. Ayurveda is more than simply a medical system of healing modalities: It is a science of living that comprehensively addresses existence by relating the life of the individual to universal principles.

As a holistic system, Ayurveda encompasses not just the treatment of disease but also the creation and maintenance of health and wellness. It is a detailed and complete system that emphasizes living in harmony with the laws of nature. As such, its principles and practices can be extended to the nonhuman members of the animal kingdom as well as to the plant kingdom.

The actual practice of Ayurveda involves the integration of the use of herbal supplements with diet, massage, exercise, and meditation in an attempt to create balance among the three elements of nature *(Doshas)* as they relate to the individual's constitution. Health in Ayurveda results from this harmonious integration of individual constitution with nature and the universe.

This chapter summarizes the background, history, and principles of Ayurvedic medicine and presents practical applications in the use of Ayurvedic herbal therapies for animals.

In present-day language, the term *Ayurveda* has assumed another meaning in addition to its textbook definition as the ancient and traditional holistic healing system of India. In the marketplace, many herbs indigenous to India are termed Ayurvedic *herbs*. Just as we can see herbs from China that are used in traditional Chinese medicine

being sold as "traditional Chinese" herbs, the term "Ayurvedic" has come to have a second meaning, namely, "from India." These herbs are not being used in the context of the indigenous holistic healing system but for their therapeutic indications.

A veterinarian need not adopt the principles and practices of Ayurvedic medicine to benefit from the use of Ayurvedic herbs from India. Many of these herbs are unique, coming from the panoply of ecosystems found in India. Ayurvedic herbs have a long and ancient history of use; thus their effects and side effects have been worked out in great detail. This history allows the practitioner a large degree of confidence in using these herbs in veterinary medical prescriptions. This chapter provides a background to the practitioner to better understand the basics of Ayurvedic thought and an introduction to some of the more important herbs of the Ayurvedic tradition.

History

India possesses one of the oldest histories of organized medicine. Ayurvedic medicine is at the root of nearly all the traditional and modern systems of medicine in the world. Early accounts of the medicinal use of plants can be found in an ancient Vedic text, the *Rigveda*. These writings originated in the period between 4500 BC and 1600 BC. The most detailed account of instructions and information to be used for the treatment or prevention of diseases is found in the text of the *Ayurveda*, which was written sometime between 2500 and 600 BC.

The *Ayurveda* comprises eight sections, each of which addresses a different aspect of medical practice:

1. Internal medicine
2. Surgery

This chapter was originally published in the 1996 Conference Proceedings of the American Holistic Veterinary Medical Association.

3. Diseases of the head and neck
4. Toxicology
5. Mental disorders, including seizures
6. Pediatrics
7. Geriatrics
8. Theriogenology and sexuality

In the *Ayurveda* and the medical texts that followed it, the *Susruta Samhita* and the *Charaka Samhita*, one can find detailed accounts of surgery, medical therapies, an Indian Materia Medica, descriptions of methods of administration of herbs (which included instructions on preparing medicines for injection), as well as a discussion of the use of anesthetics. These texts were all written and in use before the Christian era.

Ayurvedic medicine expanded its influence into Asia, contributing greatly to the roots of traditional Chinese medicine. Buddhist rulers such as Asoka and Buddhist monks practiced *Ayurveda* and planted herb gardens along their peripatetic routes while spreading Buddhist thought and political influence to the far corners of Asia. In this way, *Ayurveda* spread to Sri Lanka, Nepal, Tibet, Mongolia, Russia, China, Korea, Japan, and other parts of Southeast Asia.

The influences of Ayurvedic medicine reached as far as the empires of Egypt, Greece, and Rome. During the reign of Alexander the Great, Hindu physicians treated snakebites and other ailments among the soldiers of the Greek camp. Some authorities believe that many Greek philosophers such as Paracelsus, Hippocrates, and Pythagoras may have actually visited India and the East, learned Ayurvedic and other Eastern teachings, and brought the medicines they found back to Greece. The great Hellenic physician Dioscorides mentions many Indian plants in his work, including datura for asthma and nux vomica for paralysis and dyspepsia.

The Roman Empire also relied heavily on Indian medicines. Imports from India were so large that the famous Roman herbalist Pliny complained about the heavy drain of Roman gold for the purchase of Indian herbal medicines and spices (Kapoor, 1990).

This ancient and traditional form of healing has a broad base of followers in the modern era. Ayurveda is actively practiced in India, and the Ayurvedic practitioners can be found in increasing numbers in many countries of the modern world. In the United States, Deepak Chopra, MD, and the Transcendental Meditation movement of the Maharishi Mahesh Yogi, along with many others, have been instrumental in establishing and promulgating the concept and practice of Ayurvedic healing modalities.

Ayurvedic Concepts in Health and Disease

Because Ayurvedic thought preceded traditional Chinese medicine (TCM) and served as a basis for the development of TCM, it should be no surprise that many similarities exist between TCM and the basic structure and philosophy of Ayurvedic medicine.

For instance, the concept that *Yin* and *Yang* are the fundamental underlying substance of the Universe finds a similar concept in Ayurveda. *Purusha*, the Primal Spirit (the principle of sentience and consciousness) and the *Prakruti*, or Great Nature (the principle of creativity), are the representations of spirit and matter respectively. The union of these two produces all things. Like *Yin* and *Yang*, Purusha and Prakruti are opposite, yet complementary, concepts.

Lad (1995) describes Purusha as the male energy. It is without form or color and beyond all attributes. Purusha does not take an active role in the manifestation of the Universe. It is passive awareness without choice. Prakruti is the female energy. It has form, color, and attributes. It is divine Will. It is awareness with choice. Prakruti gives birth to the universe and all the forms in it, while Purusha bears witness to the creation.

Purusha and Prakruti are two complementary forces that are actually a single dynamic. They are continuously being created and destroyed in the same way that *Yin* becomes *Yang* and *Yang* becomes *Yin*. The joining of these two forces creates Mahat, or Cosmic Intelligence. Mahat contains all the laws of Nature and all the seeds of Manifestation (Frawley, Lad, 1988). In Eastern or Taoist philosophy the joining of the two forces of *Yin* and *Yang* creates the *Tao*, or all that is.

Another way of looking at Purusha and Prakruti is to consider Purusha the Absolute Reality from which all evolves. In other words, Purusha is consciousness without any characteristic whatsoever, beyond time, space, and causation, a single point that encompasses everything and cannot be perceived by mind or accurately described in human language. All potentialities exist within Absolute Reality in an unmanifested state (Svoboda, Lade, 1995).

Svoboda and Lade explain that Prakruti, or Relative Reality, evolves from the Absolute reality of Purusha and constitutes…a sublime creative force called Nature…. The difference between Nature and Absolute Reality is that the Absolute knows itself to be identical to Nature, whereas Nature believes itself to be different from the Absolute. The passive awareness of difference evolves into an undifferentiated Intelligence, or Mahat, the means by which this difference is actively perceived. Mahat (Intelligence) is Nature's (Prakruti) unlimited self-awareness.

Ayurveda is directed toward creating life in harmony with Mahat. For human beings this means working toward perfecting one's own consciousness to return to unity with Nature. In unity with Nature, Purusha—true Self and Spirit—is achieved. This is the spiritual background of Ayurveda, as well as that of Yoga, and serves as the basis of Ayurvedic philosophy. Ego is considered the basis for deviation from nature. Health is a natural occurrence like Prakruti, or Universal Nature. Disease is not natural—it is artificial and stems from imbalance with Mahat and Purusha. Thus most human diseases, according to Ayurveda, except those that come from the passage of time, are from the psychologic imbalance caused by the ego.

Prakruti, or Universal Nature, is further divided up into the three *Gunas*, which are basic qualities or prime attributes. These Gunas are Sattva—balance, light, perception, intelligence and harmony; Rajas—energy, activity, emotion, and turbulence; and Tamas—inertia, darkness, dullness, and resistance. Sattva is considered the ideal attribute; hence it is important to follow a sattvic lifestyle. All three of these qualities exist in nature; thus Ayurveda classifies foods and herbs according to the three Gunas.

The Five Ayurvedic elements are derived from the three Gunas. Sattva produces Ether; Rajas produces Fire; Tamas produces Earth. Sattva and Rajas combine to produce Air, and Rajas and Tamas give rise to Water. These elements correspond to the five states of matter—solid, liquid, radiant, gaseous, and ethereal. They are responsible for the physical nature of all visible and invisible matter in the universe. The Gunas also correspond to emotional states and to states of mind.

The expressions of the Five Elements as applied to the physical manifestation of Life are found in the concepts of Prana, Tejas (Subtle Fire), and Ojas (Essence). *Prana* refers to the Life Force, or the *Qi* of the body. It binds body, mind, and spirit and orchestrates their smooth interaction. Like Qi, Prana is not air. Oxygen, however, is considered one of the agents of Prana. Tejas—or Subtle Fire, the fire of the mind (Frawley, Lad, 1988)—catalyzes the transformation between the different planes of existence—physical to astral to causal. Finally, Ojas, or Essence (similar to the *Jing* of TCM), is the common ground substance that allows for the integration of body mind and spirit.

Ayurveda is a holographic and holistic system. As such, many interrelationships exist between structures and their various functions. In the ancient vedic text the *Charaka Samhita*, the Law of Microcosm and Macrocosm is stated as follows: "Everything that exists in the vast external universe, the macrocosm, also appears in the internal cosmos of the body, the microcosm, in altered form" (Kapoor, 1990).

One example of this correspondence of macrocosm to microcosm is the relationship between the Five Elements of Ayurveda and the five parts of a plant. The root is equal to the Earth, the stem and branches correspond to the element Water, the plant's flowers are considered to contain the Fire element, the leaves correspond to Air, the fruit is the element of Ether, and the seed contains all five elements.

Herbs are also categorized in Ayurveda according to the seven Dhatus, or tissue elements. The Dhatus of the plant kingdom correspond to the Dhatus of the mammalian body. These corresponding animal and plant *Dhatus* are Plasma (Juice of Leaf), Blood (Resin, Sap), Muscle (softwood), Fat (Gum, Hard Sap), Bone (Bark), Marrow and Nerve Tissue (Leaf), Reproductive Tissue (Flowers and Fruit). The Dhatus of the plants work on the Dhatus of the mammalian body. The tree is to the plant kingdom what the human being is to the animal kingdom (Frawley, Lad, 1988).

Each part of the plant is chosen for its medicinal appropriateness, taking into account its characteristics with respect to the following qualities:

- Five Elements
- Taste
- Temperature
- The Tridosha

From these selection criteria, the individualized herbal remedy is chosen to match or balance the characteristics of the Ayurvedic patient.

Critical to an understanding of Ayurvedic principles is the concept of the three Doshas (known as a group as the Tridosha), which describe the three basic characteristics, or tendencies, that result from the condensation of Prana, Tejas, and Ojas and the five elements into a more dense, material form.

In Sanskrit *Dosha* means "fault" or "error," a thing that can go wrong (Svoboda, Lade, 1995). The three Doshas are described by the elements and energies inherent in each tendency. These qualities include factors such as temperature, moisture, weight, and texture. The Tridosha represents three primal metabolic tendencies in the living organism. Each individual—be it human, plant, or animal—embodies one or a combination of two of the Doshas.

This embodiment is considered to be that organism's individual constitution, or nature (also known as *Prakruti*). Balance among the Tridosha results in health and homeostasis. Disease results from an imbalance in the three Doshas. Individual constitution also represents the type of disease to which that individual is most prone. Disease conditions different from the nature of the individual are usually easy to treat. When the disease is of the same dosha as the individual, it is more difficult to treat because the constitution of the individual reinforces the disease pattern (Frawley, Lad, 1988).

The first Dosha, Vata, which means "wind," is dry, cold, light, mobile, subtle, hard, rough, irregular, changeable, and clear. It is the principle of kinetic energy. Vata corresponds most closely to the TCM concept of *Qi* (Svoboda, Lade, 1995). It is associated with the mental phenomena of enthusiasm and concentration. Vata is concerned with processes that are activating and dynamic. It is derived from Ether and Air. Vata is the most powerful of the Doshas; it is the Life Force itself.

Vata governs all movement in the body, such as respiration, circulation, excretion, and voluntary action. It is located below the navel in the bladder, large intestine, nervous system, pelvic region, thighs, bone marrow, and legs. Its principal organ is the large intestine. When Vata is out of balance, the primary symptoms are gas and muscular or nervous energy leading to pain. In a veterinary context, dog breeds of Vata constitution are the ectomorphic ones such as the borzoi, the greyhound, and the Afghan hound. As veterinarians become more adjusted to thinking in Ayurvedic terms, further definition of the Doshas as they relate to our patients will be developed.

The second Dosha, Pitta, or "bile," is derived from Fire and an aspect of Water. It is the principle of biotransformation and balance and the cause of all metabolic processes in the body. It rules all enzymes and hormones in the body. It is most closely associated with the TCM concept of *Yang*. Pitta is associated with the mental processes of intellect with clear and focused concentration. Pitta maintains these qualities in the body: wet/oily and hot, light, intense, fluid, subtle, astringent, malodorous, soft, and clear. Pitta governs the activities of the endocrine organs. It governs body heat, temperature (thermogenesis, thermal homeostasis), and all chemical reactions.

Pitta maintains digestive and glandular secretions, including digestive enzymes and bile. It is responsible for digestion, metabolism, pigmentation, hunger, thirst, sight, courage, and mental activity. Its location in the body is between the navel and the chest in the stomach, small intestine, liver, spleen, skin, and blood. Its seat in the body is the small intestine and, to a lesser extent, the stomach. When Pitta is out of balance, its primary manifestation is acid and bile, leading to inflammation. Animals of Pitta constitution will have a mesomorphic constitution and have a tendency to hot behavior, such as that which might be found in a rottweiler, Labrador retriever, or pit bull terrier.

The third Dosha, Kapha, meaning "phlegm," is derived from Water and Earth. It is the principle of cohesion and stability and regulates Vata and Pitta. Kapha functions by way of the body fluids. It is most closely associated with the TCM concept of *Yin* (Svoboda, Lade, 1995). Kapha promotes properties that are conserving and stabilizing, such as anabolic functions. It is responsible for keeping the body lubricated and essential for maintaining the body's solid nature, tissues, strength, and sexuality. Kapha maintains substance, weight, structure, solidity, and body build. Kapha is associated with the mental properties of courage and patience. It is wet/oily and cold, heavy, slow, dull, static, smooth, dense, and cloudy. Its primary seat in the body is the chest.

Kapha integrates the structural elements of the body into stable form. It forms connective and musculoskeletal tissue. Its normal locations in the body are the upper part of the body, the thorax, head, neck, upper portion of the stomach, pleural cavity, fat tissues, and areas between joints. Kapha's principal organ is the lungs. When out of balance, Kapha manifests disease symptoms associated with liquid and mucus, leading to swelling. Discharges may or may not be present in a Kapha imbalance (Zysk, 1996). Canine patients of a Kapha constitution include the English bulldog, the Staffordshire terrier, the Newfoundland, and the Great Pyrenees.

For an organism to exist, it must embrace all three Doshas. This means it must have the following characteristics:

- Tissue structure or anabolism in its Kapha quality
- Chemical processes or metabolism in its Pitta quality
- Movement and elimination or catabolism in its Vata qualities

Without any one of these qualities life cannot exist.

Seven constitutions *(Prakruti)* are derived from the three *Doshas:*

1. Vata — Anxious, fearful, light and airy; ectomorphic; prone to Vata diseases
2. Pitta — Aggressive and impatient, fiery and hotheaded; mesomorphic; prone to Pitta diseases
3. Kapha — Stable and entrenched, heavy, wet and earthy; endomorphic; prone to Kapha diseases
4. Vata-Pitta — Blend of Vata/Pitta traits
5. Pitta-Kapha — Blend of Pitta/Kapha traits
6. Vata-Kapha — Blend of Vata/Kapha traits
7. Sama — Balanced (rare)

Box 24-1 lists the seasons and times according to Tridosha.

BOX 24-1

Seasons and Times According to Tridosha

KAPHA
Season: Spring–early summer (March–June)
Time: 6 AM (sunrise)–10 AM and 6 PM–10 PM
Life Cycle: Childhood
Digestion: Before

PITTA
Season: Midsummer–early autumn
Time: 10 AM–2 PM and 10 PM–2 AM
Life Cycle: Adulthood
Digestion: During

VATA
Season: Late autumn–winter (November–February)
Time: 2 AM–6 AM and 2 PM–6 PM
Life Cycle: Old age
Digestion: After

From Zysk KG: Traditional Ayurveda, in Micozzi, ed, *Fundamentals of complementary and alternative medicine*, New York, 1996, Churchill Livingstone.

The classifications and subclassifications in the Ayurvedic view become extremely detailed and intricate in defining and explaining body anatomy, physiology, and pathology. As mentioned earlier, seven body tissues are responsible for maintaining the normal functions of health. These Dhatus are Rasa, or tissue fluids derived from digestive food (nourishment function); Blood (invigoration function); Flesh (stabilization function); Fat (lubrication function); Bone and cartilage (support function); Marrow (bone-filling function); and Shukra, or sexual body fluids (reproduction and immunity functions) (Zysk, 1996).

The Malas are the waste products of the digested food and drink. Four categories of waste products exist: urine, feces, sweat, and the fatty secretions from the skin and intestines (e.g., earwax, nasal mucus, saliva, tears, hair, and nails).

In Ayurvedic thought, digestion is the most important function of the body. Problems with digestion are considered to be the principal cause of disease. Thus Ayurveda defines thirteen different types of Agnis, or enzymes. The Agnis assist in the digestion and assimilation of food. The enzymes are found in the mouth, stomach, and gastrointestinal tract (jatharagni), the liver (bhutagnis), and the tissues (dhatvagnis).

Ama is considered the chief cause of disease. It is formed when enzyme activity decreases or food and drink are improperly digested. Ama takes the form of a liquid sludge and travels through the Blood channels, as does the nourishing chyle from digestion. Because of its heavy nature, Ama lodges in different parts of the body, obstructing the channels and causing disease. Internal disease begins with Ama, and external diseases create Ama. The diagnosis of Ama is made on the basis of a coating on the tongue, turbid urine with a foul odor, and feces containing undigested food, a foul odor, and abundant gas.

Just as there are channels or vessels in TCM, Ayurveda has the Srotas, the vessels whereby all substances circulate through the body. Large Srotas are the large and small intestines, uterus, arteries, and veins. Small Srotas are the capillaries. Healthy bodies have open and free-flowing channels. Disease results from blockage of the channels, most commonly from the accumulation of Ama (Zysk, 1996).

In addition to the physical structures associated with the Srotas, Ayurveda recognizes that underlying the physical body are nonphysical bodies derived from higher planes of consciousness. These subtle bodies provide the energetic warp and woof that allow matter to be organized on the physical plane.

The Physical Body is also known as the Sheath of Food; it is sustained by the ingestion, digestion, and assimilation of food. The Vital Body, or Astral Body, is known as the Sheath of Prana. It connects the Sheath of Food with the highest plane of consciousness—the Sheath of the Mind. The Pranic Body allows for the smooth control and interaction between the Sheath of Food and the Sheath of Mind. The Mental Body is also known as the Causal Body and exists as the highest form of consciousness. The Sheath of Prana consists of Prana and can be sustained only by Prana itself.

The role of the Sheath of Food is to provide for the harmonization of consciousness. The Sheath of Prana activates the Sheath of Food. The Sheath of Mind works to ensure that the other sheaths remain in balance with the mind.

The Strotas provide channels for the movement of energy and fluid through the Physical Body. In the Vital Body, Prana moves through subtle channels and nodes called *Nadis* and *Chakras,* respectively. The Pranic Body affects the physical body by influencing the Srotas, which flow synchronously with the Nadis.

The Chakras are located along the most important Nadi—the Sushumna, or Central Conduit. The Central Conduit is located in the same physical location as the central sulcus of the spinal cord. Because the spinal cord and the Sushumna exist on different planes, they can occupy the same physical space simultaneously. They can also share the same sensation simultaneously through resonance of the energy in their shared physical space.

There are three causal factors for disease according to Ayurvedic principle. Diseases that originate within the body (hereditary, congenital, and *Dosha*-related or constitutional); diseases that originate outside the body (trauma, external pathogens such as bacteria and viruses); and diseases that originate from supernatural sources (seasons, planetary influences, curses, and acts of God) (Zysk, 1996).

Ayurvedic Principles of Diagnosis

Ayurveda has a well-established system of diagnosis, similar in some respects to TCM and different in others. An initial examination comprises visual observation, palpation, and interrogation. The detailed examination determines the patient's physical constitution type and mental status. The diagnostician tries to discover any indications of imbalances or abnormalities in the patient.

Pulse diagnosis is used by most Ayurvedic practitioners. The hands are positioned similarly to the TCM positioning. The radial artery of the right hand is palpated for males, and the left hand is palpated for females. Palpation of a pulse wave at the index finger that feels like a "snake" indicates Vata. If the pulse feels like a "frog" at the middle finger, it indicates Pitta. If the pulse wave at the ring finger feels like the movement of a swan or a peacock, the predominant Dosha is Kapha.

Urine examination involves the free-catch collection of the first urine midstream in a clear glass jar. The urine is examined for color and degree of transparency. Vata urine is pale yellow and oily; Pitta urine is intense yellow, reddish, or blue. Kapha urine is white, foamy, and muddy. Urine with a blackish color indicates all three

Doshas. Urine resembling lime juice or vinegar indicates Ama. After visual inspection of the urine, a few drops of sesame oil are placed in the urine and examined in the sunlight. Shape, movement, and diffusion of the oil in the urine are prognosticators. The drops will form different shapes, giving an indication of which Doshas are involved: snakelike = Vata; umbrella = Pitta; pearl-shaped = Kapha.

Visual examination of various parts of the body aid the Ayurvedic physician in diagnosis. The tongue, skin, nails, and other physical features identify the Doshas most involved in the patient's diagnosis. The physical condition of the body can be related to the Tridosha as follows:

- Vata—coldness, dryness, roughness, and cracking
- Pitta—hotness and redness
- Kapha—wetness, whiteness, and coldness

Finally, after the patient's constitution is determined, the disease itself is analyzed in a six-step process in which the following elements are studied:

1. Etiology (e.g., mental, emotional, karma, seasonal influences, diet, microorganisms, Ama and Srota blockages, imbalances in the senses)
2. Early signs and symptoms (prodromal signs and symptoms)
3. Disease signs and symptoms
4. Exploratory, or Challenge, therapy (18 different regimens of diet, herbal drugs and programs)
5. Pathogenesis (six-step process determining the manner in which a Dosha becomes aggravated and moves through the channels to create disease)
6. Prognosis (three types of diseases: easily curable, potential for palliation, incurable or difficult to cure)
- If the disease type and patient constitution are different, it will be easy to cure the disease.
- If the disease type and patient constitution are the same, the disease will be difficult to cure.
- If the disease, constitution, and season correspond to the same Dosha, the disease will be nearly impossible to cure (Zysk, 1996).

Treatment in Ayurvedic Medicine

Therapy in Ayurveda is directed toward correcting the imbalances in the Tridosha, with consideration of the constitution of the patient. Diet and herbs are used in therapy on the basis of their Tridoshic energetics. Dosha excesses are neutralized by the appropriate energetics of the herbs and food selected for the patient. Similarly, deficiencies in the Doshas are strengthened through use of the appropriate herbs and foods.

Treatment is divided into two categories in Ayurveda: prophylaxis (prevention) and disease therapy. Prophylaxis involves diet, lifestyle, herbal medicines, and regular therapeutic purification exercises. Disease therapy is further divided into three types: purification therapy, alleviation therapy, and a combination of the two.

Purification therapy, also known as *panchakarma*, consists of a fivefold approach. In preparation for receiving the five therapies, the patient is given oil internally and externally (through massage), and sweating or diaphoresis is induced. This loosens and softens the Doshas and Ama. A diet appropriate to the patient is prescribed. Finally, the five therapies are administered in a predetermined sequence over a period of a week.

First, the patient is given an emetic and made to vomit until only bile is expelled; this removes Kapha. Next a purgative is given until mucus appears on the stool; this removes Pitta. Third, an enema of oil or decocted medicines is given to remove the Vata. Fourth, head purgation is achieved with inhalation of smoke or nose drops. This will help eradicate the Doshas that have accumulated in the head and sinuses. Fifth, leeches are applied or bloodletting is performed to purify the blood.

Alleviation therapy involves basic foods such as honey, butter, or *ghee* (clarified butter), and sesame or castor oil to eliminate Kapha, Pitta, or Vata, respectively. Combinations of the two therapies are common. All five of the purification therapies can be performed, or a selection of procedures can be chosen, depending on different factors such as the physical constitution of the patient, the condition of the patient, the season, and the nature of the disease (Zysk, 1996).

Ayurveda always favors the gradual process of healing over rapid or instantaneous processes. Dietary changes are considered fundamental to the healing process in Ayurveda because most disease problems are the result of dietary indiscretions of one form or another. Panchakarma therapy is administered only if the patient is relatively strong to begin with because the purification procedure is quite intense. Each Dosha requires a specific and unique therapeutic strategy to achieve balance. For instance, Vata must be warmed and moistened because its main properties are cold and dry. When herbal remedies are used Ayurvedically, the same principles of balancing the Doshas are invoked (Zysk, 1996).

The strict application of these purification procedures may pose difficulties for most veterinarians. However, understanding the Tridosha and the other principles and diagnostics of Ayurveda can add insight to the workup of a veterinary patient's problem. For example, using the Ayurvedic herbs (discussed in the following material) according to their clinical efficacy and matching their energetics to the patient's energetics using the Ayurvedic system will increase the chances of a successful outcome for therapy.

The Herbs of Ayurvedic Tradition

Plants and the Tridosha

The *Tridosha* exist in the plant kingdom as well as the animal kingdom (Frawley, Lad, 1988). Kapha plants have lush growth, possessing abundant leaves and copious juices or sap. Like the Kapha quality they represent, they are heavy and dense. They contain quite a bit of water. All Kapha plants have certain qualities in common: they are pungent and bitter to the taste, are astringent, and have mucolytic properties. Kapha plants are most active in conditions of the stomach and lungs. Examples of Kapha plants include the following:

- Guggul *(Commiphora mukul):* for arthritis, aids in lipid metabolism
- Bayberry bark *(Myrica* spp.): liver tonic
- Clove *(Caryophyllus aromatica):* warming digestive tonic and lung remedy, used in the treatment of neuromuscular disorders
- Fenugreek seed *(Trigonella foenumgraecum):* astringent, useful in the treatment of increased blood glucose (Khalsa, 1995)

Vata plants have sparse leaves, rough, cracked bark, crooked, gnarled branches, spindly growth habits, and little sap. Vata herbs share the qualities of being nutritive with sweet, sour, and salty tastes. These plants are warm, heavy, and moist. They serve as carminative agents (prodigestion and antigas) and nervines that affect the nervous system and also assist in colon cleansing (Lung/Large Intestine—Metal/Air in TCM). Representative Vata herbs include:

- Asafetida *(Ferula asafoetida):* a digestive aid
- Ajwain seed *(Apium* spp.): antiviral, digestive aid, carminative
- Nutmeg *(Myristica fragrens):* a digestive aid and relaxant used for anxiety and insomnia
- Cinnamon bark *(Cinnamomun zeylanicum):* warming general bone tonic that enhances circulation, particularly to the joints; useful for arthritis worsened by cold and accompanied by stiffness; also used for menstrual cramps
- Bala *(Sida cordifola):* means "strength" in Sanskrit. Rejuvenating tonic useful for short-term debility and long-term stamina.
- Jatamansi *(Nardostachys jatamansi):* botanically related to the Western herb valerian *(Valeriana officinale)* with similar nervine/sedative properties (Khalsa, 1995)

Pitta plants are brightly colored, with bright flowers. They are moderate in strength and may be poisonous or create a sensation of burning when used medicinally. These plants are used for energy. Pitta plants taste both bitter and astringent. Pitta plants have the properties of being heavy, cool, and dry. In general, Pitta herbs have antiinflammatory properties and are useful for small intestine (Fire element in TCM) cleansing. Examples of Pitta plants include:

- Aloe *(Aloe* spp.): purgative and general tissue healer; antiseptic activity most potent in the small intestine
- Mint *(Mentha* spp.): cooling and soothing digestive aid; antiinflammatory

- Rhubarb root *(Rheum* spp): a relatively mild purgative
- Sandalwood *(Santalum album):* cooling
- Licorice root *(Glycerrhiza glabra):* mild laxative and general glandular and adrenal tonic used to treat dyspepsia and asthma (Khalsa, 1996)

The parts of a plant are also assigned a Dosha in addition to being related to the Five Elements. For example, the root and bark of plants (elements Earth and Water) work on Kapha conditions. The flowers (Fire) work on Pitta conditions. The leaves and fruits (Air and Ether) work on Vata (Frawley, Lad, 1988).

Ayurvedic Classification of Plants

Ayurvedic herbs are further classified according to their tastes and temperatures. Each of the six tastes is derived from two elements. The tastes are divided into sweet, sour, salty (anabolic activity), pungent, bitter, and astringent (catabolic activity). Examples of herbs and their representative tastes follow (Frawley, Lad, 1988).

Sweet (cold, wet)
- Nourishing, soothing, pleasing brain tonic; healing; antiabortifacient
- Beneficial for burning sensations, thirst, heart, skin and hair; galactagogue, antitoxin activity
- Contains carbohydrates and fats
- Kapha-increasing, Pitta-decreasing
  EXAMPLES
- Licorice root *(Glycerrhiza glabra):* calms the mind, harmonizes
- Peppermint *(Mentha piperita):* helps relieve mental and emotional tension and congestion, digestive tonic

Sour (hot, wet)
- Stimulates appetite, promotes digestive secretions and saliva, sharpens the mind, functions as an anticoagulant
- Contains acids
- Increases Pitta
  EXAMPLES
- Rose hips *(Rosa* spp.): vitamin C source, ability to influence sinus tissue, antioxidant properties
- Amla fruit *(Emblica officinalis):* single best herb for Pitta; major rejuvenator (especially good for blood, bones, liver, and heart); has the highest known food content of vitamin C, yet is heat stable and can be cooked; major ingredient in Chyavanprash; ocular tonic; potent antioxidant (Khalsa, 1995)

Salty (hot, wet)
- Digestion aid, sialogogue, expectorant, diuretic; increases water content in body, has moistening and laxative activity
- Contains minerals
- Increases Kapha and Pitta

EXAMPLES*
- Kelp *(Fucus visiculosis)*
- Garlic *(Allium sativum);* a nonseaweed herb with a pungent taste unlike anything else

Pungent (cold, dry)
- Nutrient assimilation; detoxification; nervous stimulant; resuscitative; mouth cleanser; anthelmintic; sialogogue; promotes bleeding and epiphora; causes a tingling sensation on the tongue
- Useful in dyspepsia, cardiac and skin disorders
- Promotes headaches
  EXAMPLE
- Black pepper *(Piper nigrum):* blood purifier and circulatory tonic; used for flatulence; sinus-drainage remedy (Khalsa, 1996)

Bitter (cold, dry)
- Most powerful of all the tastes
- Detoxifying, antimicrobial
- Digestive tonic when consumed before meals
- Mouth cleansing; produces xerostomia
- Anthelmintic; blood purifying; antipyretic; removes pus; discharges
- Vata and Pitta increasing
  EXAMPLES
- Fenugreek seed *(Trigonella foenumgraecum)*
- Rhubarb root *(Rheum* spp.)
- Chiretta *(Swertia chiratata):* a very bitter herb; foundation herb for the digestive and detoxifying classic formula *Mahasudarshan* (containing *Chiretta, Guduchi* [*Tinospora cordifolia*], the three-herb combination of *Trikatu* [ginger, black pepper, long pepper], and the three-herb combination of *Triphala* [*Amla, Haritaki, Bibitaki*]) (Khalsa, 1995)

Astringent (very cold, very dry)
- Dries out tissues, causes them to contract (astringency); sedative in nature; constipating; hemostatic; antidiuretic; healing; absorbent
- Produces clarity, stiffness, xerostomia, and a pulling in the tongue and throat
- Produces a sensation of heaviness; may cause discomfort in the cardiac region
- Vata-increasing
  EXAMPLE
- Turmeric *(Curcuma longa):* potent antiinflammatory; used for arthritis and dermatitis; beneficial to mucous membranes and to the intestines; used for colitis, gastric ulcers (Khalsa, 1995)

Herbs may also be classified according to their action on body temperature.

---

*Seaweeds are most representative of this category.

Hot
- Increases metabolic activity, improves circulation
- Suppresses *Kapha* and *Vata*
  EXAMPLE
- Ginger root *(Zingiber officinale):* botanically related to turmeric; has antiinflammatory properties; aids digestion; carminative (antiflatulent); dispels cold and therefore useful for cold and stiff joint disease (osteoarthritis); frequently used with turmeric (they balance each other's temperatures); effective for acute nausea, migraine onset; synergistic activity with onion (Khalsa, 1996)
- Mustard seed *(Brassica alba):* carminative; expectorant; digestive tonic; circulatory tonic; pain reliever
- Cayenne (as well as other chili peppers—*Capsicum* spp.): antiviral; circulatory tonic; beneficially influences cholesterol levels, hypertension and obesity

Cold
- Decreases metabolic activity
- Suppresses Pitta
  EXAMPLE
- Dandelion *(Taraxacum officinale):* liver tonic, diuretic
- Cardamom *(Elettaria cardamomum):* diuretic; expectorant; general tonic; benefits the heart; stimulates appetite; carminative; reduces nausea
- Peppermint *(Mentha piperita):* nervine; mild stimulant; improves digestion; cooling; diaphoretic; soothing; mentally clarifying
- Licorice root *(Glycerrhiza glabra):* reduces inflammation; counteracts heat and dryness (Frawley, Lad, 1988)

Pharmacology and Ayurveda

The classification system of Ayurveda was developed before the advent of modern theories of chemistry and predates the development of procedures used in laboratory chemical analysis (Kapoor, 1990).

For example, the term *Rasa*, which refers to the six tastes (sweet, sour, salty, pungent, bitter, and astringent), is related not just to the gustatory sensation we call taste but is also an indicator of the composition, properties, and activity of the herb. The term *Guna* refers to the physical qualities of herbs. There are ten pairs of Gunas: Heavy/Light, Dull/Sharp, Cold/Hot, Oily/Not-oily, Smooth/Rough, Dense/Liquid, Soft/Hard, Stable/Unstable, Subtle/Obvious, and Slime/Nonslime. These attributes are both physical and pharmacologic because the pharmacologic action of the herb is what determines its physical attributes.

Another concept of Ayurvedic pharmacology is that of Vipaka, the transformed state of an ingested substance after digestion. Vipaka's locus of activity is the liver, after the initial digestive process has broken the herb down in the digestive tract. In pharmacologic terms, *Vipaka* would refer to the pharmacologic effects of secondary metabolites of the herb (Frawley, Lad, 1988; Kapoor, 1990).

Drug potency is described by the Ayurvedic concept Virya, and drug action is described by the Ayurvedic concept of Prabhava. Two factors contribute to the nature of Prabhava: (1) the specificity of the chemical composition of the herb and (2) the specificity of the site of activity of the herb (drug). It is the Prabhava that defines the actual physical response of the body to the herbal therapeutic agent. An herb (drug) acting on a specific tissue, organ, or disorder is said to have Prabhava, and its action is directed toward disease, not toward Dosha. This means that herbal therapy need not be directed, therapeutically based, on the prescribing indications that result from the disease diagnosis. In veterinary use of Ayurvedic herbs, prescribing on the basis of Prabhava may be more practical than using the patient's constitution on the basis of Tridosha (Frawley, Lad, 1988; Kapoor, 1990).

The Use of Herbs in the Treatment of Disease

Ayurvedic tradition teaches that the most effective therapy is that which is adjusted according to the constitution of the patient, in addition to addressing the specific nature of the disease.

For instance, the same disease entity can occur in individuals of different constitutions. This phenomenon is also addressed in TCM and homeopathy. In the former a patient may have pruritus caused by dry skin, for example. The dry skin could be caused by the patient's Blood deficiency. Another patient may also have pruritus resulting from dry skin, but in this patient's constitution it is the weak Lung *Yin* that is the source of the problem. In homeopathy, a patient may have arthritis and fit the remedy picture of *Rhus toxicodendron*, whereas another patient may have arthritis that fits the profile of *Bryonia alba*.

In the example of Ayurveda, a patient with asthma may have unbalanced Kapha leading to excessive water in the lungs. A patient with unbalanced Vata may have a nervous hypersensitivity of the lungs, or a patient with Pitta problems may have too much damp-heat accumulation in the lungs. In each case the disease diagnosis is identical, but the patient profile and the therapeutic protocol are different (Frawley, Lad, 1988).

Ayurvedic Materia Medica

Ashwaganda *(Withania somnifera)*

Indian ginseng; winter cherry; that which has the smell of a horse; gives the energy and vitality of a horse.

Botany: Solanacea: nightshades: datura, mandragora, *Hyoscyamus niger, Lycopersicon esculentum, Nicotiana glauca, Atropina belladona*

- Root and leaves used
- Small perennial shrub 3 to 5 feet tall
- Stem and branches covered with star-shaped hairs, flowers throughout the year; one or more long tuberous roots and a short stem

Pharmacology: Contains the following:
- Sucrose, beta-sitosterol, atropine, choline, nicotine, flavones, amino acids
- Steroidal lactones: most researched constituents: withanone, withananine, withanine, somniferiene
- Withanolides: Withaferin A: antibiotic—inhibits bacteria and fungi (McCaleb, 1994)
- Glycowithanolides: Sitoindoside IX, X—immunomodulatory agents with central nervous system–stimulatory activity much like the ginseng saponins (Ghosal, 1989)

Actions: Tonic, alterative, astringent, aphrodisiac, adaptogen, nervine, sedative, diuretic *(Wealth of India)*.

Energetics:
- Bitter, astringent, sweet/heating
- Vata-, Kapha-reducing; Pitta-increasing

Target organs: Muscle, fat, bone, marrow, nerve, reproductive, respiratory.

Applications: General health tonic; restorative agent; treats general debility, exhaustion, convalescence, memory loss, skin afflictions, weak eyes (Frawley, Lad, 1988); immune modulator with potential antineoplastic activity (Ghosal, 1989); antiinflammatory; anthelmintic; senile debility; arthritis; and rheumatism.

Comments: Possesses the combined effects of Siberian ginseng and echinacea and unique properties of its own such as those relating to its influence on memory and mental alertness (Singh and others, 1982).

Research:
- Comparable antiinflammatory effect to hydrocortisone in experimentally induced degenerative joint disease (Sethi, 1970)
- Tumor inhibitory effect in mice (Devi and others, 1993)
- Antimicrobial activity (Ben-Efraim, Yarden, 1962)
- Hepatoprotective activity in mice and rats (Singh and others, 1978)

Veterinary use: Geriatric tonic, immune enhancement, antimicrobial, arthritis, stress reduction, bronchial asthma, performance enhancer.

Dosage:
- Human: 3 to 6 g/day of dried herb

• Dog: 500 mg to 1500 mg/day dried herb

Boswellia *(Boswellia serrata)*

Botany: Burseraceae
• Genus of balsamiferous trees and shrubs, including *Boswellia carteri,* the source of frankincense or olibanum
• Moderate to large branching, deciduous tree
• Bark and resinous gum used
• Secretion exuded from cut bark that becomes gumlike after exposure to the air (*Wealth of India,* 2)

Pharmacology:
• Betasitosterol
• Boswellic acids: antiinflammatory and antiarthritic effects; pentacyclic triterpene acids

Actions: Diuretic; demulcent; appetite stimulant; alterative; emmenagogue; analgesic; astringent; antiinflammatory; antirheumatic; increases blood flow to the joints by improving vascular integrity (Gupta and others, 1987).

Applications: Chronic lung diseases; diarrhea; dysmenorrhea; liver disorders; boils; ringworm; arthritis; antifungal.

Research:
• Antiarthritic and antiinflammatory activity in experimental animals without toxicity or side effects (Pachnanda and others, 1981)
• Boswellic acid improves cell-mediated immunity (Gupta and others, 1987)
• Boswellia blocked synthesis of 5-lipoxygenase products in vitro—chemical mediators of inflammation (Ammon and others, 1991)
• Boswellin significantly reduced degradation of glycosaminoglycans compared with ketoprofen (Reddy and others, 1989)

Veterinary use: Arthritis, bronchial asthma, inflammatory skin conditions.

Dosage:
• Human: 150 mg boswellic acid tid
• Dog: 150 to 200 mg bid (Sodhi, 1992)

Forskolli *(Coleus forskohli)*

Botany: Labiatae (Lamiaceae)
• Family of mints and lavenders with diterpene constituents
• Parts used: primarily the root, although occasionally the leaves are used
• Herbaceous species with a perennial root stock and erect stem 18 to 24 inches tall

Pharmacology: Forskolin, a diterpenoid compound

Mechanism of action:
• Activation of adenylate cyclase causing the increase of cyclic AMP (Seamon, Daly, 1981)
• Increased cAMP: Relaxation of smooth muscle, inhibition of platelet activation, mast cell degranulation and basophil release, increased cardiac muscle contractility, increased adipocyte lipolysis (Ammon, Muller, 1985)
• Decreased cAMP: Associated with certain degenerative diseases such as atopic dermatitis, asthma, psoriasis, angina, and hypertension (Murray, vol. 4)

Actions: Strengthens cardiac contractility; decreases blood pressure; antispasmodic and smooth muscle relaxant, especially of the uterus, heart, and intestines (Kreutner and others, 1985); anticoagulative properties; helps reduce risk of stroke and heart attack; stimulates fat metabolism and hormone production; helps nerves regenerate after injury; reduces intraocular pressure by decreasing net flow of aqueous humor, exerting a different mechanism of action than currently used antiglaucoma agents such as timolol (*Lawrence Review,* 1985; Potter and others, 1985); antiallergic properties caused by histamine release inhibition, as well as other chemical mediators of allergy (Kerouac and others, 1984); stimulates lipolysis (Okuda, Murimoto, Tsujita, 1992); increases thyroid hormone production (Roger and others, 1990); inhibits cancer metastasis (Agarwal, Parks, 1983).

Target organs: Endocrine system, heart, uterus, intestines, nerves, eyes.

Applications: Heart disease, abdominal colic, respiratory disorders, painful urination, insomnia, convulsions (Seamon, Daly, 1981); uterine cramps, asthma, angina, hypertension (Ammon, Muller, 1985); atopic allergic conditions such as bronchial asthma and allergic dermatitis (most pharmaceutical therapy is designed to increase cAMP by inhibiting cAMPase enzymes, whereas forskolin works to increase cAMP by increasing its production), acute glaucoma (*Lawrence Review,* 1985).

Comments: No adverse reactions to *Coleus forskohlii* have been cited in the literature (Ammon, Muller, 1985); however, it would be judicious to exercise caution in patients with hypotension, peptic ulcers, and with concurrent use of pharmaceuticals, especially those for asthma and hypertension, because forskolin may potentiate the effects of those agents (Murray, 1995).

Research:
• Inhibits pulmonary tumor colonization in mice; doses of 82 μg inhibited tumor metastasis in mice by more than 70% (Agarwal, Parks, 1983)
• Neutralization of concentrations by *Escherichia coli* by forskolin in the rabbit and guinea pig (Yadava and others, 1995)

• Increased blood concentrations of glucose, insulin, glucagon, and free fatty acid when given orally to healthy rats (Ahmad and others, 1991)

Veterinary use: Roots cooked in water and mixed with feed are fed to cattle with loss of appetite for food and water; green leaves cooked in water increase lactation in cattle (De Souza, Shah, 1988).

Dosage:
• Human: 50 mg bid to tid for 18% forskolin extract
• Dogs: Unknown

Guggul *(Commiphora mukul)*

Botany: Burseraceae
• Small thorny tree or shrub, 4 to 6 feet tall, same family as *Boswellia* spp.
• Closely related to myrhh
• Gum resin from the stem used

Pharmacology:
• Resin containing diverse mixture of chemical constituents, some of which are toxic and therefore requiring organic chemical extraction
• Complex of phytoketonic steroid and lipid compounds (including guggulsterol, guggulsterone, and guggulipid); contains at least 50 mg guggulsterones/g; also contains diterpenes, sterols, esters, and fatty alcohols, which, when combined, exert a synergistic effect (Murray, 1995) and is considered best fraction for medicinal purposes

Actions: Demulcent; appetite stimulant; alterative; nervine; analgesic; expectorant; antiseptic; carminative; antispasmodic; emmenagogue; menses normalizer; astringent; antiinflammatory; hypocholesterolemic and hypolipemic agent; imparts sense of well-being (psychotropic); relieves nervous pains; increases coagulation time; circulatory tonic for promoting flexibility, internal strength, and stamina (Tierra, 1988); stimulates thyroid function (Dash, 1991).

Energetics:
• Kapha- and Vata-reducing; Pitta-increasing
• Bitter, pungent, astringent, sweet/heating

TCM: Clears the channels and promotes the circulation of *Qi* and Blood.

Target organs: Activity in all tissues, especially nervous, circulatory, respiratory, and digestive systems.

Applications: Arthritis; low-back pain; gout; nervous disorders; weakness; diabetes; obesity; bronchitis; digestive disturbances; skin problems; sores and ulcers; cystitis; masses; increases white blood cell count and phagocytosis;

disinfects secretions, including mucus, sweat, and urine; catalyzes tissue regeneration (especially nervous tissue); reduces necrotic tissue; can be used as a mouth rinse for oral ulcers; better for chronic problems (Frawley, Lad, 1988; Yadava and others, 1995). Also used for hepatitis; heart problems; arthritis; obesity (Ammon and others, 1993).

Comments:
• Should be used with caution in acute kidney infection and acute stages of rashes (Frawley, Lad, 1988)
• Considered the most important resin in Ayurvedic medicine; believed to possess purifying and rejuvenating properties
• Most potent remedy against *Ama* (the accumulation of thickened mucus, cholesterol, and other waste materials associated with the aging process), which causes a variety of circulatory problems, such as atherosclerosis, arthritis, rheumatism, heart problems, high blood pressure, obesity, benign prostatic hyperplasia, and other age-associated problems
• Recommended by Ayurvedic doctors for all diseases associated with bone, joint, or nerve pain (Yadava, 1995)
• Long-term use necessary for cholesterol-decreasing effects (8 weeks); effects shown to last for as long as 3 months after discontinuation (McCaleb, 1994)

Research:
• Decreases cholesterol in human beings (Malhotra, 1973)
• Potent antiinflammatory agent compared with hydrocortisone and phenylbutazone in experimentally induced arthritis in rats (Kapoor, 1990)
• Reverses aortic atherosclerosis (Baldwa and others, 1981)

Veterinary use:
• Obesity/hypothyroid
• Arthritis (Sodhi, 1992)
• Geriatrics

Dosage:
• Human: 25 mg tid for hypercholesterolemia
• Dog: Unknown

Gymnema *(Gymnema sylvestre):* Gurmar Sugar-Destroyer

Botany: Asclepiadaceae
• Member of the milkweed family
• Climbing plant common to central and southern India
• Root and leaves used

Pharmacology: Gymnemic acid, a mixture of at least nine closely related acidic glycosides.

Actions: Astringent; stomachic; tonic; cooling; diuretic; stimulates insulin production from islet cells; regenerates pancreatic beta cells; enhances glucose control in diabetic dogs and rabbits (Murray, 1993).

Energetics:
• Kapha-reducing
• Spleen, kidney tonic

Target organs: Pancreas, gastrointestinal tract, kidney.

Applications: Diabetes (type I, type II); corrects metabolic changes in liver kidney and muscle caused by diabetes (Bone, Burgess, McLoed, 1992).

Comments:
• Known for 2000 years as a treatment of diabetes
• No published reports of human toxicity
• In addition to decreasing blood glucose, also helps repair damage to pancreas, liver, kidney, and muscle tissue (Zysk, 1996)
• Decoction of the leaves used for fever and cough
• Poultice of powdered root used for snakebite (Kapoor, 1990)

Research
• Does not increase insulin production in nondiabetic animals (Shanmugasundaram and others, 1990)
• Non–insulin-dependent diabetic patients able to reduce or eliminate conventional drug dosages (Malhotra, 1973)
• Insulin-dependent patients able to reduce insulin injections (Malhotra, 1973)
• Insulin release and beta cell formation were increased (Dash, 1991)

Veterinary use: Diabetes, obesity.

Dosage:
• Human: 20 mg/kg/day, into two doses of extract; or 30 minutes before each meal
• Animal: Same

Neem *(Azadirachta indica)*

Botany: Meliaceae
• Large evergreen tree; cultivated
• Parts used: root bark, young fruit, nut or seeds, leaves, flowers, bark, and gum

Pharmacology:
• Beta-sitosterol
• Flavonoids: kemferol, quercetin, myricetin

Actions: Anthelmintic; antiseptic; bitter; deodorant; diuretic; emmenagogue; febrifuge; antihemostatic; antibacterial; antiviral; antifungal; spermicidal; insecticidal; insect repellant; stimulant; carminative; astringent; alterative; antispasmodic; tonic; antidiabetic.

Energetics:
• Pitta- and Kapha-reducing; Vata-increasing
• Pungent, bitter, astringent, cooling

Target organs: Neem targets the epidermis and reproductive tract.

Applications: Eye disorders; persistent low fever and intermittent fever; skin diseases; peptic ulcers; wounds; blood disorders; stomach worms; galactagogue in cattle and goats; digestive aid; gum disease; intestinal helminthiasis; insect repellant *(Wealth of India);* insecticidal; antibacterial; genitourinary tract infections; natural contraceptive; abortifacient.

Research:
• Neem leaf extract showed significant and dose-dependent antiinflammatory activity in rats as well as a moderate amount of analgesic activity, with antipyretic activity at higher doses; no ulcerogenic effect on gastric mucosa was observed (Koley and others, 1994)
• *A. indica* oil had no adverse effects on the kidney and liver function of experimental animals; it was also found to be nonirritating when applied to the skin of rabbits (Tandan and others, 1995)

Veterinary use: Ectoparasites; endoparasites; gastroenteritis; wound healing; genitourinary tract infections; hepatitis; dermatologic problems; dermatophytes (Sodhi, 1992) (Caution: Possesses natural contraceptive activity and may cause abortion).

Dosage
• Human: Unknown
• Dog: 250 to 500 mg/day, for 3 weeks, of powdered leaves (Sodhi, 1992)

Phyllanthus *(Phyllanthus amarus):* Bhumy amalaki

Botany: Euphorbaciae
• Annual herb, 24 inches high
• Whole plant, leaves, and root used

Pharmacology:
• Triterpinoid compounds
• Lignans: phyllanthum, hypophyllanthum

Actions: Hepatoprotective, astringent, stomachic, diuretic, febrifuge.

Energetics: Kapha- and Pitta-reducing; Vata-increasing.

Target organs: Liver.

Applications: Leaves and roots made into poultice with rice water for edema and cutaneous ulcers; juice of the leaves used for eye disorders, constipation, gastric pain, hepatitis, edema, eczema, acne.

Research:
- Reduces the hepatotoxicity of hepatitis B virus in chronically infected patients (*Lancet,* 1988)
- An extract of *Phyllanthus* sp. found to inhibit growth of the murine P-388 lymphocytic leukemia cell line (Pettit and others, 1990)
- Significant hepatoprotection found in mice and rats treated with phyllanthus and quercitin extracted from phyllanthus when exposed to acetaminophen and alcohol (Gulati and others, 1995)

Veterinary use:
- Cholangiohepatatis, hepatitis (Sodhi, 1992)
- Hepatoprotection
- Roots helpful for camels with digestive troubles (*Wealth of India,* VIII)

Dosage:
- Human: 500 mg tid
- Dog: Unknown

Picrorrhiza *(Picrorrhiza kurroa):* kutkin

Botany: Scrophulariaceae
- Small, hairy perennial herb
- Part used: dried rhizome
- Used as a substitute for Indian gentian *(Gentiana kurroo)*

TCM: Hu Huang Lian.

Pharmacology:
- Iridoid glycosides
- Kutkin: picroside-1, kutkoside

Actions: Hepatoprotective; bitter stomachic; laxative; cholagogue; disperses heat; dries dampness; anthelmintic; antifungal.

Energetics: Kapha- and Pitta-reducing; Vata-increasing.

Target organs: Liver, spleen, lung.

Applications: Reduction in serum cholesterol; infectious hepatitis; bronchial asthma; anticoagulant; low-grade fever; hyperbilirubinemia; beneficial for edema; antimicrobial effects (*Wealth of India,* VIII); epilepsy and malnutrition in infants.

Research:
- *P. kurroa* demonstrates a protective effect against aflatoxin B hepatotoxicity in the rat (*Pharm Res,* 1993)
- Standardized extract of *P. kurroa* reduces the hepatotoxicity of various toxins and possesses anticholestatic and cholagogue properties as well as immunomodulatory and moderate antiviral activity (Dhawan, 1995)
- Androsen, a phenolic glycoside isolated from *P. kurroa,* was isolated as the active compound preventing allergen- and platelet-activating factor–induced bronchial obstruction in guinea pigs; histamine release from human polymorphonuclear cells (PMNs) in vitro was also observed to be reduced (Dorsch and others, 1991)

Veterinary use: Used to treat giardia and hepatitis (Sodhi, 1992).

Dosage:
- Human: 1 to 1.5 g/day
- Guinea pig: 10 mg/kg (Gulati and others, 1995)
- Dog: 200 mg bid (Sodhi, 1992)

Turmeric *(Curcuma longa)* (also haridra)

Botany: Zingiberacea
- Rhizome used
- Perennial herb 2 to 3 feet high with a short stem and tufted large leaves

TCM: *Jiang huang.*

Pharmacology:
- Curcumoids: curcumin, *bis*-demethoxy curcumin, demethoxy curcumin, sesquiterpenes (Kapoor, 1990), turmerones
- Zingiberone (Kapoor, 1990)

Actions: Stimulant; carminative; alterative; emmenagogue; aromatic stimulant; cholagogue; analgesic; astringent; anthelmintic; vulnerary; antibacterial; invigorates blood circulation; disperses stagnant blood; improves bile secretion; bioprotectant hepatoprotective (Kiso and others, 1983); free radical scavenger; prevents free radical formation; 5-lipoxygenase and cyclooxygenase inhibitor mediating antiinflammatory effects (Ahmad and others, 1991); antioxidant (Toda and others, 1985); antineoplastic agent (Mehta, Moon, 1991).

Energetics:
- Bitter, astringent, pungent/heating
- Kapha-reducing, Pitta/Vata-increasing
- Spleen and Liver Meridians (TCM)

Target organs: Has its greatest activity in the digestive, circulatory, and respiratory systems.

Applications: Hepatoprotection; antiinflammatory (better than nonsteroidal antiinflammatory drugs); indigestion, poor circulation; cough; pharyngitis; skin disorders; diabetes; arthritis; anemia; wound healing; bruises.

Comments: Good antimicrobial for chronically weak or ill patients; helps strengthen and stretch the ligaments; purifies the blood; improves intestinal flora; strengthens the digestion; aids in protein digestion; combined with barberry or Oregon grape root, reduces liver congestion.

Research:
- Significant value when used after surgery to reduce postoperative inflammation in human patients (*Int J Clin Pharmacol Ther Toxicol*, 1986)
- Hepatoprotective activity related to antioxidant and lipid peroxidation properties in hepatic acetaminophen toxicity in rats (Srihari and others, 1982)
- U.S. patent describing discovery that curcumin inhibits inflammatory conditions by inhibiting the formation of cyclooxygenase and 5- and 1-lipoxygenase metabolites that in turn are the proinflammatory eicosanoids (leukotrienes and certain prostaglandins). Suggested clinical uses are inflammatory bowel disease, chronic hepatitis, chronic bronchial asthma, inflammatory skin diseases (Ammon and others, 1995)

Veterinary use: Arthritis; antiinflammatory; antioxidant; free radical scavenger; pruritic or inflammatory skin disease; digestive tonic; abscesses (Sodhi, 1992); hepatoprotection, inflammatory bowel disease.

Dosage (nontoxic, a culinary herb):
- Human: 500 mg tid for curcumin
- Bromelain, an proteolytic enzyme, enhances absorption of curcumin, especially if taken 20 minutes before meals
- Curcumin in a lipid base, such as lecithin and essential fatty acids, may also increase absorption, especially when taken with meals
- A similar amount of curcumin in whole turmeric requires 8 to 60 g tid (Murray, 1995)
- Dog: 250 mg tid of curcumin; ½ tsp of whole turmeric bid (Sodhi, 1992)

Ayurvedic Herbs Common in TCM

Smilax, fennel, ginger, hemp, licorice, long pepper, rhubarb, sweet flag.

Ayurvedic Herbs Common in the West

Bayberry, barberry, calamus, onions, garlic, aloe, asparagus, barberry, cinnamon, juniper, milk thistle, gotu kola, valerian, and dandelion.

Unique Ayurvedic Herbs: Rasayanas

Special Ayurvedic formulas concerned with rejuvenation and revitalization

Shilajit

- Formed with the natural exudate of certain rocks and stones found in the Himalayas
- Resembles and smells like asphalt
- Eaten by rats and monkeys in its natural state
- High in iron and other valuable minerals
- Black in color

TCM: Kidney tonic—Kidney *Qi*, *Yin*, and *Yang*.

Preparation: The black, greasy stones are ground and boiled in water. The creamy film that results from the boiling is decanted and sun-dried.

Uses: Urinary tonic. Also useful for wasting and degenerative diseases, especially diabetes (reduces blood sugar; most effective in early stages of DM); chronic urinary tract problems; impotence and infertility; promotes bone growth; aids in fracture repair; osteoarthritis; and spondylosis (Yadava and others, 1995). For cystitis, give 100 mg bid (Sodhi, 1992).

Triphala Three Fruits

Made from equal parts of the fruit of *E. officinalis*, *T. belerica*, and *T. chebula*, three types of trees.

Actions: Rejuvenator; mild laxative and digestant; regulator of elimination and revitalizer of the entire body.

Energetically balanced formula: *E. officinalis* (Amla), Pitta- and Vata-reducing, Kapha- and Ama-regulating; *T. belerica* (Baheda), Kapha- and Pitta-reducing, Vata-regulating, both warming; *T. chebula* (Harada), cooling, rejuvenative for Vata and Kapha regulation.

Uses: Internal cleansing and detoxification; can be used by anyone, especially sensitive individuals and vegetarians; promotes normal appetite and healthy digestion; hematinic, thermogenic; relieves deficiency heat (TCM); promotes the uptake and use of B vitamins; safe, non–habit-forming bowel regulator; eyewash may be used to strengthen vision and reduce ophthalmic irritation (Yadava and others, 1991); obesity (Sodhi, 1992).

Dosage: Human: blood purifier, reducing and cleansing agent, 2 tablets tid; occasional tonic laxative, 2 to 6 tablets crushed in water at night; eye problems, 2 tablets crushed and steeped in ½ cup boiling water, strained and used as eyewash.

Chyavanprash

TCM: Spleen *Qi* and *Yang* tonic, Stomach *Qi* tonic.
- Named after the great sage who created this formula, *Chyavan*
- Made from fresh Indian gooseberries (Amla, or *T. chebula*), which are considered a major health food in India because they are the best source of easily assimilable vitamin C; the vitamin C in Amla complexed with plant tannins, which maintain the potency of the vitamin C even after heating or drying; in addition to Amla, 34 to 50 additional herbs are present in Chyavanprash

Uses: Tonic for weakness and debility; chronic bronchitis; allergies; immune weakness; fevers; emaciation; chronic cardiac problems; urinary tract problems; impotence and infertility; increases longevity and mental alertness; contributes to skin tone and complexion; promotes regular bowel movements; anthelmintic; detoxifier; aperient; digestive tonic; blood tonic for females; increases sexual strength and vigor in males; expectorant; general systemic tonic; antitussive; mild diuretic; antihypoglycemic agent; hematinic; strengthens the heart, liver, kidneys, and sensory organs (Yadava and others, 1995).

Dosage: Works best when taken over a long period of time; human: ½ to 1 tsp each morning with warm water.

References

Agarwal KC, Parks RE Jr: Forskolin: a potential antimetastatic agent, *Int J Cancer* 32:801, 1983.

Ahmad F and others: *Acta Diabetol Lat* 28(1):71, 1991.

Ammon HPT and others: *Planta Medica* 57:203, 1991.

Ammon HPT, Muller AB: Forskolin: from Ayurvedic remedy to a modern agent, *Planta Medica* 51:473, 1985.

Ammon HPT and others: Mechanism of anti-inflammatory actions in Curcumine and Boswellic acids, *J Ethnopharm* 38:113, 1993.

Ammon HPT and others: *Use of preparations of Curcuma plants*. US Patent No. 5,401,777, March 1995.

Baldwa VS and others: *J Association of Physicians of India* 29:13, 1981.

Ben-Efraim S, Yarden A: The activity of some constituents of *Withania somnifera*. I. The anti-bacterial activity of five nitrogen-free substances isolated from the leaves, *Antibiot Chemother* 12:57, 1962.

Bone K, Burgess N, McLeod D: *How to prescribe herbal medicines*, ed 2, Warwick, 1992, Mediherb.

Dash B: *Ayurvedic cures for common diseases*, ed 4, Delhi, 1991, Hind Pocket Books.

De Souza NJ, Shah V: Forskolin: an adenylate cyclase activating drug from an Indian herb, *Economic and Medicinal Plant Research* 2:1, 1988.

Devi P and others: Antitumor and radiosensitizing effects of Withania somnifera (Ashwaganda) on a transplantable mouse tumor, sarcoma-180, *Ind J Exp Biol* 31(7):607, 1993.

Dhawan BN: Picroliv: a new hepatoprotective agent from an Indian medicinal plant, Picrorhiza kurroa, *Med Chem Res* 5(8):595, 1995.

Dorsch W and others: Anti-asthmatic effects of *Picrorhiza kurroa*: Androsen prevents allergen and PAF-induced bronchial obstruction in guinea pigs, *J Int Arch Allergy Appl Immunol* 95(2-3):1128, 1991.

Effect of *Phyllanthus amarus* on chronic carriers of hepatitis B virus, *The Lancet,* October 1:764, 1988.

Evaluation of anti-inflammatory properties of curcumin in patients with post-operative inflammation, *Int J Clin Pharmacol Ther Toxicol* 24(12):651, 1986.

Frawley D, Lad V: *The yoga of herbs*, Twin Lakes, Wisc, 1988, Lotus Press.

Ghosal S and others: Immunomodulatory and CNS effects of Sitoindosides IX and X, two new glycowithanolides from Withania somnifera, *Phytother Res* 3(5):201, 1989.

Gulati RK and others: Hepatoprotective studies on Phyllanthus emblica and quercitin, *Ind J Exp Biol* 33(4):261, 1995.

Gupta VN and others: Chemistry and pharmacology of gum resin of *Boswellia serrata* (Salai guggul), *Ind Drugs* 24(5):221, 1987.

Kapoor LD: *CRC Handbook of Ayurvedic medicinal plants*, Boca Raton, Fla, 1990, CRC Press.

Kerouac R and others: Forskolin inhibits histamine release by neurotensin in the rat perfused hind limb, *Res Commun Chem Pathol Pharmacol* 45:310, 1984.

Khalsa KPS: Ayurvedic herbology in North America, *The Herbalist* 16:1, 1995, American Herbalists Guild.

Koley KM, Lal J, Tandan SK: Anti-inflammatory activity of Azadirachta indica (neem) leaves, *Fitoterapia* 65(6):524, 1994.

Kreutner W and others: Bronchodilator and anti-allergy activity of Forskolin, *Eur J Pharmacol* 111:1, 1985.

Lad V: An introduction to Ayurveda, *Alternative Therapies* 1(3):57, 1995.

The Lawrence Review of Natural Products: Forskolin, 6(4):April, 1985.

Malhotra SC: *Pharmacological and clinical studies on the effects of Commiphora mukul (guggulu) and clofibrate on certain aspects of lipid metabolism*, doctoral dissertation; All India Institute of Medical Sciences, 1973.

McCaleb RS: *Ayurvedic Medicine*, Herb Research Foundation Information Packet, p 2, 1995.

Mehta RG, Moon RC: Characterization of effective chemopreventive agents in mammary gland in vitro using an initiation-promotion protocol, *Anticancer Res* 11:593, 1991.

Murray MT, editor: Coleus forskohlii: source of a potent cell-regulating compound, *Phyto-Pharmacia Review* 4(2).

Murray MT: *The healing power of herbs*, Rocklin, Calif, 1995, Prima Publishing.

Okuda H, Morimoto C, Tsujita T: Relationship between cyclic AMP production and lipolysis induced by forskolin in rat fat cells, *J Lipid Res* 33:225, 1992.

Pachnanda and others: *Ind J Pharmacol* 13:63, 1981.

Pettit GR and others: Isolation and structure of phyllanthostatin 6, *J Nat Prod* 53(6):1406, 1990.

Pharm Res: Picroliv protects against aflatoxin B1 acute hepatotoxicity in rats, 27(2):189, 1993.

Potter DE and others: Forskolin suppresses sympathetic neuron function and causes ocular hypotension, *Curr Eye Res* 4:87, 1985.

Raw materials, *The Wealth of India* X:580-5851, 8:Ph-Re, Publications and Information Directorate, New Delhi, India, 1988.

Raw materials, *The Wealth of India* 1:504, 1988.

Raw materials, *The Wealth of India* 2:203, 1988.

Raw materials, *The Wealth of India* VIII:34 and 49, 1988.

Reddy GK and others: *Biochem Pharmacol* 38:3527, 1989.

Roger PP, Servais P, Dumont JE: Regulation of dog thyroid epithelial cell cycle by forskolin, an adenylate cyclase activator, *Exp Cell Res* 172:282, 1990.

Seamon KB, Daly JW: Forskolin: a unique diterpene activator of cyclic AMP generating systems, *J Cyclic Nucleotide Res* 7:201, 1981.

Sethi PD: *Ind J Pharmacol* 2:165, 1970.

Shanmugasundaram ERB and others: Use of Gymnema sylvestre leaf extract in the control of blood glucose in insulin dependent diabetes mellitus, *J Ethnopharmacol* 30:265, 1990.

Singh N and others: Withania somnifera (Ashwaganda), a rejuvenating herbal drug which enhances survival during stress (an adaptogen), *Int J Crude Drug Res* 20(1):29, 1982.

Singh N and others: Experimental evaluation of protective effects of some indigenous drugs on carbon tetrachloride-induced hepatotoxicity in mice and rats, *J Crude Drug Res* 16(1):8, 1978.

Sodhi T: Ayurveda in veterinary medicine. Proceedings of the Annual Conference of the AHVMA, 1992.

Srihari RT and others: *Ind J Med Res* 75:574, 1982.

Svoboda R, Lade A: *Tao and Dharma, Chinese medicine and Ayurveda,* Twin Lakes, Wisc, 1995, Lotus Press.

Tandan SK and others: Safety evaluation of Azadirachta indica seed oil, a herbal wound dressing agent, *Fitoterapia* 66(1):69, 1995.

Tierra M: *Planetary herbology,* Santa Fe, N.M., 1988, Lotus Press.

Toda S and others: Natural anti-oxidants: anti-oxidative compounds isolated from rhizome of Curcuma longa, *J Chem Pharmacol Bull* 33:1725, 1985.

Yadava and others: *Ind J Anim Sci* 1177, 1995.

Zysk KG: Traditional Ayurveda. In Micozzi M, editor: *Fundamentals of complementary and alternative medicine,* New York, 1996, Churchill Livingstone.

SELECTED READINGS

Badmaev V, Majeed M: Maintaining a healthy liver, *Health Supplement Retailer* 2(5):44, 1996.

Kiso and others: Antihepatotoxic principles of Curcuma longa rhizomes, *Planta Medica* 49:185, 1983.

Murray M: *Diabetes and hypoglycemia,* Getting Well Naturally Series, Rocklin, Calif, Prima Publishing.

Homeopathy

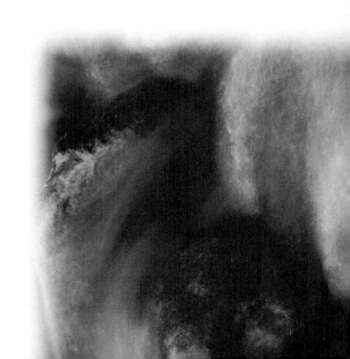

Chapter 25

Homeopathic Medicine: Principles and Research*

DANA ULLMAN

At the turn of the twentieth century, homeopathic medicine was at its apex in America. Approximately 15% of American physicians considered themselves homeopaths. There were 22 homeopathic medical schools, including Boston University, the University of Michigan, New York (Homeopathic) Medical College, Hahnemann Medical College, and the University of Minnesota. There were also more than 100 homeopathic hospitals (Coulter, 1975).

Homeopathy grew despite strong antagonism from conventional physicians and the American Medical Association (AMA). The AMA went so far as to establish within their ethics code a "consultation clause" that prohibited "regular" physicians from even consulting with homeopathic physicians. Although most other ethical violations by physicians were not enforced, the consultation clause was one of the few that was (Coulter, 1975). Homeopathy was clinically, philosophically, and economically threatening to conventional physicians. The fact that its practitioners were medical doctors further aggravated the situation.

As Nicholas von Hoffman wrote in the *Washington Post*, "Samuel Hahnemann lived from 1755 to 1843 and, although this German physician never visited the United States, for 70 years or more his ideas disturbed and divided American medicine. No single individual caused the settled and comfortable structures of this profession more trouble than Hahnemann did, and even now many of the questions he raised have not been answered" (von Hoffman, 1971).

"Homeopathy is a practice that came into being and gained widespread notoriety 'too early' in the history of medicine, at a time when it was impossible to provide any kind of explanation for it" (Bellavite, Signorini, 1995). However, a growing body of laboratory and clinical studies suggests that homeopathic medicine may have biological action and clinical efficacy, and emerging understanding of fractal, chaos, and complexity theories provides a conceptual basis for explaining the way homeopathic medicines may work.

Before attempting an explanation of homeopathic mechanisms, it is first necessary to discuss an underlying assumption—that is, that symptoms of illness are an integral part of the innate defense system of an organism.

Symptoms as Defenses

Today's animal species have survived several hundred thousand years because of the body's homeostatic ability to defend and heal itself. Although conventional medicine has created technologic miracles, they do not compare with the depth and breadth of miracles that a body creates as it continuously staves off countless pathogens and adapts to untold subtle (and not so subtle) stresses.

Many conventional physicians and veterinarians are aware of this innate wisdom but tend to ignore it and intervene more often than necessary. Inevitably, this intervention creates problems such as overprescription of drugs that lead to side effects.

A fundamental flaw in conventional medical thinking is the assumption that symptoms represent the disease itself, that they signify an abnormality with the animal's health and that these symptoms need to be controlled, managed, or eliminated. In fact, the word *symptom* is derived from Greek and means "sign," or "signal." A symptom is not a disease but a sign or signal of it. Abolishing a signal does not necessarily affect the origin of the signal. Seeking to

*Adapted from Ullman D: *The consumer's guide to homeopathy,* New York, 1996, Jeremy P. Tarcher/Putnam. Reprinted with permission.

eliminate a symptom is akin to unplugging a car's low oil warning light when it activates. Although this "treatment" may "work," it does not change the fundamental cause of the signaling.

Although symptoms may indeed suggest that an organism's health is disturbed, homeopaths and a growing number of medical scientists recognize that symptoms are adaptive responses of the organism to physiologic stress (Nesse, Williams, 1994). The emerging science of Darwinian medicine, as described by Nesse and Williams (1994), recognizes that physical, psychologic, and even genetic symptoms are innate and evolutionarily obligatory efforts on the part of an organism to defend and heal itself.

Symptoms are inherent defenses of the body, and eliminating them without addressing the source of the problem tends to suppress the body's healing responses. This suppression may inhibit resolution of disease, and because the organism seeks to defend and heal itself in the most effective way possible on the basis of the resources available to it, secondary treatments may not be as efficient as efforts to influence the original source of the problem.

For instance, a nasal discharge is a response of the body to viruses that cause upper respiratory tract disease. This nasal discharge is composed of virus and dead white blood cells. If a person with a cold takes a medication that dries mucous membranes, elimination of this dead matter is suppressed, which may lead to head and chest congestion. From a homeopathic perspective the body is not as efficient in expectorating mucus through the mouth as in discharging it from the nose, and the resulting chest congestion is more likely to lead to more serious health problems than those that occur from a common cold.

A profoundly different perspective on health and healing emerges with the realization that symptoms are actually defense mechanisms. Instead of treating, controlling, inhibiting, managing, or suppressing symptoms, as is commonly the approach in conventional medicine, therapies that augment the body's own defenses, support, and even (as discussed later) mimic them ultimately make more sense. Such is the approach used in homeopathic medicine.

Theoretical Basis of Homeopathy

Principle of Similars

Homeopathic medicine is based on the principle of similars; that is, the symptoms or syndromes a substance causes experimentally (at pharmacologic or toxic doses) are those that it may clinically resolve when given in specially prepared, exceedingly small doses to individuals who experience similar symptoms and syndromes. In fact, homeopathy derives its name from this "similars" principle. In Greek, *homoios* means similar and *pathos* means disease or suffering (Boyd, 1936). Although homeopathy was formally developed as a systematic method of applying the

similars principle in the early 1800s, the use of this healing approach is a historical pharmacologic strategy used by the ancient Egyptians, Chinese, Incas, Aztecs, and Native Americans (Boyd, 1936; Frazer, 1922).

The principle of similars may initially seem illogical. It seems logical that giving a dose of something that creates symptoms similar to those an animal is experiencing would exacerbate symptoms, not heal them. Yet because symptoms may be adaptive responses of the organism to defend against infection or stress, using small doses of a substance known to cause similar symptoms may in fact augment the defensive response. Even conventional medicine applies the similars principle in the use of immunizations and allergy hyposensitization. It is worth noting that immunizations and allergy treatment represent two of the few modern conventional medical procedures that work to augment the body's own recuperative processes, and these mechanisms essentially operate according to the homeopathic principle of similars.

An example of the body's wisdom in creating symptoms as defenses is the common fever. It is now recognized that measures to directly suppress a fever should be instituted only at very high temperatures.

Use of exceedingly small doses of medicinal agents with the capacity to cause the symptoms of fever similar to those of a febrile animal actually helps resolve fevers more quickly. Belladonna (deadly nightshade) and *Aconitum* (monkshood) are two such substances that cause fever when given in large doses and help alleviate it when given in small doses to patients who exhibit symptoms that correspond to each substance's unique characteristics.

Some evidence for the existence and value of the principle of similars is that homeopaths observe that some patients, especially those with certain chronic ailments, experience a "healing crisis," also called an "aggravation of symptoms," after taking the correctly chosen homeopathic medication. A healing crisis is a temporary worsening of symptoms before a significant improvement in the patient's health that usually leads to improvement in the primary problem, as well as in the overall health of the individual.

A healing crisis is a predictable phenomenon when it is acknowledged that symptoms of illness represent defenses of the organism to infection, stress, or both and that the therapy used mimics, rather than suppresses, the innate healing response of the organism.

Experimental Basis of Homeopathic Medicine

Every homeopathic medicine is tested for its toxicology because homeopaths have found that whatever a substance causes in overdose it can cure when prescribed in small doses. For the past 200 years, homeopaths have performed experiments called "provings" (derived from the German word *pruefung*, which means "test"), in which healthy subjects are given repeated doses of a substance from the plant, mineral, or animal kingdom. These experiments are conducted only on human subjects because human subjects are able to communicate the precise symptoms they are experiencing, and a high level of precision and detail is critical in determining the specific symptoms and syndromes that a substance causes and cures. The substances are tested only on healthy subjects because if they were tested on ill people, it would be difficult to differentiate their own symptoms from those that the substance creates.

These careful experiments have been collected in volumes of books (and now even on sophisticated software programs) that have helped establish homeopathy as the most detailed source of information on toxicology presently available. Although homeopathic literature does not provide information about the specific doses that cause a specific symptom, it describes the many common and unusual symptoms that various substances cause in greater detail than any other source.

The information from these experiments is written in homeopathic texts called *materia medica* and *repertories*. Materia medica (from the Latin, *materials of medicine*) are books with chapters on common homeopathic medicines, along with detailed descriptions of the symptoms associated with each substance. A repertory complements a materia medica, and its many chapters list thousands of symptoms with the various substances that have been found to cause or cure each symptom. Computer-minded people will not be surprised to learn that homeopathic texts have been computerized, and computer-expert systems have been developed for several programs. The impressive detail that homeopaths have collected for the past 200 years is perfect for the modern computer age.

Homeopathic provings are conducted with substances either in crude form or in homeopathic potentized dose (the definition of homeopathic potentized dose is provided later in this chapter). For example, when conducting a proving of coffee, homeopaths sometimes give repeated doses of the crude form of coffee to subjects, but more often, they will give repeated, specially prepared, highly diluted ("potentized") doses of coffee to subjects. Homeopaths collect experiences from these subjects. Although most people feel the stimulating effects of coffee, some feel restless either physically or mentally, or both; some feel anxious, some develop a headache, some experience heart palpitations, and some have idiosyncratic symptoms. The symptoms experienced by a large number of people are written in boldface letters in homeopathic texts, symptoms that are experienced by many subjects are listed in italic, and symptoms that are experienced infrequently are listed in regular type.

Subjects who volunteer for provings are never given crude doses of substances that are considered poisonous. Instead, potentized doses of these substances are tested. Subjects of provings are informed to stop taking the potentized substance once any symptoms develop, thus reducing the danger from these experiments. In fact, homeopaths have found that subjects experience health benefits from provings because these tests challenge a person's defense systems and therefore strengthen them.

Evidence that homeopathic microdoses have biologic effects is apparent not only by the clinical results of homeopaths but also by homeopathic provings. These substances may cause symptoms if taken beyond their therapeutic dose. Because so much of homeopathy is based on these experiments, homeopathic texts probably could not have developed with such consistent information if the microdoses tested acted simply as placebos.

The other lesson of homeopathic provings illustrates another basic concept of homeopathic medicine: Treatment should cease once symptoms have begun to improve. If no improvement is obvious within 48 hours in acute ailments, the homeopathic medicine was probably not the correct one. Repeating doses will not be beneficial to the patient and may in fact cause symptoms of a proving. If such symptoms develop, they rarely last long, unless the administration of the remedy is continued.

It is important to understand that homeopathic remedies are medications, not vitamins or supplements that must be taken daily. Homeopathic medicines should be taken only when an animal's symptoms match those symptoms that the substance causes.

Individualization of Care: Designer Medicine

Imagine a medical system that individualizes medicines based on the totality of unique and idiosyncratic symptoms that an animal experiences. This "designer medicine" is another concept of homeopathic medicine.

From a homeopathic perspective, diseases do not exist, only diseased animals or people. To diagnose a specific disease is too limiting because animals, like humans, experience disease syndromes in subtly and sometimes overtly different ways. One animal with liver disease may exhibit icterus, another may have ascites, and another anemia. One animal may have a coagulopathy, whereas another has hypoalbuminemia. One animal may be aggressive, and another lethargic and seemingly unattentive. One animal may seek warmth, the other may seek cool places. One may have increased thirst, the other will not. In addition to the various physical symptoms, animals experience varying behavioral changes.

Ultimately, homeopaths believe that ailing animals do not simply have a disease; they have a syndrome. This syndrome is a "bodymind" constellation of symptoms. This homeopathic perspective is considerably more modern, if not futuristic, than the limited medical model, which tends to assume that disease is somehow localized. However, conventional medicine is changing, as witnessed by the growing acceptance of psychoneuroimmunology. This field is also developing a perspective that perceives an increasing number of diseases as an integrated psychophysiologic syndrome, although it is still far from the homeopathic perspective that views all disease in this light.

From this perspective, homeopathy is a system of finding a medicine that fits the totality of physical and psychologic symptoms seen in an animal. This may at first sound like a difficult and extremely complex process, and sometimes it is, but often patients fit common patterns of symptoms that match specific remedies. Also, as practitioners study homeopathy, they learn to place more weight on certain symptoms than on others.

Individualizing a medicine to patients and their unique patterns of symptoms makes sense, and at some time in the near future it will probably seem strange that physicians ever believed they could effectively give the same medicine to patients who share only a small number of similar symptoms. The biologic individuality that geneticists have long recognized is appreciated and integrated within the homeopathic method.

Despite the emphasis on individualizing a homeopathic medicine to a sick patient, consumers today often see homeopathic remedies sold in natural food stores and pharmacies labeled to treat specific ailments of humans or animals, ranging from ear problems and arthritis to skin problems and fleas. It is easy to see that some people can be confused and wonder if these products are legitimate forms of homeopathy. Homeopathic formulas, also called *homeopathic combination remedies* or *complexes,* are mixtures of two to eight medicines, each of which may be known to be effective for treating slightly different variations of a certain ailment. These formulas are a broader-spectrum remedy, which may provide benefit to a number of animals. Although these formulas often provide relief for the acute nature of the animal's condition, they do not usually elicit a deep curative response, as do correctly chosen single medicines. Homeopathic formulas may therefore be useful when an individualized single remedy is unknown or if that single remedy is not readily available.

Potentization of Homeopathic Medicines

Those with little knowledge of homeopathy tend to know only that extremely small doses of medicines are used. However, homeopathic medicines are not simply small doses; if they were, the people of Los Angeles (or any major metropolitan area), who regularly inhale small doses of innumerable toxic substances, would probably be cured of everything.

Homeopathic medicines are specially prepared small doses that undergo a specific process of consecutive dilution and succussion (vigorous shaking). A substance is diluted 1 part to 9 parts water (1:10) or 1 part to 99 parts water (1:100), usually in distilled water, and shaken, then diluted again and shaken, and the process is repeated *(Homeopathic Pharmacopeia of the United States*).*

---

*This text is legally recognized as the source for specific guidelines that homeopathic manufacturers are to use in making homeopathic medicines.

When a substance is diluted 1:10 three times, the medicine is called "3X" ("X" is the Roman numeral for 10). When a substance is diluted 1:100 three times, the medicine is called "3C" ("C" is the Roman numeral for 100). When virtually all of the water is poured out on each dilution, a small amount of the water is assumed to adhere to the glass wall, and such dilutions are estimated as 1:50,000. These potencies are called "LM" ("L" is the Roman numeral for 50, and "M" is for 1000). When 1M or 10M is written on a homeopathic medicine, it suggests that the medicine was potentized (usually 1:100) 1000 or 10,000 times.

This pharmacologic process is called *potentization,* and homeopaths have observed from 200 years of clinical practice that the more a substance is potentized, the longer and more deeply the medicine acts and the fewer doses are necessary for treatment. Although it does not initially make sense that this potentization process would increase the clinical effect of a medication, the results have been experienced by hundreds of thousands of homeopathic physicians and tens of millions of homeopathic patients (Ullman, 1996). It is currently estimated that 39% of French physicians and 20% of German physicians prescribe homeopathic medicines, that 45% of Dutch physicians consider homeopathic medicines effective, and 42% of British physicians refer patients to homeopaths (Fisher, Ward, 1994). One interesting note about the use of small doses in homeopathy involves homeopathy's founder, Dr. Samuel Hahnemann. Dr. Hahnemann conducted his first experiments on the homeopathic principle of similars in 1790, but he did not write his first book about homeopathy until 1810, after conducting experiments for 20 years. For those first 20 years, Hahnemann primarily used medicines that were potentized very little (usually 1C to 6C).

Later in his life, as his colleagues began experimenting in higher potencies such as the 1000th, the 2500th, and higher, Hahnemann admonished them by saying, "I do not approve of your potentizing the medicines higher [than the 30th potency]; there must be a limit to the thing" (Haehl, 1971). However, after Hahnemann himself began experimenting with these highly potentized microdoses, he acknowledged that they were effective and in fact were more powerful than the lesser potentized doses. Hahnemann encouraged his colleagues to use these medicines sparingly and carefully because of their power.

Despite the initial skepticism common when people are first introduced to the concept that such extremely small doses can have any healing effect, a considerable body of literature exists from a wide variety of scientific fields that proves microdose phenomena. Many of these studies are discussed later.

Effects of Small Doses in Nature

Scientists readily acknowledge that virtually all animals have at least one sense that provides them with exquisite sensitivity to exceedingly small amounts of the substances they need for survival. For instance, sharks are known to detect small concentrations of blood in the water at a great distance, despite the large volume of water that exists in oceans. Dogs have a highly developed sense of smell. They can follow a human's trail, despite the fact that a person leaves approximately four billionths of a gram of odorous sweat per step (Droscher, 1969).

Biologists recognize that animals emit pheromones. Male night moths can locate female moths on dark moonless nights, and, if necessary, even against the wind. A male silkworm will fly many miles to find its female counterparts (Droscher, 1969). These are not exceptions—many insects can smell as little as a single molecule of their species' pheromones. This is a documented phenomenon of nature and an example of the hypersensitivity of living organisms for what they need to survive.

It is reasonable to believe that human beings are as sophisticated as most other living creatures, especially given the numerous abilities of the human brain and its cerebral cortex. Scientists acknowledge that exceedingly small doses of certain neurotransmitters in the brain can dramatically affect one's emotional, mental, and behavioral states. In addition, very small changes in hormones can have significant effects on the body. Some pituitary hormones can produce contraction of muscle tissue in doses as dilute as 1 part in 19 billion parts of water. Also, animal musk is so chemically similar to testosterone that humans can smell it in portions of as little as 0.000000000000032 (13 zeros) ounces (Ackerman, 1990).

Sensitivity to certain stimuli is often species specific. For instance, ants can smell the trails created by ants of their own species, but they cannot smell the trails created by other species. Similarly, animals can sense the pheromones from their own species but not from others.

Ultimately, this hypersensitivity may in part represent the principle of similars in nature. Homeopathy is simply the medicinal application of this natural law, and the law of similars is homeopathy's method of individualizing microdoses of a substance to a person who needs this substance and is thus hypersensitive to it. The homeopathic principle of similars may in fact be one of the important laws in nature and explains many phenomena that are presently part of nature's mysteries.

Proposed Mechanism of Action

Just as physicians do not fully understand how certain drugs work, homeopaths do not currently understand the precise mechanism of action of homeopathic medicines. Further research is necessary. Still, evaluation of research from several scientific fields provides a better sense of the ways in which microdoses used by homeopaths produce clinical effects.

Chaos Theory

Evidence from the cutting edge of current science may provide some insight into the homeopathic microdose phenomenon (Bellavite, Signorini, 1995). Modern chaos theory, for instance, recognizes the power of infinitesimal changes (Gleck, 1987). One of the basic assumptions of chaos theory is that minute changes can lead to huge differences. Another basic principle of chaos theory is that significant effects from minute changes tend to be most commonly observed in dynamic systems that are raised to high levels of energy or turbulence (what physicists call "far from equilibrium"). Theoretically the diluting and shaking process that is a vital part of the formulation of homeopathic medicines creates these high levels of energy. Because live bodies are high-energy dynamic systems, a tiny energy change from a homeopathic medicine can induce body-wide changes as a result of chaos.

Some research in health physics suggests that small doses of medicines may have a more significant effect than large doses because of a "therapeutic window" (Singer and others, 1985). This effect from small doses is more likely when an organism is in a state of "metastable excitation," a hypersensitive state that changes as soon as a specific stimulus triggers the cascade effect. For instance, large changes can occur in living organisms when specific key enzymes or hormones are activated even slightly. The homeopathic principle of similars may ultimately be the vital link to finding a substance in nature that, when individually prescribed, can trigger this avalanche effect.

Resonance Theory

All matter consists of and radiates energy. Some substances, such as radium, radiate a great deal, whereas other substances, such as a chair, radiate much less. Some objects can even store frequencies, whether it be a tape, a compact disk, or a computer disk. Homeopaths have found that water, the substance in which most homeopathic medicines are made, likewise stores frequencies (Endler and others, 1994).

All things produce their own frequencies, and like a snowflake, each substance is unique. Snow crystals, after melting, resume their previous form when they are frozen again under similar physical conditions (Bellavite, May 1996). Water stores not only frequencies but also some form of memory. Some researchers theorize that the double-distilled water used in the preparation of homeopathic medicines maintains the memory of the original substance that has been diluted in it, even when repeated dilutions of 1:10 or 1:100 have in all probability exceeded the point at which no remaining molecules of the original substance can be assumed to exist (Davenas, 1988).

Another way to understand the way repeatedly diluted water retains some form of information comes from current understanding of holograms. Holograms are high-resolution, laser-created photographs that appear three-dimensional. One feature of holograms is that if a holo-gram of, for example, a tree is broken into pieces, each small piece of the photographic plate maintains a picture of the whole tree, albeit a smaller and less clear picture of it. A similar situation of a pattern within a pattern within a pattern occurs in a phenomenon known as fractals, a frequently discussed topic in current science. A potentized homeopathic medicine may function in the same manner as a holographic fractal (Ullman, 1996).

The holographic effect may seem illogical or even impossible, but it is an accepted observation. Futhermore, genomic DNA is another example of a hologram. The complete genetic information for an individual is contained in each living cell of that individual's body. DNA is an integral part of every cell of an organism's body, and like a holograph, the DNA in each cell contains all of that organism's genetic information.

Although holograms bring to homeopathy the suggestion that some imprint or resonance of a substance will remain no matter how many times it is diluted and shaken, it still remains a mystery how or why the exceedingly small doses used in homeopathy have any effect, let alone increasingly larger effect the more times the medicine is potentized. It has previously been noted that all living and nonliving things have their own resonant frequency. As science writer K.C. Cole wrote, "Planets and atoms and almost everything in between vibrate at one or more natural frequencies. When something else nudges them periodically at one of those frequencies, resonance results" (Cole, 1985). Cole further states that resonance means to resound, to sound again, or to echo, and the power of resonance is in the pushing or pulling in the same direction that the force is already going. Synchronized small pushes can cumulatively create a significant change. A classic example of the force of resonance is the phenomenon of soldiers walking in place over a bridge and causing it to collapse from the natural resonance created.

Another point concerning resonance is the hypersensitivity that the "C" note on a piano has to other "C" notes on the piano. Even if two pianos were several hundred feet away, hitting the "C" note on one piano will cause resonance in all the "C" notes on both pianos. The "B" note immediately next to the "C" will not resonate at all. Similarly, the small doses that homeopaths use will be felt only by people who have symptoms similar to those that a substance causes.

Resonance is more powerful when some friction is present, when the force is similar to, though not exactly the same, as the initial force. The resonance becomes broader, creating something similar to a chord rather than a single note. The relationship of this concept to healing is that homeopaths find the most effective homeopathic medicine is one that in overdose creates symptoms that are the "most similar" to, not necessarily the "same" as, the symptoms the person is experiencing.

Use of small doses of the wrong substance or of the right substance at the wrong time creates no effect because no similar resonance between the substance and the individual's symptoms exists. This is the reason that incorrect homeopathic medicines generally do not have clinical effects, except when taken repeatedly by select patients who are susceptible to a "proving" of the remedy (as discussed earlier). It is similar to the lack of action when a magnet is placed near something that does not contain iron. The magnet will not draw it closer.

Homeopaths have empirically observed that when a homeopathic medication is somewhat, but not significantly, similar to the individual's pattern of symptoms, the remedy creates relatively small changes in an individual's health. Similarly a substance with a percentage of iron in it has some attraction to a magnet but less than if the substance were made entirely of iron.

Homeopaths have also observed clinically that giving a high potency (200X and higher dilutions) of homeopathic medication can sometimes create a healing crisis or a temporary aggravation of symptoms when a lower potency of the remedy was the ideal dose. This fact suggests that the substance was excessively attracted to the "magnet," causing rapid movement. Homeopaths generally find that this healing crisis is therapeutically beneficial most of the time, although the experience can be painful and discomforting to the patient. (Because of the potential for creating healing crises from high potencies, lay people are discouraged from using homeopathic medicines and professionals are encouraged to use them only after they are adequately trained in homeopathy.)

Homeopaths also have noted that homeopathic medicines can become neutralized if subjected to high temperatures or certain magnetic fields, which suggests that some type of memory or information is encoded in the water that can be erased by certain physical influences.

Scientists at the California Institute of Technology have made an observation that may shed some light on the homeopathic phenomenon. The researchers discovered magnetic particles, called *magnetite*, throughout the human brain (Maugh, 1992). The purpose and function of magnetite remain unknown, but its discovery is significant because it establishes the existence of an electromagnetic component of the brain. Perhaps the increased number of times a homeopathic medicine is diluted and shaken creates an electromagnetic state to which the magnetite in the brain is hypersensitive.

A piece of iron becomes magnetized when it is rubbed with another piece of iron. Also, a weakened magnet regains its previous magnetic field when the north and south poles of another magnet are aligned to the north and south poles of the weakened magnet. These facts about magnets may help in understanding the homeopathic process of potentizing medicines and the principle of similars. For instance, the homeopathic process of shaking a substance between each dilution may, like the rubbing of pieces of iron together to create a magnet, be a way for the substance to create its own magnetic or energetic field.

The regeneration of a weakened magnet that results from the alignment of the same poles of the magnet next to each other may illustrate the regenerative and healing effects of the principle of similars.

Homeopathic medications are derived from substances that are diluted and succussed to a "submolecular" dose (a dose that may not have any molecules of the original substance), which may be able to bypass the blood-brain barrier by an unfamiliar mechanism; perhaps each medicine develops its own electromagnetic field able to resonate with parts of the brain that are orchestrating similar symptoms as those that the substance causes. The resonance created may explain the influences that homeopathic medications have on brain physiology and subsequently disease.

In addition to the above theories, Bellavite and Signorini (1995) posit more technical theories based on recognized principles of physics—superradiance and clathrates (aggregates of water molecules)—that cannot be briefly summarized here.

The mystery of homeopathic microdoses is a serious challenge to science. However, it is not a phenomenon that should be dismissed simply because it does not correspond to the presently limited understanding of the laws of nature. The phenomenon appears to be quite real. Scientists therefore must consider ways to change or expand their present understanding of nature to incorporate the phenomenon of homeopathic medicine.

Although an understanding of the ways homeopathic medicines work is important, determination of whether they do in fact work is still more critical.

Scientific Evidence for Homeopathic Medicine

There is considerably more laboratory and clinical research on homeopathic medicine than most scientists realize. However, more research is certainly needed, not simply to answer the questions of skeptics but to help homeopaths optimize their use of these natural medications.

Some skeptics insist that research on homeopathy is mandatory because the exceptionally small doses do not make sense and these drugs have no known mechanism for action. Although homeopaths do not yet understand the ways homeopathic microdoses work, some compelling theories exist about their mechanism of action. However, pharmacologists acknowledge that the mechanism of action of some commonly prescribed medications is not completely understood either. This gap in knowledge has not stopped physicians from prescribing them, however.

Many conventional physicians express doubt about the efficacy of homeopathy, asserting that they will "believe it when they see it." It may be more appropriate for them to acknowledge that they will "see it when they will believe it." This is not meant as a criticism of conventional physicians as much as of conventional medical thinking. The biomedical paradigm has narrowed the practice of medicine to the treatment of specific disease entities with symptom-specific drugs and procedures. An integral aspect of this approach to medicine is the assumption that the larger the dose of a drug, the stronger its effects will be. Although this seems logical initially, it is not consistently true. There is a recognized principle in pharmacology called the "biphasic response of drugs" (*Health Physics*, 1987; Stebbing, 1982). Instead of a drug demonstrating increased effects as the dose is increased, research has consistently shown that exceedingly small doses of a substance may have the opposite effects of large doses. The two phases of a drug's action (hence the name *biphasic*) are dose dependent. For instance, normal medical doses of atropine block the parasympathetic nerves, causing mucous membranes to dry up, whereas exceedingly small doses of atropine cause *increased* secretions to mucous membranes (Goodman, Gilman, 1975).

This pharmacologic principle was concurrently discovered in the 1870s by two researchers, Hugo Schulz, a conventional scientist, and Rudolf Arndt, a psychiatrist and homeopath. This principle is listed as the *Arndt-Schulz law* in a medical dictionary under the definition of *law* (*Dorland's*, 1974).

These researchers discovered that weak stimuli accelerate physiologic activity, medium stimuli inhibit physiologic activity, and strong stimuli halt physiologic activity. For example, very weak concentrations of iodine, bromine, mercuric chloride, and arsenous acid stimulate yeast growth; medium doses of these substances inhibit yeast growth; and large doses kill the yeast (Oberbaum, Cambar, 1994).

In the 1920s, conventional scientists who tested and verified this biphasic response termed the phenomenon *hormesis*, and dozens of studies were published in a wide variety of fields to confirm this biologic principle (Oberbaum, Cambar, 1994; Stebbing, 1982). During the past two decades, this pharmacologic law has generated renewed interest, and now hundreds of studies in many areas of scientific investigation have verified it (*Health Physics*, 1987; Oberbaum, Cambar, 1994). Because these studies have been performed by conventional scientists who are typically unfamiliar with homeopathic medicine, the ultrahigh dilutions commonly used in homeopathy have yet to be subjected to widespread testing. However, research has consistently demonstrated significant effects from such small microdoses that even the researchers express confusion and surprise (*Health Physics*, 1987).

Research on the Arndt-Schulz law and hormesis is important for validating homeopathic research because it demonstrates evidence for the important biphasic responses and microdose effects that lie at the heart of homeopathy. Although this research is readily available to physicians and scientists, it is often ignored or misunderstood.

In Vitro Studies

Laboratory studies have demonstrated biologic activity of homeopathic medicines that cannot be explained simply as a placebo response. Although there are numerous laboratory studies of homeopathic microdoses, one interesting study used nuclear magnetic resonance, also called *magnetic resonance imaging,* to determine whether high potencies of homeopathic medicines placed in water had any measurable differences compared with controls (Demangeat and others, 1992). The study, published in an internationally respected physics journal, found that high potencies (and, therefore, high dilutions) of silicea showed a distinct difference as compared with placebo-treated water. Specifically, researchers found an increase in relaxation times T1 and in the T1/T2 ratio compared with distilled water or diluted and dynamized solutions of sodium chloride. Relaxation times, T1 and T2, are complex molecular parameters that measure proton interactions, molecular rotation and movement, and the influence of paramolecular substances (Bellavite, Signorini, 1995).

This research is of particular importance because a separate study provided evidence of a stimulatory effect on mouse peritoneal macrophages from high dilutions of silicea (Davenas and others, 1987). Bellavite notes, "This was . . . the first case in which a difference of a physical nature was rigorously demonstrated between a solvent and a high dilution of a homeopathic remedy whose biological activity was established experimentally" (Bellavite, Signorini, 1995).

In addition to the various modern studies showing biologic activity from extreme dilutions of homeopathic medicines, some important early studies are also worthy of mention. An extensive series of controlled studies was performed in 1946, 1948, and 1952 by the Scottish homeopath and scientist W.E. Boyd (Boyd, 1954). This work showed that microdoses of mercuric chloride, including potencies of 32c and greater, had statistically significant effects on diastase activity (diastase is an enzyme produced during the germination of seeds). Statistically the significance was independently found to be consistent at $p = 0.001$ in each of the 3 years of study, whereas the control results showed a normal distribution. This research was so well designed and performed that an associate dean of an American medical school commented, "The precision of [Boyd's] technique exemplifies a scientific study at its highest level" (Mock, 1969).

More than 100 studies have been conducted to evaluate the prophylactic and therapeutic effects of homeopathic doses of "toxic" substances. A collaborative effort of scientists from German research institutions and Walter Reed Hospital performed a metaanalysis of these studies (Linke and others, 1994). Like the metaanalysis described later on clinical trials, most of the studies were flawed in some way; however, of the 40 high-quality studies, positive results were found in 27 studies—50% more often than negative results. A particularly intriguing finding was that

researchers who tested doses in the submolecular range were found to have the best-designed studies and more frequently found statistically significant results from these microdoses. (Doses in the submolecular range include potencies greater than 24X or 12C because this represents the point beyond Avogadro's number, the point at which in all probability no molecules of the original substance should remain—only some type of template, resonance, hologram, or fractal.)

Specifically, several researchers administered (usually to rats) toxic doses of arsenic, bismuth, cadmium, mercuric chloride, or lead. Results showed that animals pretreated with homeopathic doses of these substances and then given repeated homeopathic doses after exposure to the crude substance excreted more of these toxic substances through urine, feces, and sweat than animals given a placebo. Furthermore, nine studies on mice that tested homeopathic doses beyond 15C demonstrated a 40% decrease in mortality compared with mice in the control group.

Homeopathic research has also explored the benefits of homeopathic medicines in protection against radiation (Khuda-Bukhsh, Banik, 1991a; Khuda-Bukhsh, Maity, 1991b). Albino mice were exposed to 100 to 200 rad of x-rays (sublethal doses) and then evaluated after 24, 48, and 72 hours. *Ginseng* (6X, 30X, and 200X) and *Ruta graveolens* (30X and 200X) were administered before and after exposure. When compared with mice given a placebo as treatment, mice given the homeopathic medicines experienced significantly less chromosomal or cellular damage.

In one study, albino guinea pigs were exposed to small doses of x-rays that cause reddening of the skin. Studies showed that *Apis mellifica* (7C or 9C) had a protective effect and a roughly 50% curative effect on x-ray–induced redness of the skin (Bildet and others, 1990). *Apis mellifica* (honeybee) is a homeopathic medicine for redness, swelling, and itching, common reactions to bee venom.

In another study, thyroxine 30X (thyroid hormone) was placed in the water of tadpoles (Endler and others, 1994). When these tadpoles were compared with tadpoles given a placebo, the study showed that morphogenesis of tadpoles into frogs was slowed for those exposed to the homeopathic thyroxine. Because thyroid hormone in crude doses is known to speed up morphogenesis, it makes sense, from a homeopathic perspective, that homeopathic doses would suppress morphogenesis. Additional investigations yielded similar results when a glass bottle of homeopathic doses of thyroid hormone was simply suspended in the water with the lip of the bottle above the waterline. This research was replicated at several laboratories, and results were consistent (Endler and others, 1994).

The implications of this study are significant, not only for verification of the biologic effects of homeopathic doses but for demonstrating that these medicines have some type of radiational effect through glass. Some unconventional approaches to homeopathy have been developed in which pupil reflex, pulse, muscle strength, and skin conductance have changed as a result of simply holding a bottle of the clinically indicated homeopathic medicine. Although this approach may seem strange to classically oriented homeopaths, research provides some basis for its application. Several studies investigating very high dilutions of histamine (>30X) on isolated guinea pig hearts demonstrate that this remedy increases blood flow through the heart. This effect was completely neutralized if high dilutions were exposed to very high temperatures (70° C for 30 minutes) or exposed to magnetic fields of 50 Hz for 15 minutes (Benveniste, 1994). It is unlikely that these microdoses could have only a placebo effect when known physical stresses to the medicine can suppress its activity.

A hematology professor at the School of Pharmacy of Bordeaux studied the effects of acetylsalicylic acid (the active ingredient in aspirin) on blood (Doutremepuch and others, 1990). Crude doses of aspirin are known to cause increased bleeding. This research demonstrated that homeopathic doses of acetylsalicylic acid decrease bleeding time in healthy subjects.

Two Dutch professors of molecular biology recently completed significant experimentation that documented the effects of homeopathic microdoses on cell cultures. These researchers exposed fibroblasts to chemical agents (arsenite, cadmium, and numerous other poisons) or a physical insult (heat) and evaluated the processes that represent recovery. They specifically confirmed the importance of heat shock proteins, whose function is to limit damage and aid recovery. For a short period the cells were exposed to a chemical agent or a change in temperature. Repeated studies showed that small doses of the stressful agent, equivalent to 6X to 7X, activated a unique pattern of synthesis of protein molecules that were specific to the agent to which the cell was exposed. The recovery of cells damaged by a stressor was activated by a low dose of the same stressor, whereas undamaged cells experienced no similar change at that low dose. The researchers also found that these microdoses are effective only when the homeopathic's principle of similars is followed (van Wijk, Wiegant, 1994).

A now famous controversial study was conducted by the French physician and immunologist Dr. Jacques Benveniste. Benveniste tested highly diluted doses of IgE on basophils. This work was replicated in six different laboratories at four different universities (the University of Paris South, the University of Toronto, Hebrew University, and the University of Milano). Although the prestigious journal *Nature* published this study (Davenas and others, 1988), it published concurrently an editorial stating that the editors did not believe the results (Maddox, Randi, Stewart, 1988). The editor insisted on going to the primary researcher's laboratory at the University of Paris South to observe the experiment personally, along with two known experts in scientific fraud (one of whom was a magician). The details of what transpired require more de-

tail and technical information than is appropriate for this book. In brief, the experiment did not show significant results, leading the *Nature* editor to pronounce that the original study was a fraud (Maddox, Randi, Stewart, 1988). However, the editor and the fraud experts were not immunologists and thus did not seem aware that many studies in immunology require considerably more replication than could be done in the short time that the *Nature* team visited.

Another problem lay in the study itself, which was technically difficult. The researchers later simplified it, provided even greater scientific controls, and noted significant results. *Nature,* however, chose not to publish these results, and this study was published instead in the *Journal of the French Academy of Sciences* (Benveniste, 1991). A detailed analysis of the limited and biased evaluation by the *Nature* team of Benveniste's work was recently published (Schiff, 1995).

Clinical Research

In 1991 three professors of medicine from The Netherlands, none of whom were homeopaths, performed a metaanalysis of 25 years of clinical studies using homeopathic medicines and published their results in the *British Medical Journal* (Kleijnen, Knipschild, ter Riet, 1991). This metaanalysis covered 107 controlled trials, of which 81 showed that homeopathic medicines were effective, 24 showed they were ineffective, and 2 were inconclusive.

The professors concluded, "The amount of positive results came as a surprise to us" (Kleijnen, Knipschild, ter Riet, 1991). Specifically, they found the following:

- 13 of 19 trials showed successful treatment of respiratory infections
- 6 of 7 trials showed positive results in treating other infections
- 5 of 7 trials showed improvement in diseases of the digestive system
- 5 of 5 showed successful treatment of hay fever
- 5 of 7 showed faster recovery after abdominal surgery
- 4 of 6 improved symptoms of rheumatologic disease
- 18 of 20 showed benefit in addressing pain or trauma
- 8 of 10 showed positive results in relieving mental or psychologic problems
- 13 of 15 showed benefit from miscellaneous diagnoses

Despite the high percentage of studies demonstrating success with homeopathic medicine, most of these studies were flawed in some way. Still, these authors found 22 high-caliber studies, 15 of which showed that homeopathic medicines were effective. Of further interest, they found that 11 of the 14 superior studies showed efficacy of these natural medicines, suggesting that the better designed and performed the studies were, the higher the likelihood that the medicines were found to be effective. Although doctors unfamiliar with research might suspect that most of the studies on homeopathy were flawed in one significant way or another, a more surprising fact is that conventional laboratory research during the past 25 years has had a similar percentage of flawed studies (Roberts, 1975).

On the basis of their research, these researchers made the following conclusion: "The evidence presented in this review would probably be sufficient for establishing homeopathy as a regular treatment for certain indications" (Kleijnen, Knipschild, ter Reit, 1991).

Different types of homeopathic clinical research exist, some of which provide individualization of remedies, which is the hallmark of the homeopathic methodology; some of which give a commonly prescribed remedy to all people with a similar ailment; and some of which give a combination of homeopathic medicines to people with a similar condition. Although positive results might be obtained by any of these methods, researchers must be aware of and sensitive to certain issues to obtain the best objective results.

For instance, if a study does not individualize a homeopathic medicine to people with a specific ailment and the results of the study show no difference existed between those given this remedy and those given a placebo, the study does not disprove homeopathy; it simply proves that this particular remedy is not effective in treating every person with that ailment, each of whom may have a unique pattern of symptoms.

In describing specifics of the following studies of homeopathic medicines, studies that allowed for individualization of medicines and those that did not are differentiated.

When the results of the following clinical studies are considered, it is important to remember that not only have homeopathic medicines been found to be effective in treating a wide variety of ailments, but they do so at a minimum cost and are considerably safer than conventional drug treatment.

Clinical Research With Individualized Care

Some people incorrectly assume that research with homeopathic medicines is impossibly complicated because each medicine must be individualized to the patient. The following studies bring into question this simplistic view.

A recent double-blind clinical trial evaluated homeopathic treament of asthma (Reilly and others, 1994). Researchers at the University of Glasgow used conventional allergy testing to determine to which allergens subjects were most sensitive. Once individual hypersensitivities were determined, the subjects were randomly assigned to treatment and placebo groups. Those patients chosen for treatment were given the 30C potency of the substance to which they were most allergic (the most common substance was house dust mite). The researchers called this unique method of individualizing remedies "homeopathic immunotherapy." (Homeopathic medicines are usually prescribed based on the patient's idiosyncratic symptoms, not on laboratory analysis or diagnostic categories.) Subjects in this experiment were evaluated by both homeopathic and conventional physicians. Subjects in the control group were given a medicine that looked and tasted exactly like a homeopathic medicine.

This study showed that 82% of the patients given a homeopathic medicine improved, whereas only 38% of patients given a placebo experienced a similar degree of relief ($p = 0.003$).

Along with this recent asthma study, the authors performed a metaanalysis, reviewing all the data from three studies they performed on allergic conditions, which totaled 202 subjects. The researchers found a similar pattern in the three studies. Improvement began within the first week and continued until the end of the trial 4 weeks later. The results of this metaanalysis were so significant ($p = 0.0004$) that the authors concluded that either homeopathic medicines work or controlled clinical trials do not. Because modern science is based on controlled clinical trials, the likelihood is that homeopathic medicines are effective. Even an editorial in *The Lancet* noted, "carefully done work of this sort should not be denied the attention of *Lancet* readers" (*Reilly's challenge*, 1994).

Another recent study, published in the *American Journal of Pediatrics*, tested homeopathic medicine for the treatment of a condition recognized to be one of the most serious public health problems worldwide today—childhood diarrhea (Jacobs and others, 1994). More than 5 million children die each year as the result of diarrhea; most of these children live in nonindustrialized countries. Conventional physicians prescribe oral rehydration therapy, but this symptomatic treatment does nothing to address the underlying cause of the diarrhea.

A randomized, double-blind, placebo-controlled study of 81 children conducted in Nicaragua in association with the University of Washington and the University of Guadalajara showed that an individually chosen remedy provided statistically significant improvement of the children's diarrhea compared with those given a placebo ($p = 0.05$). Children given the homeopathic remedy were cured of infection 20% faster than those given a placebo, and the sicker children responded most dramatically to the homeopathic treatment. A total of 18 different remedies were used in this trial; the remedies were individually chosen on the basis of each child's symptoms.

A study of the homeopathic treatment of migraine headache was conducted in Italy (Brigo, Serpelloni, 1991). Sixty patients were randomly chosen and entered into a double-blind, placebo-controlled trial. Patients regularly filled out a questionnaire on the frequency, intensity, and characteristics of their head pain. They were prescribed a single dose of a 30C remedy at 4 separate times for 2-week intervals. Eight remedies were considered, and prescribers were allowed to use any two with a patient. Although only 17% of patients given a placebo experienced relief of their migraine pain, an impressive 93% of patients given an individualized homeopathic medicine experienced good results.

A randomized double-blind, placebo-controlled trial was performed on 175 Dutch children with recurrent upper respiratory infections (de Lange de Klerk and others, 1994). Children in the treatment group were prescribed a "constitutional medicine" for their overall health, as well as symptomatic homeopathic prescriptions to treat the acute respiratory infections they developed. The study found that the children given homeopathic medicines had a 16% better daily symptom score than children given a placebo.

This study also found that the number of children given a placebo who required adenoidectomy was 24% higher than for the children given homeopathic remedies. A 54.8% reduction in the use of antibiotics in the children given homeopathic medicines was reported, whereas the children who received a placebo experienced a 37.7% reduction in antibiotic use. (This reduction in both groups was determined to be the result of the normal growth and development of the child, dietary changes [the study provided written nutritional advice to the parents], and the change in expectations as the result of being under medical care.)

The statistical possibility of these results happening by chance was 6% ($p = 0.06$). Because statistical significance in science is recognized when there is a 5% or less chance of results happening at random, the researchers concluded that homeopathic treatment seemed to add little to the course of upper respiratory tract infections. This more conservative conclusion appeared to be influenced by the fact that the authors sought and received publication of their study in the *British Medical Journal.* An alternative conclusion might be that homeopathic medicines provided benefit to children with upper respiratory tract infections, but there is a small chance (6%) that these positive results happened at random. Given the closeness of these results to 5%, the other improvements in the homeopathic group's health, the low cost of the homeopathic medicines, and the side effects associated with antibiotic usage, physicians and parents should consider seeking homeopathic care for children's upper respiratory tract infections.

Another study of individualized homeopathic care involved the treatment of 46 patients with rheumatoid arthritis (Gibson and others, 1980). Two homeopathic physicians prescribed individually chosen medicines to each patient; half of them were given the real remedy, and the other half were given a placebo. The study found that 82% of those given an individualized homeopathic remedy experienced some relief of symptoms, whereas 21% of those given a placebo experienced a similar degree of relief.

One other interesting trial of semiindividualization of care was in the treatment of primary fibromyalgia (also called fibrositis) (Fisher, 1986). Patients with fibrositis were admitted into a trial in which homeopathic physicians chose among three possible remedies, *Arnica, Rhus tox,* and *Bryonia.* Half of the patients were given one of these remedies, and the other half were given a placebo. No discernible difference appeared between these groups. However, as an integral part of the experiment's design, a panel of homeopaths who were unaware of the treatment protocol assignments evaluated the accuracy of each prescription. This analysis found that those patients whom the panel considered to have received the correct remedy experienced a statistically significant improvement in symptoms compared with those patients given the placebo.

These same researchers next conducted a more sophisticated trial in the treatment of primary fibromyalgia (Fisher and others, 1989). This double-blind, placebo-controlled, crossover trial admitted only those patients who exhibited symptoms of *Rhus tox.* The researchers found that this constituted 42% of the patients interviewed. Half of these 30 patients were given *Rhus tox* 6c during the first phase of the experiment; the other half were given a placebo. During the second phase the groups were crossed over to receive the other treatment. Researchers determined at the beginning of the experiment that improvements in pain and sleeplessness were the outcome measures most important in evaluating the results of this trial, and the results showed that 25% more of the patients experienced pain relief when taking the homeopathic remedy compared with when they were given a placebo, and almost twice as many had improved sleep when taking the remedy.

This type of crossover research design is considered sophisticated because it compares the individual under treatment with himself or herself when using a placebo. Most other research compares two supposedly similar groups of people, but researchers commonly acknowledge that it is difficult and perhaps impossible to get two exactly similar groups of people. The limitation of the crossover design for homeopathic treatment, however, is that most homeopathic medicines provide long-term benefits, so that once a person stops taking a homeopathic remedy, improvement may still continue even in the placebo stage of the trial. Low-potency medicines, such as the 6C used in the previously described experiment, generally have short-acting effects, and higher potency medicines generally have increasingly longer-term effects.

Clinical Research With Nonindividualized Care

In addition to the studies on homeopathy in which individualized remedies are prescribed, a body of research testing single remedies given to people in a nonindividualized manner also exists. Such research is potentially problematic because homeopaths acknowledge that the remedies require some degree of individualization to be effective. The results of a nonindividualized study, either positive or negative, can be misunderstood by people who do not know the basic principles of the homeopathic method.

One study of nonindividualized homeopathic treatment was sponsored by the British government during World War II and was conducted in 1941 and 1942 on volunteers whose skin was burned with mustard gas (Owen, Ives, 1982). The study showed the efficacy of mustard gas 30C as a preventative or *Rhus tox* 30C and *Kali bichromicum* 30C as therapy. The double-blind, placebo-controlled study was conducted at two centers (London and Glasgow); similarly positive results were found at both centers. The London experiments showed that those subjects given certain homeopathic medicines had significant improvement after 7 days compared with those given a placebo (mustard gas 30C [$p = 0.005$]; *Rhus tox* 30C [$p = 0.05$]; *Kali bichromicum* 30C [$p = 0.005$]). In Glasgow experiments showed that those subjects given mustard gas 30C also had significantly less severe burns after 7 days compared with those given a placebo ($p = 0.005$).

However, the researchers also tested the efficacy of opium 30C, *Cantharis* 30C, and variolinium 30C, none of which provided any noticeable benefit. If this trial had tested only these medicines, the researchers might have incorrectly concluded that all homeopathic medicines were ineffective in treating mustard gas burns. Finding the correct remedy is the key to making homeopathy work.

A controlled study on the use of homeopathy in the treatment of diabetic retinitis was conducted (Zicari and others, 1992). This double-blind, randomized, placebo-controlled study of 60 patients used *Arnica* 5C. The results of this study showed that 47% of patients given *Arnica* 5C experienced improvement in central blood flow to the eye, whereas only 1% of patients given the placebo experienced this improvement. Further, 52% of patients given *Arnica* 5C experienced improvement in blood flow to other parts of the eye, but only 1.5% of those given the placebo experienced a similar degree of improvement.

A best-selling flu remedy in France is actually a homeopathic medicine. *Anas barbariae* 200C, commonly marketed under the trade name *Oscillococcinum*, is also popular in the United States and is effective primarily at the first signs of influenza. A double-blind, placebo-controlled study of 478 patients with influenza was conducted, making this the largest trial yet of a homeopathic medicine (Ferley and others, 1989). This trial showed that almost twice as many people who took the homeopathic remedy recovered from the flu after 48 hours compared with those given a placebo.

Although this remedy was found to work for all age groups, it was considerably more effective for people under age 30. It was not effective in subjects with severe flu symptoms. In advanced cases of influenza, a more individualized homeopathic remedy may be indicated.

In addition to various studies on human health, a number of animal studies have been conducted. Such studies are useful not only for the clinical information they provide for animal health but also because they significantly reduce the chances that a placebo response is involved. British researchers have conducted trials showing that homeopathic medicines, specifically *Caulophyllum* 30C, could lower the rate of stillbirths in pigs (Day, 1984). Pigs given a placebo had 103 births and 27 stillbirths (20.8%); those given *Caulophyllum* 30C had 104 births and 12 stillbirths (10.3%).

Not all studies show efficacy of homeopathic medicines—not because they do not work but mostly because the studies were poorly designed. One such study tested a single homeopathic medicine in the treatment of osteoarthritis (Shipley and others, 1983). This study consisted of 36 patients, of whom one third were given *Rhus tox* 6C, one third were given a conventional drug (fenoprofen, a nonsteroidal antiinflammatory drug), and one third were given a placebo. Those patients given the conventional drug experienced some relief of symptoms, but those given the homeopathic remedy and the placebo had a similar lack of response to treatment. Although some might conclude that homeopathic medicines are ineffective in the treatment of osteoarthritis, this study suggests only that *Rhus tox* 6C is an ineffective remedy when given without individualization to patients with osteoarthritis.

One confounding variable in this trial was that 2 of the 12 patients given the homeopathic medicine were withdrawn from the trial because they experienced an aggravation of symptoms after taking the medicine. Because homeopathic medicines sometimes cause a temporary increase in chronic symptoms before significant improvement, the failure of the researchers to follow up is disappointing. Because this trial lasted only 2 weeks, it did not allow time for adequate evaluation. For example, if these two patients experienced the significant relief that is common after an initial aggravation of symptoms, the results of the trial would have been different. Of great significance is the fact that although *Rhus tox* is a common remedy for rheumatoid arthritis in humans, it is less common for degenerative osteoarthritis.

Clinical Research With Homeopathic Combination Remedies

Homeopathic combination remedies are formulas in which several homeopathic substances are mixed together into one remedy. This untraditional approach to homeopathic medicine is commercially popular in many countries. Although homeopaths do not consider these remedies as effective as individually chosen medicines, research has verified that they do work. However, homeopaths consistently find that single homeopathic medicines have the potential to truly cure a person's disease, whereas combination medicines at best provide safe but temporary relief of symptoms.

The same researchers who conducted the study on asthma described previously also performed a study on the treatment of hay fever (Reilly and others, 1986). This double-blind, placebo-controlled study prescribed a 30C potency of a combination remedy made from 12 common pollens. The results showed that those subjects taking the homeopathic remedy had six times fewer symptoms than those given the placebo. Both groups of subjects were allowed to use an "escape" medicine (an antihistamine) if their remedy did not work adequately. The study showed that homeopathic subjects resorted to antihistamines half as often as did those given the placebo.

Another example of significant results from a homeopathic combination remedy was in the treatment of women during their ninth month of pregnancy (Dorfman, Lasserre, Tetau, 1987). Ninety women were given the 5C potency of the following remedies: Caulophyllum, *Arnica, Cimicifuga,* pulsatilla, and *Gelsemium.* They were given doses of this combination remedy twice daily during the ninth month. This double-blind, placebo-controlled study showed that women given the homeopathic medicines experienced a 40% shorter labor than those given a placebo. Also, the women given the placebo had four times as many complications of labor as those given the homeopathic combination.

One of the limitations of research on combination remedies is that the results do not reveal whether the effective treatment came from one specific medicine or from the unique combination of remedies. A recent study of 22 healthy women in their first pregnancies tested Caulophyllum, one of the medicines used in the study cited above, which was administered in the 7C potency during the active phase of labor (one dose per hour repeated for a maximum of 4 hours). The time of labor for those women given the homeopathic medicine was 38% shorter than for women given a placebo (Eid, Felisi, Sideri, 1993). This trial was not double blind; however, the researchers recently completed a double-blind trial and confirmed their earlier results (Eid, Felisi, Sideri, 1994).

A popular homeopathic external application marketed as Traumeel has been studied for its efficacy in the treatment of acute tendonitis (Zell and others, 1988). This combination of 14 remedies in 2X to 6X potencies were given to subjects with sprained ankles. After 10 days, 24 of the 33 patients who were given the homeopathic medicine were pain free; 13 of 36 patients given a placebo experienced a similar degree of relief. This same preparation was also used in the treatment of traumatic hemarthrosis and was shown to significantly reduce healing time compared with placebo. Objective measurements of joint swelling, movement, and evaluation of the synovial fluid at injury were assessed.

A study of 61 patients with varicose veins was performed according to double-blind, placebo-controlled design (Ernst, Saradeth, Resch, 1990). Three doses of a popular German combination of eight homeopathic medicines were given daily for 24 days. Measured parameters were venous filling time, leg volume, and subjective symptoms. The study found that venous filling time improved in those given the homeopathic medicines by 44%, whereas filling time deteriorated in the placebo group by 18%. Other measures also had significant differences showing benefit from the homeopathic medicine.

In addition to the various clinical studies on human subjects, there also has been some research on homeopathic medicines to improve the health of animals. European researchers have shown that dairy cows given *Sepia* 200C at postpartum day 14 experienced significantly improved calving parameters over those given a placebo (Williamson, 1991, 1995). Low-potency (1X to 6X) combinations of *Lachesis,* pulsatilla, and Sabina, or *Lachesis, Echinacea,* and Pyrogenium, along with Caulophyllum given to pigs had preventive and therapeutic effects on mastitis and endometritis (Both, 1987).

Not all clinical studies on homeopathic combination medicines find evidence of efficacy, but there are often important factors that explain the failure. A Canadian study on the treatment of plantar warts is one such example (Labrecque and others, 1992). This randomized, double-blind, placebo-controlled trial with 162 patients prescribed three medicines to each patient. (Because the trial did not mix the remedies together, it is not completely accurate to call the use of these remedies a combination. It is more precise to consider it "polypharmacy," the use of several medicines.) The remedies used were *Thuja* 30C, antimonium crud 7C, and nitric acid 7C. *Thuja* was taken once a week, and the other two remedies were taken once a day during the 6-week trial. The results showed no noticeable difference between subjects given the homeopathic medicines and those given a placebo.

Many homeopaths may be initially surprised at the result of this trial because they consider these remedies commonly effective in the treatment of warts. However, the remedies may be effective for treating warts, but they are not necessarily effective for all types of warts or in all people. A recent study of homeopathic treatment for various types of warts found that 18 of 19 people with plantar warts were cured, on average, in 2.2 months (Gupta, Bhardwaj, Manchanda, 1991). The most common remedy was ruta, prescribed to 12 of the 19 patients. *Thuja* was prescribed for only three patients, and antimonium crud was prescribed for two patients.

This study suggests that individualization and the use of well-chosen remedies are necessary for most effective treatment.

One additional note about research using homeopathic combinations is important. The homeopathic literature refers to the fact that some remedies are antidoted by other remedies. Although the medications in the Canadian trial are not known to antidote each other, homeopaths acknowledge that the understanding of which remedies antidote each other is somewhat primitive (for a listing of which remedies antidote each other, see the appendix in *Kent's Repertory* or in the Indian edition of *Bo-*

ericke's Pocket Manual of Materia Medica with Repertory). Homeopathic research must, therefore, be aware of this possibility so that conclusions from research are not over-stated.

Summary

This review of research is not meant to be complete. Readers are encouraged to review the books listed in the References and Suggested Readings sections of this chapter for access to many other clinical and laboratory studies, as well as to theoretical foundations of homeopathic microdoses.

Despite the now strong evidence that homeopathic medicines promote biologic activity and possess clinical efficacy, there is still great resistance to their use. Recently *Lancet* published research on the homeopathic treatment of asthma (Reilly and others, 1994a). In a press release announcing this research, the authors emphasized that although homeopathic medicines may provide some benefit to people with asthma, conventional medicines offer greater benefit.

This was a puzzling statement for two reasons. First, the study did not compare homeopathic and conventional medicine; it only compared homeopathic medicine with a placebo. Any other conjecture was not founded on the data presented. Second, *Lancet* refused to openly acknowledge that homeopathic medicines may work after all.

Despite the resistance to change in general and to homeopathy specifically, it is becoming increasingly difficult for physicians and scientists to doubt the benefits that homeopathic medicines offer. Italian hematologist Paolo Bellavite and Italian homeopath Andrea Signorini's *Homeopathy: A Frontier in Medical Science* is currently the most comprehensive review of controlled studies on homeopathy. The authors conclude the following: "The sum of the clinical observations and experimental findings is beginning to prove so extensive and intrinsically consistent that it is no longer possible to dodge the issue by acting as if this body of evidence simply did not exist" (Bellavite, Signorini, 1995).

They also make the following observation: "To reject everything en bloc, as many are tempted to do, means throwing out the observations along with the interpretations, an operation which may be the line of least resistance, but which is not scientific because unexplained observations have always been the main hive of ideas for research" (Bellavite, Signorini, 1995).

To ignore the body of experimental data that presently exists on homeopathic medicines and to deny the body of clinical experience of homeopaths and homeopathic patients, one would have to be virtually blind. Presumably, this blindness is a temporary affliction—one that will soon be cured.

REFERENCES

Ackerman D: *A natural history of the senses*, New York, 1990, Vintage.

Bellavite P, Signorini A: *Homeopathy: a frontier in medical science*, Berkeley, 1995, North Atlantic.

Benveniste J: Further biological effects induced by ultra high dilutions: inhibition by a magnetic field. In Endler PC, Schulte J, editors: *Ultra high dilution*, Dordrecht, 1994, Kluwer Academic.

Bildet J and others: Demonstrating the effects of *Apis mellifica* and *Apium* virus dilutions on erythema induced by UV radiation on guinea pigs, *Berlin J Res Homeopathy* 1:28, 1990.

Boericke W: *Pocket manual of materia medica with repertory*, New Delhi, India, 1996, B. Jain.

Both G: Zur Prophylaxe und Therapie des Metritis-Mastitis-Agalactie: Komplexes des Schweines mit Biologischen Arzneimitteln, *Biologische Tiermedizen* 4:39, 1987.

Boyd L: *The simile in medicine*, Philadelphia, 1936, Boericke and Tafel.

Boyd W: Biochemical and biological evidence of the activity of high potencies, *Br Homoeopathic J* 44:6, 1954.

Brigo B, Serpelloni G: Homeopathic treatment of migraines: a randomized double-blind controlled study of 60 cases, *Berlin J Res Homeopathy* 1(2):98, 1991.

Cole KC: *Sympathetic vibrations*, New York, 1985, Bantam.

Coulter HC: *Divided legacy: the conflict between homoeopathy and the American Medical Association*, Berkeley, 1975, North Atlantic.

Davenas E and others: Human basophil degranulation triggered by very dilute antiserum against IgE, *Nature* 333:816, 1988.

Davenas E, Poitevin B, Benveniste J: Effect on mouse perineal macrophages of orally administered very high dilutions of silica, *Eur J Pharmacol* 135:313, 1987.

Day C: Control of stillbirths in pigs using homoeopathy, *Vet Rec* 114(9):216, 1984.

de Lange de Klerk E and others: Effect of homeopathic medicines on daily burden of symptoms in children with recurrent upper respiratory tract infections, *Br Med J* 309:1329, 1994.

Demangeat JL and others: Modifications des temps de relaxation RMN a 4 z des protons du solvant dans les Très Hautes Dilutions Salines de Silice/lactose, *J Med Nucl Biophy* 16:35, 1992.

Dorfman P, Lasserre MN, Tetau M: Préparation à l'accouchement par homéopathie: experimentation en double-insu versus placebo, *Cahiers de Biotherapie* 94:77, 1987.

Dorland's illustrated medical dictionary, ed 25, Philadelphia, 1974, WB Saunders.

Doutremepuch C and others: Aspirin at very ultra low dosage in healthy volunteers: effects on bleeding time, platelet aggregation and coagulation, *Haemostasis* 20:99, 1990.

Droscher V: *The magic of the senses*, New York, 1969, Harper & Row.

Eid P, Felisi E, Sideri M: Applicability of homoeopathic caulophyllum thalictroides during labour, *Br Homoeopathic J* 82:245, 1993.

Eid P, Felisi E, Sideri M: Super-placebo ou action pharmacologique? Une étude en double aveugle, randomiseé avec un remède homeopathique (caulophyllum thalictroides) dans le travail de l'accouchement. Proceedings of Fifth Congress of OMHI International Organization for Homeopathic Medicine, Paris, Oct 20-23, 1994.

Endler PC and others: The effect of highly diluted agitated thyroxine on the climbing activity of frogs, *Vet Hum Toxicol* 36:56, 1994.

Ernst E, Saradeth T, Resch KL: Complementary treatment of varicose veins: a randomised, placebo-controlled, double-blind trial, *Phlebology* 5(3):157, 1990.

Ferley JP and others: A controlled evaluation of a homoeopathic preparation in the treatment of influenza-like syndrome, *Br J Clin Pharmacol* 27:329, 1989.

Fisher P: An experimental double-blind clinical trial method in homoeopathy: use of a limited range of remedies to treat fibrositis, *Br Homoeopathic J* 75:142, 1986.

Fisher P and others: Effect of homoeopathic treatment on fibrositis, *Br Med J* 299:365, 1989.

Fisher P, Ward A: Complementary medicine in Europe, *Br Med J* 309:107, 1994.

Frazer Sir JG: *The golden bough,* New York, 1922, Macmillan.

Gleck J: *Chaos,* New York, 1987, Penguin.

Goodman L, Gilman A: *The pharmacological basis of therapeutics,* ed 5, New York, 1975, Macmillan.

Gupta R, Bhardwaj OP, Manchanda RK: Homoeopathy in the treatment of warts, *Br Homoeopathic J* 80(2):108, 1991.

Haehl R: *Samuel Hahnemann: his life and work,* New Delhi, 1971, B Jain.

Health Physics 52: May 1987.

Homeopathic pharmacopeia of the United States: Washington, DC, 1995, Homeopathic Pharmacopoeia Convention of the United States.

Jacobs J and others: Treatment of acute childhood diarrhea with homeopathic medicine: a randomized clinical trial in Nicaragua, *Pediatrics* 93:719, 1994.

Kent JT: *Repertory of homeopathic materia medica,* New Delhi, India, 1996, B. Jain.

Khuda-Bukhsh AR, Banik S: Assessment of cytogenic damage in x-irradiated mice and its alteration by oral administration of potentized homeopathic drug, ginseng D200, *Berlin J Res Homeopathy* 1(4/5):254, 1991a.

Khuda-Bukhsh AR, Maity S: Alteration of cytogenetic effects by oral administration of potentized homeopathic drug, *Ruta graveolens* in mice exposed to sub-lethal x-radiation, *Berlin J Res Homeopathy* 1(4/5):264, 1991b.

Kleijnen J, Knipschild P, ter Riet G: Clinical trials of homoeopathy, *Br Med J* 302:316, 1991.

Labrecque and others: Homeopathic treatment of plantar warts, *Can Med Assoc J* 14610:1749, 1992.

Linke K and others: Critical review and meta-analysis of serial agitated dilutions in experimental toxicology, *Hum Exper Toxicol* 13:481, 1994.

Maddox J, Randi J, Stewart W: 'High-dilution' experiments a delusion, *Nature* 334:443, 1988.

Maugh T: Magnetic particles found through the human brain, *San Francisco Chronicle* May 12, 1992.

Mock D: 1969 What's going on here, anyway?—a review of Boyd's "biochemical and biological evidence of the activity of high potencies," *J Am Inst Homeopathy* 62:197, 1969.

Nesse R, Williams G: *Why we get sick: the new science of Darwinian medicine,* New York, 1994, Times.

Oberbaum M, Cambar J: Hormesis: dose dependent reverse effects of low and very low doses. In Endler PC, Schulte J editors: *Ultra high dilutions,* Dordrecht, 1994, Kluwer Academic.

Reilly D and others: Is homoeopathy a placebo response? Controlled trial of homoeopathic potency, with pollen in hayfever as model, *Lancet* ii:881, 1986.

Reilly D and others: Is evidence for homeopathy reproducible? *Lancet* 344:1601, 1994.

Roberts RW: Good science, bad data, *NBS Dimensions* 59:32, 1975.

Schiff M: *The memory of water,* London, 1995, Harper Collins.

Shipley M and others: Controlled trial of homoeopathic treatment of osteoarthritis, *Lancet* 1:97, 1983.

Singer MV and others: Low concentrations of ethanol stimulate gastric secretion independent of gastrin release in humans, *Gastroenterology* 85:1254, 1985.

Stebbing ARD: Hormesis: the stimulation of growth by low levels of inhibitors, *Science of the Total Environment* 22:213, 1982.

Ullman D: *The consumer's guide to homeopathy,* Los Angeles, 1996, Tarcher/Putnam.

van Wijk R, Wiegant F: *Cultured mammalian cells in homeopathy research: the similia principle in self-recovery,* Utrecht, 1994, University of Utrecht.

von Hoffman N: The father of homeopathy, *The Washington Post,* July 21, 1971, p B1.

Williamson and others: A study using sepia 200c given prophylactically postpartum to prevent anoestrus problems in the dairy cow, *Br Homoeopathic J* 80:149, 1991.

Williamson AV and others: A trial of sepia 200, *Br Homoeopathic J* 84:14, 1995b.

Zell J and others: Behandlung von akuten Sprung-gelenksdistornen: Doppelblindstudie zum Wirksamkeitsnachweis eines Homoopathischen Salbenpraparats, *Fortschr Med* 106:96, 1988.

SELECTED READINGS

Banerjee DD: *Textbook of homeopathic pharmacy,* New Delhi, 1986, B Jain.

Benveniste J, Arnoux B, Hadji L: Highly dilute antigen increases coronary flow of isolated heart from immunized guinea pigs, *FASEB J* 6:7Ee e, 1992 (abstract 1610).

Benveniste J and others: L'agitation des solutions hautment diluées n'induit pas d'activité biologique specifique, *CR Acad Sci Paris* 312:461, 1991.

Bridgman PW: *The physics of high pressure,* London, 1949.

Day C: *J Am Inst Homeopathy* 4:146, 1986.

Endler PC and others: Transmission of hormone information by non-molecular means, *FASEB* 8, 1994 (abstract 2313).

Maddox J: When to believe the unbelievable, *Nature* 333:787, 1988.

Gibson RG and others: Homeopathic therapy in rheumatoid arthritis: evaluation by double-blind clinical therapeutic trial, *Br J Clin Pharmacol* 9:453, 1980.

Owen RMM, Ives G: The mustard gas experiments of the British Homeopathic Society: 1941-1942. Proceedings of the thirty-fifth International Homeopathic Congress, 1982.

Paterson J: Report on mustard gas experiments, *J Am Inst Homeopathy* 37:47, 1944.

Reilly's challenge, *Lancet* [editorial] 344:1585, 1994.

Thiel W, Borho B: Die Therapie von frischen, Traumatischen Blutergussen der Kniegelenke Hamatros mit Traumeel N Injectionslogung, *Biol Medizin* 20:506, 1993.

Zicari D and others: Valutazione dell'azione angioprotettiva de preparati di arnica nel trattamento della retinpatia diabetica, *Bolletino de Oculistica* 5:841, 1992.

RESOURCES ON HOMEOPATHIC PRINCIPLES AND PRACTICAL APPLICATIONS

Grossinger R: *Homeopathy: an introduction for beginners and skeptics,* Berkeley, 1994, North Atlantic. (This scholarly book discusses homeopathy in a historical, cultural, and scientific context in a way that helps us understand homeopathy and healing more deeply.)

Stephen C, Ullman D: *Everybody's guide to homeopathic medicine,* New York, 1997, Jeremy P. Tarcher/Putnam. (This book provides a short review of homeopathic principles and more detailed discussion on how to use homeopathic medicines for common acute ailments.)

Ullman D: *The consumer's guide to homeopathy,* New York, 1996, Tarcher/Putnam. (This book provides a comprehensive overview of what homeopathy is, what evidence exists for its therapeutic value, how consumers can treat themselves for acute disorders, and what results consumers can expect from the professional homeopathic treatment of chronic ailments.)

Ullman D: *Discovering homeopathy,* Berkeley, 1991, North Atlantic. (For skeptic or advocate of homeopathy, this book covers homeopathic principles and their application in obstetrics, pediatrics, gynecology, infectious disease, allergy, chronic ailments, mental health, sports medicine, dentistry, and more.)

Ullman D: *Homeopathic healing* (a set of six cassettes), Boulder, Colo., 1995, Sounds True. (The audiocassette series reviews homeopathic principles and practical applications for more than 30 common homeopathic medicines.)

Vithoulkas G: *The science of homeopathy,* New York, 1980, Grove. (This book describes homeopathic principles and methodology in a way that gives insight into the homeopathic process of casetaking and case analysis.)

RESOURCES ON HOMEOPATHIC RESEARCH

Bellavite P, Signorini A: *Homeopathy: a frontier in medical science,* Berkeley, 1995, North Atlantic. (This book provides the most comprehensive review of the clinical and laboratory evidence using homeopathic medicines. It also discusses the biophysics of water and chaos and complexity theories and how they provide some substantiation for homeopathy.)

British Homoeopathic Journal: 2 Powis Place, Great Ormond St, London, WC1N 3HT, England. (This journal is one of the leading resources for information about homeopathic research.)

Coulter HL: *Homoeopathic science and modern medicine: the physics of healing with microdoses,* Berkeley, 1980, North Atlantic. (A good, though dated, review of the scientific literature on homeopathy. This book includes many pre-1970s studies not discussed elsewhere.)

Doutremepuich M, editor: *Ultra-low doses,* Washington, DC/London, Taylor and Francis, 1991. (Focusing primarily on in vitro studies, this book includes a compilation of studies in the field of biochemistry, biophysics, toxicology, and cell biology.)

Endler PC, Schulte J, editors: *Ultra high dilution: physiology and physics,* Dordrecht, 1994, Kluwer Academic. (This book includes several of the specific studies mentioned by Bellavite and Signorini, but with greater detail. Articles providing provocative theories on the mechanism of action of homeopathic medicines are also included.)

IAVH, Newsletter for the International Association for Veterinary Homeopathy (formerly *Dynamis*): publisher IAVH. For more information, contact Andreas Schmidt, General Secretary, Sonnhaldenstr 24 CH-8370, Sirnach, Switzerland.

Resch G, Gutmann V: *Scientific foundations of homoeopathy,* Munich, 1987, Bartel and Bartel. (This book is a theoretic exposition of the ways homeopathic medicines may work.)

Scofield AM: Experimental research in homoeopathy: A critical review, *Br Homoeopathic J* 73(3-4): July-October 1984, pp 161-80, 211-26. (This is a critical review of the clinical and laboratory evidence for homeopathy before 1984.)

Ullman D, editor: *Monograph on homeopathic research,* vols I and II, Berkeley, Calif, 1981, 1986, Homeopathic Educational Services. (This compilation is a series of clinical and laboratory studies, before 1986.)

van Wijk R, Wiegant FAC: *Cultured mammalian cells in homeopathy research: the similia principle in self-recovery,* Urecht, 1994, University of Utrecht. (Written by molecular biologists, this book reviews their research on microdoses and the homeopathic principle of similars.)

ACCESS TO RESOURCES

Academy for Veterinary Homeopathy, 1283 Lincoln Street, Eugene, Ore, 97401. (The AVH provides training in classical homeopathy for Veterinarians, leading to certification by the AVH.)

Homeopathic Educational Services, 2124 Kittredge St, Berkeley, CA 94704. (The HES is a leading resource for homeopathic books, tapes, medicine kits, software, and correspondence courses.)

International Association for Veterinary Homeopathy, U.S. contact Susan G. Wynn, DVM, 1080 North Cobb Parkway, Marietta, Ga, 30062. (The IAVH publishes an international newsletter relating to veterinary homeopathy.)

International Foundation for Homeopathy, P.O. Box 7, Edmonds, Wash, 98020. (The IFH provides training to professionals who wish to specialize in homeopathy and publishes a bimonthly magazine.)

National Center for Homeopathy, 801 N Fairfax #301, Alexandria, VA 22314. (The NCH is the leading homeopathic organization in the United States. It publishes a monthly magazine, organizes annual conferences, coordinates homeopathic study groups, and sponsors a summer school in homeopathy.)

Chapter **26**

Veterinary Homeopathy: Principles and Practice

CHRISTOPHER DAY; research section by J.G.G. SAXTON

The use of homeopathy represents an entirely different philosophy from that of conventional medicine. The integration of the two methods is challenging. A holistic way of thinking, homeopathy involves the treatment of the patient as a whole, mind and body, and includes consideration of lifestyle, nutrition, and other interrelated factors. It does not consider the body as a collection of separate components. The concept of mind and body as one is sometimes difficult to grasp, but the mind and body are indeed an inseparable part of the individual and should be treated as such. For example, anxiety and stress have physical consequences, and a physical injury produces mental effects. All parts of the system affect all other parts and are in turn influenced by them. When this important concept is grasped, it may easily be incorporated in diagnosis and prescription. This is holistic thinking, an integral part of good homeopathy.

History

Veterinary homeopathy has a tradition almost as long as homeopathy for humans. Samuel Hahnemann, the founder of homeopathy in the late eighteenth century, lectured on the subject to the Leipzig Economic Society. The updated manuscript of this lecture resides in the cellars of the Universitäts Bibliothek of Leipzig. The text of the lecture is recorded in the journal *Classic Homeopathy Quarterly* (Kent, 1904). In his lecture, probably delivered around 1812 or 1813, Hahnemann referred to the great similarity of the method as applied to animals and humans. Thus veterinary homeopathy is at least 180 years old.

Homeopathic treatment of animals was introduced by Baron von Boenninghausen (b. 1785) (Boger, 1938). Von Boenninghausen treated various species of animals and is said to have established the principles of veterinary homeopathy.

Although the early practice of veterinary homeopathy is poorly documented, texts that survive bear witness to the continuation of the tradition throughout the intervening years. Notable historical books include those of Leath, published in Great Britain in 1851; Moore, published in Great Britain in 1857 and 1863; Lord, Rush, and Rush, published in London in 1875; Ruddock's veterinary vade mecum, third edition published in Great Britain in 1878; Boericke and Tafel, published in the United States in 1881; and Gerhardt, ninth edition published in Germany in 1912 (preface to first edition written in Baltimore in 1869).

By 1906, Humphrey's Medicine Company was producing a range of homeopathic remedies for veterinary use with accompanying booklets. The company had been serving animals since 1860.

Later authors of veterinary texts include Biddis in Great Britain in 1980; Brock and Nielsen in Denmark in 1986; Day in Great Britain from 1984 to the present; del Francia in Italy in 1985; Macleod in Great Britain from 1981 to 1994; Peker Bonnefous, in France in 1988; Quiquandon in France in 1983; Rakow in Germany in 1986 and 1987; Westerhuis in The Netherlands in 1989; Wolff in Great Britain in 1984; and Wolter in Germany in 1954 and 1989.

Veterinary homeopathy has its strongest modern tradition in Europe, particularly in Germany, France, and Great Britain. In Britain, George Macleod did more than any single practitioner to keep the philosophy alive in the latter half of the twentieth century. In fact, Macleod practiced veterinary homeopathy from World War II until his death in 1995. Macleod was one of the earliest veterinarians to address an International League Congress in 1973. Throughout the 1970s, 1980s, and 1990s, he published papers and books that have become classic works on the subject. He helped found the British Association of

Homeopathic Veterinary Surgeons in 1982 and was its president for 10 years.

Many courses are offered in veterinary homeopathy in Great Britain, Holland, and Germany and are currently being developed in other European countries. In the United States the Academy of Veterinary Homeopathy offers a course in veterinary classic homeopathy. In Great Britain the Faculty of Homeopathy, London, administers a professional qualification in veterinary homeopathy called the *Veterinary Membership of the Faculty of Homeopathy (VetMFHom).* Candidates attend a 3-year, part-time course, including live case study, and must pass written, practical, and oral examinations.

Internationally, veterinary homeopathy has never been stronger. In 1986 the International Association for Veterinary Homeopathy (IAVH) was founded in Luxembourg by veterinarians from Belgium, Germany, Great Britain, Italy, France, Luxembourg, and The Netherlands. This young and growing organization held its first congress in Oxford, England, in 1987 and has held congresses around Europe and in the United States ever since.

Scientific Basis

Various aspects of homeopathic theory are discussed in the literature. Most of this work is modern because of a recent demand for more evidence. Although findings in human homeopathy may be significant, this chapter will confine its discussion to veterinary data. Most research on veterinary homeopathy suffers from its small scale and lack of repetition by other research workers, but it nonetheless shows enough clinical trial evidence to demonstrate the efficacy of homeopathy in the treatment of farm and pet animals.

Clinical Trials and Data

Five clinical situations seem objectively to show a very good response to homeopathic medication. One is a report of a dystocia problem in a group of Friesian heifers; two others illustrate the use of mastitis nosodes in the prevention of mastitis. Other trials conducted by the author include the prevention of canine tracheobronchitis and a porcine stillbirth trial. A great deal more data would be required to prove the point beyond all doubt, but empirical evidence is difficult to obtain when practitioners are busy with the day-to-day work of general practice and when farms cannot easily be modified sufficiently to produce meaningful trials. The author has conducted a larger number of on-farm tests in many species for a wide variety of clinical problems, but even though the vast majority indicate positive results, the groups are often too small to provide analyzable data.

Friesian heifers—dystocia (Day, 1995)
Number in group: 25
At the outset of the test, 18 had calved and a great

number of serious problems had been experienced, as enumerated below.

AT OUTSET OF TEST

Number calved to date	18
Number needed assistance	18 (100%)
Number of cesareans performed	1 (5.6%) (too few judging from the figures below)
Number of calves dying at birth	7 (38.9%)
Number of maternal deaths	3 (16.7%)

OF THE SURVIVING 15 HEIFERS

Number with subsequent metritis	10 (severe) (66.7%)
Number with subsequent mastitis	9 (severe) (60%)
Number eventually held in calf again	3 (20%) (16.7% of the original group)

This situation was disastrous, with only 1 in 6 of the original 18 (16.7%) returning to the herd the following year.

After the eighteenth heifer had calved, the farmer sought homeopathic help and Caulophyllum 30C was administered via the drinking water to the remaining seven heifers. The following data were then collected.

AFTER CAULOPHYLLUM TREATMENT

Number calved	7
Number assisted	2 (28.6%—in fact, the assistance turned out to be unnecessary because the heifers calved easily)
Number of cesareans performed	0
Number of calves dying at birth	0
Number of maternal deaths	0
Number with subsequent metritis	4 (slight) (22.2%)
Number with subsequent mastitis	0
Number eventually held in calf again	7 (100%)

In this case, the only information available involved the same groups, before and after homeopathic treatment. No proper statistical control can therefore be applied. However, the possibility that another factor was involved in the group's dramatic improvement is unlikely. The lack of difficulty in calving, the resultant reduction of stress and injury to the heifers and calves, and the reduction in disease that followed all suggest that Caulophyllum had a positive effect.

This incident appears to demonstrate the ability of Caulophyllum to help in cases of calving difficulty and the effect of the traumatic births on the dams, which brought on severe metritis and mastitis problems in the untreated animals. This was not a mastitis problem *per se* but a manifestation of response to the disease situation imposed on the dams at calving. Removal of the individual's susceptibility to traumatic injury resolved the so-called mastitis problem.

Friesian cows—mastitis (Day, 1986)

A herd of 80 cows was housed in a cubicle house, split into two groups of 40 cows. The difference between this farm and the usual practice is that the groups were formed at random, not according to yield, age, or calving date. A test was conducted by administering (via the drinking water) to one side a mastitis nosode appropriate to the farm situation and to the other side an unmedicated solvent that was visually and chemically identical to the nosode except that it was unmedicated. The owner of the establishment did not know which group received the nosode and which the control.

Mastitis data were collected on specially prepared forms that contained records of date of cases, in which group they occurred, the number of quarters involved, the severity (on a scale of 1 to 3) of disease, and the number of antibiotic tubes used to treat each cow. The results appear in Table 26-1.

The nosode had a very positive effect in reducing mastitis incidence, severity, duration, and likelihood of relapse. Also, the affected cow in the treated group was affected only in the first month of the winter (there were no cases after that) and had suffered summer mastitis during her previous dry period in that quarter. That she suffered no relapse during the winter period was therefore remarkable.

This otherwise conventional farm has subsequently adopted homeopathic treatment methods. Most of the mastitis cases are now treated homeopathically in addition to other disease problems that may arise.

Mastitis in a Holstein/Friesian herd (150 cows) (Day, 1986)

Table 26-2 shows data from the season before use of mastitis nosode and the season in which it was used. Nosode was used on February 1, and unacceptable levels of mastitis at that time of year fell dramatically afterward. Again, as in the first trial described, only historical controls were available with which to compare results, but the decline in problems seems clear.

These results may require repetition before efficacy can be proved.

Canine tracheobronchitis (kennel cough) (Day, 1986)

Table 26-3 shows results obtained in a severe outbreak of canine tracheobronchitis in a boarding kennel. The terms *vaccinates* and *nonvaccinates* refer to the conventional vaccination status of dogs with respect to tracheobronchitis before admission to the kennel.

The kennel personnel recorded all signs of kennel cough occurring in inmates over this period, even minor and transient ones (e.g., a pool of mucus in the kennel one morning, a little ocular discharge, and a transient minor cough observed during exercise). The presence of these

TABLE 26-1

FRIESIAN COWS WITH MASTITIS

	SIDE A CONTROL (UNMEDICATED)	SIDE B TREATMENT (MEDICATED)
Number of cases during winter housing period	19 (10 cows only; i.e., 9 relapses)	1
Average number of quarters affected	1.6	1
Average severity (scored: 1-3)	2.16	1
Average number of tubes used to clear the mastitis (tubes were used twice daily)	9	8
Average number of days visibly affected	4.5	4
% incidence	47.5	2.5

TABLE 26-2

MASTITIS IN A HOLSTEIN/FRIESIAN HERD

	DEC	JAN	FEB	MARCH
Season before treatment Number of mastitis cases	12	8	20	20
Season of treatment Number of mastitis cases	9	20	3	4

Nosode introduced on Feb 1, 1986.

TABLE 26-3

CANINE TRACHEOBRONCHITIS

	TOTAL	VACCINATES	NONVACCINATES
BEFORE NOSODE TREATMENT			
Number of dogs in kennel	40	18	22
Number of dogs affected	37	18	19
% affected	92.5	100	86.0
AFTER NOSODE TREATMENT			
Frank disease			
Number of dogs in kennel	214	64	150
Number of dogs affected	4	3	1
% affected	1.87	4.69	0.69
Minor symptoms (transient)			
Number of dogs in kennel	214	64	150
Number of dogs affected	91	51	40
% affected	42.52	59.69	26.67

TABLE 26-4

PORCINE STILLBIRTHS

	CONTROL	TREATMENT
Number of sows in group	10	10
Number of live births	103	104
Number of stillbirths	27	12
Number of sows with stillbirths	8 (80%)	3 (30%)
% stillbirths	20.8	10.3

signs throughout the trial period suggests that the infection had not simply disappeared.

Porcine stillbirths

These results relate to a trial performed in a breeding unit of 130 sows (Day, 1984). The use of Caulophyllum 30C in this trial appears to have brought about a significant drop in the stillbirth rate (Table 26-4).

Traditional Medical Theory

Basic homeopathic principles are discussed in Chapter 25. Basic definitions of terms used in this chapter and in Suggested Reading books are discussed in Box 26-1.

Controversial Issues

Homeopathy is not a widely accepted form of therapy in veterinary medicine. This book seeks to help bridge the gap between conventional medicine and alternative medicine; to this end the controversies are discussed.

The main controversies surrounding homeopathy and therefore contributing to its fringe status involve paucity of research, the "dilution" factor, the philosophic differences from conventional science, the lack of understanding of mechanisms, and the methodology.

Research

Very few clinical trials of any worth have been performed to test the efficacy either of the homeopathic method or of specific treatments. One reason for this paucity of research is a lack of funding, no doubt because homeopathic remedies are inexpensive and offer few financial incentives to drug manufacturers. In the conventional world of chemically manufactured drugs, large sales, significant unit profit, and the ability to obtain patents generate vast sums for research. Most homeopathic research is funded by charitable groups.

Moreover, conducting trials according to conventional scientific methods is difficult in a system of medicine that relies on *individual* prescribing rather than blanket treatments. Thus for any conventionally named disease in different animals, a hundred different homeopathic medicines can be prescribed, depending on the individual patient's demeanor, conformation, and expression of signs and symptoms.

BOX 26-1

GLOSSARY

Acute disease: One that is of rapid onset and short duration. The term indicates nothing of the severity of the disease.

Aggravation: Worsening of symptoms usually associated with the administration of a correct remedy at an incorrect potency.

Allopathy: A system of medicine using agents to treat disease that are totally unrelated to the disease in their action; for example, antibiotics, which target bacteria and not the underlying disease. (This may nevertheless have a beneficial effect on the course of the disease.)

Antiopathy: System of medicine using agents whose action is opposite to the symptoms. Modern conventional medicines are often used in this way. This is palliative and suppressive in its action on signs and symptoms.

Centesimal potency: Scale of dilution of a remedy, each dilution being one in one hundred.

Chronic disease: One that is of long standing and well established, with no period of resolution. The term indicates nothing of the severity of the disease (as with acute disease).

Concomitant symptom: One that accompanies the major presenting symptom and is a useful aid to prescribing homeopathically.

Constitutional remedy: One that takes the entire makeup of the patient into account, rather than the presenting symptoms alone. It matches the pattern of an individual body's programmed response to disease. This type of remedy has a significant effect on every organ system, including the mind. (See also *Polychrest.*)

Conventional medicine: A term used in this text to describe what is presently taught in veterinary schools with regard to the use of modern drug therapy.

Cure: The total elimination of disease and restoration of health.

Decimal potency: Scale of dilution of a remedy, each dilution being one in ten.

Destructive remedy: A remedy suited to the syphilitic miasm (q.v.). The "picture" of such a remedy is one of tissue destruction.

Diathesis: Constitution or condition of the body that predisposes it to a certain type of disease reaction.

Disease: Dynamic disturbance of the harmony existing between the "vital force" in a body and the physical body itself. Literally "dis-ease."

Dynamics: A study of the activity of the body and the forces involved (as used in this book).

Heteropathy: See *Allopathy.*

Holistic: Study of the whole body and mind in the context of its environment.

Homeopathy: Treatment of disease with a substance that has the power to produce, in a healthy body, symptoms similar to those displaced by the patient.

Isopathy: Treatment of disease by the identical agent of the disease. The concept of vaccination has similarities. (See also *Nosode.*)

Materia medica: Book of provings and properties of remedies.

Miasm: A Hahnemannian philosophic term for an infective agent that underlies chronic disease. No direct definition exists in modern medical terminology. (See *Psora, Sycosis,* and *Syphilis.*)

Modality: Modification of symptoms by such influences as temperature, time, motion, and weather.

Mother tincture: Undiluted alcoholic solution obtained from the original source material of a remedy. The starting point for all potencies from soluble material (denoted by the Greek letter φ).

Nosode: Homeopathic remedies prepared from infected tissue, disease discharges, or causal organisms. (See also *Isopathy.*)

Organotropy: Affinity of a substance for a particular organ or organ system.

Palliative: Treatment aimed at directly reducing symptoms. (See *Antiopathy.*)

Placebo: Inert medicine given to humor or reassure, rather than cure, the patient. A psychologically induced cure may follow (called a *placebo effect*). This term is often used in a human context, but the technique can equally be used to humor or reassure the client who presents the animal patient, although the author does not approve of this technique.

Polychrest: One of the deep-acting, extensively applicable remedies that have a wide action on all parts of the body. Constitutional remedies are polychrests.

Potency: The dynamic principle of a remedy harnessed in the dilution and succussion (q.v.) process. Quantified by C or X (or D) and a number denoting number of dilution steps undergone.

Potentization: The above process. (See *Trituration.*)

Proving: The administration of a remedy to a healthy body sufficient to cause the symptoms noted in the materia medica. An archaic translation of the German word *Prüfung*—a test.

Psora: Hahnemann's term for the "miasm" of the "itch" (scabies). Deficient reaction of the body to disease force.

Continued

BOX 26-1

Glossary—cont'd

Repertory: Dictionary of symptoms with indicated remedies.

Side effects: The reaction of the body to antiopathic drug medication. These are unwanted effects because only the primary effect of the drug is desired and not the body's undesirable reactions to it.

Succussion: Violent shaking under controlled conditions as a part of the process of potentization (q.v.).

Sycosis: Hahnemann's term for the "miasm" of "gonorrhea." Excessive body reaction to disease force.

Syphilis: Hahnemann's term for the "miasm" of syphilis. The body's reaction to disease is "destructive" (q.v.).

Trituration: Pulverization of insoluble material with milk sugar before subsequent liquid dilution during the process of potentization (q.v.).

Furthermore, crossover studies are not suitable because homeopathy alters the whole body's way of working and immune responses, often for long periods or permanently. The result is that satisfactory results cannot be expected after stopping one line of treatment and exchanging it halfway through at trial.

Control groups can be difficult to organize on the farm because the ideal situation in a herd of pairing similar animals and maintaining them together on treatment or control regimens may somehow lead to normalization of control animals. Whether other changes in management occur simultaneously is not always clear. For example, a pig herd was studied during a stillbirth, mummification, embryonic death, infertility (SMEDI) problem. Every other sow was put on homeopathic medication, and the rest were put on a blank control medication (double-blinded). The SMEDI problem, which had plagued the herd since its inception, suddenly disappeared from the entire herd on commencement of the trial. The result is an unpublishable trial and a satisfied farmer.

Researchers must develop methods that are suitable for testing alternative medicines. Methods that do not involve the active induction of disease in experimental animals must improve. Until these problems have been addressed, research is necessarily incomplete (see Chapter 25).

Homeopathic Dilutions

Although not universal, extreme dilutions of medicines are the most common form of homeopathic remedy. The extent of dilution often appears puzzling to the conventional medical scientist, physiologist, or biochemist. How can a substance, diluted to an extent that makes the presence of even one molecule of active ingredient highly unlikely, have any worthwhile medicinal effect? Research is clearly needed to answer this question, and efforts are being made in this direction (see Chapter 25).

Water, which has an infinitely variable structure and a capacity for memory like all complex structures, is believed to be able to take on some form of energetic coding from the original substance during the stages of dilution and succussion. The fact that homeopathic provings can be conducted using such dilute medicines should serve as strong evidence for the validity of that assertion.

Molecular and atomic physics, based on Einstein's theory of relativity, suggests that energy and mass are interchangeable and what is generally considered a solid object is in reality merely an energy pattern of greater density and speed of vibration than a liquid or gaseous collection of molecules. According to this theory, energetic influence incorporated in the medicated solution is transferred to the water compartment of the body, influencing it at a rate of dispersion of approximately 1 meter per second.

Much remains to be discovered in this exciting frontier of science, and future discoveries will no doubt serve to make the homeopathic dilution phenomenon less controversial.

Philosophic Aspects

Homeopathic philosophy diverges from the teachings of conventional Western science. This divergence frequently leads to suspicion, skepticism, and lack of confidence in homeopathic remedies, but it need not.

Homeopathy is based on the following principles:

- The healthy body is one in balance and equilibrium.
- The equilibrium of internal parameters is maintained by a "life force" that corresponds to a general interpretation of the immune system. This is the energy behind the body's biochemistry that ends with the death of the organism.
- Disease is a disturbance of that equilibrium.
- The disturbance may be temporary, with balance quickly restored (acute disease), or permanent, resulting in chronic disease.
- The symptoms of a disease are *generated by the body* in its fight to regain equilibrium.
- The correct homeopathic medicine, individually chosen for the patient after close attention to detail of

demeanor, signs and symptoms (mental and physical), physique, appearance, behavior, and so on, will stimulate the life force in its fight to regain equilibrium; if the body continues a healing mechanism able to overcome symptoms, a cure is a feasible consequence of treatment.

• If no mechanism for healing the symptoms exists (e.g., in cases of kidney tissue degeneration), no cure can result and the best hope is for palliation of the condition.

This philosophic approach to medicine and disease is not difficult to comprehend, nor is it difficult to reconcile with observable facts about disease.

Mechanisms of Medical Action

The precise way the body responds to homeopathic medicines and therefore the way the medicines are able to effect a cure are not precisely known. However, a working model consistent with all observations can be devised for both the origin of symptoms and the mechanism of homeopathic action (Figs. 26-1 and 26-2).

Homeopathy works by stimulating the body's ability to fight disease, not by counteracting symptoms. By contrast, conventional (antiopathic) medicines act by counteracting symptoms (e.g., antiinflammatories, antitussives, antihistamines, antidiarrheals, antiemetics) (Fig. 26-3). The ever-present dilemma of side effects resulting from the use of conventional antiopathic medicines can be explained according to the same rationale and model (Fig. 26-4).

Methodology

Homeopathic methodology is governed by the philosophic basis of the therapy and the patient's observable responses to medication. The correct homeopathic stimulus is not just the correct remedy but also the correct dosage (potency) at the correct frequency for the correct duration. All these parameters need to be selected carefully.

Dosage is not related to body size but more to the observable dynamic of the body and the disease. The *potency* of the medicine is selected accordingly. A higher potency is selected in cases of acute disease, when the body has a robust dynamic and mental symptoms are prominent. A lower potency may be selected for chronic disease, for weaker constitutions, and for diseases in which local pathology predominates.

Frequency is determined according to the disease dynamic and the patient's response to medication. Acute serious disease generally requires more frequent dosing than chronic disease. In general, the medicine is repeated only when the effect of the first dose has worn off and symptoms persist.

The *duration* of medication is governed by the patient's response to therapy. The treatment should be given for no

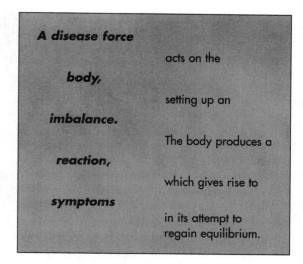

Fig. 26-1 Origin of symptoms.

longer than is necessary to achieve a return to health.

The selection of a homeopathic remedy depends not on the name of the disease but on the patient. Thus different patients with the same disease may require different homeopathic medicines. This variation can result in confusion when conventional training leads veterinarians to seek a specific drug for a specific condition. A given medicine may serve to treat many different diseases in different individuals provided that the symptoms fit the general "picture" of the remedy. For instance, the homeopathic remedy *Arsenicum album* may be selected for the treatment of gastroenteritis, peritonitis, kidney disease, skin disorders, nocturnal restlessness, asthma, and many other conditions if the picture shown by the patient fits the *Arsenicum* picture. This approach requires a philosophic change on the part of the would-be veterinary homeopath.

Practical Theory and Applications

Homeopathic medicine is a practical and pragmatic science. A practical methodology has been developed over the 200 years of its use in humans and animals.

In the application of veterinary homeopathy, the first consideration is the case history, which should be as detailed as possible. The case history must involve an interview with those caring for the animal and a close study of the animal itself. A domestic animal has feelings, motivation, desires, needs, and mental stresses in much the same way as does the human animal. The main difference between animals and humans is mental: Humans believe animals have little if any concept of the future and its concomitant anxieties, stresses, and hopes. The case study should take all these mental considerations into account just as much as the physical signs, symptoms, and complaints.

In prescribing for an animal, the veterinarian must attempt to identify the essential nature, or picture, the pa-

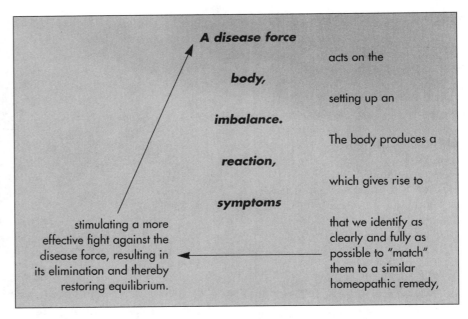

Fig. 26-2 Mechanism of homeopathic action.

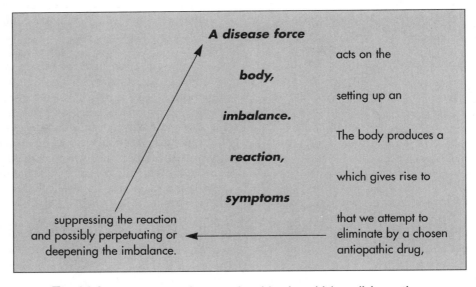

Fig. 26-3 Mechanism of conventional (antiopathic) medicine action.

tient presents and match this to the essence of a homeopathic remedy. The general picture of the case is much more important than the conventional name of the disease the patient presents. Although veterinarians must not ignore the conventional diagnosis, the true guide to the correct homeopathic prescription is the individual expression of signs and symptoms, both mental and physical.

Identifying the aspects of a case and forming a basis for the prescription involves a combination of detailed questioning and investigation (including laboratory work and radiography where necessary), which is scientific and objective, coupled with a general overview of the picture and

dynamics presented, which is more philosophic and subjective.

Veterinarians must also remember to remove any adverse influences that may have contributed to the cause of the disease or that may inhibit the patient's response to treatment and its ability to heal. Such factors are termed *obstacles to recovery* and include poor diet, environmental stressors, incorrect exercise programs, and, in the case of horses, saddling and shoeing.

The writings of Samuel Hahnemann are helpful when studying the route to a homeopathic cure. In his *Organon* (1833-1834), he wrote the following:

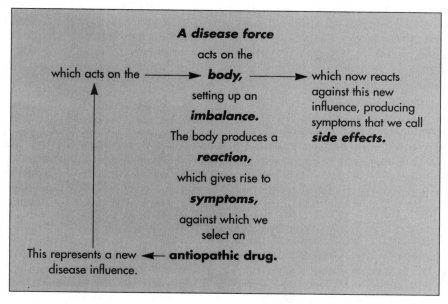

Fig. 26-4 Mechanism of side effects from the use of conventional (antiopathic) medicines.

- If the physician (veterinarian) perceives that which is to be cured in diseases;
- If he perceives what is curative in medicines;
- If he knows how to match what is curative in medicines to what he has discovered to be wrong in the patient;
- If he knows how to adjust the potency, the frequency, and the duration of the medicine;
- If he knows how to identify and remove the obstacles to recovery; then he is a *true practitioner* of the healing art.

He also makes the following observation:

- If he knows the factors that are able to derange health, and how to remove them from healthy individuals, then he is a true preserver of health.

In short, veterinarians should compose a detailed, careful, and empathic case study; match the disease picture to the remedy picture; and remove any adverse factors that may inhibit healing. Furthermore, preventive medicine is advocated via a study of factors that are likely to derange health in a healthy body.

The various components of this study include the following:

- Case study, including a scrutiny of all factors in the patient's life that contribute to the maintenance of disease (the dog will be used as an example, and other species will be discussed where relevant)
- Selection of the appropriate homeopathic medicine and its purpose (again, species differences can be studied where relevant)
- Obstacles to recovery
- Preventive medicine
- Dosage

- Administration and care of medicines

The Case Study

The case study is the foundation of good homeopathy. If the practitioner fails to establish a thorough knowledge of the patient, important aspects of the case may be lost and the subsequent remedy selection process will be flawed. It is therefore important to establish a routine in the collection of information. The veterinarian must be careful not to interrupt when the patient's caretaker is talking. These two considerations can be incompatible, but the second must take precedence so that useful, spontaneously offered material will not be missed. When questioning, the veterinarian must also refrain from asking leading questions, the answers to which may distort the picture.

Different species and problems require different procedures and areas of investigation, but the underlying principles are vital. The study can be divided into the following areas for clarity:

- Introduction to the patient
- The nature of the complaint
- The patient himself or herself
- Lifestyle, nutrition, and management

Let us first look at the dog during the initial visit to the veterinary clinic.

The Dog

Introduction to the patient
- Observe behavior from car to waiting room.
- Observe behavior in the waiting room.
- Observe entry to consulting room.

These are spontaneous offerings from the patient and should not be missed.

The nature of the complaint

WHAT IS THE PRESENTING COMPLAINT? The presenting complaint is the reason that the client has brought the animal. It should be described in the client's own words. The modern medical name of the condition should be noted when possible but must not be the controlling factor of the consultation or treatment. The disease's name is only a convenience, offering little insight into the real nature of the patient's condition.

WHAT ARE THE CHARACTERISTICS OF EACH SYMPTOM? What sort of discharge is there? What is the color and character of the mucus, pus, or diarrhea?

WHAT ARE THE MODALITIES? Modalities are the factors that affect the symptoms for better or for worse (e.g., weather, temperature, eating, drinking, and moving).

WHAT PERIODICITY DO THE SYMPTOMS FOLLOW? Is the disease worse in winter or summer, morning or evening?

FOR HOW LONG HAS EACH SYMPTOM BEEN EVIDENT? Here there is often a need to delve into the past or even to attempt to correlate seemingly unrelated symptoms or events.

WHAT HAPPENED AT THE OUTSET THAT MAY HAVE CONTRIBUTED TO THE CAUSE? The patient may have not been well since vaccination, injury, surgery, or a change of home or environment. A time span of up to 3 months before symptoms may be relevant—earlier if there is a possible chain of causes evident.

ARE THERE ANY PROBLEMS OCCURRING AT THE SAME TIME? These are the concomitant symptoms.

The patient

MEDICAL HISTORY. The complete medical history includes all known events and their outcomes.

FAMILY HISTORY, IF AVAILABLE. A breeder usually knows more than the average client, unless that client has access to family information.

MENTAL SYMPTOMS/BEHAVIOR. Like humans, animals have mental processes that are integral to the body's physiologic, biochemical, and medical processes. In some cases, the link between mental symptoms and behavior is easy to observe; in others, skill is necessary to extrapolate from behavior to the mental process behind that behavior. Sometimes, the correspondence is impossible to determine. Nonetheless, it is an important factor to consider. Is the animal shy, aggressive, friendly, impulsive, or steady? Does the animal react to criticism, music, fuss, noise, or situations?

GENERAL SYMPTOMS. General symptoms include information on build, physique, posture, movement, desires and aversions, thirst, and responses to geography, weather, seasons, and so on.

PARTICULAR (OR LOCAL) SYMPTOMS. When considering particular, or local, symptoms, the homeopath should study all the information that is obtainable from a thorough and methodical clinical examination. Details of bodily functions should also be collected at this time.

STRANGE SYMPTOMS. If present, strange symptoms are noteworthy. A recent case brought to the author was a Border collie who would insist on escaping from the garden in search of automobile exhaust fumes. Such a symptom is peculiar and therefore very important (Hahnemann, 1833-1834).

Lifestyle, nutrition, management

The veterinarian should note how the dog is kept at home, its type of bedding, to which rooms it has access, walks or exercises, how much time it spends alone, presence of animal companions, diet, type of work it does if it is a working or show dog, and any other lifestyle factors.

INTAKE FORM. A typical intake form helps ensure a complete history taking (Box 26-2). The form shown is by no means a compulsory format, and each veterinarian should design the form to match his or her own methodologies in history taking and examination of the animal patient. The most important consideration with regard to the intake form is that it must not interfere with the free flow of information from the client or dictate the pace and direction of discussion. It should serve only to ensure that, at the end of the consultation, all information has been gathered and none forgotten.

EXAMINATION FORM. The examination form (Box 26-3) lists the parts of the body and, if used, should serve merely to ensure that a thorough examination has taken place and that observations are not lost. Conducting a full and proper examination is more important than completing forms.

The Cat

With regard to the examination process, the cat differs from the dog in only a few details. Its behavior under restraint in the basket should be observed; its reaction to various stimuli in this situation and its behavior in the consulting room (if it is allowed to wander freely) all serve to complete the diagnostic picture.

Small Caged Mammals and Other Exotic Pets, Including Birds

Small caged animals are much more difficult to look at closely, but the veterinarian should take full opportunity to observe their behavior and examine them as much as possible—in each case, without causing too much shock, fear, or any physical trauma. A common error is not to carry out a proper and thorough examination because these are unusual animals. However, principles of good veterinary practice still apply, necessitating a full but careful procedure.

Farm Animals

In most cases, farm animals are production animals, with the special stresses that this role places on them. In

---

BOX 26-2

Sample Intake Form

Owner's Name: _____
Animal's Name: _____

Location: _____
Date: _____

1. *Initial Observations:*

THE PROBLEM

2. *Presenting Problem:*
3. *When Started:*
4. *Description:*
5. *Modalities:* Temperature: Weather: Rest: Motion: In/Out: Other:
6. *Periodicity:* Season: Time of Day: Female Cycle:
7. *Circumstances at Start:*
8. *Concomitant Symptoms:*

THE PATIENT

9. *Past Medical History* (General):
   Tolerance of Drugs:
10. *Vaccination:*
    Aftereffects:
11. *Past Diagnostic Efforts* (Laboratory, x-ray, etc.):
12. *Family History if Known:*
13. *Home Environment:*
    Alone?:
    Companions:
    Exercise:
    Restrictions:
    Bedding:
14. *Mental Observations:*
    Reactions to the following:
    Fuss:
    Consolation:
    Extrovert/Introvert
    People:

Scolding:
Noise:
Surrounding Activity:
Will/Manner:
Dominant/Submissive; Aggressive/Shy; Noisy/Quiet; Excitable/Docile; Impulsive/Steady; Careful/Clumsy; Gentle/Rough; Obedient/Disobedient:
Emotional Reactions:
(Jealousy, sensitivity, etc.)
Memory:

Other Dogs/Cats:
Alone/Company:
Other Fears:

15. *General Observations:*

Neat/Scruffy	Diet
Physique	Protein (source and amount)
Posture	Carbohydrate (source and amount)
Gait	Vegetable (type and amount)
Sleep	Supplements
Dreams	Treats
Female Cycle	Likes
Behavioral Quirks	Dislikes
Thirst	Feed dish material
Appetite	Water dish material

Effects/preferences: Geography: Season: Time: Travel: Outside/Inside: Temperature: Weather: Meals: Drugs:

---

many livestock cases, the obtainable history is sketchy. Again, the veterinarian must observe the patient carefully, examine the animal thoroughly, and coax as much information as possible from caregivers. The principles of treatment are the same on the farm, so quality of therapy depends on quality of information obtained. Hygiene, housing, feeding, grassland management, silage-making for cattle, dietary composition and supplementation, and medical programs must all be taken into account.

Horses

Horses are another special case because they are generally kept for work or sport, activities that place unusual demands on them. They are generally trained to be handled easily and are very sensitive and perceptive. It is important to allow time for observation and quiet, polite contact because horses will indicate their feelings under different circumstances if the veterinarian is prepared to pay attention. Shoeing, saddling (and other tack), efficiency of dentition, back alignment, and nutrition are the basis for

health and most often for disease, also, if these factors are not optimal.

Selection of the Remedy

The correct homeopathic medicine most closely matches the spectrum of symptoms found in the patient, taking into account factors such as constitutional and local symptoms and etiology. A remedy can be selected according to its symptom match:

- **At a pathologic (or causative) level**—for example, *Arnica* for injury.
- **At a local level**—of value in acute uncomplicated disease in an otherwise robust and healthy individual. A remedy can be accurately selected fairly rapidly from a few signs and symptoms, for example, gastroenteritis (Mercurius solibulus or Arsenicum) or colic (Colocynth).
- **At an organotropic level**—a remedy can be selected according to which *organ* is perceived to be under

BOX 26-3

EXAMINATION FORM

a. Head/Face
b. Eyes   Vision:
c. Nose   Smelling:
d. Ears   Hearing:
e. Mouth/Breath
f. Teeth
g. Gums
h. Tongue
i. Throat
j. Neck
k. Back
l. Forelimbs/Feet
m. Hindlimbs/Feet
n. Tail
o. Chest/Respiration
p. Heart/Pulse, etc.
q. Stomach/Abdomen
r. Bladder   Urine: Urination:
s. Rectum   Stool: Defecation:
t. Mammary Glands/Vulva   Sexuality:
u. Male Genitalia
v. Skin/Smell
w. Hair
x. Anal Glands
y. Nails
z. Nervous System
Tests: Urine Sample:

particular stress. This form of therapy is often an adjunct to other, more general, homeopathic prescriptions, as the following examples demonstrates:

Chelidonium	Liver
Euphrasia	Eye
Flor de Piedra	Thyroid
Rhus tox	Muscle

- **At a historical level**—where the veterinarian may perceive a particular historical incident to have contributed greatly to the disease. The following are examples:

Injury	Arnica
Giving birth (Day, 1985)	Caulophyllum

- **At a regulatory level**—in which one can use homeopathic potencies of a metabolite, dietary factor, or poison to facilitate metabolism, absorption, or excretion of that particular substance. The following are examples:

Ferrum	Aids iron absorption
Plumbum	Aids lead excretion
Calcarea	Aids calcium metabolism

- **At a specific level**—in which a nosode (a remedy made from disease material) may be used to treat a similar infectious disease. (The author counsels caution in the application of this method in acute serious infectious disease because the body may already be seriously weakened by the invading organism and a challenge of such isopathic nature may overwhelm or seriously disadvantage the body's defenses.)

Examples include the following:

Mastitis Nosode (Day, 1986)	Mastitis in cattle
Cat Influenza Nosode	Feline leukopenia

- **At a desensitizing level**—in which homeopathic potencies of a supposed allergen will help the body come to terms with the hypersensitivity and suffer less while a real homeopathic cure is sought.
- **At a constitutional level**—This is the most important and can be the most difficult process in homeopathic prescribing. For chronic disease, there is no substitute. Constitutional prescribing takes into account the very nature and individuality of the whole patient, including mental and physical symptoms, gait, build, and character. Homeopathic medicines suitable for prescribing for chronic disease in this manner are called *polycrests*. Polycrests are the medicines most commonly discussed in the literature. Polycrests have matching symptoms in every area and organ of the body and can be matched to the individual in his or her entirety, including the modalities of symptoms. This is true holism in action.
  - *Sulphur* suits the hot, dirty, thirsty, philosophical, cool-seeking, sweet-loving animal that usually suffers skin disease and whose symptoms are often worse in the very early morning (e.g., 3 to 5 AM).
  - *Arsenicum* suits the neat, fastidious individual who dislikes cold, has a thirst for small quantities of water, is restless, and often suffers the worst symptoms around midnight.

In the selection of a constitutional prescription, special emphasis should be placed on mental symptoms, as well as strange and peculiar symptoms (Hahnemann, 1833-1834).

Information on remedy selection is available in many books, which can be referred to as *prescribers*. The books listed at the end of this chapter contain such information. They list disease conditions and homeopathic remedies that may be suitable. There is no substitute, however, for proper selection of remedies according to the individual and his or her needs. Help is obtainable from repertories (large collections of symptoms with possible remedies listed) and computer programs. The experienced prescriber can eventually accomplish a great deal by using intuition or reasoning, prescribing without. The better the history and clinical appraisal at the outset, the better the chances of success.

Obstacles to Recovery

Medicine is most effective if supported by study and removal, correction, or mitigation of any factors that are likely to delay or obstruct healing. These factors often have played a part in or have been a significant cause of the decline in health in the first place.

The most fundamental of these factors must be diet. No study of medicine is complete without a study of diet, and no medicine should be administered without correcting or optimizing dietary factors. Of course, each species has different dietary requirements. In general, a healthy diet must consist of healthy ingredients (preferably organic), be free of potentially harmful additives, be processed as little as possible or not at all, be fresh wherever possible, and, above all, be suited to the species' needs, developed over millions of years. This applies as much to horses as to dogs and cats, and to farm animals as well as to exotics. Caution should be practiced with modern convenience diets that may contain unsuitable materials, processed foods, foods that contain artificial additives, or foods that may fail to provide an optimal diet on account of repetition rather than variety. The convenience and economy such prepared diets offer often come at a cost.

The same considerations apply to dietary supplements and treats. Quality drinking water is also important. Feed containers, storage facilities, bowls, dispensers, and mangers should also be of suitable materials and quality. Plastic or aluminum feed containers, aluminum or nonstick cooking vessels, and plastic kettles are not recommended.

Caged animals should be given adequate space and facilities. They should not be kept in isolation, especially if they belong to a gregarious species. Since they are caged, they cannot select their own environment. For this reason, cages must be kept in a comfortable and suitable environment.

Exercise routines for all species should be both appropriate to and adequate for their evolved needs.

Smoking by the animals' human companions should be avoided in a closed space in which an animal is kept. Passive smoking is likely to be as bad for animals as it is for humans.

Grazing animals should be given an adequate variety of herbage, managed under holistic husbandry techniques for both soil and sward.

Horses in particular should be correctly shod and saddled (or harnessed), and their backs and teeth should receive proper attention. Correction of saddling and shoeing problems is essential to ensure correct skeletal alignment. These factors are so important to the horse's well-being

that correcting and optimizing them may even lead to a cure, without the need for medicine in many cases.

Farm species should be housed and managed with compassion and respect, with special notice taken of their comfort, exercise, and hygiene. In dairy herds, milking facilities must be technologically and mechanically sound and properly maintained.

Handling and transport should always be carefully arranged, designed, and monitored to decrease the risk of stress or injury. In the case of animals kept for meat, their transport to slaughter, handling, and care warrants careful thought. Whether animals should be killed for food is controversial for consumers and at a global ecologic and economic level, and it is not the subject of this book. However, because the practice of using animals for food is so prevalent in modern society, the methods must be ethical and humane (Day, 1995).

Preventive Medicine

In addition to optimal nutrition, housing, and management, homeopathy may play an important part in the prevention of disease, particularly of the enzootic and epizootic infectious types. The most common and practical method is the administration of nosodes, the efficacy of which is in some part supported by the clinical trial data reported previously in this chapter. Nosodes are homeopathic remedies made from disease material, prepared in the same way as any other homeopathic remedy, by the dilution and succussion process. This method is as yet without full scientific validation, but the author uses only this method for his own animals and equine, canine, and feline patients. No ill effects have resulted from this method, and trial work in cattle and dogs (see pp. 486-488) tends to support its validity. However, the method is not yet recognized by regulatory bodies in cases where vaccination is compulsory. Veterinarians should always discuss the implications and lack of scientific evidence for this method with clients and leave the ultimate decision to them. However, in animals who reacted adversely to conventional vaccination and who appear to be suffering or likely to suffer a consequent immune disturbance, the homeopathic route is advised.

For the purpose of disease prevention, the thirtieth centesimal potency is usually used. Regimens used in preventive programs vary among prescribers but generally call for fairly frequent dosing at the outset of a program, followed by a maintenance program in which the frequency of dosing declines (e.g., every 6 months). In times of higher perceived risk, frequency can again be increased. Administration is usually oral.

A typical prevention program for dogs, cats, or horses, if used in place of conventional vaccine, might be as follows: twice daily for 3 days; followed by twice weekly for 3 weeks; followed by once monthly for 6 months; followed by a dose night and morning, every 6 months. This regimen has been used for kennel cough, distemper, hepatitis, and parvovirus in dogs; for influenza, enteritis, feline leukemia virus (FLV), feline immunodeficiency virus (FIV), and feline infectious peritonitis (FIP) in cats; and for influenza and herpes in horses. This regimen is appropriate for any epizootic (i.e., occurring in outbreaks) disease.

In cases of enzootic infectious disease, particularly in farm livestock, more regular and frequent dosing may prove necessary, depending on the prevalence of the disease in the population. In these circumstances, all possible steps should be taken to lessen disease-producing factors in management, housing, and nutrition (Day, 1995). A preventive regimen can probably never be completely abandoned once a disease is at a manageable level, because the disease-producing factors on a farm can never be entirely removed, despite improvements in management.

Dosage

Homeopathic medicines are available as liquids, powders, crystals, pillules (granules or pellets), tablets, injections, and lotions. A homeopathic remedy should be given in as small a dose as possible to produce maximal benefit. The term *dose* is used here to describe not the number of tablets, drops, quantity of powder, or size of injection but the potency, frequency, and duration.

In acute disease, in which the patient's constitution is robust, a high potency may be used. In chronic conditions or life-threatening situations, a lower potency may be used. However, different prescribers have different views and practices in this regard. The frequency should be governed by the severity of the disease and its dynamics (e.g., rapid-onset, acute disease could demand frequent dosing at short intervals; a chronic, low-grade disease may require only a single dose or infrequent doses). The duration of dosing should be governed by the patient's response to treatment. Homeopathic remedies work by stimulating the body. Once the body responds to this, the dosing should be stopped and the body allowed to make use of the stimulus as it moves toward a cure. Further doses may prove necessary if the healing process stalls. In general, acute conditions respond quickly, and chronic conditions can take a long time because they have taken a long time to develop.

Administration and Care of Remedies

Homeopathic medicines are very delicate; therefore handling should be avoided except when actually administering the dose. Handled medicine should never be returned to the bottle. Only the required dose should be dispensed from the bottle at each dosage time. The container should be tightly sealed at all times except when dispensing, and two containers of medicine should never be opened at once. Medicines should be stored away from sunlight in a cool, dark place and apart from strong-smelling substances, especially camphor, embrocations, and perfume. Homeopathic preparations should not be refrigerated or frozen. If correctly stored, homeopathic remedies can last for long periods, so do not discard unused supplies.

Pillules may conveniently be dispensed into the bottle cap before dosing. If the patient does not object, the pills may then be tossed from the cap directly into the mouth (avoiding contamination of the cap with saliva) to avoid handling of the pillules. If the patient does not accept this method, the pillules may be dissolved in a small amount of boiled, cooled water in a syringe, which provides a means of liquid dosing. Different forms of the medicine are also available, including tablets that can be crushed in paper and drops supplied in a dropper bottle.

Drops may be added to drinking water or placed directly on the tongue. Cats frequently lick a few drops of the medicine off their noses without stress. In birds, drops can be applied to the upper beak area. A typical dose is generally between 1 and 3 drops.

Powders can be poured directly into the mouth from the paper. These are not recommended for birds.

Homeopaths disagree about the efficacy of injections, another form of administration. However, they are widely used by veterinarians with apparent success. The author has often used this method in cattle because oral dosing can be problematic.

The veterinarian must ensure that the dose is either swallowed or retained in the mouth for 30 seconds; thereafter, it may be ejected without diminished effect. When more than one medicine has been prescribed, the doses should be administered at different times. If possible, the veterinarian should allow at least a 5-minute interval between prescriptions and avoid giving medication within 15 minutes of food. For farm species and horses, this is not possible, but the veterinarian should warn the animal's caregiver to prevent the animal from eating compound feeds at least 5 minutes before and after dosing. Medicines can be given to horses in a very small amount of bland food (such as grated apple or a tiny piece of bread). In the case of caged birds and other small pets, pillules may be added to the drinking water, freshly prepared each day. They do not need to be seen to dissolve to be effective. Animals should not receive strong-smelling sweets (such as peppermints) while they are on medication, and aromatherapy oils may be counterproductive to homeopathic medication in some instances.

Clinical Indications

Small Animal

Homeopathy is clearly indicated in all medical conditions of small animals, especially conditions of a chronic nature that have failed to prove amenable to conventional drug therapy. Although few controlled studies have been conducted (and the special difficulties such studies in homeopathy would involve could be the subject of another book), clinical efficacy in practice demonstrates that homeopathy can be extremely beneficial in the treatment of chronic and acute disease conditions. Whereas conventional medicine may only palliate and alleviate symptoms in chronic disease, homeopathy can often lead to cure of dermatologic, autoimmune, gastrointestinal, musculoskeletal, and neurologic conditions. When accompanied by good nutrition and management, homeopathy offers a real chance of cure. The positive healing effect of homeopathy is seen not only in the alleviation of symptoms but also in the deeper well-being of the patient.

Homeopathy is also beneficial in acute disease. Homeopathy has been used successfully in cases of acute gastroenteritis, infectious tracheobronchitis, feline influenza, acute injury-related disease, all cases of injury, and acute infectious diseases of all types. All these have proved amenable to homeopathy, which in most cases results in rapid, gentle resolution of the problem. For instance, canine tracheobronchitis often responds in only 3 or 4 days under correct homeopathic prescribing, whereas the condition often persists as long as 3 weeks with conventional medication.

In all cases, success depends on the following factors:

- Satisfactory removal of the obstacles to recovery
- Correct remedy selection (depending on a good history and examination)
- The ability of the body to heal

The last item is particularly crucial because there are certain diseases in which one cannot reasonably expect a cure in the real sense of the word. (For a definition of cure as used in this text, see Box 26-1.) Diseases such as kidney degeneration cannot be fully healed because the body cannot replace lost kidney tissue. Some injuries may be too violent and extensive for full recovery. Chronic degenerative radiculomyelopathy (CDRM) in the German shepherd cannot be expected to heal entirely because the body has no known mechanism for reconstruction of the degenerated nerve tissue and myelin sheaths.

The author uses homeopathy, along with other natural therapies such as acupuncture and herbs, to the almost total exclusion of conventional drug therapy in his practice. This approach often obviates the need for surgical intervention.

Equine

Homeopathy offers a realistic and effective treatment for all acute infectious diseases of the horse and for all injuries that do not lead to death or permanent incapacity (under which unfortunate circumstances homeopathy will still provide help and comfort). Colic, too, can improve with homeopathic remedies, usually either Nux vomica or Colocynth or both, depending on the symptoms. Con-

ventionally trained clinicians are often surprised to see this serious problem improved by natural treatment and usually without conventional spasmolytic drugs.

As with dogs and cats, horses can respond to homeopathic remedies, and a complete cure is a realistic aspiration. Conditions that are especially susceptible to homeopathy include laminitis, allergic dermatitis and urticaria, chronic obstructive pulmonary disease (COPD), navicular disease, and degenerative joint disease.

Laminitis

Laminitis is a distressing and dangerous problem for the horse. It causes a great deal of pain and can cause serious deformity of the feet. If the patient does not have a long history of suppressive antiinflammatory drug treatment before homeopathic medication, the long-term prospects are extremely good.

Navicular disease and other bone and joint diseases

Arthritis, degenerative joint disease, navicular disease, sprains, and strains can all respond to correct homeopathic prescriptions, especially if the nutrition and management of the horse are optimal. Success rates are good with bone and joint diseases, despite the grave prognoses outlined in conventional veterinary texts or discussions. The veterinarian should remember, however, that the patient is being treated, not the disease. With a basic foundation for health and freedom from obstacles to recovery, the body is able to reverse many pathologic changes. This reversal is due to the regular turnover and replacement of tissues in the body (including bone), which allows for replacement of diseased tissues with healthy structures. This basic foundation for health is created by optimizing management, diet, saddling, riding, shoeing, back alignment, and tooth function.

Allergic dermatitis/hypersensitivity (sweet itch)

Allergic dermatitis is amenable to homeopathic remedies. Sensitivity to sun, grass, or midge is a function of immune imbalance, and the application of appropriate homeopathy can resolve the problem over a period, often totally.

Urticaria (hives)

As with other allergic types of reactions, urticaria can often be cured by homeopathic desensitizing measures and a constitutional prescription.

Chronic obstructive pulmonary disease (COPD)

Chronic respiratory allergies respond well to homeopathic prescribing over time. A constitutional approach is imperative to achieve a cure, and homeopathic or isopathic desensitizing efforts may also be pursued in the hope that the violent allergic response can be modulated while a proper constitutional homeopathic cure is being sought.

Horses often exhibit residues of medicines in their tissues and blood. This can create problems for horses involved in certain sporting endeavors and horses who will later be used as food for humans. Homeopathic medications do not create residues; the veterinarian can prescribe them without facing legal or ethical problems.

Horses respond well to homeopathy and acupuncture. The speed of response and the extent of healing are excellent, provided the nutrition, saddling, shoeing, teeth, and back are maintained in an optimal condition.

Food Animals

With cattle, sheep, pigs, goats, and poultry, one important consideration applies to veterinary medicine: Do the medicines affect the value of the animals for meat purposes or the value of eggs, milk, or milk products sold from the animals? In all cases, homeopathic medicine presents no danger of residues and therefore no fear of contamination of meat or milk. This removes the possibility of ethical and legal problems for the prescriber and farmer alike.

Homeopathic medicine has a great deal to offer on the farm, whether it is for the maintenance of fertility in breeding females, the treatment or prevention of mastitis, or the treatment of many diseases often considered incurable (such as septic feet/foot joints in cattle). Herd problems often prove amenable to homeopathic medication. Problems such as warts; keratoconjunctivitis (pink eye); foul in the foot; pneumonia; ringworm (dermatophytosis); ketosis; mastitis, metritis, or agalactia in sows; and contagious pustular dermatitis (orf) in sheep and goats prove to be much less of a problem under homeopathic management and respond quickly to homeopathic therapy.

In many of the farms at which the author conducted routine herd fertility and management visits, the farmers are now effectively prescribing and treating according to their own knowledge and experience, resulting in better herd health, better profitability, and a healthy decrease in routine veterinary involvement.

The welfare of animals is of paramount importance in all veterinary endeavors. The medical necessity for reducing stress and other obstacles to recovery has been mentioned often in this chapter. However, veterinarians also have an ethical obligation to reduce stress. This can be particularly problematic in farm and herd situations. Even well-managed farms have certain fundamental properties that contribute to disease and can only be mitigated, not removed. Such factors include fencing, housing, concrete, production-stress, milking machines, removal of calves, and many others. Along with the need to move, manipulate, transport, dehorn, and milk, these stressors can jeopardize the welfare of farm animals. Because of its ability to provide relevant and effective treatments for stress, injuries, minor ailments, chronic disease, and acute disease without lessening the economic value of animals, homeopathy is an excellent way to safeguard the welfare of farm animals. Furthermore, animals who are considered appropriate candidates for conven-

tional treatment because of poor prognoses and the loss of salvage value if drugs are used can be treated homeopathically. In addition to these important considerations, the use of homeopathy on the farm results in a more congenial, sensitive, and compassionate way of management, which has positive effects on the welfare of farm animals.

Exotics

The most salient problems facing the conventional veterinarian in the treatment of exotic pets—be they birds, reptiles, fish, or mammals—are the unpredictability of idiosyncratic drug effects, the wide variations in needs among various species, the plethora of diseases that remain untreatable, and the possible stress of treatment. Because not all conventional drugs can be administered orally, injection may be necessary. The palatability of oral drugs can also be a problem and may result in decreased food or water intake.

The use of homeopathy solves most of these problems. Homeopathic medicines are safe and offer a real chance of cure in many conditions that are unresponsive to conventional therapy. Effects seem consistent among species, and the medications can be administered without stress or discomfort.

The same principles of remedy selection used for the major domesticated species are appropriate for exotic pets. Injuries, skin diseases, respiratory disorders, musculoskeletal problems, gastrointestinal upset, acute infectious diseases, and many other conditions are amenable to homeopathic therapy. Diet, management, housing, and lifestyle are important considerations, as well as the individual species' evolved needs.

Many species are not suited to caged domestication, which may prevent proper cure. It is hoped that people will eventually recognize the folly of keeping these animals as pets.

Veterinary Homeopathic Aide-Mémoire

Box 26-4 is a brief guide and aide-memoire to trained veterinarians for selection of helpful homeopathic remedies in common veterinary situations. It is not comprehensive and is designed to be used as a guide only. Owing to their seriousness and the importance of diagnosis, many of the conditions listed are not amenable to home treatment or treatment by nonveterinarians.

Incorporation Into Veterinary Practice

Feeling Your Way

As with any new therapeutic skill, the introduction of homeopathy into the veterinary practice should be gradual. Because of the widespread demand for natural thera-

BOX 26-4

GUIDE TO HELPFUL HOMEOPATHIC REMEDIES

ABRASION
See Injury

ABSCESS
Belladonna: if peracute, red, hot and painful
Calc. sulph.: if discharging yet not healing
Hepar sulphuris: if acute and painful
Pyrogenium: if accompanied by septic fever
Silica: if chronic

ACETONEMIA KETOSIS (BOVINE)
Lycopodium will usually help constitutionally
Senna may alleviate symptoms

ACNE (FELINE)
Constitutional prescription; for example, *Graphites, Natrum muriaticum, Sulphur*

ACCIDENTS
See Injury

ALOPECIA (ESPECIALLY FELINE)
Arsenicum or *Natrum muriaticum* according to constitution plus, as an adjunct, potencies of *Pituitary*, with *Folliculinum* or *Testosterone*, depending on the gender of the neutered animal

ANESTHETIC—DELAYED RECOVERY
Nux vomica

ANAL GLANDS
Silica: if chronically filling; see above if abscessation

ANAPHYLAXIS
Aconitum: in acute phase
Apis mellifica: if swelling of face and dry mucous membranes

APPETITE LOST OR REDUCED
Ignatia, Lycopodium, Nux vomica

APPETITE VARIABLE
Pulsatilla

ARTHRITIS
Apis mellifica: if red, swollen, improved by cold bathing
Bryonia: if worse for any movement. Patient prefers to be motionless. Worse in warm weather
Calc. fluor.: if exostoses or result of growth problems
Causticum: in the older, weaker dog or cat. Restless at night, improved by warmth and warm damp weather
Ledum: especially in the small joints, worse in hot weather
Rhus tox: worse for cold, damp weather, worse rising from rest, worse first movement, improved by warmth and by continued moderate movement, worse from overexertion

Ruta grav.: similar to above. Especially after sprains and strains

BACK PROBLEMS
See Arthritis, Disk, Injury

BEHAVIORAL AND MENTAL PROBLEMS
Anticipated fear and "show fright": *Gelsemium*
Sudden fright or panic: *Aconitum*
Bereavement with hysteria: *Ignatia*
Bereavement with moroseness: *Natrum muriaticum*
Cowed: *Natrum muriaticum, Silica, Staphisagria*
Difficult if left alone: *Phosphorus, Pulsatilla*
Panics if left alone: *Arsenicum album*
Excitement: *Belladonna, Nux vomica*
Fear of dark: *Carbo vegetabilus, Phosphorus, Stramonium*
Fear of thunder/sudden noise: *Belladonna, Gelsemium, Nux vomica, Phosphorus*
Hysteria, especially young pups: *Belladonna, Chamomilla*
Hysteria generally: *Aconitum*
Jealousy: *Lachesis*
Irritability: *Chamomilla, Nux vomica*
Panic: *Aconitum*
Resentment: *Staphisagria*
Sexual excitement: *Gelsemium, Staphisagria, Tarentula hisp.*
Show fright: see Show fright
Urine spraying (inappropriate): see Spraying

BEREAVEMENT
See Behavioral and mental problems

BIRTH DIFFICULTIES
Caulophyllum: helps all stages of the birth process

BITES
See Injury

BLEEDING
See Injury

BLOAT (TYMPANY) (BOVINE)
Colchicum: if rumen contents are frothy
Nux vomica: if there is also constipation

BONE INJURY
See Injury

BOVINE VIRUS DIARRHEA
Mercurius solubilis

BREATH BAD
See Teeth, Mouth, Worms, Kidneys, Liver, Throat

BRUISING
See Injury

Continued

BOX 26-4

Guide to Helpful Homeopathic Remedies—cont'd

BURNS/SCALDS
See Injury

CANKER
See Ears

CAR SICKNESS
See Travel

CAT INFLUENZA
Aconitum: in acute, very early stages
Arsenicum album: sneezing, burning discharge, sore nose, worse from cold
Euphrasia: sore runny eyes, discharge is excoriating
Kali bich: ropy, tenacious mucus, yellow discharges, ulcerated nostrils
Natrum muriaticum: constant sneezing, runny eyes and nose, seeks solitude
Pulsatilla: greenish, yellowish discharges, thirstless, seeks company
Silica: chronic stopped-up nose and sinuses

CHILLING
Aconitum: sudden onset
Calc. phos.: if diarrhea
Gelsemium: weakness, paresis

COLIC
Chamomilla: if seeks solace constantly
Colocynthis: griping, cramping pains causing animal to curl up or, in the case of the horse, roll over and draw hind legs up, kicking out at intervals
Lycopodium: with bloated abdomen
Nux vomica: after rich food, constipation, knotty feces

COLLAPSE
Carbo vegetabilis

CONCUSSION
See Injury, Head

CONJUNCTIVITIS
See also eyes
Aconitum or *Euphrasia:* from cold winds
Mercurius solubilus: if photophobic
Pulsatilla: purulent green-yellow discharges; thirstlessness (see also Cat influenza)

CONSTIPATION
Nux vomica: small, knotty feces
Sulphur: dry feces exuded with much effort

CONVALESCENCE (TO SUPPORT THE SYSTEM IN ITS RECOVERY PHASE)
Cinchona (medium potency, e.g., 30c), *Phosphoric Acid* low potency

COWED
See Behavioral and mental problems

COUGH
Aconitum: constant short, dry cough, from cold exposure. Sudden onset
Bryonia: harsh, dry cough, worse for movement and from cold dry weather. Wants to be alone
Causticum: hard cough with mucus difficult to expel
Hepar sulphurus: coughing spells, aggravated by cold
Kali bich.: cough with plugs in nose. Ulcerated nostrils
Nux vomica: dry cough with gagging. Worse in the cold Oversensitive patient. Hoarse in the morning
Phosphorus: exhausting cough; thirst for cold water, which is soon vomited
Pulsatilla: annoying dry cough, thirstless. Worse in warm room in the evening
Spongia: if heart is involved

CRUSH INJURY
See Injury

CUTS
See Injury

CYSTITIS
Aconitum: sudden onset, very painful
Cantharis: blood, constant urging, can cry out
Sarsaparilla: if accompanied by stones or plugs

DANDRUFF
Constitutional prescription; for example, *Arsenicum, Kali sulphuricum, Natrum muriaticum, Sulphur*

DIARRHEA
Arsenicum album: usually chilly patient, often vomits too, some blood, thirst for small quantities, restless, worse around midnight. Dry mouth
Mercurius corrosivus: thirsty, chilly, wet mouth. Much straining with blood
Mercurius solubilus: less dramatic than *Mercurius corrosivus,* similar symptoms
Nux vomica: after too much rich food, worse in the early morning
Pulsatilla: variable consistency, worse in the evening, thirstlessness
Sulphur: worse in the early morning, especially about 5 AM. Worse in hot weather

DISK DISEASE
Hypericum and *Nux vomica:* Acupuncture is particularly helpful in this condition

EARS
Belladonna: if acute, red, hot, painful

BOX 26-4

*G*UIDE TO *H*ELPFUL *H*OMEOPATHIC *R*EMEDIES—cont'd

Calc. sulph.: watery, yellow discharge
Graphites: weeping, smelly, sore
Hepar sulphuris: purulent discharge, painful
Mercurius solubilus: foul, purulent discharge
Sulphur: if not itchy, smelly

ECZEMA
See Skin

ENTERITIS
See Diarrhea

EXCITEMENT
See Behavioral and mental problems

EYES
See also Conjunctivitis
Cornea ulcerated: *Mercurius corrosivus*
Ulcerated, chronic: *Conium*
Photophobia: *Aconitum, Euphrasia, Mercurius corrosivus*
Entropion: *Rhus tox*
Injury (orbital): *Symphytum;* (corneal): *Ledum*

FALSE PREGNANCY
Mild, sweet natured, thirstless, "nursing": *Pulsatilla*
Bad tempered, moody: *Sepia*
Milk production: *Urtica* (in very low potency)
If element of hysteria: *Ignatia*

FEAR
See Behavioral and mental problems

FEATHER PECKING IN BIRDS
Ignatia: when upset, bereaved, excitable
Sepia: when moody and broody
Sulphur: if too hot, itchy (ensure adequate humidity and even temperature, reduce boredom factors)

FELINE UROLOGIC SYNDROME
Hydrangea: helps dissolve deposits
Sarsaparilla: helps relieve obstruction
Lycopodium: if there is a tendency

FELON (SEPTIC TOENAILS)
Hepar sulphuris: painful, acute, suppurating
Silica: chronic, brittle nails

FLATULENCE
Carbo vegetabilus: chilly, poor vitality, fear of darkness
Lycopodium: distended abdomen, with rumbling bowels, bloated
Nux vomica: after rich food, overeating, hard knotty feces

FOOD POISONING (ESPECIALLY IN CATS)
Arsenicum

Baptisia

FOREIGN BODY (TRAUMATIC, IN TISSUES)
Silica: prolonged treatment to promote rejection

FOUL IN THE FOOT (BOVINE)
If acute: *Hepar sulphuris, Kreosotum, Tarentula cubensis*
If chronic: *Silica*

FRACTURES
See Injury

GINGIVITIS
See Mouth

GROWTH PROBLEMS
In heavy-framed animal: *Calc. carb.*
In light-framed animal: *Calc. phos.*
If bone abnormalities: *Calc. fluor.*

GUMS
See Mouth

GUNSHOT WOUND
See Injury

HEMORRHAGE
See Injury, Bleeding

HAIR BALL
Nux vomica

HAIR LOSS
Arsenicum: restless, chilly type
Sulphur: hot, itching, smelly skin

HALITOSIS
See Teeth, Mouth, Worms, Kidneys, Liver, Throat

HEAD INJURY
See Injury

HEART PROBLEMS
Digitalis: in low potency, helps to strengthen the heartbeat and smooth irregularities
Crataegus: supports the heart in case of cardiac insufficiency
Spongia: if there is a congestive cough

HEATSTROKE
See also Sunstroke
Aconitum: if dramatic symptoms
Glonoinium: if stupor and exhaustion

HICCOUGH
Nux vomica

HIT BY CAR
See Injury, Road Accident

Continued

BOX 26-4

Guide to Helpful Homeopathic Remedies—cont'd

HYSTERIA
See Behavioral and mental problems

INCONTINENCE, FECAL
Causticum: in aged
Gelsemium: if nervous, weak type
Phosphorus: if paralysis

INCONTINENCE, URINARY
Causticum: in aged

INFECTION
See Injury

INFLUENZA
See Cat influenza

INJURY
Abrasions/grazes/scratches: *Calendula*
    If painful: *Hypericum/Calendula lotion* topically
    If infected: *Hepar sulphuris* internally
Bites (cat/dog): *Arnica* and *Ledum*
    If infected: *Hepar sulphuris*
Bites/stings (insect):
    Apis: if swollen and improved by cool applications
    Cantharis: if hot, blistered
    Ledum: if improved by cool applications
    Urtica: if improved by warm applications
Bites (snake):
    Cedron: if malarial types of symptoms
    Crotalus: rattlesnake
    Golondrina: if blood toxin
    Guaco: if nerve toxins
    Lachesis: Surucucu snake—purpling of tissues
    Naja: Cobra
    Beware of using the isopathic venom in severe cases. It is more helpful in the recovery phase.
Bleeding (hemorrhage): *Arnica, Phosphorus*
Bruises: *Arnica*
Burns/scalds: *Cantharis, Urtica*
Crushing injury: *Arnica, Hypericum*
Cuts: *Staphisagria, Calendula lotion*
Eye injury: see Eye
Fractures/bone injury: *Symphytum* (and obtain immobilization of fracture if appropriate)
Gunshot wounds: *Ledum, Staphisagria*
Head injury: *Aconitum, Arnica, Belladonna, Glonoinium*
Lacerations: *Arnica, Hypericum, Hypericum/Calendula lotion*
Puncture wounds: *Ledum*
Road accident: *Aconitum* and *Arnica*
Septic infection: *Hepar sulphuris, Calendula lotion*
    If chronic: *Silica*
Shock: See Shock

Spinal injury: *Hypericum, Phosphorus*
Sprains: *Arnica, Ruta*
Surgical injury: *Staphisagria*
Tail or foot injury: *Hypericum*
Always remember *Arnica* cannot be wrong in any injury and will always help. Do not use topically on open wounds. The sooner it is given, the better it will help

IRRITABILITY
See Behavioral and mental problems

JEALOUSY
See Behavioral and mental problems

KIDNEYS
Mercurius solubilus, Natrum muriaticum, Phosphorus, Kali chloratum

LABOR
See Birth Difficulties

LACERATIONS
See Injury

LACTATION
Urtica: high potency (30C and above) if insufficient milk flow
Urtica: low potency (6C and below) to help "dry up"
Pulsatilla, Cyclamen, Aristolochia: may help in cases of lactatio falso

LAMINITIS (EQUINE)
Aconite: if sudden onset
Belladonna: if sudden onset with heat and throbbing in the feet
Hypericum: longer term
Silica or *Graphites:* in chronic cases

LIVER
Lycopodium: if bloated, poor appetite, likes sweet food, prefers lukewarm water
Nux vomica: if irritable, toxic, dull in mornings

MANGE
See Skin

MASTITIS
If hot, red, swollen, painful: *Belladonna*
If unwilling to move: *Bryonia*
If hard, knotted: *Phytolacca*
If chronic: *Silica*
If abscessation: *Hepar sulphuris*
If suppressed milk flow: *Urtica*

MENTAL PROBLEMS
See Behavioral and mental problems

BOX 26-4

GUIDE TO HELPFUL HOMEOPATHIC REMEDIES—cont'd

METRITIS
Caulophyllum: will help clear postpartum discharges
Sabina and *Secale:* may be helpful for more chronic cases

MOUTH
Bleeding gums: *Phosphorus*
Smelly breath, much saliva, swollen gums: *Mercurius solibulis*
Dry mouth, sore gums: *Arsenicum*

MUD FEVER/GREASY HEEL (EQUINE)
Constitutional treatment is necessary but consider especially: *Arsenicum, Graphites, Hepar sulphuris, Antimonium crudum*

NAILS
Abnormal growth of nails or hooves should be helped by constitutional prescribing but consider especially: *Graphites, Silica, Thuja*

NETTLE RASH
Apis mell.: better cold applications
Urtica: better warm applications

NEW FOREST EYE (BOVINE/OVINE) (ALSO LISTERIA EYE)
If acute: *Kali iodatum, Mercurius corrosivus*
If chronic: *Silica*

OBESITY
Dietary measures may be necessary but consider: *Calcaera carbonica, Thyroid* (low potency), *Iodum, Graphites*

OILING
Contamination of fur or feathers with oil, diesel, or petrol: *Petroleum* (in addition, the animal needs careful washing, avoiding dangerous solvents)

PANIC
See Behavioral and mental problems

PARALYSIS
Causticum, Gelsemium, Hypericum, Phosphorus

PINING
See Behavioral and mental problems

POISONING
Nux vomica and *Echinacea:* In general, these remedies will help support the system and eliminate toxins. Other symptoms should be noted and appropriate remedies selected accordingly

POSTOPERATIVE CARE
See also Shock
Arnica: helps the body to recover from surgical trauma
Staphysagria: helps the body to come to terms with the interference

Phosphorus: helps excessive bleeding
Strontia and *Hamamelis:* help seepage in the wound
Aconitum: if there is shock or sudden hemorrhage

PREGNANCY
It is useful to support the dam and fetus homeopathically
Calcarea phosphorica aids the calcium metabolism for both; give one dose weekly during pregnancy
Caulophyllum one dose twice weekly for the last 3 weeks prepares for parturition (i.e., six doses in all)

PREGNANCY TOXEMIA (OVINE)
Lycopodium, Senna: if ketosis
Cicuta: if torticollis

PREOPERATIVE CARE
Treat any mental symptoms (see Behavioral and mental problems)
Use *Arnica* twice daily for 2 days before and during the surgery

PROSTATE
Thuja

PROSTRATION
See Collapse

PUNCTURE WOUNDS
See Injury

PYOMETRA
Sepia

RESENTMENT
See Behavioral and mental problems

RESPIRATORY PROBLEMS
Aconitum: Sudden onset, cough, rapid breathing
Arsenicum: Asthmatic with thirst, worse around midnight
Lycopodium: Sudden onset, very ill

RHEUMATISM
Treat as with Arthritis

RINGWORM
Bacillinum: the first-line remedy to help this problem
Kali arsenicum, Kali sulphuricum, Sepia, Tellurium: other possible remedies to consider if *Bacillinum* fails

ROAD ACCIDENT
See Injury

RODENT ULCER (FELINE)
Kali bichromicum
Nitric acid

BOX 26-4

GUIDE TO HELPFUL HOMEOPATHIC REMEDIES—cont'd

Natrum muriaticum

SCRATCHES
See Injury

SEXUAL EXCITEMENT
See Behavioral and mental problems

SHOCK
Aconitum, Arnica
Postoperative: *Phosphorus, Staphisagria*

SHOW FRIGHT
Gelsemium: if there is anticipatory anxiety
Aconite: if there is panic
Argentum nitricum: if fear leads to diarrhea

SINUSITIS (FELINE/EQUINE)
Acute: *Euphrasia, Sabadilla, Allium cepa, Aconite*
Chronic: *Kali bichromium, Silica, Hydrastis*

SKIN (ECZEMA, ITCHINESS, SORES, MANGE, ALLERGY, ATOPY, PYODERMA)
Apis mell.: urticarial rash, edema, improved by cool applications
Arsenicum: much hair loss, chilly type, worse in spring, worse at or about midnight
Cantharis: hot, blistered, appearance of having been burnt
Graphites: seeks warm but is worse in warmth. Clear, sticky discharges. Worse in bends of limbs. Ears discharging
Hepar sulphuris: purulent discharges
Mercurius corrosivus: purulent, smelly discharges
Natrum muriaticum: thirsty, chilly type, hair loss, odor, licks human hands and feet, seeks salt
Psorinum: chilly type, seeks covers
Sulphur: hot, smelly type, worse warmth
Urtica: itchiness, urticarial rash, worse in cold environment

SPINAL INJURY
See Injury

SPLINT (EQUINE)
Hekla lava.

SPRAINS
See Injury

SPRAYING OF URINE (FELINE)
Cantharis, Staphisagria

STINGS
See Injury

SUNBURN/SUNSTROKE
See also Heatstroke
Aconitum: if dramatic symptoms
Cantharis: if sores
Glonoinium: if stupor

SURGERY
See Injury

SWEET ITCH (EQUINE ALLERGIC DERMATITIS)
Constitutional treatment is necessary but consider especially: *Apis, Arsenicum, Graphites, Sulphur, Natrum muriaticum*

TEETH
Hepar sulphuris: abscessation
Mercurius solubilus: loose, much saliva, pyorrhea

THROAT SORE
Mercurius solubilus: thirsty, much saliva
Phytolacca: glands hard, swollen, difficulty in swallowing
Pulsatilla: thirstless, gentle type

TRAUMA
See Injury

TRAVEL SICKNESS
Petroleum

URTICARIA
See Nettle rash

VOMITING
Arsenicum: with diarrhea, restlessness, worse around midnight
Mercurius corrosivus: repetitive, watery mucus, vomits after drinking
Mercurius solubilus: as above but yellowish vomitus
Phosphorus: soon after food

WARTS
Causticum, Thuja

WORMS
Herbal treatment may help or may substitute for modern chemicals. No homeopathic medicine has yet been proven (by proper tests) to eliminate worms. Remedies that have the reputation are:
Abrotanum, Cina: Roundworms
Filix max, Granatum: Tapeworms

WOUNDS
See Injury

pies and holistic treatment, the temptation to satisfy clients beyond one's own capabilities can be strong. At any stage in development, veterinarians should recognize that admitting their shortcomings is safer and wiser than attempting unfamiliar techniques.

First-aid accident and trauma remedies are a useful, convincing, and easy way to start using homeopathy. The fact that conventional medicine, unlike homeopathy, has little to offer by way of internal medicines to treat some problems such as bruising makes homeopathy particularly attractive. The medicines are harmless, alleviate the patient's discomfort, improve healing, and increase the patient's chance of survival, often by a wide margin. A good example here is *Arnica*. The author has often noted surgical colleagues' surprise at the lack of hematoma formation after bone fracture or the speedy recovery from surgery in patients treated with Arnica before surgery.

Once prescribers are confident that the extreme dilutions of homeopathic remedies can be effective, they will feel more secure in branching out into the treatment of medical problems in general. Acute disease (e.g., gastroenteritis) that represents a temporary disturbance of an otherwise robust constitution is much less difficult to treat at an acute, local, or pathologic level than is chronic disease. The treatment of chronic disease (which demands constitutional prescribing) requires a much greater depth of understanding and knowledge, both of disease and of homeopathy, to achieve good results. Therefore the treatment of chronic disease should be the ultimate aim of the practitioner, not the first target.

Homeopathy is not a substitute for surgery, fluid therapy, or mineral and vitamin supplementation, but it can markedly reduce the need for such procedures. Homeopathy does not kill bacteria and is therefore not a substitute for antibiotics, but it can eliminate the need for antibiotics in most cases by stimulating the body's defense processes. Experience is required, however, before embarking on such a serious endeavor.

Interaction With the Public

Because of the growing increase in demand for homeopathy, beginners are finding it difficult to learn at their own pace. However, they should always recognize their own capabilities and share that knowledge with clients. It is better in the beginning not to encourage referrals or second opinion cases from outside the practice but to concentrate on developing skills safely and gradually at home. Clients who know that veterinarians are beginners trying to develop skill in natural medicine are often understanding and supportive. On the other hand, veterinarians who pretend to have skills that exceed their actual capabilities risk not only losing their discerning clients but being sued when failures occur.

Interaction With Colleagues in a Practice

When beginning to use homeopathy, practitioners must be sensitive to the reactions of colleagues both within a practice and within a community. Jealousy, anger, hatred, respect, animosity, friendliness, support, and obstruction are possible reactions from veterinary colleagues. This must not be allowed to affect professional ability or responsibility, nor should it deflect practitioners from the perceived correct path in any given case. However, in the patient's and client's best interests, differences should be minimized during consultations. Close follow-up of cases is essential. Because the practice of homeopathy is still considered unconventional, the practitioner must be particularly careful to shield the patient from any possible ill effects.

Professional communication with colleagues is essential and in the patient's best interests. It will also encourage greater friendliness and respect and may in fact increase interest among colleagues in the long term.

Conclusions

Homeopathy now stands at a watershed. There is, on the one hand, a demand for greater scientific proof of efficacy and, on the other, a rapidly burgeoning demand from the public. It also faces opposition from commercial, professional, and scientific interests that threaten to marginalize homeopathy.

Conventional medicine has followed a mechanistic and reductionist (Cartesian) approach to medicine and disease. For this reason, it tends to favor surgery, vaccination, antibiotics, antiopathic (antisymptomatic) medication, and the study of organs, tissues, cells, and biochemistry. Homeopathy, on the other hand, follows a holistic pathway, taking into account the effect of any influence on the whole body and, likewise, the reaction of the whole body to any influence. Homeopathy is less concerned with the mechanics of individual processes and the effects on any single organ or structure and more concerned with the integrated reaction of all organs and systems taken together and the effects that all organs or components have on each other. The gulf between the two modalities is wide, but it is not insurmountable.

Curiously, research published to date has done little to convince most conventionally trained veterinarians of the efficacy and value of homeopathy. It is possible that not only are the conventional research procedures inappropriate for holistic, homeopathic methodology, but also that the conventional approach makes interpretation of results difficult. Further research is clearly necessary, but the direction it should follow is unclear.

Animal experimentation is the research tool most widely respected in modern medicine. The double-blind, crossover trial is also a bastion of modern scientific methodology. Neither method is appropriate to homeopathic research. Animal experimentation is problematic for several reasons—particularly because of the ethical dilemma it poses for veterinarians and the artificial situations that the laboratory creates. Given the holistic concept that lifestyle, nutrition, and other intrinsic influences are all vital factors in disease processes, the laboratory environment is a poor substitute for the home or farm. Furthermore, artificially induced disease is a poor mimic of naturally occurring equivalents.

The double-blind, crossover trial is not always appropriate for the following reasons:

- Homeopathy does not treat all individuals as if they were the same.
- Crossover of treatments between groups is not possible because the homeopathic remedy has a long-lasting effect on healing processes that does not stop on withholding the medication.

What is needed is a large number of clinical trials conducted under field conditions without the full benefit of a scientific control group. The control group may have to consist of historical controls or be supplied by the background population on other units, which is either treated conventionally or not treated at all. Also, vast numbers of individual clinical cases, managed homeopathically and carefully documented, will supply a wealth of important clinical material, and this weight of data should be taken into account when assessing the therapy. Control data would be available from other similar cases treated conventionally or left untreated. The combined experience of the veterinary profession in formulating prognoses for animals suffering from particular clinical conditions will provide a backdrop against which to evaluate response to homeopathic therapy.

None of these data will be easy to collect, nor will small-scale studies offer results equivalent to those produced by a more conventional approach to research. Homeopathic research is therefore both expensive and time consuming. However, it is infinitely more meaningful and more appropriate to the homeopathic method.

Clients who turn to veterinary homeopathy and veterinarians using homeopathy in practice, however, are convinced of the value of this therapy despite the lack of ideal research programs. No doubt they have all witnessed at least one convincing case of recovery that surpasses conventional expectations.

However, proper study is the only route to consistent success and ethical practice of homeopathy. There are no shortcuts. For this reason, a wide reading of homeopathic theory, philosophy, and practice is important for each veterinarian who decides to study homeopathy. Attendance at conferences and seminars is also an essential part of learning, bringing the added dimension of discussion with like-minded colleagues, both expert and novice.

Research in Veterinary Homeopathy*

Contrary to the view expressed by many in the conventional medical and veterinary establishments, much work has been and is being done at all levels to investigate and validate homeopathy. The draft report on nonconventional medicine by the European parliament states, "conclusive proof of the effectiveness of homeopathy is piling up, even if the orthodox scientific community is not yet convinced." The same report also states, "numerous medical practices validated by [conventional medicine] have been so on the basis of the opinions returned by the medical profession rather than on the basis of rigorous scientific studies" (Lannoye, 1995). That is not to say that rigorous scientific studies should not be performed, but there is more in life and research than the double-blind trial on which sections of the scientific community seem to depend.

A paper in the *Lancet* (Reilly and others, 1994) concludes that

> for today's science, the main barrier to acceptance of homeopathy is the issue of serially vibrated dilutions that lack any molecules at all of the original substance. Can water or alcohol of fixed biochemical composition encode differing biologic information? Using current metaphors, does the chaos inducing vibration, central to the production of homeopathic dilution, encourage biophysically different fractal-like patterns of the diluent, critically dependent upon the starting conditions? Theoretical physicists seem more at ease with such ideas than pharmacologists, considering the possibilities of isotopic sterodiversity, clathrates, or the resonance and coherence within water as possible modes of transmission, while other workers are exploring the idea of electromagnetic changes. Nuclear magnetic resonance changes in homeopathic dilutions have been reported and, if reproducible, may be offering us a glimpse of a future territory.

It is true that many of our colleagues in allied professions have less difficulty than our medical partners with the concepts of homeopathy. A biophysical model for homeopathy has been postulated (Towsey, Hasan, 1995) in the context of energy medicine and current biophysical theory. Water exists in a crystalline hexagonal geometry, and ice formed from different potencies forms different crystalline patterns at dilutions beyond the Avogadro's constant, although ultrasound techniques have failed to detect any differences between "normal" and "potentized" water (Silvo, Arnaldo, 1990). However, measurement of the electrical resistance of homeopathic dilutions has shown marked differences between various potencies of the same remedy (Bourkas, 1996). Topologic studies of the ethanol-water system have shown that succussion produces potentized molecules mimicking the properties of the drugs used (Singh, Chhabra, 1993). The action of homeopathic medicines can now be explained in terms of new concepts of matter (Poitevin, 1995). Stochastic reso-

---

*J.G.G. Saxton wrote this section.

nance has been suggested as a possible mode of action (Torres, Ruiz, 1996). From such theoretic starting points, researchers have confirmed the requirements for homeopathic medicines that Hahnemann proposed on the basis of practical experience 200 years ago.

The difficulties in publishing homeopathic research may contribute to the relative paucity of documented work. One example of this difficulty can be found in an episode surrounding the work of Jacques Benveniste, a respected immunologist who developed an interest in homeopathic research. A detailed discussion of this incident is beyond the scope of this section; the reader is referred to *The Memory of Water* (Schiff, 1995) for more information about this controversial episode in homeopathic research.

The difficulties researchers may encounter in devising protocols for trials are discussed elsewhere in this chapter. Homeopathy emphasizes individualization in natural conditions, whereas conventional science values randomization and clear-cut results. A double-blind trial involving Baryta Carb and hypertension (Bignamini and others, 1987) illustrates this fundamental difference. Toxicology, an important source of information in homeopathic pathogenesis, has shown that arterial blood pressure rises in cases of poisoning with barium salts. The trial was undertaken to evaluate the effectiveness of Baryta Carb, a common homeopathic treatment for hypertension, and explore the validity of the assumptions underlying its choice. Analysis of the randomized groups as a whole revealed no significant differences, but analysis that took account of the suitability of the patient for the remedy favored homeopathy. A similar study on the treatment of warts, in which individual remedies were selected by experienced practitioners, showed positive results for the homeopathic treatments (Gupta, Bhardwag, Manchanda, 1991). Consideration of in vitro studies can be found in Chapter 25.

Clinical trials have shown that homeopathic remedies can produce physiologic effects. Using Chelidonium Majos on healthy provers (a group of people who test the effects of homeopathic remedies), researchers documented a 58% increase in serum globulins (Vakil, Vakil, Nanabhai, 1989), whereas another study with the same remedy demonstrated a 25% decrease in serum cholesterol compared with controls in rabbits after cholesterol feeding (Baumans and others, 1987). Baptisia tincture produced marked leukopenia in rabbits (Engineer, Valik, Engineer, 1990) in a study that failed to demonstrate antibody production. Hypericum perforatum produced a significant antiinflammatory effect in induced arthritis with albino rats (Varma and others, 1988). Positive antiinflammatory action has also been described for Arnica Montana using induced edema in rats' paws (Desai and others, 1992). Homeopathic histamine has been shown to protect against histamine-induced edema of rats' paws (Conforti, Signorini, Bellavite, 1993). The administration of zinc in homeopathic form to healthy rats resulted in a marked increase in histamine release (Harish, Kretschmer, 1988).

Silica demonstrated a positive wound-healing effect in a mouse model compared with controls (Oberbaum and others, 1992, 1995). Silica also increased platelet activating factor (PAF) in mice (Davenas, 1987). The homeopathic preparation Gelsemium has also been shown to produce a significant increase in PAF production potential.

In the field of toxicology, studies involving arsenic and bismuth in homeopathic dilutions showed increased elimination in artificially posioned rats (Cazin and others, 1991; Lapp, Wurmser, Ney, 1955). The studies demonstrated a specificity in the effect. In homeopathic dilution, phosphorus and carbon tetrachloride have been shown to protect rat livers against tetrachloride-induced hepatitis (Bildet and others, 1984). Phosphorus has also been shown to decrease the mortality of rats from liver intoxication induced by α-amonitine (Guillemain, 1987). The authors concluded that the mode of action was in accordance with homeopathic principles. X-ray–induced skin symptoms can be prevented by the use of Apis, a homeopathic preparation containing bee products (Bildet and others, 1990). The ability of a homeopathic preparation of disease material (nosode) to protect against that disease has been illustrated (Jonal and others, 1991). Testing Tularemia nosode in a model of *Tularemia* infection, with mortality as the criterion, a series of 15 experiments demonstrated a significant positive effect after administration of the homeopathic remedy. In chickens the restoration of immune response was demonstrated after bursectomy by the administration of homeopathic dilutions of bursin (Youbicier-Simo and others, 1993; Bastide, 1994). Catalepsy in mice has been used to investigate the effects of *Agaricus muscarius* in homeopathic dilutions (Sukul, Battacharyya, Bala, 1987). In one study involving restraint-induced catalepsy, *Agaricus* enhanced the cataleptic effect. In another, haloperidol-induced catalepsy was suppressed by orally administered *Agaricus* 30c but not when given by the peritoneal route (Sukul and others, 1995). Later work has shown the effect to be dose related (Sukul, Ghosh, Sinhababu, 1996).

Two themes that commonly merge in much of the work related to homeopathy are the phenomenon of organ- or system-specific effects for both ultradilute and undiluted substances and an inversion of effect, with a dilution creating the potential to interfere with the action of the original substance. Recognition of both these phenomena is necessary in the development of a valid theory of the mode of action in homeopathy.

Increasing numbers of clinical trials are proving the efficacy of homeopathic treatments. The beneficial effects of Caulophyllum on the duration of labor in women have been shown, with a mean reduction in labor time of 90 minutes (Eid, 1993). This labor-facilitating effect has also been demonstrated in cattle and pigs (Day, 1985). In a clinical study involving parturition problems, high calf mortality, and mastitis, Caulophyllum 30c administered via the drinking water produced significant reductions in all conditions. A group of 18 heifers monitored before the administration of the remedy had all required assistance with calving, resulting in three maternal deaths (16.7%) and seven calf deaths (38.9%). Of the surviving heifers, 10 developed metritis and nine developed mastitis; all cases were classified as severe. Only three animals were held in calf again. A subsequent group of seven treated with Caulophyllum 30c had two requiring minimal calving assistance, no deaths, no mastitis, four cases of mild metritis, and all seven in calf again. Although only small numbers were involved in a noncontrolled situation, other management factors were constant, the only change being the use of the remedy. Although the most dramatic difference was in the ease of parturition, researchers believe that the resultant reduction of stress produced a beneficial influence in other areas.

Similar results were obtained in a pig unit. A trial using control and treatment groups of 10 sows each showed the treatment group having 30% of sows with stillbirths and 10.3% of stillbirths in the group as a whole, compared with 80% with stillbirths in the controls and a stillbirth percentage of 20.8%. In this case Caulophyllum was administered orally to each sow. A double-blind placebo-controlled trial in France involving Caulophyllum and Arnica confirmed these effects (Grandmontagne, 1995). Several practices were involved with 50 bitches, all selected using the same criteria, split randomly into two equal groups. Caulophyllum 9C and Arnica 7C were given on alternate days starting 15 days before expected whelping. The overall duration of labor was 6.96 hours in the controls, compared with 5.04 hours in the treated group. The first stage of labor was shortened from an average of 3.15 hours to 1.71 hours. Survival of pups was also favorably influenced. The same workers also investigated the effect of a complex of Caulophyllum 30C, Sepia 6X, and Cocculus 6X on labor times and piglet survival rates in a pig breeding unit. In this work, 101 sows received the mixture in food for 5 days before their expected delivery dates. Stillbirths in the control group were 20%, compared with 10% in the treated group. A beneficial effect on 48-hour survival times can also be attributed to the decrease of stress during labor.

A survey of British farms using nosodes for the control of mastitis concluded that no significant effect could be attributed purely to the nosode in most cases (Stopes, Woodward, 1988). However, several interesting and valuable conclusions were drawn. First, most farmers introduced to homeopathy also tend to try other holistic management techniques. Second, record-keeping under normal farm conditions was generally inadequate for the purposes of scientific study, which underscores the need for properly planned and recorded trials. Third, the possibility of a passive placebo effect is indicated because those farmers most committed to homeopathy produced the most glowing reports of the effects of the nosodes. This raises the possibility that a positive attitude on the part of an animal keeper influences the outcome of a treatment. Likewise, a positive or negative expectation on the part of a researcher can influence the outcome of a study.

Homeopathy has a favorable effect on bovine mastitis. A trial in England using a mixed nosode administered via the drinking water (Day, 1986) reported significant reductions in both clinical cases and cell counts. The herd was randomized into groups of 40. Comparison of the two groups showed a reduction in overall incidence from 47.5% to 2.5%, with a corresponding improvement in other parameters in the group treated homeopathically as compared with controls. No significant reduction occurred in the treatment time for cases that did develop. Another study with encouraging results involved a herd of 150 cows who were examined over two seasons. From December to March in the first year, the average monthly incidence of mastitis was 15 cases. This was confirmed in the second year, when in December and January the incidence was 14.5 cases. After the introduction of nosode on February 1, the monthly average in February and March was 3.5 cases. Work in Mexico using the remedies Phytolacca, Phosphorus, and Conium similarly produced significant reductions in both clinical and subclinical mastitis (Searcy, Reyes, Guajardo, 1995). This study involved 26 animals in two groups of 13. The California Mastitis Test was used on all quarters. The difference in affected quarters between the control and treatment groups was 68% compared with 32%. As in the English trial, no practical reduction occurred in the treatment time required for clinical cases. A pilot using Sepia for anestrus in 101 dairy cows (Williamson and others, 1991) gave encouraging results. The animals were split into three groups: untreated controls, a group treated with Sepia 200C on day 14 postpartum, and a group treated with Sepia 200C on day 21. The group given Sepia on day 14 showed positive results. This was followed by a full controlled trial involving 120 cows (Williamson, 1995). In this, animals were randomly split into four groups: untreated controls, placebo controls, Sepia given 24 to 48 hours postpartum, and Sepia given 14 days postpartum. One dose of Sepia 200C was given to the latter two groups at the relevant time. This gave statistically significant results in favor of Sepia given at 14 days postpartum; the criteria used were percentage holding to first service, calving to conception interval, total percentage in calf, and mean number of services required.

Encouraging early results were obtained using homeopathy in the prevention of respiratory disease in pigs and the treatment of rectal prolapse in the same species. Podophyllum and Phosphorus were used, both in the 200C potency. One problem with treating a control group in this latter study was the attitude of the supervising veterinary surgeon on the farm. Initially skeptical, he subsequently would not allow any affected animal to go without homeopathic treatment on ethical grounds (Searcy, Guajardo, 1994). Homeopathic remedies as growth promoters have been investigated in two studies. The effect of

Sulphur 200C was assessed in a blind placebo-controlled trial (Guajardo, 1996). The remedy was administered via food every 10 days to pregnant sows. Weight was monitored from birth to weaning. A statistically significant improvement in weight gain occurred in subsequent litters. A study of the effect of Barium Carbonicum LM1 on pigs with retarded growth gave positive results. No effect was noted in groups given Calcium Carbonicum and Calcium Phosphoricum in the same trial (Briones, 1989). This study followed good results with various calcium salts in broiler chickens and pigs of normal weight.

A pilot double-blind study of diarrhea in neonatal calves showed that the rate of recovery was accelerated by using Arsenicum Album 30C in conjunction with conventional treatment compared with conventional treatment on its own (Kayne, Rafferty, 1994). Although this involved only 16 animals, plans for a larger study are being considered.

Canine tracheobronchitis was the subject of a study using nosode to control an epidemic situation (Day, 1987). Positive results included a reduction in clinical disease, on a before-and-after basis, from 92.5% to 1.87%. The study also calls into question the effectiveness of conventional vaccination methods. The use of nosode as a means of controlling canine distemper in a stray kennel has been reported (Saxton, 1991). Nosode was administered via the drinking water to a total of 11,749 dogs over a period of 36 months. Significant reduction of clinical distemper was observed, compared with a prenosode sample of 1275 dogs over 5 months; the level of clinical distemper was reduced from 11.67% to 4.36%.

One study examined a homeopathic remedy as a disease preventative in batches of calves being transported before slaughter (Mahe, 1987). The group was considered as a single animal, and from a homeopathic repertory, a remedy was selected by the classic prescription method, using rubrics that fit the overall situation. The indicated remedy was Nux Vomica, which was given to each batch of calves before starting the journey. This treatment resulted in a marked reduction in weight loss, faster recovery, and improvement of carcass quality.

Homeopathy has proved useful in many different clinical situations. Further research is necessary, but the parameters and protocols must take account of the intrinsic difference between this modality and conventional scientific approaches.

JOURNALS

British Homoeopathic Journal
2 Powis Place
Great Ormond St.
London WC1N 3HT
England

Journal of the American Holistic Veterinary Medical Association
2214 Old Emmorton Road
Bel Air, MD 21015
phone: 410-569-0795
FAX: 410-569-2346

Newsletter for the International Association for Veterinary Homeopathy
Dr. Andreas Schmidt
Sonnhaldenstr. 18
CH-8370 Sirnach
Switzerland
phone: 41 (73) 26 14 24
FAX: 41 (73) 26 58 14

USEFUL ADDRESSES FOR FURTHER INFORMATION

American Holistic Veterinary Medical Association (AHVMA)
2214 Old Emmorton Road
Bel Air, MD 21015

British Association of Homeopathic Veterinary Surgeons
Hon. Sec.: Alternative Veterinary Medicine Centre
Chinham House
Stanford in the Vale
Faringdon, Oxon, SN7 8NQ

International Association for Veterinary Homeopathy (IAVH)
(Veterinary Courses in Europe apart from UK)
Peter Andresen
16 Route de la Forêt
F-78125 Hermeray, France

Faculty of Homeopathy
Hahnemann House
2 Powys Place
Great Ormond Street
London, WC1N 3HR

Liga Medicorum Homeopathica Internationalis (LMHI)
Sandra Chase, USA

Academy of Veterinary Homeopathy
1283 Lincoln Street
Eugene, Oregon, 97401, USA

Alternative Veterinary Medicine Centre
Chinham House
Stanford in the Vale
Faringdon, Oxon, SN7 8NQ

Homeopathic Physicians Teaching Group
(UK Veterinary Courses)
28 Beaumont Street
Oxford, OX1 2NP

REFERENCES

Barthel H: *Synthetic repertory: psychic and general symptoms of the homeopathic materica medica,* Heidelburg, Germany, 1981, Haug Verlag.

Bastide M: Immunologic examples on ultra high dilution research. In Endler PC, Schulte J, eds: *Ultra high dilutions,* Dordrecht, Germany, 1994, Klumer Academy.

Bastide M, Doucet-Jaboeuf M, Daurat V: Activity and chronopharmacology of very low doses of physiological immune inducers, *Immunol Today* 6:234, 1985.

Baumans V and others: Does Chelidonium 3x lower serum cholesterol? *Br Homeopathic J* 76:14, 1987.

Biddis K: *Homeopathy in veterinary practice,* London, 1980, British Homeopathic Association (pamphlet).

Bignamini M and others: Controlled double blind trial with Baryta Carb 15cH versus placebo in a group of hypertensive subjects confined to bed in two old people's homes, *Br Homeopathic J* 76:114, 1987.

Bildet J and others: Demonstrating the effects of apis mellifica and apium virus dilutions on erythema induced by u.v. radiation on guinea pigs, *Berlin J Res Homeopathy* 1:28, 1990.

Bildet J and others: Resistance de la cellule hepatique du rat apres une intoxication infintesimale au tetrachlorure de carbon, *Homeopathie Francais* 72:175, 1984.

Boericke W, Tafel: *A manual of homeopathic veterinary practice,* New York, 1881, Boericke & Tafel.

Boericke W: *Materia medica with repertory,* ed 9, Philadelphia, 1927, Boericke & Runyon.

Boger CM: *Boenninghausens characteristics and repertory,* New Delhi, India, 1938, B Jain.

Bourkas P: The measurements of the homeopathic remedies, *Eur J Classical Homeopathy* 1:34, 1996.

Boyd H: *Introduction to homeopathic medicine,* Beaconsfield, England, 1981, Beaconsfield Publishers.

Briones F: Effect of Barium Carbonicum LM11 and the combination of Calcium Carbonicum LM1 and Calcium Phosphoricum LM11 on the weight of pigs with retarded growth, *Int J Veterinary Homeopathy* 4:2, 1989.

A trial of Sepia 200c, *Br Homeopathic J* 84:14, 1995.

Brock K, Nielsen J: *Veterinær homøopati,* Copenhagen, Denmark, 1986, DSR Forlag.

Burt WH: *Physiological materia medica,* ed 3, New Delhi, India, 1882, B Jain.

Cazin J and others: A study of the effect of decimal and centesimal dilutions of arsenic on the retention and mobilization of arsenic in the rat, *Hum Toxicol* 6:315, 1991.

Clarke JH: *A dictionary of practical materia medica,* Saffron Walden, England, 1900, Health Science Press.

Conforti A, Signorini A, Bellavite P: Effects of high dilutions of histamine and other natural compounds on acute inflammation in rats, *Omeomed 92 Editrice compositori Bologna* 163, 1993.

Davenas E and others: Effect on mouse peritoneal macrophages of orally administered very high dilutions of silica, *Eur J Pharm* 135:313-319, 1987.

Day C: Isopathic prevention of kennel cough, *Int J Veterinary Homeopathy* 2:57, 1987.

Day C: Control of stillbirths using homeopathy, *Veterinary Record* 114:216, 1984.

Day C: Clinical trials in bovine mastitis using nosodes for prevention, *Int J Veterinary Homeopathy,* 1:15, 1986.

Day C: Dystocia prevention, *Proceedings of LMHI Congress,* Lyon, France, 1985.

Day C: *Homœopathy first aid for horses,* London, JA Allen & Co (in press).

Day C: *Natural remedies (for horses),* Addington, Buckingham, England, 1996, Kenilworth Press.

Day C: *Homeopathic treatment of small animals,* ed 2, Saffron Walden, England, 1990, CW Daniel.

Day C: In Andrews AH: *Bovine medicine,* Oxford, 1992, Blackwell Scientific Publications.

Day C: *Homeopathic treatment of beef and dairy cattle,* Beaconsfield, England, 1995, Beaconsfield Publishers.

Day C: *Natural remedies for your cat,* London, 1994, Piccadilly Press.

Day C: *Homeopathy, first aid for pets,* Stanford in the Vale, England, 1992, Chinham Publications.

del Francia F: *Omeopatica veterinaria,* Italy, 1985, Studio redazionale.

Desai V and others: *Antiinflammatory activity of Arnica on carragenen induced rat paw oedema,* 3rd IAVH Congress, Munster, 1992.

Eid P and others: Applicability of homeopathic *Caulophyllum thalictroides* during labour, *Br Hom J* 82:245, 1993.

Engineer S, Valik S, Engineer L: A study of antibody formation by Baptista tinctoria φ in experimental animals, *Br Hom J* 79:109-113, 1990.

Gerhardt A: *Handbuch der Homöopathie,* Leipzig, Germany, 1912, Wilmar Schwabe.

Guajardo-Bernal G, Searcy-Bernal R, Soto-Avila J: Growth promoting effect of Sulphur 201c in pigs, *Br Hom J* 85:15-21, 1996.

Guillemain J and others: Pharmacologie de l'infinitesimal. Application aux dilutions homeopathiques, *Homeopathie* 4:35, 1987.

Gupta R, Bhardwaj O, Manchanda R: Homeopathy in the treatment of warts, *Br Homeopathic J* 80:108, 1991.

Hahnemann CFS: *Organon of medicine,* eds 5 and 6, New Delhi, India, 1833-1834, B Jain.

Harish G, Kretschmer M: Smallest zinc quantities affect the histamine release from peritoneal mast cells in the rat, *Experientia* 44:761, 1988.

Hering C: *Condensed materia medica,* ed 4, New Delhi, India, 1884, B Jain.

Hunter F: *Homeopathic first aid treatment for pets,* London, 1988, Thorsons.

Jonas WW and others: Prophylaxis of tularemia infection in mice using agitated ultra high dilutions of tularemia infected tissues, Proceedings of the fifth GIRI meeting, Paris, ABS 21, 1991.

Kaiser D: A rediscovered manuscript of one of Hahnemann's basic writings, *Classical Homeopathy Q* 4:66, 1991.

Kayne S, Rafferty A: The use of Arseicum Album 30c to complement conventional treatment of neonatal diarrhea ("scours") in calves, *Br Homeopathic J* 83:202, 1994.

Kent JT: *Repertory of the homeopathic materia medica,* ed 6, London, 1991, Homeopathic Book Service.

Kent JT: *Lectures on homeopathic materia medica,* New Delhi, India, 1904, B Jain.

Koehler G: *Handbook of homeopathy,* Wellingborough, Northamptonshire, England, 1986, Thorsons.

Lannoye: European Parliament. Draft report on the status of non-conventional medicine, DVC no EN/PR/289/289543, 1995.

Lapp C, Wurmser L, Ney J: Mobilization de l'arsenic fixe chez le cobaye sous l'influence des doses infintesimales d'arseniate, *Therapie* 10:625, 1955.

Leath J, ed: *Veterinary homeopathy comprising rules for the general treatment of all domestic animals,* London, 1851, James Leath.

Lord RPG, Rush J, Rush W, editors: *The veterinary vade mecum,* London, 1875, The Homeopathic Publishing Co.

Macleod G: *A veterinary materia medica,* Saffron Walden, England, 1994, CW Daniel.

Macleod G: *Pigs: the homeopathic approach to the treatment and prevention of disease,* Saffron Walden, England, 1994, CW Daniel.

Macleod G: *Cats: homeopathic remedies,* Saffron Walden, England, 1990, CW Daniel.

Macleod G: *Dogs: homeopathic remedies,* Saffron Walden, England, 1983, CW Daniel.

Macleod G: *Goats: homeopathic remedies,* Saffron Walden, England, 1991, CW Daniel.

Macleod G: *Homeopathy for pets,* London, 1981, HDF (pamphlet).

Macleod G: Scour in calves and the rational approach to treatment, *Homeopathy* 24:1974.

Macleod G: *The treatment of cattle by homeopathy,* Saffron Walden, England, 1981, CW Daniel.

Macleod G: *The treatment of horses by homeopathy,* Saffron Walden, England, 1977, CW Daniel.

Mahe F: Evaluation of the effect of a collective homeopathic cure on morbility and the butchering qualities in fattening calves, *Int J Veterinary Homeopathy* 2(1):13, 1987.

Moore J: *Outlines of veterinary homeopathy,* London, 1857, H Turner.

Oberbaum M and others: Wound healing by homeopathic dilutions of silica in experimental animals, Proceedings of the fifth GIRI meeting. Paris ABS 23, 1992, 1995.

Peker J, Bonnefous L: *Dictionnaire des médecines douces pour chiens et chats,* France, 1988, Rocher.

Poitevin B: Mechanism of action of homeopathic medicines, *Br Homeopathic J* 38:32, 1995.

Quiquandon: *Homéopathie vétérinaire,* France, 1983, Editions du Point Vet.

Rakow B: *Der Homöopatische Katzendoktor,* Germany, 1986-1987, Kosmos.

Rakow B, Rakow M: *Bewährte Indikationen der Homöopathie in der Veterinärmedizin,* Germany, 1988, Sonntag.

Reilly D and others: Is evidence for homeopathy reproducible? *Lancet* 344:1601, 1994.

Ruddock EH, Reud Lade G: *The pocket manual of homeopathic veterinary medicine,* ed 3, London, 1878, The Homeopathic Publishing Co.

Saxton J: Use of distemper nosode in disease control, *Int J Veterinary Homeopathy* 15:8, 1991.

Schiff M: *The memory of water,* Wellingborough, Northamptonshire, England, 1995, Thorsons.

Schroyens F, editor: *Synthesis repertorium homeopathicum syntheticum,* London, 1993, Homeopathic Book Publishers.

Searcy R, Guajardo G: Papers on homeopathic research, Proceedings of the American Holistic Veterinary Medical Association Congress, Orlando, Fla, 1994.

Searcy R, Reyes O, Guajardo G: Control of subclinical bovine mastitis. Utilization of a homeopathic combination, *Br Homeopathic J* 84:67, 1995.

Silvo M, Arnaldo P: Ultrasonic study of homeopathic solutions, *Br Homeopathic J* 179:212, 1990.

Singh P, Chabra H: Topological investigation of the ethanol/water system and its implication for the mode of action of homeopathic medicines, *Br Homeopathic J* 82:164, 1993.

Stopes C, Woodward L: The use and efficacy of a homeopathic nosode in the prevention of mastitis in dairy herds: a farm survey of practicing users, *Int J Veterinary Homeopathy* 3:35, 1988.

Sukul N and others: Haloperidol induced catalepsy in mice suppressed by orally pre-administered potentized agaricus, *Br Homeopathic J* 84:6, 1995.

Sukul N, Ghosh S, Sinhababu S: Dose dependent suppression of haloperidol induced catalepsy by potentized agaricus mascarius, *Br Homeopathic J* 185:141, 1996.

Sukul N, Bhattacharyya B, Bala S: Differentiation of potencies of agaricus muscarius by experimental catalepsy, *Br Homeopathic J* 76:122, 1987.

Torres J, Ruiz M: Stochastic resonance and the homeopathic effect, *Br Homeopathic J* 85:134, 1996.

Towsey M, Hasan M: Homeopathy—a biophysical point of view, *Br Homeopathic J* 34:218, 1995.

Tyler ML: *Homeopathic drug pictures,* England, 1942, Health Science Press.

Vakil A, Vakil Y, Nanabhai A: Elevation of serum globulin levels in Chelidonium majus provers, *Br Homeopathic J* 78:97, 1989.

Varma P and others: A chemo-pharmacological study of Hypericum Perforatum, *Br Homeopathic J* 77:27, 1988.

Vithoulkas G: *Homeopathy, the dawn of the new man,* London, 1985, Thorsons.

Vithoulkas G: *The science of homeopathy,* London, 1986, Thorsons.

Westerhuis AH: *Hond en Homeopathie,* The Netherlands, 1989, Homeovisie.

Williamson A and others: A study using sepia 200c given prophylactically post partum to prevent anoestrus problems in the dairy cow, *Br Homeopathic J* 80:149, 1991.

Williamson AV and others: A trial of sepia 200, *Br Hom J* 84(1):14-20, 1995.

Wolff HG: *Homeopathic medicine for dogs,* London, 1984, Thorsons.

Wolter H: *Kompendium der Tierärztlichen Homöopathie,* Germany, 1989, Enke.

Wolter H: *Klinische Homöopathie in der Veterinärmedizin,* Heidelberg, Germany, ed 2, 1968, Haug Verlag.

Youbicier-Simo B and others: Effects of embrionic bursectomy and in ovo administration of highly diluted bursin on adenocorticotropic and immune response of chickens, *Int J Immunotherapy* 9:169, 1993.

Chapter 27

*H*omeopathy in Food Animal Practice

C. EDGAR SHEAFFER

Therapeutic programs for livestock farms must be safe, economical, and easy to implement. Homeopathic medicines not only fulfill these requirements but are useful for prevention of illness, as well as for treatment of individual sick animals. They can also be used in prevention and treatment of illness in entire herds. The use of alternative therapies such as homeopathy must abide by Food and Drug Administration (FDA) regulations.

This discussion of the use of homeopathy in food animal practice is based on clinical experience as well as the literature. A comprehensive review of alternative and complementary approaches to food animal practice is beyond the scope of this chapter. For more information on sustainable agriculture, refer to the reference list at the end of this chapter.

As with most complementary therapies, homeopathy requires attention to nutritional status. Nutritional manipulation is the subject of intense study among conventional veterinarians and scientists, and the veterinarian must stay current with the science of nutrition to optimize food animal performance through the efficacy of homeopathic treatment (Dunn, Moss, 1992; Hurley, Doane, 1989).

Most dairy farmers readily accept a low-cost program that is easy to implement. Education and on-farm experience are necessary for the veterinarian and herdsman. Both caregivers must realize that accuracy in prescription and frequency of dosing is a learning process. Once all persons involved become familiar with applications early in the course of disease, short-term results are generally positive. If the herdsman continues to incorporate the medicines into the health program, long-term benefits will be apparent.

Homeopathic medicines are a viable alternative to the use of crude drugs. Compassionate and responsible caregivers realize that the welfare of the individual animal and the herd or flock takes priority over convenience. Sick livestock must be cared for humanely; failure to do so violates the Hippocratic oath. The choice between conventional drugs and homeopathic medicines is determined by experience and knowledge. Regardless of the therapy chosen, the animal must be treated or humanely salvaged.

The reasons for choosing homeopathic medicines are as follows:

- They are an effective alternative to crude drugs
- They complement vitamins and probiotics
- They are economical to purchase and store
- They are easy to administer to individual patients or herds and flocks
- They are nontoxic at normal potencies—6X, 6C, 12X, 12C, 30X, 30C, 200X, and 200C.
- They require no withdrawal time before milk, meat, or eggs can be used
- They may relieve suffering in patients with chronic disease
- They may be administered by the farmer for acute illness or accident until the veterinarian arrives

All caregivers are advised to take classes on the use of homeopathic remedies before they prescribe them. Together the herdsman and veterinarian choose a prescription based on their knowledge of keynote symptoms in livestock. For example, a prominent symptom indicating the use of *Hypericum perfoliatum* is injury to toes (hooves), tails, and tips of ears and teats. Another defining symptom is numbness of a limb after nerve injury. Persons using homeopathic medicines have learned which symptoms can be relieved by 20 to 30 different remedies. In addition, various materia medicas list keynote symptoms in bold print.

Monitoring animals from birth through their life stages can be helpful in the learning process. The information in this chapter may be applied to lambs, calves, kids, cria, and foals. The indications describe "symptom pictures." For a more complete description of homeopathic prescribing based on the symptom picture, see Chapters 25, 26, and 28.

Homeopathic Repertory for Food Animal Practice

Homeopathic Remedies for Neonates

Arnica montana—dystocias; bruising from head, neck, and musculoskeletal trauma; 30C every 5 to 10 minutes to effect.

Aconitum napellus—shock at birth, apnea with rapid heart rate and feeble pulse, 30C every 5 to 10 minutes to effect.

Apis mellifica—swelling and edema with anuria on the first day of life, 12X or 30C hourly doses to effect, follows arnica or aconite when indicated.

Supportive therapy—colostrum for probiotics and vitamins A, D, E, and K.

Homeopathic Remedies for Patients on a Milk Diet

Calcarea phosphoricum—important in the development of bones, joints, and teeth; 12X, 30C, or 30X weekly for prevention; for treatment of limb or dental deformities, daily with 12X or 30X for 2 weeks.

Belladonna—sudden febrile attacks with delirium and threatened convulsions; 2 or 3 200C doses every ½ hour to effect; follow-up medicines that follow: bryonia, calcarea, phosphorus, and sulphur.

Chamomilla—colic or diarrhea during teething; stool with chopped spinach appearance; swollen, red, and painful gums; refusal of warm milk and preference for cool drinks; 12X, 30X, or 30C dose 4 times daily; compatibility with belladonna and pulsatilla.

Supportive therapy—probiotics; balanced electrolytes provided in drinking water or by stomach tube.

Homepathic Remedies for Weanlings

Calcarea carbonica—diarrhea, constipation, or muscle laxity with a potbellied appearance; 12X, 30X, or 30C once or twice a day until effect. (Transition diets require a change in the animal's ability to digest different foods.)

Arscenicum album—diarrhea from stress, including parasites and coccidia, with weakness and dehydration; 12X, 30X, or 30C doses 2 or 3 times daily until effect.

Mercuris corrosivus—chronic enteritis with poor growth and low weight gain, nonformed stools, and frequent straining.

These medicines may be given twice daily for 10 days; potency should be 12C or 30X.

Supportive therapy—high-quality forage with high digestibility, free of molds and mycotoxins; acetylated glucosamine supplements. (Do not overfeed grain or pelleted grain by-products.)

Homeopathic Remedies for Yearlings

Chenopodium—strongyles and tapeworms; 3X and 6X potencies daily for 14 days.

Abrotanum—ascarids and oxyurids, same dosage and potencies as for chenopodium.

Ferrum metallicum—anemia from the effects of internal parasites, 6x dose twice daily for 7 days.

Supportive therapy—highly digestible forage, kelp supplement or multivitamins and minerals from natural sources.

Homeopathic Remedies for Breeding Animals

Pulsatilla—anestrus or delayed first estrus after verification of proper age and weight gain; 30C or 30X doses daily for 1 week.

Ovarian—anestrus in patients with small, underdeveloped ovaries; effective in low potencies from 5C to 30C given for 1 week.

Palladium—anestrus in patients with swollen painful right ovary (not a cystic condition); 30C potency dose daily for 5 days.

Folliculinum—underdeveloped follicles or prolonged estrus with delayed ovulation; effective in low potencies from 5C to 30C until follicle matures.

Natrum muriaticum—deranged cycles with tendency for ovarian cyst formation; 30C or 200C potency daily for up to 10 days.

Supportive therapy—kelp or vitamins and minerals from natural sources; adequate pasture (not overgrazed); spacious shelter, especially during the winter.

Homeopathic Remedies for Infertility in the Male

Lycopodium clavatum—physically underdeveloped animal with low libido, recommended dosage for most species: 200C once every 20 to 25 days.

China officionalis—exhaustion of potency from breeding excesses, debility from loss of body fluids, dosage: 12C or more daily for 10 days.

Sepia—aversion to breeding from pain, falling asleep during act of breeding (a rare and peculiar symptom) (Kent, 1945), dosage: 30C or more weekly for 1 month.

Supportive therapy—clean stall, adequate daily nutrition, and proper immunity to diseases prevalent in the herd and region; limiting the number of females to be serviced.

Care of the Expectant Mother

Once pregnancy has been established, management and nutrition become even more important. Adequate exercise, potable water, and balanced nutrients should be provided. Homeopathic medicines useful in pregnant animals are *Calcarea phosphorica*, *Magnesia phosphorica*, *Sepia*, and *Cimicifuga racemosa*. The potency and frequency of dosage should be based on the individual patient and farm situation.

Calcarea phosphorica—fetal development, prevention of milk fever, and eclampsia.

Magnesia phosphorica—prevention of grass tetany and milk fever, amelioration of cramping pains of pregnancy.

Sepia—prevention of miscarriage and uterine prolapse.

Cimicifuga racemosa—relief of pelvic discomfort, prevention of first- and second-trimester miscarriage.

Labor and Delivery

Caulophyllum—daily 12C or 30C dose for the last 2 weeks of gestation.

Pulsatilla—abnormal presentation of the fetus and inertia of the uterus with excitement, potencies of 30C and higher until delivery occurs.

Arnica montana—bruising of the birth canal, swelling of the perineum and udder, three times daily for 3 days using the 30C dose.

Bellis perennis—administered after *Arnica* for deep bruising of soft tissue, potencies of 30C or 200C twice daily for 5 days.

Calendula—topically and orally for tears in the cervix or vagina, 30C three times daily for 5 days, 5% to 10% saline infusions once daily for five days.

Retained placentas

Retained placentas may be managed by the use of four remedies:

Caulophyllum—relaxation of the cervix.

Pulsatilla—involution and expulsion of membranes.

Sabina—excess bleeding accompanied by membrane retention, making infection likely.

Sepia—possible metritis with retention, most useful in the warm weather months. ("If you can smell it, use sepia.")

These medicines are generally given as a 30C twice daily for 3 to 5 days. All vital signs should be monitored throughout the postpartum period for accompanying signs of illness. Temperature increases, loss of appetite, mastitis, or diarrhea should be addressed immediately.

Echinacea and *Pyrogenium* are helpful in the prevention and treatment of metritis. Selection of the medicines is determined by the total symptom picture. Echinacea is useful when general sepsis accompanies uterine infection. Pyrogenium is indicated in toxemias when the patient's temperature and pulse are opposite from one another: for example, a rapid pulse with a subnormal temperature or a sluggish pulse with a high fever.

Supportive therapy—sternal position to avoid bloating, probiotics to restore gastrointestinal tract function, high levels of vitamin C 2 to 4 times daily to reduce the effects of sepsis and toxemia.

Metabolic disorders

Metabolic disorders occur frequently in lactating animals consuming processed feeds. Both ketosis and displacement of the abomasum may be prevented with judicious use of the following medicines:

Phosphorus—increased thirst and fear, depressed appetite, soft manure.

Nux vomica—constipation, depressed appetite and thirst, sensitivity to stimulation (noise, touch).

Lycopodium—small amounts of feed eaten and remainder refused, trapped gas with alternating bouts of loose and solid manure.

Carbo vegetabilis—bloating, with inability to belch and tendency to collapse; ruminants, distention on the left side of the body in the carbo vegetabilis state.

These remedies work best in the 30C to higher potencies given once or twice daily for metabolic conditions. Supportive measures include probiotics and antacids, if indicated. Changes in diet are highly recommended: feeding more long-stem, good-quality roughage, while decreasing the concentrate and silage.

Mastitis

Mastitis causes the largest economic loss for the dairy industry. Homeopathic remedies give the dairy producer an effective treatment alternative to antibiotics. Each of the following remedies can be given in the 12X, 30X, or 30C potencies 3 or 4 times daily until symptoms improve. Frequent stripping of the affected quarter has also proven helpful.

Phytolacca—the most common homeopathic remedy for mastitis, swelling and sensitivity of the mammae with clots of milk or blood in the secretion. (The lactating animal resents washing and stripping and may kick or try to run away.)

Bryonia alba—general swelling in patients that do not want to move. (The bryonia patient is commonly found lying on the inflamed portion of the udder.)

Apis mellifica—udder that is edematous, red, and hot; prepartum ventral edema. (The animal welcomes cold applications.)

Thiosinaminum-rhodallin—scar tissue on mammary gland from recurrent inflammations, fibroma of the streak canal.

The full range of potencies available to homeopathic practitioners has been useful in the treatment of mammary disorders. Topical massage with arnica and phytolacca ointments is useful in acute flare-ups. Chronic disorders with induration may respond to external applications of bryonia ointment.

Nosodes

The term *nosode* may be defined as a homeopathic remedy developed from a disease product. Veterinarians and pharmacists may prepare nosodes from any secretion or body fluid. The first recorded use of veterinary nosode was by Wilheim Lux, a German veterinarian who conceived the idea in 1831 of making a 30CH dilution of a drop of nasal mucus from an animal inflicted with glanders to subsequently treat other glanders sufferers (AAHP and AHVMA, 1991). One indication for nosode use is in the lactating animal with mastitis. A nosode made from a culture of mastitic milk has been clinically beneficial to the affected individual animal and the herd. Most nosodes are autogenous; that is, originating from the patient. Herd nosodes are beneficial in the prevention and control of specific disease conditions within a herd. Nosodes are much more effective for preventing problems than they are for treating sick animals. Prescriptions for the sick individual or the sick herd should always be based on the total symptom picture rather than the diagnosis alone. Excellent presentations of nosode use in livestock have been given by Day (1995) and Macleod (1981, 1991, 1994).

Research in Homeopathic Treatment of Food Animals

Most homeopathic research in livestock has been performed using clinical field trials. Christopher Day (1986) studied bovine mastitis using five homeopathically prepared bacterial nosodes. This double-blind study involved 82 cows: 41 received the combined mastitis nosode, and 41 received the unmedicated solvent. The results were dramatic—the incidence of mastitis in the treatment group was 2.5%, and that for the control group was 25%. Day reported two additional studies in the same paper: dystocia in Friesian dairy heifers and somatic cell counts in a herd divided by previous mastitis history into a high-risk group and a low-risk group. Both studies produced positive results, documenting the beneficial effects of nosodes.

Searcy and Guajardo (1994) studied rectal prolapse in 12 pigs after unsuccessful steroid therapy. Homeopathic medications were given to eight, with four left as controls. Seven of the eight were cured in a mean time of 13.1 days. In this small trial, homeopathic remedies proved to be helpful (Guajardo-Bernal, Searcy-Bernal, Soto-Avila, 1995). This group has continued research in swine, comparing antibiotics and homeopathic combinations in the prevention of porcine respiratory disease. They have found statistically significant results $p < .05$. A third swine study looked at weight gain in nursing and weaned piglets whose mothers had been given 200C sulphur every 10 days during the previous pregnancy. Litters from treated sows had a higher daily weight gain than those of untreated sows ($p < 0.05$) (Searcy, Guajardo, 1994).

Other studies in cattle measured the homeopathic effect on clinical and subclinical bovine mastitis. Cattle were matched by age, lactation status, and clinical and subclinical mastitis status. Measurable clinical mastitis was 7.1% for the treatment group compared with 42.8% for the placebo group ($p > 0.05$) (Searcy, Guajardo, 1994).

Day (1984) investigated the use of homeopathy in the treatment of stillbirths in swine. Caulophyllum 30C was given twice weekly to alternate sows; the controls did not receive treatment. In controls the stillbirth rate was 20.8%, compared with 10.3% for treated sows. Later in the trial, when the entire herd received caulophyllum treatment twice weekly during pregnancy, the stillbirth mortality fell to 1.9%.

Williamson and others conducted ongoing clinical trials from 1987 through 1990, assessing the use of 200C sepia given postpartum for the prevention of anestrus. The results of several double-blind trials indicated that timing may be as important in homeopathic therapy as in conventional prostaglandin treatments. The overall cull rate for infertility problems in this herd was 10%, out of which those cows receiving the sepia on day 14 had the largest proportion (Williamson and others, 1995). However, the cows receiving the sepia on day 21 postpartum had a consistently higher conception rate and a lower culling rate. Clinically, herds outside of this study validate these findings that sepia given after day 21 postpartum results in improved conception rates and shorter calving intervals (Mackie and others, 1990; Williamson and others, 1991, 1995).

Homeopathic medicines form the basis for the holistic approach used in food animal practice. For the health care program to succeed, all farming and management practices must be compatible with the three basic tenets outlined by Samuel Hahnemann (O'Reilly, 1996) and the principles of cure outlined by Constantine Hering (1865). Proper farming and management practices remove obstacles to cure, thus enabling each patient to exhibit a curative response to the homeopathic medicines administered. The welfare of each animal and of the herd is our priority. The second goal follows closely, that is, the improvement of health, production, and longevity. The natural outcome of these goals is better quality milk and meat for human consumption.

References

American Association of Homeopathic Pharmacists and the American Holistic Veterinary Medical Association: *The place of homeopathic remedies in veterinary medicine*, 1991, the Associations.

Boericke F: *Homeopathic materia medica with repertory*, ed 9, Philadelphia, 1927, Boericke and Runyon.

Boericke F, Tafel A: *A manual of homeopathic veterinary practice designed for horses, all kinds of domestic animals and fowls*, Philadelphia, 1881.

Clarke J: *Dictionary of materia medica*, vols 1-4, 1900.

Day C: Control of stillbirths in pigs using homeopathy, *Vet Record* 114:216, 1984.

Day C: Clinical trials in bovine mastitis, *Br Homeopathic J* 75:11, 1986.

Day C: *The homeopathic treatment of beef and dairy cattle,* Beaconsfield, Bucks England, 1995, Beaconsfield Publishing.

Dunn TG, Moss GE: Effects of nutrient deficiencies and excesses on reproductive efficiency of livestock, *J Animal Sci* 70:1580, 1992.

Guajardo-Bernal G, Searcy-Bernal R, Soto-Avila J: Growth-promoting effect of sulphur 201 c in pigs, *Br Homeopathic J* 85:15, 1996.

Hering C: Hahnemann's three rules concerning the rank of symptoms, *Hahnemann Monthly* 1:5-12, 1865.

Hurley WL, Doane RM: Recent developments in the roles of vitamins and minerals in reproduction, *J Dairy Science* 72:784, 1989.

Kent J: *Repertory of the homeopathic materia medica,* New Delhi, 1945, B Jain Publishers.

Mackie W and others: A study model with initial findings using sepia 200 c given prophylactically to prevent anoestrum problems in the dairy cow, *Br Homeopathic J* 79:132, 1990.

Macleod G: *The treatment of cattle by homeopathy,* Saffron Walden, 1981, CW Daniel Co.

Macleod G: *Goats: homeopathic remedies,* Saffron Walden, 1991, CW Daniel Co.

Macleod G: *Pigs: the homeopathic approach to the treatment and prevention of disease,* Saffron Walden, 1994, CW Daniel Co.

O'Reilly W: *Organon of the medical art by Dr. Samuel Hahnemann,* Redmond, Wash, 1996, Birdcage Books.

Searcy R, Guajardo G: Three papers on homeopathic research. Proceedings of the American Holistic Veterinary Medical Association Annual Conference, 1994, p 93.

Williamson A and others: A study using sepia 200 c given prophylactically postpartum to prevent anoestrus problems in the dairy cow, *Br Homeopathic J* 80:149, 1991.

Williamson A and others: A trial of Sepia 200, *Br Homeopathic J* 84:14, 1995.

*S*ELECTED READINGS

Boericke W: *Homeopathic materia medica with repertory,* ed 9, Philadelphia, 1927, Boericke and Runyon.

Boericke F, Tafel A: *A manual of homeopathic veterinary practice designed for horses, all kinds of domestic animals, and fowls,* Philadelphia, 1881, Authors.

Clarke J: *Dictionary of materia medica,* vols 1-4, Saffron Walden, Essex, England, 1900, Health Science.

Guajardo-Bernal G, Searcy-Bernal R, Soto-Avila J: Swine rectal prolapse treated with homeopathy, *Dynamis,* 8:20, 1995.

Kayne S: Homeopathic veterinary prescribing, *Br Homeopathic J* 8:28, 1992.

Neatby E, Stonham T: *A manual of homeo-therapeutics,* ed 3, London, 1948, Stables Press.

Schmidt A: Homeopathy: a field of work for the veterinarian, *Schweizer Archiv fur Tierheilkunde* 135:257, 1993.

Chapter 28

Homeopathy in Equine Practice

PEGGY FLEMING

Homeopathic preparations are becoming increasingly popular in the equine product market. The list of available products includes pills promoting relief from arthritis, pastes for relaxation, and lotions for skin disease. More often than not, consumers do not fully understand the way these medications work, and most people assume they are similar to herbs in their action. Even more disturbing, many practitioners prescribe homeopathics without understanding the basic and unique principles that differentiate this medicinal paradigm from the traditional concepts studied in veterinary school.

Homeopathy can be a powerful and effective mode of healing. Recent scientific research is beginning to demonstrate this fact (Bellavite and others, 1996). Unfortunately, it is often dismissed as ineffective by the veterinary community. The failures of homeopathy early in a prescriber's career are usually caused by an attempt to dispense these medications as if they were conventional pharmaceuticals. The practitioner must thoroughly understand the basic principles of homeopathy before using this complicated mode of therapy.

Literature Review

Veterinary medicine, as a whole, views homeopathy with skepticism. Much of this attitude is based on the assumption that "valid" research on the efficacy of this modality is lacking. In this context, *valid* is defined as the use of double-blind studies, controlled clinical trials, and repeatable results.

This definition has several drawbacks, however, with regard to homeopathy. The first problem involves the fundamental difference between homeopathy and allopathic medicine. Homeopathy is based on the susceptibility of the individual rather than the diagnosis of a disease. According to Hahnemann's laws, it is an illusion to label a disease such as diabetes: There are only individuals in whom some diabetic-type symptoms manifest. Depending on their unique mental and general symptoms and their previous history, individuals probably need different remedies. In addition, as treatment progresses toward a cure, remedies generally must be changed. Thus this form of prescribing does not lend itself to double-blind, controlled data gathering. Second, some practitioners may consider double-blind studies unethical in a clinical situation. Most physicians would find it difficult to allow half their patients to suffer while the other half receives treatment.

The best approach to this dilemma seems to involve testing the homeopathic treatment rather than the remedy itself. A logical methodology in a clinical setting would be to compare the outcomes of patients who received conventional treatment with those of patients who received homeopathic therapy. This approach is especially feasible in veterinary practice, where there is more freedom to opt for alternative approaches.

Despite these stumbling blocks, veterinary research is playing a critical role in validating homeopathy. Conventional practitioners of human medicine argue that any significant improvement in a patient receiving a homeopathic remedy is due to the placebo effect. This argument is inappropriate when applied to research conducted on laboratory animals (an environment devoid of even the placebo-like nurturing of a caring owner). Veterinary research in toxicology has produced interesting results about the efficacy of isopathy and nosode administration in counteracting the resultant disease state. Ideally, future research will focus on nonharmful strategies.

All experimental studies begin with a hypothesis. The two primary areas of contention regarding homeopathy are based on the "law of similars" and the principle of dilution. It is necessary in this technologic age not only to verify the efficacy of homeopathy but to search for the mechanisms by which this modality operates. As our understanding of quantum physics increases, so does our knowledge of homeopathic concepts and the likelihood that this 200-year-old system of medicine will be an accepted part of modern science. For example, experts now confirm that information can be stored in water molecules as frequencies of molecular dipoles (superradiance). Biochemists are beginning to realize that homeopathic remedies activate homeostasis systems via mechanisms other than those activated by endogenous mediators. These drugs seem to act as substitutes for an endogenous regulatory signal that may be ineffective because the system is no longer sensitive to it—being blocked by the disease itself (Bellavite and others, 1996). These are plausible hypotheses that might explain the positive results found in the studies discussed here.

Several significant veterinary scientific studies have proved the efficacy of highly diluted substances in treating the disease state induced by the same substance given at toxic levels. Research has shown that dilute solutions of 7C arsenic (10-14 molar) can increase the urinary elimination of this toxin when given to laboratory rats (Cazin and others, 1987; Lapp and others, 1955; Wurmser and others, 1955). The difference in these rats versus those given dilutions of water alone was highly significant. Other studies have shown that renal toxicity caused by high levels of cadmium was found to be reduced by the administration of the homeopathic form of this metal (Bascands and others, 1990). A similar study found that 9C Mercurius protected rats against the nephrotoxic effects of the concentrated form of this substance.

Research has also shown that similar substances (i.e., causing a similar disease), as well as identical diluted substances, may exert a protective effect against toxins. In a study in which rats were injected with carbon tetrachloride to induce hepatitis, researchers found that 7C phosphorus (a hepatotoxic agent when given in large doses) significantly reduced mortality (Bildet and others, 1975; Bildet and others, 1984). In a similar study, rats treated with lethal doses of hepatotoxic α-amanitine responded favorably to the administration of Phosphorus 15C, again demonstrating that small doses of similar substances can treat disease (Guilleman and others, 1987). Hahnemann's law of similarity was further substantiated by a study using the homeopathic remedy Apis. Apis is a substance derived from the venom of the honey bee that is commonly used by homeopaths for the treatment of hypersensitive skin reactions such as hives and edema. Guinea pigs subjected to radiation pretreated with 7C Apis showed a 50% reduction in skin lesions compared with those left untreated (Bastide, Aubin, Baronnet, 1975; Bildet and others, 1990; Poitevin and others, 1988).

Further veterinary research has provided insight into the way homeopathy might induce these kinds of results. Silicea, a remedy derived from sand, has long been used in homeopathy for the treatment of inflammatory-type reactions such as abscesses and chronic nonhealing ulcers. In one study, 9C dilutions (1.66×10^{-19} M) of Silicea were given to a colony of mice for 25 days. The peritoneal macrophages of these mice showed up to a 60% increase in production of platelet-activating factor compared with those of the mice in the control group. This effect could not be seen in mice given nonrelated homeopathic remedies such as Gelsemium (Davenas and others, 1987). Homeopathic preparations of interferon increase T-cell response and production of plaque-forming cells (Bastide and others, 1987). Homeopathic Zinc (12X = 0.025 pg) significantly increases the release of histamine by peritoneal mast cells in rats given this metal for 7 days (Harish, Kretschmer, 1988). Further immune research shows that homeopathic preparations of antigens (6C and 7C) are capable of inducing specific IgM and IgG responses. The conclusion is that homeopathic preparations of extremely dilute substances are enough for immunomodulation (Bentwich, 1993; Weisman and others, 1991).

Other modes of action include the excitation of nerve tissue. In one study, rats fed high-salt diets were given homeopathic sodium chloride. Microelectrodes implanted in the hypothalamus of each rodent showed that discharge frequencies of this organ's neurons were significantly decreased (Sukul and others, 1993). In another study researching the effect of homeopathic copper on gastrointestinal motility, mice pretreated with Neostigmine (an intestinal stimulant) showed a return toward normal rates compared with mice in the control group (Santini and others, 1990).

Homeopathy appears to exert a significant influence on developing embryos. In chick embryos a hormone called *bursin* is necessary to complete immunologic development. Embryos devoid of this hormone develop a normal immune system when given highly diluted levels of the same substance (beyond the Avogadro constant) (Bastide, 1994; Yubicier, 1993). In tadpoles, thyroxine is known to accelerate metamorphosis. Research has shown that 30X Thyroxine actually inhibits this metamorphosis (Endler and others, 1994).

Valid clinical studies are less prevalent than those of laboratory research. However, two of significant merit should be mentioned. The positive therapeutic effects of various homeopathics have been shown in the treatment of metritis, mastitis, and diarrhea in pigs (Both, 1987), and dairy cows benefited from the postpartum administration of Sepia (cuttlefish ink) at a 200C dilution (Williamson and others, 1991).

The studies demonstrate that homeopathic preparations do seem to exert biologic activity. In addition, this biologic activity is specific and related closely to the activity exerted by pharmacologic levels of the same or similar substances. Furthermore, the resultant activity often appears to be the antithesis of the activity induced by the homeopathic's pharmacologic counterpart.

The precise nature of this phenomenon is not understood. Perhaps the answer lies in the study of solvent behavior. Resistance to homeopathic research may stem not from scientific invalidity but from the challenge homeopathy represents to the claim that the molecular paradigm is the only way of interpreting biologic reality (Bellavite and others, 1996). Clearly, new hypotheses regarding the physiochemical principles of nature are necessary to stimulate further research.

Principles

To understand homeopathy is to understand its roots. At the beginning of the nineteenth century, a German physician named Samuel Hahnemann developed a new form of medicine as a viable alternative to the invasive conventional medical methods of his day (Hahnemann, 1796). He called this form of healing *homeopathy*, a Greek word meaning "similar suffering" (Weiner, 1996). Hahnemann presented the system as a complete therapeutic method of healing based on clinically demonstrable laws and principles.

The primary law of this modality is the "law of similars," which is based on the assumption that the symptoms expressed by the patient are not the disease but rather the positive reactions of the organism under stress in an attempt to regain physiologic balance. To help the patient reestablish order, the physician assists and strengthens these reactions (symptoms) instead of suppressing them. The correct homeopathic remedy is selected based on its ability to produce those symptoms in a healthy individual. The ill patient is extremely susceptible to such a remedy, and his symptoms are temporarily strengthened to evoke a cure. The same remedy that produces those symptoms of illness in the healthy subject heals the sick one.

Health to a homeopath represents harmony between the entire body and a vigorous life force. This life force is capable of restoring equilibrium by producing strong symptoms that quickly and efficiently remove any insult. A sudden and high fever, for example, is a sign of a strong vital force. The object of giving a remedy that produces the same symptoms is to stimulate that vital force to effect a cure. This is in sharp contrast to allopathy, which views symptoms as the disease; consequently symptoms are suppressed, and the vital force of the patient is compromised. Homeopathy does not view disease in terms of invading factors but in terms of the patient's susceptibility. Homeopathy seeks to strengthen these lines of susceptibility to help a patient resist morbid influences.

Disease to a homeopath is viewed as an unsuitable or disproportionate reaction to an initial insult. An organism's first reaction to an insult begins with a mental state. The body then responds at the level of the neuroendocrine

axis. Therefore a pathogenic factor initially causes a central disturbance (mental and neuroendocrine reaction). The mental symptoms may manifest as fear and anxiety to compel the organism into action. The neuroendocrine system then reacts, for example, with inflammation. If this strategy is unsuccessful or out of proportion, less important parts of the body are sacrificed and pathology ensues (Sankaran, 1995). A strong general reaction is a sign of health, as often seen in young children in whom little physical pathology is seen. A weak general reaction is seen in more chronically diseased individuals in whom physical pathology is prominent yet a general reaction appears to be minimal. Homeopathic remedies are intended to stimulate the central reactions to deal with the insult appropriately.

According to Hahnemann's second law, only one similimum (exact remedy) exists at the moment of treatment that can effect a cure (Hahnemann, 1796). A cure is defined as the restoration of equilibrium without further treatment. Every patient is treated as a unique individual. No remedy exists for navicular disease or equine protozoal myelitis because homeopaths do not treat symptoms. The practitioner is treating the patient's vital force, and the way in which one horse reacts to a pathogen may be completely different from another horse's reaction. The practitioner is not interested in removing the presenting complaint but in permanently restoring the patient's health.

Detailed history taking is the cornerstone of successful prescribing. Most patients are afflicted with a complex layering of lifelong symptoms that reflect their reactions to a singular chronic disease (Coulter, 1976). The deepest layer (termed *psora*) comprises the weaknesses the patient inherits, and the more superficial layers are a combination of current morbid influences (miasms) and previous suppression with conventional medication (i.e., corticosteroids). In most cases, practitioners are only able to prescribe according to presenting symptoms. Obtaining a detailed history is particularly difficult in the treatment of horses. One remedy is used, those symptoms begin to subside, and a new disease picture emerges. A new single remedy is selected based on the new information. Remedies should never be casually prescribed or changed too frequently (Hahnemann, 1994). This precaution is important in treating acute disease as well as chronic.

Hahnemann began exploring his theories by administering full-strength extractions of various plant, animal, and mineral substances. He discovered that after an initial violent reaction, the diseased patient would recover fully. He later discovered that if he diluted the remedy and succussed (forcibly tapped the solution against a solid object) it in water and alcohol, he actually "excited" the latent curative force of the substance and removed the physical toxicity. This process, known as *potentization*, reduced the initial aggravation and increased the stimulation of the vital force (Ullman, 1991). For example, if a substance is diluted 1 part to 99, it is called 1C (centisimal) in potency. If one part of that solution is then diluted again to 99, it is called 2C, and so on. The more times this procedure is performed, the greater the energetic healing power of the remedy is when released into the solution, and the more the physical characteristics are removed. The tenfold dilution system is signified with an X, whereas the thousandfold dilution system carries an M (the most potent dilution) (Vithoulkas, 1990). The action of the remedy is brief, perhaps seconds, but the reaction of the vital force may be lengthy, depending on the potency given. As long as the vital force is reacting, the remedy should not be repeated. An initial aggravation of symptoms, along with a sensation of increased well-being, is soon followed by an alleviation of symptoms. This type of response is considered curative. An often misleading situation can occur with the administration of a remedy: The immediate disappearance of symptoms occurs without aggravation; however, the disease quickly returns without continuous administration of increasing doses of medication. This is termed *palliation* and is not considered a curative reaction (Hahnemann, 1994). Palliation is a common practice in Western medicine (corticosteroids for skin disease), but it can also occur in homeopathy, particularly when combination remedies are used.

The third law involves the nature of a cure, which follows a particular and predictable pattern. First, symptoms tend to move down the body from head to extremities. Healing begins in the mind and moves to the body (Ullman, 1991). A curative reaction is always heralded by an improvement in the mental state. For example, a client may remark that even though his horse's skin disease has worsened after administration of a remedy, the horse has more energy. In homeopathy, this response is considered an initial favorable reaction, especially when the primary complaint is external. Second, symptoms tend to move from the deeper parts of the body toward the surface as the body casts out the disease. Often a complete cure is preceded by the appearance of an old skin lesion. This healing symptomatic reaction must not be suppressed with medication. Third, old symptoms that have been suppressed may return, generally in the reverse order of their original occurrence.

Prescribing the Correct Remedy

The homeopathic materia medica is a record of the effects of active substances on healthy human beings (Murphy, 1994). Under each remedy a list of symptoms is categorized according to parts of the body affected (e.g., extremities, head, face, mental symptoms) and generalities (unique modalities of the symptoms). A generality may include phraseology such as "worse with cold," "worse at night," "better with rest." Usually a symptom has a unique characteristic (keynote symptom) that suggests a certain remedy. For example, a keynote mental symptom for the homeopathic substance phosphorus is fear of thunderstorms. As a rule, priority is given to the mental symptoms and generalities. If a particular remedy fits a physical symptom but does not match the mental picture, it will usually be ineffective in curing the condition (Sankaran, 1995).

Many human materia medicas are available (see the list of commonly used materia medicas and suppliers at the end of the chapter). Some have been transcribed to computer software. Veterinary materia medicas are also available, but they are not as complete as their counterparts in human medicine.

The physician records all symptoms, both past and present, paying particular attention to peculiar symptoms, mental state, and generalities. The physician then selects the appropriate remedy through a process called *reportization* and researches the symptoms in a book called a *repertory*. A repertory catalogues all symptoms according to parts of the body. Next to each symptom is the list of remedies that would create that symptom in a healthy individual *(proving)*. Through the process of elimination a selection of remedies is made that would elicit all the symptoms. The potential remedies are then researched in a materia medica to determine the one that most closely matches the patient's disease picture.

After selecting the remedy, the practitioner must determine the correct potency. Potency depends on the strength of the patient's vital force, the degree of physical pathology, and the chronicity of the disease (Hahnemann, 1994). The stronger the vital force, the higher the potency employed (e.g., young horses can be given higher potencies). The greater the tissue pathology, the lower the potency (kidney failure versus cystitis). The higher potencies tend to exert their influence on the vital force for a greater period of time (a 1M potency can last a month, whereas a 30C potency may last only a week). If the prescription for the case is clear and the pathology not severe, 200C or higher can be used. Higher concentrations may be advantageous because the higher the potency, the more clearcut the reaction. If the pathology is significant, concentrations should remain below 200C. A diseased organ may not be able to adjust to a strong aggravation. If the patient is old and weak, concentrations of 30C or below are advised. If the case is clear with strong mental symptoms, high potencies must be used to stimulate the mental level of disease. If the case is unclear, low potencies are recommended (Pitcairn, 1992).

As long as the patient feels relief, the remedy should not be repeated. The single most common error in prescribing is overmedication. Remedies come in both pilule and liquid form. The number of pilules taken in a single dose is relatively unimportant: It is the potency that is critical.

Homeopaths advise against the use of certain substances when administering a homeopathic remedy. Strong aromatic products such as camphor should be avoided (Weiner, 1996). Similarly, concomitant administration of allopathic medication creates unclear results and often counteracts any benefit the remedy might have produced. Practitioners should be careful not to touch homeopathic substances with their hands, to keep the substances from sunlight and electromagnetic radiation, and to administer them on an empty stomach. For some horses, applying pilules in the commissure of the lip is the simplest way to administer the remedy; for more head-shy patients, dispensing the liquid form via dose syringe works well.

Acute Versus Chronic Disease

There are two approaches to prescribing homeopathics, depending on whether the disease is in an acute or chronic state. Many homeopaths theorize that most apparently acute disease is actually a partial manifestation of a deep-seated, "hidden," chronic disease, the result of generations of suppression (Hahnemann, 1994). Therefore the differentiation between acute and chronic is negligible, and the diseases are treated the same way. In other words, the practitioner looks at the entire history of the horse to determine the pattern of his singular disease and prescribes a remedy according to not only his current symptoms but all previous ones he has manifested. These chronic, all-encompassing remedies are called *constitutional remedies* and cover a wide range of symptoms. Often, homeopaths will study the patient's bloodline because chronic disease is usually inherited. Warmbloods tend to be constitutionally different from thoroughbreds. Because constitutional treatment builds up the patient's resistance to attacks of acute disease, as well as clearing chronic conditions, constitutional prescribing is both a preventive and a curative approach.

Many remedies are not as inclusive as constitutional homeopathics. In some situations, as in mechanical injuries, the indications for a remedy are purely physical. This does not mean that the remedy itself has no mental symptoms in its provings, but simply that in the case described, the remedy can be determined on physical indications alone. In other situations the mental component is of primary importance or serves to distinguish between conditions calling for different remedies. For example, several remedies exist for blunt trauma to the head, but arnica has the mental symptom "fear of touch" that may lead to its homeopathic employment, even months after the trauma has apparently healed.

In acute first-aid prescribing a complete symptom image of the patient is not always available. Often the remedy is given based on only the presenting symptoms. This may appear to be a departure from the homeopathic principle of looking at the patient as a whole. However in first-aid situations the symptomatic condition of the patient depends to a large degree on the nature of the acute ailment. The employment of these remedies stabilizes the patient's condition and hastens recovery. Often, after these initial "acute" remedies are administered, the initial crisis is resolved and a more clear-cut constitutional picture emerges.

Recommended dosages for first aid and acute illness vary somewhat, but generally 30C is preferred (Weiner, 1996). As a rule of thumb, the remedy should be repeated every 30 minutes for three treatments. If no response is seen, the remedy should be reevaluated. The remedy should never be repeated, however, if the patient is showing an active positive response. In the treatment of chronic disease, the length of action of a remedy depends on its potency. Generally, 30C lasts for several days to a week, 200C exerts its influence for several weeks, and a 1M potency may stimulate a curative reaction for months.

Equine Materia Medica

Before discussing the uses of each specific remedy, it is important to clarify the term *remedy picture*. As mentioned previously, a homeopathic remedy can be used in the treatment of both acute and chronic ailments; however, when chronic disease is treated, patients must be considered in their entirety (Hahnemann, 1994). In other words, attention is given not only to the presenting complaint but to all facets of the patient's being.

To illustrate this concept, the reader is asked to imagine several artists painting a scene of a particular forest. Picasso may render this picture very differently from Monet, yet the scene remains the same. We can view a symptom such as diarrhea in the same way. The symptoms may at first appear similar, but in actuality the disease for one horse may be entirely different from that of another, depending on the specific mental and general symptoms of the individual. This concept is based on the holistic approach of combining mind, spirit, and body with the realization that insults at the mental level have ramifications on the physical plane. For example, a sensitive and nervous filly sent to the track at an early age may be stressed to the point of developing diarrhea after one outing on the backside, whereas an aggressive colt may develop similar symptoms only after exceeding his unique mental stress level, which might be overrestraint in a workout. In homeopathic prescribing, one must determine the means and the reason that each individual's neuroendocrine axis is triggered into action.

The way in which individual horses fall into a pattern of disease depends on their remedy pictures. Their symptoms reflect the way they deal with life. Diarrhea may be the outcome of this reaction, but the origin of the insult depends on the mental state of the individual. When the animal's symptom picture is clear, the remedy that best matches it is prescribed for that animal.

Some descriptions of constitutional remedies may appear subjective. Readers may ask if practitioners can truly distinguish between a "sensitive" horse and an "aggressive" one. The practice of homeopathy requires this leap of faith because it is the essence of this medical system. This is not to say that a practitioner cannot successfully prescribe a remedy without grasping the mental state of the patient; in fact, in first-aid prescribing, this knowledge is often unnecessary. However, to truly understand the power and effectiveness of this medicine in increasing the well-being of the patient, the practitioner must attempt to understand the patient's mental state (Sankaran, 1995).

The following sections are just a few among thousands of substances used as homeopathics. These are the remedies that are of major benefit in an equine practice and should be present in a basic emergency kit. The substance from which the remedy is derived is listed in parentheses.

Aconitum (Monk's Hood)

Aconitum, along with Belladonna, is one of the best-known fever remedies in the materia medica. It is most effective at the first signs of an acute illness, before its development into distinctive pathology. The Aconitum state, or symptom picture, is one of intense anxiety, restlessness, nervous agitation, fear, and excitement.

In the horse, Aconitum is useful in the beginning stages of laminitis, when a high fever is present, and in the first stages of a respiratory viremia. Aconitum is useful both in the prevention of stress-related illness and in the treatment of such conditions. Therefore it can be given during long shipping excursions to prevent shipping fever (Macleod, 1992). Fright is a keynote symptom of this remedy. It can be used for chronically fearful horses, especially if they have a history of trauma, and it is often successful in high potency to alleviate "show jitters" (Shaw, 1994).

Apis (Honey Bee)

Like the insect it is derived from, Apis can cause (and in homeopathic preparation, cure) rapid swelling and inflammation (Murphy, 1994). Apis is an excellent treatment for insect bites and stings, especially when hive formation is present. It is also useful for edematous swellings that pit on pressure, and it can stimulate healing of pulmonary edema.

Apis horses are irritable, suspicious, and hard to please. However, like the honey bee, they desire the open air and dislike being alone. Their conditions are worse with touch, heat, and pressure and better with cold application (Shaw, 1994).

Apis is also useful in mares with right ovarian cysts who display the above temperament and generalities (Day, 1993).

Arsenicum (Arsenic)

Arsenicum is one of the major constitutional remedies of horses, particularly thoroughbreds. Its hallmark is restlessness, with the patient always appearing to be in a state of motion, as often seen in weavers and stall-walkers (Murphy, 1994). During the disease state, the Arsenicum horse may have watery, acrid discharges, either in the eye, from the nose, or in the form of diarrhea. In fact, Arsenicum is often used in food poisoning and has been used successfully for diarrhea caused by excessive dosing of antibiotics (Macleod, 1992). A keynote symptom of Arsenicum is desire for water, especially in frequent, small sips. A familiar picture is the distressed horse continuously dropping his head in his water bucket but only imbibing a small amount.

Arsenicum is an excellent remedy for allergic asthma and chronic obstructive pulmonary disease, especially with a concomitant dry and scaly skin disease. Often the client will complain that the horse's wheezing and strong coughing attacks occur more frequently at night.

The Arsenicum horse is elegant and refined and tends to be on the chilly side, faring poorly in winter without the warmth of a barn or blankets (Shaw, 1994).

Belladonna (Deadly Nightshade)

Belladonna is comparable to Aconitum as one of the great fever remedies (Murphy, 1994). Onset is often sudden and violent, accompanied by symptoms associated with inflammation, such as heat, redness, pain, and swelling. Belladonna is a useful remedy in convulsions. A keynote symptom is bilateral dilation of the pupils. Therefore this remedy may be considered in acute encephalitis and severe heatstroke. The bounding pulse of acute laminitis responds well to repeated doses of Belladonna (Macleod, 1992).

The mental state of Belladonna is one of rage, excitement, and fear. These horses worsen with touch or sudden jarring motions and improve in a dark, quiet stall. Along with the intense heat of this patient is a strong thirst with a concomitant dry mouth.

Although obviously an acute remedy, Belladonna has its chronic state. Its employment is often successful in improving the disobedient and quarrelsome horse who displays irrational behavior (Shaw, 1994).

Bellis Perennis (Daisy)

Bellis perennis is a great remedy to have in an equine practice because it is used for deep bruising of tissue, especially in the pelvis (Murphy, 1994). This remedy is often effective months and even years after a horse experienced a fall that subsequently damaged his back (Shaw, 1994).

Any bruising or strain that does not respond to Arnica may respond to this remedy. Because of its affinity to the pelvic region, Bellis is useful postpartum to reduce bruising and pain.

The Bellis horse is stiff and unwilling to move but improves with continued motion. Symptoms improve with cold applications rather than warm ones. These horses dislike being touched on the distressed region.

Bryonia (Wild Hops)

Bryonia is often called the *grumpy-bear remedy* because the mental state is one of a dull irritability. Imagine the horse that prefers to be left alone, hates going out on trail, and with any opportunity turns toward the barn (Shaw, 1994).

A keynote generality of Bryonia is "worse from least motion and better from rest" (Sankaran, 1994). It is another important equine remedy because of effectiveness in treating lameness. Most Bryonia-susceptible lamenesses are deep-seated and slow in appearance, becoming more severe over a long period (Morgan, 1988). This is often seen in many cases labeled as *navicular disease*. These horses hate the warmth of summer, and often their symptoms worsen at this time. When winter comes, everything seems to improve.

Bryonia can be used in tendinitis as well as synovitis. The affected joint is hot and swollen, improving with the application of ice boots and pressure bandages. This remedy is also useful in many equine respiratory ailments, particularly pleurisy. Patients are reluctant to move but prefer pressure on the chest; therefore they are often found lying in their stalls on the affected side.

Calcarea Carbonica (Oyster Shell)

Calcarea carbonica is an important equine constitutional remedy, particularly for warmbloods. This remedy is wide ranging in its actions and frequently employed in an equine practice.

The mental state can alternate between a stubborn aggressiveness mingled with moments of inattentive spookiness and tenacious adherence to a rigorous training schedule. These horses are often distinguished by their phlegmatic shape. Coarsely boned and often portly, they exhibit a hearty appetite. Their insatiable oral fixation often leads to a desire for indigestible things and manifests in the equine as wood chewing and the grazing of weeds and plants in preference to grass (Shaw, 1994).

Calcarea carbonica is related to bone formation in the horse, and as youngsters these equines often develop growth abnormalities such as osteochondritis dessicans (OCD) and epiphysitis (symptoms are worse with exertion). Exostosis is a common symptom, seen often in the warmblood, and Calcarea carbonica is useful for ringbone and splint formation. Dentition is also affected, and Calcarea carbonica is often successful when caps do not shed.

Calcarea carbonica is a useful respiratory remedy (Murphy, 1994). It can be helpful in treating bleeders, especially when the mental state and generalities fit. The Calcarea carbonica cough is dry and irritating and exacerbated by eating. The expectoration, when present, is thick and yellow.

The skin can be affected, often manifesting as hyperkeratosis along the chest, belly, and face. Calcarea carbonica is often useful for the treatment of facial warts. Calcareas are always worse in wet weather and with washing, so the skin is usually not improved with bathing.

Calcarea Fluorica (Fluoride of Lime)

Calcarea fluorica is a powerful tissue remedy with a tendency to form exuberant and disproportionate growths in the face of injury (Murphy, 1994). This seems to be a predominant disease state in the horse. Surgeons are familiar with the equine susceptibility to scar formation after cataract surgery, adhesion formation after colic surgery, and exostosis after bone surgery. Calcarea fluorica can do a great deal to allay these sequelae.

Calcarea fluorica also has an affinity for blood vessels that are enlarged and pathologic (navicular disease) and those that have been damaged or caused by toxins (laminitis).

Overall, this is a powerful remedy for chronic bone disease in the horse. Osselets, ringbone, chronic navicular disease, chronic laminitis, and all other conditions in which excessive bone remodeling is occurring may be helped by this remedy. The stony hardness of this remedy can also be found in the skin, and the remedy may be effective in the treatment of horses with a tendency to display nodular necrobiosis.

Horses that respond to Calcarea fluorica are worse when they begin to move but seem to improve somewhat with continued motion. Weather changes and cold weather cause an increase in symptoms, whereas warmth and massage ameliorate the condition (Murphy, 1994).

Calcarea Phosphorica (Phosphate of Lime)

Calcarea phosphorica is another constitutional remedy of the horse, sharing some of the properties of both Calcarea carbonica and Calcarea phosphorus. The Calcarea phosphorica horse resembles the Calcarea carbonica horse with respect to size. The former tends to be much leaner and more restless than the latter (Shaw, 1994). This remedy picture often appears in the fast-growing quarter horse yearling on a diet of oats and alfalfa hay who shakes and knuckles on his forehand, in the throes of a continual case of epiphysitis.

The horse's lower jaw is lined with the bony enlargements of the dental roots, and the submaxillary glands are in a state of continual lymphadenopathy. This horse may suffer from a low-grade, chronic, suffocative cough and mild colic attacks after eating. The Calcarea phosphorica horse is worse when the weather is damp and cold and better in a warm, dry atmosphere.

Calendula (Marigold)

Any wound that requires healing may benefit from this remedy, and considering the amount of wound trauma horses inflict on themselves, this remedy is an essential part of a homeopathic equine emergency kit.

This remedy promotes granulation and rapid healing. The pure tincture can be applied locally or added to other healing salves (Macleod, 1992). A diluted form can be used as an intrauterine lavage in cases of endometritis, and ophthalmic lotions can be prepared for eye injuries and after surgery.

Carbo Vegetabilis (Vegetable Charcoal)

Carbo vegetabilis is a remedy that reflects the great weakness and debility following a chronic disease state (Day, 1993). This horse is often seen in the equine hospital, lifeless and lethargic, head lowered, with a distant gaze and a dropping lip. Respiration is rapid, pulse is weak, and limbs are cold. A low vital force creates an increased susceptibility to sepsis. This mental state is common after prolonged surgery, excessive administration of drugs, and blood loss. However, after the emergency has been dealt with and the patient discharged, this horse never seems to fully recover. In these cases, Carbo vegetabilis can aid in stimulating full recovery. This mental state of sluggishness may also be helpful in treating the mental state of otherwise healthy horses.

Carbo vegetabilis is a good colic remedy when intestinal gas is a predominant feature (Murphy, 1989). Anterior enteritis appearing shortly after eating, with the characteristic putrid reflux, often responds well to this remedy. The Carbo vegetabilis state is worse in dampness and when the animal is walking and better in the open air and when the horse is reclining (Murphy, 1989).

Causticum (Potassium Hydrate)

The Causticum state can be seen in the chronic and debilitating conditions found in the older horse (i.e., joint deformity, progressive loss of muscular strength, tendinous contracture, and progressive paralysis). This state, however, is not reserved for geriatric patients; it can appear in younger patients, especially when this condition is preceded by severe fright, worry, or grief (Murphy, 1994).

Many types of paralysis are susceptible, especially facial paralysis of the right side. A keynote symptom of Causticum is unsteady walking and a tendency to fall. Equine protozoal myelitis (EPM) patients and wobblers often display this symptom. Causticum might be applicable in these cases if there is also a history of severe stress. The Causticum state is worse in dry, cold winds; clear weather; and the morning and is better in damp, wet weather and warmth (Murphy, 1994).

Colocynthis (Squirting Cucumber)

Colocynthis is an excellent acute remedy for colic that appears suddenly, especially after eating or drinking. The mental state is one of intense irritability, anger, and impatience. The abdominal pain causes patients to drop suddenly, rolling, twisting, and contorting their bodies in the process (Macleod, 1992). This abdominal pain can also be caused by ovarian activity in mares, and Colocynthis is suitable for irritable fillies who tend to exhibit colic or tie-up during their heat cycles (Shaw, 1994).

The Colocynth state is made worse by anger, eating, and drinking. It also tends to worsen in the evening. It is improved by a recumbent position and application of hard pressure (Murphy, 1994).

Cuprum Metallicum (Copper)

Cuprum metallicum is one of two remedies (Magnesium phosphorus being the other) that should always be considered in treating horses with a tendency to develop myositis.

Spasmodic affections and cramps are the main expressions of the action of this remedy, particularly in the extremities and after overexertion and heat exhaustion (Morgan, 1988).

The mental state is one of rage or fear of approach with the horse preferring solitude. The condition is worse in cold air and with touch and better with perspiration (Murphy, 1989).

Euphrasia (Eyebright)

Euphrasia is the primary remedy to consider when treating horses with eye disorders. Conjunctivitis, corneal abrasions, and uveitis can be treated with this remedy both orally and topically (Macleod, 1992). Characteristically the eyes water profusely, especially in the sun.

Ferrum Phosphorus (Phosphate of Iron)

Ferrum phosphorus is an acute febrile remedy, useful for alleviating early inflammatory conditions that fail to respond to Aconitum. The anxious restlessness of Aconitum is replaced by a more anxious exhaustion (Weiner, 1996). A keynote symptom is bright hemorrhage from an orifice. Therefore ferrum phosphorus may be prescribed for bleeders with a nervous, sensitive, and anemic disposition.

Gelsemium (Yellow Jasmine)

Gelsemium is an effective remedy for both acute and chronic equine conditions. In acute flulike states, gelsemium is used in cases that develop slowly (Weiner, 1996). The horse is listless and may prefer to lie quietly in the stall. He usually displays no thirst, has a poor appetite, and appears weak and uncoordinated in his extremities.

Gelsemium is used for several chronic states. The mental state is one of emotional excitement and fear that can lead to physical disease. Gelsemium is often employed in horses with a tendency toward "stage fright." Often the manure of these horses softens and increases in frequency in the face of a frightening situation. Paralysis is a prominent physical symptom, and Gelsemium is useful in treating local paralysis, as well as the muscular incoordination of various spinal afflictions, especially when excessive trembling is also present. Entrapped epiglottis and recurrent laryngeal hemiplegia also may be susceptible to this remedy (Macleod, 1992).

The Gelsemium state is worse during damp weather and emotional excitement and is better when the horse is peaceful and in open air (Murphy, 1989).

Hepar Sulphuris Calcareum (Calcium Sulphide)

The most prominent feature of the Hepar state is one of suppuration. It is the first remedy recommended to abort abscess formation in the early stage of infection or to promote drainage of abscesses after their formation (Murphy, 1989). This remedy aids in the healing of hoof abscesses, injection reactions, septic sinusitis, guttural pouch empyema, pyometra, and strangles abscesses (Macleod, 1992).

Hepar sulphuris calcareum has a strong affinity for the respiratory tract. These horses may have either a dry, hoarse cough or a loose, rattling, choking cough, worse in dry, cold air and better in damp (Murphy, 1989). The mental state is one of oversensitivity. These horses cannot stand to be touched, are irritable on approach, and are usually quarrelsome with other horses (Shaw, 1994).

Hypericum (St. John's Wort)

Hypericum is considered the most important first aid remedy for puncture wounds, especially in regions rich in nerve endings such as the caudal pastern and hoof. Extreme nerve pain is a prominent symptom, with excessive sensitivity to the injured area. Painful sacral and coccygeal injuries also respond well to Hypericum, and its successful use for this condition can occur even years after the original injury (Morgan, 1988).

The Hypericum state is worse with motion and touch and better by being left alone (Murphy, 1989).

Lachesis (Surukuku Snake Poison)

The mental state of Lachesis represents a deceivingly silent yet surprisingly reactive individual (Sankaran, 1995). This horse is extremely jealous. He is also suspicious, with a careful and methodical approach to the outstretched hand. The snake suffocates and tightens, and this too can be seen in the mental state as an aversion to constrictive devices such as girths, cribbing collars, and blankets (Shaw, 1994).

The disease states susceptible to Lachesis mimic the symptoms inflicted by the venom of the deadly creature from which it is derived. Septicemia, purpura, and hemorrhagic cellulitis are all symptoms. Lachesis has a special affinity for the throat region (the Achilles' tendon of the snake) and the left side of the body (Murphy, 1994). Chronic, dry coughs, worse with the application of pressure to the throat, are often helped by this remedy.

The Lachesis horse is always worse in the spring. The disease state is often the result of suppressed discharges. When the discharge is relieved, the condition improves. Anhidrosis in this type of horse can be helped with this remedy (Day, 1993).

Ledum (Marsh Tea)

Ledum is commonly referred to as the "homeopathic tetanus" of the materia medica and has been said to allay this disease if given 3 times a day for 5 days after the injury (Murphy, 1989). Along with Hypericum, Ledum is used as a first aid treatment for the effects of any kind of puncture wound, including those inflicted by insects, animal bites, and veterinary injections (Macleod, 1992). The unique symptom of these wounds is that they are cold to the touch but can be relieved by applying cold.

Ledum is an excellent remedy for arthritic pain of the joints of the extremities, especially the hock (Day, 1993). In these cases the joints often chronically crack on movement. The joint pain of Ledum improves with cold application and worsens with warmth (Murphy, 1994).

Lycopodium (Club Moss)

Lycopodium is a constitutional remedy predominantly involving the gastrointestinal, renal, and hepatic systems (Murphy, 1994). This horse is kind and intelligent, although often lacking in self-confidence. His build is light, often on the thin side, with a somewhat dry hair coat.

His weakness lies in his digestive system. He easily goes off feed, his manure becomes dry and slimy, and he develops intestinal gas. Many cases of low-grade colic respond favorably to this remedy (Macleod, 1992).

Many respiratory symptoms fall under Lycopodium. This remedy should be considered in cases of neglected pneumonia (Murphy, 1994). A keynote symptom is the flaring of the nasal alae, independent of the respiratory rate. Mucous rales may be present, and expectoration may vary in color from gray to bloody.

Lycopodium has an affinity for the right side of the body, and most of its symptoms intensify between the hours of 4 and 8 PM and with heat.

Nux Vomica (Poison Nut)

Nux vomica is considered the great detoxification remedy of the homeopathic world. It is used to counteract the injurious effects of repeated medication, low-grade toxins, and an overtaxing lifestyle (Murphy, 1994). In humans, it is a remedy for type-A personality types. The stereotype is the corporate executive who works late nights and drinks too much coffee and too many martinis, with little regard for his health. The equine counterpart is often found on the racetrack. Repeated medication and a training schedule that is unnatural to his way of existence makes the racehorse a likely beneficiary of this remedy. The mental state of Nux vomica is one of irritability, anger, and hypersensitivity (Weiner, 1996). He is prone to biting and usually exhibits addictive behaviors involving food or cribbing.

Most cases considered for homeopathy often have a history of extensive allopathic medication. Therefore Nux vomica is a good remedy with which to begin many cases. Often it will help to distinguish the true disease state from that created by previous medication.

Because of his greedy eating habits, Nux vomica horses are prone to colic and laminitis. They are always worse in the morning and may show symptoms of colic only after the morning meal. In fact, Nux vomica is one of the best remedies to give to a horse with colic when the symptoms occur after eating (Macleod, 1992). These horses feel better when recumbent and are often found asleep in their stalls during the day.

Nux vomica is useful for both constipation and diarrhea, especially if symptoms appeared after some form of drugging or poisoning. This remedy is also used in treating certain horses with chronic obstructive pulmonary disease. The cough and dyspnea are worse in the morning or after eating.

Phosphorus (Phosphorus)

Because Phosphorus is one of the major constitutional remedies of the horse, it is frequently applied in an equine practice. The Phosphorus constitution in the horse is unmistakable. He is the bright, friendly chestnut whom everybody loves. Usually tall and slender, his facial features show a state of constant alertness, displaying an oversensitivity to external expressions. He may spook at a loud noise or on spotting a distant shadow, and he fears being alone. He will be the one calling for his departed stable mates. Despite his eccentricities, he loves everyone and quickly endears himself to those around him.

As youngsters, these colts are all legs. Often they will develop the associated growing pains of epiphysitis accompanying a fast growth rate. They are prone to respiratory infections, and Phosphorus is an excellent remedy for chronic hacking coughs, pneumonia, and epistaxis (Murphy, 1994). In fact, Phosphorus is a remedy for many types of bleeding, especially when the blood is bright red.

Diarrhea is often amenable to Phosphorus treatment. The manure painlessly and uncontrollably projects from the anus (Murphy, 1994). It has a watery consistency and often has a fetid odor.

The sensitive Phosphorus individual is worse during weather changes and often dreads thunderstorms. Symptoms, including fear, always increase in the evening. He improves with the calming strokes of his owner and with eating.

Pulsatilla (Windflower)

Pulsatilla is a predominantly female remedy and is useful for gentle mares with a tendency toward shyness. These individuals are in desperate need of support, whether from the herd or their owners. This horse is seldom aggressive. Rather than disobey, she will readily submit to the demands of her trainer, but her feelings are sometimes hurt in the process. Pulsatilla horses are almost always thirstless and are prone to colic, respiratory tract infections, endometritis, and irregular heat cycles. Even though they are susceptible to cold, they prefer to be outdoors and often feel better after they are turned out.

Her discharges are thick and yellow. If she has a respiratory tract infection, she always develops a nasal discharge. Pulsatilla is an excellent acute remedy for horses with influenza when a thick, yellow nasal discharge is also present. Her eyes are prone to conjunctivitis with the same thick, yellow characteristics, and if she develops endometritis, the same keynote symptom is present. The Pulsatilla filly often has an immature reproductive system. Pulsatilla may help stimulate estrus in these cases.

Rhus Toxicodendron (Poison Ivy)

Rhus toxicodendron *(Rhus tox)* is one of the most common homeopathic medicines used in the treatment of sprains (Morgan, 1988). However, in order for this remedy to be effective, the mental state and general symptoms, especially keynote symptoms, must agree (Morgan, 1988).

The mental state of *Rhus tox* can be illustrated by a person with a recent case of poison ivy. Extreme restlessness with continued change of position is a keynote symptom of this remedy. The more these patients move, the better they feel; thus the characteristic symptom is improvement with motion. A *Rhus tox* responsive injury is always worse during and after rest (Murphy, 1994). This is in contrast to the remedy Bryonia, which improves injuries that worsen with movement. Therefore horses who need *Rhus tox* may constantly change their stance. They may appear unwilling to leave their stalls in the morning, but they seem to improve with activity.

A peculiarity of this plant is that it becomes more toxic in the absence of sunlight and in damp weather (Murphy, 1994). Therefore the symptoms often worsen at night and on cold, wet, and cloudy days. Often an initial lameness can be traced back to a day when the horse was ridden in a wet environment.

Rhus tox markedly affects fibrous tissue (joints and tendons) as well as the skin. This remedy also has an affinity for the nerves and spinal cord, and it can be used to treat paretic-type patients with concomitant stiffness of the muscles and joints that improves with movement (e.g., some cases of Lyme disease).

Back pain as the result of overuse responds well to rhus tox, as well as the worn and torn fetlock joint or carpus that has degenerated from the constant trauma of racing. Skin diseases responsive to this remedy produce symptoms similar to those of poison ivy. Itching is intense, and the lesions may vary from urticaria to cellulitis or vesicle formation. In all cases the skin worsens when wet. Some cases of dermatitis with a pattern of eruption along sweat lines may improve with this remedy, as well as lesions that are aggravated when the horse is left in the rain.

Ruta Graveolens (Bitter Wort)

Ruta graveolens is one of the chief remedies for injured joints, tendons, bones, and especially bruised bones. The mental state of Ruta is one of intense and painful weariness. There is a tendency for these horses to develop deposits on the periosteum, tendons, and about the joints, and ruta is therefore useful for horses with large splints, thick tendons, and knobby ankles.

Ruta is not a remedy to consider at the onset of the injury, when more symptom-specific remedies are appropriate. It is effective after use of Arnica in joint and tendon injuries and after Symphytum use in bone injuries. Ruta is also useful after *Rhus tox* and is best employed following a reduction in swelling and pain or following any remedy that has failed to improve the condition within a reasonable time (Morgan, 1988). A keynote symptom of Ruta is that the injury is neither definitely worse by motion nor significantly improved by continued movement (Morgan, 1988).

Sepia (Cuttlefish Ink)

Sepia is a remedy affecting the female pelvis that has proved useful in the prevention of abortion, uterine prolapse, and retention of placenta in mares susceptible to this remedy. The mental state of Sepia is one of indifference. Often these mares give lackluster performances at the racetrack or in the hunter ring. This same apathy carries over to breeding and motherhood; these brood mares show little interest in their foals. This horse may also exhibit irritability. After foaling, she may chase away people and pasture mates but still hate to be left alone in the barn (Shaw, 1994).

Sepia can treat infertility, anestrus, endometritis, and abortion in these types of mares (Macleod, 1989). It can also cover gastrointestinal symptoms, especially gas and impaction colic when the internal rectum protrudes from the anus on straining.

As a rule, the Sepia mare is chilly and weak, worsening with rest and improving with strong activity.

Silicea or Silica (Flint)

The main action of Silicea is on the bone, especially of the extremities, where it is capable of causing caries and necrosis. This remedy, however, covers suppuration in any area of the body, especially after acute symptoms have passed and a chronic state has arisen (Macleod, 1989). Silicea ripens abscesses, heals chronic fistulas and slow-healing wounds, and promotes the absorption and remodeling of excessive scar tissue. It is an excellent remedy for hoof abscesses, pedal osteitis, vaccine abscesses, sequestrum, corneal ulcers, and exuberant granulation tissue (proud flesh).

The silicea constitution is one of nervousness and timidity. Silicea horses usually have poor self-confidence and may suffer illnesses resulting from anticipation (Shaw, 1994). Refined and delicate, these horses are constitutionally prone to worm infestation. Often the foal appears malnourished and wormy despite a good feed-management program. The belly is large and round, and the limbs are crooked. On the chilly side, this foal is prone to chronic respiratory tract infections, especially when exposed to cold weather.

Sulphur (sulphur)

Sulphur is a deep-acting constitutional remedy for individuals in whom chronic disease manifests as symptoms on the skin. A key to many of the conditions responsive to Sulphur is found in an irregular distribution of the circulation. This is manifested as hot and reddened skin, profuse sweating or patchy sweating, and inflammation with effusion (Murphy, 1994). A second prominent symptom of the Sulphur constitution is a feeling of emptiness, particularly in the stomach. Horses may exhibit a ravenous appetite or the desire to crib. Sulphur types are usually unable to assimilate food effectively; despite their strong appetite, they remain thin. Sulphur horses are always worse in the heat and after a bath. They dislike being enclosed in the barn and resist the repetition and boredom of a schooling ring, preferring the stimulation of an open trail ride. They are generally irritable, lazy, and obstinate, with a strong tendency to take long afternoon naps (Shaw, 1994).

The skin of a Sulphur horse is dry, itchy, and inflamed. Scratching temporarily relieves the itching. Sulphur also works well for skin disease that has been suppressed with previous administration of corticosteroids or disease that seems to improve almost completely before a relapse occurs.

The Sulphur constitution tends toward constipation, with hard and dry manure. Sometimes the tendency to constipation alternates with diarrhea.

Symphytum (Comfrey)

A common name for the plant comfrey is *knitbone,* and appropriately this remedy is considered the orthopedic "specific" of homeopathic medicine (Murphy, 1994). Symphytum is of great use in wounds penetrating to the perineum, and accelerates healing of both fresh fractures and nonunion fractures as well as injuries to the cartilage of the joints.

Symphytum is also useful in eye injuries, especially when blunt trauma is involved. Its action in this area exceeds that of Arnica (Murphy, 1994).

Thuja (Arbor Vitae)

Thuja is the primary remedy for the negative effects of vaccination in the horse. Vaccinosis appears on the skin and in the hooves and is always worse in wet weather;

therefore thuja is useful in treating many forms of skin and hoof disease that worsen in the rainy season. This is especially true when the symptoms appear to worsen a few weeks to a few months after vaccination.

The mental state of thuja is one of marked irritability and is especially prevalent among mares. Thuja horses tend to fight and kick at other horses. Primarily a left-sided remedy, Thuja is effective in many left-sided complaints. Thuja can cure left-sided nasal discharges occurring after vaccination (Pitcairn, 1992). It is also useful in left-sided cataracts.

Thuja is the primary remedy for the treatment of warts and other pedunculated masses on the skin such as sarcoids. In these cases Thuja is administered both internally and topically (Macleod, 1989). These pedunculated masses may appear elsewhere in addition to the skin; polyps in the throat may be also cured with this remedy (Murphy, 1989).

Vaccinosis

No discussion of equine homeopathy would be complete without the mention of vaccination. It has provoked intense controversy because of the harmful side effects many associate with use of these products. The incorporation of homeopathy into a conventional practice cannot be responsibly advocated without warning prescribers of the often counteractive effects of vaccine injection on homeopathic treatments.

All new insights begin with clear and objective observation. Homeopathy is not necessarily antagonistic to vaccination; however, since Hahnemann's time, practitioners have observed that vaccination produces certain undesirable side effects in addition to its well-known benefits. Injection of sizable quantities of foreign protein into the body can cause adverse effects (Miller, 1994). In addition, the artificial stimulation of specific immune reactions can jeopardize the body's immune balance and interfere with its protective functions. Experiencing natural disease early in life boosts the organism's overall immunity (Coulter, 1988). Vaccines "trick" the body into focusing on only one aspect of the many complex and integrated strategies normally available to the immune system. Diseases contracted naturally are ordinarily filtered through a series of immune defenses. However, when the vaccine is injected and absorbed directly into the blood and lymphatic systems, it gains access to all the major tissues and organs of the body without the body's normal advantage of a total immune response. In other words, the body must learn to be ill, and the immune system benefits from a certain amount of stress caused by disease at a young age. Some have speculated that lowered physical defenses created by early vaccination may be responsible for a new breed of autoimmune diseases (Miller, 1994).

Vaccinosis therefore refers to the indirect symptoms created in those individuals vaccinated in the face of a weakened or stressed immune system. Homeopaths have observed that symptoms such as dermatitis, arthritis, and various autoimmune diseases may be the result (Day, 1993; Pitcairn, 1992).

The benefits of vaccination cannot be completely dismissed until these suspected side effects have been thoroughly researched and reliable alternatives (i.e., nosodes) adequately documented. However, strategies to limit hazards might be included in a vaccination protocol. These should include restricting the use of vaccinations to life-threatening diseases such as encephalitis and exploring the feasibility of routinely measuring antibody titers for these diseases (instead of automatic vaccine schedules).

If the decision is made to vaccinate, several homeopathic procedures can minimize the ill effects of the vaccine. Hypericum can be administered in medium potency before the injection, thus minimizing damage to the central nervous system. The day after injection, Ledum can be administered to reduce the effects of a puncturelike wound. Thuja is then given for 1 week to avert any future ill effects.

Conclusion

Modern medicine dismisses homeopathy as an archaic doctrine. Today's scientists adhere to a model that treats the patient as fragmented. Despite the development of spectacular drugs and techniques, evidence suggests that horses are not healthier. Equine protozoal myelitis, for example, has reached epidemic proportions and certainly suggests a disease founded in immunodeficiency. Still, veterinarians continue to search for the wonder drug that will rid their patients of the "evil germ." Louis Pasteur claimed initially that all disease was caused by external microbes, but later conceded that the internal environment was the key (Weiner, 1996). Unfortunately, his earlier ideas endured.

Many physicians do not understand the way that a substance diluted hundreds of times can exert an effect on a living organism. Recently the field of ultramolecular medicine has provided insights into the way this could happen (Bellavite and others, 1996). All substances in nature have a unique energy field, a magnetic blueprint that maintains its identity in the absence of that substance in a material sense. Homeopathy, as currently practiced, may be only a crude precursor to what we will ultimately discover is the best method for maintaining health. Perhaps someday we will perfect another way of imparting the energetic pattern of a substance to a neutral medium. Such speculation can be validated only with the passage of time.

Thus the advocates of modern medicine continue to argue that homeopathy is unscientific. However, as the mysteries of the universe continue to unfold, these skeptics may discover that this field of healing is more consistent with scientific theory than any other form of medicine—and more important, more humane.

References

Bascands JL and others: Pretreatment with low doses of cadmium protects rat mesangial cells against the direct toxic effect of cadmium, JOMHI 3:9, 1990.

Bastide M: Immunological examples on ultra high dilution research. In *Ultra high dilution*, Dordrecht, Germany, 1994, Kluwer Academic Publishers.

Bastide M and others: Immunomodulatory activity of very low doses of thymulin in mice, *Int J Immunotherapy* 3:191, 1987.

Bastide P, Aubin B, Baronnet S: Etude pharmacologique d'une préparation d'apis mel vis-à-vis de l'érytheme aux rayons U.V. chez le cobayes albinos, *Ann Hom Fr* 17(3):289, 1975.

Bellavite P and others: *Homeopathy: a frontier in medical science*, Berkeley, Calif, 1996, North Atlantic Books.

Bentwich Z: Specific immune response to high dilutions of KLH; transfer of immunological information. In *Omeomed 92*, Bologna, Italy, 1993, Editrice Compositori, p 9.

Bildet J and others: Demonstrating the effects of Apis and apium dilutions on erythma induced by U.V. radiation on guinea pigs, *Berlin J Res Homeopathy* 1:28, 1990.

Bildet J and others: Etude de l'action de différentes dilutions de phosporous sur l'hépatite toxique du rat, *Ann Hom Fr* 17(4):425, 1975.

Bildet J and others: Etude au microscope électronique de l'action de dilutions de phoshorus 15c sur l'hépatite toxique du rat, *Homeopathie Francaise* 72:175, 1984.

Both G: Zur prophylaxe and therapie des metritis-mastitis-agalactie komlexes des schweines mit biologischen arzeneimitteln, *Biologische Tiermedizin* 4:39, 1987.

Cazin JC and others: A study of the effect of decimal and centisimal dilutions of Arsenic on the retention and mobilisation of arsenic in the rat, *Human Toxicol* 6:315, 1987.

Coulter H: *Guida alla Medicina Omeopatica*, Milan, 1976, EDIUM Editrice.

Coulter C: *Portraits of homeopathic medicines*, vol 2, Berkeley, Calif, 1988, North Atlantic Books.

Davenas E and others: Effect on mouse peritoneal macrophages of oral administration of very high dilutions of silica, *Eur J Pharmacol* 135:313, 1987.

Day C: Advanced homeopathy seminar, Minneapolis, 1993, IVAS Congress.

Endler PC and others: The effect of highly diluted agitated thyroxine on the climbing activity of frogs, *Vet Hum Toxicol* 36:56, 1994.

Guilleman and others: Pharmacologie de l'infinitésimal application aux dilutions homeopathiques, *Homeopathie* 4:35, 1987.

Hahnemann C: *Organon of medicine* (edited from the fifth and sixth editions), Haifa, 1994. Homeopress.

Hahnemann C: Essay on a new principle for ascertaining the curative powers of drugs, and some examinations of the previous principles, *Hufland's Journal* 2:391, 1796.

Harish G, Kretschmer M: Smallest zinc quantities affect the histamine release from peritoneal mast cells, 1988.

Lapp C and others: Mobilization de l'arsenic fixe chez le cobaye sous l'influence des doses infinitésimales d'arséniate, *Therapie* 10:625, 1955.

Macleod G: *A veterinary materia medica and clinical repertory*, Saffron Waldon, Great Britain, 1992, CW Daniel.

Miller N: *Vaccines: are they really safe and effective?* New York, 1994, New Atlantean Press.

Morgan L: *Homeopathic treatment of sport injuries*, Rochester, Vermont, 1988, Healing Arts Press.

Murphy R: *Lotus materia medica*, Pagosa Springs, Colo, 1994, Lotus Star Academy.

Pitcairn R: Course notes in Certification Course for Veterinary Homeopathy, Eugene, Ore, 1992.

Poitevin B and others: In vitro immunological degranulation of human basophils is modulated by lung histamine and apis mellifica, *Br J Clin Pharmacol* 25:439, 1988.

Sankaran R: *The spirit of homeopathy*, Santa Cruz, 1995, Homeopathic Medical Publishers.

Santini R and others: Incidence d'un traitement homéopathique par cuprum 4 C sur le transit intestinal de la souris: étude preliminaire, *CR Soc Biol* 184:55, 1990.

Shaw S: *Homeopathy for horses*, Nelson, British Columbia, 1994, Fie Ships Literary Co.

Sukul NC and others: Hypothalmic neuronal responses of rats to homeopathic drugs. In *Omeomed 92*, Bologna, Italy, 1993, Editrice Compositori, p 1.

Ullman D: *Discovering homeopathy: medicine for the 21st century*, Berkeley, Calif, 1991, North Atlantic Books.

Vithoulkas G: *The science of homeopathy*, New York, 1990, Grove Press Inc.

Weiner M: *The complete book of homeopathy*, Berkeley, Calif, 1996, Avery Publishing Group.

Weisman Z and others: *Immunomodulation of specific immune response to KLH by high dilution of antigen*, Procedures of the 5th GIRI Meeting, Paris, 1991, (Abstract 19).

Williamson AV and others: A study using Sepia 200c given prophylactically postpartum to prevent anoestrus problems in the dairy cow, *Br Hom J* 80:149, 1991.

Wurmser L and others: Mobilisation de l'arsenic fixe chez le cobaye, sous l'action de doses infinitésimales d'arséniate de sodium, *Therapie* 10:625, 1955.

Yubicier BJ: Effects of embrionic bursectomy and in ovo administration of highly diluted bursin on adrenocorticotropic and immune responses in chickens, *Int J Immunother* 9:169, 1993.

Suggested Materia Medicas and Repertories on Homeopathy

Allen HC: *Keynotes and characteristics with comparisons of some of the leading remedies of the materia medica*, ed 6, New Delhi, 1977, Jain Publishing.

Boericke W: *Pocket manuel of homeopathic materia medica*, ed 9, New York, 1927, Boericke & Runyon.

Kent JT: *Lectures on homeopathic materia medica*, New Delhi, 1972, Jain Publishing.

Kent JT: *Repertory of homeopathic materia medica*, New Delhi, Jain Publishing.

Macleod G: *A veterinary materia medica and clinical repertory*, Saffron Waldon, Great Britain, 1992, CW Daniel Co.

Murphy R: *N.D. homeopathic materia medica*, Pagosa Springs, Colo, 1994, Lotus Star Academy.

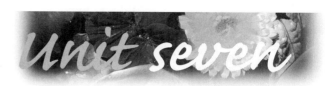

Miscellaneous Therapies

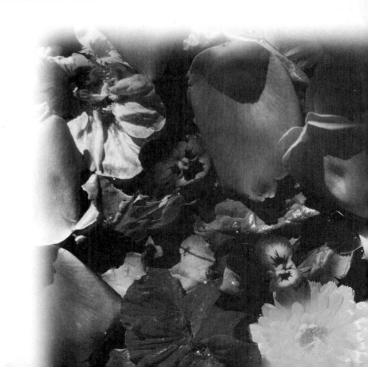

Chapter 29

Environmental Medicine for Veterinary Practitioners

SHERRY A. ROGERS

Introduction and Historical Perspective

Environmental medicine evaluates and identifies potential environmental exposures that may lead to numerous disease syndromes. Therapeutic approaches are aimed at eliminating the cause and resolving symptoms through nutritional support and attention to the total load of body stressors. The goal is to reverse pathology and resolve symptoms without further medications.

According to some sources, the field of environmental medicine began in 1951, when Dr. Theron Randolph of Chicago realized that everyday household chemicals could cause symptoms that eluded diagnosis or treatment. Others say that it had a quiet inception over the last two decades as practitioners combined knowledge about xenobiotic detoxification (foreign chemical metabolism), a multitude of immunologic and nonimmunologic hyperreactive states, and nutritional biochemistry to heal conditions that hitherto had been considered incurable. It could be argued that Dr. Albert Rowe's appreciation in the 1970s that food sensitivities could masquerade as nearly any symptom heralded the era of environmental medicine. However, thousands of years earlier, Hippocrates warned, "Let food be thy medicine and medicine be thy food."

Foods, chemicals, and dust, mold, pollen and dander sensitivities, as well as nutrient deficiencies, are now known to have a bearing on triggering symptoms. For example, in the 1970s, when hundreds of thousands of people retrofitted their homes with urea foam formaldehyde insulation, physicians specializing in environmental medicine discovered that formaldehyde can cause varied insidious symptoms. These cases enhanced knowledge of environmental medicine. One of the facts that emerged was that often the entire household (including pets) was affected by this formaldehyde poisoning, but no two patients had the same symptoms. Biochemical individuality was one of the paradigm shifts that countered the conventional assumption that everyone reacting to one chemical would have the same symptoms. Biochemical individuality became one of the many new principles to be learned and has been proven over and over again.

When the Environmental Protection Agency (EPA) installed 28,000 square feet of carpeting in one of their Washington mall offices in 1988, a large number of diverse health complaints by employees surfaced. Out of 2000 workers, 126 developed symptoms, and no two people had the exact same symptoms.

Later, when one of the diagnostic and therapeutic techniques for chemical, food, and inhalant sensitivities was published in the National Institutes of Health medical journal, *Environmental Health Perspectives*, skeptics insisted that these patients were malingerers. Because animals are affected by sensitivities to pollens, dusts, foods, chemicals, and molds, the next study used horses suffering from chronic obstructive pulmonary disease (COPD) in place of humans with asthma; obviously, the equine subjects could not be accused of malingering and the results of both studies were consistent (Rogers, 1988).

The veterinary field is beginning to recognize the importance of environmental medicine concepts. Dye and Costa (1995) recently described typical indoor air pollutants and published recommendations to reduce exposures for pets.

What Is Environmental Medicine?

Environmental medicine can be understood as a philosophy or a causal approach to medical problems that differs considerably from the current approach. In conventional medicine a history, physical examination, and laboratory tests are generally performed to determine a diagnostic label. Once that label is attained, practice guidelines usually include a variety of medications or surgery. Aside from the use of antibiotics for infections, cure is rarely established, and patients often face a lifetime of treatments to manage or suppress symptoms of chronic diseases such as arthritis, colitis, and allergies. Very seldom is medication temporary; on the contrary, chemical treatment becomes chronic. Cure is so rare that to even suggest that it is possible in many conditions borders on quackery. Medicine is practiced as though arthritis were a deficiency of antiinflammatory drugs.

In contrast, in an environmental medicine workup the diagnostic work begins where the workup in conventional medicine ends. After a history, physical examination, and pertinent laboratory tests and x-rays are done, the cause of the symptoms is pursued. Clues gathered by the preliminary workup may suggest whether hidden environmental food, chemical, or mold sensitivities might be relevant, for example. A biochemical workup to determine deficiencies of vitamins, minerals, essential fatty acids, amino acids, and hormones may be in order, or the practitioner may investigate intestinal triggers such as intestinal dysbiosis or intestinal hyperpermeability.

Not all these parameters need to be considered, because properly trained physicians become proficient in prioritizing the possibilities. Often, causes can be found and corrected for syndromes that were thought incurable or chronic. The goal is to render the patient free of both symptoms and medications. Research supports the concepts that coronary artery plaque is reversible, metastatic end-stage cancer may regress, and rheumatoid arthritis is reversible. To the uninitiated, these ideas sound preposterous, but once the actual mechanism of disease is understood, the mystery of cure vanishes.

Definitions

Certain terms related to environmental medicine must be defined before proceeding. A *xenobiotic* is a foreign chemical, something that does not belong in the body, at least in amounts that can cause toxicity (for instance, the body makes small amounts of formaldehyde). *Detoxification* is the process the body uses to reduce a foreign chemical to a form that the body can more easily depurate or excrete. The detoxification system is extremely elaborate and complicated, consisting of scores of enzymes and processes. Usually only a few are used on any one xenobiotic, however. This is fortunate in view of the large range of chemicals that the body detoxifies daily.

Enzymatic detoxification systems probably evolved originally to aid in eliminating dietary compounds. Xenobiotic detoxification enzymes probably developed phylogenetically as needed (Netter, 1994).

The enzymatic detoxification systems consist of the phase I (oxidative) and phase II (conjugative) systems.

Oxidative mechanisms involve activity of the microsomal mixed function oxidase system; cytochrome P-450 is the hemoprotein catalyst central to this system. Although P-450 is a well-conserved protein, over 150 different genes have been described. In humans, genetic variation in xenobiotic handling has been noted.

Several types of conjugative reactions exist. Glucuronidation, sulfation, and acetylation are the most thoroughly studied. Interestingly, glucuronidation may lead to active products, as well as inactivation (Netter, 1994).

Research difficulties are caused by many factors. For one, many pathways can be used by the body to metabolize specific chemicals. If one pathway is used one day, the chemical may produce no symptoms. However, on another day, when that pathway is overloaded from other exposures and its enzymes are being used elsewhere, the chemical can be metabolized through a different pathway, creating different metabolites and different symptoms. This difference partially accounts for the varying symptoms that have made many doubt the credibility of patients. Sometimes the body is unable to metabolize the chemical at all, whereupon the chemical is stored in lipids only to equilibrate later by leaking back into the bloodstream after the overload exposure has ended. This, likewise, creates symptoms that can be confusing without an understanding of environmental medicine. Sometimes, the normal oxidation pathway, which is often the first step in detoxification, creates a more toxic compound than the original parent compound. This heightened toxicity occurs with many types of pesticides (Klaasen, 1986).

The *total load* refers to the total body burden of stressors that lead to the package called disease. For example, removing foods implicated in the development of arthritis does not, as a singular treatment, resolve the intestinal hyperpermeability leading to autoantibody production or correct a magnesium deficiency contributing to muscle spasm.

For example, a human patient may complain of bloody diarrhea. Once the label of ulcerative colitis is made through colonoscopy, intestinal x-rays, and blood tests, various medications are prescribed to suppress the symptoms, beginning with anticholinergics and progressing to sulfa derivatives, prednisone, and sometimes chemotherapeutic drugs. These drugs are designed not to cure the problems but to mask them. Masking drugs are characterized by the recurrence of symptoms when the substances are withdrawn. If drugs fail to control the bleeding, surgical resection of a portion of the gut may be in order. Rarely are complete diagnostic diets a part of the workup. In fact, most patients are told that diet has no bearing on their symptoms—in spite of the scores of papers that show hidden food sensitivities as a sole or contributing cause.

An Environmental Medicine Scenario

In conventional medicine, drugs and surgery are most commonly prescribed for arthritis, regardless of the many papers on the benefits of finding the causes of the arthritis (Felder, de Blecourt, Wuthrich, 1987; Panush and others, 1983). In fact, the major drugs used (nonsteroidal antiinflammatory dugs [NSAIDs] and steroids) actually promote and hasten the underlying pathology (Doube, Collins, 1988; Rogers, 1996b). For example, NSAIDs deplete xenobiotic detoxification nutrients, including magnesium, which can be a cause of muscle spasm associated with arthritis. In human medicine the average American diet provides only 40% of the magnesium needed in a day, yet 90% of doctors fail to check for a magnesium deficiency, even when patients are hospitalized from its effects. When underlying deficiencies are not corrected, a spreading phenomenon emerges wherein, for example, the undiagnosed magnesium deficiency that is contributing to the arthritis pain may cause hypertension, depression, high cholesterol, migraines, asthma, and over 40 different symptoms. Eventually, when the undiagnosed magnesium deficiency worsens, atrial fibrillation and sudden cardiac arrest may result because the original cause was never recognized or treated appropriately.

Worse, NSAIDs can cause intestinal hyperpermeability. This "leaky-gut syndrome" can foster the development of food allergies, autoimmune diseases, impaired nutrient absorption, and chemical sensitivity symptoms, all of which can then masquerade as nearly any symptom. Intestinal hyperpermeability may begin as irritable bowel syndrome or colitis, and the patient is referred to the gastroenterologist for a battery of tests and drugs. As more specialists are consulted and more medications are recommended, the true cause of the disease remains hidden. Every added medication can hasten the depletion of detoxification nutrients.

As the nutrient chemistry becomes progressively more unbalanced, the ability to properly metabolize cholesterol may become jeopardized; however, the physician usually prescribes cholesterol-lowering drugs. 3-hydroxy-3-methyl-glutamyl (HMG) coenzyme A (CoA)-blocking drug, lowers the cholesterol so well that a relative cholesterol deficiency may develop. Cholesterol is necessary for the synthesis of sex hormones such as testosterone, the adrenal stress hormones such as dehydroepiandrosterone (DHEA), and the brain membranes and neurotransmitters. Soon the patient develops poor libido, poor energy, and poor memory, none of which concerns the physician because they do not constitute a recognized disease or syndrome. However, the scientific literature documents a heightened death rate for suicide and accidents resulting from the deficiency of cholesterol in brain and hormone synthesis pathways. Recent studies suggest that patients taking cholesterol-lowering drugs have a higher rate of cancer (Newman, Hulley, 1996).

In addition, numerous "undiagnosable" and "untreatable" arthritic, musculoskeletal, metabolic, renal, hepatic, and malignant diseases occur because of the ingestion of hydrogenated polyunsaturated oils containing trans-fatty acids (Enig, 1995). Many people and animals have a total package of food, chemical (e.g., pesticide, hydrocarbon), and inhalant (e.g., pollen, dust, mold, danders) overloads as their triggers in addition to the biochemical defects.

Still, when patients continue to worsen, practitioners seldom consider environmental and biochemical causes. Instead, they recommend a change in drugs and eventually surgery. However, very common causes of arthritis, which in many cases can be completely eliminated without drugs or surgery, are unsuspected food, chemical, and mold sensitivities, as well as undiagnosed nutrient deficiencies. Environmental medicine looks for the environmental triggers, nutritional deficiencies, and metabolic or biochemical defects causing the symptoms so that they can be eliminated, not controlled. Avoiding the use of drugs for an indeterminant amount of time can result in untold health and economic benefits.

Environmental Medicine: A Paradigm Shift

A paradigm is a model, a way of conceptualizing something. As knowledge grows, paradigms often lose applicability and, until corrected, actually prevent further growth of knowledge. Unfortunately, paradigms, having been in use for so long, are slow to die. Many examples of paradigm shift exist in the history of science.

The integration of the current medical paradigm into the era of molecular and environmental medicine is essential. Invisible chemicals, foods, molds, inhalants, electromagnetic fields, and nutrient deficiencies are just a few causes of ubiquitous symptoms.

In one study, bakers and pastry chefs with wheat allergies were treated with 20 months of immunotherapy to wheat; they not only achieved subjective symptom improvement but also experienced a significant decrease in hyperresponsiveness to methacholine, skin sensitivity, and specific IgE (Armentia, 1990). However, the American Academy of Allergy still maintains that one cannot hyposensitize with food antigens. Vitamin C significantly increased the FEV_1 (forced expiratory volume over 1 second) on the pulmonary function of allergic patients 1 hour after treatment (Bucca, 1990). In spite of improved lung function, vitamin C supplementation is still not recommended by conventional allergists.

Some professionals still believe that everyday chemicals cannot cause disease states such as lupus. Hydrazine, for example, may cause systemic lupus erythematosus (SLE)-like symptoms. Approximately 52% of the population are genetically "slow acetylators" (i.e., they do not metabolize certain chemicals as well as the other 48%) and are susceptible to induction of lupus with the appropriate stimulus and total load (Reidenberg and others, 1983).

Genetic variations are one of the less well-understood components of environmental illness (EI); individual variability in the response to environmental stressors contributes to the slow accumulation of knowledge about this field. For example, the craving for alcohol is genetically determined and not a matter of willpower (Blum and others, 1990). Tools are available to diagnose and treat these individual underlying causes. Resistance is not due to a lack of data.

Environmental medicine can identify environmental triggers, metabolic defects, and biochemical deficiencies, thus resolving often untreatable symptoms. The purpose of this chapter is to introduce veterinarians to the comprehensive approach of environmental medicine and offer resources for further information.

Total Load

Tools are now available to identify the environmental and nutritional triggers for most diseases. If the principles of environmental medicine are used early, prevention is even more cost effective. Any disease that has no known cause and no known cure, such as scleroderma, can serve as an example. When the environmental possibilities are considered, it becomes clear that everything has a cause.

To find these sometimes obscure causes, the total burden of stressors must be considered to sufficiently unload the body and allow it to heal. If someone has a motorcycle accident and sustains lacerations filled with road dirt, simple suturing is not adequate treatment. The total load is decreased as much as possible to allow optimal healing. The area may be anesthetized, decontaminated, and radiographed for fractures; the patient may be boosted for tetanus; and an antibiotic may be prescribed.

Likewise, when one deals with multiple symptoms and tries to identify a cause, a more precise history is needed. Specialized allergen testing, preferably with the fine-tuned titration method, may be appropriate. Because food sensitivity can mimic nearly any symptom as well, various dietary elements should be evaluated. Food testing and injections are used only if necessary.

Nutrient deficiencies should be evaluated because they also can mimic any symptom. Intestinal dysbiosis may be the underlying cause for many systemic and organ-specific symptoms, from Crohn's disease to rheumatoid arthritis (Doube, Collins, 1988; Jenkins and others, 1987; Pearson and others, 1982; Rogers,1996b). Hormone imbalances and general standard medical conditions should be ruled out.

Finally, a myriad of chemical sensitivities can mimic any symptom. Pesticides are among the most surreptitious, yet ubiquitous, of these chemicals. Identifying and avoiding these or taking measures to improve their detoxification can reduce symptoms.

Likewise, undetected pesticide exposures can rapidly deplete cellular mechanisms, and "enzyme induction can increase the overall rate of biotransformation of a chemical, which can in turn lead to an excess production of reactive intermediates" (Rea, 1992). These doses need not be large for detoxification pathways to be compromised.

Nontoxic doses of a xenobiotic can now result in cellular injury. In other words, if possible chemical culprits are not sought, a variety of metabolic defects can worsen with "undiagnosable" and "untreatable" symptoms (Sipes, Gandolfi, 1986).

Many conditions have no known cause or cure. Chemical exposures trigger the conditions (Black, Welsh, 1988). Nutritional deficiencies may determine the vulnerability. One consideration for total load is the integrity of the intestinal tract because it is responsible for the absorption and assimilation of nutrient intake.

Intestinal Dysbiosis and Intestinal Hyperpermeability

Diet, antibiotics, hormones, and other factors can significantly alter the intestinal flora. The flora is important in determining the integrity of the intestinal barrier. For example, if organisms (even those that are not normally pathogenic) are present in abnormal amounts, they can inflame the intestinal lining. Likewise, undetected food allergies can also cause inflammation of the intestinal lining. Food antigens can leak across a hyperpermeable gut and trigger food allergy, another vicious cycle of disease that can be interrupted only by an environmental medicine approach (Buist, 1983; Jackson and others, 1981; Reinhardt, 1984; Walker, 1988).

When this lining is inflamed, several events occur. Large food particles that normally do not cross the intestinal barrier are allowed through interstitial spaces into the bloodstream (Reinhardt, 1984). When the body is exposed to these foreign antigenic substances, it mounts a defensive attack and antibodies are formed. New food allergies can arise, and autoimmune antibodies may be formed, which leads to autoimmune diseases. If similar antigenic sites exist on the thyroid gland, in joint spaces, or in the lung, for example, an autoimmune episode can occur whenever a particular antigen is ingested.

Arthritis may represent a common cycle of this type. It can become initiated by food allergens, NSAIDs, or dysbiosis causing the leakage of food allergens (Doube, Collins, 1988; Jenkins and others, 1987; Strobel, 1991; Wilcox and others, 1994). The conventional treatment for arthritis is the very drug category that is capable of initiating it. The sick necessarily get sicker as the gut becomes more permeable and other pathogenic mechanisms progress. Intestinal hyperpermeability has been associated with other diseases as well. It matters little what the end target organ is (Pearson and others, 1982).

Likewise, a major part of the detoxification pathway of the body lies in the lining of the intestine. This includes phase I pathways of the cytochrome P-450 system and conjugates of phase II. Furthermore, some of the intestinal flora play a role in xenobiotic detoxification. When the surface of the intestinal lining becomes inflamed, a major part of the detoxification capability is lost and chemical sensitivity, arthritis, autoimmune diseases, and other conditions can develop.

The third major problem caused by intestinal inflammation is that the carrier proteins, which normally bind minerals and carry them into the bloodstream, can be lost or damaged. Therefore nutrient deficiencies occur, which then can lead to other symptoms and diseases.

Furthermore, a hyperpermeable gut can allow the absorption of toxins that can cause fatigue and body achiness, neurologic disturbances (Iwata and others, 1976), and other symptoms. Therefore practitioners should test for intestinal dysbiosis and abnormal amounts of organisms, whether they are considered pathogenic or not, such as the yeast *Candida albicans.* A leaky or hyperpermeable gut signifies damage to the intestinal mucosa, and the repercussions frequently cause illness by the mechanisms previously explained.

Furthermore, having the proper probiotics (e.g., species of *Lactobacillus acidophilus*) in the intestine has many advantageous effects that help improve health (Mott and others, 1973; Shahini, Friend, 1973). For example, bifidobacteria enhance immunity, lower cholesterol, suppress tumors, improve hepatic function, and decrease free phenols (Mitsuoka, 1990).

The intestine contains hundreds of bacteria and fungi for many reasons. Some bacteria help nourish the intestinal lining, and some help manufacture vitamins such as K and B_{12}, but most help break down food into smaller molecular pieces so that it is easily absorbed.

Oral antibiotics do not kill all intestinal organisms. Some organisms are resistant (e.g., *C. difficile, Helicobactor pylori, C. albicans*), so when some of their competition is eliminated, they grow unencumbered and multiply rapidly (Seelig, 1966). These organisms can consequently irritate the intestine, impair immunity, and by many mechanisms lead to many diagnostic disease labels, including cancer.[*]

C. albicans is an opportunistic fungus or yeast that may be a significant factor in human medicine, and anecdotal evidence suggests animals may be susceptible as well. It has been observed microscopically to cross into the bloodstream from the gut (Deitch and others, 1991), it inhibits leukocyte proliferation (Nelson and others, 1984; Witkin, Yu, Ledger, 1983; Witkin, 1985), and it causes chronic urticaria (James, Warrin, 1971) and allergies (Kerdelko, 1971; Liebeskind 1962). Likewise, overgrowth of bacteria such as *H. pylori (Campylobacter pylori)* can cause duodenal and gastric ulcers and gastric cancer in humans.[†] Clearly

the health of the gut must be considered when a diagnostic dilemma surfaces.

Sometimes the overgrowth is of a certain species of mold (or fungi or yeasts) that is particularly resistant to antibiotic therapy. When this happens (as in a host that is especially compromised by undetected nutrient deficiencies), the molds are also capable of producing toxins that cause hyperpermeability of the gut, leading to leaky-gut syndrome and food allergies, autoimmune antibodies, and more.

Also, the host (patient) may become sick from the toxins produced by molds. They may damage the immune system and other systems in a myriad of ways and mimic many diseases. In fact, some mycotoxins (toxins produced by molds, such as aflatoxins) are known to be strong carcinogens, and only extremely small amounts are needed to initiate cell transformation and possible cancer.

Stool cultures can identify these yeasts, intestinal hyperpermeability can be tested, diets that foster the health of the gastrointestinal tract can be implemented, and products can be prescribed to decrease the growth of these abnormal amounts of normally harmless molds and other intestinal dysbiotic organisms.

Again, if intestinal dysbiosis occurs or abnormal amounts of organisms are present, whether they are normally considered pathogenic does not matter, because bacteria, yeasts, protozoa, and other organisms usually considered commensal may become more pathogenic with increasing host susceptibility. Nutrient status should always be considered for recalcitrant infections. For example, women with recurrent yeast vaginitis, exhibited significantly lower levels of beta-carotene compared with disease-free women in a control group (Mikhail and others, 1994). It stands to reason that an additional factor (or several factors) must be present for the enhanced vulnerability to occur (Mikhail and others, 1994).

Not surprisingly, the health of the rest of the family can offer clues about the symptoms of the household pet. Whether the patient is human or animal, advanced diagnostic and therapeutic approaches now exist to treat environmentally induced disease.

For veterinarians interested in learning more about this approach to medical problems, recommended reading can be found in the resources section at the end of this chapter. Because the guiding principles are similar and assessing nutrient levels in animals is costly, veterinarians should consider reading human medical literature and applying it to their animal patients.

Nutrition

Nutritional Deficiencies Are Common

Numerous factors contribute to nutrient deficiencies. For example, every drug causes a loss of nutrients in the work of detoxification (Brown, 1995). Food processing is

---

[*]Fedotin (1993); Forbes and others (1994); Gumkowski and others (1987); James, Warrin (1971); Liebeskind (1962); Nelson and others (1984); Rogers (1996b); Suzuki and others (1993); Tamura and others (1993); Ward and others (1989).

[†]Boren and others (1993); Fedotin (1993); Forbes and others (1994); Parsonnet (1993); Rex (1994); Suzuki and others (1993); Tamura and others (1993).

changing the biochemistry of both humans and animals. Schroeder, Nason, and Tipton (1969) have shown that processing brown rice to bleached white rice causes the loss of many minerals, some by as much as 80%. Chief among the deleterious food-processing effects have been the introduction and widespread use of hydrogenated oils (Enig, 1995). These substances are capable of causing widespread physiologic disturbances that initiate common degenerative diseases in animals and humans.

For example, the hydrogeneration of oils may expose them to temperatures in excess of 400° F, which causes the molecule to twist from the natural *cis* isomer to the *trans* isomer. When this abnormal *trans* isomer is incorporated in cell membranes, it acts like a broken key, inhibiting the incorporation of beneficial constituents and inhibiting normal chemistry functions. Because this chemistry is pivotal to all body functions, nearly every disease from arteriosclerosis to cancer can be produced by substituting trans-fatty acids in the diets (Enig, 1995; van Tol and others, 1995). Correcting essential fatty acid deficiencies may correct many dermatologic, psychologic, and metabolic diseases, most notably seborrhea, psoriasis, learning disabilities, cardiac disease, chemical sensitivities, and more (Ganzales, 1995).

Essential fatty acids not only control the inflammatory response but also have the potential to influence whether the body develops allergies, arthritis, autoimmune diseases, chemical sensitivity, cancer, or arteriosclerosis. Essential fatty acids are major constituents in the cell membrane, which houses the cellular ion pumps, hormone receptors, and antibody receptors; secretes enzymes; and protects the nuclear membrane and cell organelles.

Studies from the *New England Journal of Medicine* (Mensink, Katan, 1990) show that ingested hydrogenated oils (the main oils in processed foods such as fried foods, breads, eggs substitutes, salad dressings, margarines, and commercial pet and livestock foods) actually displace the preferred essential fatty acids (e.g., eicosapentaenoic acid) and accelerate the chemistry that fosters arthritis, arteriosclerosis, hypercholesterolemia (van Tol and others, 1995), unexplained renal and hepatic dieases (which are escalating), brain and retinal disease (Neuringer, Connor, 1986), chronic fatigue (Gray and others, 1994), schizophrenia and other psychoses (Dohan, 1966; Rudin, 1981), and other disorders, including cancer (Enig, 1995; Rose and others, 1995). Many pet foods are baked in ovens with temperatures in excess of 400° F, which can lead to the formation of trans-fatty acids. More animals ingest these acids because their owners are also eating more processed "convenience" foods. Even wild birds and other animals suffer as humans feed them pretzels, white bread, corn chips, and other fast foods containing hydrogenated oils.

Unfortunately, hydrogenated oils are replacing the membrane lipids of animals and humans, ushering in an era of more undiagnosable or untreatable diseases, all because we choose to mask symptoms instead of finding and fixing the biochemical defects, nutritional deficiencies, and environmental triggers (Enig, 1995).

This brief scenario illustrates the way the ecology of humans and animals slowly changes, predisposing us to increased illness and making treatment more difficult. Changes in the essential fatty acids and the resultant changes in the cell membranes have far-reaching health effects. The membrane is the computer keyboard of the cell, the mitochondrial membrane affects the efficiency of energy metabolism, the endoplasmic reticular membrane affects the efficiency of xenobiotic detoxification, the nuclear membrane affects the fate of the cell and organism, and so on. Scores of papers show that slight deficiencies of essential fatty acids can cause "undiagnosable" problems within general systems (e.g., renal, hepatic, cardiovascular, musculoskeletal) (Siegel, 1994).

The current generation is the first to eat so many processed foods lacking in nutrients and the first to be exposed to so many artificial chemicals. The average person has to detoxify over 500 chemicals in the average home and office environments. The work of detoxifying chemicals that outgas from furniture, carpet, clothes, toiletries, business supplies, paper products, machines, construction materials, industrial and auto exhaust, and other sources actually depletes nutrients.

Every time we walk through a grocery store, an office building, or a pesticide-treated lawn, we use certain detoxification nutrients for every molecule of pesticide we detoxify. For example, every molecule of pesticide detoxified depletes one molecule of glutathione. Magnesium, phosphatidyl choline, and many other nutrients are lost as well. This accentuates the depletion of nutrients. Household pets and young children (who both inhabit the lower third of the living space) face increased risks from substances such as new household carpeting and pesticides. Young children and animals not only sustain greater exposure but also have detoxification systems that are immature or genetically unsuited for this type of detoxification.

Correction of Nutrient Deficiencies Treats Symptoms

Nutrient deficiencies can be compounded by the use of medications that also deplete detoxification nutrients because every medication is also a foreign chemical requiring metabolism or detoxification. Medication drives the detoxification system even further toward depletion, subjecting the patient to new illnesses and worsening the existing illnesses.

To give a simplified example of the way most drugs and other chemicals are detoxified, a popular pathway for phase I detoxification in the body is the mixed-function oxidase system of cytochrome P-450 enzymes. This system serves to switch electrons around to allow the xenobiotic to proceed to phase II detoxification, using primarily oxidation or hydrolysis. Next, a large molecule such as the conjugating tripeptide glutathione attaches to the xenobiotic. This serves to make the xenobiotic larger, heavier, and more polar so that it can then be dragged out into the bile and excreted with the stool.

The problem is that for every molecule of xenobiotic that the body detoxifies, the body loses a molecule of glutathione. Other nutrients are also lost, but the details of the myriad of xenobiotic pathway biochemistry of particular nutrient losses are beyond the scope of this work.

The ultimate detoxification of any xenobiotic is its complete removal from the body. However, this is not always possible because of the nutrient status, diet, and environment of the host. Sometimes it is stored (usually in lipid substances, hence the increasing prevalence of neurologic and dermatologic diseases). In other situations the body actually produces a more toxic compound, as often happens with some pesticides that are carcinogenic.

The integrity of the xenobiotic detoxification system hinges on nutrient repleteness (Anderson, Kappas, 1991; Bland, Brally, 1992; Yuesheng and others, 1992). In the following section, magnesium exemplifies the way one nutrient can cause multiple symptoms.

Magnesium as an Example of the Diverse Symptoms One Mineral Deficiency Can Cause

The current generation is the first to be continually detoxifying such a great number of daily chemicals (over 500 on average). Add to that the fact that the work of detoxification depletes nutrients, and it is indeed a tribute to the design of the human body that it does so well. A Food and Drug Administration study analyzing 234 foods over 2 years found that the average American diet had less than 80% of the recommended daily allowance (RDA) of one or more of the nutrients calcium, magnesium, iron, zinc, copper, and manganese (Pennington, Young, 1986).

In the following example, magnesium (one of the more than 40 known essential nutrients) illustrates the prevalence of nutritional deficiencies and the degree to which they are underdiagnosed. The example also shows the importance of nutrients in disease progresssion.

About 90% of physicians do not routinely test for magnesium deficiency despite the fact that over half of the population is at risk and a significant number of patients actually die from its sequelae. In one paper, over 54% of the subjects were found to have low levels of magnesium (Whang, Ryder, 1990). In this study, researchers used a less expensive magnesium assay (serum) known to miss a significant number of subjects who are deficient in magnesium (only 1% of total body magnesium is in the serum) (Seelig, 1989; Rhinehart, 1988). Furthermore, government studies show that the average American diet provides less

than 40% of the daily requirement for magnesium (*New misgivings about magnesium*, 1988). Many studies demonstrate the effects of this deficiency (Marier, 1986; Pennington, Young, 1986; Roubenoff and others, 1987).

Studies show that magnesium deficiency can cause bronchial spasm and asthma. It can cause the abnormal metabolism of cholesterol and therefore cause hypercholesterolemia. It can lead to spasm in the gut and irritable bowel syndrome. It can cause or contribute to fatigue (Cox, Campbell, Downson, 1991). It can cause or exacerbate chemical sensitivity (Rea and others, 1986; Rogers, 1991a), cystitis, chronic back problems, hypertension (Seelig, 1989), cardiac arrhythmia, premenstrual syndrome (PMS), sudden death and cardiac arrest (Cannon and others, 1987; Leary, Reyes, 1983; Purvis, Cummings, 1994; Singh, Cameron, 1982), refractory hypokalemia (Seelig, 1989), and many other conditions (Marino, 1991; Nicar, Pak, 1987). By viewing disease biochemically instead of as a drug deficiency, specialists in nutritional biochemistry can resolve chronic disorders without the use of drugs. Drugs usually mask biochemical defects, as in the common use of calcium channel blockers for hypertension, cardiac arrhythmia, and angina. Magnesium is nature's calcium channel blocker (Iseri, French, 1984).

The relevance for animals is that magnesium deficiency stimulates histamine release (as well as irritability), thereby exacerbating allergies, especially pruritic skin conditions. In some cases, merely correcting an underlying magnesium deficiency may correct severe itching or pruritic dermatoses even when no attempt was made to isolate and remove the offending cause.

Hundreds of articles in the literature describe various conditions that improve after magnesium deficiency is discovered and corrected. Likewise any single disease is accompanied by mutiple nutrient deficiencies whose diagnoses and corrections have led to the termination of the symptoms. For practitioners the bottom line is the extent to which this knowledge furthers therapeutic goals. Following are some additional examples.

Other Nutrients

Circumstances similar to those surrounding magnesium exist for more other nutrients; for example, government studies show the average American gets less than 1 mg of copper a day, although the requirement is 2 to 4 mg a day (National Research Council, 1980). Copper is in 21 enzymes, and deficiencies are prevalent (Holden, Wolf, Mertz, 1979; Klevay, Reck, Barcome, 1979), leading to aneurysms, depression, hypoglycemia, fatigue, chemical sensitivity, high cholesterol, arthralgia, poor postsurgical and posttrauma wound healing, and other problems.

Likewise, zinc is in over 90 enzymes and is commonly deficient (*Zinc: a public health problem*, 1992). Zinc deficiencies lead to a broad range of effects, from digestive and metabolic problems to cancer and chemical sensitivity (Rogers, 1990).

The literature often shows that patients with asthma are low in magnesium, vitamin B_{12}, and omega-3 essential fatty acids. High cholesterol can be caused by the inability to properly metabolize cholesterol; this problem is often preceded by deficiencies of chromium, manganese, magnesium, copper, and many other substances. Obviously, broad multisystem and multimetabolic problems such as chronic fatigue and chemical sensitivity can be associated with a host of deficiencies. The diagnosis of fatigue alone warrants a full investigation of all potential nutrient deficiencies.

Amino acids are also critical. Taurine has corrected cardiac failure, chronic inflammatory conditions, retinal diseases, cardiac arrhythmias, and seizure disorders. This stands to reason because taurine is the most plentiful amino acid in the heart, brain, and retina. One reason it is so commonly deficient (aside from frank dietary insufficiency) is that cysteine (its metabolic precursor in the body) is depleted with the work of detoxification, an ongoing process during the life of an organism.

Chemical sensitivity reflects an inability to metabolize everyday chemicals as efficiently as the average person. People with chemical sensitivities have this problem because they are deficient in the nutrients that control the detoxification pathways. Animals can also have this problem. For example, researchers have noted increased infertility in humans and animals during the last few decades. This increase is due to multiple factors, chief among which are environmental pollutants and biochemical deficiencies (Rea, 1992).

To assay some of the key minerals, at the very least a red blood cell (RBC) manganese, RBC zinc, RBC copper, and a magnesium loading test are necessary. An RBC potassium test may also be helpful. When this sensitive indicator is abnormally low, it suggests that the potassium pump has been damaged. This damage sometimes results from years of exposure to trans-fatty acids or simple antihistamines (Rogers, 1986). Because the potassium pump lies in the cell membrane, it indicates further damage in the cell membrane, which, like the computer keyboard of the cell, orchestrates many disease states and symptoms such as allergies, autoimmune phenomena, arteriosclerosis, and cancer.

A biochemical approach to symptoms can lead to vastly improved health and productivity and other economic benefits. This approach is relevant to nearly all problems, even cancer. For example, after receiving every conventional treatment for certain types of bladder cancers, 80% of patients have a recurrence of their cancer within 2 years. However, for those given four simple vitamins, the recurrence rate dropped from 80% to 40%, or in half (Lamm and others, 1994). In many humans and animals, end-stage metastatic cancers that had foiled all that medicine can offer have completely cleared as a result of inexpensive, easily accessible environmental medicine principles (Rogers 1992, 1994, in press).

In another study of patients admitted to an acute medical service, 23% to 50% were found to have undiscovered deficiencies, and this was not a sophisticated analysis (Roubenoff and others, 1987). Studies have demonstrated magnesium deficiency in more than 50% of the population (Rea and others, 1986; Rogers, 1991; Whang, Ryder, 1990), and even the most seemingly minor of symptoms, such as anxiety or insomnia, can signal a deficiency of magnesium or other nutrients that may eventually disrupt arterial and cardiac integrity, consequently increasing vulnerability to life-threatening events (Seelig, 1989). However, if symptoms are masked with a seemingly harmless tranquilizer or hypnotic, the opportunity to prevent more serious sequelae is lost or, at best, delayed.

Summary

- Deficiencies are so common that they are the rule, not the exception.
- The average processed diet and daily exposure to chemicals are among the primary causes of deficiencies.
- Deficiencies of nutrients are behind many symptoms that are customarily masked with medications.
- When symptoms are masked, the opportunity to find their cause is lost.
- Drugs are often unnecessarily prescribed over a subject's lifetime.
- Ignoring the cause of symptoms invariably causes further symptoms and diseases.

In the current drug-oriented system, the sick get sicker—and more quickly.

Accessory Nutrients

A host of "nonessential," accessory, or conditionally essential nutrients have extremely important properties. Study after study reports their many important benefits, and the fact that they are neither known nor used in conventional medicine is difficult to understand. For example, L-glutamine can inhibit the gastrointestinal changes that result from radiation to the gut during treatment of malignancies (Jan-Klimberg and others, 1990). Carnitine has reversed congestive heart failure when conventional cardiovascular drugs have failed, as has taurine (Furlong, 1996).

Vitamin A, retinoic acid derivatives, and butyric acid have reversed and actually cured certain types of leukemias. Butyric acid has also caused differentiation* (or return to normal) of certain types of colon cancer cells. Butyric acid also induces colon cancer cells to undergo apoptosis; thus it actually induces and selects for cancer cell death. It may cause differentiation of neoplastic colon

---

*Gope, Gope (1993); Hague and others (1993a); Ho and others (1994); Hutt-Taylor and others (1988); Schroy and others (1994).

cells and render them capable of secreting alkaline phosphatase and mucin, as do normal colon cells.

Butyrate also increases the radio-resistance of colon cells (Jan-Klimberg and others, 1990, Leith, 1988), which is important in sparing the gut when the abdomen is treated (as has also been found for glutamine). Like vitamin A and its analogues, butyrate has reversed some leukemias. Because bacterial fermentation of bowel fiber produces butyrate, another reason that a high-fiber diet correlates inversely with health problems such as cancer is appreciated (Anderson, 1986; Hague and others, 1993b). Scientists have long assumed that the benefits of a high-fiber diet result from a reduction of the time that carcinogens are in contact with luminal cells. Butyrate chemistry is one example of a rarely discussed but nonetheless important accessory nutrient.

Minerals, Vitamins, Amino Acids, and Essential Fatty Acids Are Essential to Body Biochemistry

The previous sections have provided examples of common deficiencies in the typical diet, the prevalence of such deficiencies, the ability of these deficiencies to cause many symptoms, and the extent to which such deficiencies underlie nearly all diseases and symptoms.

Magnesium was used as an example because it is essential in the function of over 300 enzymes. Government studies show that the average person does not get even half of the daily requirement (*New misgivings about magnesium*, 1988). If humans are generally deficient, animals are also likely to experience similar deficiencies. Humans and animals are ingesting progressively more processed foods (versus whole foods) and foods grown on increasingly nutrient-depleted soils fertilized with artificial chemicals. These foods are treated with pesticides, shipped, fumigated, and altered in a myriad of secret ways.

All nutrients could be explored in similar fashion. The bottom line is that if people have a deteriorating nutrient status, as scores of scientific papers report, animal chemistry may not be very different. This is true whether they eat table food or commercial foods.

Intestinal Hyperpermeability Syndrome

Leaky gut syndrome is a common problem that does not necessarily manifest as gastrointestinal symptoms. It is a common cause of food allergies, chemical sensitivities, autoimmune diseases, and uncorrectable nutrient deficiencies, all of which may produce a variety of symptoms. Leaky gut syndome is commonly caused by an imbalance of abnormal intestinal organisms, such as the overgrowth of *C. albicans* caused by an excess of antibiotics, or *Klebsiella* or *Proteus*. Leaky gut syndrome is also caused by nonsteroidal antiinflammatory drugs, steroids, food additives, and food allergies.

L-Glutamine is one of many inexpensive, nonprescription nutrients that are used to treat leaky gut syndrome but rarely used in medicine, veterinary or human. Studies demonstrate its potency, yet it remains unknown in medicine (Rogers, 1996). For example, when radiation must be administered to the abdomen in the treatment of cancer, the bowel can become so damaged with radiation-induced necrosis that the failure of the gut to survive can kill the patient (Jan-Klimberg, 1990). Glutamine has been shown to exhibit a protective effect against radiation-induced gastrointestinal mucosal damage. Glutamine may also be extremely useful for healing ulcers (Klein, 1990; Shrive and others, 1957) rather than using aluminum-laden antacids or H$_2$ blockers that turn off stomach acid secretion, thus further compromising absorption of nutrients (Shrive and others, 1957).

Glutamine also plays an important role in immune functions, healing the gut to such an extent that hospitalization is reduced and recovery is faster (Pastores and others, 1994). Clearly, it is much less expensive than most prescription medications and possibly more effective because, unlike most drugs, it actually heals rather than merely masks symptoms.

Nutrient Deficiencies Are a Component of Chemical Sensitivity

Victims of chemical sensitivity have impaired xenobiotic detoxification (metabolism or processing). Correcting this impairment can allow them to recover.

Jakoby describes the major detoxification enzymes of phase 1 and phase 2, including alcohol dehydrogenases, aldehyde oxidase, cytochrome P-450, superoxide dismutases, glutathione peroxidase, and monoamine oxidases. The conjugation pathways are also discussed (Jakoby, 1980).

Hathcock describes the ways vitamins E and A contribute to the stability of membranes, which, of course, include endoplasmic reticular membranes, where the work of chemical (xenobiotic) detoxification occurs. The role of vitamin C as a major detoxification agent protecting against hydrocarbons, pesticides, and heavy metals, decreasing carcinogenicity and toxicity and improving drug metabolism is also described (Hathcock, 1987). For example, vitamin B$_3$ supplies the reducing equivalent to cytochrome P-450 (NADPH). Vitamin B$_1$ is important in carbohydrate metabolism; for example, in people with chronic fatigue, as well as those with mental symptoms, heavy metal disease, and pesticide toxicity, vitamin B$_6$ is important in enhancing drug detoxification to decrease toxicity. One role is the transamination of amino acids used as conjugates for phase II detoxification; it also is useful to detoxify carbon tetrachloride and other chemicals that can be included as part of the inert ingredients of pesticides and also are common solvents in the industrial workplace, as well as industrial and incinerator effluents into air and ground water. Vitamin B$_{12}$ is important in the detoxification of cyanide, which is a common component of pesticides.

Nutrients are interrelated (Caldwell, Jacoby, 1983). For example, vitamin A protects vitamin E; vitamin C is important for the regeneration of minerals into the active or reduced form (recycling them for further use) and does the same with vitamin E, reducing it to the active tocopherol form again. Lipid peroxidation can lead to damaged cellular membrane function, and without antioxidants to protect these membranes, endoplasmic reticular detoxification membranes are compromised. The organism exhibits the "spreading phenomenon," wherein it gets progressively sicker via many routes.

The continual loss of nutrients adversely affects the work of detoxification, as with the loss of glutathione and phosphatidylcholine (Feuer, de la Iglesia, 1985).

Nutrient Deficiencies Should Be Explored for Every Symptom and Disease

In the interest of brevity, thousands of references have been omitted. The main points that these papers support are the following:

- Nutrient deficiencies are the rule, not the exception.
- Every symptom or disease has biochemical (nutrient) deficiencies associated with it.
- Taking medication further depletes nutrients.
- Nutrient deficiencies cause symptoms and classifiable diseases that are treated with drugs.
- Correction of these deficiencies can correct symptoms if the deficiency alone is a major cause. Otherwise the other contributing factors must be considered.
- Each nutrient is responsible for specific enzymes and pathways. One nutrient deficiency alone can cause over 40 different symptoms.
- Because of individual biochemistry, the same symptoms are not caused by the same deficiencies and the same deficiencies do not cause the same symptoms in every individual.
- The medical literature to date supports the importance of investigating the nutritional biochemistry before resorting to chronic drug therapy. Aside from producing side effects, drugs potentiate the underlying cause of symptoms and foster the development of new symptoms because they deplete nutrients essential to detoxification.

Household pets are at great risk because their diets often include processed foods and table scraps, but no animals are immune; commercial livestock foods are heavily laden with hydrogenated oils (to retard rancidity and spoiling) as well. Even the wild animal cannot escape pesticides, artificial fertilizers, and industrial contamination of soil and waterways. A great deal of data suggests the deleterious effects of food additives, dyes, coloring, pesticides, preservatives, emulsifiers, stabilizers, and other common substances.

Food Allergy

In conventional medical and veterinary practice, food allergy is not considered a common cause of many symptoms; however, many problems, including arthritis, allergies, angina, diabetes, nephrotic syndrome, migraine, colitis, and metastatic end-stage cancers, have been resolved with a mere diet change (Karjalainen and others, 1992; Panush and others, 1990; Rogers, 1992, 1994; Rowe, Rowe, 1965a,b).

Food allergy is a known cause for multiple undiagnosable or treatment-refractory symptoms. Food allergy is also an important, treatable cause of many disease states that are commonly treated with drugs or assumed to be untreatable. In fact, it is unusual to find a patient with treatment-resistant or recalcitrant symptoms whose symptoms are not exacerbated by one or more foods. This allergy is not restricted to IgE- or IgG-mediated sensitivities because foods can cause symptoms by many different mechanisms and diet trials are the least expensive way to diagnose many of them.

This knowledge of the many guises of food allergy is not new and seemingly knows no disease boundaries, because it has been observed to be a factor in rhinitis (Davis, 1951; Derlacki, 1955; Piness, Miller, 1931; Rowe, Rowe, 1965a,b), migraines (Egger and others, 1983; Monro and others, 1980), asthma (Hoj and others, 1981; Ogle, Bullock, 1980; Rowe, Young, 1959), recurrent infections, fatigue, colitis, arthritis (Felder, de Blecourt, Wuthrich, 1987; Kjeldsen-Kragh and others, 1991; Panush and others, 1983; Van de Loar, Van der Korst, 1991), Meniere's disease (Endicott, Stucker, 1977), emphysema and chronic bronchitis (Rowe, Rowe, 1965a), epilepsy (Adamson, Sellers, 1933; Dees, 1951; Fein, Kamin, 1968), prostatitis or cystitis (Pastineszky, 1959; Powell and others, 1972), nephrosis (Labo, 1977; Sandberg and others, 1977), nephrotic syndrome (Law-Chin-Yung, Freed, 1977), many neurologic conditions (Campbell, 1973), diabetes (Karjalainen and others, 1992; Maclarren, Atkinson, 1992), fatigue, depression, chemical sensitivity, and many other recalcitrant conditions (Brostoff, Challacombe, 1987).

One of the more common problems food allergies can cause is the buildup of middle ear fluid in young children, which can lead to recurrent infections and hearing loss (Green, 1983; Nsouli, 1994). A common treatment involves insertion of tympanostomy tubes, or polyethylene pressure-equalizing (PE) tubes. These tubes can actually cause hearing loss. It makes more sense to identify the hidden food sensitivities causing these symptoms and eliminate them.

Food allergy can cause a variety of syndromes. In spite of this, specialists who treat these conditions do not routinely rule out food allergy as a cause of symptoms. Although ruling out this common cause of recalcitrant disease can be challenging, the rewards are great when the outcome of this simple and natural approach is successful.

Therapeutic Diets

Elimination diets are invaluable in the diagnosis and treatment of food allergy. Certain diets require a great deal of instruction, patient education, and time. Therefore providing clients with books in addition to counseling in the office is often less expensive and more efficacious.

Many books for human patients describe diets, which are a necessary adjunct to treatment, because patient education and responsibility are a hallmark of non–drug-oriented medicine (Randolph, 1987; Rapp, 1991; Rogers, 1996a).

In veterinary medicine, consideration should be given to the overall quality of the diet and the ingredient listing. Because it is often not possible to state with confidence that a commercial diet has a restricted food allergen content or is free of pesticides and preservatives, home-prepared diets may be necessary. Organic foods, or foods that are chemically less contaminated (and therefore put less of a toxic burden on the body), are recommended. Furthermore, studies have shown that organic foods have up to 2½ times the nutrient value as foods grown on commercial soils (Smith, 1993). Also, groups eating organic, pesticide-free foods had unexpectedly higher sperm counts compared with control groups who ate pesticide-treated foods (Abell and others, 1994).

Although a thorough discussion of biochemistry is beyond the scope of this chapter, the biochemistry of cellular membranes has significantly changed with the introduction of such substances as trans-fatty acids into the food supply. A host of daily chemical exposures in air, food, and water have reduced the nutrient base, as has the processing of foods. The combination has resulted in changes in mitochondrial, endoplasmic reticular, and nuclear and cellular membranes, which explains a vast amount of symptomatology. The reader who is cognizant of this can understand the reason that a change in diet may slow the course of disease progression and in some cases reverse diseases not thought to be reversible (Rogers, 1996b).

For example, if men with prostate cancer avail themselves of all the treatments conventional medicine has to offer (e.g., chemotherapy, surgery, hormones, radiation), the median survival is 6 years. If, however, they do not do this (and thereby save tens of thousands of dollars and avoid impotence and urinary incontinence, among other problems) but instead adopt a strict macrobiotic diet for a minimum of 3 months, median survival increases from 6 years to 19 years (Carter and others, 1993). Likewise, patients with other types of cancer showed marked increases in survival. For example, patients with pancreatic cancer had a 500% increase in survival, despite the fact that patients with this disease rarely survive longer than 3 months when treated according to conventional methods.

The macrobiotic diet, which relies heavily on whole grains and beans (preferably organic) and sea and land vegetables, has helped many people with multiple chemical sensitivities, asthma, eczema, chronic sinusitis, and many undiagnosable or seemingly untreatable conditions such as chronic fatigue, fibromyalgia, lupus, rheumatoid arthritis, and sarcoiditis. Many patients have documented their reversal of cancer with these diets after exhausting conventional resources (East West Foundation, 1991; Nussbaum, 1986; Rogers, 1991b, 1992, 1994). Many mechanisms explain the successful recovery of health, but they all support the xenobiotic detoxification system through nutrients, phytochemicals, and pH balance (Anderson, Kappas, 1991; Rogers, 1990b; Yuesheng and others, 1992).

The macrobiotic diet is the basis for the book *Dr. Dean Ornish's Program For Reversing Heart Disease* (Ornish, 1990b). When traditional medical practices fail, including high-tech bypass surgery, cholesterol-lowering drugs, antiangina drugs, and antiarrhythmia drugs, diet is the only way to reverse coronary artery disease, as shown on positron-emission tomography (PET) scans and symptom scores a year later (Ornish, 1990b). Many books explain the various diagnostic and macrobiotic diets available (Rogers, 1992a).

Food Allergy Injections

Food allergy testing by injection is similar to serial dilution endpoint titration (SDET), which is used for diagnosing and treating inhalant (dust, mold, pollen, dander) allergies. Instead of several antigens being tested at once, only one antigen is tested at a time. This technique can provoke symptoms and has been called the *provocation-neutralization* technique because once the symptom is provoked, the dose can often be lowered by one logarithm of five dilutions to neutralize it. However, this technique does not always provoke a symptom.

Regardless of whether a symptom is provoked, food allergy injection testing is a useful way to find the exact treatment dose to administer. Testing for and treating food allergies has been efficacious for people, especially children, whose food sensitivities are not controlled with diets alone.*

Food allergy can mimic many symptoms and can be diagnosed and treated, depending upon severity, with diets, skin testing and injections, or both.

Inhalant Allergies

In 1969, when Ishizaka discovered the reaginic or allergic IgE antibody, one mechanism for allergy and its treatment became clear. When mammals inhale or breathe certain antigens such as grass pollens or ragweed, they make IgE or allergic antibody if they have the genetic propensity to do so. When this antibody meets the antigen to which it was directed, the IgE becomes attached to specific cells and triggers the release of histamine and other

*Draper (1972); King and others (1978a, 1978b); Miller (1972, 1978, 1980, 1981); Morris (1969); Rapp (1978a, 1978b, 1978c, 1978d, 1978e,f); Rea and others (1984).

cell mediators. This results in the myriad of symptoms possible from any such exposure, depending on the body tissues that have become the allergic target organs.

The route of exposure can be inhalation, ingestion, dermal contact, or inoculation. A wide range of target organs is also possible. If the IgE is primarily directed toward the nose, rhinitis results. In dogs and cats the principal target organ is the skin (Baker, 1990). If the lung is targeted, bronchitis or asthma may result. If it is the brain, mood swings, depression, seizures, migraine, transient ischemic attacks (TIA; small strokes), and many other symptoms are possible (Rogers, 1996b). Any symptom is possible depending on the target organ predilection of the host, which results from a combination of factors, including genetics, environment, nutritional status, and previous trauma or injury.

Potential antigens that can be inhaled include pollens of trees, grasses, and weeds, as well as dusts, danders, mites, cockroaches, and other insects. The most important inhaled antigens, however, are those provoked by molds. Molds, yeasts, and fungi come in a variety of forms, from spores to mycelia, and thousands of species exist. Small doses of these antigens can be used for treatment and intradermal skin testing. Contact allergens may not even require intradermal injection because patch tests may be used. As with any allergen, after identification of the offender the first line of treatment is avoidance. This involves a variety of environmental controls, from cleaning household surfaces to the air itself.

Allergies to certain fungi can be recalcitrant to treatment if the organism is "wearing" the mold to which it is allergic. A gut full of *C. albicans* from antibiotic treatment, a yeast overgrowth in the lungs from steroids, or a fungal dermal infection can exacerbate asthma and other allergic reactions to molds until the host source is eradicated. As Pasteur pointed out, the initial vulnerability to become a host for the organism depends heavily on the metabolic integrity or nutrient status of the host. Mold allergies have been implicated in asthma (Licorish and others, 1985; Schwartz, Ward, 1995; Ward and others, 1989), rhinitis (Gumkowski and others, 1987), urticaria, and angioedema (Platts-Mills and others, 1987).

The mechanism of hyposensitizing injections has been known since Ishizaka discovered the reaginic antibody IgE, which is responsible for some types of hypersensitivity. With an injection of a minuscule amount of the antigen to which the patient is sensitive, the body makes the protective or blocking antibody IgG. This attaches to the IgE receptor site on the cell, thereby blocking access of the IgE. Hence, exposure to this antigen no longer produces symptoms. Of course, the success of the injection is dose related, but it is the basis of many immunizations.

To evaluate the need for treatment and its subsequent success, culture plates must be exposed to assess mold persistence. Because mold is a living organism that can regrow, eradication may not be permanent. The plates must be exposed while symptoms are at their worst, because

species have specific times of peak sporulation. For example, *Hormodendrum (Cladosporium),* the most common fungus in the world, has a peak sporulation time around noon, whereas *Sporobolomyces* (of the class *Basidiomycetes*) has a peak time around midnight. Sporulation also depends on many other factors, such as light and dark cycles, temperature, and humidity. Extensive work on molds has been performed to establish the optimal growing media, exposure techniques, and incubation periods for recovery (Rogers, 1982, 1983, 1984).

Testing Procedure: Serial Dilution Endpoint Titration

Immunotherapy fosters the production of IgG-blocking antibody, and symptoms gradually lessen and often disappear entirely. To merely treat symptoms with drugs is to invite further problems in other target organs. For example, prescription antihistamines can trigger potentially fatal cardiac arrhythmias, compromise the xenobiotic detoxification system, and inhibit the potassium pump in the cardiac muscle cells (Good, Rochwood, Schad, 1994).

Iatrogenic side effects are a significant cause of hospitalization and illness. A recent study showed that several antihistamines such as astemizole (Hismanal), loratadine (Claritin), and hydroxyzinc hydrochloride (Atarax) have the potential to promote cancer growth, even in low doses (*Physician's Desk Reference,* 1994). Therefore the immunotherapy route has several advantages beyond merely masking allergic symptoms with drugs.

Traditionally, allergists test patients with one or a few strengths of an antigen and use this as a conclusive determination of a patient's sensitivity to the antigen. Then the dose of each injection is arbitrarily raised until an end point is determined—sometimes by a severe reaction or even death. Determining the maximum tolerated dose for each antigen within the safety of the allergist's office is therefore recommended.

Titration involves testing with several strengths to find the optimum (and safest) dose. In serial dilution end point titration (SDET) testing, the dilutions are the logarithm of five of the preceding strength. The second dilution would be 5 times weaker than the preceding one, the third dilution would be 5 times weaker than the second, and so on. The different strengths are tested to obtain the highest dose that can be given without precipitating adverse reactions; hence, it is a titration. The last dose not to cause a wheal-and-flare reaction is the end point. If no reaction occurs at a specific dose, testing for that antigen is stopped and the patient is considered nonreactive. However, if the patient demonstrates a wheal-and-flare reaction, titration continues until the first nonreactive or safe treatment dose is found.

SDET is currently the most precise in vivo quantitation of the body's immune system that the practitioner can easily, safely, and inexpensively perform. Clearly, the conventional practice of administering the same dose to all patients is potentially more dangerous, less accurate, and less scientific. It does, however, require less time and skill and remains the only form endorsed by the American Academy of Allergy (AAA) (Bosquet, Michel, 1994). In fact, conventional immunotherapy without titration has been so risky that "when these potent extracts were used, allergen injections initially resulted in a greater number of systemic reactions" (Locky and others, 1987).

Based on one study using ragweed and cat dander antigens, the Council on Scientific Affairs stated the following:

> Skin test endpoint titration provides a useful and effective measure of patient sensitivity. Controlled studies have shown that the intradermal method of skin test endpoint titration is effective for quantifying sensitivity to ragweed pollen extract and for identifying patients highly sensitive to ragweed. This method provides reliability comparable to that of in vitro leukocyte histamine release and radio allergosorbent test (RAST). Controlled studies have shown that the prick test method of skin test endpoint titration can be used as a measure of response to immunotherapy with cat extract (Council on Scientific Affairs, 1987).

The American Medical Association (AMA) and the American Academy of Allergy and Immunology (AAAI) have recommended the use of this technique with highly dangerous Hymenoptera (stinging insects) and cat antigens (Van Metre and others, 1988). The American Academy of Allergy and Immunology Training Program Director's Committee published a list of "unproven techniques," but SDET was not included (AAAI Training Program Director's Committee Report, 1994).

There are currently no papers refuting the value of SDET that do not have errors in methodology. However, scores of papers show the benefit of this technique (Boris and others, 1983; Lee and others, 1969; O'Shea and others, 1981; Rapp, 1978a,b,c; Rogers, 1991d, 1994). It is the very foundation of pharmacologic research: to find the optimum dose of each substance for each organism.

The official position of the American Academy of Allergy on testing by titration versus arbitrarily defined standard doses is that insufficient data exist for titration; therefore, titration is not recommended or taught. However, titration offers the following advantages:

- It is the basis of all scientific quantitation.
- It is safer, because no deaths have been reported in contrast to the many recorded deaths with the conventional standardized-dose technique.
- It is used by the AAAI when safety is particularly critical, as with stinging insect allergy.
- It is supported by the AMA.
- It compensates for the lack of standardization and variability in commercial extracts.
- It has been successfully used for diagnosing and treating food, chemical, and inhalant sensitivities by thousands of physicians for more than 30 years.
- It has many double-blind studies to support it, and all the studies purporting to discredit it were fraught with methodologic errors.

For veterinarians who deal with animals ranging in weight from less than 1 lb to over 1000 lb, titration is the preferred way to safely and effectively treat allergies that could be life threatening. Food, chemical, and inhalant allergies in humans and animals can mimic many recalcitrant symptoms, for which there exist no more suitable treatments. For several decades, physicians have successfully used this technique* and many have elaborated on the mechanisms (Ali and others, 1983; Rocklin and others, 1976).

Clinical Applications

An example of an application in veterinary practice follows. This published case involves a double-blind study on a horse with such severe COPD that he could not be ridden for 6 years. Just sitting on his back and walking him around the paddock resulted in paroxysmal coughing and severe dyspnea.

Within 2 weeks of the injection therapy (taught to the owner), the horse could be ridden and later galloped. A 2-year follow-up revealed that he was still being ridden. This study was preserved on video tape (Rogers, 1987/1988).

Chemical Sensitivity

Medical physicians still do not routinely include chemical sensitivity in their differential diagnosis. Testing for chemical sensitivity should not be as difficult a paradigm shift for the veterinarian, who tends to be more involved with chemicals, especially pesticides. The role of chemical sensitivities in illness can be recognized by the significant increase in malignancies, autoimmune phenomena, and other recalcitrant illnesses in animals over the last few decades.

Significant awareness of chemical sensitivity began in the 1970s, when people developed bizarre symptoms overnight after installing urea foam formaldehyde insulation in their homes. Those cases made it easy to identify cause and effect, but because the symptoms were so diverse and unusual and contradicted the current medical paradigm, much controversy arose.

Subsequent studies showed that these levels of chemical (xenobiotics) were not different from ambient levels in many homes and offices. However, victims who suffered insidious symptoms (either from low-level chronic exposure or individual genetic and biochemical susceptibility), received psychiatric diagnoses.

Emerging studies progressively substantiate the principles of environmental medicine. For example, because of the increased use of latex to prevent the spread of acquired immunodeficiency syndrome (AIDS), extensive data have

---

*Mandell, Conte (1982); Miller (1977); Rinkel (1963a, 1963b); Rogers (1987/1988); Van Niekerk, DeWet (1987); Williams (1969, 1971); Willoughby (1969, 1973, 1974, 1979).

been collected over the last few years on latex sensitivity. However, only a few years ago, when reactivity to latex was suggested, the idea was dismissed because latex was thought to be inert. Now studies document dozens of symptoms, some caused by mere proximity to latex products (Jeager and others, 1992; Latex allergy—an emerging healthcare problem, 1995). Despite the data, many physicians still do not test for latex sensitivity, partly because of influence from the food, chemical, manufacturing, and pharmaceutical industries.

Chemical sensitivity can mimic literally any disease or symptom, including hepatotoxicity (Zimmerman, 1978), glomerulonephritis (Ravenskov, Forseberg, Skerfving, 1979), heart disease (Magos, 1981), scleroderma (Black, Welsh, 1988), acidosis (Voigts, 1983), balance and memory problems (Kilburn, Warshaw, Thornton, 1987), and cancer (Swenberg and others, 1983).

Many books and papers have been written on chemical sensitivity, only a small sample of which can be discussed here.

Organic Solvents

Organic solvents are used in paints, fuels, adhesives, pesticides, glues, and cosmetics. They are also used in the manufacture of numerous products, most importantly construction materials and furnishings. Millions of workers experience chronic low-level exposures throughout their professional lives. Consumers using the various products containing solvents occasionally sustain adverse effects from exposure—even when the products are used according to their directions. Accidental overexposure also occurs. In addition, the entire populace is exposed to organic solvents that contaminate air, water, and food.

Recently, Wallace analyzed breath samples from 350 New Jersey residents and found benzene, perchloroethylene, and trichloroethylene in 89%, 93%, and 29% of the samples, respectively (Wallace and others, 1986). Many other organic solvents were also detected. The long-range effects of low levels of these potential carcinogens are not known. However, low-level solvent exposure may be a contributing factor in the rising cancer rate in the United States, and it definitely contributes to chemical sensitivity.

Solvent exposure can cause significant depression of the central nervous system (CNS) (Rogers, 1997). Trichloroethylene, for example, was once used as an anesthetic gas. Often the symptoms of CNS depression occurring on either a short-term high-level or chronic low-level basis result in nonspecific, vague symptoms.

Indeed, organic solvents are known to cause cancer (Davis, Magee, 1978; National Toxicology Program, 1982), and chlorinated aliphatic hydrocarbon solvents are known to be hepatotoxic (Zimmerman, 1978). Scientists have known for over 100 years that chloroform damages the liver. Stimulation of liver enzymes by some solvents

can cause adverse responses to ethanol and other drugs. Moreover, occupational and home exposure to solvents can alter immune system responses and cause lymphocytosis. A brief exposure to a mixture of solvents was shown to suppress lymphocyte function among workers (Denkhaus and others, 1986).

Halogenated alkanes (trichloroethylene, fluorocarbons, 1,1,1-trichloroethane, perchloroethylene, and others) cause cardiac arrhythmias (Magos, 1981; Reinhardt and others, 1973) and sudden death (King, 1985) by altering cardiac sensitivity to endogenous catecholamines. Sudden death has been reported from inhaling typewriter correction fluid containing 1,1,1-trichloroethane (Anderson and others, 1985; Garriott and others, 1980). Likewise, kidney disease (Emmerson, 1985; Mutti and others, 1992), such as glomerulonephritis (Ravenskov, Forseberg, Skerfving, 1979), acute tubular necrosis after diesel oil exposure, and Fanconi's syndrome (renal tubular acidosis) after glue sniffing, have been reported (Voigts, 1983).

Xenobiotics can cause bizarre neurologic symptoms (Feldman, Ricks, Baker, 1980; Lazar and others, 1983) and dermatoses (Orris, Tesser, 1982), and many target organs are subject to their deleterious influence. Unfortunately, the thresholds for exposure were arbitrarily determined before the vast scope of chemical sensitivity was understood (The American Conference of Government Industrial Hygienists, 1984).

Common sources of solvent exposure include chemicals used in dry cleaning and carpet products. Dry-cleaning fluids outgas the following chemicals, which can be measured in the bloodsteam of someone working in a room with a recently cleaned carpet, or wearing recently dry-cleaned clothes: tetrachlorethylene, trichlorethylene, 1,1,1,-trichloroethane, ethylene dichloride, and mineral spirits. Household pets have the opportunity to inhale even more carpet chemicals.

Likewise, paints outgas toluene, xylenes, acetone, methyl ethyl ketone, methyl isobutyl ketone, and mineral spirits. Gasoline fumes can outgas benzene, toluene, xylenes, ethylene dibromide, ethylene dichloride, and many other chemicals. Furthermore, common household cleansers, adhesives for furniture, and carpet backings outgas toluene, xylenes, methyl ethyl ketone, methyl isobutyl ketone, 1,1,1,-trichlorethylene, P-dichlorobenzene, and many other substances. Some of these, such as benzene and vinyl chloride, outgas from plastics and are known carcinogens.

Because most laboratories do not have the means to measure these compounds or their metabolites in patients, solvent toxicity is not widely recognized. These compounds can be assayed in a number of ways. For example, benzene can be measured as total phenol (its main metabolite) in the urine. Styrene from plastics can be measured as mandelic acid in urine or phenylglyoxylic acid in urine. Toluene from household and office paints can be measured as hippuric acid in urine, and unconjugated toluene is measured directly in venous blood. Intradermal testing of certain chemicals is also possible and can often duplicate the symptoms that exposures precipitate. Special hepatic function tests (caffeine, benzoate, and acetaminophen clearance) may help localize a biochemical defect in the detoxification pathway of the xenobiotic. This enables the practitioner to improve its function with manipulation of key nutrients for details that are necessary to do a thorough evaluation (Rea, 1992; Rogers, 1990b, 1996b).

Because many of the aforementioned studies were performed on animal subjects, their relevance to veterinary medicine is apparent.

Perchloroethylene

Perchloroethylene (PCE), also known as tetrachloroethylene or "perc," is a chlorinated hydrocarbon solvent commonly used in the dry-cleaning industry and in metal degreasing. Factory workers and people who wear dry-cleaned clothes are often exposed to this, as well as people working in places where this solvent is used to clean carpets. Chronic low-level exposure is known to cause impaired brain function, decreased memory, cancers, malaise, dizziness, headache, increased perspiration, fatigue, and incoordination (Axelson and others, 1977; Sittig, 1981). Likewise, animals exposed to newly cleaned carpets often exhibit a variety of bizarre cerebral and body symptoms.

Toluene

Toluene, also known as methylbenzene, is an aromatic hydrocarbon solvent widely used in industry. It is also used in the manufacture of benzene, which is used in the production of detergents, fuels, pharmaceuticals, dyes, paints, textiles (which are worn and put on furniture and walls), plastics, and many other substances. Again, low-level chronic exposure can cause CNS depression, decreased memory, headache, dizziness, fatigue, muscular weakness, drowsiness, incoordination, ataxia, skin paresthesia, and other conditions (Axelson and others, 1977; US EPA, 1980).

Toluene outgases from plastics, paints, adhesives used for furnishings, carpeting, and many other common products (Rea, 1994; US EPA, 1980). Toluene can be measured in the blood or as hippuric acid in the urine. Many prescription medications interfere with the metabolism of toluene and vice versa. When the body does not properly metabolize all the toluene to which it is exposed daily, the toluene is stored in body fat and slowly released when the body is able to do so (Angerer, 1979; Carlsson, Ljungquist, 1982; Dossing and others, 1984). Pets in a newly painted or carpeted room or cows in a newly painted milking parlor are potentially as vulnerable as humans.

Trichloroethylene

Trichloroethylene (TCE) is a chlorinated hydrocarbon solvent in widespread use as a metal degreaser and solvent. TCE addiction can occur and can cause peripheral neuropathy with chronic low-level exposure, decreased memory, impairment of the CNS, and cancer (Rea, 1994). TCE is stored in the fat when the body is unable to detoxify it because of nutrient deficiency states in the detoxification pathway or other reasons.

For example, a deficiency of zinc in the enzyme alcohol dehydrogenase impairs the ability of the body to detoxify TCE (Reynolds, 1990a). Furthermore, when the body is not able to fully detoxify TCE, the brain funnels it into a different chemical pathway where it manufactures chloral hydrate, commonly known as "Mickey Finn" or "knockout drops." This substance is often responsible for "brain fog" or toxic encephalopathy, an inability to concentrate that is common in people with chemical sensitivity (Reynolds, 1975). This symptom fluctuates depending on exposure to the chemical, the ambient level of the chemical, other chemicals in the air competing for metabolic resources, other chemicals in the diet, and the nutrient status of the body. As with other volatile hydrocarbons, TCE has a plethora of effects (Axelson and others, 1977; Sittig, 1981) and an even greater number of metabolic pathways, depending on the victim's total environmental load and individual detoxification biochemistry.[*]

Formaldehyde

Probably one of the most widely studied hydrocarbons is formaldehyde. Previous sections have discussed its deleterious effects in the form of urea foam formaldehyde insulation. Since then the sources of formaldehyde have been studied extensively[†]. The potential symptoms cover nearly every target organ.[‡]

Formaldehyde sensitivity can mimic allergic symptoms (Gamble, 1983; Morgan, Patterson, Gross, 1983). With the increase in allergies in both human and animal populations, sensitivity to formaldehyde may be an overlooked diagnostic clue. Just as the symptoms know no boundaries,

---

[*]Apfeldorf, Infante (1981); Ertle and others (1972); Fernandez and others (1977); Monster, Boersma, Duba (1979); Muller, Spassovski, Henschler (1974); Vesterberg, Astrand (1976).
[†]Acheson and others (1984); Dally, Hanrahan, Woodbury (1981); Gupta, Ulsamer, Preuss (1982); Konipinski (1985); National Academy of Sciences (1982); Stock, Mendez (1985); Woodbury, Zenz (1983).
[‡]Beall, Ulsamer (1984); Bernstein and others (1984a,b); Blair and others (1984); Broder and others (1988); Gupta (1984); Horvath and others (1988); Kilburn, Warshaw, Thornton (1987); NIOSH (1981); Olsen, Dossing (1982); Scott, Margosches (1985); Ulsamer and others (1984); EPA (1987); Zimmerman (1988).

the mechanisms by which formaldehyde can initiate symptoms are equally varied.*

Animals may be exposed to the following potential sources of formaldehyde: foam insulation, wood or fiber products, carpets, upholstery, and draperies (Dye, Costa, 1995).

Organophosphate Pesticides

Organophsophate pesticides have been a mainstay of flea control products for many years. Malathion and chlorpyrifos are two such chemicals commonly found in commercial products. Organophosphate pesticides are powerful inhibitors of cholinesterase, the enzyme responsible for the metabolism of acetylcholine. Acetylcholine is the neurotransmitter at parasympathetic and myoneural junctions, in autonomic ganglia, and in the brain. Poisoning occurs when the inhibition of cholinesterase leads to accumulation of acetylcholine at the nerve synapses, resulting initially in overstimulation and then paralysis of neural transmission. Symptoms can be difficult to diagnose and distinguish from those of many other illnesses. In humans, symptoms may include chest tightness, headache, weakness, sweating, nausea, vomiting, abdominal pain, asthma, muscle twitching, anxiety, irritability, anorexia, paresthesias, memory loss, restlessness, confusion, staggering, bradycardia, and hypotension (Hayes, 1982).

Chlorpyrifos (O,O-diethyl O-[3,5,6-trichloro-pyridyl] phosphorothioate, commonly known as Dursban) is not only commonly encountered by the average person, but veterinarians and their staff and pet owners have even higher potential exposure. It is a common ingredient in flea collars, flea and tick sprays, powders, dips, and shampoos. Pets, especially those that roam freely in houses where corners and wall-floor margins are sprayed for roaches and fleas, are exposed to even higher levels.

Similarly, pets that are allowed to roam outside can be exposed to pesticide-treated lawns. For example, cats can develop a delayed neuropathy from accumulated exposure (Fikes and others, 1992). Another problem with pesticides and other pollutants is that they can occupy hormone receptor sites and alter the function of hormones in the body. This alteration can initiate a variety of symptoms, not the least of which is cancer (Raloff, 1995).

Chlorpyrifos has been extensively researched and can cause many symptoms in the animal and the owner. Some of the most perplexing symptoms are cerebral, with depression, mood changes, irritability, dizziness, and neuropathies (Rogers, 1996b).

Every animal is not affected to the same degree by an exposure. Within a given genetic class of animal, researchers have observed variations as great as thirteen fold

---

*Batelle Columbus Laboratory (1981); Broughton, Thrasher (1988); Casanovea, Heck (1987); French, Edsall (1945); Swenberg and others (1983); Thrasher, Broughton, Micevich (1988); Wilhelmsson, Homlstrom (1987).

in the serum enzyme paraoxonase, which detoxifies Dursban (Li, Furlong, 1993).

If that were not enough, the supposedly inert ingredients used as the transport vehicles of pesticides are trade secrets and often contain other pesticides, as well as any or all of the chemicals described. Furthermore, pesticides are ubiquitous in modern life. Many people and animals do not have sufficient capacity to detoxify all the chemicals to which they are exposed daily through air, food, and water. Therefore their bodies store the unmetabolized portions. These xenobiotics slowly leak into the system by a myriad of pathways, damaging and poisoning enzymes and resulting in chronic low-level undiagnosable symptoms.

Our air and water have been so polluted that animals and humans need not spend most of their time in an office, home, or vehicle to have symptoms of chemical sensitivity. Numerous studies show that outdoor industrial pollutants trigger far more than respiratory problems. For example, diesel exhaust (e.g., cars, trucks, tractors, factories) can trigger autoimmune antibodies leading to diseases of any body organ, such as kidney disease, cardiac disease, diabetes, infertility, immune system vulnerability, recurrent infections, and cancer (Klaasen, 1986).

Other Chemical Classes

Briefly, some epidemiologic evidence suggests that dogs exposed to 2,4-D–treated lawns show higher than normal incidence of lymphoma (Hayes, 1991). More recently, the insect growth regulator fenoxycarb and many other chemicals are slowly coming under EPA scrutiny as possible carcinogens.

Chemicals Usher in a New Era in Medicine

Clearly, the topic of chemicals is too enormous for more than a spotty overview. Whole books have been written solely on the toxic effects of carpets (Beebe, 1991). Infants and household pets have a more concentrated exposure. Phenylcyclohexane (4-PC) was the carpet chemical that caused 126 out of 2000 EPA workers to become ill when a new carpet was installed in the EPA mall office. Later, Anderson Laboratories showed, on television, dead mice that were merely exposed to the carpet remnants in a jar overnight.

Many books and articles have documented the plethora of home chemicals (Gosslin, Smith, Hodge, 1984; Rea, 1992; Sterling, 1985; Thrasher, Broughton, 1984) and the symptoms they can cause (Ashford, Miller, 1991; Rea, 1992; Rogers, 1992, 1995; Samet, Marbury, Spengler, 1987; Shusterman, Blanc, 1992). Mobile homes (Riche, Lehnen, 1987; Thrasher and others, 1987), plastics (Thrasher and others, 1989), and even paper products (LaMarte, Merchant, Casale, 1988; Marks and others, 1984) seem to represent significant exposure hazards.

Once awareness of chemical sensitivity is acquired, it is easy to appreciate what others have observed for over a decade: Anyone can react to any chemical and any target organ can be affected—at any time. Indeed, chemical sensitivity can trigger diseases of the skin, lung, and musculoskeletal, gastrointestinal, hepatic, renal, cardiac, endocrine, immune, and nervous systems. The practitioner should always consider the possibility of chemical sensitivity when investigating any medical condition.

Testing Chemicals: Provocation/Neutralization

Because the provocation/neutralization technique is useful in diagnosing chemical sensitivity, and because phenol or glycerine sensitivity is very common in chemically sensitive people, testing for these antigens is necessary to determine whether patients can tolerate the preservatives and stabilizers used in injections. Phenol sensitivity was first recognized when people reacted to titrated injections. When the preservative was omitted, they experienced no problems. In 1987 the National Institutes of Health published a description of the provocation/neutralization technique (Rogers, 1987). The EPA also listed this technique in its *Indoor Air Reference Bibliography* (US EPA, 1990).

Provocation/neutralization is similar to serial end point titration. The difference is that only one antigen is tested at a time. Often a symptom can be provoked or triggered by the wrong dose and then neutralized by the correct one. Numerous books and peer-reviewed journals (Boris and others, 1983; Rogers, 1987/1988, 1989, 1990c,d, 1991d,e) document the technique as effective for diagnosing chemical sensitivity, and it was featured in several symposiums (Rogers, 1986, 1987, 1988, 1989, 1990c).

The only paper refuting the technique contained significant methodologic problems; the dose that was supposed to neutralize symptoms was actually the dose required to trigger symptoms (Jewett, Fein, Greenberg, 1990). Because they were unfamiliar with the technique, these researchers stated that the technique was invalid (AAAI, 1994). However, many publications support the use of the technique.* Many rebuttals and critiques have addressed the erroneous assumptions about the technique (Finn, Battcock, 1985; Forman, 1981; Podell, 1983; Rapp, 1987).

The Occupational Hazards of Veterinary Practice

A thorough discussion of all the occupational hazards of the veterinary profession would fill an entire book. However, some of these hazards must be considered because they are particularly important in the lives of veterinarians, veterinary technicians, and their families, as well as the animal owners. Pesticides cause some of the most devastating chemical sensitivity syndromes. This chemical class includes all substances used to kill insects, nematodes, molluscs, fungi, weeds, and other life forms.

Pesticides have caused Parkinson's disease, multiple sclerosis, lupus, depression, memory loss, cancer, immune dysregulation, and a host of undiagnosable symptoms that mimic other diseases (Rogers, 1996b). The symptoms merely depend on which target organ was the most vulnerable and easily damaged. Although pervasive in air, food, and water, pesticides cause even higher exposures for the veterinarian and staff in the workplace. Family members of the veterinary staff can also be affected because these pesticides can linger on clothes. Children who play with animals wearing flea collars or flea-bath solution are at risk.

Organophosphate Pesticides

Organophosphate pesticides are powerful inhibitors of cholinesterase, the enzyme responsible for the metabolism of acetylcholine. Acetylcholine is the neurotransmitter at parasympathetic and myoneural junctions, in autonomic ganglia, and in the brain. Poisoning occurs when the inhibition of cholinesterase leads to accumulation of acetylcholine at the nerve synapses, resulting initially in overstimulation and then paralysis of neural transmission. For example, an insect dying of pesticide poisoning often twitches markedly before dying.

Symptoms in humans can be bizarre or nebulous, such as chest tightness, headache, weakness, sweating, nausea, vomiting, abdominal pain, asthma, muscle twitching, anxiety, irritability, memory loss, restlessness, confusion, staggering, bradycardia, and hypotension. Veterinarians need only read the fine-print precautions on the labels of flea and tick collars, sprays, dips, and oral flea-prevention products to recall the toxicity of these ubiquitous chemicals.

These chemicals are stored in the body when detoxification processes cannot keep pace with accumulation. The chemicals leak out and cause chronic, low-level, undiagnosable symptoms later, when the body is able to metabolize them.

Pesticides are but one of the many chemicals to which people are daily exposed that can cause variable levels of damage. Chemical sensitivity can trigger diseases of the skin and respiratory, musculoskeletal, gastrointestinal, hepatic, renal, cardiac, endocrine, and nervous systems. No medical condition or symptoms are exempt.

The Interrelatedness of It All

Pet owners and veterinarians and their technicians, office staff, and families are at risk of the insidious effects of pesticide poisoning, which can mimic any disease. The pet is not exempt, either. Certainly the health of the owners

---

*Boris and others (1987); Boris, Schiff, Weindorf (1985, 1988); Brostoff, Scadding (1986); King and others (1988a, 1988b); Lee and others (1969); Lee, Williams, Binkley (1960); Miller (1981, 1987).

and the family reflect their diet (which may be passed on to the pet) and their environment (which the pet may also share). A brief evaluation of the family's health problems, pesticide schedules, diet, and environmental changes may be particularly revealing. For example, pesticide treatment of kitchens is commonly concentrated at floor margins and under cabinets—exactly where many pets forage for crumbs. Certainly, if a household animal has a mysterious illness, the rest of the family should be questioned about symptoms such as headaches, body aches, stomach problems, depression, and mood swings. The cause may be as simple as a faulty heating system, caused by natural gas or incompletely combusted fuel oil products backwashing down a cold flue or stack. Alternately the family might have recently completed a new family room with glued carpet, a highly toxic combination that has caused a host of animal and human ills (Rogers, 1990b). Pets are closest to the source. An environmental approach explores the interrelatedness of these factors. Just as the human's diet and environment affect the health of the animal, so can the pet's flea collar, shampoo, intestinal parasites, and allergenic dander affect its owner. Likewise, the health of the owners can provide just as much information about the cause of the animal's symptoms as the overall health of the pet may reveal about the health of the owners.

Veterinarians are familiar with the symptoms of pesticide poisoning, but what about a client's 3-year-old child, who may watch television with his head nestled in the pet's flea collar and subsequently develop mysterious behavior problems?

Chronic fatigue, depression, poor memory, chronic musculoskeletal pains leading to drug dependence or alcoholism, and irrational mood swings are all maladies that may eventually be referred to a psychiatrist. Practitioners should first consider an environmental medicine workup, which seems preferable to a lifetime prescription for antidepressants.

Multiple causative factors invariably emerge when disease is fully investigated. A harried lifestyle leads to the consumption of more processed foods that are low in nutrients. Chemical exposure further depletes the body of detoxification nutrients, leaving the victim tired and depressed because of an inadequate supply of nutrients to synthesize beneficial hormones in the brain (Rogers, 1997). This phenomenon further makes the individual more vulnerable to the hidden effects of repeated pesticide exposure. The high levels of sugar, caffeine, alcohol, fermentation products, and chemical additives in the diet can exacerbate problems with cerebral metabolism. In addition, new furnishings, paint, carpet, construction materials, pesticides, commercial cleaning fluids, and other substances common in the home and office environments can increase the total load of stressors that require environmental or biochemical intervention.

When they ignore the environmental approach to medicine, practitioners miss a number of opportunities to identify the cause and resolve the problem. They must learn to consider the patient's air, food, water, and nutrient status. By practicing some simple principles of environmental medicine, practitioners for all species may achieve new levels of therapeutic success.

REFERENCES

AAAI Training Program Director's Committee Report: Topics related to controversial practices that should be taught in an allergy and immunology training program, *J Allergy Clin Immunol* 93:955, 1994.

Acheson ED and others: Formaldehyde in the British chemical industry, *Lancet* 1:611, 1984.

Adamson WB, Sellers ED: Observations on the incidence of the hypersensitive state in one hundred cases of epilepsy, *J Allergy* 5:315, 1933.

Ali M and others: Serum concentration of allergen specific IgG antibody in inhalant allergens; effect of specific immunotherapy, *Am J Clin Pathol* 80:290, 1983.

Anderson HR and others: Epidemiology: deaths from abuse of volatile substances: a national epidemiological study, *Br Med J* 290:304, 1985.

Anderson KE, Kappas A: Dietary regulation of cytochrome P450, *Annu Rev Nutr* 11:141, 1991.

Anderson JW: Fiber and health: an overview, *Am J Gastroenterol* 81:892, 1986.

Angerer J: Occupational chronic exposure to organic solvents: VII metabolism of toluene in man, *Int Arch Occup Environ Health* 43:63, 1979.

Apfeldorf R, Infante P: Review of epidemiologic study results of vinyl chloride related compounds, *Environ Health Perspect* 41:221, 1981.

Armentia A: Baker's asthma: prevalence and evaluation of immunotherapy with a wheat flour extract, *Ann Allergy* 65:265, 1990.

Ashford NA, Miller CA: *Chemical exposures low level high stakes*, New York, 1991, Van Nostrand Reinhold.

Axelson O and others: Current aspects of solvent related disorders. In Zenc C, editor: *Developments in occupational medicine*, St Louis, 1977, Mosby.

Baker E: *Small animal allergy: a practical guide*, Malvern, Penn, 1990, Lea & Febiger.

Battelle Columbus Laboratory: *A chronic inhalation study in rats and mice exposed to formaldehyde: final report for the chemical industry institute of toxicology, vols 1-4, CIIT Docket No 10922*, Raleigh, NC, 1981, Chemical Industry Institute of Toxicology.

Beall JR, Ulsamer AG: Formaldehyde and hepatotoxicity: a review, *J Toxicol Environ Health* 13:1, 1984.

Beebe G: *Toxic carpet III*, Cincinnati, 1991, Author.

Bernstein RS and others: Inhalation exposure to formaldehyde: an overview of its toxicology, epidemiology, monitoring and control, *Am Ind Hyg Assoc J* 45:778, 1984a.

Bernstein RS and others: Nonoccupational exposures to indoor air pollutants: a survey of state programs and practices, *Am J Public Health* 74:1020, 1984b.

Black CM, Welsh KI: Occupationally and environmentally induced scleroderma-like illness: etiology, pathogenesis, diagnosis, and treatment, *Intern Med* 9:135, 1988.

Blair A and others: Mortality among industrial workers exposed to formaldehyde, *J Natl Cancer Inst* 76:1071, 1984.

Bland J, Brally A: Nutritional up-regulation of hepatic detoxification enzymes, *J Appl Nutr* 44:2, 1992.

Blum K and others: Alleic association of human dopamine D2 receptor gene in alcoholism, *JAMA* 263:2055, 1990.

Bosquet J, Michel FB: Specific immunotherapy for asthma: is it effective? *Allergy Clin Immunol* 94:1, 1994.

Boren T and others: Attachment of *H. pylori* to human gastric epithelium mediated by blood group antigens, *Science* 262:1892, 1993.

Boris M, Schiff M, Weindorf S: Antigen-induced asthma attenuated by neutralization therapy, *Clin Ecol* 3:59, 1985.

Boris MN, Schiff M, Weindorf S: Injection of low-dose antigen attenuates the response to subsequent bronchoprovocative challenge, *Otolaryngol Head Neck Surg* 98:539, 1988.

Boris M and others: Late phase response treated with neutralization therapy, presented at the 21st Scientific Session of the American Academy of Environmental Medicine, Oct 31, 1987, Nashville, Tenn.

Boris M and others: Bronchoprovocation blocked by neutralizing therapy, abstracted, *J Allergy Clin Immunol* 71:92, 1983.

Broder I and others: Comparison of health of occupants and characteristics of houses among control homes and homes insulated with urea formaldehyde foam. II. Initial health and house variables and exposure-response relationships, *Environ Res* 45:156, 1988.

Brostoff J: A double-blind crossover placebo-controlled study of neutralization, presented at the 20th Advance Seminar of the American Academy of Environmental Medicine, Oct 27, 1986, Clearwater, Fla.

Brostoff J, Challacombe SJ: *Food allergy and intolerance,* Philadelphia, 1987, Bailliere Tindall.

Brostoff J, Scadding G: Low dose sublingual therapy in patients with allergic rhinitis due to house dust mite, *Clin Allergy* 16:483, 1986.

Broughton A, Thrasher JD: Antibodies and altered cell mediated immunity in formaldehyde exposed humans, *Comments on Toxicology* 2:155, 1988.

Brown C: Drug and nutrient interactions, *Perspect Appl Nutr* 3:10, 1995.

Bucca C: Effect of vitamin C on histamine bronchial responsiveness of patients with allergic rhinitis, *Ann Allergy* 65:311, 1990.

Buist R: The malfunctional "mucosal barrier" and food allergies, *Int Clin Nutr Rev* 3:1, 1983.

Caldwell J, Jacoby WB, editors: Impact of nutrition on detoxication. In Caldwell J, Jacoby WB, editors: *Biological basis of detoxication,* New York, 1983, Academic Press.

Campbell MB: Neurologic manifestations of allergic disease, *Ann Allergy* 31:485, 1973.

Cannon LA and others: Magnesium levels in cardiac arrest victims: relationship between magnesium levels and successful resuscitation, *Ann Emerg Med* 16:1195, 1987.

Carlsson A, Ljungquist E: Exposure to toluene: concentration in subcutaneous adipose tissue, *Scand J Work Environ Health* 8:56, 1982.

Carter JP and others: *J Am Coll Nutr* 12:209, 1993.

Casanovea M, Heck Hd'A: Further studies of the metabolic incorporation and covalent binding of inhaled [3H]-and [14C] formaldehyde in fischer-334 rats: effects of glutathione depletion, *Toxicol Appl Pharmacol* 89:105, 1987.

Council on Scientific Affairs: In vivo diagnostic testing and immunotherapy for allergy. Report I, part I, part II, Report II of the Allergy Panel, *JAMA* 258:1363, 1987.

Cox IM, Campbell MJ, Dowson D: Red blood cell magnesium and chronic fatigue syndrome, *Lancet* 337:757, 1991.

Dally KA, Hanrahan LP, Woodbury MA: Formaldehyde exposure in nonoccupational environments, *Arch Environ Health* 36:277, 1981.

Davis DL, Magee BH: Cancer and industrial chemical production, *Science* 206:1356, 1978.

Davison HM: The role of food sensitivity in nasal allergy, *Ann Allergy* 9:568, 1951.

Dees SC: Allergic epilepsy, *Ann Allergy* 9:446, 1951.

Deitch EA and others: Bacterial translocation from the gut impairs systemic immunity, *Surgery* 109:269, 1991.

Denkhaus W and others: Lymphocyte subpopulations in solvent-exposed workers, *Int Arch Occup Environ Health* 57:109, 1986.

Derlacki EL: Food sensitization as a cause of perennial nasal allergy, *Ann Allergy* 13:682, 1955.

Dohan FC: Wartime changes in hospital admissions for schizophrenia, *Acta Psychiatr Scand* 42:1, 1966.

Dossing M and others: Effect of ethanol, cimetidine, and propanol on toluene metabolism in man, *Int Arch Occup Environ Health* 54:309, 1984.

Doube A, Collins AJ: Is the gut intrinsically abnormal in rheumatoid arthritis? *Ann Rheum Dis* 47:617, 1988.

Draper WL: Food testing in allergy, *Arch Otolaryngol* 95:169, 1972.

Dye J, Costa D: A brief guide to indoor air pollutants and relevance to small animals. In *Current Veterinary Therapy XII,* Philadelphia, 1995, WB Saunders.

East West Foundation: *Cancer-free, 30 who triumphed over cancer naturally,* New York, 1991, Japan Publishers.

Egger J and others: Is migraine food allergy? A double-blind controlled trial of oligoantigenic diet treatment, *Lancet* 2:865, 1983.

Emmerson B: Toxic nephropathy. In Wyngarden JB, Smith, editors: *Textbook of medicine,* ed 17, Philadelphia, 1985, WB Saunders.

Endicott JN, Stucker FJ: Allergy in Meniere's disease related to fluctuating hearing loss. Preliminary findings in a double-blind crossover clinical study, *Laryngoscope* 87:1650, 1977.

Enig MG: *Trans fatty acids in the food supply: a comprehensive report covering 60 years of research,* Silver Spring, Md, 1995, Enig Associates.

Ertle T and others: Metabolism of trichloroethylene in man, *Arch Toxicol* 29:171, 1972.

Fedotin MS: *Helicobacter pylori* and peptic ulcer disease, *Postgrad Med* 94:38, 1993.

Fein BT, Kamin PB: Allergy, convulsive disorders and epilepsy, *Ann Allergy* 26:241, 1968.

Felder M, de Blecourt ACE, Wuthrich B: Food allergy in patients with rheumatoid arthritis, *Clin Rheumatol* 6:181, 1987.

Feldman RG, Ricks NL, Baker EL: Neuropsychological effects of industrial toxins: a review, *Am J Ind Med* 1:211, 1980.

Fernandez JG and others: Trichloroethylene exposure: simulation of uptake, excretion and metabolism using a mathematical model, *Br J Ind Med* 34:43, 1977.

Feuer G, de la Iglesia FA: *Molecular biochemistry of human disease, vol I,* Boca Raton, Fla, 1985, CRC Press.

Fikes JD and others: Clinical, biochemical, electrophysiologic, and histologic assessment of chlorpyrifos induced delayed neuropathy in the cat, *Neurotoxicology* 13:663, 1992.

Finn R, Battcock TM: A critical study of ecology, *Practitioner* 229:883, 1985.

Folkers K and others: Biochemical evidence for a deficiency of vitamin B_6 in the carpal tunnel syndrome based on a cross-over clinical study, *Proc Natl Acad Sci USA* 75:3410, 1978.

Forbes GM and others: Duodenal ulcer treated with *H. pylori* eradication, *Lancet* 343:258, 1994.

Forman R: A critique of evaluative studies of sublingual and intracutaneous provocative tests for food allergy, *Med Hypotheses* 7:1019, 1981.

French D, Edsall JT: The reactions of formaldehyde with amino acids and proteins, *Adv Protein Chem* 2:278, 1945.

Furlong TH: Acetyl-L-carnitine: metabolism and applications in clinical practice, *Altern Med Rev* 1(2):85-93, 1996.

Gamble J: Effects of formaldehyde on the respiratory system. In Gibson JE, editor: *Formaldehyde toxicity*, New York, 1983, Hemisphere Publishing Co.

Ganzales MJ: Fish oil, lipid peroxidation and mammary tumor growth, review article, *J Am Coll Nutr* 14:325, 1995.

Garriott J and others: Death from inhalant abuse: toxicology and pathological evaluation of thirty-four cases, *Clin Toxicol* 16:305, 1980.

Good AP, Rochwood R, Schad P: Loratadine and ventricular tachycardia, *Am J Cardiol* 74:207, 1994.

Gope R, Gope ML: Effect of sodium butyrate on the expression of retinoblastoma (RB1) and P53 gene and phosphorylation of retinoblastoma protein in human colon tumor cell line HT29, *Cell Moll Biol (Noisy-le-grand)* 39:589, 1993.

Gosslin RE, Smith RP, Hodge HC: *Clinical toxicology of commercial products*, ed 5, Baltimore, 1984, Williams & Wilkins.

Gray JB and others: Eicosanoids and essential fatty acid modulation in chronic disease and chronic fatigue syndrome, *Med Hypotheses* 43:31, 1994.

Green RG: Diet and otitis media, *Can Family Physician* 29:15, 1983.

Gumkowski P and others: Chronic asthma and rhinitis due to *Candida albicans, Epidermophyton*, and *Trichophyton, Ann Allergy* 59:48, 1987.

Gupta K: *Health effects of formaldehyde*, Washington, DC, 1984, US Consumer Product Safety Commission.

Gupta K, Ulsamer AG, Preuss PW: Formaldehyde in indoor air: sources and toxicity, *Environment International* 8:38, 1982.

Hague A and others: Sodium butyrate induces apoptosis in human colonic tumor cell lines in a p53-independent pathway: implications for the possible role of dietary fibre in the prevention of large-bowel cancer. *Int J Cancer* 55:498, 1993b.

Hague A and others: Escape from negative regulation of growth by transforming growth factor beta and from the induction of apoptosis by the dietary agent sodium butyrate may be important in colorectal carcinogenesis, *Cancer Metastasis Rev* 12:227, 1993a.

Hathcock JN, editor: Micro nutrients in detoxication. In Hathcock JN, editor: *Nutritional toxicology*, Orlando, Fla, 1987, Academic Press.

Hayes WJ: *Pesticides studied in man, organic phosphorus pesticides*, Baltimore, 1982, Williams & Wilkins.

Ho SB and others: Stable differentiation of a human colon adenocarcinoma cell line by sodium butyrate is associated with multidrug resistance, *J Cell Physiol* 160:213, 1994.

Hoj L and others: A double-blind controlled trial of elemental diet in severe perennial asthma, *Allergy* 36:257, 1981.

Holden JM, Wolf WR, Mertz W: Zinc and copper in self selected diets, *J Am Diet Assoc* 75:23, 1979.

Horvath EP and others: Effects of formaldehyde on the mucous membranes and lungs, *JAMA* 259:701, 1988.

Hutt-Taylor SR and others: Sodium butyrate and a T lymphocyte cell line-derived factor induce basophilic differentiation of the human promyelocytic leukemia cell line HL-60, *Blood* 71:209, 1988.

Iseri LT, French JH: Magnesium: nature's physiologic calcium blocker, *Am Heart J* 108:1, 1984.

Iwata K and others: Studies on the toxins produced by *Candida albicans* with special reference to the etiopathological role. In Iwata K, ed: *Yeasts and yeast-like microorganisms in medical science*, Tokyo, 1976, University of Tokyo.

Jackson P and others: Intestinal permeability in patient with eczema and food allergy, *Lancet* 1285, 1981.

Jakoby WB: *Enzymatic basis of detoxication, vols I -II*, London, 1980, Academic Press.

James J, Warrin RP: An assessment of the role of *Candida albicans* and food yeasts in chronic urticaria, *Br J Dermatol* 84:227, 1971.

Jan-Klimberg VA and others: Prophylactic glutamine protects the intestinal mucosa from radiation injury, *Cancer* 1:66:62, 1990.

Jeager D and others: Latex-specific proteins causing immediate-type cutaneous, nasal, bronchial, and systemic reactions, *J All Clin Immunol* 89:759-768, 1992.

Jenkins RT and others: Increased intestinal permeability in patients with rheumatoid arthritis: a side effect of oral NSAID therapy? *Br J Rheumatol* 26:103, 1987.

Jewett DL, Fein G, Greenberg MH: A double blind study of symptom provocation to determine food sensitivity, *N Engl J Med* 323:429, 1990.

Johnston CS, Martin LJ, Cai X: Antihistamine effect of supplemental ascorbic acid and neutrophil chemotaxis, *J Am Clin Nutr* 11:172, 1992.

Karjalainen J and others: A bovine albumin peptide as a possible trigger of insulin-dependent diabetes mellitus, *N Engl J Med* 302, 1992.

Kerdelko NM: Allergy in chronic monilial vaginitis, *Ann Allergy* 29:95, 1971.

Kilburn KH, Warshaw R, Thornton JC: Formaldehyde impairs memory, equilibrium, and dexterity in histology technicians: effects which persist for days after exposure, *Arch Environ Health* 42:117, 1987.

King WP and others: Provocation/neutralization: a two-part study, part I. The intracutaneous provocative food test: a multi-sensor comparison study, *Otolaryngol Head Neck Surg* 99:263, 1988a.

King WP and others: Provocation/neutralization: a two-part study, part II. Subcutaneous neutralization therapy: a multi-center study, *Otolaryngol Head Neck Surg* 99:272, 1988b.

King GS: Sudden death in adolescents resulting from the inhalation of typewriter correction fluid, *JAMA* 253:1604, 1985.

Kjeldsen-Kragh J and others: Controlled trial of fasting and one-year vegetarian diet in rheumatoid arthritis, *Lancet* 338:899, 1991.

Klaasen CD, Amdur MO, Doull J, eds: *Casarett and Doull's toxicology*, ed 3, New York, 1986, Macmillan.

Klein S: Glutamine: an essential nonessential amino acid for the gut, *Gastroenterology* 99:279, 1990.

Klevay LM, Reck SJ, Barcome DP: Evidence of dietary copper and zinc deficiencies, *JAMA* 241:1916, 1979.

Konopinski VJ: Seasonal formaldehyde concentrations in an office building, *Am Ind Hyg Assoc J* 146:65, 1985.

LaMarte FP, Merchant JH, Casale TB: Acute systemic reactions to carbonless copy paper associated with histamine release, *JAMA* 260:248, 1988.

Lamm DL and others: Mega-dose vitamins in bladder cancer: a double-blind clinical trial, *J Urol* 21:76, 1994.

Latex allergy—an emerging healthcare problem, *Ann All Asthma Immunol* [editorial] 75:19-22, 1995.

Law-Chin-Yung L, Freed DLJ: Nephrotic syndrome due to milk allergy, *Lancet* 1:1056, 1977.

Lazar RB and others: Multifocal nervous system damage caused by toluene abuse, *Neurology* 33:1337, 1983.

Leary WP, Reyes AJ: Magnesium and sudden death, *S Afr Med J* 64:697, 1983.

Lee CH and others: Provocative testing and treatment for foods. *Arch Otolaryngol* 90:113, 1969.

Lee CH, Williams RI, Binkley EI, Jr: Provocative inhalant testing and treatment, *Arch Otolaryngol* 90:81, 1960.

Leith JT: Potentiation of x-ray sensitivity of combinations of sodium butyrate and buthionine sulfoximine, *Int J Radiat Oncol Biol Phys* 15:949, 1988.

Li WF, Furlong CE: Serum paraoxonase status: major factor in determining resistance to organophosphates, *J Toxicol Environ Health* 40:337, 1993.

Licorish K and others: Role of *Alternaria* and *Penicillium* spores in the pathogenesis of asthma, *J Allergy Clin Immunol* 76:819, 1985.

Liebeskind A: *Candida albicans* as an allergic factor, *Ann Allergy* 20:394, 1962.

Locky RF and others: Fatalities from immunotherapy and skin testing, *J Allergy Clin Immunol* 79:660, 1987.

Maclarren N, Atkinson M: Is insulin-dependent diabetes mellitus environmentally induced? *N Engl J Med* 327:348, 1992.

Magnesium deficiency: a new risk factor for sudden cardiac death, *Intern Med World Rep* 5:9, 1990.

Magos L: The effects of industrial chemicals on the heart. In Balazs T, editor: *Cardiac toxicology*, Boca Raton, Fla, 1981, CRC Press.

Mandell M, Conte A: A role of allergy in arthritis, rheumatism and polysymptomatic cerebral, visceral and somatic disorders: a double-blind study, *J Int Acad Prev Med* 7:5, 1982.

Marier JR: Magnesium content of the food supply in the modern-day world, *Magnesium* 5:1, 1986.

Marino PL: The hidden threat of magnesium deficiency, *Intern Med* 12:32, 1991.

Marks JG and others: Contact urticaria and airway obstruction from carbonless copy paper, *JAMA* 252:1038, 1984.

Mensink RP, Katan MB: Effect of dietary trans-fatty acids on high-density and low-density lipoprotein cholesterol levels in healthy subjects, *N Eng J Med* 323:439-445, 1990.

Mikhail MS and others: Decreased beta-carotene levels in exfoliated vaginal epithelial cells in women with vaginal candidiasis, *Am J Reprod Immunol* 32:221, 1994.

Miller JB: Hidden food ingredients, chemical food additives, and incomplete food labels, *Ann Allergy* 41:93, 1978.

Miller JB: Intradermal provocation-neutralizing food testing and subcutaneous food extracr infection therapy. In Brostoff J, Challacombe SJ, editors: *Food allergy and intolerance*, London, 1987, Bailliere Tindall.

Miller JB: *Food allergy*, Springfield, Ill, 1972, Charles C Thomas.

Miller JB: Management of food allergy. In Gerrard JW, editor: *Food allergy*, Springfield, Ill, 1980, Charles C Thomas.

Miller JB: Rapid relief of varicella and infectious mononucleosis through immunotherapy, *Ann Allergy* 47:135, 1981.

Miller JB: A double-blind study of food extract injection therapy: a preliminary report, *Ann Allergy* 39:185, 1977.

Mitsuoka T: Bifidobacteria and their role in human health, *J Ind Microbiol* 6:263, 1990.

Monro J and others: Food allergy in migraine: study of dietary exclusion and RAST, *Lancet* 2:1, 1980.

Monster AC, Boersma G, Duba WC: Kinetics of trichloroethylene in repeated exposure to volunteers, *Int Arch Occup Environ Health* 42:282, 1979.

Morgan KT, Patterson DL, Gross EA: Formaldehyde and the nasal mucociliary apparatus. In *Formaldehyde: toxicology, epidemiology, mechanisms*, New York, 1983, Marcel Dekker.

Morris DL: Use of sublingual antigen in diagnosis and treatment of food allergy, *Ann Allergy* 27:289, 1969.

Mott GE and others: Lowering of serum cholesterol by intestinal bacteria in cholesterol-fed piglets, *Lipids* 8:428, 1973.

Muller G, Spassovski M, Henschler D: Metabolism of trichloroethylene in man, *Arch Toxicol* 32:283, 1974.

Mutti A and others: Nephropathies and exposure to perchloroethylene in dry-cleaners, *Lancet* 339:1131, 1992.

National Academy of Sciences: Report of the Federal Panel on Formaldehyde, *Environ Health Perspect* 43:139, 1982.

National Institute of Occupational Safety and Health: Formaldehyde: evidence of carcinogenicity, *Current Intelligence Bulletin* 34, 1981.

National Research Council: *Recommended dietary allowances*, Washington, DC, 1980, National Academy of Sciences.

National Toxicology Program: *Third annual report on carcinogens*, Washington, DC, 1982, US Dept of Health and Human Services.

Nelson RD and others: Two mechanisms of inhibition of human lymphocyte proliferation by soluble yeast mannan polysaccharide, *Infect Immun* 43:1041, 1984.

Netter KJ: The role of nutrients in detoxification mechanisms. In Kotsonis, Mackey, Hjelle, editors: *Nutritional toxicology; target organ toxicology series*, New York, 1994, Raven Press.

Neuringer M, Connor WE: N-3 fatty acids in the brain and retina: evidence for the essentiality, *Nutr Rev* 44:285, 1986.

New misgivings about magnesium, *Science News* 133:32, 1988.

Newman TB, Hulley SB: Carcinogenicity of lipid-lowering drugs, *JAMA* 275:55-60, 1996.

Nicar MJ, Pak CYC: Oral magnesium deficiency, causes and effects, *Hosp Pract* (Off Ed) 116A, 1987.

Nsouli T: Role of food allergy in serous otitis media, *Ann Allergy* 73:215, 1994.

Nussbaum E: *Recovery*, New York, 1986, Japan Publishing.

Ogle KA, Bullock JD: Children with allergic rhinitis and/or bronchial asthma treated with elimination diet: a five year follow-up, *Ann Allergy* 44:273, 1980.

Olsen JH, Dossing M: Formaldehyde induced symptoms in day care centers, *Am Ind Hyg Assoc J* 43:366, 1982.

Ornish D: *Reversing heart disease*, New York, 1990a, Random House.

Ornish D: Can lifestyle changes reverse coronary heart disease? The Lifestyle Trial, *Lancet* 336:624, 1990b.

Orris L, Tesser M: Dermatosis due to water, soaps and solvents. In Maibach H, Gellin G, editors: *Occupational and industrial dermatology*, St Louis, 1982, Mosby.

O'Shea JA and others: Double-blind study of children with hyperkinetic syndrome treated with multi-allergen disabilities, *J Learning Disabilities* 14:189, 1981.

Panush RS and others: Diet therapy for rheumatoid arthritis, *Arthritis Rheum* 26:462, 1983.

Parsonnet J: *H. pylori* as a risk factor for gastric cancer, *Eur J Gastroenterol Hepatol* 5 (suppl 1):S103, 1993.

Pastinszky I: The allergic diseases of the male genitourinary tract with special reference to allergic urethritis and cystitis, *Urol Int* 9:288, 1959.

Pastores SM and others: Immunomodulatory effects and therapeutic potential of glutamine in the critically ill surgical patient, *Nutrition* 10:385, 1994.

Pearson A and others: Intestinal permeability in children with Crohn's disease and cardiac disease, *Br Med J* 285:20, 1982.

Pennington JA, Young BE: The selected minerals in food surveyed from 1982 to 1984, *J Am Diet Assoc* 86:876, July 1986.

Physician's desk reference, ed 51, Montvale, NJ, 1997, Medical Economics.

Piness G, Miller H: The importance of food sensitization in allergic rhinitis, *J Allergy* 2:73, 1931.

Platts-Mills TAE and others: Serum IgE antibodies to trichophyton in patients with urticaria, angioedema, asthma and rhinitis: development of a radioallergosorbent test, *J Allergy Clin Immunol* 79:45, 1987.

Podell R: A critical review of intracutaneous and sublingual provocation and neutralization, *Arch Clin Ecol* 2:13, 1983.

Powell NB and others: Allergy of the lower urinary tract, *J Urol* 107:631, 1972.

Purvis JR, Cummings DM: Effect of oral magnesium supplementations on selected cardiovascular risk factors in non-insulin-dependent diabetics, *Arch Fam Med* 3:503, 1994.

Raloff J: Beyond estrogens. Why unmasking hormone-mimicking pollutants proves so challenging, *Science News* 148:44, 1995.

Randolph T: *An alternative approach to allergies,* New York, 1987, Bantam Books.

Rapp DJ: *Is this your child?* New York, 1991, WM Morrow.

Rapp DJ: Critique of the literature concerning sublingual provocation and neutralization. In Brostoff J, Challacombe SJ, editor: *Food allergy and intolerance,* London, 1987, Bailliere Tindull.

Rapp DJ: Chronic headache due to foods and air pollution, *Ann Allergy* 40:289, 1978a.

Rapp DJ: Hyperactivity and food allergy: are they related? *Ann Allergy* 40:297, 1978b.

Rapp DJ: Herpes progenitalis responding to influenza vaccine, *Ann Allergy* 40:302, 1978c.

Rapp DJ: Food allergy treatment of hyperkinesis, *J Learning Disabilities* 19:42, 1978d.

Rapp DJ: Weeping eyes in wheat allergy, *Trans Am Soc Opthalmol Oto Allergy* 18:149, 1978e.

Rapp DJ: Double-blind confirmation and treatment of milk sensitivity, *Med J Aust* 1:571, 1978f.

Ravenskov U, Forseberg B, Skerfving S: Glomerulonephritis in exposure to organic solvents, *Acta Med Scand* 205:575, 1979.

Rea WJ: *Chemical sensitivity, vol 1 and 2,* Boca Raton, Fla, 1992, CRC.

Rea WJ: *Chemical sensitivity, vol 2,* Boca Raton, Fla, 1994, Lewis.

Rea WJ and others: Elimination of oral food challenge reaction by injection of food extracts, *Arch Otolaryngol* 110:248, 1984.

Rea WJ and others: Magnesium deficiency in patients with chemical sensitivity, *Clin Ecol* 4:17, 1986.

Reidenberg MM and others: Lupus erythematosus-like disease due to hydrazine, *Am J Med* 75:365, 1983.

Reinhardt C and others: Epinephrine-induced cardiac arrhythmias potential of some common industrial solvents, *J Occup Med* 15:953, 1973.

Reinhardt M: Macromolecular absorption of food antigens in health and disease, *Ann Allergy* 53:597, 1984.

Rex DK: An etiologic approach to management of duodenal and gastric ulcers, *J Fam Pract* 38:600, 1994.

Reynolds ES: Hepatotoxicity of chloride and 1,1-chloroethylene, *Am J Pathol* 81(1):219-231, 1975.

Rhinehart RA: Magnesium metabolism: a review with special reference to the relationship between intracellular content and serum levels, *Arch Intern Med* 148:2415, 1988.

Richie IM, Lehnen RG: Formaldehyde-related health complaints of residents living in mobile and conventional homes, *Am J Public Health* 77:323, 1987.

Rinkel HJ: Inhalant allergy, part I: the whealing response of the skin to serial dilution testing, *Ann Allergy* 7:625, 1949.

Rinkel HJ: The management of clinical allergy, *Arch Otolaryngol* 77:50, 1963a.

Rinkel HJ: The management of clinical allergy, part II: etiologic factors and skin titration, *Arch Otolaryngol* 7:42, 1963b.

Rocklin RE and others: Generation of antigen-specific suppressor cells during allergy desensitization, *N Engl J Med* 30:1378, 1976.

Rogers SA: Diagnosing the tight building syndrome, *Environ Health Perspect* 76:195, 1987.

Rogers SA: Zinc deficiency as a model for developing chemical sensitivity, *Int Clin Nutr Rev* 10:253, 1990a.

Rogers SA: Unrecognized magnesium deficiency masquerades as diverse symptoms. Evaluation of an oral magnesium challenge test, *Int Clin Nutr Rev* 11:117, 1991a.

Rogers SA: *Depression cured at last!,* Sarasota, Fla, 1997, Sand Key Publishing.

Rogers SA: *Tired or toxic?* Sarasota, Fla, 1990b, Sand Key Publications.

Rogers SA: A thirteen month work, leisure, sleep environmental fungal survey, *Ann Allergy* 52:338, 1984.

Rogers SA: A comparison of commercially available mold survey services, *Ann Allergy* 50:37, 1983.

Rogers SA: In-home fungal studies, methods to increase the yield, *Ann Allergy* 49:35, 1982.

Rogers SR: *The E.I. syndrome, revised,* Sarasota, Fla, 1996a, Sand Key Publications.

Rogers SA: *The scientific basis for selected environmental medicine techniques,* Sarasota, Fla, 1994, Sand Key Publications.

Rogers SA: *The cure is in the kitchen,* Syracuse, NY, 1992a, Prestige Publications.

Rogers SA: *You are what you ate,* Sarasota, Fla, 1991b, Sand Key Publications.

Rogers SA: *Chemical sensitivity,* New Canaan, Conn, 1995, Keats Publications.

Rogers SA: Chemical sensitivity: breaking the paralyzing paradigm, *Intern Med World Rep* Part I 7:3, 1992b; Part II 7:6, 1992c; Part III 7:8, 1992d.

Rogers SA: Resistant cases: response to mold immunotherapy and environmental and dietary controls, *Clin Ecol* 8:115, 1987.

Rogers SA: Indoor fungi as part of the cause of recalcitrant symptoms of the tight building syndrome, *Environ Internat* 17:271, 1991.

Rogers SA: Provocation-neutralization of cough and wheezing in a horse, *Clin Ecol* 5:185, 1987/1988.

Rogers SA: Case studies of indoor air fungi used to clear recalcitrant conditions. In Berglund B, Lindvall T, Mansson LG, editors: *Healthy buildings, '88,* Stockholm, 1988, Swedish Council for Building Research.

Rogers SA: Diagnosing the tight building syndrome. In Seifert B, Esdorn H, Fischer M, Ruden H, Wegner J, editors: *Indoor air '87,* Proceedings of the 4th International Conference on Indoor Air Quality and Climate, West Berlin, 1987, Institute for Water, Soil, and Air Hygiene.

Rogers SA: Indoor air quality and environmentally induced illness, a technique to revoke chemically induced symptoms in patients, *Proceedings of the ASHRAE Conference,* Atlanta, Ga, 1986, American Society for Heating, Refrigeration, and Air Conditioning Engineers.

Rogers SA: A practical approach to the person with suspected indoor air quality problems, *Int Clin Nutr Rev* 10:253, 1991d.

Rogers SA: Diagnosing the tight building syndrome or diagnosing chemical hypersensitivity, *Environment International* 15:75, 1989.

Rogers SA: Diagnosing chemical hypersensitivity: case examples, *Clin Ecol* 4:129, 1990c.

Rogers SA: *A practical approach to the person with suspected indoor air quality problems,* Toronto, Canada Mortgage and Housing Corporation, 5:345, 1990d.

Rogers SA: Diagnosing the tight building syndrome, an intradermal method to provoke chemically induced symptoms. In Brassser LJ, Mulder WC, editors: 1989, the Hague, Netherlands, Society for Clean Air.

Rogers SA: *Diagnosing the tight building syndrome, an intradermal method to provoke chemically induced symptoms,* In Berlund B, Lindvall T, Mansson LG, editors: 1988, Stockholm, Swedish Council for Building Research.

Rogers SA: *Wellness against all odds,* Syracuse, NY, 1994, Prestige.

Rose DP and others: Influence of diets containing eicosapentaenoic or docosahexaenoic acid on growth and metastasis of breast cancer cells in nude mice, *J Natl Cancer Inst* 87:587, 1995.

Roubenoff R and others: Malnutrition among hospitalized patients: problem of physician awareness, *Arch Intern Med* 147:1462, 1987.

Rowe AH, Young EJ: Bronchial asthma due to food allergy alone in 95 patients, *JAMA* 169:1158, 1959.

Rowe AH, Rowe A: Food allergy: its role in emphysema and chronic bronchitis, *Dis Chest* 48:609, 1965a.

Rowe AH, Rowe A Jr: Perennial nasal allergy due to food sensitization, *J Asthma Res* 3:141, 1965b.

Rudin DO: The major psychoses and neurosis as n-3 essential fatty acid deficiency syndrome: substrate pellagra, *Biol Psychiatry* 16:837, 1981.

Samet JM, Marbury MC, Spengler JD: Respiratory effects of indoor air pollution, *J Allergy Clin Immunol* 79:685, 1987.

Sandberg DH and others: Severe steroid-responsive nephrosis associated with hypersensitivity, *Lancet* 1:388, 1977.

Schroeder JA, Nason AP, Tipton IH: Essential metals in man, magnesium, *J Chron Dis* 21:815, 1969.

Schroy PC and others: Growth and intestinal differentiation are independently regulated in HT29 colon cancer cells, *J Cell Physiol* 161:111, 1994.

Schwartz HJ, Ward GW: Onychomycosis, *Trichophyton* allergy and asthma—a causal relationship? *Ann Allergy Asthma Immunol* 74:523, 1995.

Scott CS, Margosches EH: Cancer epidemiology relevant to formaldehyde, *J Environ Sci Health* 3:107, 1985.

Seelig CB: Magnesium deficiency in hypertension uncovered by magnesium load retention, *J Am Clin Nutr* 8:5, 1989.

Seelig M: Cardiovascular consequences of magnesium deficiency and loss: pathogenesis, prevalence, and manifestations—magnesium and chloride loss in refractory potassium repletion, *Am J Cardiol* 53:4g, 1989.

Seelig MS: Mechanisms by which antibiotics increase the incidence and severity of candidiasis and alter the immunological defenses, *Bacteriol Rev* 30:442, 1966.

Shahini KM, Friend BA: Nutritional and therapeutic aspects of lactobacilli, *J Appl Nutr* 37:136, 1973.

Shrive E and others: Glutamine in treatment of peptic ulcer, *Tex J Med* 53:840, 1957.

Shusterman DJ, Blanc PC: Occupational medicine: state of the art reviews, *Unusual Occupational Diseases* 7:3, 1992.

Siegel E: *Essential fatty acids in health and disease,* Brookline, Mass, 1994, Nutrek Inc Press.

Singh RB, Cameron EA: Relation of myocardial magnesium deficiency to sudden death in ischaemic heart disease, *Am Heart J* 103:3, 399, 1982.

Sipes G, Gandolfi AJ: Biotransformation of toxicants. In Klaasen CD, Amdur MD, Doul J, editors: *Casarett & Doull's toxicology,* ed 3, New York, 1986, Macmillan.

Sittig M: *Handbook of toxic and hazardous chemicals,* 1981, Noyes Publications.

Smith R: Organic foods versus supermarket foods, *J Appl Nutr* 45:35, 1993.

Sterling DA: Volatile organic compounds in indoor air: an overview of sources, concentrations and health effects. In Gammage RB, Kaye SV, Jacobs VA, editors: *Indoor air and human health,* Chelsea, 1985, Lewis Publishers.

Stock TH, Mendez SR: A survey of typical exposures to formaldehyde in the Houston area, *Am Ind Hyg Assoc J* 46:313, 1985.

Strobel S: Mechanisms of gastrointestinal immunoregulation and food induced injury to the gut, *Eur J Clin Nutr* 45 (suppl):1, 1991.

Suzuki M and others: *H. pylori* elicits gastric mucosal cell damage associated with neutrophil-derived toxic oxidants, *Eur J Gastroenterol Hepatol* 5(suppl 1):S35, 1993.

Swenberg JA and others: The effect of formaldehyde on cytotoxicity and cell proliferation. In *Formaldehyde: toxicology, epidemiology, mechanisms,* New York, 1983, Marcel Dekker.

Systemic reactions from allergen immunotherapy, *J Allergy Clin Immunol* 567, 1992 (editorial).

Tamura K and others: Ammonia produced by *H. pylori,* related to superoxide generation in situ, as a major factor in acute gastritis, *Eur J Gastroenterol Hepatol* 5(suppl 1):S51, 1993.

Thrasher J, Broughton A: *The poisoning of our homes and workplaces,* 1984, Antigen Assay Labs.

Thrasher JD and others: Building-related illness and antibodies to conjugates of formaldehyde, toluene diisocyanate and trimellitic anhydride, *Am J Ind Med* 15:187, 1989.

Thrasher JD and others: Evidence for formaldehyde antibodies and altered cellular immunity in subjects exposed to formaldehyde in mobile homes, *Arch Environ Health* 42:347, 1987.

Thrasher JD, Broughton A, Micevich P: Antibodies and immune profiles of individuals occupationally exposed to formaldehyde: six case reports, *Am J Ind Med* 14:479, 1988.

Ulsamer AG and others: Overview of health effects of formaldehyde. In *Hazard assessment of chemicals: current developments, vol. 3,* New York, 1984, Academic Press.

US Environmental Protection Agency: *Formaldehyde health risk assessment,* Washington, DC, 1987, US Environmental Protection Agency.

US Environmental Protection Agency: *Indoor air referenced bibliography,* Washington, DC, July 1990, Office of Health and Environmental Assessment.

US Environmental Protection Agency: *Toluene, health and environment effects,* Profile No 160, Washington, DC, April 30, 1980, Office of Solid Waste.

Van de Loar MAFJ, Van der Korst JK: Rheumatoid arthritis, food and allergy, *Semin Arthritis Rheum* 21:12, 1991.

Van Metre TE and others: Immunotherapy for cat asthma, *J Allergy Clin Immunol* 6:1055, 1988.

Van Niekerk CH, DeWet JI: Efficacy of grass-maize pollen oral immunotherapy in patients with seasonal hay fever: a double-blind study, *Clin Allergy* 17:507, 1987.

van Tol A and others: Dietary trans fatty acids increase serum cholesterylester transfer protein activity in man, *Atherosclerosis* 115:129, 1995.

Vesterberg O, Astrand I: Exposure to trichloroethylene monitored by analysis of metabolites in blood and urine, *J Occup Med* 18:224, 1976.

Voigts A: Acidosis and other metabolic abnormalities associated with paint sniffing, *South Med J* 76:443, 1983.

Walker W: Transmucosal passage of antigens. In Schmidt E, editor: *Food allergy,* New York, 1988, Raven Press.

Wallace L and others: Concentration of 20 volatile organic compounds in air and drinking water of 350 residents of New Jersey compared with concentrations in their exhaled breath, *J Occup Med* 38:603, 1986.

Ward GW and others: Trichophyton asthmas: sensitization of bronchial and upper airways to dermatophyte antigen, *Lancet* 859, 1989.

Whang R, Ryder KW: Frequency of hypomagnesemia and hypermagnesemia, requested versus routine, *JAMA* 2634:3063, 1990.

Wilcox and others: Gastrointestinal hemorrhage and the use of NSAIDS, *Arch Intern Med* 154:42, 1994.

Wilhelmsson B, Homlstrom M: Positive formaldehyde-rast after prolonged formaldehyde exposure by inhalation, *Lancet* 2:164, 1987.

Williams RI: Skin titration: testing and treatment, *Otolaryngol Clin North Am* 4:3, 1971.

Williams RI: Technique of serial dilution antigen titration, *Arch Otolaryngol* 89:109, 1969.

Willoughby JW: Serial dilution titration skin tests in inhalant allergy: a clinical quantitative assessment of biologic skin reactivity to allergenic extracts, *Otolaryngol Clin North Am* 7:579, 1974.

Willoughby JW: Diagnosis of allergy by serial dilution skin end-point titration, *Cont Ed Fam Physicians* 11:21, 1979.

Willoughby JW: *Intracutaneous serial dilution titration in clinical allergy.* Printed privately for the postgraduate course in clinical allergy, April 1973, Kansas City, Mo.

Witkin SS, Yu IR, Ledger WJP: Inhibition of *Candida albicans*-induced lymphocyte proliferation by lymphocytes and sera from women with recurrent vaginitis, *Am J Obstet Gynecol* 147:809, 1983.

Witkin SS: Defective immune responses in patients with recurrent candidiasis, *Infections in Medicine,* pp 129-132, May/June 1985.

Woodbury MA, Zenz C: Formaldehyde in the home environment: prenatal and infant exposures. In Gibson JE, editor: *Formaldehyde toxicity,* New York, 1983, Hemisphere Publishing Corp.

Yuesheng W and others: A major inducer of anticarcinogenic protective enzymes from broccoli. Isolation and elucidation of structure. *Proc Natl Acad Sci USA* 89:2399, 1992.

Zimmerman H: Environmental hepatotoxicity. In *Hepatotoxicity,* New York, 1978, Appleton-Century-Crofts.

Zimmerman N: The carcinogenic potential of formaldehyde, *Comments on Toxicology,* June, 1988.

Zinc: a public health problem, *Nutrition and MD* 18:4, 1992.

*R*ESOURCES

NOTE: Most of the references, with discussion (and our papers in toto), can be found in the following books:

Rogers, SA: *Depression cured at last!*

Rogers SA: *Tired or toxic?*

Rogers SA: *Wellness against all odds*

Rogers SA: *The scientific basis for selected environmental medicine techniques*

Rogers SA: *The E.I. syndrome, revised*

Rogers SA: *You are what you ate*

Rogers SA: *The cure is in the kitchen*

Gallinger SG, Rogers SA: *Macro mellow*

Rogers SA: *Total Health* (monthly subscription newsletter, featuring new findings, referenced).

All these books are available from Sand Key Publishing, Box 40101, Sarasota, FL 34278, or 1-800-846-6687, or Prestige Publishing, Box 3161, Syracuse, NY 13220.

Also available are the formaldehyde spot test (for testing home and office supplies, textiles, furnishings, etc.), and special petri dishes or mold plates for culturing airborne molds and body secretions, and scheduled phone conversations with the author.

Chapter **30**

Aromatherapy

SUSAN G. WYNN, MICHAEL D. KIRK-SMITH

Aromatherapy is the therapeutic use of volatile essential oils to effect a psychologic or physiologic response. The oils are administered in a number of ways: by diffusion or nebulization, with massage or by topical application, and, rarely, orally. Aromatherapy is similar to herbal therapy in that natural plant substances are used medicinally. Unlike herbal therapy, however, volatile oils are used because of their ready absorption through the nasal mucosa or skin. Herbal therapy also makes use of whole plant derivatives, which include aqueous components excluded in essential oil preparation. Aromatherapy is probably an ancient therapy, although it is not well known today. The practice is experiencing a renaissance, however, especially in France and England (in fact, French medical schools sometimes include it in the curriculum) (Lavabre, 1990).

History

Aromatic plant combustion, or fumigation, was probably used early in human history; in fact, the word *perfume* is derived from the Latin terms *per*, for "through," and *fumus*, for "smoke." Fragrant oils and spices were used thousands of years ago in the Middle East and Egypt, before the Christian Era. One reason for the major international trade in these oils was their medicinal value (Doty, 1995b). Essential oil isolation was not described until Herodotus mentioned distillation of turpentine beginning about the fifth century BC (Guenther, 1948). Distillation was commonly used by the Arabs in early medieval times, and refinement of the techniques occurred around the thirteenth century, when pharmacies prepared "remedy oils" and began to compile pharmacopoeias to record their actions (Bauer and others, 1990). The description of essential oil actions by Paracelsus (1493-1541) probably accounts for the name "essential" oil; he theorized that the "quinta essentia" (quintessence) represents the "last possible and most sublime extractive" and that this isolation should be

the goal of pharmaceutical preparation (Guenther, 1948). The medicinal properties of various essential oils were catalogued by Lemery in his *Pharmacopée Universalle* in 1697 (Doty, 1995b). The term *aromatherapy* was not coined until Gattefosse turned his attention to the use of essential oils in medicine with the publication of his novel work in 1937 (Gattefosse, 1937). Gattefosse compiled the work of a number of scientists in the field at that time by characterizing the chemistry of the oils, as well as their traditional medical uses. He concluded that "besides their antiseptic and bactericidal properties . . . essential oils possess anti-toxic and antiviral properties, have a powerful vitalizing action, an undeniable healing power and extensive therapeutic properties" (Gattefosse, 1937).

Today the flavor and fragrance industry is responsible for most new findings in essential oil chemistry. The trend in scientific investigations is to identify characteristic aromatic substances that occur in large and small amounts to produce "nature identical" and synthetic essential oils (Bauer and others, 1990). Aromatherapy is presently gaining a commercial reputation along with its medicinal reputation; it is commonly used by companies in the United States to create a "mood" in customers, to encourage increased purchases in stores, and to encourage productivity (Griffin, 1992). Researchers at the Taste Treatment and Research Foundation have even found that Las Vegas slot machines took in almost 45% more money when patrons were dosed with attractive odors (*Your Health*, 1992).

The use of aromatherapy in veterinary medicine is largely unexplored. Accounts of veterinary disease management by inhalant therapy are found rarely in the historical literature. One description of a treatment for glanders in horses recommended that animals with pulmonary symptoms be made to inhale origanum vapor (probably oregano) daily for 3 days. The vapor was produced by heating an earthenware pot over a charcoal fire, a form of "dry fumigation." Aspyrte wrote in the fourth century that treatment of horses with fumigations was an ancient practice (Blancou, 1994).

A report on traditional veterinary medicine in Sri Lanka also claims that fumigation is a common practice. Again, heat is used to cause aromatic plants to burn, producing scented smoke. Elephants are commonly treated in this manner, often cloaked by mats or gunny bags to retain the smoke. Clinical indications for fumigation include indigestion, constipation, colic, bloat, anuria, and myiasis. Plants used in fumigation include *Cuminum cyminum* (seed), *Cinnamonum zeylanicum*, *Piper longum*, *Piper nigrum*, *Vitex negundo*, *Oeinum locilicum*, and *Azadirachta indica* (Wasantha Piyadasa, 1994).

Modern descriptions of the use of essential oils are sparse. Gattefosse experimented with certain oils for intrauterine and intravesical injection for their anesthetic and "calmative" properties on membranes (Gattefosse, 1937). Only one book published to date is devoted entirely to veterinary aromatherapy (Grosjean, 1994), but the oil mixtures and indications are derived entirely from traditional human uses. Clinical indications for essential oil prescriptions in animals are not yet well characterized. More original research is necessary to determine the best use of aromatherapy in veterinary medicine.

Essential Oil Chemistry

Description

Essential oils are volatile, lipophilic substances obtained from plant materials by distillation, mechanical separation (pressing), or solvent extraction. The oils are mainly hydrocarbon metabolites of monoterpenes and sesquiterpenes, phenylpropanoids, amino acids, and fatty acids. Volatility is largely a function of molecular mass. Molecular weights of about 200 are found most commonly in essential oils. In perfumery the "top notes" are often the most volatile, changing in composition the most during evaporation, whereas the "middle notes" and "end note," or "dry out," are less volatile and longer lasting (Bauer and others, 1990). Odor descriptions are listed in Box 30-1.

Sources

Essential oils are obtained from the flowers, buds, fruits, peel, leaves, bark, wood, roots, seeds, and resins of plants. The composition of any oil can vary widely with plant source. Geographic location, plant cultivation techniques, soil structure, and climate heavily influence the essential quality in any plant species (Bauer and others, 1990). Aromatherapists generally agree that only organically grown plants should be used for essential oil production. Therapists claim that organically grown plants are of better quality, but an additional concern is the amount of organic pesticide and herbicide that survives the distillation of extraction processes. One worldwide problem is

BOX 30-1	
ODOR DESCRIPTIONS	
Aldehydic	Long-chain fatty aldehydes (e.g., sweat, ironed laundry, seawater)
Animalic	Typical notes: musk, castoreum, skatol, civet, ambergris
Balsamic	Heavy, sweet odors (e.g., vanilla, cocoa, cinnamon)
Camphoraceous	Camphor
Citrus	
Earthy	Similar to humid earth
Fatty	Similar to animal fat
Floral, flowery	
Fruity	
Green	Freshly cut grass
Herbaceous	Complex herbal odors (e.g., sage, mint, eucalyptus)
Medicinal	Phenol, lysol, methyl salicylate
Metallic	
Minty	
Mossy	Forests, seaweed
Powdery	
Resinous	Tree exudate
Spicy	
Waxy	Similar to candle wax
Woody	Cedarwood, sandalwood

Modified from Bauer K and others: *Common fragrance and flavor materials*, New York, 1990, VCH.

monitoring claims of "organic" plant production processes. Confirming a manufacturer's claims regarding organic essential oils is currently difficult, if not impossible. Aromatherapists point to food contamination as a source for much greater levels of "biocides" than those encountered in essential oil therapeutics (Tisserand, Balacs, 1995).

Synthetic essential oils are widely available and probably constitute a large proportion of many commercially available brands. Most components of natural essential oils are common to many plant species. For instance, pinene, camphor, and limonene are found in many different oils. Some authorities have stated that as few as 500 compounds account for 90% of the constituents in essential oils in most species (Adams, 1989). Natural medicine practitioners argue that natural-source essential oils are too complex to be reproduced synthetically and that their unique therapeutic effects result from this complexity. Differences in oil composition are responsible for the different "chemotypes" within a plant species (Tisserand, Balacs, 1995). One advantage to synthetic oils is purity and absence of pesticide contaminants. Synthetic oils would be superior for research purposes because a degree of standardization of active components is possible.

Preparation

Essential oils are isolated in one of three ways. Steam distillation is most commonly used to separate volatile components. Distillates may contain more thermolabile components, which are only released from the plant under distillation conditions. Solvent extraction is used if nonvolatile components are desired or if the plant material is of low yield (e.g., from blossoms or resins). Pressing is also used if certain nonvolatile components are desirable. Citrus peel, for example, yields dyes, waxes, and furocoumarins, as well as the characteristic volatile substances stored in small oil glands in the peel (Bauer and others, 1990; Tisserand, Balacs, 1995).

Selection of Oils

Because purity and composition cannot yet be guaranteed, certain precautions should be borne in mind when purchasing essential oils. A common admonishment is to buy from reputable suppliers, but even aromatherapists cannot agree as to who these suppliers are (Mackereth, 1995). One therapist recommends that a buyer closely examine the price range of all oils offered in a line. Prices that do not vary widely raise suspicions of adulteration because oil sources range from the extremely precious (linden, frankincense) to the very common (pine, lavender) (Clayton, 1992). Aromatherapists tend to be suspicious of synthetic oils because of the holistic, "vitalist" associations inherent in this treatment modality (Engen, 1991). When examining the label, consumers should ensure that the entire botanical name—genus and species—is listed because different species within a genus may contain different active components. Some exploration and experimentation will be necessary before large essential oil investments are made. Some large suppliers are listed in the resources section at the end of the chapter.

Olfactory Physiology and Transnasal Systemic Medication

The potential for direct psychologic and physical effects becomes clear when the anatomy of the olfactory system is examined. In the nasal mucosa, chemoreceptors give rise to axons that synapse on the olfactory bulb. Olfactory neurons run through the olfactory tract to the olfactory cortex. Behavioral reactions to scent are mediated by direct connections to the limbic system. Dog and cat olfactory nerve function is routinely assessed by exposure to alcohol, cloves, xylol, benzol, or fish-flavored cat food. The nasal mucosa is innervated by the olfactory and trigeminal nerves (Oliver, Lorenz, 1983).

Chemosensory research has determined that different chemicals stimulate different nerve endings in the nasal mucosa. For instance, substances termed "pure odorants" are those whose action focuses on the olfactory nerve alone, whereas "impure odorants" tend to stimulate trigeminal nerve endings. One study demonstrated that some "impure odorants" produced "augmented inspirations without altering respiration per se." In one large study, people with neither trigeminal nerve function nor olfactory function alone could detect various scents as well as normal subjects. Because essential oils may contain a variety of "pure" and "impure" components, essential oil therapeutic action would tend to be mediated by both trigeminal and olfactory nerves (Doty, 1995a).

Although the human olfactory system is sensitive enough to distinguish thousands of chemicals at lower concentrations than are detectable by most analytic instruments (Doty, 1995b), differences among species probably exist. Differences in relative proportions of olfactory sensory tissue, as well as increased folding of the turbinates, may account for increased deposition of inhaled particles, leading to increased olfactory sensitivity or discrimination in some species, especially in the dog (Lewis, Dahl, 1995).

The rich vasculature and large surface area of the nasal mucosa are well recognized, so drug absorption through the membranes has great therapeutic potential. Intranasal drug delivery for the treatment of sinus congestion and diabetes insipidus has been used for years. Other drugs administered intranasally include propranolol, hydralazine, atropine, and vaccines such as influenza, polio, measles, respiratory syncytial virus (Bond, 1987), canine infectious tracheobronchitis, and feline infectious peritonitis. Nebulization as a drug delivery vehicle is becoming increasingly popular for a number of reasons in veterinary medicine. It is less stressful for certain species, such as exotic birds, reptiles, and lab animals, and it allows for rapid drug absorption with documented systemic therapeutic blood levels. When gastrointestinal complications such as drug stability or hepatic first-pass metabolism exist, intranasal drug administration is an accepted alternative to oral administration for certain drugs. Intranasal administration of lipophilic drugs has resulted in blood levels similar to those observed by IV administration in dogs, rats, and humans (Chien, 1985).

Volatile or topical elements can affect the body in a number of ways. For instance, absorption directly from the nasal mucosa can effect physiologic change by pharmacologic means. Chemoreceptor stimulation may directly supply information to the olfactory cortex and the limbic system. Alternatively, axoplasmic transport of some substances may cause different signals at higher levels in the brain. In fact, numerous studies have demonstrated that olfactory manipulation, including bulbectomy, anesthesia, and ablation, can change mating and copulatory behaviors in various species (Doty, 1995a). The direct connections to neuroendocrine and limbic structures suggest that some relationships between odor and psychologic state may be hardwired (Kirk-Smith, Booth, 1987). Although this concept carries much potential for the treatment of human psychologic states, the neurologic meaning of certain odors for animals is unclear.

Physical and Social Implications of Odor in Domestic Animals

Certain mammalian scent glands came to the attention of perfumers early in history. Musk is produced in the preputial gland of the musk deer, *Moschus moschatus.* Civet is produced in the anal glands of *Viverra civetta,* and castor is a product of castor glands of the beaver *(Castor canadensis).* Ambergris, produced in the intestines of the sperm whale, has been used since antiquity as a source of scent. Darwin speculated that scent glands and odors in animals serve defense and reproduction functions. Another function since postulated is that of social recognition. Compared with mammals, birds have fewer scent glands and, sometimes, brighter coloring. The greater variety of scent glands found in mammals may therefore represent a unique evolutionary strategy for intraspecies communication (Brown, 1979).

The attempt to decipher olfactory communication among animals has been compared to the attempt to translate a foreign language "based on the order and abundance of words, but with little inkling of their (chemical) spelling and even less of their meaning" (Macdonald, Brown, 1984). Although the functions of the different glandular secretions among domestic animals remain unclear, certain signals seem promising as communication vehicles. The domestic dog, *Canis familiaris,* uses anal sacs, supracaudal glands, perioral cheek glands, foot glands, saliva, urine, and feces. *Felis catis,* the domestic cat, probably uses anal sacs, subcaudal glands, supracaudal glands, saliva, urine, and feces to communicate (Macdonald, Brown, 1984). Horses may use circumanal, circumoral, perineal, vomeronasal, flehmen, and feces as a means for communication (Moehlman, 1984). Many glandular secretions from these species vary among individuals, and in an individual the secretions may be influenced by hormonal or possibly even emotional states (Macdonald, Brown, 1984).

The term *pheromone* was coined to describe ectohormones, the function of which is intraspecies communication. "Whether a behavioral or physiologic response is elicited depends on the nature of the odor and the ability of the receiver to extract information about the sender from the odor" (Brown, 1979). An allomone, on the other hand, is a chemical signal that evokes an interspecies response favorable to the emitter of the odor (Macdonald, Brown, 1984). Plant allomones may exert some effect on animals. Some animal steroids are found in plants (Cooke, 1994), and essential oils, although a metabolic by-product of plants of incidental importance to the plant, seem to have

functions similar to those of animal pheromones (i.e., reproduction and defense) (Guenther, 1948). It is tempting to view this coevolution of the pheromone strategy as a natural opportunity to exploit a wider range of signals in the treatment of our animal patients.

Given the important role of odor in animal communication, not to mention the potential for therapeutic use of scents, practitioners should remember that an anosmic animal will not fully respond to aromatherapy. Although anosmia is difficult to document, possible causes include upper respiratory tract viral infections, head trauma, and nasal and sinus disease (Doty, 1995a).

The subject of communication through pheromones relates to odors produced by the animals themselves. The remainder of this chapter gives examples of possible uses of the pharmacologic, physiologic, and psychologic effects of plant essential oils and other odors in veterinary practice.

Potential Clinical Use of Aromatherapy

Antibacterial and Antifungal Effects

The pharmacologic use of plant extracts (i.e., phytopharmacognosy) is a long-established academic discipline. Similarly the antibacterial and antifungal properties of many plant essential oils are well established (Deans, Ritchie, 1987). Indeed, plants produce the oils to defend themselves against invading microorganisms; one might argue that they have had more time to evolve effective defenses than mammals. In recent years interest has been renewed in naturally occurring, wide-spectrum antimicrobial agents, especially given the development of resistance of microorganisms to single chemicals. Two examples are given here to suggest the range and efficacy of these effects.

Tea tree
Some of this attention has focused on tea tree oil, the essential oil of the Australian plant *Melaleuca alternifolia.* Tea tree oil, which is produced by steam distillation of the freshly harvested leaves and terminal branchlets of *Melaleuca alternifolia,* is a pale-yellow viscous liquid with a distinctive pungent odor that is composed of a complex mixture of monoterpenes, 1-terpinen-4-ol, cineole, and other hydrocarbons (Carson, Riley, 1993), with the main active antimicrobial ingredient being 1-terpinen-4-ol (Williams, Home, 1995). Gas chromatography has revealed 97 components (Brophy and others, 1989), with 1-terpinen-4-ol and seven others demonstrating in vitro antimicrobial activity against a range of microorganisms, including *Candida albicans, Lactobacillus acidophilus, Enterococcus faecalis,* and *Staphylococcus aureus* (Carson, Riley, 1995). The antimicrobial activity of tea tree oil was originally identified and used by the Australian aborigines in tinctures and poultices; however, clinical use began with the extensive research into its disinfectant and antiseptic properties since the 1920s (Carson, Riley, 1993). In vitro

tests show activity against *Escherichia coli, Mycobacterium smegmatis, Clostridium perfringens, L. acidophilus, Bacteroides fragilis, S. aureus, Serratia marcescens, B. subtilis,* and *C. albicans* (Carson, Riley, 1994a). The susceptibility of 32 strains of *Propionibacterium acnes* to tea tree oil was also examined using a broth dilution method. The minimum bactericidal concentration of tea tree oil for five strains was 0.25% or less, whereas for the remainder it was 0.50% (Carson, Riley, 1994b). Shapiro and others (1994) found tea tree oil to be active against a range of anaerobic oral bacteria (obligate and capnophilic microaerophiles and facultative anaerobes), inhibiting their growth at concentrations of less than 0.6%. As mentioned previously, essential oils are broad-spectrum antibiotics, presumably because many components are active and also may act synergistically. Essential oils may be used when resistance to conventional antibiotics has developed. For example, Carson and others (1995) found that all 66 isolates of *S. aureus* were killed by tea tree oil in in vitro tests. Of these, 64 were methicillin-resistant *S. aureus,* and 33 were mupirocin resistant. The minimal inhibitory concentration (MIC) and MBC for 60 Australian isolates were 0.25% and 0.50%, respectively.

Clinically, tea tree oil has been used to treat vaginal infections. Blackwell (1991) reports a woman with bacterial vaginosis who used a 5-day course of tea tree pessaries; standard clinical testing revealed a complete cure after 28 days. Pena (1962) gives an anecdotal account of 130 patients who had various vaginal complaints and reported clinical cures among 96 patients with trichomonal vaginitis after using tampons saturated with tea tree oil and daily douches with 0.4% oil. Belaiche (1985) used vaginal capsules containing tea tree oil applied daily in his study of 28 patients with vaginal candidiasis and claimed that after 30 days of treatment, 23 patients exhibited a complete cure based on biologic and clinical examination. Another clinical application is for treatment of onychomycosis, which is the most frequent cause of nail disease (prevalence from 2% to 13%). Buck and others (1994) assessed the efficacy and tolerability of 6 months of twice-daily topical application of 1% clotrimazole solution (CL) versus tea tree oil (TT) for the treatment of toenail onychomycosis. This double-blind, randomized, controlled trial had 117 cases. The results showed that the treatments were similarly effective in terms of culture cure (CL = 11%, TT = 18%), and clinical assessment documented partial or full resolution (CL = 61%, TT = 60%). Three months later, about half of each group reported continued improvement or resolution (CL = 55%, TT = 56%).

The antifungal activity of tea tree oil may be selective. Tong and others (1992) compared the treatment of tinea pedis by 10% weight to weight (w/w) tea tree oil cream compared with 1% tolnaftate and placebo creams in a randomized, double-blind trial. Tolnaftate-treated patients (85%) showed a significant absence of the fungus by the end of therapy compared with patients treated with tea tree oil (30%) and a placebo (21%). However, both treatment groups showed similar significant clinical improvements when compared with the placebo group. Under the conditions of the study, tea tree oil appears to reduce the clinical signs but not the underlying infection.

Finally, tea tree oil must be used carefully because reports exist of allergic contact eczema possibly caused by components such as *d*-limonene (Knight, Hausen, 1994) or cineol (DeGroot, Weyland, 1994). Tea tree oil toxicosis has also been reported when the oil was applied in inappropriately high doses topically to dogs and cats for dermatologic conditions. However, treatment of the clinical signs of depression, weakness, incoordination, and muscle tremors combined with supportive care allowed recovery within 2 to 3 days (Villar and others, 1994).

Thyme

The essential oil of thyme has been traditionally used for its antiseptic action, and many anecdotal claims have been made for various medicinal effects (Price, 1993). Good in vitro evidence supports these claims. For example, Deans and Ritchie (1987) tested the antibacterial properties of thyme oil in plate inhibition tests of 50 plant essential oils against 25 genera of bacteria, including *Escherichia coli, Salmonella pullorum, Yersinia enterocolica, Streptococcus faecalis,* and *Staphylococcus aureus.* Thyme had the greatest overall inhibitory effect of all plant oils. Indeed, the only bacterium of the 25 tested that did not show inhibition was *Clostridium sporogenes,* the only anaerobe tested. Juven and others (1994) found that the inhibition of *Salmonella typhimurium* and *S. aureus* were both greater under anaerobic conditions. These authors suggest that the likely bactericidal effect of thyme involves the action of a main phenolic, thymol, in complexation reactions with the bacterial membrane proteins, because addition of serum albumin (Desferal) neutralized the antibacterial action of thymol, presumably through the proteins' ability to bind to phenolic compounds with their amino and hydroxylamine groups. The phenolic composition of thyme oil means that it has to be used carefully to avoid skin irritation.

The antioxidative effect of thyme oil may also have applications. Aging is associated with a peroxidative reduction in polyunsaturated fatty acids (PUFAs) Deans and others (1994) showed that drinking 720 µg of thyme oil per day for 19 weeks significantly increased the levels of major PUFAs in aging mice. In mice fed thyme oil over 5 months, arachidonic and docosahexanoic acid levels in aged mice rose higher than those in young mice. In vitro tests suggest that the most active components were linalool, thujone, camphene, carvacrol, and thymol. with aging, PUFA levels decline, and a concomitant loss of cellular function and integrity is noted. Thyme appears to protect tissues with a high PUFA content. Thyme also exhibited the best in vitro antifungal activity of four essential oil concentrations in inhibiting *Saprolegnia ferax.* This finding may also be a membrane phenomenon because thyme's phenolic components, carvacrol and thymol, were also effective (Perucci and others, 1995). Thyme occurs in many "chemotypes"; the chemical composition varies widely both between and within strains. Most thyme oils on the market are rich in thymol; however, some chemotypes are rich in compounds such as linalool and contain little or no thymol. These latter compounds are thus unlikely to be as active against bacteria or to cause skin irritation. For example, the most common thyme, *Thymus vulgaris,* has different chemotypes that may be rich in either thymol (32% to 63%), cineol (>70%), geraniol (>41%), linalool (65% to 70%), or *p*-cymene (>44%). The thymol chemotype, if used undiluted, can severely irritate mouse or rabbit skin, although a 12% solution produces no irritation in humans. Thymol should not be used at more than 1% concentration on mucous membranes or on diseased or damaged skin (Tisserand, Balacs, 1995).

The sensitivity to skin may account for the long popularity of thyme and thymol as antiseptics in oral and dental preparations such as mouthwashes and toothpastes (Meeker, Linke, 1988). Shapiro and others (1994) found that thymol was active against a large number of bacterial strains implicated in dental disease. The concentration ranges needed for effect in vitro were narrow (MIC, 0.02% to 0.09% weight to volume [w/v]; MBC, 0.04% to 0.18% w/v). They suggest that this general bactericidal effect is consistent with the action of thymol in perturbing and destabilizing bacterial membranes.

Pharmacologic Effects

As mentioned previously, intranasal drug treatments have become widespread. Ambient odors such as lavender oil may also be considered a form of intranasal drug treatment. The main components of lavender oil are the lipophilic terpenoids, linalool, and linalyl acetate. Terpenoids suppress cell action potentials through interaction with cell membranes, possibly by closing ion channels (Teuscher and others, 1990). This damping of cell electrical activity suggests the possibility of a light sedative or anesthetic effect. Buchbauer and others (1991, 1993) found a 78% decrease in the motility of mice after inhalation of ambient lavender oil for 1 hour, with similar effects for linalool (73%) and linalyl acetate (63%). When mice were first agitated by caffeine injection, inhaled lavender oil reduced motility even more significantly (92%). Plasma levels followed the reduction in motility. The authors comment that inhalation of lavender oil leads to a serum level comparable to an intravenous injection and that this effect is likely to be caused by rapid absorption by both the nasal and lung mucosa (Buchbauer and others, 1991). Lavender oil, linalool, and linalyl acetate were the most effective of 42 different oils and their components tested as ambient odors. Paradoxically, isoeugenol, a common component in essential oils, had an activating effect except when the mice were already aroused with caffeine, in which case it had a strong sedative effect, second

only to lavender oil. Essential oils may therefore have interactions with other drugs and states.

Applied studies have not been performed with other species, although Hardy and others (1995) found clinically relevant effects in insomniac psychogeriatric patients receiving long-term drug treatment (temazepam, promazine, clomethiazole [Heminevrin]). After 2 weeks of sleep monitoring, patients were taken off the drug regimen for 2 weeks. For a final 2 weeks an unobtrusive level of lavender oil was introduced using an odor diffuser for three 1- to 1½-hour periods each night. As expected, patients slept less when the drugs were taken away. However, after introduction of the ambient lavender oil, sleep returned to the same level as with medication. The same results with lavender oil as with conventional drugs suggest a strong enough effect for veterinary uses. This sedative effect might be used to calm anxious animals and reduce obtrusive behaviors such as barking in commercial kennels. Apart from the ease of administration, lavender oil may also mask unpleasant odors, which may be beneficial to staff and may dampen the stimulating effects of the animals' own odors in enclosed environments.

Other ambient odors are known to have similar physiologic effects. Warren and others (1987) patented the use of a nutmeg-based fragrance to reduce stress as measured by reduction in blood pressure and self-ratings. Humans were stressed by mental arithmetic and sentence completion tasks under a fragrance with and without nutmeg oil. With nutmeg oil, systolic blood pressure from the stressors was reduced by 9 mm Hg, and subjects rated themselves as more calm and less anxious. These effects might be due to myristicin and elemicin, two ingredients of nutmeg that convert to the mood-altering hallucinogens trimethoxy-amphetamine and methoxy-methylene-dioxy-amphetamine. The authors note that high ambient concentrations (13 to 1000 mg) were used in the test, which might restrict clinical uses.

These studies suggest that ambient odors are powerful enough to produce pharmacologic effects and that the effects can be evaluated relatively easily. Buchbauer's study (1993) suggests other compounds that might be tested for clinically relevant sedative and alerting effects on animals (e.g., the interaction of isoeugenol with caffeine).

Odor Conditioning

Immune response

Classical (or pavlovian) conditioning is the presentation of a neutral object before a stimulus. After several presentations the neutral object begins to elicit the same reaction as the original stimulus. Classical conditioning usually relates to the pairing of a neutral object with an emotional or physiologic reaction, such as liking, fear, and salivation. In the 1930s, Russian psychologists discovered that taste and smell could be paired with viruses, albumin, parasites, and bacterial vaccines and later elicit similar immune responses. In the past 15 years, American researchers have been reexamining these responses. In several studies on mice, saccharine has been paired with cyclophosphamide, an anticancer drug that causes various types of immunosuppression. After one or a few pairings, presentation of saccharine suppressed the levels of antibodies and natural killer cells (NKCs) and reduced graft rejection and tumor resistance (Ader and others, 1991). Similarly, saccharine, previously paired with cyclophosphamide, boosted the drug effect in delaying the development of an autoimmune disease such as systemic lupus erythematosus (SLE) in mice bred with the disorder (Ader, Cohen, 1982).

One intriguing clinical application, albeit in a human patient, has been reported. Olness and Ader (1992) adapted Ader and Cohen's (1982) animal conditioning protocol to treat severe SLE in a 13-year-old girl. She was already being treated with corticosteroids, phenobarbital, antihypertensives, and diuretics. Frequent bleeding and intermittent heart failure caused by antibodies to blood coagulating factor II meant that cyclophosphamide was needed to reduce antibody levels. However, her physicians believed that the doses required would be fatal. She sipped cod liver oil as cyclophosphamide was infused intravenously into her foot over 5 minutes with simultaneous presentation of rose oil. Cod liver oil was chosen because it was previously unknown to the patient, who found it unpleasant and thus unforgettable. Rose oil was used to provide additional conditioning. This pairing of cod liver oil and rose oil with drug infusion continued once monthly for 3 months. For the next 9 months the cod liver and rose oils were paired with the drug for 1 month and then presented by themselves for the next 2 months. Thus over a period of 12 months, the girl received six rather than twelve treatments, delivering only half the dose of the cytotoxic drug. The clinical outcome appeared to be the same as if 12 treatments had been given, except that she survived. No conclusions can be drawn from a single case because the conditioning may have had nothing to do with her improvement. However, many animal studies on conditioned immune suppression suggest that formal evaluation in veterinary trials should be considered.

Classical conditioning can also be used to increase the immune response. NKCs are involved in natural immunity against lymphoid and other tumors and in antiviral and antibacterial responses. They also help regulate antibody production. Their activity is enhanced by interferons and polyinosinic:poly-cytidylic acid (polyI:C). Solvasan and others (1988) placed a glass container with camphor dissolved in mineral oil on top of a mouse cage for 1 hour before injecting beta-interferon or polyIC. This pairing needed to be done only once. Later introduction of camphor increased NKC activity, as measured by the attack of the NKC on radiolabeled tumor cells.

Fever, a defensive response of the body to infection, can also be elicited by camphor after pairing with fever induc-

tion (Hiramoto and others, 1991). Camphor conditioned to polyIC may also increase resistance to cancer directly. Ghanta and others (1987) implanted myeloma cells in mice and 2 days later injected the mice with polyIC just before 4 hours of exposure to camphor. The mice were then reexposed to camphor every third day. These mice had a median survival time of 43 days, compared with 38, 37, and 34 for those in control groups. The conditioning may also be specific to certain cells rather than a general NKC response. Hiramoto and others (1993) found that injected spleen cells induce specific cytotoxic T lymphocytes (CTLs) against them. Camphor odor paired with their injection for 1 hour elicited CTLs 1 week later. The simplicity of the method suggests ready adaptation to veterinary practice.

Hiramoto and others (1993) point out that conventional classical conditioning using visual and auditory stimuli requires many pairings and that the stimuli must be presented close together. In contrast, conditioning of NKC, fever, and CTL to camphor needs only one pairing and can have an interstimulus interval as long as 2 days. The implication is that the central nervous system is sensitive to these stimuli and is able to link these events to immune responses 2 days later. The authors comment that these robust properties indicate a long-established link between the olfactory and the immune systems and the singular importance of this communication for species survival.

Although the effects are well established, the mechanisms underlying the conditioning of immune suppression and augmentation are unknown. Olfactory projections to the hypothalamus may be involved, acting via the hypothalamic-pituitary-adrenal axis and involving the production of corticotropin-releasing factor (CRF), adrenocorticotropic hormone, and glucocorticoids or catecholamines (Dunn, 1995). The effect might also be under the neural control of the hypothalamus, such as through the release of immune-related cells from the bone marrow into the bloodstream via the autonomic system (Miyan and others, 1996).

The sense of smell has similar limbic and neuroendocrine projections across species; therefore the procedures may be easily generalized to other species. For example, they may be used to reduce the amounts of toxic immunosuppressive drugs used to treat autoimmune diseases. The use of olfactory and taste stimuli to condition resistance to autoimmune, cancer, and other diseases has the advantage of simplicity, strength, and robustness; however, evaluation on model systems in veterinary practice remains to be carried out.

Aversive conditioning

Before examining veterinary applications of olfactory conditioning, clinicians should be aware of the ease with which taste and odor can pair with illness, especially in species with naturally wide diets. One possibility is that an odor may become associated with the consequences of an illness rather than its treatment. The brain appears to be hardwired through evolution to associate certain stimuli more easily with other stimuli; that is, some things are more conducive to conditioning than others. In this respect, taste is more easily associated with internal pain and illness than other sensory stimuli because the nervous pathways of taste and the gastrointestinal system converge at the top of the brainstem (Palmerino and others, 1980). In contrast, visual and auditory stimuli are more easily associated with external stimuli such as electric shock.

Aversive taste conditioning is common in humans, with a 40% to 65% incidence (Bernstein, 1991); however, the ease with which such associations are made varies across species. A single pairing of the taste and smell of a food with illness can be sufficient, even though several hours may have elapsed since eating. Such aversions are relatively permanent; they are hard to unlearn. This difficulty arises in part because organisms simply avoid a food in the future and thus never have the opportunity to learn that the food does not always cause illness. Although taste conditions to internal illness better than odor, if taste and odor are paired together with the illness, the aversions to the odor are even more aversive than the taste (Palmerino and others, 1980). This makes evolutionary sense: Once poisoned by a food, the animal is better off avoiding it through aversion to the odor rather risking toxic effects by tasting it again. Taste and odor aversions also develop to the internal illness or stress caused by toxic effects of drugs and allergies. Indeed, such paired aversions are a sensitive measure of toxicity. Bernstein (1991) suggests that pairing food with the pain of chronic illness may result in general food aversions and low appetite. These findings have led to various clinical applications. Patients with cancer frequently have poor appetite and consequent weight loss. The causes of cancerous cachexia have not been well understood despite decades of research, and its management remains a serious problem. However, patients readily acquire food aversions as a consequence of chemotherapy treatments (Bernstein, 1991). In effect, the last meal eaten gets the blame for the nausea caused by the drug, leading to a loss of appetite for normal food. "Scapegoat" foods, such as sweets given between a meal and chemotherapy treatment, have a significant protective effect (Broberg, Bernstein, 1987).

Conditioning analgesia

The following speculative application arises from the particular affective characteristics of odor conditioning. In humans, placebo effects are important in the control of pain; however, classical conditioning is more powerful than persuasive instruction in creating analgesia. In other words, a stimulus paired with pain reduction leads to the ability to reduce the perceived pain (Voudouris and others, 1990). The easy conditionability of odor to internal states allied with pain suggests that odor may be an effective stimulus for such pairing in animals.

A clinical trial might involve the presentation of a taste and odor as an administered analgesic takes effect, so that the pain relief is associated with these stimuli. Later pre-

sentation of the odor would be expected to maintain or augment the analgesic effect of the drug, as assessed by a reduction in the amount of drug required to achieve the same behavioral signs of reduced pain. The mechanism may be analogous to the development of preferences for particular foods. Eating a high-calorie food relieves the discomfort of hunger. The taste and smell of this food become paired with the relief of this pain, and thus the food is preferred (Booth and others, 1982). In addition, the initial combination of taste and smell potentiates the later effect of smell alone, as observed in flavor aversion. This possibility of odor-conditioned analgesia remains to be clinically evaluated; however, if effective, it would reduce the cost and effort of administering conventional analgesics.

Conditioning behavior

Wider affective aspects of odor conditioning also have therapeutic implications. The conditioning of odor to emotional states may be hardwired, like taste, through the projections of the olfactory system to the limbic system. Emotional responses are essentially source oriented, guiding the organism on whether to approach or avoid the source. Odors therefore may be little more than carriers of the meaning of their source; they evoke both recognition of the source and any emotion that may be associated with it, with the concomitant approach or avoidance behavior. Accordingly a neutral odor can be easily paired with an emotional state (often in a single session) so that the odor will evoke the same emotional state in another circumstance at a later time (Kirk-Smith and others, 1983). The ease with which this can be done suggests clinical uses: Pairing an odor with, for example, a calm or relaxed state may calm the animal when the odor is reintroduced under stressful circumstances. Alternately, an odor might be paired with an aversive stimulus so that the odor is avoided. The odor might then be used to prevent behaviors. For example, the animal will avoid areas or boundaries where the smell is present (similar to the aversive effect of competitor scents on territorial boundaries).

So far this discussion has dealt with the investment of a previously neutral odor with evaluative meaning. A naturally aversive odor can also be used in conditioning to reduce unwanted behaviors. According to Juarbe-Diaz and Houpt (1996), a dog collar that gave off a lemon smell (Fig. 30-1) in response to barking reduced barking in 8 of 9 dogs and was more effective than an electric shock collar. They suggest that the strange odor may be less tolerated than the presumably painful shock stimulus, given dogs' sensitive sense of smell. The direct aversive effect may have less to do with the odor than with the unexpected stimuli of the odor and the startling hiss of its release (Houpt, 1996). The dogs quickly learned not to bark when the collar was put on; that is, the collar quickly became the conditioned stimulus. One might envisage a similar apparatus being worn by the male of a herd, with the aversive scent produced when a certain boundary line is crossed; this information could be programmed into a small global posi-

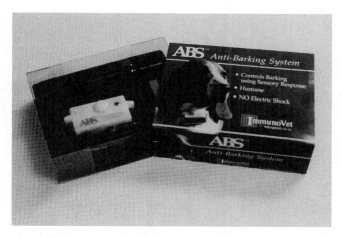

Fig. 30-1 The Anti-Barking System (ABS) by Animal Behavior Systems, Inc. The collar is equipped with a sensor that is activated by a bark. When activated, the collar emits a citronella spray. (Courtesy Animal Behavior Systems, Inc.)

tioning sensor (GPS) receiver worn by the animal, thus saving the cost of fencing the herd's range.

Healing Effects of *Centella asiatica*

Centella asiatica (CA) (also called *Hydrocotyle asiastica,* Indian pennywort, or Gotu Kola) is a slender, creeping plant that grows commonly in swampy areas of India, Sri Lanka, Madagascar, South Africa, and the tropics. It has long been used in these areas for healing. An (ethanol) extract or fraction of the triterpenes asiatic acid, asiaticoside, and madecassic acid is usually used in treatment because these are the active components. This mixture directly stimulates fibroblasts to produce collagen and fibronectins, but it does not seem to affect cell proliferation, total protein synthesis, or the biosynthesis of proteoglycans (Tenni and others, 1988). Asiatic acid has been found to be the only component responsible for the stimulation of collagen synthesis, although all three components increased the intracellular free proline pool; this effect was independent of the stimulation of collagen synthesis (Maquart and others, 1990). The asiaticoside is transformed into asiatic acid in vivo, so it will also add to the production of collagen (Grimaldi and others, 1990). In in vitro studies the extract also enhanced attachment of fibroblast cells and increased their tPA production (Kim and others, 1993). It is these fibroblast-stimulating properties that give CA its healing effect. A major internal use is improvement of venous flow through improvement of the vascular walls. The resulting reduction in capillary permeability and increased microcirculation lead to improved venous sufficiency overall (Belcaro and others, 1990b). Studies using doses of 60 to 120 mg/day of the CA triterpene extract over 1 to 2 months have shown significantly reduced lower limb edema and concomitant lowered leg pain (Belcaro and others, 1990a; Pointel and others, 1987).

In another application, CA extract reduced the size of stress- and cold-induced gastric ulcers in rats from 20 to 7.2 mm, compared with 6.2 mm with famotidine (an H_2 inhibitor) and 10 mm with pretreatment with sodium valproate (Chatterjee and others, 1992).

Finally, because the raw and triterpene extracts of CA are extremely weak skin sensitizers in guinea pigs (Hausen, 1993), the risk of acquiring contact sensitivity to this useful plant or its constituents is low, even when it is applied to damaged skin.

Clinical Use of Essential Oils and Forms of Treatment

Aromatherapy for human use may be administered by massage, diluted in a base of almond or other high-quality neutral oil; as a perfume, diluted in alcohol or base oil; in water, as a scented bath; or by diffusion, through heating devices or humidifiers. Oral administration is becoming less common for safety reasons and is never recommended for veterinary patients. Topical administration of essential oils, although difficult in veterinary patients, may have some application.

In veterinary medicine, essential oils are most easily administered by diffusion to scent an entire room. Diffusers used in the home may be as simple as a candle that heats a small bowl containing diluted oils. More expensive and effective models are heated electrically, and the volatilized oils diffused by fan. These diffusers may vary in strength to disperse the volatile oils throughout rooms of various size. This method may not be an advantage in a hospital, where individual patients may need different treatments. One solution is to soak a cotton ball with diluted oil and affix it to the inside of the patient's cage. Essential oils for topical use or diffusion in close quarters may be diluted in a base of vegetable oil at a rate of three to eight drops per teaspoon. Essential oils for flea control can be diluted in water (perhaps 10 to 20 drops per pint), shaken well, and administered as a spray or dip.

These concentrated oils may be toxic in small amounts if administered orally. Special consideration should be given to the tendency for veterinary patients to lick and ingest topically applied oils. When designing oil prescriptions, practitioners should also remember the cat's unique sensitivity to chemicals of the phenol class. Aromatherapists tend to mix oils with similar properties for a synergistic effect in much the same way as herbalists use combinations, but combinations are also advantageous in reducing potential toxicity from any single oil.

Pharmacopeia

The actions listed in this section are those reported by traditional aromatherapists. Although these indications may have been confirmed by years of clinical experience, little experimental support exists for these uses; exceptions are cited in the text. All toxicity data are derived from the text *Essential Oil Safety: A Guide for Health Care Professionals* (Tisserand, Balacs, 1995). The proposed clinical indication and traditional "property" for which the oil is known are derived from a number of comprehensive aromatherapy resources (Lawless, 1996; Tisserand, 1977). This list is intended to provide the practitioner with a starting point for clinical experimentation.

Aniseed *(Pimpinella anisum)*

Constituents: Trans-anethole, 80% to 90%.

Clinical use: Aniseed is used in the treatment of gastroenteritis, flatulence (carminative), bronchitis, and pneumonia (expectorant). Anise oil decreases the specific gravity of respiratory tract fluid when administered by steam inhalation but only in concentrations that produced inflammatory lesions (Boyd, Sheppard, 1968).

Toxicity or contraindications: *Trans*-anethole has estrogenic effects.

Basil *(Ocimum basilicum)*

Constituents: Estragole, 40% to 87%; minor amounts of linalool.

Clinical use: Gastroenteritis (carminative, digestive), lethargy (nervine, tonic).

Toxicity or contraindications: Because estragole may be carcinogenic, oils with low (5% or less) estragole content are recommended.

Bergamot *(Citrus bergamia)*

Constituents: Linalyl acetate, 36% to 45%; limonene, 28% to 32%; linalool, 11% to 22%; bergapten, 0.3% to 0.4%.

Clinical use: Lethargy (antidepressant, stimulant), topical for wounds (vulnerary).

Toxicity or contraindications: Phototoxic (bergapten increases photosensitivity of treated skin); photocarcinogenic in presence of UV light. (Bergapten-free bergamot oil, known as FCF, is available.)

Birch *(Betula lenta)*

Constituents: Methyl salicylate, 98%.

Clinical use: Topical analgesic, antiinflammatory.

Toxicity or contraindications: Highly toxic if taken internally. Reports of cases of human poisoning from trans-

dermal absorption. For topical use only. Should be used with extreme caution. Contraindicated for use in cats.

Camphor *(Cinnamomum camphora)*

Constituents: Camphor, 15% to 50%; cineole, 50%; safrole, 10% to 20% (in some fractions).

Clinical use: Camphor is used to treat bronchitis and pneumonia (expectorant). It is also used as a mild topical analgesic and dental antiseptic. Camphor significantly reduced experimentally induced cough frequency and increased cough latency when aerosolized to guinea pigs (Laude and others, 1994). The oil significantly inhibited the growth of *Trichophyton rubrum* and *Microsporum gypseum* in vitro (Kishore, Mishra, Chansouria, 1993). Camphor oil was found to be miticidal against *Psoroptes cuniculi* in vitro (Perucci and others, 1994). Camphor induces hepatic p-450 and glutathione-s-transferase (hepatic microsomal enzymes associated with xenobiotic detoxification processes) at an oral dose of 300 mg/kg (Banerjee and others, 1995).

Toxicity of contraindications: Neurotoxic, convulsant in high concentrations. May be carcinogenic and hepatotoxic (because of safrole).

Cardamom *(Elletaria cardamomum)*

Constituents: Terpinyl acetate, cineol, limonene, sabinene, linalool, linalyl acetate, pinene, zingiberene, others.

Clinical use: Cardamom is used to treat gastroenteritis and nausea (digestive). Cardamom increased levels of hepatic acid–soluble sulfhydryls in mice when administered orally and decreased cytochrome p-450 levels (Banerjee and others, 1994). The oil also suppressed formation of carcinogenic metabolites from aflatoxin B1 in vitro (Hashim and others, 1994).

Toxicity or contraindications: Not toxic.

Cedar *(Cedrus atlantica, Juniperus ashei,* or *Juniperus virginiana)*

Constituents: Atlantone, caryophyllene, cedrol, cadinene, cedrene, thujopsene, depending on the species used.

Clinical use: Cedar is used to treat bronchitis, pneumonia (expectorant, antiseptic), and dermatitis (antiseptic, antifungal). It is also used as an insect repellant. Cedar leaf oil produced a dose-dependent decrease in specific gravity and an increase in total solids and insoluble mucus in respiratory tract fluid when volatilized for steam inhalation in rabbits (Boyd, Sheppard, 1968). Cedarwood oil was cercaricidal against *Schistosoma mansoni* cercariae in one study (Naples and others, 1992).

Toxicity or contraindications: Not toxic.

Chamomile—German (*Matricaria chamomilla*)

Constituents: Chamazulene, farnesene, bisabolol oxide, en-yndicycloether, caprylic acid, possibly others.

Clinical use: Chamomile is used to treat dermatitis (antiinflammatory, vulnerary), anxious behaviors (sedative), and gastroenteritis. Chamazulene was found to block peroxidation of arachidonic acid and suppress leukotriene formation in vitro, supporting its use as an antiinflammatory bowel and topical skin treatment (Safayhi and others, 1994).

Toxicity or contraindications: Not toxic.

Chamomile—Roman (*Anthemis nobilis*)

Constituents: Angelic acid ester, tiglic acid ester, pinene, farnesol, nerolidol, chamazulene, pinocaarvone, cineol, possibly others.

Clinical use: Nervous or anxious behaviors (sedative), dermatitis (vulnerary, cicatrizant). Similar to German chamomile.

Toxicity or contraindications: Not toxic.

Cinnamon (*Cinnamomum zeylanicum*)

Constituents: Eugenol, 70% to 90%; cinnamaldehyde, 3%; linalool; safrol.

Clinical use: Cinnamon is used to treat patients with external parasites (mites, dermatophytes), dental problems (antiseptic), and pneumonia (antimicrobial). It is also used as a circulatory stimulant. Volatilized cinnamon oil was found to possess antibacterial activity against *E. coli, S. aureus, Salmonella typhi, S. faecalis,* and *Mycobacterium avium* in vitro (Maruzzella, Sicurella, 1960). Cinnamaldehyde inhibited growth of food-borne *Staphylococcus, Micrococcus, Bacillus,* and *Enterobacter* species in vitro as well (Moleyar, Narasimham, 1992). Cinnamon oil inhibited clinical dermatophyte isolates in vitro (Lima and others, 1993). Fungicidal activity against *Aspergillus flavus* has also been documented for cinnamaldehyde (Mahmoud, 1994).

Toxicity or contraindications: Dermal and mucous membrane irritant; should not be used undiluted.

Citronella (*Cymbopogon nardus*)

Constituents: Geraniol, citronella, geranyl acetate, limonene, camphene.

Clinical use: Insect repellant, stimulant.

Toxicity or contraindications: Not toxic.

Clove (*Eugenia caryophyllata*)

Constituents: Eugenol, eugenyl acetate, caryophyllene.

Clinical use: Clove is used to treat skin infections (antiseptic) and gastroenteritis (antiemetic, carminative, antimicrobial). It is also a dental analgesic. Eugenol (a primary constituent of clove oil) is a potent antibacterial agent against oral anaerobic bacteria (Shapiro and others, 1994). One study demonstrated that eugenol, given orally to rats with experimentally induced arthritis, significantly suppressed swelling (Sharma and others, 1994). Clove oil has also been found to inhibit platelet aggregation and thromboxane synthesis (Saeed, Gilani, 1994). Eugenol is a free radical scavenger (Tsujimoto and others, 1993).

Toxicity or contraindications: Dermal and mucous membrane irritant, hepatotoxic.

Eucalyptus (*Eucalyptus globulus*)

Constituents: Cineol, pinene, limonene, cymene, phellandrene, terpinene, aromadendrene.

Clinical use: Eucalyptus is used in the treatment of pneumonia, bronchitis, sinusitis, upper respiratory tract infections (antiseptic, decongestant, expectorant), and urinary tract infections (urinary antiseptic). Eucalyptus decreased the specific gravity of respiratory tract fluid when administered by steam inhalation but only in concentrations that also produced inflammatory lesions (Boyd, Sheppard, 1968). Eucalyptol has been found to induce liver microsomal enzymes when administered as an aerosol; this finding may have implications for the metabolism of other drugs given concomitantly (Jori and others, 1969), as well as for xenobiotic toxification potential.

Toxicity or contraindications: Not for internal use. Signs of toxicity in children after ingestion of as little as 2 ml of eucalyptus oil (Tibballs, 1995).

Fennel (*Foeniculum vulgare*)

Constituents: Trans-anethole, 52% to 86%; limonene; phellandrene; pinene; anisic acid; anisic aldehyde; camphene; estragole; perhaps fenchone; others.

Clinical use: Enteritis, colic, borborygmus (carminative), estrogenic.

Toxicity or contraindications: Not for internal use. Estrogenic, possibly carcinogenic (because of estragole), dermal sensitizer.

Fir Needles *(Abies alba)*

Constituents: Santene, pinene, limonene, bornyl acetate, lauraldehyde, others.

Clinical use: Fir needles are used for arthritis and musculoskeletal disorders (analgesic). They also have antimicrobial properties. One study examined rumen microbial activity in sheep and deer who ate Douglas fir needles as part of their diets. Individual oil components either promoted or inhibited rumen microbial activity selectively, but at the highest concentrations tested the net effect was inhibitory. The greatest inhibitory effect was seen in sheep, whose normal diet contained no fir needles. Deer rumen microbes had apparently become habituated to the presence of the fir needles (Oh and others, 1967).

Toxicity or contraindications: May be a dermal irritant.

Garlic *(Allium sativum)*

Constituents: Allicin (diallyl thiosulphinate), allylpropyl disulfide, diallyl disulfide, diallyl trisulfide, citral, geraniol, linalool, phellandrene, others.

Clinical use: Garlic is one rare exception to the admonition against internal use. Garlic oil is available in capsules for oral administration. Garlic is a hypolipemic, anticoagulant, detoxicant (binds heavy metals and other toxins), antioxidant, nonspecific immune stimulant, antineoplastic, and antimicrobial (Abdullah, 1988; Resch, Ernst, 1995).

Toxicity or contraindications: Prolonged use may cause anemia in small animals because garlic is a member of the onion family, which has been known to cause Heinz body anemia. Garlic has been associated with thyroid disease (inhibits iodine metabolism) and coagulation disorders. It may cause dermal irritation.

Geranium *(Pelargonium odontantissimum)*

Constituents: Citronellol, geraniol, linalool, isomenthone, menthone, phellandrene, sabinene, limonene, others.

Clinical use: Skin disorders (astringent, antiinflammatory, cicatrizant), antidepressant, antiseptic.

Toxicity or contraindications: Not toxic.

Ginger *(Zingiber officinale)*

Constituents: Gingerin, gingenol, gingerone, zingiberine, linalool, camphene, phellandrene, citral, cineol, borneol, others.

Clinical use: Ginger is useful in the treatment of vomiting (antiemetic), depression, and arthritis (antiinflammatory). One study demonstrated that ginger oil, given orally to rats with experimentally induced arthritis, significantly suppressed swelling (Sharma and others, 1994). The oil also suppressed formation of carcinogenic metabolites from aflatoxin B_1 in vitro (Hashim and others, 1994). Components of ginger are known to inhibit the cyclooxygenase and lipoxygenase inflammatory pathways (Flynn and others, 1986; Kiuchi and others, 1982).

Toxicity or contraindications: Phototoxicity.

Hyssop *(Hyssopus officinalis)*

Constituents: Pinocamphone, isopinocamphone, estragole, borneol, geraniol, limonene, thujone, myrcene, caryophyllene, others.

Clinical use: Skin trauma and inflammatory lesions (astringent, antiseptic, vulnerary, cicatrizant), stimulant. Fungistatic against *Aspergillus fumigatus* (Ghfir and others, 1994).

Toxicity or contraindications: Pinocamphene may have convulsant action and is contraindicated for animals with a history of seizures.

Juniper *(Juniperus communis)*

Constituents: Pinene, myrcene, sabinene, limonene, cyrmeme, terpinene, thujene, camphene, others.

Clinical use: Diuretic, urinary antiseptic.

Toxicity or contraindications: Not toxic.

Lavandin *(Lavandula X intermedia)*

Constituents: Linalyl acetate, linalool, cineol, camphene, pinene, others.

Clinical use: Similar to true lavender (see next section).

Toxicity or contraindications: Camphor may endow neurotoxicity. It is contraindicated in animals with a history of seizures.

Lavender *(Lavendula angustifolia)*

Constituents: Linalyl acetate, linalool, lavadulol, lavandulyl acetate, terpineol, cineol, limonene, ocimene, caryophyllene, others.

Clinical use: Lavender is used as an antidepressant and tranquilizer. It is also helpful in the treatment of inflammatory skin disease or lesions. Lavender oil reduced motility in mice after a 1-hour inhalation period (Buchbauer and others, 1993) and may have anticonvulsant activity (Yamada and others, 1994). Linalool was miticidal against *P. cuniculi* in vitro (Perucci and others, 1994).

Toxicity or contraindications: Lavender is not considered toxic.

Lemongrass *(Cymbopogon citratus)*

Constituents: Citral, myrcene, dipentene, methylheptenone, linalool, geraniol, nerol, citronellal, farnesol, d-limonene, others.

Clinical use: Lemongrass is used in the treatment of infections, particularly of the skin. It also has insecticidal properties. Lemongrass oil was bactericidal against *E. coli* and *B. subtilis* (Onawunmi, Ogunlana, 1986) and inhibited clinical dermatophyte isolates in vitro (Lima and others, 1993). Lemongrass also significantly inhibited the growth of *T. rubrum* and *M. gypseum* in vitro and produced mycologic cures of experimentally infected guinea pigs when applied as an ointment of 1 ml oil into 100 g of petroleum jelly (Kishore, Mishra, Chansouria, 1992). Some components of the oil are believed to act as anticarcinogens by inducing glutathione-s-transferase in a variety of tissues (Zheng and others, 1993).

Toxicity or contraindications: Glaucoma (citral may cause a rise in ocular pressure). Prostatic hyperplasia (prolonged administration caused benign prostatic hyperplasia in rats) (Servadio and others, 1986). May cause hypersensitivity reactions when administered topically (because of d-limonene).

Marjoram *(Origanum marjorana)*

Constituents: Terpinene, terpineol, sabinene, linalool, carvacrol, linalyl acetate, ocimene, cadinene, geranyl acetate, citral, eugenol, others.

Clinical use: Sedative, specifically for a hyperactive libido (anaphrodisiac); analgesic for musculoskeletal disorders.

Toxicity or contraindications: Marjoram is not considered toxic.

Melissa *(Melissa officinalis)*

Constituents: Citral, citronellal.

Clinical use: Topically, for skin lesions. May have androgenic and estrogenic effects. Virucidal against herpes simplex when used as an extract in vitro (Dimitrova and others, 1993).

Toxicity or contraindications: Glaucoma (may cause a rise in ocular pressure). Prostatic hyperplasia. May cause dermal sensitization.

Orange (*Citrus aurantium* or *Citrus sinensis*)

Constituents: d-Limonene, 89% to 96%; bergapten; auraptenol.

Clinical use: Its best use may be as an insecticide because of a high d-limonene content; the desiccant action strips insect cuticles of oil (Greek, Moriello, 1991).

Toxicity or contraindications: Although orange oil used alone reportedly causes only phototoxicity, d-limonene dips have produced toxic reactions in dogs and cats. Hooser and others (1986) examined the effects of a commercial d-limonene in concentrations greater than those recommended by the manufacturer. At these levels cats exhibited hypersalivation, ataxia, and muscle tremors; some exhibited excoriation of the skin. No ill effects were seen at recommended treatment concentrations. A dog was reported to have an idiosyncratic reaction of erythema multiforme major and disseminated intravascular coagulation that resulted in death (Greek, Moriello, 1991). Other idiosyncratic reactions in dogs and cats include hypothermia, hypotension, perineal dermatitis, vomiting, mydriasis, and, rarely, death.

Pennyroyal

Constituents: Pulegone, menthone, *iso*-menthone, octanol, piperitenone, *trans*-isopulegone.

Clinical use: Externally, diluted, for insect repellant properties only.

Toxicity or contraindications: Pennyroyal is fatal if ingested (hepatotoxic). It also has abortifacient properties. Pennyroyal oil proved fatal to one dog who was treated topically with undiluted oil (Sudekum and others, 1992).

Peppermint *(Mentha piperita)*

Constituents: Menthol, menthone, menthyl acetate, menthofuran, limonene, pulegone, cineol, others.

Clinical use: Peppermint is used in the treatment of gastroenteritis, colic, inflammatory bowel disease (carminative, antispasmodic), bronchitis, and asthma. It is also an effective anesthetic. Peppermint oil was determined to be bactericidal for fastidiously and facultatively anaerobic oral bacteria (Shapiro and others, 1994) and mildly antibacterial against *S. aureus*. Volatilized peppermint possessed antibacterial activity against *E. coli*, *S. aureus*, *S. typhi*, *S. faecalis*, and *M. avium* (Maruzzella, Sicurella, 1960). The oil was bacteriostatic against *Salmonella enteritidis* and *Listeria monocytogenes* in food (Tassou, Drosinos, Nychas, 1995). The potential for use of peppermint oil in the treatment of enteric diseases such as inflammatory bowel disease is partially supported by observations that it relieves colon spasm during sigmoidoscopy and barium studies (Leicester and Hunt, 1982; Sparks and others, 1995). Peppermint is often used for headaches in humans; one study found a significant analgesic effect for headaches when peppermint was administered topically with ethanol to areas of the head (Gobel and others, 1994). Menthol, a major constituent of peppermint oil, significantly reduced experimentally induced cough frequency and increased cough latency when aerosolized to guinea pigs (Laude and others, 1994).

Toxicity or contraindications: Neurotoxic (respiratory depressant, convulsant), dermal irritant, cardiac dysrhythmias.

Rosemary *(Rosmarinus officinalis)*

Constituents: Pinene, camphene, limonene, cineol, borneol, camphor, linalool, terpineol, octanone, bornyl acetate, others.

Clinical use: Rosemary is a neurologic stimulant that is also useful for dry, erythematous skin. Administration of rosemary oil by inhalation increased locomotor activity in mice (Kovar and others, 1987).

Toxicity or contraindications: Rosemary is contraindicated in epilepsy (convulsant).

Tarragon *(Artemisia dracunculus)*

Constituents: Estragole, 70% to 87%; methyleugenol; capillene; ocimene; nerol; phellandrene; thujone; cineol; others.

Clinical use: Estrogenic, gastroenteritis (antispasmodic, carminative).

Toxicity or contraindications: Possibly carcinogenic, hepatotoxic.

Tea Tree *(Melaleuca alternifolia)*

Constituents: Terpinene-4-ol, cineol, pinene, terpinene, cymene, sesquiterpenes, sesquiterpene alcohols, others.

Clinical use: Tea tree is used in the treatment of dermatophytosis (fungicidal) and bacterial skin lesions. Tea tree is reportedly effective against a variety of bacteria and fungi (Carson, Riley, 1993; Raman and others, 1995). One study examined tea tree fungicidal activity against tinea pedis. Tea tree oil reduced the symptoms, but was no more effective than the placebo in eradicating the mycologic infection (Tong and others, 1992).

Toxicity or contraindications: Oral ingestion of topically applied melaleuca oil has resulted in cases of toxicity (Villar and others, 1994); oral ingestion is therefore discouraged.

Terebinth *(Pinus palustris)*

Constituents: Terpineol, estragole, carene, fenchone, fenchyl alcohol, borneol, others.

Clinical use: Bronchitis, pneumonia, sinusitis (expectorant).

Toxicity or contraindications: Dermal irritant.

Thyme *(Thymus vulgaris)*

Constituents: Thymol, carvacrol, cymeme, terpinene, camphene, borneol, linalool, others.

Clinical use: Thyme is useful in the treatment of pneumonia, gastroenteritis, and skin and oral infections (antimicrobial). Volatilized thyme oil was found to possess antibacterial activity against *E. coli*, *S. aureus*, *S. typhi*, *S. faecalis*, and *M. avium* (Maruzzella, Sicurella, 1960). Thymol and carvacrol possess antibacterial activity against common oral bacteria (Didry and others, 1994). Fungicidal activity against *A. flavus* has also been documented (Mahmoud, 1994).

Toxicity or contraindications: Dermal and mucous membrane irritant.

Turmeric *(Curcuma longa)*

Constituents: Tumerone, ar-tumerone, atlantones, zingiberene, cineol, borneol, sabinene, phellandrene.

Clinical use: An antiinflammatory with a variety of uses, curcuma has antioxidant properties (Selvam and others, 1995) and is effective in the treatment of chronic ulcers and scabies in humans (Charles, Charles, 1992). The oil significantly inhibited the growth of *T. rubrum* and *M. gypseum* in vitro (Kishore, Mishra, Chansouria, 1992).

Toxicity or contraindications: Not toxic.

Valerian *(Valeriana officinalis)*

Constituents: Bornyl acetate, isovalerate, caryophyllene, pinene, valeranone, ionone, eugenyl isovalerate, borneol, patchouli alcohol, valerianol.

Clinical use: Although the sedative effects of the valerian herb are well recognized, one study of the essential oil showed little effectiveness in reducing the motility of mice after a 1-hour inhalation period (Yamada and others, 1994).

Toxicity or contraindications: Probably not toxic.

Controversies

Experiments with aromatherapy have demonstrated that clear pharmacologic effects are difficult to document. One possible explanation is that therapeutic blood concentrations of essential oil components are difficult to attain; the environment in which we treat animals (home, hospital, or open air cages) makes saturation of ambient air difficult, in contrast to the experimental situation using a mouse cage. In addition, dogs and cats are larger animals, so larger amounts of essential oil components are necessary to reach therapeutic concentrations because of the larger blood volumes of these animals. The study by Warren and others (1987), described previously, reflects this difficulty in the pharmacologic treatment of larger subjects.

Another difficulty in using essential oils to evoke positive psychologic responses is in identifying scents that are pleasant to animals. One has only to watch dogs investigate stools, urine, and decayed food to realize that human standards do not apply to animals. It may be possible to evoke positive responses from humans, such as relaxation or stimulation, with the addition of lavender or lemon to the environment; these scents may elicit pleasant memories, such as being in "grandmother's attic" (lavender) or remembering childhood summer days behind a lemonade stand (lemon). To dogs and cats, these scents may be irritating. Likewise, dogs and cats sometimes react positively to valerian oil, a notoriously unpleasant scent for humans.

Another important point is animal sensitivity to odor. Two issues are of concern. Domestic animals are certainly more sensitive to odor than are people, so ambient odors may be too concentrated for animal comfort. The second issue involves the communication signal; we are not yet ready to use intraspecies communication tools such as urine and feces as therapeutic interventions, and our commonly used scents may contain hidden signals about which we are unaware. Because domestic animals use odor as a communication tool, our attempts to manipulate them with scent may result in confusing and possibly overstimulating messages.

Conclusions

The potential for pharmacologic interventions using aromatherapy is still unclear; however, the use of aromatherapy to condition physiologic and behavioral responses appears promising. It seems logical that if animals depend so heavily on scent to communicate and if scent is a powerful signal that can be used sparingly and effectively, the safety and power of aromatherapy will make it an important addition to the practitioner's treatment options. If conditioned responses to odors allow the practitioner to reduce the dose or frequency of potentially toxic drugs or the trainer to use harsh corrections less often, the value of aromatherapy will be evident.

Further Reading and Resources

Useful Texts

Gattefosse R-M: *Gattefosse's aromatherapy,* Essex, England, 1937, CW Daniel.

Lawless J: *The encyclopedia of essential oils,* Rockport, Mass, 1996, Element.

Tisserand R, Balacs T: *Essential oil safety: a guide for health care professionals,* New York, 1995, Churchill Livingstone.

Tisserand RB: *The art of aromatherapy,* Rochester, Vt, 1977, Healing Arts Press.

Valnet J: *The practice of aromatherapy: a classic compendium of plant medicines and their healing properties,* Rochester, Vt, 1990, Healing Arts Press.

Journal

The International Journal of Aromatherapy, Robert Tisserand, Editor, Aromatherapy Publications, PO Box 746, Hove, East Sussex, BN3 3XA United Kingdom (Phone: 0273-772479; Fax: 0273-329811)

Suppliers

Oshadhi Oils, supplied by RJF, Inc, 32422 Alipaz, Suite C, San Juan Capistrano, CA 92675 (Phone: 714-240-1104; Fax: 714-489-4854)

Butterbur and Sage, 894H Route 52, Beacon, NY 12508 (Phone: 914-833-4340)

Aura Cacia, PO Box 399, Weaverville, CA 96093 (Phone: 800-437-3301)

Essentially Oils, Ltd. 8 Mount Farm, Junction Road, Churchill, Chipping, Norton, Oxfordshire OX7 6NP, United Kingdom (Phone: 44-1608-658544; Fax: 44-1608-659566)

$\mathcal{R}$EFERENCES

Abdullah TH and others: Garlic revisited: therapeutic for the major diseases of our times? *J Nat Med Assoc* 80(4):439, 1988.

Adams RP: *Identification of essential oils by ion trap mass spectroscopy,* New York, 1989, Harcourt Brace Jovanovich.

Ader R, Cohen N: Behaviorally conditioned immunosuppression and murine systemic lupus erythematosus, *Science* 215:1534, 1982.

Ader R and others: *Psychoneuroimmunology,* San Diego, 1991, Academic Press.

Banerjee S and others: Influence of certain essential oils on carcinogen-metabolizing enzymes and acid-soluble sulfhydryls in mouse liver, *Nutr Cancer* 21:263, 1994.

Banerjee S and others: Modulatory influence of camphor on the activities of hepatic carcinogen metabolizing enzymes and the levels of hepatic and extrahepatic reduced glutathione in mice, *Cancer Lett* 88(2):163, 1995.

Bauer K and others: *Common fragrance and flavor materials,* New York, 1990, VCH.

Belaiche P: Treatment of vaginal infections of *Candida albicans* with the essential oil of *Melaleuca alternifolia, Phytotherapy* September(15):13, 1985.

Belcaro GV and others: Capillary filtration and ankle edema in patients with venous hypertension treated with TTFCA, *Angiology* 41(1):12, 1990a.

Belcaro GV and others: Improvement of capillary permeability in patients with venous hypertension after treatment with TTFCA, *Angiology* 41:533, 1990b.

Bernstein IL: Flavor aversion. In Getchell TV: *Smell and taste in health and disease,* New York, 1991, Raven Press.

Blackwell AL: Tea tree oil and anaerobic (bacterial) vaginosis, *Lancet* 337:300, 1991.

Blancou J: Early methods for the surveillance and control of glanders in Europe, *Rev Sci Tech Off Int Epiz* 13:545, 1994.

Bond S: Intranasal administration of drugs. In Ganderton D, Jones T: *Drug delivery to the respiratory tract,* Lichester, England, 1987, Ellis Horwood.

Booth DA and others: Starch content of ordinary foods associatively conditions human appetite and satiation, indexed by intake and eating pleasantness of starch-paired flavors, *Appetite* 3(2):163, 1982.

Boyd EM, Sheppard EP: The effect of steam inhalation of volatile oils on the output and composition of respiratory tract fluid, *J Pharmacol Exp Ther* 163:250, 1968.

Broberg DJ, Bernstein IL: Candy as a scapegoat in the prevention of food aversions in children receiving chemotherapy, *Cancer* 60:2344, 1987.

Brophy JJ and others: Gas chromatographic quality control for oil of *Melaleuca* terpinen-4-ol type (Australian tea tree), *J Agri Food Chem* 37:1335, 1989.

Brown R: Mammalian social orders: a critical review. In Rosenblatt JEA: *Advances in the study of behavior,* New York, 1979, Academic Press.

Buchbauer G and others: Aromatherapy: evidence for sedative effects of the essential oil of lavender after inhalation, *Zeitschrift fur Naturforschung c-a, Journal of Biosci* 46c:1067, 1991.

Buchbauer G and others: Fragrance compounds and essential oils with sedative effects upon inhalation, *J Pharm Sci* 82:660, 1993.

Buck DS and others: Comparison of two topical preparations for the treatment of onychomycosis: *Melaleuca alternifolia* (tea tree) oil and clotrimazole, *J Fam Practit* 38:601, 1994.

Carson CF, Riley TV: Antimicrobial activity of the essential oil of *Melaleuca alternifolia, Lett Appl Microbiol* 16:49, 1993.

Carson CF, Riley TV: The antimicrobial activity of tea tree oil, *Med J Austral* 160:236, 1994a.

Carson CF, Riley TV: Susceptibility of *Propionibacterium acnes* to the essential oil of *Melaleuca alternifolia, Lett Appl Microbiol* 19(1):24, 1994b.

Carson CF, Riley TV: Antimicrobial activity of the major components of the essential oil of *Melaleuca alternifolia, J Appl Bacteriol* 78:264, 1995a.

Carson CF and others: Susceptibility of methicillin-resistant *Staphylococcus aureus* to the essential oil of *Melaleuca alternifolia, J Antimicrob Chemother* 35:421, 1995b.

Charles V, Charles SX: The use and efficacy of *Azadirachta indica* ADR ("Neem") and *Curcuma longa* ("Turmeric") in scabies: a pilot study, *Trop Geogr Med* 44(1-2):178, 1992.

Chatterjee TK and others: Effects of plant extract *Centella asiatica* (Linn) on cold restraint stress ulcer in rats, *Ind J Exp Biol* 30:889, 1992.

Chien Y: *Transnasal systemic medication,* New York, 1985, Elsevier Science.

Clayton V: Aroma as therapy, *Let's Live* June:70, 1992.

Cooke M: Fragrance: its biology and pathology, *J R Coll Phys London* 28(2):133, 1994.

Deans SG, Ritchie G: Antibacterial properties of plant essential oils, *Int J Food Microbiol* 5:165, 1987.

Deans SG and others: A new type of approach to modify lipid patterns in aging mice: natural anti-oxidants of plant origin. In Knook DL, Hofecker G: *Aspects of aging and disease,* Ninth Weiner Symposium on Experimental Gerontology, Vienna, 1994, Facultatas, Universtatsverlag.

DeGroot AC, Weyland JW: Contact allergy to tea tree oil, *Contact Dermatitis* 27:279, 1994.

Didry N and others: Activity of thymol, carvacrol, cinnamaldehyde, and eugenol on oral bacteria, *Pharm Acta Helv* 69(1):25, 1994.

Dimitrova Z and others: Antiherpes effect of *Melissa officinalis* L. extracts, *Acta Microbiol Bulgarica* 29:65, 1993.

Doty R: Intranasal trigeminal chemoreception. In Doty R: *Handbook of olfaction and gustation,* New York, 1995a, Marcel Dekker.

Doty R: Introduction and historical perspective. In Doty R: *Handbook of olfaction and gustation,* New York, 1995b, Marcel Dekker.

Dunn AJ: Interactions between the nervous system and the immune system. In Bloom FB, Kuper DJ: *Psychopharmacology: the fourth generation of progress,* New York, 1995, Raven Press.

Engen T: *Odor sensation and memory,* New York, 1991, Praeger.

Flynn DL and others: Inhibition of human neutrophil 5-lipoxygenase activity by gingerdione, shogaol, capsaicin, and related pungent compounds, *Leukot Med* 24:195, 1986.

Gattefosse RM: *Gattefosse's aromatherapy,* Essex, England, 1937, CW Daniel.

Ghanta VK and others: Influence of conditioned natural immunity on tumor growth, *Ann NY Acad Sci* 496:637, 1987.

Ghfir B and others: Effect of essential oil of *Hyssopus officinalis* on the lipid composition of *Aspergillus fumigatus, Mycopathologia* 126:163, 1994.

Gobel H and others: Effect of peppermint and eucalyptus oil preparations on neurophysiological and experimental algesimetric headache parameters, *Cephalgia* 14(3):228, 1994.

Greek JS, Moriello KA: Treatment of common parasiticidal toxicities in small animals, *Feline Pract* 19:11, 1991.

Griffin K: A whiff of things to come, *Health* Nov/Dec: 34, 1992.

Grimaldi R and others: Pharmacokinetics of the total triterpenic fraction of *Centella asiatica* after single and multiple administrations in healthy volunteers: a new assay for asiatic acid, *J Ethnopharmacol* 28(2):235, 1990.

Grosjean N: *Veterinary aromatherapy*, Essex, England, 1994, CW Daniel.

Guenther E: *The essential oils*, New York, 1948, D Van Nostrand.

Hardy M and others: Replacement of chronic drug treatment of insomnia in psychogeriatric patients by ambient odour, *Lancet* 346(8976):701, 1995.

Hashim S and others: Modulatory effects of essential oils from spices on the formation of DNA adduct by aflatoxin B1 in vitro, *Nutr Cancer* 21(2):169, 1994.

Hausen BM: *Centella asiatica* (Indian pennywort): an effective therapeutic but weak sensitizer, *Contact Dermatitis* 29(4):175, 1993.

Hiramoto RN and others: Conditioning fever: a host defence response, *Life Sci* 49:93, 1991.

Hiramoto RN and others: Conditioning the allogeneic cytotoxic lymphocyte-response, *Pharmacol Biochem Behav* 44:275, 1993.

Hooser SB and others: Effects of an insecticidal dip containing *d*-limonene in the cat, *JAVMA* 189:905, 1986.

Houpt KA: Personal communication, 1996.

Jori A and others: Effect of essential oils on drug metabolism, *Biochem Pharmacol* 18:2081, 1969.

Juarbe-Diaz SV, Houpt KA: Comparison of two anti-barking collars for treatment of nuisance barking, *J Am Animal Hosp Assoc* 32:231, 1996.

Juven BJ and others: Factors that interact with the antibacterial actions of thyme essential oil and its active constituents, *J Appl Bacteriol* 76:626, 1994.

Kim YN and others: Enhancement of attachment on microcarriers and tPA production by fibroblast cells in a serum-free medium by the addition of extracts of *Centella asiatica*, *Cytotechnology* 13(3):221, 1993.

Kirk-Smith MD, Booth DA: Chemoreception in human behaviour: experimental analysis of the social effects of fragrances, *Chemical Senses* 12:159, 1987.

Kirk-Smith MD and others: Unconscious odour conditioning in human subjects, *Biological Psychol* 17:221, 1983.

Kishore N, Mishra AK, Chansouria JPN: Fungitoxicity of essential oils against dermatophytes, *Mycoses* 36:211, 1993.

Kiuchi F and others: Inhibition of prostaglandin biosynthesis from ginger, *Chem Pharm* 30:747, 1982.

Knight TE, Hausen BM: *Melaleuca* oil (tea tree oil) dermatitis, *J Am Acad Dermatol* 30:423, 1994.

Kovar KA and others: Blood levels of 1,8-cineole and locomotor activity of mice after inhalation and oral administration of rosemary oil, *Plant Medica* 53:315, 1987.

Laude EA and others: The antitussive effects of menthol, camphor and cineole, in conscious guinea pigs, *Pulmonary Pharmacol* 7(3):179, 1994.

Lavabre M: *Aromatherapy workbook*, Rochester, Vt, 1990, Healing Arts Press.

Lawless J: *The encyclopedia of essential oils*, Rockport, Mass, 1996, Element.

Leicester RJ, Hunt RH: Peppermint oil to reduce colonic spasm during endoscopy, *Lancet* 2(8305):989, 1982.

Lewis J, Dahl A: Olfactory mucosa: composition, enzymatic localization and metabolism. In Doty R: *Handbook of olfaction and gustation*, New York, 1995, Marcel Dekker.

Lima EO and others: In vitro antifungal activity of essential oils obtained from officinal plants against dermatophytes, *Mycoses* 36:333, 1993.

Macdonald D, Brown R: Introduction: the pheromone concept in mammalian chemical communication. In Brown R, Macdonald D: *Social odors in mammals*, New York, 1984, Oxford University Press.

Mackereth P: Aromatherapy—nice but not "essential," *Complementary Therapies Nursing Midwifery* 1:4, 1995.

Mahmoud AL: Antifungal action and antiaflatoxigenic properties of some essential oil constituents, *Lett Appl Microbiol* 19(2):110, 1994.

Maquart FX and others: Stimulation of collagen sythesis in fibroblast cultures by a triterpene extracted from *Centella asiatica*, *Connective Tissue Res* 24(2):107, 1990.

Maruzzella JC, Sicurella N: Antibacterial activity of essential oil vapors, *J Am Pharm Assoc* 49:692, 1960.

Meeker HG, Linke HA: The antibacterial action of eugenol, thyme oil, and related essential oils used in dentistry, *Compendium* 9(1):32, 1988.

Miyan J and others: Neural control of release of cells from the bone marrow, in preparation, Manchester, England, 1996, University of Manchester Institute of Science and Technology.

Moehlman P: The odd-toed ungulates: order Perrisodactyla. In Brown R, Macdonald D: *Social odors in mammals*, New York, 1984, Oxford University Press.

Moleyar V, Narasimham P: Antibacterial activity of essential oil components, *Int J Food Microbiol* 16:337, 1992.

Naples JM and others: *Schistosoma mansoni*: cercaricidal effects of cedarwood oil and various of its components, *J Trop Med Hygiene* 95:390, 1992.

News item, *Your Health*, Globe International, Inc., Montreal, Quebec. Dec29:7, 1992.

Oh HK and others: Effect of various essential oils isolated from Douglas fir needles upon sheep and deer rumen microbial activity, *Appl Microbiol* 15:777, 1967.

Oliver J, Lorenz M. *Handbook of veterinary neurologic diagnosis*, Philadelphia, 1983, WB Saunders.

Olness K, Ader R: Conditioning as an adjunct in the pharmacotherapy of lupus erythematosus, *Dev Behav Pediatr* 13(2):124, 1992.

Onawunmi GO, Ogunlana EO: A study of the antibacterial activity of the essential oil of lemon grass, *Int J Crude Drug Res* 24(2):64, 1986.

Palmerino CC and others: Flavor-illness aversions: the peculiar role of odor and taste in the memory for poison, *Science* 208:753, 1980.

Pena EF: *Melaleuca alernifolia* oil: its use for trichomonal vaginitis and other vaginal infections, *Obstet Gynecol* 19:793, 1962.

Perucci S and others: Acaricidal agents of natural origin against *Psoroptes cuniculi*, *Parassitologia* 36(3):269, 1994.

Perucci S and others: In vitro antimycotic activity of some natural products against *Saprolegnia ferax*, *Phytother Res* 9(2):147, 1995.

Pointel JP and others: Titrated extract of *Centella asiatica* (TECA) in the treatment of venous insufficiency of the lower limbs, *Angiology* 38(1):46, 1987.

Price S: *Practical aromatherapy*, London, 1993, Diamond Books.

Raman A and others: Antimicrobial effects of tea-tree oil and its major components on *Staphylococcus aureus*, *Staph. epidermidis*, and *Propionibacterium acnes*, *Lett Appl Microbiol* 21(4):242, 1995.

Resch KL, Ernst E: Garlic *(Allium sativum)*—a potent medicinal plant (German), *Fortschritte der Medizin* 113:311, 1995.

Saeed SA, Gilani AH: Antithrombotic activity of clove oil, *J Pakistan Med Assoc* 44(5):112, 1994.

Safayhi H and others: Chamazulene: an antioxidant-type inhibitor of leukotriene B4 formation, *Planta Medica* 60:410, 1994.

Selvam R and others: The antioxidant activity of turmeric *(Curcuma longa), J Ethnopharmacol* 47(2):59, 1995.

Servadio C and others: Early stages of the pathogenesis of rat ventral prostate hyperplasia induced by citral, *Europ Urol* 12:195, 1986.

Shapiro S and others: The antimicrobial activity of essential oils and essential oil components towards oral bacteria, *Oral Microbiol Immunol* 9(4):202, 1994.

Sharma JN and others: Suppressive effects of eugenol and ginger oil on arthritic rats, *Pharmacology* 49:314, 1994.

Solvasan HB and others: Conditioned augmentation of natural killer cell activity, *J Immunol* 140:661, 1988.

Sparks MJ and others: Does peppermint oil relieve spasm during barium enema? *Br J Radiol* 68:841, 1995.

Sudekum M and others: Pennyroyal oil toxicosis in a dog, *JAVMA* 200:817, 1992.

Tassou CC, Drosinos EH, Nychas GJE: Effects of essential oil of mint *(Mentha piperita)* on *Salmonella enteritidis* and *Listeria monocytogenes* in model food systems at 4o and 10o, *J Appl Bacteriol* 78:593, 1995.

Tenni R and others: Effect of triterpenoid fraction of *Centella asiatica* on macromolecules of the connective matrix in human skin fibroblast cultures, *Ital J Biochem* 37(2):69, 1988.

Teuscher E and others: Untersuchungen zum Wirkungsmechanismus atherischer Ole, *Zeitschrift fur Phytotherapie* 11:87, 1990.

Tibballs J: Clinical effects and management of eucalyptus oil ingestion in infants and young children, *Med J Austral* 163(4):177, 1995.

Tisserand RB: *The art of aromatherapy*, Rochester, Vt, 1977, Healing Arts Press.

Tisserand RB, Balacs T: *Essential oil safety: a guide for healthcare professionals*, New York, 1995, Churchill Livingstone.

Tong MM and others: Tea tree oil in the treatment of tinea pedis, *Australasian J Dermatol* 33(3):145, 1992.

Tsujimoto Y and others: Superoxide radical scavenging activity of phenolic compounds, *Int J Biochem* 25:491, 1993.

Villar D and others: Toxicity of melaleuca oil and related essential oils applied topically on dogs and cats (review), *Vet Human Toxicol* 36(2):139, 1994.

Voudouris NJ and others: The role of conditioning and verbal expectancy in the placebo response, *Pain* 43:121, 1990.

Warren CB and others: Method of causing the reduction of physiological and/or subjective reactivity to stress in humans being subjected to stress conditions, U.S. Patent No. 4671959, 1987.

Wasantha Piyadasa HD: Traditional systems for preventing and treating animal diseases in Sri Lanka, *Rev Sci Tech Off Int Epiz* 13:471, 1994.

Williams L, Home V: A comparative study of some essential oils for potential use in topical applications for the treatment of the yeast *Candida albicans*. NHAA International Conference Proceedings, 1995.

Yamada K and others: Anticonvulsive effects of inhaling lavender oil vapour, *Biol Pharm Bull* 17:359, 1994.

Zheng G and others: Potential anticarcinogenic natural products isolated from lemongrass oil and galanga root oil, *J Agri Food Chem* 41(2):153, 1993.

Chapter 31

Bach Flower Therapy: A Practitioner's Perspective*

STEPHEN R. BLAKE, JR.

Overview

Flower essence therapy is a healing modality based on the clinical findings and philosophy of Edward Bach, an English physician. The proposed mode of action does not use pharmacologic means but influences the patient by manipulating "energy," affecting the mental, emotional, and physical balance of the individual. Although the scientific basis of this approach is unclear, Dr. Bach proposed that this method of treatment relies on the transfer of the "Life Energy Forces" from the plants to the patient to help balance the individual's "vital force." For a more detailed discussion of the vitalist philosophy of medicine, other literature is available on the subject (Coulter, 1973-1977). When an animal is ill, a change in behavior may accompany changes in physical function. The psychoemotional state of the animal may influence the immune and endocrine systems by altering various neurotransmitters and cytokines (Ader and others, 1995). Use of the essences balances the psychoemotional state, thereby helping the animal reach homeostasis. The flower essence method addresses the patient on an energetic basis, and is a noninvasive means of positively altering behavior patterns. This therapy is based on the concept that correction of emotional (mind) dysfunction can help heal physical (body) dysfunction.

Flower essence therapy complements any form of medicine. It can enhance the efficacy of either conventional or alternative medicine without interfering with concurrent

*English flower essence therapy is gaining popularity among pet owners and veterinarians. However, the efficacy of flower essence therapy has not been documented, nor have preparations and dosages been standardized. Practitioners are cautioned to discuss all aspects of this type of therapy with clients and use sound clinical judgment when employing English flower essences in their practices. This chapter is included to educate veterinarians, not necessarily to validate this approach.

therapies. Currently, flower essence therapy is used more extensively in humans than animals, although many veterinarians have used this system on animals with positive results for over 50 years.

Bach described a treatment system unfamiliar to the medical establishment; his system still uses philosophies and substances that are unique among the complementary therapies. He described the essence of his philosophy as follows:

> The action of these remedies is to raise our vibrations and open up our channels for the reception of the Spiritual Self; to flood our natures with the particular virtue we need, and wash out from us the fault that is causing the harm. They are able, like beautiful music or any glorious uplifting thing which gives us inspiration, to raise our very natures, and bring us nearer to our souls and by that very act to bring us peace and relieve our sufferings. They cure, not by attacking the disease, but by flooding our bodies with the beautiful vibration of our Higher Nature, in the presence of which, disease melts away as snow in the sunshine (Sheffer, 1986).

After reading Bach's description, many veterinarians may wonder whether they give short shrift to the higher natures of their animal patients. Flower essence therapy may have a unique place in veterinary medicine.

History

Bach identified the 38 English flower essences used in the treatment method he discovered. As Casualty Medical Officer at University College Hospital London, Bach became frustrated by the nature of a busy medical practice and the fact that healers were too busy to consider patients as individuals rather than collections of disease patterns. This frustration led him into immunology, and he became a published author and specialist in bacteriology (Teale, Bach, 1920a, 1920b, 1920c). Eventually, his attitudes about the holistic nature of disease led him to homeopathy. A pioneer in combining schools of healing, Bach sought to overcome "the prejudice amongst the homeopaths against mixing, as they thought, orthodoxy with the pure principles of Hahnemann" (Weeks, 1972). His lasting contribution to homeopathy is that of the so-called bowel nosodes, or homeopathic preparations of intestinal bacteria, which he successfully used in the treatment of many classes of human disease. Bach eventually became disenchanted with homeopathy because he was convinced that illness could—and should—be treated with nontoxic substances alone. In 1930, he gave up his medical practice to focus his efforts on finding nontoxic plant remedies and perfecting their preparation (Weeks, 1973).

Flowers of wild plants, bushes, and trees compose 37 of the remedies, and water the last; Bach found all necessary ingredients in the English countryside. These plants were selected from species that were nontoxic in their natural states. He thoroughly studied various methods of preparation and came to believe that the plants, together with local environment, time of year, and other factors, contributed to the therapeutic power of his remedies. He finally developed a method of harvesting flowers at the height of their "energetic" power, when the flowers were freshest and dew still present. The properties were extracted by decocting in spring water in full sun. The decoctions were then filtered and mixed with brandy for stability. Bach perceived the therapeutic properties of these plants by "feeling" them and not by any traditional herbal healing properties known at that time. Bach was said to have a developed sixth sense—he often cured patients by laying hands on them, and his perception of the healing powers from these plants was purely intuitive on his part.

Traditional Theory

Flower essences are not homeopathic, herbal, or aromatic in their preparation. They are similar to homeopathics in that they are vibrational in nature and physically dilute, but flower-essence actions were not determined by provings (see Chapter 24) and are generally used only in 1:10 or 1:100 dilutions. Bach did not prescribe remedies according to the simillimum, as classic homeopathy requires. Because Bach's therapies are plants prepared by decoction, they may be considered by some to act as herbal remedies. In fact, Bach called himself an *herbalist* (Weeks, 1973). These preparations do not have the same pharmacologic activities as more concentrated forms of the same plants; in fact, the most salient feature of these diluted herbs is their ability to work on a different plane than the pharmacologic one. They are usually considered an energy medicine, and their sphere of action is on the "emotional body." Bach once described disease as "a kind of consolidation of a mental attitude" and said that "it

is necessary to treat the mood of a patient, and the disease will disappear" (1979). Bach theorized that negative psychoemotional states suppress the healing process and are the primary cause of disease. He perceived patients as representing certain patterns of emotional dysfunction, and flower essences were prescribed to patients based on emotional state only. He identified 12 pathologic emotional states that, left untreated, would inevitably lead to physical disease (Box 31-1).

Do animals have emotional states that affect physical conditions? Bach said that "behind all disease lies our fears, our anxieties, our greed, our likes and dislikes" (1979). Most pet owners and veterinarians would agree that behavioral problems are a major concern. They often accompany or precede physical disease as well. Connections between the immune, endocrine, and nervous systems clearly support this seemingly foreign theory of disease. Established connections exist between cytokine levels and the hypothalamic-pituitary-adrenal axis, and lymphocytes and macrophages contain receptors for many neurotransmitters (Ader and others, 1995). Perhaps Bach's theory that "there is no true healing unless there is a change in outlook, peace of mind, and inner happiness" (Sheffer, 1986) is not so foreign after all.

The flower essence practitioner who sees human patients might start an interview with a general question about the patient's health. This approach is obviously unsuited to veterinary patients, but best results are obtained when the practitioner is aware of the emotional state of the animal; in this case, the prescription fits the individual and not the pathologic state. A committed doctor-client-patient relationship is essential for correct prescribing. Practitioners should also be aware that patients often reflect their caretakers. Clients frequently respond to case taking with statements such as "that sounds just like me!" or "will that help me, since I have the same symptoms?"

BOX 31-1

PATHOLOGIC EMOTIONAL STATES

1. Fear
2. Terror
3. Mental torture or worry
4. Indecision
5. Indifference or boredom
6. Doubt or discouragement
7. Overconcern
8. Weakness
9. Self-distrust
10. Impatience
11. Overenthusiasm
12. Pride or aloofness

An appropriate response might be that the remedies are also used in human medicine, and if clients want to explore their use for self-care, they should contact their health care providers.

Flower essence use in animals has no scientific support at this time. Double-blind studies have not been accomplished in animals because of lack of funding, lack of interest by the scientific community, and the fact that mechanism of action is unknown. The fact that the remedies have been effective with this author's patients for over 10 years suggests that they are not placebos. The dramatic positive changes in the animals' behavior demonstrates the effectiveness of the noninvasive way the remedies work. The 38-remedies system is a gentle, nontoxic, and noninvasive means of alleviating the emotional stresses in veterinary patients. Using the remedies in combination with the total patient program provides an excellent complement to consider for all clinical cases.

To prepare English flower essences (EFE) for patients, mix 2 drops of each EFE, up to a maximum of 7 EFEs per patient, in a 1-ounce bottle. The only exception to the 2-drop method is in the five-flower combination Stress formula, when 4 drops are used and counted as one remedy. Place these tinctures in a 1-ounce amber glass bottle with a glass dropper and add 3 parts spring water to 1 part alcohol (vodka, brandy, or Purol). Shake well, and instruct the owner to shake it each time it is used. Store in a cool place out of direct sunlight, microwaves, heat, or x-rays.

Dosage depends on the animal's response, but a general rule is 3 drops 1 to 4 times per day as needed. I have discovered many ways to administer the EFE over the years and found most to be effective. With dogs and horses the remedies can be administered orally. Cats and birds are best treated by adding the essences to drinking water at a dose of 1 to 3 drops per day, depending on taste acceptance. I have mixed it in food, massaged it into the skin, and rubbed it in the ears with equal success. Another technique involves mixing the essences in a spray bottle and misting kennels, barns, stalls, pens, and clinic intake and exhaust ducts to treat large areas. Essences can also be mixed in a tub of water to soak animals, or in the case of horses, sponged on them. One dropperful is the recommended strength in whatever the volume of water used. In acute situations, give 3 drops orally every few minutes until the condition stabilizes, then repeat as needed. If bleeding occurs during surgery, the Trauma formula, given every 30 seconds until the situation is resolved, can be very useful.

When prescribing for any patient, the practitioner should consider similarities between owner and patient. Animals often respond in kind to their caretakers, resulting in added stress that disturbs homeostasis of the body. If the owner is interested in knowing more about this, the practitioner can provide a self-help handout and suggest further investigation of the modality with the medical practitioner.

Materia Medica

The following is a materia medica of the essences. This listing of emotional symptoms is derived completely from books in the human field. Many practitioners may be resistant to the subjective nature of the symptoms listed, but in flower-remedy therapy, inference to animal emotions must be based solely on the practitioner's judgment. Practitioners will find it helpful to review the many texts available on animal behavior, and listen carefully to the client's assessment of the pet's emotional state when prescribing flower remedies.

Agrimony

Animals who may respond to agrimony are sensitive and easily distressed when owners argue or quarrel. The owners may perceive them as "peacemakers." They are often stoic. They do not like to be alone, and are restless. They may develop skin problems, arthritis, and gastrointestinal disturbances when stressed. Agrimony is also effective for urinary incontinence.

Aspen

Aspen is an excellent remedy for fear, especially when animals are afraid of anything unfamiliar. These animals spook easily and become nervous for no obvious reason. Aspen is an excellent remedy to give animals before storms, firecrackers, thunder, and trips to the veterinarian. Many bladder and kidney problems may improve with administration of aspen. Separation anxiety is often very responsive to this essence.

Beech

Beech is for the intolerant pet who complains vocally. These pets usually tolerate only their master or immediate family and do not like other animals or people. Beech is often indicated when a first pet rejects a new pet. These pets can also be selective eaters and are intolerant of insects, pollen, pollution, heat, cold, and changes in barometric pressures. This remedy is an excellent way to reduce territorial aggression and may also be effective in the treatment of arthritic conditions and allergies.

Centaury

Centaury fits the timid, quiet animal who is easily dominated by other animals. These animals are usually subservient and eager to please. They allow themselves to be pushed aside, without defending themselves. Centaury is a good remedy for the runt of the litter who gets pushed away from the teat or is ill after birth. Fear of other dogs and submissive urination are problems responsive to this essence.

Cerato

Cerato is for the animal who is easily distracted, particularly during training. These animals are usually vocal and restless and may be considered "discipline problems." This essence should be considered for chronic barkers.

Cherry Plum

Cherry plum is for fear of losing control. One example is the cat who panics and becomes vicious when restrained because he feels he is not in control. This can manifest as incontinence when excited, self-mutilation, and fear-related aggression. These animals seem to know that they have misbehaved after biting or scratching.

Chestnut Bud

Chestnut bud is an excellent way to help animals learn basic skills and break bad habits. This remedy is indicated for use in training and prevention of future mistakes. Chestnut bud can be used with any form of behavior modification.

Chicory

Chicory is for dominant animals who think they own the house and everything in it. They demand attention, and food and may be overly protective of the family. They may try to dominate particular individuals in the family and can be jealous. They often follow the owner around and are constantly underfoot or in the owner's lap.

Clematis

Clematis may be helpful for the pet who is distracted, indifferent, inattentive, and preoccupied, which makes it useful in training. It is excellent for hastening recovery after surgery or trauma. It is also good for patients who have had drug overdoses, debilitating colic, and exhaustion from whelping. It is one of the flowers in the five-flower Emergency formula. Clematis can also be used in vestibular disease when the patient is weak.

Crab Apple

Crab apple is a cleansing remedy that should be used for "toxic" states in which the body exudes discharge or odor. It is excellent for wounds, body odor (e.g., during estrus), unhealthy coats, any form of dermatitis, poisoning by drugs or chemicals, and infections. It is also effective for cats who are extremely fastidious. The essence can be used both orally and topically to treat infections.

Elm

Elm is indicated for the animal who is overwhelmed by a demanding situation, such as travel, competition, or even a trip to the veterinarian or groomer. It is a good remedy for show animals at competitions, where they become overly anxious.

Gentian

Gentian can be given to the animal who appears depressed or discouraged, either emotionally or physically. Situations when an animal seems depressed because of illness, work, loss of a friend, chronic disease, rehabilitation, or a bad experience are indications for gentian. This remedy is often used when detoxifying animals to make the healing process easier on their systems.

Gorse

Gorse is indicated for pets who appear hopeless. They refuse food, and improvement from chronic illness may be inordinately slow. Gorse helps encourage patients to make renewed efforts to heal.

Heather

Heather is indicated for the animal who demonstrates excessive attention-getting behavior, vocalizes constantly, and worsens when alone. This animal is often friendly to the point of being obnoxious.

Holly

Holly can be used to treat animals that are aggressive, jealous, and suspicious. These animals tend to bite and anger easily. When these animals release anger, the positive aspect is that they can be loving, tolerant, and happy. If no single remedy seems clearly indicated, holly may ease the transition to the next indicated remedy. Wild oat is also good if the prescription is unclear or when the animal is not angry. Holly is a good choice for most cases of aggression.

Honeysuckle

Honeysuckle is indicated for animals with anxious behavior. Kennel stays, separation from home or family, and hospitalization are all possible indications for honeysuckle. These animals may exhibit grief with illness. Honeysuckle may also be helpful in weakness caused by loss of blood or illness.

Hornbeam

Hornbeam is indicated in cases of mental and physical exhaustion. It is effective for animals who have lost interest in life or show animals who appear fatigued during work.

Impatiens

Animals to be treated with impatiens are best described as impatient, irritable, and nervous. This remedy should be considered for neurologic conditions accompanied by nervousness, shaking, or seizures made worse by excitement. These are generally anxious animals, especially during feeding time. Impatiens is another remedy for show animals who are anxious during competition. It is also one of the remedies in the Emergency formula because it may alleviate pain in general.

Larch

Larch is for the animal who cowers in submission. This remedy is excellent for abused animals.

Mimulus

Mimulus is indicated for animals who have specific fears that can be identified. These animals may hide in the presence of visitors and sometimes become aggressive when cornered. This is an excellent remedy for fear of thunder, lightning, people, animals, abandonment, noise, and air balloons. Inappropriate urination caused by fear may also be treated with this remedy.

Mustard

Mustard is a good remedy for animals who suddenly become depressed, prefer solitude, and stay in one place. It is also excellent for animals who have been chronically ill and have apparently given up hope of recovery.

Oak

Oak is a great remedy for animals who are struggling to overcome a disability. These animals may appear despondent, but they continue their effort. This remedy helps rebuild the strength of the animal after any physically stressful situation. It is excellent for endurance competitions that require stamina. It is also excellent for animals who have lost a body function (e.g., limb paralysis, loss of elimination functions).

Olive

Olive is indicated for mental and physical exhaustion. These animals are worn down from chronic illness. This remedy is indicated for detoxification when the animal is weak and for support during the cleansing process. This remedy enhances stamina during endurance competition. It is also indicated for any condition that includes loss of function.

Pine

Pine can be used with patients who are devoted to their owners despite poor treatment. These animals may cower when people are upset and make constant attempts to please their owners.

Red Chestnut

Red chestnut is appropriate for when an animal seems afraid for those it loves. These animals may stand at the window, waiting for owners to return. They appear overly anxious about their young and do not tolerate separation well. Red chestnut is a good remedy for the pet who must be separated from its owner.

Rock Rose

Rock rose is another fear remedy. It is also a component of the five-flower Emergency remedy and is indicated for terror, panic phobias, and extreme fear. This remedy is excellent for the animal who destroys the house out of fear when left alone or during thunder, lightning, fireworks, and loud noises.

Rock Water

Rock water is made not from plants but from water (which can wear away the hardest rock). Rock water therefore represents a hard, intractable nature and is used for stubborn animals who resist breaking old habits. These animals tend to have routines and may also have physical stiffness of joints and muscles. Rock water can also be helpful when a new pet or family member moves into the household. Degenerative arthritis sometimes responds to rock water.

Scleranthus

Scleranthus is indicated for loss of balance, lack of co-ordination, hormonal imbalances, and any neurologic condition. It is often helpful in the treatment of strokes, hemiparesis, and monoparesis. These animals may have severe mood swings. Scleranthus may also be helpful for motion sickness accompanied by vomiting with salivation. It is also helpful in vestibular syndrome in both dogs and cats.

Star of Bethlehem

Star of Bethlehem is indicated for any form of mental or physical shock. It is also one of the remedies in the five-flower Emergency remedy. These animals may appear withdrawn. Star of Bethlehem is also helpful for situations in which the animal's emotional or physical trauma appears to cause paralysis or loss of a biologic function. It is also excellent for kenneling, loss, weaning, and change of environment, such as a move to a new home. Separation anxiety may respond to this remedy.

Sweet Chestnut

The indication for sweet chestnut is best described by a quote from Dr. Bach's writings: "It is the hopeless despair of those who feel they have reached the limit of their endurance" (Bach, 1979). This emotional state is exemplified by the wild animal in captivity who paces back and forth. This remedy may also help competitive animals obtain access to the extra reserves of energy necessary to finish a competition that requires endurance.

Vervain

Animals who respond to vervain are usually high-strung, hyperactive, and intense. They have a great deal of nervous energy and may pace, jump, and bark. This remedy may help calm animals who seem to have inexhaustible energy. Vervain may also help in roaming and escaping tendencies.

Vine

Vine is used in animals who are dominant, inflexible, and strong-willed quick thinkers. They are difficult to train.

Walnut

Walnut is the "transition remedy" that helps protect the patient during any state of change, such as a move, new owner, travel, surgery, and loss of a body part. It is recommended to aid the patient in the healing process. This remedy is also useful for training.

Water Violet

Water violet is appropriate for aloof animals who prefer solitude when ill. They tend to be antisocial with other animals and people. This remedy fits many cats because they are often aloof, intelligent, and indifferent to others around them. Water violet is an excellent remedy for animals who become aloof during grief over a loss.

White Chestnut

White chestnut is indicated for anxious animals. It helps them focus during any form of training and abandon old behaviors.

Wild Oat

Wild oat is for animals who appear depressed from boredom. Oat is good for animals who retire after enjoy-

able competition. These animals may exhibit signs of separation anxiety, such as destruction of the house or corral, chewing, and feather picking.

Wild Rose

Wild rose is indicated for animals who seem to lack energy and motivation. This is an excellent remedy for patients who appear apathetic, but it may also be used for animals who seem overly serious and tense.

Willow

Willow's keynote indication is resentment. These animals often show their displeasure by urinating, defecating, and destroying the house. Willow may help in all cases of destructive behavior in which resentment appears to be the underlying cause.

General Remarks

In most cases the transition from the disease state to homeostasis should be smooth. In some cases the emotional or physical detoxification process can result in a brief "healing crisis" in which symptoms worsen. This normally lasts only a few hours and then passes. If this should occur, practitioners are recommended to allow their patients to pass through the process without interference. If the crisis persists more than 24 hours, the remedy should be discontinued and gentian and five-flower emergency formula administered. Once the problem is resolved, the five-flower and gentian are stopped and the original remedy or combination may be continued. Some hypersensitive patients cannot take the remedies at the usual concentration and require dilutions of 2 drops in 4 to 16 ounces of water, at a dose of 3 drops. The concentration is then gradually increased until the remedy can be given in its original strength. Sometimes the remedy can be rubbed into the animal's ears instead of being orally administered.

Flower Essence Repertory

Box 31-2 lists formulas that may help in specific conditions and situations. Flower essence practitioners regard these physical conditions as emotionally based, but appropriate physical treatments should always be considered simultaneously.

BOX 31-2

*F*lower *E*ssence *R*epertory

Anemia: Walnut, chestnut bud, olive, star of Bethlehem, gentian

Animals that do not get along: Walnut, chestnut bud, beech, willow, holly

Barking excessively: Chestnut bud, cerato, heather, vervain

Car sickness: Walnut, chestnut bud, scleranthus, mimulus, five-flower formula

Cystitis caused or aggravated by fear: Walnut, chestnut bud, aspen, mimulus, rock rose

Dermatitis: Crab apple, walnut, chestnut bud, five-flower formula

Detoxification: Crab apple, walnut, chestnut bud, olive, gentian

Diarrhea: Walnut, crab apple, olive, star of Bethlehem, five-flower formula

Epilepsy: Walnut, cherry plum, scleranthus, larch, olive

Fear: Walnut, chestnut bud, mimulus, aspen, rock rose, larch

Grieving: Star of Bethlehem, walnut, honeysuckle, chestnut bud, gentian

Greeting formula for patients in exam room: Five-flower formula, elm, aspen, mimulus, sweet chestnut

Immune disorders: Walnut, chestnut bud, scleranthus, olive, star of Bethlehem, and crab apple

Incontinence: Walnut, chestnut bud, olive, agrimony

Infections: Crab apple, walnut, olive, gentian, five-flower formula

Kenneling: Walnut, chestnut bud, honeysuckle, star of Bethlehem, olive, gentian, white chestnut; sweet chestnut for the owner who worries about the pet during a stay in the kennel

Lack of confidence: Walnut, chestnut bud, centaury, larch

Negative stress environment: Mixture of walnut, mustard, wild rose, crab apple sprayed in area

Newborn remedy for new mother: Red chestnut, five-flower formula, walnut, larch, gentian, olive

Paralysis: Walnut, chestnut bud, star of Bethlehem, gentian, olive, scleranthus

Trailering (horses): Walnut, chestnut bud, mimulus, aspen, rock rose, scleranthus

Training: Walnut, chestnut bud, olive, clematis, impatiens, wild oat

Trauma: Walnut, crab apple, gentian, olive, star of Bethlehem, five-flower formula

Vestibular syndrome: Walnut, scleranthus, olive, cherry plum, chestnut bud, star of Bethlehem

Vomiting: Five-flower formula, walnut, crab apple, olive, star of Bethlehem

*R*EFERENCES

Ader R and others: Psychoneuroimmunology: interactions between the nervous system and the immune system, *Lancet* 345:99-103, 1995.

Bach E, Wheeler FJ: *The Bach flower remedies,* New Canaan, Conn, 1979, Keats Publishing Inc.

Coulter H: *Divided legacy: a history of schism in medical thought,* vol 1-4, Washington, 1973-1977, Wehawken Book Co.

Sheffer M: *Bach flower therapy theory and practice,* Rochester, Vt, 1986, Thorsons Publishers Inc.

Teale FH, Bach E: The fate of "washed spores" on inoculation into animals, with special reference to the nature of bacterial toxaemia, *J Path Bacteriol,* 1920a.

Teale FH, Bach E: The nature of serum antitrypsin and its relation to autolysis and the formation of toxins, *Proceedings of the Royal Society of Medicine,* 1920b.

Teale FH, Bach E: The relation of the autotryptic titre of blood to bacteria infection and anaphylaxis, *Proceedings of the Royal Society of Medicine,* 1920c.

Weeks N: *The medical discoveries of Edward Bach, physician,* New Canaan, Conn, 1973, Keats Publishing Inc.

*S*ELECTED READINGS

Baker MD: *Bach flower remedy repertoires parts one and two,* Wellingborough, Northants, 1979, Thorsons Publishers Ltd.

Bear J: *Practical uses and applications of the Bach flower remedies,* Las Vegas, 1989, Balancing Essentials Press.

Chancellor PM: *Dr. Philip M. Chancellor's handbook of the Bach flower remedies,* New Canaan, Conn, 1980, Keats Publishing, Inc.

Cunningham D: *Flower remedies handbook,* New York, 1992, Sterling Publishing.

Kaminski P, Katz R: *Flower essence repertory,* Nevada City, Calif, 1994, The Flower Essence Society.

Wood M: *Seven herbs: plants as teachers,* Berkeley, Calif, 1987, North Atlantic Books.

*S*OURCES

Ellon USA, Inc 800-423-2256
Flower Essence Pharmacy 619-299-8166
Flower Essences Services 800-548-0075
Homeopathic Educational Services 800-359-9051
Jessica Bear, N.D. Balancing Essentials 702-598-0727
Nelson Bach, USA 800-314-2224
Standard Homeopathic 800-624-9659

Integration into Veterinary Practice

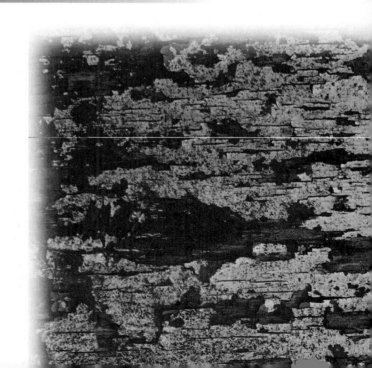

*I*ncorporating Complementary Veterinary Therapies into Conventional Small Animal Practice

ALLEN M. SCHOEN

Introduction

Small animal veterinary practice is evolving and expanding into new therapeutic arenas as the demand for other areas seems to decrease. A paradigm shift is beginning to occur wherein the public is no longer satisfied with conventional approaches to veterinary medicine, just as they are becoming dissatisfied with the limitations of conventional medicine and surgery for themselves (Eisenberg, 1993). The incorporation of new and emerging therapeutic modalities into conventional practice also makes economic sense. Procedures such as ovariohysterectomies and castrations are performed more frequently by humane societies and spay-and-vaccination clinics. The scientific basis of vaccination protocols and their potential side effects are currently being reevaluated (Smith, 1995). These procedures, neuterings, and vaccinations often form the economic basis of many small animal practices. As these economic foundations weaken, replacement with other procedures and therapies that are beneficial to animal health is essential. A broad range of complementary therapies are available to small animal veterinarians that will enhance their practices as well as their perspectives on health. However, the veterinarian must receive adequate postgraduate training in these therapies to perform them properly. A paradigm shift is often necessary in practitioner philosophy before a comprehensive perspective on these new approaches can develop. Some of these therapies may be quite different from the conventional medical model in which veterinarians have been trained. Now is an excellent time for veterinarians to explore, develop, and

incorporate emerging concepts into their own practice philosophy.

There are many approaches to incorporating complementary and alternative veterinary medicine (CAVM) into a conventional small animal practice. This chapter discusses educational requirements, American Veterinary Medical Association (AVMA) guidelines, and legal considerations concerning this incorporation. Examples of different approaches to incorporating these therapies into practice are offered, as well as techniques to educate staff, colleagues, and clients. Conflicts and contraindications are also discussed.

Education Requirements

Many avenues and approaches may be used to incorporate CAVM into a conventional small animal practice. Veterinarians must complete appropriate professional postgraduate educational programs before they can be considered competent in any of these therapies; at this time, no veterinary school in the United States offers such a program. Postgraduate certification courses are being offered in certain therapies, although no AVMA board-certified specialty in any of these therapies exists. The International Veterinary Acupuncture Society (IVAS) offers a postgraduate certification course in both veterinary acupuncture and Chinese herbal medicine. The American Veterinary Chiropractic Association offers postgraduate certification in veterinary chiropractic care, and the Academy of Veterinary Homeopathy offers training in veterinary homeopathy (see Appendix). The American Holistic Veterinary Medical Association has an annual conference to introduce veterinarians to holistic medicine. In addition, many national and international conferences now offer introductory lectures in the various therapies.

Veterinarians must also abide by the AVMA guidelines on alternative therapies (AVMA, 1997; see Box 1-1) when incorporating these therapies into a small animal practice. The AVMA offers guidelines on alternative therapies—including ultrasound diagnosis and therapy, magnetic field therapy, holistic medicine, homeopathy, chiropractic, acupuncture, and laser therapy—that were approved in 1996.

Holistic Medicine

The AVMA guidelines (1997) define holistic veterinary medicine as follows:

> Holistic veterinary medicine is a comprehensive approach to health care involving alternative and conventional diagnostic and therapeutic modalities.
>
> In practice, holistic veterinary medicine incorporates, but is not limited to, the principles of acupuncture and acutherapy, botanical medicine, chiropractic, homeopathy, massage therapy, nutraceuticals, and physical therapy, as well as conventional medicine, surgery, and dentistry. It is recommended that holistic veterinary medicine be practiced only by licensed veterinarians educated in the modalities employed. The modalities of holistic veterinary medicine should be practiced according to the licensure and referral requirements concerning each modality. The public should be informed in advance by the practitioner that holistic veterinary medicine currently is considered unconventional.

Many so-called holistic modalities are being practiced by various lay individuals with questionable training. For the public to receive the optimal care for their animal companions, veterinarians must receive appropriate training before incorporating these modalities into their practices. If a veterinarian is not interested in incorporating these therapies, he or she is advised to learn at least enough about these modalities to make an appropriate referral to a properly trained colleague. Veterinarians should also consult local state guidelines concerning the practice of these therapies. Review of Chapter 42 is also advised.

Another important goal is that veterinarians have excellent skills practicing conventional medicine before practicing any of the CAVM therapies. Although this prerequisite may seem obvious, it is important to emphasize: If a practitioner is not competent in conventional veterinary diagnostics and therapy, he or she may not be able to offer the client and patient the absolute best options for appropriate care. Clients may seek out a "holistic" practitioner without really understanding what this entails; they may not even have an appropriate diagnosis. The veterinarian who ventures into CAVM must also incorporate Western medical conventional training and explore all appropriate options for diagnosis and treatment, including Western medicine.

Incorporation into Practice: Examples

After veterinarians have received the appropriate training, the next step is to decide how these therapies are to be incorporated into practice. Because CAVM is a relatively new field of practice in veterinary medicine, veterinarians are incorporating these therapies in various ways. For example, practitioners may decide to incorporate only one therapy into a conventional practice, such as acupuncture, and use it to treat only certain conditions they believe to be responsive to this therapy with their level of training. Other veterinarians may undertake every advanced training course offered in many of the different therapies and dedicate their practices solely to alternative therapies. Many possibilities between these two examples also exist. Veterinarians may begin with one particular therapy, such as acupuncture, and slowly incorporate it into a practice. As they become comfortable using that therapy, they may decide to take advanced training in another therapy and then incorporate that one, continuing their training as appropriate. Training and proficiency are imperative before any modality is incorporated into a practice.

After receiving appropriate training, veterinarians also ensure that hospital staff receive education concerning their roles in these therapies and in client education. If practitioners are considering advertising these therapies and accepting referrals, they should educate local colleagues about this additional training and the conditions that are appropriate for referral. These concepts are discussed in more detail.

Diagnostic Examination

Practitioners may incorporate these therapies into the diagnostic examination and therapy. As in Western medicine a comprehensive history is critical. In addition to the conventional history, a historical questionnaire relating to each particular modality is beneficial. With modalities such as acupuncture and homeopathy the history is usually extremely detailed, recording details such as response to weather conditions, behavior patterns (e.g., preference for warm or cold areas), food preferences, and behavior toward other animals. For example, an acupuncture or homeopathic history may include references to symptoms that worsen in various weather conditions. Different behavior patterns are also significant. For example, the preference for ambient warmth (such as that obtained by lying near a heater) and the preference for cold (such as that obtained by lying on a cold tile floor) suggest completely different homeopathic remedies. If practitioners are concerned about potential exposure to environmental toxins or food allergies, they should include questions regarding potential exposure into a comprehensive questionnaire.

Chapter 29 suggests diagnostic lines of inquiry. For example, practitioners may ask whether the symptoms began when a new carpet was installed or new house construction initiated. The significance of such simple questions is highlighted in the following example. A 6-year-old female spayed domestic short-hair cat had a history of generalized pruritus and abdominal alopecia. A previous veterinarian made a tentative diagnosis of allergic dermatitis and prescribed corticosteroids. The animal responded but had side effects; when the steroid dosage was reduced, the pruritus and alopecia recurred. A second veterinarian diagnosed feline endocrine alopecia and prescribed Ovaban (megestrol acetate, Schering-Plough, Kenilworth, NJ). The animal again responded but then developed diabetes as a sequela. When the medication was stopped, the diabetes fortunately resolved, but the symptoms also recurred. The owner then contacted this author regarding a more holistic approach. I first asked, "Was there a change in the environment within the previous few weeks before the onset of symptoms?" The owner replied that new wall-to-wall carpeting had just been installed in her home, and within days, the cat began to show signs.

My first recommendation was to remove the cat from the possible environmental irritant. After this was done, all symptoms resolved without further treatment. The cat was kept away from the carpeting for 2 months to evaluate if it was just the potential initial outgassing that occurs in new carpets or if it was the carpet material itself. Fortunately for the owner, it was merely the outgassing, and the symptoms never recurred. This is only one example of the importance of a comprehensive environmental questionnaire in a holistic approach. Other potential questions are listed in Box 32-1.

Veterinarians should also review the dates and types of previous vaccinations. As is evident from Chapter 40 and the article on potential vaccine reactions (Smith, 1995), the possibility of a potential reaction to a vaccine may not occur for a few weeks after vaccination.

If only one modality is being practiced, the questionnaire may be limited to questions relevant to that particular therapy. If veterinarians are using a comprehensive holistic approach that incorporates many therapies, different sections of the questionnaire may be designed to reflect each modality.

BOX 32-1

Holistic Environmental Questionnaire

1. When did signs/symptoms first appear? DATE: _____
   SEASON: Spring _____ Summer _____ Autumn _____ Winter _____
2. Did any dietary changes occur before onset of the condition?
   a. Changes in diet? _____
   b. Additional medications? _____
   c. Additional supplements? _____
3. Did changes in the indoor or outdoor environment occur?
   a. Indoor: 1. New carpeting _____
               2. New furniture _____
               3. New housecleaning detergents _____
               4. New cat litter _____
               5. New hair sprays, deodorants, or other chemicals _____
               6. Other _____
   b. Outdoor: 1. Seasonal changes _____
               2. Outdoor chemicals: pesticides, fungicides _____
               3. Outdoor paints, sprays _____
               4. Antifreeze exposure _____
               5. Other _____
4. Vaccination History
   1. Dates of last vaccinations and types of vaccines _____
   2. Obvious reactions to vaccinations _____
5. Miscellaneous:
   1. Any other changes of concern before onset of problems?
   _____
   _____
   _____

During the diagnostic examination, veterinarians must perform a thorough conventional physical examination. In addition, appropriate conventional diagnostic tests are beneficial. Western medicine has excellent diagnostic tools that should not be ignored. With the appropriate examination and diagnostic tests, a physical examination may be included. This examination should be based on the therapies in which the practitioner has received training. Acupuncture, chiropractic care, and physical therapy all require additional diagnostic examination techniques. For example, an acupuncture physical examination may include analysis of the pulse and tongue for diagnoses based on traditional Chinese medical theory (TCM). The Eastern and Western diagnostic techniques may be combined to yield a diagnosis based on both paradigms. In a chiropractic examination, both static and motion palpation diagnostic techniques, along with palpation for various misalignments and fixations, may be performed (see Chapter 12).

After making a diagnosis on the basis of history, physical examination, appropriate diagnostic tests, and appropriate diagnostic examination findings according to the various alternative therapies incorporated, the practitioner may then select the best approach for the individual patient.

Therapeutic Options

The various CAVM therapies may be incorporated as a sole therapeutic option or integrated into a comprehensive approach. Some therapies actually complement each other, whereas others may counteract one another. Veterinarians may find it difficult to determine the modality that is working when a combination is being used. This is a reasonable concern. As their expertise in the various modalities increases, veterinarians are better able to anticipate results and often experienced enough to distinguish the effects of particular modalities. Until then, veterinarians are advised to limit themselves to one or two approaches at a time. Occasionally, however, clients may request that everything possible be done at once because of the severity or rapid progression of a condition. This request may not be unreasonable, and if the comprehensive approach does work, the veterinarian can elucidate the effects of the individual approaches later.

Certain therapies complement each other well. Acupuncture, Chinese herbal medicine, nutritional supplements, acupressure, and physical therapy have been used together for thousands of years. Acupuncture and chiropractic care also complement each other extremely well. Classically trained homeopaths sometimes argue that homeopathy should be used with no therapy other than mild nutritional changes. Traditional homeopaths believe that any other therapy, be it conventional medication or surgery, acupuncture or herbs, may jeopardize the practitioner's ability to determine the response to the homeopathic remedy prescribed. Other homeopaths may use individual remedies with other alternative therapies. Use of a particular remedy and evaluation of its response are ideal. However, situations are not always ideal; clients may be impatient and demand a more comprehensive approach immediately. Also, exceptions exist if the patient is critically ill and time is limited.

The key principle for incorporating these therapies into practice is the improvement of patients' health as a foundation for their general well-being, as well as the treatment of specific conditions, rather than the palliation of symptoms. When the general health of the patient is improved, treatment of the specific condition is generally easier. Rather than relief of symptoms, the goal of many alternative therapies is resolution of the underlying cause whenever possible. For example, rather than using steroidal and nonsteroidal antiinflammatory agents that may have significant side effects in the treatment of arthritis, a holistic practitioner would explore the possible causes of the condition, evaluating the possibility of food allergies and drug reactions, as well as using nutritional supplements to support joint function. These supplements might include additional vitamins, minerals, and chondroprotective agents, as well as acupuncture and chiropractic, to assist the body in its own homeostatic mechanisms. Suggestions for incorporating the individual therapies into practice are discussed specifically in each therapy chapter.

Nutrition and Nutritional Supplements

Nutrition and nutritional supplements are the simplest approach to incorporate into a conventional small animal practice. Many practitioners already recommend supplements, and many holistic veterinarians have individual preferences regarding nutrition and supplements. Some holistic veterinarians recommend a homemade balanced diet for their patients, believing that it has more fresh ingredients essential to good nutrition. Some have ranked pet foods on a scale of 1 to 10, 10 being the best. A rating of 10 is reserved for a well-balanced, homemade, fresh diet comprising fresh organic grains, meats, and vegetables with a high-quality vitamin and mineral supplement. The lowest rating, 1, is reserved for a homemade, unbalanced diet. If owners tend to eat TV dinners, processed foods, candy, and carbonated beverages, their perspective on a homemade diet may actually make it the worst option. Generic, poorer-quality pet foods are then rated 2 through 5, with slightly better quality foods rated 6 and 7. The higher-quality processed pet foods that incorporate human-grade ingredients with a minimum of artificial flavors, colors, and preservatives are usually rated between 8 and 9. Some holistic veterinarians may offer these higher-quality pet foods and snacks in their office as a convenience for their clients. Specific nutritional recommendations for specific conditions may also be suggested.

Quality nutritional supplements are a necessary component of a holistically oriented practice. They may include many of the supplements discussed in Chapters 3 and 4: digestive enzymes, chondroprotective agents for degenerative joint disease, and supplements for dermatologic conditions. These products are readily available to veterinarians, and more are being developed every year.

Botanical Medicine (Phytotherapeutics, Herbal Medicine)

Botanical medicine, or phytotherapeutics, is commonly known as *herbal medicine*. Herbal medicines have been used in animals for thousands of years in various cultures. They may be incorporated relatively easily into a conventional veterinary practice. Many clients are already familiar with herbal remedies and may be using them on their pets. Clients are often reluctant to discuss their use with the veterinarians for fear of being ridiculed. Likewise, evidence suggests that human patients hesitate to discuss their personal use of alternative therapies with their physicians (Eisenberg and others, 1993).

When clients are aware that veterinarians are knowledgeable in this field, opportunities for further discussion increase. After receiving advanced training in botanical medicine, veterinarians can write brochures explaining phytotherapeutics and herbal medicine, the AVMA guidelines, their personal philosophies, and suggestions for use for their patients. Education of veterinary staff on ways to incorporate herbal medications may also be beneficial.

Both Western and Oriental herbal medicines are being used in small animal practice for many conditions (see Chapters 20 and 23). Western herbs being used include valerian root as a mild sedative and antianxiety herb; garlic, echinacea, and goldenseal for infections; ginger for motion sickness and gastrointestinal disorders; hawthorn berry for cardiovascular conditions; topical pennyroyal as a flea repellant; milk thistle for liver conditions; and red raspberry leaves for reproductive conditions. These herbs may easily be incorporated as an adjunct to conventional therapy. Clients are usually grateful for the additional support. Knowledge of these herbs is important, as suggested by the report concerning pennyroyal toxicity in dogs (Sudekum and others, 1992).

Chinese herbal formulas are an excellent support for many conditions, including chronic degenerative conditions, arthritis, and dermatologic, immunologic, and gastrointestinal conditions. They may also be used as an adjunct to conventional medicine or for conditions in which conventional drugs are not working or are causing side effects. For example, an herbal formula known as polyporous combination (Sunten) is an excellent formula for chronic recurring feline urinary tract infections. An herbal formula containing bupleurum has been clinically effective in the treatment of various hepatopathies. Certain herbal formulas may be used postoperatively in the geriatric patient to improve recovery. Chapter 23 contains further recommendations on the use of Chinese herbal formulas in small animal practices. Clients should be informed that the use of herbal remedies is considered unconventional. Release forms may be appropriate.

Acupuncture and Chiropractic Care

After the practitioner receives the appropriate certification training in veterinary acupuncture or chiropractic care, these therapies may be easily incorporated into a conventional practice. They may be used as an adjunct to conventional treatment, individually or simultaneously. Acupuncture may be beneficial in the treatment of various musculoskeletal, gastrointestinal, neurologic, dermatologic, reproductive, respiratory, and cardiovascular conditions. Chiropractic may be used for similar conditions but is primarily used for musculoskeletal problems at this time. Details concerning further indications are reviewed in Chapters 10 and 12, as well as in Schoen (1994).

Acupuncture or chiropractic care may be practiced in a regular or extended office visit. Acupuncture may also be used for postoperative analgesia and in cardiovascular emergencies. Chiropractic may also be beneficial after surgery for any anesthetized patient. Brochures in the waiting room explaining the indications and limitations of these procedures are beneficial. Staff education is also helpful in promoting these therapies.

Veterinarians are often surprised by the great number of clients who visit acupuncturists and chiropractors and are elated to learn that their veterinarian has received training in these therapies and is now offering them as part of the practice. New clients may be searching specifically for these therapies. Most veterinarians gradually incorporate these therapies into their conventional practices. However, some continue to study these approaches and then develop practices limited to these therapies. They may limit the practice to small animals or to both small and large animals. Some veterinarians may practice acupuncture and invite a chiropractor trained in animal chiropractic into the practice. The legality of this practice depends on individual state practice acts.

Veterinarians ready to accept referrals for acupuncture or chiropractic care should contact colleagues by letter or telephone. Lectures to local veterinary associations educating members about these therapies are an important component of developing a referral practice in these therapies.

Homeopathy

Of the alternative therapies, homeopathy is the most challenging to incorporate into a conventional practice. Homeopathic principles often contradict conventional medical philosophy. The AVMA guidelines (1997) state the following:

> Veterinary homeopathy is a medical discipline in which conditions in nonhuman animals are treated by the administration of substances that are capable of producing clinical signs in healthy animals similar to those of the animal to be treated. These substances are used therapeutically in minute doses. Research in veterinary homeopathy is limited. Clinical and anecdotal evidence exists to indicate that veterinary homeopathy may be beneficial.

This research is reviewed in Chapters 25 through 28. Further research should be conducted in veterinary homeopathy to evaluate efficacy, indications, and limitations (AVMA, 1997).

Because some of the substances may be toxic when used at inappropriate doses, the AVMA believes that "veterinary homeopathy should be practiced only by licensed veterinarians who have been educated in veterinary homeopathy" (AVMA, 1997).

Advanced training in veterinary homeopathy is essential before practitioners can be considered competent because the principles, philosophy, and practice of homeopathy are so different from those of conventional medicine. In addition, many different approaches and philosophies exist within homeopathy itself. Depending on the homeopathic philosophies the practitioner espouses, homeopathy may be integrated into a practice in various ways. After receiving appropriate training, traditional homeopaths often limit their practice to classical homeopathy. This practice may develop as an outpatient clinic, house-call service, or telephone consultation practice. The legality of practicing homeopathy by telephone consultation across state lines should be evaluated (see Chapter 42). In any homeopathic practice, clients must be informed of the AVMA guidelines concerning homeopathy, and consent forms are recommended; they should be a common part of administrative practice.

In a classical homeopathic practice a detailed history is essential, particularly one that includes questions regarding classical homeopathic pictures of particular remedies and constitutional types (see Chapter 26). Occasionally, homeopaths use dietary recommendations and nutritional supplements. However, traditional homeopaths rarely recommend using homeopathy with other modalities, including acupuncture, chiropractic, or conventional medications. Their concern is that the other techniques may interfere with the response to the remedy. Other, less traditional homeopaths may use individual remedies or combination remedies. Combination treatments are also used in various human homeopathic practices. The efficacy of these different approaches depends on the expertise of the individual practitioner. Few double-blind studies and clinical efficacy trials of homeopathic approaches in animals have been conducted. Unfortunately, most results are still based on anecdotal reports and individual case reports.

Further research and documentation must be conducted for the use of veterinary homeopathy to advance and become a common part of practice.

Some veterinarians choose to limit the use of homeopathy to acute prescribing in their practice rather than committing to the time-consuming challenge of practicing constitutional classical homeopathy. This approach may be incorporated into a holistic practice much more easily. For example, a combination remedy or a single remedy may be used to treat a simple complaint such as motion sickness. The remedies cocculus, petroleum, and tabscum are often useful in this condition. Combination remedies from various manufacturers are also available, such as homeopathic motion-sickness medicine (P & D, 1995). In addition, remedies may be used for specific conditions such as anxiety, cystitis, and thunderstorm or noise phobias. This is a simplified approach to homeopathy that does not address the long-term goal of resolving the problem completely. Other veterinarians use constitutional homeopathy only when the client requests it or the veterinarian feels confident that it may be the best approach. For example, a 10-year-old spayed female cat had a history of recurring rodent ulcer lesions on the upper lip, as well as inappropriate urination throughout the house. Appropriate conventional medications were prescribed without any response. The client requested a classical homeopathic approach. After completion of a detailed history a low-potency remedy was prescribed for daily use; both conditions improved but did not resolve. After administration of one high dose of the constitutional remedy, all signs resolved completely, and the attitude and general behavior of the animal returned to normal. Such results can be rewarding; however, the practitioner must take the time to interpret the homeopathic picture and determine the constitutional remedy. For further details of this approach, see Chapter 26.

Physical Therapy, Low-Level Laser Therapy, Electromagnetic Therapy

Physical therapy, laser therapy, and electromagnetic therapy may be incorporated relatively easily as adjuncts to conventional practice. They may be used as part of a comprehensive rehabilitation program for postoperative or geriatric patients. These techniques are often practiced by licensed veterinary technicians under the auspices of veterinarians with advanced training in these areas. For example, postoperative rehabilitation may be beneficial for dogs after dorsal laminectomy for acute posterior paralysis resulting from an intervertebral disk disease episode. Swimming, hydrotherapy, and massage may be used to exercise muscles, as may laser therapy to stimulate acupuncture points or accelerate healing of decubital sores. Electromagnetic therapeutic beds may be used in practice for postoperative pain relief. For further details on these therapies, see Chapters 17 and 18.

Geriatric Medicine

CAVM therapies are well suited to incorporation into geriatric medicine. According to a 1991 AVMA survey, 13.9% of dogs and 11% of cats treated were more than 11 years old and considered geriatric (AVMA, 1991). Preventive wellness programs, including a comprehensive physical examination, complete blood count, complete serum chemistry profile, thyroid profile, urinalysis, and possibly electrocardiographic, ultrasound, or radiographic evaluation, can be of excellent diagnostic value. Combining these therapies with a history based on traditional Chinese medical diagnosis, homeopathic evaluation, chiropractic evaluation, and an environmental questionnaire can make the wellness program even more comprehensive. Early diagnosis of the many diseases that appear in geriatric patients yields a broader selection of therapeutic options, including nutrition, acupuncture, chiropractic, physical therapy, and Eastern and Western botanical medicine.

Medications such as nonsteroidal antiinflammatory drugs, aminoglycosides, steroids, and barbiturates can produce serious side effects in animals with age-related dysfunction. Alternatives to these medications are available and should be considered, especially for geriatric patients.

It is not uncommon for several serious conditions to be treated with drugs that may cause adverse interactions. Practitioners must examine all the problems present in the geriatric subject and develop a proactive program not only to treat the specific condition but to improve the overall health of the pet. According to traditional Chinese medical theory, most geriatric patients are Spleen *Qi* deficient and would benefit from several Chinese herbal formulas. The goal of most CAVM approaches is to improve the general health of the geriatric patient, not merely to treat the symptom.

Incorporation into Conventional Practice: Client Education

In incorporating alternative therapies into a conventional practice, veterinarians must educate clientele, staff, and colleagues about the basis of these therapies, their indications and limitations, and the practice philosophy. Such education may be conducted with appropriate brochures, educational videos, and staff communication (Boxes 32-2 and 32-3). The International Veterinary Acupuncture Society and the American Veterinary Chi-

---

BOX 32-2

*V*ETERINARY *A*CUPUNCTURE *C*LIENT *E*DUCATION *B*ROCHURE

Acupuncture is one of a variety of therapies that a veterinarian may use to treat your animal. Most simply stated, acupuncture (*acus*, needle; *punctura*, puncture) is the stimulation of specific points on the body that have the ability to alter various biochemical and physiologic conditions to achieve the desired effect. It is a means of helping the body heal itself. Acupuncture has been used successfully for nearly 4000 years on animals, as well as human beings. As a matter of fact, it is still the treatment of choice for one quarter of the world's population for many problems. It is now being utilized by an increasing number of veterinarians for various conditions. It is not a panacea, or cure-all, but where it is indicated it works well.

QUESTIONS MOST FREQUENTLY ASKED:

What conditions respond to acupuncture?

Acupuncture bridges a gap between medicine and surgery. In the Western world acupuncture is used primarily when medications are not working or are contraindicated because of possible side effects or when surgery is not feasible. In China, it is often used as the primary treatment before conventional medicines and surgery.

In small animals acupuncture is most commonly used for:

1. **Musculoskeletal problems:**
   a. Hip dysplasia
   b. Arthritis
   c. Intervertebral disk disease
   d. Long-term injuries
2. **Skin problems**
   a. Lick granulomas
   b. Sensory neurodermatitis
3. **Nervous disorders**
   a. Traumatic nerve injury
   b. Certain types of paralysis
4. **Respiratory problems**
   a. Feline asthma

Many other conditions have responded to acupuncture as well.

In horses acupuncture is most commonly used for:

1. **Musculoskeletal problems**
   a. Back problems
   b. Navicular disease
   c. Laminitis
   d. Tendinitis
   e. Numerous other lamenesses
2. **Nervous disorders—traumatic nerve injury**
3. **Analgesia—for surgery**
4. **Respiratory problems—heaves "bleeders"**

Continued

BOX 32-2

*V*ETERINARY *A*CUPUNCTURE *C*LIENT *E*DUCATION *B*ROCHURE—cont'd

How does it work?

Acupuncture is now known to affect all major physiologic systems. It works primarily through the central nervous system, affecting the musculoskeletal, hormonal, and cardiovascular systems. It does more than relieve pain. How it works depends on the condition being treated and the points used. Acupuncture increases circulation, causes a release of many neurotransmitters and neurohormones (some of which are endorphins, the "natural pain-killing" hormones), relieves muscle spasms, stimulates nerves, and stimulates the body's defense systems, among many other beneficial effects.

It is interesting to note that according to Chinese philosophy, disease is an imbalance of energy in the body. Acupuncture therapy is based on balancing the energy correcting the flow of energy and thereby healing the animal.

Is it painful? How will my animal react?

Acupuncture is often performed with sterilized thin stainless steel needles. There is occasionally a brief moment of sensitivity as the needle penetrates the skin in certain sensitive areas. Once the needles are in place, most animals relax, often falling asleep during treatment.

Is it safe?

Acupuncture is one of the safest therapies available if practiced by a competent acupuncturist. Side effects are rare. Occasionally an animal's condition may deteriorate temporarily before results are evident. However, if the body's own system of healing is allowed to work and no chemicals are administered, complications rarely, if ever, develop.

How often and for how long does one treat?

Treatments may last from 10 seconds to 30 minutes depending on the condition treated and the method used. There are many ways of stimulating acupuncture points, including needles, electroacupuncture, aquapuncture (injecting a solution into the point), moxibustion (heating the point), and laser acupuncture. Patients are often treated 1 to 3 times a week for 4 to 6 weeks. A positive response is often noticed within the first four to six treatments, sometimes earlier, depending on the condition treated.

If you have further questions, ask your veterinarian or write the International Veterinary Acupuncture Society, David Jaggar, M.R.C.V.S., Executive Secretary, 5139 Sugar Loaf Road, Boulder, CO 80302.

BOX 32-3

*V*ETERINARY *C*HIROPRACTIC *C*ARE *C*LIENT *E*DUCATION *B*ROCHURE

WHAT IS CHIROPRACTIC CARE?

Chiropractic care is a holistic approach to many of the health and performance problems of the horse and dog. Chiropractic does not replace traditional veterinary medicine and surgery but provides an alternative method of care. Chiropractic focuses on the health and proper functioning of the spinal column.

The spinal column

The spinal column of the horse is a complex structure made up of bones, ligaments, muscles, and nerves. The spine provides many crucial functions to the body.

The functions of the spine are as follows:
1. Framework of support
2. Muscle attachment
3. Protection of the central nervous system
4. Protection of internal organs

What is a subluxation?

Chiropractors use the term *subluxation* to describe a specific problem or disease of the spinal column. A *subluxation* is defined as a misaligned vertebra that is "stuck" or unable to move correctly. When movement between two vertebrae is restricted, the animal will not have total flexibility of the spine. Stiffness, resistance, and lack of ability result. These symptoms then lead the client to seek veterinary help for the patient.

Subluxations also cause problems in the nervous system, especially at areas where nerves exit between two vertebrae. Misaligned vertebrae cause problems in nerves by interfering with nerve transmissions. Nerves are the communication lines of the body, carrying information back and forth between the brain and the cells. Subluxations may be pictured as pinching off or altering that flow of information. Depending on the area

BOX 32-3

VETERINARY CHIROPRACTIC CARE CLIENT EDUCATION BROCHURE—cont'd

and amount of nerve interference, problems may then develop in the body.

Every movement from simple swishing of the tail to the piaffe in dressage requires a constant synchronization of muscles in contraction and relaxation. If proper nerve messages to muscles are obstructed, this coordination will falter. Minor interferences may result in only slight changes in performance. In high levels of competition, however, even these slight changes may affect performance success. Lack of muscle coordination can cause missteps, resulting in damage to the joints and tendons of the legs. Nerve pressure can also result in pain. Pain also prevents horses from working at optimal potential.

Subluxations in the spine may cause the animal to compensate in movement or posture. The animal may attempt to avoid pain of a subluxation by shifting weight or avoiding certain movements. When the spine is not functioning correctly in one area, stress is placed on other vertebral joints. Secondary subluxation can occur in other areas of the column, further complicating the problems.

What causes subluxations?

Traumatic and stressful situations present themselves daily to the performance horse. Saddles, riders, confinement, and sustained vigorous exercises can all cause problems in the spinal column.

How are subluxations corrected?

When subluxations are identified in the spine, a veterinary chiropractor will attempt a correction of the misalignment. This is called an *adjustment*. An adjustment is a short, rapid thrust onto a vertebra in the direction that will return it to normal position.

Chiropractic is very specific, and adjustments are made on vertebrae directly. Jerking on legs or tails is not a chiropractic adjustment. An examination before the adjustment will identify all the subluxations of the spinal column.

An adjustment uses a controlled force. Simply because horses are large does not mean that abnormally large forces are needed to adjust them. The joints of the spine are moveable, and if the correct angle is used, the adjustment is relatively easy and low in force. Veterinary chiropractors may also manipulate the joints of the legs, as well as the jaw.

Chiropractic is a diverse field, and many different types of techniques are used. Most veterinary chiropractors use only their hands to adjust the vertebrae of horses. This is possible by using leverage of vertebrae that are distinctive in size and shape. Some doctors use a small impacting device, called an *activator*, to move the vertebrae. The device is effective because of its specificity and speed. Some individuals use mallets that are struck onto pads over the vertebrae. This technique can be effective if used by skilled practitioners but can create more problems if used by the unskilled.

The adjustment releases the "stuck" vertebra and restores alignment, thus eliminating nerve pressure. The body can then repair tissues and restore function.

The most common misunderstanding concerning chiropractic care involves the need for several adjustments. The purpose of an adjustment is to realign the spine. The muscles and ligaments of the horse must be able to maintain the correct spinal alignment. When an orthodontist works to straighten teeth, he applies a rigid brace directly to the teeth. Chiropractors cannot do this for the spine. Several adjustments may be needed until the body accepts and maintains the correct alignment. Most horses show significant improvement in one to four adjustments. However, chronic spinal problems take longer to respond. Horses that are basically sound, with a conformation suited to the desired performance, respond quickly to adjustments and maintain spinal alignment longer.

Examining the horse for subluxations

Chiropractors are trained to locate and correct subluxations. However, trainers, riders, and owners may check to see if their horses have problems with the spinal column. **Examination of the spine before purchase is just as important as examination of the extremities.**

Gait and performance

The owner should mentally review the current performance of the horse.

1. Has the horse recently changed behavior, or is it working below its ability?
2. Does an obscure or shifting lameness exist?
3. Is the rider having difficulty staying centered?
4. Is the rider or trainer noticing subtle shifts or difficulties in gaits without apparent lameness?
5. Is the horse dragging toes or showing unusual shoe wear?

The following may cause subluxations:

1. Trauma
2. Conformation traits
3. Trailers
4. Birth
5. Confinement
6. Performance type
7. Rider ability
8. Equipment
9. Age
10. Shoeing

Continued

BOX 32-3

Veterinary Chiropractic Care Client Education Brochure—cont'd

What are the symptoms of a subluxation?

Subluxations of the spinal column may produce many symptoms. The most common problem is pain. Animals in pain compensate in gait or posture and may resist or refuse to perform. Compensatory movements may cause other problems, such as added stress on joints. The following is a list of symptoms that **may indicate pain from a subluxation:**

1. Abnormal and varying posture when standing
2. Discomfort when saddling
3. Discomfort when riding
4. Evasions such as extending head and neck or hollowing back
5. Wringing of tail and pinning of ears
6. Refusal or unwillingness over jumps
7. Refusal or resistance in performance such as lateral or collected movements
8. Development of unusual behavior patterns
9. Facial expression of apprehension or pain
10. Sensitivity
11. Stiffness, resistance to movement

Subluxations may cause **changes in muscle coordination and flexibility** that affect the performance ability of the horse or dog.

Possible symptoms are as follows:

1. Lack of coordination in gaits
2. Unusual, perhaps indefinable gait abnormalities that vary from limb to limb and change depending on gait
3. Stiffness coming out of stall
4. Stiffness in lateral movements of neck or back
5. Muscle atrophy
6. Shortened stride in one or two limbs
7. Inability to engage rear quarters
8. Inability to lengthen top line
9. Improper frame
10. Decreased strike length
11. Difficulty flexing at the poll
12. Lameness
13. On line or pulling on one rein
14. Inability of rider to sit centered on horse
15. Unwillingness to use the back in movement (leg movers)

Subluxations **may cause problems in the nerves** that supply other cells, such as those of the skin, glands, and blood vessels. Possible symptoms are as follows:

1. Unusual body or tail rubbing
2. Increased sensitivity to heat or cold
3. Asymmetric sweating or lack of sweating

Range of motion

The horse should move freely in all ranges of motion with no tension, both under saddle and from the ground.

1. Ask the horse to bend its head and neck to touch its nose to the cinch area on each side. Does the horse resist more on one side? This could indicate a subluxation of the neck.
2. Test the lateral bend of the horse's back by pulling on the tail with one hand as the other hand rests on the tops of the vertebrae. Is one side stiffer than the other?
3. Apply moderate downward pressure on the back. The back should flex slightly and not feel tight and rigid.

Muscle palpation

Examine the major muscles of the horse for pain, tone, and symmetry. Horses in condition should display muscles of good tone that are symmetric from one side to the other. The muscles should be firm without being too hard or soft. Muscles should not be painful to moderate pressure of palpation.

Bone palpation

Palpate down the spine for prominent elevations or bumps. Compare the two prominences at the top of the hips; they should be level. Notice any bumps in the neck.

Spinal health care

Because proper functioning of the back and neck is vital to performance, care of the horse's back should be a major concern for equestrians.

Conformation

The conformation of the horse should be considered when selecting a horse for a particular use. Horse breeds have been selectively modified to function best in a variety of performance types. Selection of breed or halter conformation is not a guarantee of successful athletic function. Study those horses that are winning consistently. What are their characteristics? Horses with long backs are more prone to muscle and ligament injuries, and straight shoulders predispose to front leg problems.

Massage

Massage and muscle therapy is beneficial in the continued spinal health of a horse. Massage increases blood supply that brings nutrition to muscles as well as carrying away waste toxins. Massage relaxes tight, tense muscles, allowing for better function. Massage is helpful in the healing of tissues to remove adhesions and speed removal of fluid.

*V*ETERINARY *C*HIROPRACTIC *C*ARE *C*LIENT *E*DUCATION *B*ROCHURE—cont'd

Conditioning

Horses are more prone to subluxations and spinal trauma when soft tissues such as ligaments, tendons, and muscles are not conditioned for work. Interval training, adequate warm-up periods, and variation in the type of activity help condition the equine athlete.

Veterinary chiropractic care

Chiropractic care can be a cost-effective way to maintain the performance ability of the horse. Chiropractic works to eliminate the source of the pain or potential problem.

If you believe that your horse may benefit from the services of an animal chiropractor, how do you choose a practitioner?

Always have your veterinarian examine the horse first to determine if problems exist that require medical or surgical attention.

The certified animal chiropractor

The American Veterinary Chiropractic Association trains and certifies veterinarians in the art and science of animal adjustment. Veterinarians with certification in animal chiropractic may be called to see your horse without a referral.

When selecting a chiropractor for your horse, be wary of exaggerated claims. Performance horses often have many problems and many compensations. Some problems are permanent and some diseases are progressive despite the best health care. Have realistic expectations. Do not expect the veterinary chiropractor to solve long-standing or multiple problems with one adjustment. Healing takes time.

For more information on animal chiropractic and certified animal chiropractors please write or call:
American Veterinary Chiropractic Association
P.O. Box 249
Port Byron, IL 61275
Phone: 309-523-3995

---

ropractic Association offer client education brochures on these therapies. Staff meetings dedicated specifically to education regarding the various therapies is important. When the staff members are familiar with the therapies, they can discuss them with clients over the telephone or in the reception area. Staff members may recommend introductory books about holistic medicine, which can be loaned or sold to clients. Excellent books on holistic veterinary medicine for both the veterinary staff and clients include *Dr. Pitcairn's Guide to Natural Health for Dogs and Cats* (Pitcairn, 1995) and *Love, Miracles, and Animal Healing* (Schoen, Proctor, 1995). When referrals are accepted for various therapies, these therapies should be discussed with colleagues on a one-to-one basis over lunch or dinner or through lectures at a local veterinary association. Education of breeders and various kennel and cat clubs is also beneficial. A practice newsletter may devote a section to advances in CAVM. Every promotional method for the practice can also be used to promote alternative therapies. However, practitioners should take care not to identify themselves as specialists because no current board certification in these therapies exists.

Complications and Contraindications

Many of these therapies can be easily incorporated into a conventional practice. Homeopathy is the one alternative therapy that is the most difficult to integrate, as previously discussed. Appropriate client communication, educational brochures, staff education, and release forms are an essential foundation for incorporation of these therapies. They should not be used in practice without appropriate professional training for veterinarians and, where appropriate, their licensed technicians. If veterinarians choose to limit their practices to alternative therapies, they should keep current on the latest advances in conventional medicine as well so they can be confident that they are offering the best alternatives to their patients. Veterinarians who limit themselves to alternative therapies without considering appropriate conventional options make themselves vulnerable to legal action. Practitioners should consult local state practice acts and consider legal implications before practicing any CAVM therapy.

The major limitation to CAVM is the lack of double-blind controlled studies and clinical efficacy trials. (The problems with this type of research are discussed in Chapter 2.) However, if we wait for these studies, many animals will not benefit from these therapies, which are based on hundreds of years of clinical efficacy and numerous studies on other species, such as mice, rats, and humans. This problem may be adequately addressed through discussion with clients during the office visit and provision of appropriate release and consent forms.

Implications

The future of veterinary medicine is incorporation of the best complementary and alternative therapies along with conventional medical and surgical procedures. Veterinarians should be able to offer, either through their own practices or through referrals to appropriately trained veterinarians, the best options to their clients and patients to provide comprehensive animal health care. Clients will appreciate the vast scope of veterinary modalities and the number of services beyond medications and surgery that their veterinarians have to offer. The designation *veterinary medicine* must expand to include these emerging approaches. As other areas of practice decline, CAVM presents an excellent opportunity for veterinarians to extend the parameters of their practices. A paradigm shift is occurring in the public perception of medical care, with increased interest in CAVM for humans and their animals. The future of veterinary medicine involves the incorporation of these modalities into a more comprehensive approach to animal health care. For this to be successful, further research must be conducted to document the indications, limitations, and efficacy of the various modalities in small animal practice. As veterinary medicine progresses and incorporates these therapies, clients and patients will be offered new hope for the resolution of conditions that were previously untreatable. As a result, public appreciation of the profession and its many important contributions to our animal companions will increase.

REFERENCES

AVMA Directory: *Guidelines for alternate therapies,* Schaumburg, Ill, 1997, American Veterinary Medical Association.

AVMA: 1991.

Eisenberg DM and others: Unconventional medicine in the United States, *N Engl J Med* 328:246, 1993.

Littman M: Why I don't vaccinate for Lyme disease, *JAHVMA* 14(2):11, 1995.

Pitcairn R: Dr. Pitcairn's guide to natural health for dogs and cats, Emmaus, Penn, 1995, Rodale Press.

Schoen AM: *Veterinary acupuncture: ancient art to modern medicine,* St Louis, 1994, Mosby.

Schoen AM, Proctor P: *Love, miracles, and animal healing,* New York, 1995, Simon & Schuster.

Smith C: Are we vaccinating too much? *J Am Vet Med Assoc* 207(4):421-425, 1995.

Sudekum M and others: Pennyroyal oil toxicosis in a dog, *J Am Vet Med Assoc* 200(6):817, 1992.

Chapter 33

Holistic Approach to Equine Practice

JOYCE C. HARMAN

Holistic medicine is particularly applicable to the performance horse for several reasons. Holistic equine medicine considers the evaluation of the horse in its environment, including the rider, saddle, conformation, shoeing, training, and nutrition. This complementary approach to medicine not only accelerates healing times but restores the horse to optimal performance and health. The holistic modalities produce minimal or no side effects and no drug residues that would cause the horse to test positive in competitions and racing jurisdictions. With this approach, horses can reach their full potential because the whole animal may become healthier, not just a single part (the target for most conventional interventions). Horses can last much longer in competition because they are healthy and moving correctly. As the price of acquiring and maintaining horses increases, most owners keep their horses longer and do not treat them as disposable commodities. Currently, most leading equine athletes last 1 to 3 years in competition before they disappear or are downgraded significantly. Owners also wish to keep their horses longer for emotional reasons; more people seem to be connected to their animals on a deeper level or are at least acknowledging their emotional attachment as the "new age" movement gains momentum. This is evident as one reviews the lay magazines and books, which provide information on holistic approaches to health care, management, and training (Barnes, 1996; Bromily, 1994; Grosjean, 1993; Knight, 1996; *Practical Horseman,* 1995a, 1995b, 1996). Two veterinary periodicals also feature a column on alternative therapies (Jones, 1995-1996; Harman, 1994a, 1995, 1996).

In the racing industry, wastage through lameness and respiratory disease has been well documented (Jeffcott and others, 1982; Rossdale and others, 1985). In all of the horse industry, including racing, an enormous and largely undocumented wastage of horses results from performance problems. Many horses in all sports are bought as expensive prospects or are purchased while at an acceptable level of performance that later deteriorates. The traditional approach is to treat the horses with drugs and hope they improve; however, these horses rarely return to maximal performance and are usually sold at a reduced price. Many talented horses end up as school horses or in sale barns because of perceived behavior or performance problems. The results are losses of significant amounts of money, as well as frustrated owners.

A truly holistic approach to health requires making many changes, but the rewards are great. The weekend pleasure horse must be viewed as an athlete, as is the weekend rider. A complete holistic program for the horse involves the rider as well. Riders who are unhealthy or in pain may negatively influence their horses. Encouraging riders to heal themselves is often the most difficult part of the holistic health program, but it can also be rewarding. Practitioners must not forget to look at the whole horse and its environment.

Nutrition

Nutrition is the foundation of any holistic program. Without correct balance and availability of all nutrients, no horse can achieve maximal performance. The topic of feeding horses is generally surrounded by tradition, mystique, and many exaggerated claims. Horse owners have varying opinions on the type of feed to provide, but they are all still feeding the same equine species with the same digestive tract. Because horses are not food-producing animals, little money has been spent on equine nutrition research. As for equine nutrition from a holistic perspective, virtually nothing has been published and little research has been performed. One of the difficulties in conducting nutrition research from a holistic perspective is the complex interaction of nutrients. For example, in some cases, low calcium may be caused by another mineral deficiency or excess or the individual animal's ability to absorb calcium. Basic studies of single nutrients improve our understanding of each nutrient, but more complex studies should examine the interactions between them. However, these studies will be costly and difficult to perform.

Horses evolved as foraging animals, grazing on whatever scrub, grass, and weeds were available. While foraging, horses move constantly, except for relatively short periods spent sleeping. If they became ill, a wide selection of herbs (weeds) were available to help solve their health problems. Today, commercialization of nutrition needs and rich, cultivated pastures have changed equine nutrition habits from rough forage to processed feeds and rich grass. Predictably, domestication and increasing levels of confinement for the horse occurred as humans became more "civilized." Moreover, increasing interest in new equine sports has created new demands on horses' bodies and minds.

Physiology of Equine Digestion

In horses, food is processed through acid digestion in the stomach and fermentation in the cecum (Clarenburg, 1991; Swenson, 1977). The acid stomach absorbs water and begins protein digestion, mainly through the action of pepsin. Evidence suggests that some microbial fermentation of carbohydrates takes place in the stomach and small intestine (Alexander, Davies, 1963; Kern and others, 1974). The acid environment also ionizes minerals such as calcium, magnesium, manganese, and iron (Kimbrough, Martinez, Stolfus, 1995) to make them absorbable by the body; consequently, when acidity is reduced through the use of alkalinizing agents, those minerals are not readily absorbed (Hunt, Johnson, 1983; Mahoney, Hendricks, 1974; Mahoney, Holbrook, Hendricks, 1975; Oliver, Wilkinson, 1933). The acid changes pepsin to pepsinogen and triggers secretin, which triggers the release of pancreatic enzymes. The small intestine then hydrolyzes protein, fat, and carbohydrates into their final form for absorption. The fermentation vat, the cecum, is perhaps the most important part of the equine digestive tract. The cecum is designed to break down and ferment long-stem fiber and, through bacterial action, to produce vitamins and fatty acids. When the horse is fed mostly concentrates in the form of grain and little long-stem fiber such as hay, the incidence of colic is higher (Clarke, 1990; White and others, 1993). Horses should be fed frequently to keep the digestive tract full because they evolved to graze continually in the wild; the common practice of feeding twice a day can create digestive-tract illnesses and behavioral problems. Feeding meals primarily based on heavy grains causes significant fluid shifts, acid-base shifts, and changes in the microbial flora similar to those that occur in the rumen when excessive carbohydrates are fed (Clarke, 1990).

The intestinal tract contains bacteria and protozoa designed to digest food, manufacture vitamins, and make minerals available. These bacteria use dietary fiber in the digestive tract (Folino, McIntyre, Young, 1995) as an energy source. They live on the fiber and not in the intestinal wall; consequently, when fiber is deficient, the bacterial population is not healthy. The normal pH of the intestinal tract is acidic in the stomach and upper small intestine, becomes more neutral in the lower small intestine, and becomes close to neutral in the large intestine (Swenson, 1977), with microbial balance helping keep the pH in the correct range. Because bacteria inhabiting the intestinal tract are pH specific in their requirements for growth, they are found in places where the pH is correct for each bacterial species. The large intestine has a different vascular supply than the small intestine. The large intestine in the horse is basically a fermentation vat for the digestion of complex carbohydrates and a place for absorption of water and electrolytes (Swenson, 1977). "Pathogenic" bacteria normally inhabit the large intestine, but the immune system, along with mucus and fluids present in the large intestine, prevents these bacteria from becoming pathogenic in this location.

The small intestine is acidic and inhabited in part by the acidophilic lactobacillus species, a bacterium that controls its own reproduction by the excretion of lactic acid. If the environment becomes too acidic as a result of bacterial overgrowth or poor digestion, replication is slowed until the pH returns to optimum level (Clarke, 1990). If the pH stays too acidic, the lactate-consuming bacteria are adversely affected, causing an increase in lactic acid and consequent damage to the intestinal mucosa (Lupton, Coder, Jacobs, 1985; Moore and others, 1979). In the small intestine the vascular supply is much greater and mucus is produced as cytoprotection for the intestinal walls (Cepinskas, Specian, Kvietys, 1993), because this is the area for digestion and absorption of nutrients (Swenson, 1977). The tissues here are adapted to the acidic environment (Cepinskas, Specian, Kvietys, 1993).

When the digestive tract microflora become unbalanced, bacteria are not present in the correct proportions and incomplete digestion occurs. With incomplete digestion and poor-quality feeds, the pH can change, frequently becoming more alkaline. Motility can also change, allowing pathogenic bacteria to ascend from the large intestine, where the pH is alkaline, into the acidic small intestine. Intestinal mucosa may be irritated by gram-negative lipopolysaccharides, causing diarrhea. Alternatively, if the pH of the large intestine becomes more acidic and the acidophilic bacteria move down, the colonic mucosa may become irritated and produce pathologic signs (Mackowiak, 1982; Rolfe, 1984; Simon, Gorbach, 1986).

Much of the key to good nutrition is keeping the bacteria balanced in their proper places in the digestive tract. Just replacing bacteria in the form of a probiotic may not be the whole answer; if the pH is incorrect for the incoming bacteria, they will not be able to repopulate the gut as effectively. Substrates for bacterial growth and replication are supplied by a good natural diet high in insoluble fiber. The intestinal environment is a miniature ecosystem in which each player has a place and a job, and if any piece is out of place, the whole is affected.

Natural raw food has all the bacteria and enzymes needed to aid digestion; however, the processing of food may alter them. The healthy digestive tract, when functioning normally, can still digest high-quality processed food because healthy indigenous bacteria and enzymes already present in the digestive tract will continue to function. The unhealthy digestive tract has more problems functioning with poorer-quality feed. Live foods also appear to have other, as yet undefined, advantages that cannot be packaged or processed into a ration; overall health and hair coat quality are consistently better when animals are fed live foods as opposed to processed foods.

Anything that upsets the natural balance of the intestinal tract flora affects digestion and direct use of food. A course of oral antibiotics upsets the digestive flora balance and should be used only in specific, appropriate situations (Midtvedt and others, 1986; Schmidt and others, 1993). Overuse of antibiotics and nonsteroidal antiinflammatory drugs has been shown to increase intestinal permeability, allowing food antigens and fragments of bacteria to enter the bloodstream; in some cases the resulting immune response leads to inflamed and arthritic joints (Bjarnason, So, Levi, 1984; Bjarnason, Peters, 1989; Darlington, 1991; Meilants and others, 1991). Antibiotics may also alter the immune system. Tetracycline inhibits the phagocytic ability of white blood cells, sulfonamides inhibit antimicrobial activity of white cells, and trimethoprim-sulfamethoxole inhibits antibody production, according to a study carried out at the Stanford University School of Medicine (Hauser, Remington, 1982). Decreased thyroid function has been noted in dogs treated with trimethoprim-sulfamethoxazole (Hall and others, 1993). Reducing a fever pharmacologically may lead to slower recovery from infections (Doran and others, 1989; Jaffe, 1987). In cattle, oral antibiotics decrease the digestible energy (DE) of the diet by increasing the rate of passage of organic matter into the small intestine (Zinn, 1993).

A probiotic supplement with enzymes, bacterial substrate, and yucca should be given concurrent with or after any antibiotic therapy. The best probiotics are either a fermented product or a high-quality broad spectrum of live cultures. Few available live-culture products contain a good range of quality bacteria; consequently, many people believe probiotics are not helpful. However, overall health improves significantly with the use of appropriate probiotics.

Other factors that appear to disturb the normal digestive flora are frequent use of dewormers, illness, confinement, the stress of being worked during pain (a common occurrence today), and changes of diet. Dietary changes are in fact common because most feed manufacturers use least-cost programs to formulate feed, which means quantities of certain grains vary depending on cost. The final formula is still balanced for protein, vitamins, and minerals as listed on the label, but the proportion of each particular grain has changed. Prolonged stress may cause hypertrophy of the adrenal cortex, atrophy in the lymphatic system, and decreased intestinal integrity (Jefferies, 1991). Stress increases susceptibility to upper respiratory tract infections (Cohen, Tyrrell, Smith, 1991), depletes vitamin C, and increases urinary excretion of calcium, manganese, and pantothenic acid. The more horses are confined, stressed, and managed by humans, the more nutritional deficiencies and imbalances the observant veterinarian will find.

Water

Water is the nutrient fed in highest proportion to any animal and the most often overlooked component in the nutritional program. By weight, horses consume 2 to 3 times as much water as food. If the water contains toxins, high levels of minerals, or any other unbalanced agent, nutritional problems will result. As has been widely reported in the media, water quality throughout the nation is suspect, even that of rural wells and springs far from polluted cities (*Consumer Reports*, 1990, 1993, 1996; Ritter and others, 1995; Worsnop, 1994). The quality of bottled water is often suspect as well; there have been reports of contamination and the marketing of municipal water as spring water (*Consumer Reports*, 1992).

Herbicides and pesticides are designed to kill plants or insects. A quart of one of these agents can treat many acres of land after it has been diluted; a product so dilute could be acting similarly to a homeopathic reagent. The dilution process involves much mixing (sucussing), and the solution is driven around in a tank through a bumpy field, shaking it up even more. The runoff then gets into our waterways and is mixed or sucussed more as it flows downstream. The waterways become large vats for these diluted combinations of herbicides and pesticides mixed together, and yet little is known about the effects of these chemicals in combination. A recent study showed that just mixing two environmental chemicals that function as estrogens (dieldrin and endosulfan) had 160 to 1600 times as much strength as either chemical by itself (Arnold and others, 1996). This study marks the beginning of our understanding of multiple chemical interactions.

Many horses live in areas with urban water supplies. Some stables give horses water considered unpotable for people. Increasingly, people are drinking bottled water; however, this is not practical for horses. However, use of excellent nutrition and detoxifying agents can help horses cope with the toxins. Clays such as bentonite absorb toxins in the gut (Schell and others, 1993, a,b). Nutritional supplements, as well as herbal and homeopathic treatments, can aid in the detoxification process. New products are coming on the market daily to help humans and animals adjust to our polluted world; however, most of these products have not been evaluated sufficiently to prove their efficacy.

Chloride is an important nutrient that has been found in excess in much of the water supply, most certainly in urban chlorinated sources (Troianskaia and others, 1993). Chloride is used in water disinfection. Evidence is mounting that chlorinated water is toxic and may contribute to or cause cancer in people (Flaten, 1992; Jansson, Hyttinen, 1994; Morales Suarez-Varela and others, 1994; Nelemans and others, 1994). No specific data are available involving its effects on horses yet, but similar associated disease is probable. Water consumption is influenced by mineral content—in particular, chlorine, potassium, and sodium—as the animal tries to maintain homeostatic balance (Brocks, 1995; Jordhal, 1995). Horses may not consume enough water for healthy hydration if the water is contaminated.

Water frequently contains excesses of a particular ingredient such as nitrates (*Consumer Reports*, 1990, 1996; Kross and others, 1993; Ritter and others, 1995; Worsnop, 1994). Nitrates can affect vitamin A and selenium absorption. Without vitamin A the metabolism of vitamins D, E, and the B complex vitamin is incomplete. Nitrates are implicated in some infant diseases and cancer (Senft, 1995). High nitrates are converted to nitrites in the cow's rumen, converting hemoglobin to methemoglobin and creating an anemic state. In the monogastric swine, high nitrates may be irritating to the digestive tract. Neither of these effects have been documented in the horse; however, any substance that causes significant toxicity in one species probably causes some degree of toxicity in other species.

The best way to manage the potability of the water source is to test for toxins and high levels of minerals and chloride. Testing can be done through standard water analysis. Water filters of many sorts can be used, from simple charcoal filters attached at the spigot to complex systems attached to the main water intake for the farm. *Consumer Reports* (1993) published an excellent review of different systems.

Vitamins

A healthy digestive tract will manufacture water-soluble vitamins—the B vitamins and vitamin C. Because many equine digestive tracts are unbalanced, they cannot manufacture sufficient water-soluble vitamins. This leaves the horse deficient and consequently more susceptible to illness. According to human and veterinary literature, stress also depletes the water-soluble vitamins (Gross, 1992), and certainly today most of our horses are under a great deal of stress. However, the answer is not just to start feeding a massive amount of these vitamins, because if the digestive tract is functioning poorly, the vitamins may not be used properly. Vitamins are also lost in the processing of feed (Pickford, 1968). As the horse industry moves

more towards extruded and pelleted foods, more dietary deficiencies may become apparent.

Fat-soluble vitamins for horses are supplied mostly from food, except for vitamin D, which comes mainly from exposure to sunlight. Horses kept in stalls 24 hours a day and fed poor-quality hay may be vitamin D deficient because the main sources of vitamin D are sunshine, good-quality hay, and supplementation (Abrams, 1979). However, vitamin D is sufficiently inexpensive to manufacture that almost all supplements contain some; if supplements are combined, an excess of vitamin D may result. Excessive vitamin D causes prolonged hypercalcemia by accelerating intestinal calcium absorption and bone resorption (Morita and others, 1993). Vitamin D increases intestinal calcium and phosphate absorption. Vitamin D regulates the coabsorption of other essential minerals, such as magnesium, iron, and zinc, as well as toxic metals including lead, cadmium, aluminum, and cobalt and radioactive isotopes such as strontium and cesium (Moon, 1994). Vitamin D may contribute to the pathologies induced by toxic metals by increasing their absorption and retention.

Vitamin supplements commonly contain plenty of vitamins and minerals that are inexpensive to manufacture (vitamins A and D for example) and low levels of more expensive ones (phosphorus). Balance is the key to proper supplementation, and natural sources are better than artificial ones because they are closer in composition to the food naturally eaten by animals. A few supplement lines meet these criteria; however, more are becoming available. Many of the higher-quality supplements combine quality vitamins, minerals, enzymes, probiotics, and herbs to achieve balance.

Minerals

Mineral balance is perhaps even more critical than vitamin balance in the equine diet. A complex interaction occurs among many minerals; even a slight excess of one mineral in a diet may disrupt metabolism of other minerals (Fig. 33-1). Many of the trace minerals act as catalysts to help transform the major minerals into a form that can be used. Plants are good sources of trace minerals, and horses may seek out certain plants for their trace mineral content. Chemically fertilized soils that are farmed repeatedly (as most of our farms are) become depleted of trace minerals, so the grains grown on these soils and fed to horses are also depleted (Walters, Fenzau, 1996). Mineral nutrition then becomes extremely important.

A new branch of science called *zoopharmocognosy* involves the study of animals and their natural ability to select plants and herbs according to their needs and particular illnesses (DeMaar, 1993; Jisaka and others, 1993; Lipske, 1993; Robles and others, 1995). Horses naturally select from free-choice minerals as long as they are not too sick to sense their needs through instinct and odor recognition. Although conventional nutrition research reports

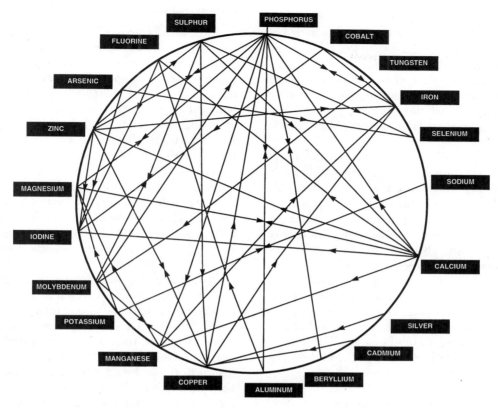

Fig. 33-1. Mineral interaction chart. Arrows pointing together mean that minerals interact; both are required for either to be available. Arrow pointing toward the other one means that the second mineral requires the first one.

that no species can accurately select free-choice minerals, some early research indicates that animals and children can self-select nutrients successfully (Al-Grecht, 1945; Barrows, 1977; Davis, 1934; Richter, 1943). Also, careful observation reveals that seasonal variations in mineral and vitamin consumption are significant. For example, when large areas of the Midwest were flooded in 1993, horses with free-choice selections of minerals and vitamins ate large quantities of B vitamins during the summer, when they would normally get most of the B vitamins they needed from the pasture. When horses' hair coats change in the spring and fall, horses offered free-choice sulfur along with other free-choice minerals eat extra sulfur, which is used in hair production (sulfur-containing amino acids). In the spring, when the grass is growing rapidly and is low in magnesium, horses consume extra free-choice magnesium, but they do not do this during any other time of the year.

Free-choice minerals should be fed with salt (provided separately from the salt supply). If both are fed together with salt in a mineralized salt block, the salt may limit the mineral intake. The average salt block, whether mineralized or plain, is designed for the rough tongues of cows. The mineralized block is generally 95% salt. If horses need minerals but not salt, they will not eat the mineralized

block any more readily than a person would eat oversalted food. When horses are given plain minerals, the quantity they eat is often astounding (2 to 3 times normal intake) for a few months, until they have balanced out their minerals; then the amount consumed tapers off to a maintenance level of $\frac{1}{2}$ to 1 ounce per day. For successful free-choice products, artificial flavorings, salt, and molasses should not be used because they may affect the intake of the nutrient.

One of the least understood minerals is calcium. Calcium is often given in excess to "help build strong bones." Calcium is also present in high levels in alfalfa hay. Still, many people want to add more calcium to a diet high in alfalfa. When a diet contains excess calcium, calcium metabolism is modified, leaving calcium in the bones and not absorbing it from the gut. Then, when the horse needs extra calcium (e.g., when performing in an endurance competition), the mechanism for supplying extra calcium from the bones is inoperative, causing calcium-deficient signs such as "thumps" or synchronous diaphragmatic flutter. Calcium is a key mineral; however, a so-called "calcium deficiency" problem may actually be caused by the level of available phosphorus. Phosphorus is an expensive mineral and therefore often deficient in supplements, whereas calcium is cheap and therefore commonly added as a processing agent in soybean meal to improve the flow. As a processing agent, calcium does not need to be included in the ration formulation, so the true amount of calcium in a ration may not be reflected by the calcium itself on the label. If the calcium added to the soybean meal was balanced properly with phosphorus, the cost of the phosphorus would be prohibitive. When phosphorus is added to the diet, calcium becomes more available in the blood as it is removed from bones.

A high concentration of iron in the water has an indirect effect on calcium and phosphorus. High iron levels impede the use of phosphorus, which in turn affects the availability of calcium. Therefore a calcium deficiency can actually be a phosphorus or iron problem. Moreover, because the transport of iron depends on a copper enzyme, low copper levels can prevent iron from being mobilized from its liver stores, causing anemia (Lee and others, 1969).

Balancing for deficiencies by adding an ingredient is a relatively simple procedure, but balancing for excesses is costly and requires extensive technical experience. Other ingredients must be increased to balance the one that is in excess. Steps can be taken to bind excesses, but few are successful. Clay can sometimes be of help by adsorbing minerals in the intestinal tract, allowing excess minerals to pass out in the manure.

In the author's opinion, the best way to approach mineral nutrition is through a free-choice system, with the salt and mineral separated. Few companies provide a plain mineral supplement; usually, salt will be in the top half of the ingredient list. Avoid unbalanced single minerals or combinations of just a few minerals unless they are given free-choice (and are palatable for that purpose). Many products are formulated based on human requirements, which may not be appropriate for the nutritional needs of the horse. Racehorses are constantly given iron tonics to "build their blood," although most horses have normal iron levels. Several other mineral imbalances that can be important include (1) excess iron, which can tie up calcium; (2) calcium, which can inhibit zinc absorption; and (3) zinc, which can inhibit calcium absorption (Argiratos, Samman, 1994; Schryver, Hintz, 1982). Racehorses have more bone problems than other types of horses, and most are in a growth and remodeling stage of bone development (Schryver, Hintz, 1994), so deranged calcium metabolism could prove particularly detrimental.

Minerals occur in nature in all forms (acetates, citrates, sulfates) and are best if fed in varied forms. Chelated minerals are fashionable in mineral nutrition; however, they consist of a central metal atom and are absorbed by the body using only one mechanism. Complexing involves incorporating a mineral into the crystalline lattice of another substance that is not a metal. Absorption of a complex requires a different biochemical pathway. Although the terms *chelation* and *complexing* are often confused, the use of both in a formula is advisable, as well as all other types, such as citrates.

Antioxidants

Antioxidants are receiving a great deal of press because considerable research in human nutritional medicine suggests the benefits of these nutrients. Free radicals are extremely reactive compounds containing an unpaired electron, and they have short half-lives. Free radicals readily bind with any available electron to become more stable; the available electrons may be found in the double bond in fatty acids of the phospholipid bilayer of the cell wall. The fatty acid then becomes a radical and requires another electron, which it acquires from the next fatty acid in the cell wall. This process eventually ends in cell membrane rupture and death of the cell (Toohey, Kreutle, 1995). Free radical damage from lipid peroxidation leads to brittle tissues, including loss of blood vessel integrity, poor circulation, and swelling of the legs. In some cases the lack of response to a well-selected treatment regimen may be attributed to a free-radical damage that leaves the tissue unable to heal properly. Refractory cases may respond clinically to coenzyme Q_{10} and other antioxidants (Ward, 1995). When free radical scavengers are added to nutritional programs, the body gains valuable ingredients to support recovery from diseases involving pathologic inflammation (Nockels, 1988). Free-radical scavengers and antioxidants include MSM; vitamins A, E, and C; the carotenoids; superoxide dismutase (SOD); pycnogenol; coenzymne Q_{10}; selenium; tumerin; and zinc (Toohey, Kreutle, 1995). Some horses need just one of these nutrients, whereas others may need all the antioxidants to affect the entire oxidation cascade.

Glandulars

Glandulars are nutritional supplements made from actual glandular tissue, often prepared with supporting nutrients. In small animal and human medicine, glandulars are used as replacement therapy for organs functioning suboptimally and as support for organs that show evidence of inflammatory or degenerative processes. Because glandulars are produced from animal sources, it is not "natural" for the herbivorous equine to eat glandulars, and some horses will refuse them. However, glandulars can be useful in equine nutrition and should be considered instead of synthetic hormone replacement, as in thyroid therapy or as support for other organs, such as the pituitary gland. Many glandulars are costly, especially for horses, which contributes to their infrequent use in equine medicine. For more information on glandular therapy, see Chapter 6.

Enzymes

Enzymes are present in organic, whole, raw foods in the correct amounts needed to digest that food. The problem comes when the food is grown under suboptimal conditions, processed, cooked, or otherwise altered. Most foods for horses have been grown on mineral-depleted, heavily fertilized soils and have been processed to some degree, denaturing many native proteins and enzymes. In a normal, healthy intestinal tract, enzymes are produced by indigenous bacteria (Mitsuoka, 1992), and the enzyme reserves are sufficient for normal digestive processes to handle cooked or processed food. Because many horses exhibit suboptimal digestive function, equine patients often improve significantly when digestive enzymes are added to their diets.

The addition of enzymes to the food is controversial, because many nutritionists believe that enzymes are digested in the stomach and cannot reach the small intestine where they function. However, some research suggests that peptides and some intact proteins are passed through the stomach and absorbed from the gut in active form (Gardner, 1988; Sanderson, Walker, 1993; Walker, 1981). One study of chickens fed an enzyme-supplemented diet showed higher apparent ileal digestibility of organic matter, crude protein, starch, fat, and dietary fiber, indicating the efficacy of enzymes (Frigard, Pettersson, Aman, 1994).

Enzymes may prove helpful in the treatment of certain viral conditions such as herpes zoster in immunosuppressed patients (Jaeger, 1990), and the immune deficiency of AIDS has been ameliorated with enzymes (Stauder and others, 1988; Wolf, Rosenberg, 1972). Enzyme supplementation is routinely used in the treatment of pancreatic disorders, mainly insufficiency problems (Goldberg, 1992) but is now being investigated for a wider variety of uses (Prochaska, Piekutowski, 1994). Many veterinarians have also seen improvements in skin conditions, especially in atopic dogs. At this writing, no controlled studies of enzyme therapy in horses have been reported, although enzyme supplementation has been used for horses with poor hair coats and digestion, with good results. Enzymes tend to be expensive supplements, although they are valuable in selected cases.

Protein

According to National Research Council (NRC) nutrition tables, adult horses require only 7.5% to 12% protein in their total diet, including all grain, hay, and forage. The lowest percentage of protein in commercial feed available is 10%, and protein levels of 14% to 16% are common. Because horses have evolved to eat mainly roughage, no physiologic reason exists for these high protein levels. High-performance horses are routinely fed more grain, so an accompanying increase in simple volume of food usually provides for any extra protein requirements in this population. Some horses, especially older animals, do seem to have a greater protein requirement and may benefit from its addition to their diet.

Besides being expensive, providing excess protein is one of the more harmful practices in feeding horses. In the cattle industry the ill effects of excess protein have been well studied, yet farmers still feed too much of it. In cattle fed

excess protein, ulcers and poor digestion result, and although ulcers have not been studied in relation to protein levels in the horse, this association may merit further study.

In the horse industry, people spend a lot of money trying to combat the ill effects of excessive protein in horses. Some of the ill effects include anxiety or tenseness, difficulty in riding, swollen hind legs, problems with maintaining weight, liver and kidney disease, soft feet and frogs, and a poor hair coat. Research has documented many ill effects of excess protein intake in the horse (Box 33-1). Increased water intake, urine volume, sweating, urea in sweat and urine, plasma urea levels, and postexercise orotic acid excretion have been noted (Freeman, 1985; Hintz, 1980, 1987; Meyer, 1987; Miller-Graber and others, 1991; Slade and others, 1975). Because of these factors, early dehydration and thirst may limit endurance performance (Glade, 1989). No beneficial—and some detrimental—effects in the performance of racehorses and endurance horses are seen, including higher heart and respiratory rates in endurance competition, early fatigue in endurance horses, and slower racing times in thoroughbreds (Glade, 1983; Hintz, 1980; Miller, Lawrence, Hank, 1985; Slade and others, 1975; Smith, 1986). Lower muscle glycogen concentrations and increased blood ammonia concentrations are also seen with excessive protein in the diet (Meyer, 1980; Miller, Lawrence, Hank, 1985; Pagan, Essen-Gustavson, Lindholm, 1987). Increased urinary calcium and phosphorus loss with excess protein (Glade, 1985) may contribute to some of the develop-

---

BOX 33-1

*E*FFECTS OF *E*XCESSIVE *P*ROTEIN *I*NTAKE

- Increased water intake
- Increased urea in sweat
- Higher plasma urea levels
- Increased postexercise orotic acid excretion
- Lower muscle glycogen concentrations
- Increased urinary nitrogen excretion adversely affecting respiratory health
- Increased sweating
- Higher heart rates in endurance competition
- Higher respiratory rates in endurance competition
- Increased urine volume
- Increased urinary nitrogen
- Slowing racing times in thoroughbreds
- No beneficial effects in performance of racehorses or endurance horses
- Increased blood ammonia concentrations
- Early fatigue in endurance horses
- Increased urinary calcium and phosphorus loss
- Early dehydration and thirst, which may limit endurance performance

mental bone diseases seen in horses; many young horses are fed extremely high levels of protein.

Plant protein byproducts such as soybean meal are energy deficient because the oils are removed through a toxic solvent process. Feeding soybeans may contribute to incomplete digestion. Urea breaks down instantly, whereas soybean meal takes longer; both can be toxic to horses when fed in excess.

Alfalfa hay is extremely high in protein (15% to 22%, average 17%), perhaps because excess nitrates (nitrogen) are used as fertilizer on the fields. A level of 12% is considered poor quality, although this is a healthy level for alfalfa; 20% or higher is considered good, but it is dangerously high for horses. Recall that the equine dietary requirement for protein is 7.5% to 12%. If samples of alfalfa hay are taken from the field in the early morning to test for nitrogen content, the plant is still covered with nitrates from its own overnight metabolic process. It is not until the sunlight converts the nitrates into plant tissues that a true reading is obtained. The laboratory analysis may show the hay as up to 5% higher in protein than it really is. Feeding alfalfa hay from nitrogen-fertilized fields makes it extremely difficult to achieve a correct protein level in the diet.

Energy

Horses eating good-quality pasture grass or hay generally take in all the nutrient energy they need from forage. Concentrates (grain) are needed only to provide extra energy (calories) required by the horse to perform stressful work and maintain weight. Owners have an obsession with feeding grain, even to fat horses, on the basis of the mistaken belief that grain is necessary to balance the diet. However, provision of grain is necessary only to maintain a healthy weight. Balance can easily be achieved without grain by using forages and a balanced supplement, although a small amount of grain is an excellent way to persuade a horse to come to the barn regularly. A horse at proper weight should have barely visible ribs; most show horses are well over 100 pounds overweight.

Much information is available concerning the overfeeding of foals and the resulting developmental orthopedic diseases. It is common practice to start a foal's life by creating obesity. Foals receiving proper nutrition, especially with regard to minerals, are better able to tolerate being overfed without developing problems and are much less likely to develop problems if they are not overfed.

Sources of Food

Horse feeds are becoming more and more processed, to the extent that some extruded feeds resemble dog food and probably have as many nutritional problems as commercial dog food. Many feed companies use "least cost" means to select ingredients, so quality and content can change from batch to batch. Cleanings and fines from cracked corn make up a portion of the grain used in commercial feeds, and molasses is added to reduce dust, satisfy the demand of horse owners for a sweet feed, and increase palatability of ingredients such as soybean meal.

Sugar is as bad for horses as it is for any other species, and horses may exhibit mood swings similar to those seen in humans. In my clinical experience, horses calm rapidly and consistently after molasses-sweetened feeds are removed from their diets. Molasses also contains chemical preservatives and often propylene glycol as a surfactant. If sensitive to preservatives or propylene glycol but not to the sugar content of molasses, the horse may eat human food-grade organic molasses with no problems. Some other chemicals allowed as preservatives to guard against fermentation of sugars in feed-grade molasses are sodium benzoate, calcium propionate, and acetic acid, in levels from 2 to 20 pounds per ton depending on weather conditions. One study showed a significant rise in blood sugar after the consumption of sweet feed, with a corresponding drop in blood pH (Ralston, 1992). Although the authors drew no conclusions as to the effects of these fluctuations, such changes might have significant effects on the horse's body and behavior.

Pelleted feeds are used as an alternative to sweet feeds and do not cause the characteristic increase in blood sugar of sweet feeds. However, poor-quality feeds are easily disguised in pellet form. Some horses eat pellets too rapidly and may choke; others may be slightly dehydrated, causing pellets to form a blockage in the esophagus.

The best feeds are oats, barley, and corn with no added molasses and, perhaps, beet pulp. Availability of quality grains is a problem, especially with barley, which is used in England as a staple equine food. Corn may contain aflatoxins in certain areas. A mixture that works well consists of 25% large cracked or flaked corn; 30% steamed, rolled barley (the only form available in bulk); and 45% oats (large racehorse oats or crimped oats). Any combination can be used in a given area of the country. Contrary to popular belief, corn has the lowest heat of digestion of any grain because corn contains less fiber and more DE than any other grain (National Research Council, 1989). Corn is an excellent summertime horse feed, particularly for equine athletes requiring endurance because of the low heat of digestion. Beet pulp is a useful food and can be substituted for bran in the commonly used bran mash. Beet pulp is a good source of minerals, carbohydrates, and fiber (National Research Council, 1989).

Fats are commonly added to equine diets. Most fats in horse feed are probably preserved with chemicals routinely used in dog foods and are extracted with a solvent processes. Holistically minded owners should be encouraged to buy cold-pressed corn oil to supplement the feed. The best source of vegetable oils is from the plant itself, and providing a bit of extra corn is an inexpensive way to feed oils.

Pasture need not be lush and chemically fertilized to provide the energy needed for horses. Excellent grazing can be obtained from pasture with herbs (weeds) mixed with the grass; this combination allows the horse to select plants other than grass for both nutritional and medicinal reasons. Horses with all-day access to lush pastures tend to be fat. On the other hand, many horses are never turned out to pasture. These horses miss not only the movement that helps digestion and the sunlight necessary for vitamin D formation, but also the chiropractic benefits of stretching, rolling, swatting flies, and the like. Perhaps the biggest benefit of pasture time is the mental relaxation.

Hay forms the bulk of the horse's diet in winter and, in some areas of the country, year-round. Fiber stimulates the intestinal mucosa and muscle in the presence of healthy intestinal flora (Goodlad and others, 1995). The horse's "fermentation vat" (cecum) needs long-stem fiber and not chopped fiber such as that provided by finely chopped hay cubes. Digestion of short-stem fiber takes place primarily in the small intestine, leaving the cecum less full than it should be. Some parts of the country have only alfalfa hay, which is too high in protein and calcium. A variety of hay is the best, combining some grasses with some legumes; balance is the key. A horse is meant to eat long-stem roughage for about 20 hours a day, not in two small meals of rich hay. Ideally, herbicide-free hay grown in mineral-rich soil should be fed.

Horses receiving adequate nutrition have fewer health problems, recover from disease faster, are more resistant to contagious illnesses, and are better able to maintain physical condition.

Evaluation

Environmental Evaluation

Horses are herd animals and move 20 hours a day in nature; when a horse is confined to a stall for 23 hours a day, ridden for 1 hour, and returned to the stall, behavioral and health problems may result. Some horses exhibit repetitive-motion disorders such as cribbing and weaving. Most horses with these disorders behave normally when they have access to open fields and companionship, although some persist in their bad habits. Most show horses in all disciplines express their dissatisfaction with over-confinement by being tense, nervous, or difficult to ride. Other horses become aggressive or difficult to manage. Most horse-show clients are looking for drugs or, more recently, natural products to slow their horses down and make them manageable because they refuse to turn them out to play and persist in feeding too much grain, often laced with molasses.

The horse's environment, feeding habits, water situation, and turnout should be carefully observed. Horses who are bored or infrequently fed are more likely to experience problems. Choking from eating too fast and colic are much more common in stall-kept horses (White and others, 1993).

Stable air quality is another way in which the environment may affect horses adversely. Ammonia is often present at toxic levels, but owners and stable help become accustomed to the smell and may not notice it. People generally notice air and odors more in the aisleway of the barn because they do not smell the bedding at ground level, especially after a horse has spent 12 or 15 hours in the stall. Horses spend a lot of time with their head on the ground, even those fed from a manger. Ammonia is toxic to lung tissue at a level of 10 parts per million (ppm) (do Pico, 1992). This is the level at which an odor can just be detected. At 30 ppm a person's eyes will water. Ammonia in the air has been shown to increase bacteria and fungi in lungs (Kastner, 1989; Walthes, Johnson, Carpenter, 1991). Air-circulation studies in English barns point to increased ammonia and dust as significant factors in the development of allergic lung disease such as heaves (McPherson and others, 1979). Ammonia levels are much higher in urine from horses fed excessive amounts of protein (Hintz, 1987; Lawrence, 1994); consequently, high-protein feeds can increase the odor and toxicity of ammonia in the air. High-nitrogen urine can be identified by the appearance of yellow, dead grass at each urination spot.

Horse owners frequently install overhead automatic fly-control systems designed to spray insecticides at regular intervals. Some of these units are set to spray every 15 minutes, filling the air and covering feed, hay, and water with insecticide. Under these conditions, horses are not only breathing the insecticides but also ingesting them. These pesticides are for use in non–food-producing animals, so the long-term effects of these compounds have not been thoroughly investigated. Humans are exposed to the pesticides as well; most barn owners using these systems stand directly underneath the sprayers, not realizing the potential for adverse effects. People may leave the barn to get relief, but horses are confined to their stalls and are forced to breathe the chemical mist.

Barns are kept closed for human comfort. New barns are often built and covered with Tyvex (house wrap) to seal out all drafts; ammonia buildup occurs rapidly in this situation. The ideal barn has stalls open to the outside, wide spacious aisles with good air circulation, and partial doors, gates, or stall guards to allow air circulation at the most critical place—the floor. Other ways to improve existing structures are as follows:

- Open doors and windows, closing them only long enough to do barn chores. If the weather is bad, open the door opposite the prevailing wind so air can circulate without causing the contents of the aisle to blow away.
- Clean the urine spot out of the stall every day. Many people let the urine build up, then strip the stall occasionally. Ammonia builds up at floor level but may not be detectable to humans.
- Consider the bedding. Straw is not absorbent; consequently, ammonia levels become toxic in a few

hours. A base of shavings or other absorbent material may help. Shavings are absorbent and, if kept fresh, can be good bedding. Sawdust is absorbent but may be extremely dusty.

- If rubber mats are on the stall floor, many people use only a thin layer of bedding. The thin layer may be acceptable for cushioning, but it may not absorb enough ammonia.
- Cross-ventilation is an effective technique for reducing ammonia odor. Stall guards or screens are valuable, especially with full-length doors and small windows. The air must circulate at the floor level to carry the ammonia odor away from the horse's nose.
- In the winter an extra lightweight blanket (generally weighing only 4 to 6 pounds) can keep horses warm if they are clipped and need additional warmth. This allows more airflow in the barn.
- Lime or soft rock phosphate can be put in the urine spots when the stalls are cleaned, but neither substance will cover up heavy ammonia odors; good management is needed for maximal benefit.
- Odor-controlling products can be used, but adding a stronger smell to cover up the ammonia odor does not eliminate ammonia and may increase the amount of chemical irritation in the horse's lungs. A homeopathic odor-controlling formula is available that appears to control odors by preventing the release of nitrogenous gases. The research for this product was accomplished in the livestock industry, where odors are often more intense than in horse operations. I have found that regular use of the product yields a noticeable decrease in ammonia odor after application. Decreasing the ammonia odor helps reduce the fly population.
- Monitor the fly population; flies are attracted to ammonia. If manure piles are close to the barn, ammonia levels will be higher and the flies will be worse.

Horses kept outside (with shelter from the wind and rain) and given extra hay in extremes of cold weather are consistently healthier than horses living inside. However, pasture may not be available, and some horses prefer to live inside. Some horses are best kept in stalls at least part of the day because they are not accustomed to living outside.

Horses are often sensitive to dust, molds, and other environmental contaminants, as can be seen by the high incidence of allergic respiratory disease. Ammonia damages the lungs and may be a factor in the development of allergic conditions, although no studies have shown such a relationship. In my experience, barns with detectable levels of ammonia in the air have a higher incidence of respiratory disease in both the horses and the caretakers. In some barns the dust level is high because of the type of bedding used. Other barns are damp and moldy with poor air circulation, and molds levels are high. Horses living in damp environments are more prone to arthritic conditions.

Horses evolved as grazing animals to eat from the ground, and the practice of feeding grain, water, and hay from buckets and mangers at chest height or higher may prevent removal of irritants from the lungs. This important consequence is evident after a horse has been in a trailer for several hours, eating from an elevated hay net; many horses have a significant nasal discharge for several hours after a trailer ride.

Essential oils of various herbs such as citronella, pennyroyal, eucalyptus, and cedarwood are being used successfully in hand-held fly sprayers, although at this writing no similar products are available for overhead sprayers. Most natural products or homemade mixtures work reasonably well in repelling flies and seem to last about the same length of time as the chemical fly sprays without adverse effects. If essential oils are used with an overhead system, some caution is advisable; 12- to 24-hour exposure to these concentrated compounds has not been thoroughly investigated. On the other hand, a controlled population of flies may be something of an advantage; swatting flies is good for the horse's spine because it keeps the muscles stretched and the vertebrae moving.

Air pollution, runoff from agricultural products (herbicides, pesticides, and nitrates), and ambient temperatures and humidity are factors over which horse owners have little control. If a horse is sensitive to any of these factors, moving may be the only solution.

Conformation Evaluation

Everyone in the equine world spends a great deal of time studying and examining conformation. Most believe that by selecting the perfectly conformed horse, the owner will win at the chosen sport. Looking for a correctly conformed horse is appropriate, but many "incorrectly" conformed horses have won championships and races.

Some horses are able to perform at high levels of competition because of proper conformation and positive mental attitude. When horses perform at a level of skill that is comfortable for them, they have significantly less pain than when performing at their maximal level of skill. Horses with significant conformation faults put excessive stress on certain parts of the body to compensate. For example, a horse with long, low pasterns is more prone to bowing tendons than is a horse with more normal conformation, and a horse with a relatively long back is more prone to back problems, especially when carrying a heavy rider. This long-backed horse tends to stress the hocks and stifles, compensating for soreness through the back. This certainly does not mean that every horse with long pasterns will bow a tendon or that every horse with a long back will be sore, but the likelihood is greater. Horses with conformation problems need more regular therapy than well-conformed horses or may need to be directed to another sport.

A swaybacked topline is often manmade and is generally caused by pain. Swaybacked horses often regain normal conformation once pain is relieved with acupuncture and chiropractic. Horses are rarely born swaybacked. An old broodmare who has carried many heavy foals and has not been properly conditioned to maintain her abdominal muscles may become swaybacked, but in many horses the condition develops as a result of back pain. Horses ventroflex the spine (i.e., dip down in the center) in an attempt to evade pain by trying to prevent movement and subsequent spasms of the longissimus dorsi. Horses who are 4 to 6 years of age commonly carry their backs 2 to 3 inches lower than normal. When a horse's back is ventroflexed, or swayed, the hindquarters cannot easily engage and the neck is not carried correctly. With the use of acupuncture and chiropractic, in combination with abdominal "belly lifts" (to tone up the rectus abdominis) and improved training, the back can be returned to the natural position (Fig. 33-2).

Conformation needs to be examined in relation to the sport because a deviation might be acceptable in one sport but less desirable in another. For example, a flat croup from the sacroiliac joint to the tail head might be accept-

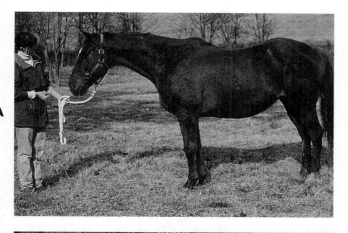

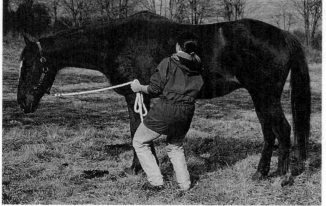

Fig. 33-2. **A,** The mare in this picture is swaybacked, or in permanent ventroflexion. Note the angles of her hips, loin, and neck, as well as the relaxed rectus abdominis. **B,** The same mare with the rectus abdominis contracted. Note the change in the angles of the hips, loins, and neck.

able in a driving horse but could create problems in a cutting horse or dressage horse. A short-backed horse may be strong but a large Western saddle may be too long for that horse's back, leading to significant back pain. A cutting horse with sickle hocks or a race horse with a turned-out leg may be more prone to injury; however, if that same horse moves efficiently, the conformation fault may not be a problem. If horses were allowed to compete pain free with correctly fitting saddles and good riders who did not interfere with their movements, many so-called conformation faults would never become problems. If the rider uses training methods that force the horse into unnatural frames such as the low-head carriage of the Western pleasure horse or the head-high, hollow-back frame of the show-jumper, the conformation faults contribute to the unnatural stress and lameness problems may result.

Most equine enthusiasts evaluate conformation while the horse stands still. Evaluation of conformation during movement is also appropriate to visualize the way the joints move together. Pain affects posture and, consequently, both standing and moving conformation. Many conformation analysts seem unaware of the relationship of pain to body shape. The science of chiropractic involves the study of motion between joints, the restoration of normal motion between joints, and consequently the alteration of posture and conformation. The addition of acupuncture, chiropractic care, muscle work, saddle fit, and correct shoeing relieves pain and can improve and correct the way a horse stands and moves (Willoughby, 1991).

Several examples of potentially correctable conformation faults include ewe necks and uneven shoulders and pelvises. Other horses stand with their legs underneath their bodies, and still others have choppy gaits and hit the ground hard with their heels. Ewe-necked newborn foals are rarely seen, yet many exhibit ewe necks by the time they are 6 months old; in others ewe necks develop when the horses are fully grown. Shoulders often become uneven from muscle tension (Fig. 33-3), spasms, and pain, leading to slightly uneven gaits and differing foot shape (or vice versa, because uneven shoeing may result in uneven shoulders and subsequent muscle spasms). Sacroiliac asymmetries often develop because of muscle tension and altered gait and probably lead to remodeling of bone. The loss of normal motion in the sacroiliac joint is sometimes opposite the visually high side (Haussler, Stover, 1995); however, many practitioners incorrectly believe the high side is the abnormal side. Horses shod with long toes and low heels, who have acquired pain in their upper body, may stand with their front feet under the body until the shoeing is corrected and the muscle pain that accompanies that position is relieved. In many horses, restricted motion develops. One way to observe this phenomenon is to monitor the growth and development of normal foals. Foals injure themselves easily, resulting in multiple chiropractic subluxations. A foal that was previously a good mover may subsequently lose normal, fluid movement and begin to ap-

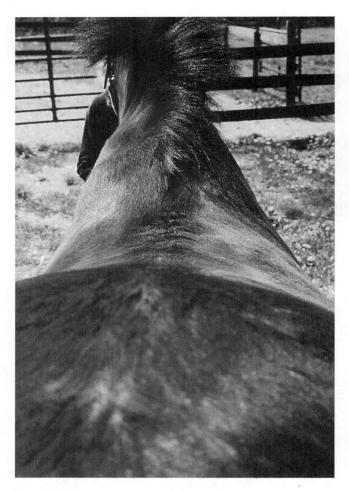

Fig. 33-3. Uneven shoulders. Horse must be standing squarely on level ground.

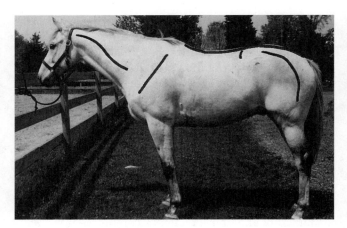

Fig. 33-4. Reflex test. A blunt object such as a needle cap is passed along the lines shown and the degree of involvement of the horse's body noted.

pear swaybacked, short-strided, and, often, ewe-necked. With appropriate chiropractic care the conformation may return to the previous normal shape within a few weeks.

A more dynamic way of evaluating the horse's ability to perform does exist. This method tests neuromuscular coordination, combined with movement evaluation. The test has not been scientifically evaluated but seems to be clinically useful to assess the flexibility and responsiveness of the horse. The neuromuscular test of the reflexes (Harman, 1992; Scullin, 1986) can be conducted in all horses, regardless of training or age, although the horse should be receptive to handling. A blunt object, such as a needle cap or the round side of a plastic pen, is traced along the horse's body; the reflex reaction indicates the type of neuromuscular coordination for that individual. This test also reveals areas of pain or restricted joint movement and can be quite uncomfortable if the horse has significant pain. Caution should be exercised when examining a sore horse.

Light pressure with the blunt object should be used along the side of the neck, beginning approximately at the level of the atlas and continuing to the base of the neck (Fig. 33-4). The normal reaction is to tip the nose away and bend the neck in a snakelike fashion toward the tester. The tester should then proceed along the scapula, from dorsal to ventral. The normal reaction is to move the shoulder away and bend the neck around toward the examiner, sometimes bringing the nose around far enough to reach the shoulder. The instrument is then applied along the top of the spinous processes, beginning at the withers and continuing toward the tail head. The normal reaction is to ventroflex the back, flatten the croup, and tuck the tail. The top of the middle gluteal muscle and the groove just lateral to the semitendinosus (ending just above the gastrocnemius) should then be tested. The normal reaction is to flatten along the croup and then move away from the tester, bending the spine through the lumbar area. In another test, the needle cap is placed in the lumbar muscle approximately 4 to 6 inches off the spine (at approximately Bladder-22 or -23 for acupuncturists). The needle cap should be held still, and the degree and extent of gentle muscle fasciculation observed. The farther forward the muscle fasciculation goes, the more responsive the horse will be to the leg of the rider.

Interpretation of the test takes some practice. Some athletic horses require a great deal of pressure with a blunt object to obtain the reflex movements. Such horses require a great deal of strength from their riders, especially when the rider is using the legs for aids. Horses who respond to a light touch with the needle cap ride lightly and are quite responsive to the leg. Examiners should start with a light touch and increase pressure if there is no response. If a horse is not responsive to heavy pressure, the reflexes are probably limited. Before recommendations are made on the basis of this test, examiners should practice it on a variety of horses. If the interpretation is correct, riders should confirm that the results of the test correspond to their observations. A high degree of correlation exists between the test finding and the rider's assessment of the horse.

Signs of pain and stiffness can also be determined with the reflex test. As practitioners become practiced in performing the reflex test, they are better able to determine the pain responses. A normal test should not be uncomfortable to the horse. Areas of muscle spasm may exhibit less motion or appear stiff. When vertebrae are not moving correctly, in some areas the reflex appears to stop and that part of the body stays stiff; the reflex movement then resumes on the other side of the stiff locus. An acupuncture and chiropractic examination is helpful at this stage to confirm areas of pain. Many horses find the test uncomfortable because they are in pain, so it is preferable mainly in prepurchase examinations or when clients want to assess the horse's potential to move up to higher levels of competition. Many horses believed to be incapable of advancement are restricted by pain, poor saddle fit, and shoeing problems. These are sometimes compounded by the rider's lack of ability or training methods that do not allow the horse to move properly.

Movement is the next step of the conformation evaluation. Each horse should be observed in motion. The horse is best examined without a rider, either lunged or freely moving around a paddock, because pain or a poorly fitting saddle changes the movement picture. Finally, if the horse is old enough to ride, it should also be observed while it is being ridden.

Performance Problems

Performance problems may be due to physical pain, as well as mental attitude. Most horses who are pain free perform to the best of their ability, and if specific behaviors remain after relief of pain, such as fear of jumping, boredom in dressage, or nervousness around cows, it may be time to reassess the best career for the horse. "Enjoyment" is difficult to evaluate and quantify. Sometimes there is no way to know in advance whether a horse can cope with the stress of high levels of competition. A horse who enjoys its sport appears more relaxed and consequently has less pain and tension than a horse who is not content. However, horses in pain do not enjoy anything they do or perform well.

Performance and behavioral problems are often the result of soft-tissue pain in the neck or back area. One of the most frequent causes is saddle-induced pain, either from a poor fit or improper positioning of the saddle. Other causes are poor rider balance resulting from the rider's own pain; lack of rider skill; training techniques that inhibit the natural movement of the back; unbalanced hooves; and mouth pain from sharp teeth, rough hands, and a harsh bit. Any of these factors may cause a horse to hollow its back, invert its neck, and constantly attempt to evade the rider. Lower-leg lameness may cause chronic back soreness or, more commonly, can be a result of back soreness. In many cases, lower leg lameness disappears when the back problem is cleared up, and it will not recur unless the back pain returns. Muscle pain from injuries caused either in the pasture (extremely common) or while being ridden (also common) is also common.

Back and neck muscles can become sore for a variety of reasons. However, practitioners must also remember that the horse can be its own worst enemy. Horses inflict a great deal of damage on themselves, both in the pasture and in the stall. The forces exerted on the body of a horse are great if two horses are playing and slip or fall down. One thousand pounds of falling horse weight is analogous to a person experiencing an automobile accident. Like an auto-accident victim, the horse sustains repercussions over the months that follow. Vertebrae are subluxated in a fashion similar to that of humans after an accident (see Chapter 12). Muscles, tendons, and ligaments are pulled and gradually become tighter over time unless the spasms are relieved. When the accident is forgotten, 6 months or a year later, chronic back pain has developed and performance problems may become severe. Becoming cast, a frequent problem in horses that spend a lot of time in their stalls, can also put a large amount of torque on the musculoskeletal system. The owner usually does not see the accident but simply notes that the horse's performance is deteriorating; in many cases the decrease in performance starts almost overnight.

Evaluation of the Back

The horse's back is central to the function of the musculoskeletal system and the ability to carry a rider (Bennett, 1988; Harris, 1993; Willoughby, 1991). Biomechanically the head, neck, back, and hindquarters are connected and move together, so if a horse carries its neck in a raised, hollow position, the back is hollow. The hollow position of the back alters the position of the pelvis, making it impossible to engage the hindquarters correctly underneath his body. For the horse to use its back properly, the rectus abdominis muscles, iliopsoas, tensor fasciae latae, and quadriceps (all protractor muscles of the hind limbs) must contract. Contracture of the longissimus dorsi ventroflexes the back, and if it is contracted from pain, the muscle is usually in spasm and motion is prohibited. The contraction of the lower half of the "circle, or ring, of muscles" (Fig. 33-5) (Bennett, 1988; Harris, 1993), including the abdominals and small muscles of the pelvis and neck, raises the back, allowing the longissimus dorsi to relax and contract selectively, which then allows the back to move freely.

As the horse's back becomes hollow or stiff, the hind legs cannot engage properly and the front feet tend to hit the ground heel first. Essentially the horse is in a stretched or "parked-out" position similar to that of a gaited horse. This stance is an exaggerated example of the way a horse with a hollow back looks and moves; with hind legs positioned behind the body, the horse has difficulty performing a dressage test or negotiating fences. A cutting or roping

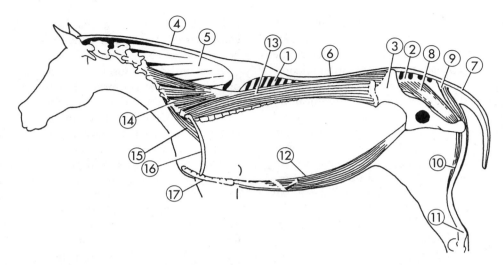

Fig. 33-5. The ring of muscles actually is composed not only of muscles but also of bones, tendons, and ligaments. The anatomic parts include the following: *1,* Dorsal spinous process; *2,* sacrum; *3,* pelvic bone (ileum); *4,* nuchal ligament, a cablelike portion that forms the crest of the neck; *5,* nuchal ligament, a sheetlike portion that connects withers and crest to the vertebrae; *6,* dorsal ligament of the back; *7,* dorsal ligament of the tail; *8,* sacrosciatic ligament, a sheet of elastic tissue that connects the sacrum to the pelvis; *9,* semitendinosus, upper part, which connects the sacrum to the pelvis; *10,* semitendinosus, lower part, which connects the ischium to the hock; *11,* point of the hock (the semitendinosus ends at the Achilles' heel just above it); *12,* rectus abdominis, which connects the pelvic bone to the sternum; *13,* longissimus dorsi, the largest single muscle in the body; *14,* division of the longissimus dorsi, found at the root of the neck; *15,* scalenus muscle, which connects the first rib to the neck; *16,* first rib; *17,* sternum. (Courtesy Dr. Deb Bennett.)

horse coming to a sliding stop in this hollow position puts extreme force on the front legs, and the rider is severely jarred. Unnatural strain is placed on the stifles and hocks, creating lameness or soreness and leading to resistance. The front legs in the hollow-backed horse are working slightly in front of the vertical position rather than truly under the horse. Some of these horses have an attractive headset with a motionless back and relaxed abdominal muscles. The feet and tendons endure the stress of this position and can become sore or strained. Most horses in all sports today are performing with hollow backs, at all levels of training and competition, from backyard pleasure to the Olympics. The horse that uses the lower half of the circle of muscles is the exception. The performances of these horses appear effortless in all sports. The cutting horse who shifts its weight rapidly and fluidly, the dressage horse who appears to lift the rider off its back and float though the motions, the open jumper who makes a 5-foot course look like a pony hunter course—all of these horses are using the lower half of the circle of muscles.

Good dressage training has traditionally been aimed at strengthening the abdominal muscles to give the lift and suspension so desirable in that sport. Dressage horses need especially strong abdominal muscles to allow true engagement of the hindquarters, lifting of the back, and lightness of movement. The abdominal muscles should be used correctly in all sports because the horse needs to lift its

back and engage its hindquarters to carry a rider properly, whether the sport is cutting, Western pleasure, or endurance. Strong abdominal muscles and engagement of the hindquarters are crucial to the jumping horse as the source of power for the jump. They are also responsible for the lightness on its feet that helps prevent fatigue, especially in the cross-country phase of an event.

To illustrate the effect of the abdominal muscles, the practitioner should try this exercise with a horse. A finger (or fingernails or a plastic pen, if the horse is not sensitive) that is run down the midline of the horse's abdomen from the girth area to just before the umbilicus causes most horses to raise their backs. The rectus abdominis contracts, the back rises, the longissimus dorsi relaxes, the neck lowers and stretches forward, and the pelvis moves into the correct position. With abdominal muscles contracted, the back can move freely while still carrying the weight of a rider. If the horse is pain free and has well-developed abdominal muscles with strength and freedom to move its back, the exercise will cause a flatter topline, similar to that of a young horse.

The practitioner may perform the following exercise to illustrate the consequences of a rigid back: Stand on one foot, hollow the back, and lift the other leg as high as possible, leaving the knee bent. Then round the back and see how much farther the "hind leg" can come—almost to the chest. Note the freedom the "hind leg" has with the back rounded and the stiffness in the "hind leg" when the back is hollow.

Evaluation of the Rider

The rider has enormous influence on the horse's back. The integral relationship between the rider and the horse has been brought to light in recent years in part through the writing and teaching of Sally Swift and her trade-marked concept of Centered Riding (Swift, 1985). Swift has demonstrated that if the rider is stiff in any area, such as the back or right shoulder, that stiffness is directly re-flected in the horse, in this case manifesting as stiffness in the horse's back and right shoulder. Most riders have some degree of back pain and stiffness that they transfer directly to the horse. To compound the problem, many training methods are detrimental to the freedom of the horse's back. For example, in dressage training the rider is often asked to sit back behind the vertical and drive the but-tocks into the saddle and the horse's back. This posture results in riders moving behind the motion of the horse, thereby inhibiting movement of the back and pushing all their weight onto the back muscles, stopping all move-ment of the longissimus dorsi.

In the average Western saddle, riders are placed in a chair-seat position, with their legs in front of the vertical axis of the rider's body. This automatically places riders behind the motion of the horse and all their weight at the back of the saddle, freezing the longissimus dorsi in the same manner as the dressage rider described above. It is not until riders become centered or balanced, with their legs and feet lined up with the pelvis, rib cage, shoulders, head, and neck, that horse and rider can move freely as a unit. Often it is the rider's style or the saddle's design that creates back pain in the rider. The pain is caused by the rider's inability to move with the horse, causing muscle tenseness. For veterinarians, making suggestions to riders is the most difficult aspect of treatment because most rid-ers do not want to hear that they need to change; they have hired the veterinarian to treat their horses. Riders must be handled carefully because if they are offended, they will not only not listen but look elsewhere for veteri-nary treatment.

The Horse's Mouth

Horses with mouth pain often behave like horses with back pain. When experiencing mouth pain, the natural in-stinct of a horse is to throw the head up, which hollows the back. In general, the horse pulls harder, rushes onto the forehand, becomes unbalanced, and may appear to be trying to escape the pain. The source of mouth pain is of-ten pinching of the lip between the bit and the sharp sec-ond premolars, but it can also result from bits that are harsh, rough hands on the part of the rider, and accessories or training aids such as an incorrectly fitted drop nose-band. Browbands are often too tight, creating head pain and sometimes mimicking mouth pain. Wolf teeth or first premolars, especially those buried beneath the gum line, are also sometimes overlooked as a source of pain by both veterinarians and "lay equine dentists."

Fitting the correct bit to the mouth is also important (*Practical Horseman*, 1995). The shape of the mouth, the sport the horse is performing, and the rider's hands must be taken into consideration. In dressage and many other English sports, the trend is toward thick, fat-mouthed snaffle bits, but many horses' mouths are much too small for such bits, and the horses experience a great deal of dis-comfort as a result. The commonly used snaffle bit exerts a downward force on the tongue, preventing the horse from swallowing when rein contact is being taken. Horses often try to escape this tongue pressure by either putting their noses slightly up in the air or ducking behind the bit to swallow (Myler, 1997). Horses who constantly fight the bit can be heard to swallow when they succeed in freeing their tongues. Bits made with an extra joint in the center, as in the "French" snaffle, allow easier swallowing, and bits made with ports allow complete freedom for swallowing. Western horses are traditionally shown in bits with ports and have fewer problems opening their mouths during competition. English horses are shown with more rein contact and have severe problems opening their mouths and fighting the bit, which sometimes causes riders to re-sort to cruelly tight nosebands. When horses are given as much tongue freedom as they want, they leave their mouths closed and perform with significantly more free-dom of movement (see Resources section). Compounding the bit situation, many riders place the bit too high or, oc-casionally, too low in the mouth. Either placement causes discomfort and can be a major source of irritation or pain. The bit should sit comfortably in the mouth, just wrin-kling the corners of the mouth, depending on the size and shape of the horse's mouth.

The improved performance afforded by allowing the tongue freedom is partly due to the relationship of the tongue to the hyoid apparatus, the muscles from the hyoid apparatus to the sternum, and the origin of some nerves of proprioception located in the hyoid and temporo-mandibular area. As discussed previously, horses must use the ventral half of the circle of muscles to carry their backs correctly. The muscles from the sternum to the hyoid ap-paratus (sternohyoideus, omohyoideus, sternothyroideus) are an important part of this circle. Tension in the tongue can lead to tension through the sternum, abdominals, and into the circle of muscles.

A bit with some unique characteristics is that used by the TTEAM practitioners (see Chapter 15). The outward appearance is that of a large Western bit with a copper roller in the mouthpiece, with two sets of reins (as with a Pelham bit). The bit balances the horse's head and neck, in part because its construction allows the tongue freedom, which encourages the temporomandibular joint (TMJ) and hyoid apparatus to loosen. Proprioception and movement can be seen to improve significantly. With just the bit, no reins attached, and the horse on a lunge line, the horse relaxes at the poll and loosens its jaw. This bit is designed to be ridden with light hands, and English riders, who usually object to its appearance, can use it just for training, going back to their traditional bits for competitions.

Proper floating of teeth can dramatically affect performance, yet veterinarians have traditionally not been taught the proper way to finish the second premolar. The bit and the corner of the lip must contact a smooth surface; that being the most important part of the floating job for the performance horse. Quality dentistry should be performed regularly and the teeth checked as part of all performance examinations.

TMJ pain is another cause of mouth or head pain that can mimic back pain and performance problems. This joint is critical to the proprioceptive system, the hyoid apparatus, and the normal motion of the entire spine (Ridgway, 1995). Pain or loss of normal motion in the TMJ affects the motion of the whole body because high-speed cameras show that the mouth is in constant motion in all species. A dog videotaped galloping before and after picking up a lightweight cloth disk lost its free stride completely. The spinal movement changed from graceful and flowing to stiff, with the head in the air and the tail held stiff. No matter what type of object the dog held in its mouth, its gait changed in the same manner (Clothier, 1995). The implications in equine medicine are great; in English riding the trend is to fasten the noseband as tight as possible. Some riders make the noseband so tight that padding must be added to prevent sores. Most horses open their mouths because the bits are inhibiting their normal swallowing, not because they need a tighter noseband. The rider then wonders why the horse's movement is poor and the horse is not using its back.

Equine dentists and veterinarians often file large amounts off the incisors to realign the bite. Many of them are poorly trained and may be doing more damage than good because the uneven bite may be the result of loss of normal TMJ mobility. Once the incisors are partially removed, restoration of the incisor alignment may take a long time, and because most of these horses do not receive chiropractic adjustments to the TMJ, the original problem is never corrected. Some horses seem immediately better after the realignment, but the long-term damage may not become apparent until the rest of the body becomes sore as a result of compensating. The bite realignment may be useful in selected cases to keep a damaged or painful TMJ functional or when the procedure is performed correctly in conjunction with an adjustment.

Hoof and Shoe Evaluation

A correctly shod foot is critical to the musculoskeletal system, especially to the spine and related musculature (see

Chapter 12). Many farriers try to correct back pain from the foot up. Although a correctly balanced foot does help the back, some of the degree pads and creative shoeing techniques perpetuate the cycle of back pain and behavioral problems. The horse's musculoskeletal system is balanced on top of four small feet. A slight change in the balance of a foot is magnified many times by the time it reaches the shoulder, hips, and back.

The ideal way to shoe a horse is to have the foot in natural balance with the rest of the leg and the body. This balance is not always possible because of conformation, injuries, and previous poor shoeing. However, many of the most successful farriers adhere to the basic principle of balancing the foot as nearly as possible to the natural way the food should go. Each time a foot is trimmed or shod out of balance in an attempt to correct some other problem, the upper part of the body must compensate. Over time the horse becomes chronically sore, but the pain is seldom directly linked to the shoeing. This chapter does not discuss the details of correct shoeing because much literature is available on the subject (Butler, 1985; Confield, 1968; Hunting, 1988; War Department, 1941; Wiseman, 1977).

Equine orthotics are being used by some farriers and veterinarians around the country. Orthotics are pads, wedges, or shims added to a single foot or pair of feet to balance the upper body or correct movement problems. The addition of orthotics can be useful, although many equine acupuncturists and chiropractors find that when the pain or loss of spinal motion is corrected, the horse no longer requires orthotics. Some horses need them for a short time, perhaps just a few shoeings, while the muscles adjust to a new way of moving, whereas other horses may need them forever. Some horses need orthotics added once or twice a year to maintain balance and comfort. Each horse should be evaluated individually and reevaluated periodically throughout the treatment schedule.

Additional Management Factors Influencing Horse Comfort

Many other management and training practices affect the horse's comfort level and consequent performance (Box 33-2). Taking the whole horse into consideration means looking at all these factors.

Ponying racehorses
Ponying racehorses with their heads torqued around to the lead pony's rider physically pulls the muscles and vertebrae in the neck, causing serious chiropractic subluxations and stiff, sore neck muscles. The rest of the horse's body gallops at an angle down the racetrack, putting torque on the thoracic, lumbar, and sacral vertebrae and straining muscles throughout the back and hindquarters. Unnatural stress is also placed on the joints and tendons in the lower leg, contributing to many of the injuries that are so common on the racetrack. Tracks in other parts of the world—notably, England, Ireland, and Hong Kong—use

Management and Training Practices that Strain the Horse's Body

- Ponying racehorses
- Lungeing
- Training devices
- Muscles neglected after exercise
- Failure to observe warm-up and warm-down measures
- Use of mechanical hot-walkers
- Excessive use of swimming to condition
- Blankets that are too tight

ponying on only the most unruly horses. In the United States, almost every horse is ponied to the starting gate—routinely during racing and often during training.

Lungeing

Lungeing, especially for long periods, causes stress to the horse's entire musculoskeletal system, including the lower legs. The horse must constantly hold its body in the same position with the head and neck bent in one direction. Some good trainers have recognized this problem and have found other ways to teach horses. Many horses at shows are lunged for hours to calm them, but in reality, they stay much more relaxed with minimal lungeing when they are no longer experiencing pain from sore backs and poorly fitting saddles. Herbal relaxation formulas are also good substitutes for lungeing.

Training aids

The number of training aids on the market is endless, ranging from benign to abusive. If one joint is locked up, the rest of the spine loses normal motion, and training devices always cause at least one joint to brace against the device or lose normal motion. Most training devices are not needed when back and neck pain is gone and the rider learns to move with the horse instead of against it. However, because of the variable quality of trainers, most riders never achieve freedom of movement along with freedom from pain.

Unfortunately, training aids are not going to disappear, so if owners cannot be persuaded to stop using them, the veterinarian may be able to teach owners to use them in a more educated way. One of the major faults in the use of these devices is that horses are kept in the same unnatural position for long periods. Muscles fatigue quickly when held in the same position for even a few minutes. No human training method in common practice uses the same motion over and over again for up to an hour or more, as is done routinely with training devices. The best way to use some of the training devices is to connect them for

only a few minutes, release them, and then reconnect them after a few minutes of rest or movement without them. This is commonly known as *interval training* and is an effective method of training in many sports, both human and equine.

Appropriate muscle work

Most horse owners and veterinarians spend an inordinate amount of time with the horse's legs and little time with the muscles of the upper body. Human athletes have learned that an important way to decrease injuries is to take care of the muscles before and after exercise. Football players come off the field and get massaged, sit in the whirlpool, and generally loosen up before going home; marathon runners routinely get quick massages at each pit stop to prevent muscle knots and tension from becoming problems. All horse owners can learn a few basic stretches to do with their horses, and the motivated ones can help their horses enormously every day by learning more about massage and stretching.

Warming up and warming down

Warming up and warming down play an important role in keeping the muscles loose and free from soreness. One study (Marlin and others, 1991) showed that horses trotted for 20 minutes after maximal exercise cleared lactic acid from their blood significantly faster than horses who were walked or held still. Human athletes have practiced this for a long time, and horses in all sports can also benefit. Endurance horses are often warmed up on the trail; however, the fast early pace requires a warmed-up muscle to prevent injuries. Horses shown only in flat classes should also be warmed up for maximal performance, although sufficient preparation rarely occurs unless the horse was ridden before showing to calm him.

Mechanical hot-walkers

For safety reasons, mechanical hot-walkers place the horse in a hollow position with the head and neck up in the air, causing the back to hollow also. Hot-walking is done immediately after exercise, when the horse needs most to stretch its muscles, not tighten and shorten them. Old-fashioned hand-walking works much better, but if that is not possible, the horse should be allowed to stretch after use of the hot-walker. Hot-walkers with individual stalls in which the horses do not need to be tied are becoming more available.

Swimming

Swimming has a prominent place in the rehabilitation of horses. Swimming acts as a break in the normal routine and keeps horses fit when they do not need stress placed on their legs. However, horses swim in a hollowed-out position, which can cause muscles of the neck and back to develop in a hollow position, with strong shoulder muscles from pulling through the water. This activity does not generally cause strong development of the hindquarters because water offers little resistance. This can cause a horse to travel in a hollow position under saddle. Owners should be encouraged to use swimming judiciously.

Blanketing

Blanketing can be a source of problems for horses. "Cut-back" blankets that do not touch the withers cause a viselike tightness between the back of the withers and the points of the shoulders. The cranial thoracic vertebrae, with their long dorsal processes, may become subluxated, as can the attachments of the first few ribs to the sternum. The shoulder muscles become compressed, and the stride shortens significantly. To compensate, the horse tightens up the entire back. Many horses use short strides to move around stalls and fields over winter. By the time spring arrives, clinical lameness appears. Blankets should be selected to fit as loosely over the shoulder as possible so that after the horse has been turned out all night, the buckles should still be easy to open. To achieve this, the most effective shape is a blanket that comes over the withers and up onto the neck slightly. This style tends to hang well, leaving the shoulders free to move. Because many new lightweight, durable materials are available, weighing 4 to 6 pounds per blanket, there is no need to have 20 to 30 pounds of material hanging on the horse's back 24 hours a day. An old blanket can sometimes be improved by the addition of darts in the center of the neck area that cause the blanket to hang away from the shoulder (Harman, 1996).

Back and Neck Pain Diagnosis

Painful muscles are extremely common but infrequently recognized. Many veterinarians examine for back pain by running their fingers down the longissimus dorsi, but cervical examination is not as common. If the touch used is light and gently probing, the reaction can be subtle. The touch may also elicit the normal reflex response of ventroflexion of the back, followed by dorsiflexion of the pelvis. Sometimes this response can be mistaken for soreness when it is actually normal. A more accurate evaluation of back pain can be obtained from palpating the inner Bladder acupuncture meridian about 4 inches lateral to the spine. The reaction along this meridian can offer more specific information as to the true degree of pain in relation to the function of the horse's back. A complete chiropractic examination of the motion in the spine and muscle gives additional information. The details of the examination are discussed in Chapter 12.

Pain reactions vary from mild contracture of the surrounding muscle at a few places to severe sinking from the pressure accompanied by a hardening of the longissimus dorsi. The common reaction of "splinting" (bracing the back muscles so they do not move) is a frequent response in many horses because the pain is decreased when the painful muscle is held rigid. Splinting is sometimes misinterpreted as not painful because the horse does not ap-

pear to sink away from pressure. Some horses splint their backs so severely that they almost buck. These horses often buck when ridden, especially during the warm-up. Neck pain can be observed by palpation with one or two fingers along the verebral column to search for tight or sore places. The horse may flinch only slightly; however, muscle tightness and hardness are significant. Neck soreness may be caused by vertebral subluxations, muscle pain, or pain along the acupuncture meridians that traverse the neck or referred from other areas.

Performance Problem Evaluation

Back pain accounts for a long list of both performance and behavioral problems (Box 33-3). The list encompasses most of the problems that are commonly associated with training; however, veterinarians are often called on to help these horses. For holistic practitioners, these complaints account for a large portion of their practice because alternative therapies often offer more answers for treating

---

BOX 33-3

PERFORMANCE PROBLEMS

- Objection to being saddled
- "Cold-backed" during mounting
- Slowness to warm up or relax
- Resistance to work
- Resistance to or need for training aids
- Hock, stifle, or obscure hind-limb lameness
- Front-leg lameness, stumbling, or tripping
- Excessive shying
- Lack of concentration on rider and aids
- Rushing to and from fences; refusing jumps
- Rushing downhill or pulling uphill with front legs; inability to use hind end
- Inability to travel straight
- Inability to round back or neck
- Annoying habits (e.g., swishing tail, pinning ears, grinding teeth, tossing head)
- Hypersensitivity to being brushed or touched
- Poor attitude
- Difficulty becoming collected or maintaining impulsion
- Twisting over fences
- Bucking or rearing regularly
- Decreased speed on the racetrack
- Slowness out of the starting gate
- Ducking out of turns
- Starting ride well but becoming resistant later
- Not moving or bucking, rolling excessively in field
- Difficulty in shoeing

chronic pain and consequently improve performance problems.

Although some horses learn to overcome these pain-related performance problems, others do not and are usually sold. When horses are treated for back pain and saddles are fitted properly, these training problems can resolve, often overnight. In many cases, however, training techniques and rider balance must also be changed and the mouth and foot problems corrected, or the back pain and behavior problems may return.

Signs of saddle-induced injuries (Box 33-4) found in the physical examination indicate a past or present problem with a saddle. If a poorly fitted saddle has been used on a horse for any length of time, residual back pain and, probably, subluxations of the thoracic and lumbar vertebrae are evident. Residual back pain will probably require treatment with acupuncture and chiropractic; saddle-induced pain and general back pain often persist for many years if not treated.

Indications of Poor Performance

Performance problems can result in anything from mild protest about being saddled to an unridable bucking bronco. The reactions seen are listed in Box 33-3 and discussed in more detail in the following sections. Many, if not most, of the difficulties encountered in training horses can be traced to back pain or a combination of back and neck pain.

Objection to being saddled

Many horses object to being saddled or girthed. Most performance horses have sore backs, and many have problems originating from poor saddle fit. Time after time, when the proper saddle is fitted, the protests stop. Moreover, the horse immediately resumes protesting if the original, ill-fitting saddle is put on. Sometimes a narrow or uncomfortable girth, especially an incorrectly fitted short dressage girth, can cause discomfort at saddling time. Many horses are sore in the pectoral area, and any type of girth bothers them. The weight of the rider must be considered as well, although a heavy but good rider exerts less

---

BOX 33-4

*S*addle-*I*nduced *I*njuries

- Obvious sores
- White hairs under the saddle
- Swellings—temporary (after removing saddle) or permanent
- Scars deep in the muscle
- Atrophy of muscles on sides of withers

---

pressure on a horse's back than a light but poor rider (Harman, unpublished data).

"Cold-backed"

Some horses sink down when being mounted or tighten and hump their backs during the first few minutes of being ridden. Some may actually buck early in the ride, then settle down after warming up. Correct saddle fit and treatment of the horse's pain generally eliminate the problem.

Slowness to warm up or relax

Some horses are tense or stiff for the first part of the ride and seem to have difficulty warming up. Certainly, slowness to warm up may be due to arthritis, navicular syndrome, or some other bone or joint ailment, but the problem often disappears when the back pain is cleared up, the saddle is fitted, and the other issues are resolved. In some instances the back is the main problem; in others, resolution of the back problem allows the horse to travel more easily and thus compensate for other physical problems.

Resistance to work

Most riders and trainers find that all horses show resistance to training at different stages, and some horses appear resistant by nature. This is simply not true. Sometimes the horse may not understand the messages or aids given by the rider, but horses are not naturally resistant. Almost all horses are agreeable and willing to do as they are told if they are able. Being able means being free of pain and not being inhibited by the rider.

Resistance to training aids; requires aids to perform

Training aids or gadgets such as draw reins, side reins, chambons, gags, tiedowns, and various tight nosebands are used either to shortcut training time or solve resistance problems. However, in the long run the horse's neck is usually locked into a "frame" or a specific position with these devices; consequently, the back is locked rather than moving freely. The setting of the head and neck starts the same stiff, hollow-backed reaction that other sources of back pain produce, and more pain is caused from lack of normal motion. The one difference is that the horse often has a head set that looks correct and hides the real problem of a fixed or locked back.

Hock, stifle, and obscure rear-leg lameness

When horses are free of pain and can use their backs more normally, common manifestations of hock and stifle pain improve and often resolve without routine antiinflammatory treatment or joint injections. The lamenesses occur because the hind legs cannot engage or come underneath the body in a normal strong movement. The hind legs tend to trail behind the horse, causing excessive stress and concussion in the joints of the hind leg. Obscure lameness that cannot be blocked in a routine veterinary examination often originates in the back or hip and gluteal area.

Front-leg lameness, stumbling, or tripping

Perhaps the most common saddle problem is placement of the saddle that is too far forward. The rider is trying to sit over the horse's center of gravity; however, when the saddle is too far forward, the tree, which is generally totally inflexible, rests on top of the shoulders. A significant part of the weight of the rider is now sitting on the shoulder blades, preventing the shoulder from moving freely and the front legs from moving fluidly. The problem then becomes a shortened stride and increased concussion of the foot on the ground. This limited movement can lead to fatigue and often contributes to front-leg lameness, such as suspensory and chronic foot problems, as well as frequent stumbling or tripping. Sometimes the treatment can be as simple as moving the saddle back. In addition, horses traveling in the hollow-backed position hit the ground harder with the heels of their front feet than horses traveling with a free, loose back. A hollow back can lead to heel pain, commonly referred to as "navicular syndrome," but the origin may be in the function of the back.

Excessive shying and lack of concentration on the rider and aids

Shying and lack of concentration can be grouped together. A horse in pain cannot concentrate on the rider or the exercise. Lack of concentration can show up as short attention span or as shying. People in pain often become extremely irritable and difficult to deal with, and they have trouble focusing. Horses are no different, and most unfocused horses become amenable to training when their pain is relieved.

Rushing to or from fences; refusing jumps

A horse who anticipates that a certain action, such as jumping, will cause pain, frequently rushes to finish that task. This is normal "fight-or-flight" behavior because the horse's normal response to discomfort is flight. If the horse experiences pain during jumping, it may rush into the fence or come to the fence slowly, jump carefully, and rush away afterward. Some refuse to jump at all or may become chronic stoppers. These horses cannot use their backs properly during some phase of jumping and are in a great deal of pain. In general, this type of jumping problem is written off as a training issue, and increasingly severe methods are applied to force the horse to behave when simply removing the pain generally stops the negative behavior. Of course, some horses simply do not like to jump, but they generally do not show the pain reactions described here.

Rushing downhill or pulling uphill with front legs

Many horses rush downhill. This behavior is generally regarded as a training and balance problem. Indeed, that can be true, especially if the horse is just learning to carry a rider. Many times, however, when the pain is addressed, the horse naturally handles the downhill straighter and more slowly, with the hind legs engaged; this is less stressful to both horse and rider. Horses who pull themselves along with their front legs, especially going uphill, are generally unable to use their backs or hind legs properly. The hollow position of the back leaves the hind legs behind the horse rather than in a strong pushing position underneath him.

Inability to travel straight

Some horses are seemingly incapable of traveling in a straight line, even on flat ground, and are worse going downhill. These horses may have neck, lower-back, or hip pain. A poorly fitted saddle or a saddle with a twisted or broken tree can cause this problem. Some issues involving the rider, feet, and teeth may also contribute.

Unwillingness to round the back or neck; traveling on forehand

Resistance to the training mandate to "become round" and use the back and hindquarters properly is common in all sports. Minor problems are acceptable while the rider learns to communicate and the horse learns to respond, but the horse who will become round and engage the hindquarters only for a few strides is common, as is the horse who will not become truly round or engaged at all. Trying to force a horse into a round frame by holding the head only creates back pain and more resistance.

Annoying habits

Horses who habitually pin their ears, swish or wring their tails, grind their teeth, toss their heads, or exhibit other repetitive behaviors are definitely trying to alert their riders to a problem. The origin may be poor saddle fit, back pain, the use of gadgets creating discomfort, or other sources of pain.

Hypersensitivity to brushing

Many horses do not like to be brushed or touched. Horses with musculoskeletal pain may be superficially sensitive as well. When these horses stop hurting, they suddenly enjoy being groomed and touched.

Poor attitude

Horses considered to have poor attitudes are often reacting to pain or fear. Some horses need different education techniques (e.g., TTEAM approaches) as well as the usual evaluation for sources of pain (see Chapters 12, 15).

Difficulty becoming collected or maintaining impulsion

When horses are not engaged and pushing from behind, maintaining collection is difficult because they will start to pull themselves along with their front end. Discomfort in the hind legs or back is usually the source.

Twisting over fences

Twisting over fences comes from pain or inability to jump the requested height. Some high-level open jumpers are thought to have a style of jumping that involves back twisting; however, most of these horses are simply sore and twist to avoid pain.

Bucking or rearing regularly

Habits such as bucking or rearing may be caused by pain resulting from poor riding, saddle fit, or any of the other causes of pain described in this chapter.

Decreased speed on the racetrack

Many promising horses start their career showing a great deal of speed, only to go slower and slower as time goes by. After treatment for chronic pain the poor performance often improves.

Slowness out of the starting gate

If a horse cannot crouch or "sit down" and propel itself from the rear end, the performance out of the starting gate will be poor. Back pain is a primary cause of poor starting-gate performance; neck, back, and hip pain can also contribute to this problem.

Ducking out of turns

Ducking can occur in all sports and is due to discomfort, poor balance, or poor riding. Young horses who have not learned to balance with a rider may duck out of turns, but they can usually be helped easily; older horses often need bodywork.

Starting ride well, but becoming resistant later

As discomfort increases, the horse becomes less tolerant of the work rather than warming up and working better.

Not moving, bucking, rolling excessively in field

Horses with excessive behaviors in the pasture or stall are trying to adjust themselves (bucking or rolling) or are too sore to move.

Difficulty in shoeing

A horse in pain has a great deal of trouble standing with one leg in the air and its back torqued. Horses are often unfairly disciplined for misbehaving with the farrier when they are actually in pain.

These signs are messages from the horse that something is not right. Surely other signs exist that horses may demonstrate. Once the origin of a problem is discovered and a solution implemented, the improved level of performance is rewarding.

Saddle Fit

The Effects of Saddles on Backs

Saddles are the necessary evil of the competition horse. A saddle is a rigid structure that connects the dynamic structures of the horse with the rider. The fit and position of the saddle affect the movement of the horse and the ability of the rider to communicate with the horse. Soft-tissue pain created by saddles contributes significantly to the poor-performance syndrome, as well as to many of the behavior and lameness problems seen in horses in every sport. Saddle-induced pain is one of the most frequent causes of back pain, resulting from poor fit or improper positioning. If saddle-induced injuries are present, residual back pain results; tissue is damaged every time a poorly fitted saddle is used.

The saddle industry has not used any system to aid in saddle fitting, manufacturing, design, or quality control. Saddles are sold with little consideration for fit and even less knowledge about the consequences of poor fit. Manufacturing defects abound, many of which are detrimental to the horse. A computerized saddle-pressure measurement device is now in use (SaddleTech), bringing science and technology to the saddle industry (Harman, 1994b). The equipment can measure pressures exerted on the horse's back by the weight-bearing saddle and give a multiple-color scan similar in appearance to a thermogram. Pressure-sensing equipment has permitted compilation of information about pressures under saddles. With comparison of data from the saddles with data from human hospital-bedsore research, it is possible to estimate the amount of damage that is occurring.

The blood pressure in the arterial capillaries of humans and dogs is 35 mm Hg, or about 0.75 pounds per square inch (psi). In the capillary beds the pressures are as low as 10 mm Hg, or less than 0.25 psi on the venous side (Guyton, 1986). Pressure of 32 mm Hg (0.68 psi) lasting more than 2 hours causes significant tissue damage in these species (Madsen and others, 1984; Todd, Thacker, 1994). Saddles create much greater pressures (up to 4 psi, or 140 mm Hg) over long periods, compressing the capillaries and causing tissue damage and pain. This in turn causes a decrease in performance. Because tissue trauma is a factor of pressure over time, many people are not aware that damage is occurring unless they ride for several hours and see swelling (which is actually reactive hyperemia) (Holloway and others, 1975) after removing the saddle. Performance is affected long before serious tissue damage results; however, further clinical studies are necessary to determine the precise amount of pressure necessary to affect performance and the length of time required to damage tissue under a saddle.

Pressures are transferred through muscle tissue to the underlying bone. The measured pressures at the level of the bone are significantly greater than at the skin surface (Madsen and others, 1984). Surgical evidence in human medicine suggests that subcutaneous necrosis begins closer to the bone before cutaneous redness and ulceration are apparent (Todd and others, 1994). The effect of the saddle on the skin beneath it can be compared with the effect of a wheelchair on the human back. In the horse the trapezius muscle and longissimus dorsi muscles are compressed by the saddle. Extrapolation from human data suggests that pressures near the vertebrae may be higher than those measured by the computerized saddle pad. In most cases the addition of a thick pad increases the pressure readings at the skin, so the pressure may continue to increase closer to the bone. The use of pads can be helpful if the saddle and pad are fitted together so that the saddle is wide enough across the withers to allow room for the pad. However, the use of pads can also be detrimental. In an ideal world, computerized fitting of the saddle and pad would permit the best combination for each horse.

Saddle-Induced Injuries

Saddle-induced injuries are listed in Box 33-4. Several ways of evaluating saddle fit are discussed later in the chapter. The SaddleTech unit can now define the areas where pressure injuries are occurring. A direct correlation exists between known pressure places in the saddle and the scans produced with the computer unit (Harman, unpublished data). With practice, the correlation can be easily observed with basic palpation of the saddle on the horse's back and observation of the shape and symmetry of the panels. The use of the computer allows evaluation of the fit during movement and the accurate evaluation of the effects of pads.

Sores

Sores on a horse's back are a clear indication of a saddle or rider imbalance problem. A rider who has moderate to severe pain on one side of the body cannot ride in a balanced manner and is as likely to cause sores as an ill-fitting saddle.

White hairs

White hairs can be insidious in onset and often do not appear until a coat change, in either spring or fall. The white hairs result from saddle pressure and may be the only visual sign that a problem exists. Saddle pressure alters the follicle, resulting in pigment changes in the hair. If the damage is not too severe and the pressure is removed, the white hairs may disappear at the next coat change; however, the damage may be permanent. The only solution is to change the saddle fit.

Temporary swelling

Temporary swellings that appear immediately after a saddle is removed are frequently referred to as *heat bumps* because they often appear after the horse is ridden for a long time. Temporary swellings are actually edema from damaged tissue and represent a saddle or rider problem.

Scars

Scars can occur deep in the muscle on either side of the withers. Although not always visible, scars can be felt by palpating deeply into the muscle. Superficial scars directly caused by saddles are frequently seen in endurance and Western-ridden horses but can occur in all sports and with all types of saddles. The skin and sweat glands at these superficial scars are often so damaged that areas without sweat marks will be evident even when a correctly fitted saddle is used.

Muscle atrophy

Many horses show signs of muscle atrophy on their backs, manifesting as depressions on either side of the withers. These pockets are often formed by saddles that are too narrow or thick saddle pads that compress the withers. When a correctly fitted saddle is put on the horse, these hollow areas fill out. Sometimes this occurs in a matter of weeks.

Saddle Evaluation

In the evaluation of a potential saddle problem, the saddle should be examined on and off the horse. Ideally the saddle should be used for 20 minutes, allowing the horse to warm up and begin to move its back. Watching the rider in the saddle is important, and the rider can have most of the warm-up done before the veterinarian arrives. Saddle fit should be considered as important as, and similar to, shoe fit in a person. The basic factors to be considered when examining a saddle include the following:

- The structure of the saddle
- The position of the saddle on the back
- The contact of the panels against the horse's back and the presence or absence of bridging
- Whether the panels are wide enough for good support
- Whether the gullet is wide enough to clear the spine completely ($2\frac{1}{2}$ to 3 inches)
- The fit of the tree to the horse's back, especially across the withers
- Whether the saddle sits squarely in the center of the back
- The levelness of the seat
- The placement and shape of the girth

Structure

Although the structure of the saddle is extremely important, saddle manufacture has seldom included quality control. Therefore new saddles may have serious defects, such as twisted trees or panels and flaps installed asymmetrically. The initial cost of the saddle seems to have no bearing on the number or severity of structural defects to be found. The saddle should be examined carefully from all angles to check for balance and symmetry (Figs. 33-6 and 33-7).

Position

The position of the saddle on the back is the most critical aspect of saddle fit. The most common mistake is placement of the saddle too far forward. This position places the rigid tree over the top of the scapula, significantly restricting the movement of the front legs. If the

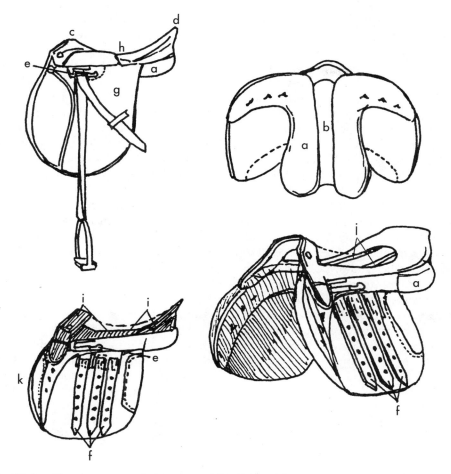

Fig. 33-6. Top, bottom, and side view of English saddle, showing saddle parts. *a,* Panel; *b,* gullet; *c,* pommel; *d,* cantle; *e,* stirrup bar; *f,* billets; *g,* flaps; *h,* seat; *i,* tree; *j,* spring of tree; *k,* knee roll. (Illustrations by Susan Harris.)

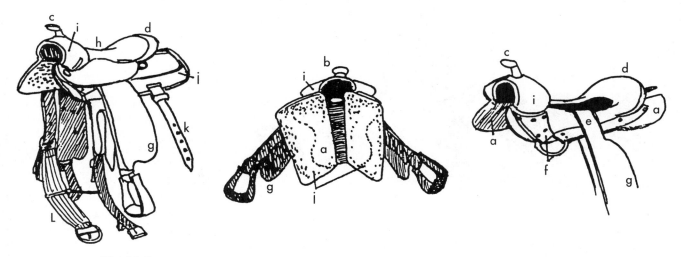

Fig. 33-7. Top, bottom, and side view of Western saddle, showing saddle parts. *a,* Bars; *b,* gullet; *c,* horn; *d,* cantle; *e,* stirrup leather around bars; *f,* rigging; *g,* fender; *h,* seat; *i,* fork; *j,* skirt; *k,* flank bullet; l, girth.

saddle is moved back to the correct position, the stride generally lengthens immediately. If the saddle does not fit, regardless of type, no change in position will correct the problem.

When an English saddle is placed too far forward, the pommel is too high, causing the seat to slope down toward the cantle and placing the rider's legs too far forward in an unbalanced position. The rider then tries to level the seat with pads under the back of the saddle, which causes more pressure at the front, over the shoulders. When a properly fitting saddle is in the correct position, the seat is level.

Western saddles, when placed too far forward, exert enormous pressure on the top of the scapulae, but the seat is often balanced as a result of design. Moving the saddle back to the correct position frees the scapulae. When some Western saddles are moved off the shoulders, the seat becomes better balanced; with others, however, the rider will be tipped forward. Also, it is common for the pommel to become too close to the withers. Compact style saddles, such as those used in barrel racing and those designed for Arabians, are easier to move into the correct position but may be more difficult to ride because they are designed for a specific type of riding.

Panels

Moving the saddle back (off the withers) also increases the contact area between the panels (underside) and the horse's back. When the saddle is too far forward, a bridge is created with pressure on the shoulders and the back of the saddle. The rider's weight becomes distributed on four points, one on each side of the withers/shoulder blades and one on each side of the back at the rear of the saddle, rather than evenly along the horse's back. This misalignment causes the horse to stiffen its back. Many saddles, English and Western, have this bridge between the front and the back caused by poor construction or poor fit, even when the saddle is in the correct position (Fig. 33-8). Bridging must be avoided; however, in an ideally fitting saddle, the contact with the horse's back should be slightly less in the center to allow the horse to raise its back while moving. To evaluate the amount of clearance a horse needs, the examiner should raise its back slightly while the saddle is in place and be sure that even contact occurs on the panels. Most of the new flexible-panel endurance saddles are too long for the horse's back, creating pressure points on the shoulder and loins. Then the flexible center of the panels offers no support, and the same type of bridging is created.

The panels should be wide enough to offer good support without losing the contour needed to fit the horse's back. The gullet should be wide enough (2½ to 3 inches) to allow the spine complete freedom from pressure and allow the spine to bend slightly laterally during movement. In some saddles, especially dressage saddles, pressure points occur under the area of the stirrup bars because manufacturers design saddles to be wide through the front

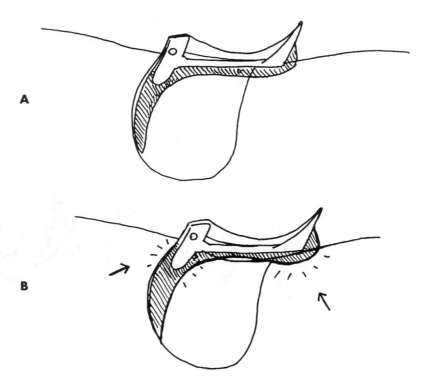

Fig. 33-8. **A,** Saddle fitting correctly with the panels almost flat against the back. **B,** Bridging in an English saddle showing the areas of high pressure *(arrows)*. (Western saddles bridge in the same manner.)

of the tree to clear the scapulae. The wide front leaves the saddle tight near the area of the stirrup bar. The tight area can be caused by a narrowing of the gullet or sometimes by the stirrup bars angling inward toward the spine.

The angle of the panels should follow the angle of the horse's back under the cantle. Many Western or English saddles have too acute an angle, which puts pressure on the outer corner of the panel and creates pain at the center of the longissimus dorsi muscle.

English saddles should be reflocked (restuffed) every year or even more frequently to maintain good contact with the horse's back. Wool stuffing is resilient, offers a smooth surface for the horse's back, and can be adjusted slightly to conform to the horse's back. Foam-stuffed panels are hard to replace, and some foam begins to lose its memory in just a few months. However, a good-quality foam will hold its shape, and if the shape conforms to the horse's back, the saddle will fit much better over a longer period. Wool-stuffed panels should be reflocked by a competent saddler once every 6 months to 1 year for the saddle to maintain its shape and should not be overstuffed.

The saddle must sit squarely down the middle of the back and be supported by the panels because the spine is not designed to carry weight directly. No muscle covers the spinous processes; therefore nothing cushions the hardness of the saddle from the spinous processes. Pressure can cause bone pain and degeneration of the ligament that runs along the top of the spine. Some preliminary diagnostic ultrasound data from England indicate that damage to this ligament may be common and may be an important factor in back pain (Barnes, unpublished data).

Position and shape of the girth

The girth always ends up in the narrowest point of the thoracic cage and is perpendicular to the ground. Because the girth is attached to the saddle, the girth must drop naturally down into the narrowest part of the thorax or the saddle will move either forward or back as the girth finds its natural spot. Some horses' girth spots are just behind the elbows, whereas others are 1 to 2 hand-breadths behind the elbow. An otherwise well-fitting saddle can become a poorly fitting saddle just by having the girth attached in the wrong place, which causes the saddle to shift to an incorrect position.

Short girths (both Western and short dressage girths) can cause discomfort just behind the shoulders and elbows. The correct length for the girth is so it ends just below the saddle, just out of the rider's way and as long as possible for the horse.

Trees

The tree of the saddle, as it crosses the withers, must fit the horse without the use of pads. In fact, a bare tree with no leather should conform to the horse's back. If the tree is too narrow for the withers, pressure points or sores will be created and the pommel will sit up too high, unbalancing

the rider. In this situation, if pads are placed under the back of the saddle to raise it, more pressure is placed on the withers. If the saddle is too wide across the withers, the rider is tipped forward and the saddle contacts the withers.

Many saddles are poorly designed through the withers area and have built-in pressure points. Western saddles frequently have large, slightly raised areas at the front of the tree where contact with the withers area occurs. When saddles are new, this is not apparent, but after the leather is broken in these areas become painful pressure points. English close-contact saddles often have an outward flare to the tree along the withers. This flare causes a small and painful pressure point because the horse's withers are flat at this point. Most horses do not tolerate pressure points well and shorten the stride and hollow the back. Other saddles have pressure points underneath the stirrup bars or attachments.

Exercise saddles at the racetrack are designed to be light and small; however, they do not spread the rider's weight out evenly and contribute significantly to poor-performance pain syndromes. The American-style exercise saddle has a half-tree, the rear points of which poke into the horse's back if the horse is well-muscled. If the horse has a narrow back or a spine that sticks up above the muscle, the center of the saddle sits directly on the spine. The SaddleTech system has been used to demonstrate the problems associated with exercise saddles (Harman, unpublished data). The full-tree exercise saddle may be only slightly better; they still have no significant gullet or panels to spread the rider's weight and protect the back. The degree of back pain that occurs in racehorses as a result of the poor design of the saddles costs the industry a great deal of money. A new exercise saddle (The Performer; see Resources) is available to help solve many of the fitting problems; initial clinical results show significant changes in performance, and SaddleTech is being used to test it at each stage of development.

A relatively new saddle is the "treeless" saddle (Sport Saddle; see Resources). It features a piece of a tree at the pommel and cantle, with leather and neoprene everywhere else. The rigging for the girth and the stirrups hangs from the pieces of the tree so that when a rider sits in the saddle, it almost folds in the middle, lifting the two ends up to minimize pressure on the horse's back. The saddle has no gullet, so horses with prominent spines require a pad with a gullet built in. Horses with spines below the longissimus dorsi (e.g., certain quarter horses) do not need a special pad. The placement of the girth and the shape of the pommel do not allow the saddle to fit every horse, but this saddle is versatile for general riding and even Western showing. Western styles are available, as are endurance styles.

Saddles come in all different tree widths and shapes. Some brands have a range of sizes, whereas others have only one size. As with shoe fit, some saddles tend to be wide, whereas other brands with the same width on the label run narrow. Knowledge of saddle fit is uncommon in tack shops, and the truth is that a saddle cannot be sold as being correctly fitted for a horse without actually being tried on the horse. Many saddles are sold as "one-size-fits-all"; however, all breeds of horses have different sizes of withers, and variations also occur within the breeds.

The complicating factor is that horses do change shape across the withers—rapidly, at times—particularly with changes in the demands of performance, level of nutrition, or the seasons. Horses in hard competition change shape basically three times throughout the competitive season. They start out heavy and wider when they are unfit, lose weight and become average midseason, and become thinner late in a hard season. This is when saddle fit becomes a complicated issue. Eventually, an adjustable-tree saddle will be made that will solve these problems, but those now on the market do not work well and are not durable.

Level seat

An important aid in determining saddle fit is the levelness of the seat when viewed from the side. If the seat is not level, the rider will be unbalanced and unable to help the horse or ride correctly. The rider may be totally unaware of the problem. A saddle that is too narrow sits too high at the cantle because the tree is too narrow to follow the contours of the withers. The rider's weight is pitched toward the cantle and the rider's legs forward, one of the most common rider faults. If the saddle fits well but needs significant restuffing, it slopes down toward the cantle. A saddle that is too wide tips forward or down at the pommel, pitching the rider forward and the rider's legs behind the vertical position.

Locating pressure points

If white hairs are appearing under the saddle, that location is a pressure point. On a Western saddle the sheepskin covering of the panels becomes worn down over the pressure points. Another way to locate pressure points is to ride with a thin, clean white saddle pad. Where dark spots appear on the pad after 15 or 20 minutes there are generally pressure points. Light areas and areas with no sweat are generally exempt from pressure, but reevaluation may reveal that these are also caused by excess pressure, which decreases the amount of sweat produced.

Measuring the back

A plaster cast of the back can be made fairly easily with the use of 6-inch fast- or ultra–fast-drying plaster. The horse must stand on all four feet evenly while the plaster is setting. If the horse is in pain, this may be difficult, and some horses require light tranquilization to stay still for a sufficient time. Casting requires at least six rolls of plaster cut into approximately 20-inch lengths depending on the size of the horse. Each layer is laid in a different direction; in other words, the first layer is laid across the back, the next layer lengthwise along the back, then across again. After the plaster sets it is carefully removed. The cast will withstand shipping and the weight of a saddle but not the weight of a rider. The plaster cast cannot indicate the placement of the girth line or the appearance of the horse in motion, but it is a cheap and relatively easy project.

Another, much less satisfactory way of measuring the horse's back for some assistance in saddle fitting is with the use of a flexible ruler from a stationery store. This tool can be molded to the shape of the horse's withers where the points of the tree would lie and at 4-inch intervals along the horse's back to the rear of the saddle. After each measurement is taken, the shaped ruler is placed on a piece of cardboard; the inside of the curve is traced, then each piece is cut out. This method yields a pattern that can then be held up to the bottom of the saddle, giving a general idea of whether the saddle fits the shape of a particular horse. This is not an exact method, but it approximates the shape of the horse's back.

A new measuring device for mapping the shape of the horse's back (Lauriche Back Graph) is available. The device consists of a set of calibrated vertical posts in a horizontal frame. The Back Graph is placed on the horse's back, the posts are adjusted to the shape of the horse, and the numbers are recorded. The Graph can be reset to measure different horses. The advantage of this system is that the shape of the back can be recreated anywhere. Data can be gathered regarding the shape of the back and the way it may change during treatment, training, and conditioning.

Therapeutic pads

Therapeutic pads are often used in an attempt to solve problems with saddle fit. Pads may provide only temporary relief and ultimately cause more problems than they solve. The addition of the pad to a saddle is analogous to the addition of an extra sock to a person's shoe. If the tree of the saddle is wide enough, the pad may help. If the tree is already too narrow—the most common scenario—the addition of the pad creates more pressure on the withers. Muscles atrophy along each side of the withers after long use of thick pads. Extra pads, such as pommel pads, compress the withers even more. Because the addition of most therapeutic pads narrows the space available for the withers, the pommel sits higher in front, as it does when the tree is too narrow. This puts the rider off balance and creates the need for more pads under the back of the saddle, which lifts the back and drives more pressure onto the withers.

Frequently the addition of a pad causes a dramatic improvement in a horse's performance. This may last for several months or only a few days, but the same problems usually return because the pad changes the fit of the saddle and slightly moves the pressure points. The intensity of the pressure point is also changed by the addition of the pad but is seldom eliminated, and the pressure is often increased. Over time, the pressure continues to work its way through the pads, and the previously undamaged skin and muscle becomes bruised and painful, creating new pressure points. The creation of new pressure points results in an endless search for pads to help correct the problem. The computerized device measures pressure on the skin under the pad. Individualized fit is important because one pad may help the fit of a saddle and another may make the situation worse (Harman, 1994). If the computer reveals a pressure point before the addition of a pad, that same pressure point will exist after use of the pad and will often be larger.

Shims are thin pads placed under parts of a saddle in an attempt to correct a problem with fit or to balance a rider. More research in shim design is necessary to explore their use as a temporary or permanent correction. Shims must be made carefully to prevent new pressure points. Shims can be a valuable tool for the rider to see the way a correctly balanced saddle feels.

Treatment of Performance Problems

Treatment of performance problems requires a whole-horse approach to be consistently successful. The saddle sits on one third to one half of the acupuncture Bladder meridian association points; consequently the rider and the saddle have a significant effect on the flow of *Qi*, or energy, through the body. *Qi* affects the health of many parts of the body. For example, pressure points often occur at the cantle, caused by the saddle or the rider. These points put pressure on some of the association points related to the meridians that traverse the hind leg (BL-18 through 22). Many horses with chronic back pain have hind-leg lameness or stiffness, and treating the problem locally, whether with conventional therapy or with acupuncture, only palliates the problem. Using a whole-horse approach reduces the need for many repeat treatments. Failing to examine all aspects of the horse and rider is one reason that acupuncture and chiropractic have the reputation of providing only temporary results.

Conclusion

The rewards of looking at the whole horse are great. The challenge is to determine the pieces of the puzzle that need attention and then whether the pieces can work together. When the practitioner considers the whole horse, corrects saddle fit, analyzes the rider's position, and helps the horse learn new behaviors, the results often far exceed expectations and last for a long time. Owners are pleased, and practitioners are rewarded not only with faithful clients but also with many referrals.

Suppliers

Saddle Equipment

The Performer by Blake Kral
5300 N US Highway 27
Ocala, FL 34482

352-622-2522
Exercise saddle for racehorses

SaddleTech
Equitech
Woodside, CA 94062
415-851-4636
Computerized pressure-measurement equipment

Lauriche Back Graph
Lauriche Saddlery
22 Station St. Walsall
West Midlands, England WS2 952
+01922-26430
Measurement device for saddle fitting

Mylers Bits, Inc.
Rt. 3, Box 31D1
Marshfield, MO 65706
800-354-3613
417-859-7468
Bits that relieve tongue pressure

Sport Saddle
Horse Works
4917 Cairo Rd
Paducah, KY 42001-9117
502-443-1505
Treeless saddle

Natural Products

Advanced Biologic Concepts
301 Main St.
Osco, IL 61274
800-373-5971
Fax 309-522-5570
Food supplements, probiotics

Cell Tech
1300 Main St.
Klamath Falls, OR 97601
800-800-1300
Blue-green algae and other food supplements

Equilife Products
PO Box 5005
Glendale, CA 91221-1005

Equilite, Inc.
20 Prospect Ave.
Ardsley, NY 10502
914-693-2553
Herbal products

Espree Animal Products
PO Box 167707
Irving, TX 75016-7707
Natural fly spray

Hilton Herbs
US Distributor: Echo Publishing, Inc.
PO Box 23294
Santa Fe, NM 87502
505-989-7280
Herbal products

JBR
840 South Park Rd.
Slate Hill, NY 10973
914-355-2607
Herbal products

Matol Botanical International, Ltd.
111 46th Ave.
Lachine, Quebec H8T 3C5
Canada
514-639-0730
Km, herbal tonic

Nutrimax Laboratories, Inc.
5024 Campbell Blvd.
Baltimore, MD 21236
800-925-5187
Nutriceuticals and supplements

NutriWest
PO Box 5
Douglas, WY 82633
800-443-3333, 307-358-5066
Glandulars; naturopathic, and other supplements

Thousand Mile Chinese Herbs
3065 Center Green Dr., Suite 140
Boulder, CO 80301
800-481-4433, 303-541-0778
Chinese herbs and nutritional supplements

Vetri Science
20 New England Dr.
Essex Junction, VT 05453
800-882-9993
Neutriceuticals and natural supplements

Washington Homeopathic Products
4914 Delray Ave.
Bethesda, MD 20814
800-336-1695, 301-652-1695
Primary Spray Conditioner—homeopathic odor control and complete line of homeopathics

ACKNOWLEDGMENTS

I would like to thank Jim Helfter for this assistance in researching equine nutrition and Ann Harman for editing and proofreading the manuscript.

REFERENCES

Abrams JT: The effect of dietary vitamin A supplements on the clinical conditions and track performance of racehorses, *Bibl Nutr Dieta* 27:113, 1979.

Alexander F, Davies EM: Production and fermentation of lactate by bacteria in the alimentary canal of the horse and pig, *J Comp Pathol* 73:1, 1963.

Arnold SF and others: Synergistic activation of estrogen receptor with combinations of environmental chemicals, *Science* 272:1489, 1996.

Argiratos, V, Samman S: The effect of calcium carbonate and calcium citrate on the absorption of zinc in healthy female subjects, *Eur J Clin Nutr* 48:198, 1994.

Barrows GT: Research efforts have lagged in free-choice feeding, *An Nutr Health* 5:150, 1977.

Barnes M: Myofascial release and the equine athlete, *Dressage and CT* 113(276):23, 1996.

Bennett D: *Principles of conformation analysis I*, Gaithersburg, Md, 1988, Fleet Street Publishing Corp.

Bjarnason I, Peters TJ: Intestinal permeability, non-steroidal anti-inflammatory drug enteropathy and inflammatory bowel disease: an overview, *Gut* 30S:22, 1989.

Bjarnason I, So A, Levi AJ: Intestinal permeability and inflammation in rheumatoid arthritis: effects of non-steroidal anti-inflammatory drugs, *Lancet* 2:1171, 1984.

Brocks PH: Water must be seen as a nutrient, *Feedstuffs* Jan 1995.

Bromily M: *Natural methods for equine health*, Oxford, England, 1994, Blackwell Scientific Publications.

Cepinskas, G, Specian RD, Kvietys PR: Adaptive cytoprotection in the small intestine: role of mucus, *Am J Physiol* 264:(5)G921, 1993.

Clarke LL: Feeding and digestive problems in horses. *Vet Clin North Am Eq Pract* 6(2):433, 1990.

Clothier S: *Your athletic dog: A functional approach*, video. Stanton, NJ, 1995, Flying Dog Press.

Cohen S, Tyrrel D, Smith A: Psychological stress and susceptibility to the common cold, *N Engl J Med* 325:606-612,1991.

Darlington LG: Dietary therapy for arthritis, *Nut Rheum Dis/Rheum Dis Clin North Am* 17(2):273, 1991.

Davis C: Studies in the self-selection of diet by young children, *J Am Dental Assoc* 21:636, 1934.

DeMaar TW: Zoopharmacognosy: a science emerges from Navajo legends, *Ceres* 25(5):5, 1993.

Flaten TP: Chlorination of drinking water and cancer incidence in Norway, *Int J Epidemiol* 21:6, 1992.

Frigard T, Pettersson D, Aman P: Fiber degrading enzyme increases body weight and total serum cholesterol in broiler chickens fed a rye based diet, *J Nutr* 124(12):2422, 1994.

Gardner ML: Gastrointestinal absorption of intact proteins, *Annu Rev Nutr* 8:329, 1988.

Getting in touch, *Practical Horseman* 23(4):43, 1995b.

Glade MJ: Nutrition and performance of racing thoroughbreds, *Eq Vet J* 15:31-36, 1983.

Glade MJ and others: Dietary protein in excess of requirements inhibits renal calcium and phosphorus in young horses, *Nutr Res Intern* 31:649-660, 1985.

Glade MJ: Nutrition for the equine athlete. In Jones, ed: *Equine sports medicine*, Philadelphia, 1989, Lea & Febiger.

Grosjean N: Veterinary aromatherapy, Saffron Waldon, England, 1993, CW Daniel Co.

Gross WB: The effects of ascorbic acid on stress and disease in chickens, *Av Dis* 36(3):688, 1992.

Hall IA and others: Effect of trimethoprim/sulfamethoxazole on thyroid function in dogs with pyoderma, *J Am Vet Med Assoc* 202(12):1959, 1993.

Harman JC: Selecting the optimum horse for your sport: Can your horse do what you want it to do? *TTEAM News International,* June 1992.

Harman JC: Homeopathy in equine practice, *Eq Pract* 16(1): 1994a.

Harman JC: Practical use of a computerized saddle pressure measuring device to determine the effects of saddle pads on the horse's back, *J Eq Vet Sci* 14:11, 1994b.

Harman JC: Homeopathic case report, *Eq Pract* 17(3):32, 1995.

Harman JC: Does your blanket fit? *Practical Horseman,* 115, Dec 1996.

Harris SE: *Horses' gaits, balance and movement,* New York, 1993, Howell Book House.

Hauser WE, Remington, JS: Effects of antibiotics on the immune response, *Am J Med* 72(5):711, 1982.

Haussler KK, Stover SM: Survey of anatomic variations and pathologic findings in the lumbosacral spine of the thoroughbred racehorse, *Proc Assoc Eq Sports Med* p 41, 1994/1995.

Healthier hocks with natural supplements? *Practical Horseman* 24(1):40, 1996.

Hunt JN, Johnson C: Relationship between gastric secretion of acid and urinary excretion of calcium after oral supplements of calcium, *Dig Dis Science* (28)417, 1983.

Hunting W: *The art of horseshoeing,* New York, 1988, William R. Jenkins.

Into the mainstream, *Practical Horseman* 23(4):80, 1995a.

Jaeger CB: Polymer encapsulated dopaminergic cell lines as "alternative neural grafts," *Prog Brain Res* 82:41-46, 1990.

Jansson K, Hyttinen JM: Induction of gene mutation in mammalian cells by 3-chloro-4-(dichloromethyl)-5-hydroxy-2(5H)-furanone (MX), a chlorine disinfection by-product in drinking water, *Mutation Res* 322(2):129, 1994.

Jeffcott L and others: An assessment of wastage in thoroughbred racing from conception to four years of age, *Eq Vet J* 14:185-198, 1982.

Jefferies WM: Cortisol and immunity, *Med Hypoth* 34:198, 1991.

Jisaka M and others: Antitumoral and antimicrobial activities of bitter sesquiterpene lactones of Vernonia amygdalina, a possible medicinal plant used by wild chimpanzees, *Biosci Biotech Biochem* 57(5):833-834, 1993.

Jones W: Regular monthly column on alternative medicine, Wildomar, Calif, *Eq Vet Data* 1995-1996.

Jordhal G: Personal communication, Tama, Iowa, Agro Systems, 1995.

Kern DL and others: Ponies vs steers: microbial and chemical characteristics of intestinal ingesta, *J Anim Sci* 38:559, 1974.

Kimbrough DR, Martinez N, Stolfus S: A laboratory experiment illustrating the properties and bioavailability of iron, *J Chem Educ* 72(6):558, 1995.

Knight C: Alternative healing for horses, *Western Horseman* 61(1):30, 1996.

Kross BC and others: The nitrate contamination of private well water in Iowa, *Am J Public Health* 83(2):270, 1993.

Lipske M: Animal, heal thyself, *National Wildlife* 32(1):46, 1993.

Mackowiak PA: The normal microbial flora, *N Engl J Med* 307:83, 1982.

Madsen El KM and others: An in-depth look at pressure sores using monolithic silicon pressure sensors, *Plast Recontr Surg* 74:745, 1984.

Mahoney A, Hendricks DG: Role of gastric acid in the utilization of dietary calcium by the rat, *Nutr Metab* 18:375, 1974.

Mahoney A, Holbrook RS, Hendricks DG: Effects of calcium solubility on absorption by rats with induced achlorhydria, *Nutr Metab* 18:310, 1975.

Marlin DJ and others: Influence of post exercise activity blood lactate disappearance in the thoroughbred horse. In Gillespie JR, Robinson NE, editors: *Equine exercise physiology II,* Davis, Calif, ICEEP Publications, 1991.

Meilants H and others: Intestinal mucosal permeability in inflammatory rheumatic diseases. II, Role of disease, *Can J Rheumatol* 18(3):394, 1991.

Meyer H: Nutrition of the equine athlete, *Proc 2nd Int Conf Equine Exer Physiol* 2:644, 1987.

Midtvedt T and others: Influence of peroral antibiotics upon the biotransformatory activity of the intestinal microflora in healthy subjects, *Eur J Clin Invest* 16:11, 1986.

Mitsuoka T: Intestinal flora and aging, *Nutr Rev* 50(12):438, 1992.

Moon J: The role of vitamin D in toxic metal absorption: a review, *J Am Coll Nutr* 13(6):559, 1994.

Moore JN and others: Intracecal endotoxin and lactate during the onset of equine laminitis: a preliminary report, *Am J Vet Res* 40:722, 1979.

Morales Suarez-Varela and others: Chlorination of drinking water and cancer incidence, *J Environ Pathol Toxicol Oncol* 13(1):39, 1994.

Morisco C, Rimarco B, Condrelli M: Effect of coenzyme Q10 therapy in patients with congestive heart failure: a long-term multi center randomized study, *Clin Invest* 71:S134, 1993.

Morita R and others: Hypervitaminosis D: a review, *Nippon Rinsho— Jpn J Clin Med* 51(4):984, 1993.

Myler D: Personal communication, 1997.

Nelemans PJ and others: Swimming and the risk of cutaneous melanoma, *Melan Res* 4(5):281, 1994.

Nockels CF: The role of vitamins in modulating disease resistance, *Vet Clin North Am Food Anim Pract* 4(3):531, 1988.

National Research Council (NRC): *Nutrient requirements of horses,* ed 5, Washington DC, 1989, National Academy Press.

Oliver TH, Wilkinson JF: Critical review achlorhydria, *Q J Med* 2:431, 1933.

Pickford JR: The effect of mill processing on vitamin levels in diets. In Swan H, Lewis D, editors: *Proc 2nd Nutr Conf Feed Mfrs Univ Nott,* London, 1968, Churchill.

Prochaska LJ, Piekutowski WV: On the synergistic effects of enzymes in food with enzymes in the human body: a literature survey and analytical report, *Med Hypoth* 42(6):355, 1994.

Ralston SL: Effect of soluble carbohydrate content of pelleted diets on post-prandial glucose and insulin profiles in horses, *First European Conference on Nutrition of the Horse,* Pferdeheilkunde, Sonderausgabe, 3(4):112, 1992.

Richter C: Total self-regulatory functions in animals and human beings, *Harvard Lecture Series* 38:63, 1943.

Ridgway K: Equine performance deficits associated with temporomandibular joint disease, *Am Hol Vet Med Assoc Proc* p 127, 1995.

Ritter WF and others: Drainage and water quality in northern United States and eastern Canada, *J Irrigat Drain Engin* 121(4):296, 1995.

Robles M and others: Recent studies on the zoopharmacognosy, pharmacology and neurotoxicology of sesquiterpene lactones, *Planta Med* 61:199, 1995.

Rolfe RD: Interactions among microorganisms of the indigenous intestinal flora and their influence on the host, *Rev Infect Dis* 67:S59-S73, 1984.

Rossdale PD and others: Epidemiological study of wastage among racehorses 1982-1983, *Vet Rec* 116:66-69, 1985.

Sanderson IR, Walker WA: Uptake and transport of macromolecules by the intestine: possible role in clinical disorders (an update), *Gastroenterology* 104:622, 1993.

Schell TC and others: Effects of feeding aflatoxin-contaminated diets with and without clay to weanling and growing pigs on performance, liver function and mineral metabolism, *J Anim Sci* 71(5):1209, 1993a.

Schell TC and others: Effectiveness of different types of clay for reducing the detrimental effects of aflatoxin-contaminated diets on performance and serum profiles of weanling pigs, *J Anim Sci* 71(5):1226, 1993b.

Schmidt MA and others: *Beyond antibiotics*, Berkeley, Calif, 1993, North Atlantic Books.

Schryver HF, Hintz HF, Lowe JE: Calcium metabolism, body composition and sweat losses of exercised horses, *Am J Vet Res* 39(2):245, 1978.

Schryver HF, Hintz HF: Trace elements in horse nutrition, *Comp Cont Ed Pract Vet* 4:5534, 1982.

Scullin R: Personal communication, 1986.

Senft D: Cleaner well water, *Agr Res* 43(7):16, 1995.

Simon GL, Gorbach SL: The human intestinal microflora, *Dig Dis Sci* 31(9):147S, 1986.

Slade LM and others: Nutritional adaptations of horses for endurance performance, *Proc Nutr Physiol Symp* 4:114, 1975.

Stauder G and others: The use of hydrolytic enzymes as adjuvant therapy in AIDS/ARC/LAS patients, *Biomed Pharmacother* 42:31, 1988.

Swenson M, editor: *Dukes' physiology of domestic animals*, Ithaca, NY, 1977, Cornell University Press.

Swift S: *Centered riding*, North Pomfret, Vt, 1985, David & Charles.

Swistock BR, Sharpe WE, Robillard PD: A survey of lead, nitrate and radon contamination of private individual water systems in Pennsylvania, *J Environ Health* 55(5):6, 1993.

Todd BA, Thacker JG: Three-dimensional computer model of the human buttocks, in vivo, *J Rehab Res Develop* 31(2):111, 1994.

Toohey L, Kreutle S: *Nutritional physiology: clinical applications and scientific research*, Fort Collins, Colo, 1995, HealthQuest Publishing.

Troianskaia AF and others: The use of summary indices for assessing organochlorine compounds in water, *Gigiena i Sanitariia* (12):12, 1993.

Walker WA: Intestinal transport of macromolecules. In Johnson LR, editor: *Physiology of the gastrointestinal tract*, New York, 1981, Raven Press.

Walters C: *Weeds, control without poison*, Kansas City, Mo, 1991, Acres USA.

Walters C, Fenzau CJ: *Eco-farm*, Kansas City, 1996, Acres USA.

Walthes CM, Johnson HE, Carpenter GA: Air hygiene in a pullet house: effects of air filtration on aerial pollutants measured in vivo and in vitro, *Br Poult Sci* 32(1):31, 1991.

War Department: *The horseshoer*, War Department Technical Manual, (2):220, 1941, Washington, DC.

Ward M: A holistic approach to laminitis, *Am Hol Vet Med Assoc Proc*, p 130, 1995.

White NA and others: Equine colic risk assessment on horse farms: a prospective study, *Proc Am Assoc Eq Prac* 39:97, 1993.

Willoughby SL: *Equine chiropractic care*, Port Byron, Ill, 1991, Options for Animals Foundation.

Wiseman RF: *The complete horseshoeing guide*, Stillwater, Okla, 1977, University of Oklahoma Press.

Worsnop RL: Water quality: should safety standards for drinking water be tougher in the US? *CQ Res* 4:(6)140, 1994.

SELECTED READINGS

Butler D: *The principles of horseshoeing II*, Marysville, Mo, 1985, self-published.

Clarenburg R: *Physiologic chemistry of domestic animals*, St Louis, 1991, Mosby.

Cleave TL: *The saccharine disease*, New Caanan, Ct, 1978, Keats.

Confield DM: *Elements of farrier science*, Middle Tennessee State University, Albert Leo, Minn, 1968, Enderes Tool Co., Inc.

Consumer Reports: Water treatment, Yonkers, NY, Consumers Union, 1:41, 1990.

Consumer Reports: Carbonated waters, Yonkers, NY, Consumers Union, 9:569, 1992.

Consumer Reports: Water treatment devices, Yonkers, NY, Consumers Union, 2:73, 1993.

Consumer Reports buying guide: Water treatment, Yonkers, NY, 1996, Consumers Union.

Do Pico GA: Hazardous exposure and lung disease among farm workers, *J Clin Chest Med* 13(2):311, 1992.

Doran and others: Acetaminophen: more harm than good for chickenpox? *J Pediatrics* 114(6):1045, 1989.

Folino M, McIntyre A, Young GP: Dietary fibers differ in their effects on large bowel epithelial proliferation and fecal fermentation–dependent events in rats, *J Nutr* 125(6):1521, 1995.

Freeman DW: Nitrogen metabolism in the mature physically conditioned horse. II. Response to varying nitrogen intake, in *Proceedings of the Ninth Nutrition and Physiology Symposium*, East Lansing, Mich, 1985.

Goldberg DM: Enzymes as agents for the treatment of disease, *Clin Chim Acta* 206:45, 1992.

Goodlad RA and others: Dietary fiber and the gastrointestinal tract: differing trophic effects on muscle and mucosa of the stomach, small intestines and colon, *Eur J Clin Nutr* 49:S178, 1995.

Guyton AC: *Textbook of medical physiology*, Philadelphia, 1986, WB Saunders.

Hintz HF: Effects of protein levels on endurance horses, *J Anim Sci* 51:202, 1980.

Hintz HF: Feeding programs. In Robinson NE, editor: *Current therapy in equine medicine*, ed 2, Philadelphia, 1987, WB Saunders.

Holloway GA Jr and others: Effects of external pressure loading on human blood flow measured by ^{133}Xe clearance, *J Appl Physiol* 40(4):597, 1975.

Jaffe DM: High fever: is early antibiotic treatment useful? *N Engl J Med* 317:1175, 1987.

Kamikawa T and others: Effects of coenzyme Q10 on exercise intolerance in chronic stable angina pectoris, *Am J Cardiol* 56:247, 1985.

Lee GR and others: The effect of caeruloplasmin on plasma iron in copper-deficient swine, *Clin Res* 17:152, 1969.

Lupton JR, Coder DM, Jacobs LR: Influence of luminal pH on rat large bowel epithelial cell cycle, *Am J Physiol* 249:G382, 1985.

McPherson EA and others: Chronic obstructive pulmonary disease (COPD) in horses. Aetiological studies: responses to intradermal and inhalation antigenic challenge, *Eq Vet J* 11:159, 1979.

Miller PA, Lawrence LM, Hank AM: The effect of exhaustive exercise on blood metabolites and muscle glycogen levels in horses, *Proc 9th Nutr and Physiol Symp*, East Lansing, Mich, 1985.

Miller-Graber PA and others: Dietary protein level and energy metabolism during treadmill exercise in horses, *J Nutr* 121:1462, 1991.

Pagan JD, Essen-Gustavson B, Lindholm A: The effect of energy source on exercise performance in standardbred horses. In Gillespie JR, Robinson NE, editors: *Equine exercise physiology II*, Davis, Calif, 1987, ICEEP Publications.

Sampson S: Does his bit fit? *Practical Horseman* 23(10):60, 1995.

Smith FH: Nutritional aspects associated with poor performance in the racehorse, *Ir Vet J* 40:87-89, 1986.

Wolf M, Ransberg K: *Enzyme therapy*, New York, 1972, Biological Research Institute.

Zinn RA: Influence of oral antibiotics on digestive function in Holstein steers fed a 71% concentrate diet, *J Anim Sci* 71(1):213, 1993.

Chapter 34

Incorporating Holistic Medicine into Equine Practice

JOYCE C. HARMAN

The most appropriate term for the alternative modalities is *complementary medicine. Complementary,* in this case, means that all forms of medicine are valid. It is up to the practitioner to pick the modality most appropriate for the case, one that is also the least invasive and kindest to the horse's body. Most of the so-called alternatives are noninvasive, cause minimal (if any) side effects, and promote the healing of the entire horse, not just a single part. Many conventional forms of medicine are invasive (surgery), have side effects (drugs), or are focused on healing only the dysfunctional part or system. In most cases, the entire animal is involved, and in the treatment of only the "sick" part, the rest of the horse is left to some extent compromised. For example, if musculoskeletal pain is only partially resolved, equine practitioners are accustomed to seeing compensatory lamenesses in other parts of the body; in contrast, if the immune system is only partially addressed, most practitioners do not recognize slow deterioration of the other systems as connected to the original disease.

When all types of medicine are embraced and the least invasive and most complete form of treatment selected, maximal healing can be achieved. Complementary medicine offers many options from which to choose. Practitioners need not practice all forms of medicine, but they should be able to recognize indications for treatment and make referrals for particular forms of therapy. Just as there are specialists in conventional medicine, some practitioners limit their practices to alternative medicine, although no board certification exists at the time of this writing. Many more practitioners incorporate alternative therapies into their practices as part of their normal treatment repertoires. Practitioners derive great personal satisfaction in helping animals respond without side effects and the anxiety associated with conventional treatments. Learning about these new modalities is challenging and rewarding in itself; general equine practice can become fairly routine.

Clients now demand alternative therapies much more frequently. Many equine practices are experiencing financial difficulties because the economy in some areas has led to a changing horse population. Some parts of the country are overflowing with equine practitioners; expanded facilities and specialized education may give an individual practitioner needed competitive advantages. Alternative forms of medicine may be offered to maintain optimal health and performance, as well as to allow practitioners to see good clients on a more regular basis.

Some clients are beginning to question the validity of vaccines. The controversies concerning vaccines are addressed in Chapter 40. Vaccinations are a primary strategy used in conventional preventive medicine, and many equine clients know they can buy vaccines less expensively from catalog companies. How many of us went to veterinary school to wander the countryside vaccinating horses? Most veterinarians, given the choice, would prefer the challenges of working up a complex case or performing a maintenance acupuncture treatment that really enhances the performance of a horse.

Much of an equine veterinarian's practice is centered on treating chronic problems, many of which are difficult to solve. In conventional medicine, chronic disease often requires progressively stronger and potentially toxic drug treatment. Holistic therapies are generally beneficial in treating chronic diseases. In fact, holistic therapies may slow the progress of a disease or even reverse it. The disease may not be reversed if it is long-standing and severe, in which case the horse can retire or function as a pleasure horse. Holistic medicine provides an excellent variety of treatments for chronic diseases in young and old horses.

As holistic modalities are incorporated into an existing practice, some clients may choose to find another practitioner. However, such losses are usually amply offset by the numbers of clients interested in holistic therapies. Clients who leave may come back in time, when they hear of the successes of holistic medicine.

Incorporating holistic modalities into the equine practice is not only rewarding but also an excellent practice builder. Holistic medicine adds another option in solving a variety of cases, especially chronic ones that may be refractory to conventional treatments.

Recognizing True Health and Chronic Disease From a Holistic Perspective

Health is defined as freedom from disease. In conventional medicine, "normal" chronic conditions are accepted as healthy, as long as the horse is considered free from devastating illness. In other words, many signs of chronic disease, when not life threatening, are accepted as normal health. True health, in holistic terms, is freedom from any sign of disease; it includes the ability to acquire common, self-limiting diseases and mount adequate immune responses such that the illness is short lived and requires little medication to help the subject recover. Healthy horses should have a strong reaction to an infectious disease, often running a high fever (up to 105° F) for a short period of time, followed by a quick recovery. The hair coat of healthy horses is deep and rich in color and does not bleach out in the sun.

According to these principles, many domesticated horses are not truly healthy. Many horses have low-grade problems that few conventional practitioners regard as signs of ill health; practitioners simply treat each symptom as it appears (Harman, Shaefer, Ward, 1994). A horse, by nature, is a prey animal, lives in areas with scrub-type vegetation, moves for 20 hours a day eating, and spends about 4 hours sleeping. We expect horses to adapt to our ways of living, eating, and exercise; for the most part, horses do this very well. However, some of the conditions encountered in equine medicine must be examined in the context of evolutionary equine behavior. Horses are willing to depend on people for emotional support and caring—this is part of the reason they have allowed themselves to be domesticated. As the basic signs of chronic disease are presented in this section, the reader is encouraged to consider new ways of looking at patterns of disease and experiment with management from a more holistic perspective.

The signs discussed below are an introduction to the signs of chronic disease. They are presented to stimulate thought about the current state of equine health and familiarize the practitioner with the conditions that might be treated with complementary medicine. The conditions presented can often be treated when the chronic disease is addressed with the appropriate therapy (homeopathy, acupuncture, chiropractic, herbal medicine, and others), nutrition, and management changes.

How to Recognize Signs of Chronic Disease

Chronic disease may manifest as excessive fear, which is consistent with the equine role as a flight animal (as in "fight or flight"). However, excessive fears of every new addition to the environment or change in treatment is abnormal. Horses with repetitive behaviors such as weaving, stall-walking, self-mutilation, and cribbing appear addicted to these behaviors and are probably not dealing with the stresses of confinement very well. Many horses' repetitive behaviors are corrected if the animal is turned out for at least 12 hours a day in a large field. However, if increased turnout times are not feasible, other ways of treating mental problems may need to be considered.

In general, horses who are either consistently underweight or overweight have a problem with chronic disease. Underweight horses may have trouble digesting or using food, or chronic stress may contribute to the problem. Chronically overweight horses, especially those with fat deposits and "cresty" necks with thickened, hard fat, have metabolic problems such as hypothyroidism and Cushing's syndrome, or may just be overfed, sometimes on grass that is too rich for a gastrointestinal system designed to eat scrub.

The respiratory system is the horse's main target system for the expression of allergies, although cutaneous manifestations are being seen much more frequently, particularly in warm climates. Horses are also showing allergic reactions by flipping their noses in a way that suggests intense pain. Both respiratory and dermatologic systems fall into the same family based on the five-element theory in Chinese medicine—metal. Treatment of the skin phase of allergies is difficult, but the respiratory phase of allergic disease seems more responsive. Chronic infections are common throughout the respiratory tract. Many horses who acquire a simple respiratory tract infection are treated with antibiotics. They may take months to recover to their previous level of performance, if they ever do. Permanent damage is not uncommon, especially in form of a chronic cough, yet an upper respiratory tract infection should be an acute, self-limiting disease. Many speed horses (race, event, steeplechase) bleed from the lungs, a sign of weakness in the respiratory tract. Foals are considered normal if they have upper respiratory mucous discharge for long periods, and some of those foals end up with long-term respiratory damage from what should be a self-limiting infection. Holistic treatments are often successful in treating respiratory illness refractory to conventional treatments.

Skin is the largest organ in the body, and the skin and hooves reflect internal health and nutritional state. Dry, dull, bleached hair coats are best treated from the inside out with a complete holistic approach. Allergies, especially pruritic eruptions, are signs of chronic immune-mediated problems (Dodds, 1993), and although skin allergies are difficult to manage with any form of medicine, the holistic approach is often successful. Seemingly simple conditions such as dermatophilis (e.g., "rain rot") are signs of subtle disease because all horses on a given property may be exposed to the causative agent and yet only a subset of the horses are susceptible to the infection. As horses are cured of chronic diseases, skin conditions such as warts, sarcoids, oily or sticky sweat, discharges from the sheath, poor wound healing, and excessive production of scar tissue tend to clear up.

Feet are an adaptation of the skin structures, and the old adage "no foot, no horse" is as true today as when it originated. Poor nutrition, chronic disease, and weather conditions play important roles in the health of the foot, as does the quality of the farrier's work. Quality varies greatly by area, and even when good work is available, the owners, for personal reasons, may not be willing to change from a poor farrier to a good one, even when their horses have severe problems. Cracked, brittle, or dry feet—as well as soft or crumbly feet—can be signs of chronic disease. Thrush, odor without obvious pathology, white-line disease, abscesses, and seedy toe should be addressed from a holistic standpoint and considered subtle signs of disease. Troublesome hoof conformation, particularly thick walls and soles or thin walls and soles, can sometimes be corrected with the holistic approach.

Laminitis is generally the result of chronic disease, unless the horse has eaten a large quantity of feed. Laminitis from overeating can be considered acute; however, many horses who have well-balanced diets and are otherwise healthy do not have the urge to overeat as severely as a horse who is not healthy. Chronic pain in the foot, resulting from a tendency to bruise easily or any form of arthritis, may be the result of shoeing or chronic disease.

Gastrointestinal disorders are an important disease entity; colic is the primary killer of horses. However, most places where colic is common have identifiable management problems, especially when horses' natural grazing and exercising habits are taken into account. Insufficient roughage is one of the main causes of colic; the horse's gut is designed for long-stem roughage and not concentrates (see Chapter 33). The stress of confinement contributes to colic, as does the overuse of antibiotics and dewormers. Horses with chronic digestive-tract problems may exhibit signs as diverse as dry or soft feces; ulcers; sensitivity to change in diet or weather; odoriferous stools; failure to digest food completely; cravings for dirt, salt, or wood; fussy eating; and various mouth problems. These conditions respond well to holistic healing.

The reproductive system is affected by nutrition, management, heredity, and chronic disease. Horses are selected for desirable performance, not for reproductive health as they are in the wild. Many problems, both physical and behavioral, are associated with mares' heat cycles. Many of these estrus-related problems are probably related to pain in the ovaries and uterus. Infertility of the male and female—including lack of libido, sterility, ovulation problems, and chronic uterine infections of all types—can often be corrected holistically.

Eye disorders can be a sign of internal imbalances. Horses often injure their eyes. Sometimes the trauma originates from itching or some form of pain; however, trauma is usually dismissed as an acute problem. The presence of nonresponsive ulcers, bilateral ulcers, and unresponsive infections suggests an internal problem with the defense systems, or in traditional Chinese medicine (TCM), with the Liver meridian, a common meridian for equine problems. Chronic drainage from the eye and periodic ophthalmia are also signs of chronic disease.

Because lame horses cannot perform their jobs well, the musculoskeletal system is the system practitioners are most often called to evaluate. Muscle stiffness and azoturia, as well as weak tendons and ligaments, may have a nutritional or chronic-disease origin. Arthritic changes in the joints, including navicular syndrome, can result from an ill-fitting saddle, improper shoeing, poor nutrition, or chronic disease. Splints appearing in young horses (especially those in light work) and bucked shins may result from poor training techniques, but frequently the bone is weak as a result of chronic disease and unbalanced nutrition. According to TCM, constant swelling or stocking up of the legs indicates poor digestion (Xie, 1994).

Holistic therapies can become valuable tools in the treatment of chronic disease. By observing horses consistently recovering from these syndromes and leading healthy lives without frequent recurrences, the practitioner learns the relationship of the problem to chronic disease. Until studies can confirm the details of holistic practitioners' findings, results (in the form of healthy horses) must speak for themselves.

History and Physical Examination as a Basis for All Therapies

Training in holistic diagnostics consistently leads to improved history-taking, palpation, and observation skills. The history and physical examination are the most important roles of diagnostic decision making and must be mastered completely for success. Other diagnostic tools, such as blood tests and radiographs, are helpful in diagnosis but must be put into perspective, with the history and physical examination findings taking priority in most cases. For example, a horse with liver disease may improve clinically from a homeopathic treatment, but the blood work may show high concentrations of liver enzymes for 3 to 6 months before resolution is demonstrated. The reason for this phenomenon is not clear; it may be related to improvements in the "energy systems" of the body first, with the physical body second.

Each modality emphasizes different signs, but all require a complete history; the process is like gathering all the clues to a puzzle. Many veterinarians take only a cursory history and will need to adjust to the time required for a lengthy history (see the section on practice management). Holistic medicine requires more detailed information than conventional medicine for the individualized treatment of the patient rather than the disease.

Practitioners can use routine physical, lameness, and prepurchase examinations to practice these new palpation and examination techniques. Generally clients appreciate the thoroughness of the examination even if the practitioner chooses not to explain the techniques or results. Any chronic illness or lameness offers the practitioner repeated opportunities to examine the same horse and observe the subtle changes that can occur. For example, changes in drinking habits, skin and coat texture, desire for company, and other subtle signs become important to the holistic practitioner. The practitioner should begin the examination by standing back and looking at the horse from both sides, front and back, and in motion (Box 34-1). Next is palpation, beginning with a light touch and moving deeper if needed. All the information must be recorded for future reference, on either a piece of plain paper or a complete invoice with diagrams (Fig. 34-1) for musculoskeletal, acupuncture, or chiropractic cases. Many experienced practitioners are willing to share their forms, and organizations that teach courses all have forms available to use as guides.

Many experienced acupuncturists and chiropractors do not go through the entire in-motion examination for an average poor-performance case because they are only going to perform acupuncture on the meridians they feel need to be treated or give a chiropractic adjustment where they observe a loss of normal motion in the spine. However, in the beginning the practitioner will learn much

---

BOX 34-1

General Physical Exam

OBSERVE
Stand back and observe entire animal at rest
   Stance, symmetry, respiration
   Dorsal view of shoulders, pelvis, spine
Walk and trot the horse in hand or on lunge line
Perform flexion tests
Check while ridden, if appropriate
Examine skin and coat
Assess weight
Examine eyes

LISTEN
Listen to heart, lungs, digestive tract
Take history

PALPATION
Use a light touch over the entire body
Palpate acupuncture points
Perform a chiropractic examination
   Static palpation
   Motion palpation
   Carrot stretch
   "Belly lifts"
Perform a muscle palpation

---

more by being thorough, and in reality, experienced practitioners should always watch horses in motion.

Western diagnostics have much to offer, including radiography, ultrasound, scintigraphy, and blood work. These tools should all be used as needed. However, this information should serve only as data in the complete history and physical examination findings. Every equine practitioner has seen lame horses with no radiographic changes and completely sound horses with radiographic changes so severe the horse should not be performing well.

Observation

The horse should be observed while standing at rest and wearing no equipment. The natural stance of the horse is noted because many horses develop a compensatory positioning of the legs at rest, when pain is present. Some horses stand stretched out (or "parked out") to rest their backs, whereas others stand with their legs underneath their bodies. The practitioner should determine whether the horse is splinting its abdomen, holding its neck in an uncomfortable position, or tilting its head. The shoeing should also be observed because unbalanced feet lead to alterations in stance, foot pain, and upper-body pain. The practitioner should determine whether the horse always rests one foot or places one foot in a certain position. Many horses are not able to stand square because of discomfort.

The horse should be examined for symmetry from all angles. Many horses' shoulders are uneven. The practitioner stands the horse squarely on level ground and examines the points of the shoulders, knees, and slope of the pasterns, as well as the shape of the feet. The practitioner stands directly behind the horse, noting asymmetries in the pelvic structure, muscle mass over the hindquarters and in the gaskins, and the shape of the feet. The practitioner places a stool behind the horse and stands above the horse's back, looking down. The horse must be standing square, although discomfort may prevent a square stance in front and behind at the same time. If the horse cannot stand square, the front and the rear should be examined separately. The shoulders are often positioned asymmetrically (see Chapter 33). The horse may stand crooked and be unable to straighten its neck or have a spinal deviation that will not correct itself even when the horse is repositioned.

The horse can be observed while walking and jogging in hand, while being lunged, with a rider mounted, and in traditional flexion tests. Many horses move freely on the lunge line but change their movement in some way (usually adversely) while carrying a rider. Significant changes in movement with the rider's weight indicate back pain, which may originate in a poorly fitting saddle, musculoskeletal trauma, poor riding technique, or training aids that position horses into artificial "frames" or head positions.

A horse with a serious internal medical condition will not be ridden but should be evaluated for willingness and

HARMANY EQUINE CLINIC, Ltd
Joyce C. Harman, DVM MRCVS
PO Box 8, Washington, VA 22747
540-675-1855

Name_____
Address_____
_____

Phone (h)_____ (w)_____

Barn_____Date_____ Veterinarian_____Farrier_____

Horse_____Age____Sex____Breed_____Color_____Use_____
History_____
_____
_____
_____
_____

Current Tx_____Teeth_____Blankets_____

Acupuncture Treatment

Meridians
BL13 Lung ___
BL14 Pericard ___
BL15 Heart ___
BL16 Gov. Ves. ___
BL17 Con. Ves. ___
BL18 Liver ___
BL19 Gall Bl. ___
BL20 Spleen ___
BL21 Stomach ___
BL22 Tri. Heat. ___
BL23 Kidney ___
BL24 Sea o'Energy ___
BL25 L. Intes. ___
BL26 Local ___
BL27 S. Intes. ___
BL28 Bladder ___

Body Points
Head_____
Neck_____
Ft. legs_____
Chest_____
Abd._____
Back_____
H. legs_____
_____
_____

Foot Points
PC ___ KI ___
HT ___ BL ___
SI ___ GB ___
TH ___ ST ___
LI ___ SP ___
LU ___ LV ___

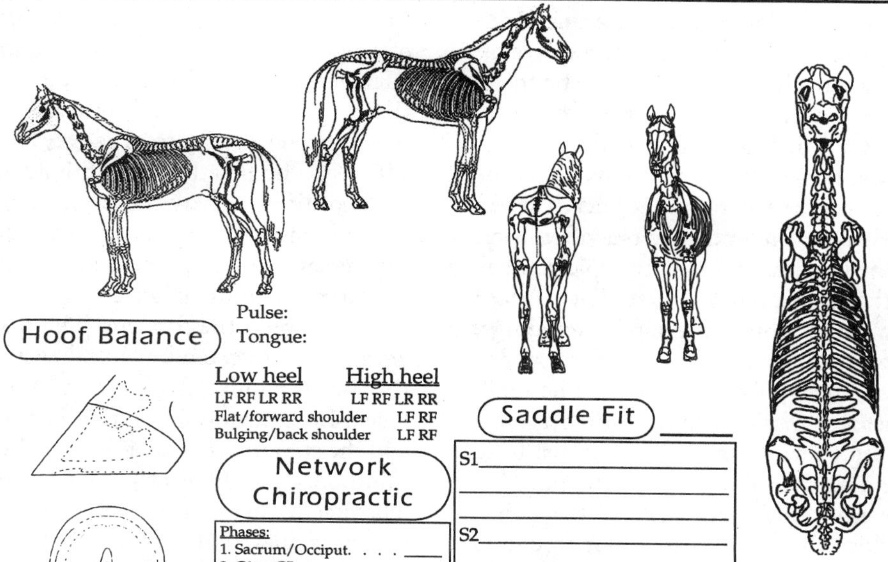

Musculoskeletal Exam
areas of pain, muscle spasms, injuries, scars, muscle atrophy, asymmetry of hips, shoulders, conformation

Hoof Balance

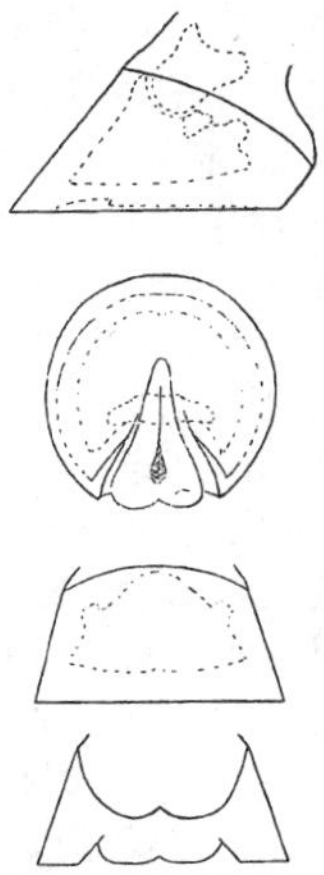

Pulse:
Tongue:

Low heel	High heel
LF RF LR RR	LF RF LR RR
Flat/forward shoulder	LF RF
Bulging/back shoulder	LF RF

Saddle Fit _____

Network Chiropractic
Phases:
1. Sacrum/Occiput. . . . ___
2. C1 or C5 . . . . . . ___
3. Sacrum/Ilium . . . . ___
4. C2 or C3. . . . . . . ___
5. Coxxyx/C5. . . . . . ___
Sacrum/Axis. . . . . ___

S1_____
S2_____
_____
_____
Instr._____

Instructions

___**Carrot stretches**
(eat carrot at hip, stifle and lower; between ft. legs)
___**Belly lifts**
(gently tickle midline starting at elbows)
___**Non-stretch leg stretches**
(use gentle releases - hold leg in a comfortable position like picking feet, and wait for releases to happen)
___**Leg circles**
(hold leg in flexed position, draw circles with hoof or leg, 4 - 5 times in each direction)
___**Hair analysis** (no chg-results-call in 2 wks)

Herbs _____
Bach flowers _____
Homeopathics _____

Nutritional supplements _____

Movement Evaluation

Walk:
Trot: Foot
                        Path
Back movement:
Hips:
Shoulders:
Toe dragging:
Head carriage:
Engagement:
Symmetry:

Chiropractic Treatment

Jaw_____
Occ_____
C1 _____
C2 _____
C3 _____
C4 _____
C5 _____
C6 _____
C7 _____
Sternum

Ft.L _____

T1 _____
T2 _____
T3 _____
T4 _____
T5 _____
T6 _____
T7 _____
T8 _____
T9 _____
T10 _____
T11 _____
T12 _____
T13 _____
T14 _____
T15 _____
T16 _____
T17 _____
T18 _____
L1 _____
L2 _____
L3 _____
L4 _____
L5 _____
L6 _____
LS _____
Sacral _____
Ba _____
Ap _____
Pelvis _____
SI _____
Il _____
Hd.L _____
Logan

Stance

CHARGES:
Stable visit _____
Initial treatment _____
Follow-up/wellness _____
Nutritional suppl. _____
Homeop./herbs _____
Consult._____ _____
TOTAL _____
TOTAL (other pgs) _____
Prev. balance _____
Paid _____
TOTAL DUE _____

Fig. 34-1 Complete examination form and invoice.

ability to move. Some horses demonstrate pain on the first movement, then move more freely; some seem to feel better with movement; and some appear to feel worse with movement. These differences may become important in the prescription of certain complementary therapies.

The skin and hair coat should be observed. A healthy horse has soft, supple skin with a deep, rich color and a good shine. Any discoloration, bleeding, dryness, brittleness, or excessive greasiness is a sign of chronic disease. If skin lesions are present, the practitioner must look carefully at their current appearance and ask about their original appearance, before ointments or steroids were used. The horse's weight should be assessed and the owner questioned about the diet used to maintain that weight.

The horse's eyes should be examined for expression and the presence of discharge. Discharges are important in determining whether chronic disease is present. Expression of the eyes can be revealing when planning a holistic treatment. Many horses are fearful or worried, and others are devoid of significant emotional response. Sometimes the owners are aware of the horse's emotional state, but competitive owners often neglect their animal's needs when they conflict with their own. Endurance horses often "shut down" to cope with the overtraining and multiple competitions common in that sport. These horses have vacant expressions and show little interest in their surroundings. Racehorses are under an enormous amount of stress. Because they receive little turnout time, they become tense and often exhibit repetitive-motion behaviors such as cribbing and weaving. High-level show horses receive little turnout time and are often handled by staff who have little concern with the emotional well-being of the horse. These horses often lose their emotional attachment to people and their ability to experience pleasure. By looking at a horse's expression, the practitioner can determine whether the horse is coping well with its environment or whether some form of stress reduction is needed.

Listening

For a nutritional consultation or an internal medicine case, the practitioner should listen to the heart, lungs, and digestive tract. Listening is also important in poor-performance cases, although most of these horses function normally unless true exercise intolerance is present.

Besides listening carefully to the history, the practitioner should phrase questions in an open-ended manner so the owner really answers the question and does not simply agree with the practitioner. Owners often unknowingly reveal important information in a chance remark.

Palpation

The first palpation is a gentle passing of the practitioner's hand over the entire neck, back, thorax, and legs in a search for muscle tension, sensitivity, flinching, discomfort, and changes in temperature. A light touch often reveals more than a heavy one, and practice is required to develop it.

The next stage is the acupuncture diagnosis, which involves palpation of the acupuncture meridians for pain or tension (see Chapters 9, 10, and 11). As the practitioner gains experience palpating for acupuncture points, subtle changes can be found. Sensitivity at specific acupuncture points can be used diagnostically, not only for meridian imbalances or back or neck pain but also for distal limb lameness (Schoen, 1994). Changes in skin temperature, such as cold extremities or hot ears, should be noted. Tongue and pulse diagnosis should also be conducted (Schoen, 1994).

The next stage involves chiropractic examination (see Chapter 12). All joints in the body, including those of the spine, should move smoothly through their entire ranges of motion. Many horses have lost normal motion throughout their spine, resulting in stiffness and pain. To examine the range of motion, the practitioner gently moves the spine through its normal range, looking and feeling for stiffness. The practitioner can hold a carrot by the horse's hip and stifle and between the front legs to check neck and back mobility (the "carrot stretch") and then raise the back by pressing on the ventral midline to contract the rectus abdominis. A normal horse can reach its hip and stifle and down between the forelegs. The back should rise easily, with the horse extending and lowering its neck. If raising the back is painful, the horse will not do so with a rider in place. Loss of normal motion at the junction of the ribs and the sternum or loss of motion through the withers and midthorax usually produces pain when the back is raised. The practitioner then applies a specific motion palpation of the individual joints of the spine and extremities, looking for restrictions. Healthy joints move freely and exhibit spring, whereas problem joints often feel stiff.

Muscle palpation is also important, starting with a light touch and moving deeper to assess muscle quality. Healthy muscle feels soft and springy, and the horse will not object to the palpation. Muscle under tension feels tight and hard, with little spring. Muscle spasms and fasciculation may be seen locally and at a distance from the palpation site. Muscle in spasm is more likely to become injured and will take longer to warm up because blood flow through the spasm is diminished (Beck, 1994; Meagher, 1980). Sometimes a horse will "splint" the back, or hold it rigidly in place, while being examined to avoid moving it. This action reflects pain, which practitioners sometimes miss because the horse has not moved away from the palpation.

Specific History and Physical Examination Questions for the Various Modalities

Acupuncture

The acupuncturist needs information on the vitality, texture of the skin, secretions and excretions, body type and appearance, and odor (Box 34-2). The acupuncturist inquires whether the symptoms change with weather con-

BOX 34-2

Acupuncture-Specific Questions and Examinations

Body type and constitution
Spirit or vitality
    Positive outlook, happy, soft "liquid" look to eye
    Personality that suits body type and constitution
Effects of weather
Environment
Hair coat color and texture
    Deep, rich hair coat color; soft skin texture
Discharges
    Color, odor
Manure and urine
    Color, odor, texture
Tongue and gums
    Color, moisture, coating, size, shape
Pulse
    Depth, strength, rate, quality

BOX 34-3

Chiropractic-Specific Questions and Examination

Behavior changes
Movement changes
Accidents ("never been the same since")
Musculoskeletal problems
Mysterious lameness
Stiffness, resistance to work

ditions or environment. Some practitioners use Five-Element diagnosis; others use the Eight Principles or a combination of the two. For more information on Chinese diagnosis, the reader is referred to Chapter 9 and other texts (Schoen, 1994; Xie, 1994; Youbang and others, 1987).

Good vitality is present when the horse is in good spirits; has a happy, positive attitude; and has a soft "liquid" look to its eye. A horse who is dull or inattentive to its environment or who has a worried, unhappy look to the eye may be in pain or have a deep illness that is difficult to treat. Sometimes people believe they own a dull, quiet animal only to find after acupuncture or other holistic therapy that the horse is much more lively.

The whole body is examined to yield a picture of internal health. Body type or appearance indicates the constitution and personality of the horse. A fine-boned thoroughbred tends to have a hotter personality, a higher metabolic rate, and often a weaker constitution than a heavier-boned draft horse or quarter horse.

The color of discharge is also carefully observed. A thick, yellow discharge is a sign of a "Heat condition," according to TCM principles, whereas a thin, clear discharge indicates a "Cold syndrome" (Xie, 1994). In TCM, the odors of discharges, manure, and urine suggest internal health and the type of condition present. Foul-smelling manure may indicate a Damp-Heat condition, whereas the sour smell of stomach reflux indicates poor digestion and food retention.

Tongue and pulse diagnosis are frequently used in TCM as important parts of the diagnostic technique. Both methods require practice but can be extremely useful

in equine medicine. When the tongue is examined, gum color and moisture are recorded, as are tongue size, shape, and color. The tongue can be a useful visual indicator to explain the significance of the problem being treated and to allow client monitoring of the horse's progress. Tongue color in horses can be more difficult to observe than in other species because most horses have a very thin tongue coating unless their acupuncture meridians are significantly imbalanced. Also, horses do not like to have their tongues examined. A thin, moist, whitish coat is normal, whereas a thick yellow coat indicates a heat condition (Xie, 1994).

The pulse is traditionally felt over the horse's carotid artery, just cranial to the shoulder under the jugular vein (Xie, 1994). For acupuncture diagnosis, each individual meridian is represented by a different feel to the pulse under the practitioner's fingers. Changes in the pulse may be appreciated during the course of the acupuncture treatment, and the point locations changed according to the changes felt in the pulse. The pulse for herbal diagnosis is felt as a single pulse in the same location or possibly on the facial, femoral, or radial artery, although these locations are not traditionally used in China. The quality and character of the pulse are determined, and along with the tongue findings the practitioner can identify the TCM syndrome present and determine an herbal formula (Xie, 1994). The tongue and pulse may be rechecked to determine the effectiveness of the treatment.

Chiropractic

The details of the chiropractic examination are covered in Chapter 12 and in the previous section's description of a complete physical examination. Most of the problems treated by chiropractic are musculoskeletal in origin, so history-taking centers on the musculoskeletal system (Box 34-3) and behavior because many so-called behavior problems are actually caused by pain (see Chapter 33). Changes in behavior and movement when the horse is mounted frequently indicate chiropractic problems, as do signs of stiffness and subtle lameness. A common scenario is that a horse has never been the same after a specific event, such as a fall, a night in an unfamiliar stall, or simply a visit to the pasture one day. Although no accident was observed, trauma cannot be ruled out.

Many practitioners believe the spine is not worth checking unless a musculoskeletal problem is being examined; however, every cell in the body has a nerve supply originating in the central nervous system (Gray, 1974). The nerve supply is therefore important to the health of all organ systems, and a chiropractic examination is advised for every patient.

Homeopathy

The medical history required for homeopathic treatment is extensive and includes conditions encountered since birth (Box 34-4). Unfortunately, most people have owned their horses for only 2 to 6 years, and few purchase their horses before they are 3 or 4 years old; therefore valuable information for a homeopathic prescription is lost. Learning to prescribe homeopathic remedies accurately de-

---

BOX 34-4

HOMEOPATHIC-SPECIFIC QUESTIONS AND EXAMINATIONS

Complete history
Coat, color, texture, whether color bleaches out easily
    Length of hair, ease of shedding
Problems noticed since birth (if available)
Specific description of lesions
    Original and current appearance
Discharges
    Original and current appearance
Amount and type of pain
Frequency of problem
Modalities
    Conditions that worsen or improve the problem
    Cold, hot, pressure, touch, motion, weather, time
        of day
    Sun or shade
Personality and any changes since illness began
Body type, hoof structure
Drinking habits
Appetite, sensitivity to changes in diet
Digestive tract upsets, colic
Skin temperature
Sensitivity or lack of sensitivity to palpation
Sensitivity to insects, flies
Skin problems, past or present
Previous or current drug therapy
Vaccination history
This is just a sampling of the questions to ask. More details on any area that applies to the case will be extremely helpful.

---

pends largely on learning to take a good history. Chapter 27 contains detailed information on equine homeopathy.

Basic first-aid homeopathy is fairly straightforward. Required information includes appearance, amount of pain, colors of discharges, odors, and modalities (or the conditions that influence the animal or affected body part for better or worse—cold, hot, pressure, touch, motion, weather) (Day, 1984). Clients easily learn to check for temperature preference by putting hot or cold packs on the affected part or hosing the horse with hot or cold water.

Treating chronic disease with homeopathy, often called *constitutional treatment*, requires a complete history. With a complex case, this process may take up to an hour (see Practice Management), although often only a limited history is available. Many horse owners see their horses only once a day; consequently, they do not know the time of day horses are worse or better or have a complete picture of the problem. All body systems must be covered completely. The pathologic condition must be described in great detail, especially the modalities, or the patient's response to hot, cold, touch, motion, and weather.

Small details are important, such as whether the horse prefers to be in the sun or the shade and whether these characteristics have changed since the illness began. Relevant questions include the following: Was an aloof horse previously affectionate or vice-versa? Does the horse who previously liked to go to shows now stand in the back of the stall when the trailer pulls up? Does the horse have diarrhea with each change of food, frequent low-grade colics, frequent respiratory tract infections, or an allergic cough? A change in drinking habits (e.g., from regular drinking to little interest in water) can be an important guide to finding a remedy. However, when discussing laminitis, for example, owners do not generally volunteer information such as whether their horse has a long coat, has had frequent bouts with colic, or is more attractive to flies than his pasture mates.

In the physical examination, seemingly minor details are of major importance. The practitioner may ask the following questions: What is the horse's condition? How long has it been excessively fat or too thin? How long has its coat been dull and dry or bleached out? What is the skin temperature of the extremities (warm or cold), and is it normal for this horse? How alert to its surroundings is the horse, and how does it respond to palpation of the affected area? Detailed progress notes are essential because, as treatment progresses, changes in all the symptoms are important in evaluating the response to the remedies.

Herbs

Treatment with Chinese herbs requires a different approach than treatment with American and European herbs. A complete history and physical examination are important, and modalities such as those used in homeopathy are useful but not critical to herbal treatments. Because herbs are usually quite safe and tend to act slowly, the practitioner usually has sufficient time to evaluate the horse as it heals.

Chinese herbal treatments require a history and physical examination similar to those described for acupuncture. Tongue and pulse diagnosis are important in the choice of Chinese herbs. However, some general formulas can be used safely for specific conditions in a wide range of animals. Chinese herbs work according to principles similar to those of acupuncture and are complementary to acupuncture.

American and European herbalists tend to work with the more familiar Western diagnoses, symptoms, or conditions, so the history and physical examination require less detail than the previously described systems; still, much more extensive historical and physical data are collected than is commonly done in conventional practice.

Incorporating Specific Modalities

Incorporating Acupuncture into Your Practice

Since 1975 the International Veterinary Acupuncture Society (IVAS) has trained and certified veterinarians in all parts of the world in acupuncture. Any veterinarian interested in incorporating acupuncture into their practice should enroll in the IVAS course. For veterinarians interested in an overview of acupuncture principles, introductory weekend courses are held around the country; these weekends may help the practitioner decide whether to take the complete course. As in any other area of expertise, education is the key to good, consistent results. State boards may begin requiring extra education for veterinarians practicing acupuncture, although at the time of this writing no specific laws require continuing education.

Certification in acupuncture also promotes credibility among both clients and colleagues. Because acupuncture is considered new (even though it is 3000 years old), credibility and quality are particularly important. Practitioners will find that they get more satisfaction and more consistent results with a solid educational foundation.

The beginning acupuncturist should choose cases that seem straightforward and clients who seem receptive. Cases that generally respond well include (but are not limited to) mild nondescript lameness, many cases of known back pain, performance problems (see Chapter 33), laminitis, eye problems, arthritic conditions such as bone spavin, allergic coughs, chronic obstructive pulmonary disease (COPD), and tying up, either acute or chronic.

When acute cases such as laminitis or colic are treated, acupuncture can be added to the normal treatment regimen; often the horse responds more quickly than expected. In the treatment of chronic cases, acupuncture should be performed with no other changes in the medication regimen until several treatments have been accomplished. As the horse's condition improves, a decrease in medications

may be possible, and if the horse is doing well, the client may stop medication before the next examination.

The newly certified acupuncturist is advised to tell the client who presents a chronic or complicated case to wait until the practitioner gains experience. If the client insists on trying acupuncture anyway, the practitioner should explain that it may take four to eight treatments to help the horse. The client should then understand that acupuncture may not work on the first treatment; it is better to err on the conservative side than create unrealistic hopes.

All equine practitioners should learn saddle fitting and all equine acupuncturists should make it a major part of their practice. Because the saddle sits on one third to one half of the Bladder meridian Association points, the saddle has a major influence on the success of acupuncture (see Chapter 33). If a saddle puts pressure on one of the acupuncture association points, it will continually irritate that point and cause the same blockage every time the saddle is put on the back. Lack of proper saddle fit and placement may account for complaints about the short duration of results obtained by acupuncture. Saddle fitting is exactly like shoe fitting; no athlete would dare go into competition with ill-fitting shoes.

Legal aspects

Because acupuncture is considered a relatively recent technique in conventional equine medicine, practitioners must be especially careful to apply it in a professional manner. A few precautions are necessary for the best interests of the horse and for legal reasons. In several states, treatment of a racehorse within 48 hours of racing is illegal, so local tracks should be consulted before a treatment is administered; the owners may not know the law or may not care to be accurate. Moreover, horses may become relaxed and not run true to form after a treatment; a trainer may take advantage of this to manipulate handicappers.

In some sports, such as endurance racing, officials are considering the prohibition of acupuncture just before or during a competition for two reasons: First, it may give an individual an unfair advantage; second, certain diagnostic signs may be masked by the release of endorphins that occurs with acupuncture, thereby allowing a horse to pass a veterinary check and collapse or even die on the trail. The Fédération Equestrie International (FEI) international competition in endurance does not permit acupuncture; other sports may or may not follow this example. The veterinarian is advised to consult the appropriate authorities. At the time of this writing, state boards are generally undecided about holistic therapies. The state boards tend to adopt the American Veterinary Medical Association (AVMA) guidelines, and American Association of Equine Practitioners (AAEP) guidelines, which read as follows:

> Veterinary acupuncture and acutherapy involve the examination and stimulation of specific points on the body of nonhuman animals by use of acupuncture needles, moxibustion, injections, low-level lasers,

magnets, and a variety of other techniques for the diagnosis and treatment of numerous conditions in animals. Veterinary acupuncture and acutherapy are now considered an integral part of veterinary medicine. These techniques should be regarded as surgical and/or medical procedures under state veterinary practice acts. It is recommended the educational programs be undertaken by veterinarians before they are considered competent to practice veterinary acupuncture (*J Am Vet Med Assoc,* 1996).

Many states are not enforcing this policy, but as the rules continue to change, the practicing veterinarian must assume responsibility in monitoring these changes.

Incorporating Chiropractic into the Equine Practice

Chiropractic, more than any other holistic modality, has acquired a bad name in the horse world because of the numbers of untrained people, lay and professional, who are adjusting horses with the use of violent techniques. Research has shown that very little force, directed in the wrong way, can damage a joint (Leach, 1994; Sandoz, 1976) and adjustments must be performed carefully to restore normal motion between the joints and avoid injury. Most untrained people, even veterinarians and chiropractors, believe they must use 10 times as much force to adjust a horse's bones as a human's. This is not the case (see Chapter 12), and long-term joint damage may result. Short-term improvements are often seen, but the long-term damage to the joints begins with the first incorrectly applied adjustment.

Veterinarians should complete a comprehensive chiropractic course offered by the American Veterinary Chiropractic Association (AVCA). Formal training is necessary, not only to learn the physiology of adjusting and correct techniques but to gain credibility among colleagues and clients. Chiropractors spend 4 years in chiropractic college learning the correct adjusting techniques, so it is unlikely a practitioner will learn correct technique in a day or a weekend.

Clients may be skeptical of chiropractic therapy because they have heard horror stories of horses being handled roughly by untrained individuals. Educating clients about correct technique alleviates fears and promotes trust.

As practitioners begin to learn chiropractic skills, they should incorporate motion palpation and a chiropractic examination into each routine examination, even if the case is judged inappropriate for chiropractic treatment. Lameness and prepurchase examinations are excellent opportunities to begin examining supposedly normal horses. If acupuncture has been learned first, all acupuncture cases should be motion palpated even before the practitioner feels ready to begin adjusting. Practitioners will be interested to note that most horses who have been in work have sustained some loss of motion between some joints. Many unbroken horses have significant loss of motion be-

tween their joints as a result of pasture accidents, becoming cast, or being halter-broken.

In selecting cases for treatment, veterinarians should focus on horses with problems that are likely to respond well; this builds both practitioner and client confidence. Horses with performance problems (see Chapter 33) and horses who seemed fine until an accident occurred but have not been the same since are excellent choices for the beginning practitioner. Other horses appropriate for chiropractic treatment are those with painful backs or "cold backs" or who present difficulty during shoeing. All mares and foals should be checked; foals are prone to falling, with consequent spinal trauma. Foals that are adjusted regularly grow up moving more freely and appear easier to train than foals that have not been adjusted.

The new practitioner should initially look for simple cases in which loss of motion in certain joints is easily appreciated and the owners are open to trying chiropractic. Horses with back problems and subtle or difficult-to-diagnose lameness are good candidates. While palpating the horse, the practitioner can tell the clients about the findings of the examination. Clients may be aware of stiffness in an area that appears abnormal during the examination. Often, clients ask about ways to reduce or correct the stiffness, thereby becoming interested in chiropractic.

The combination of chiropractic with acupuncture and saddle fitting produces the most complete and long-lasting results. Acupuncture quickly releases muscle spasms and pain, as does chiropractic if it is repeated several times in a row. The two therapies complement each other well. Improper saddle fit and placement cause many clients to assume mistakenly that the effects of chiropractic are short-lived. Saddle fitting is essential for maximal performance.

Chiropractic is an excellent way to build a veterinary practice because it includes preventive care after the initial problem is solved. One chiropractic study with human athletes demonstrated that performance increased with regular chiropractic adjustments, when results of a standardized exercise test were compared with a control group in which no adjustments were done (Lauro, Mouch, 1991). The implication for the equine athlete is that performance can increase with regular chiropractic care.

Legal aspects

Chiropractic is considered unconventional in veterinary medicine, and although it is gaining acceptance slowly, many veterinarians still consider it invalid. Chiropractic treatment must be performed in the most professional manner possible. Although no lawsuits resulting from poor-quality chiropractic care are known of this writing, the possibility certainly exists. If chiropractic is conducted by an educated, certified chiropractor, the chances of a lawsuit are minimal because chiropractic is statistically safe (Dvorak and others, 1992; Dvorak, Orelli, 1985).

State boards are currently undecided with regard to chiropractic. Chiropractic boards may not want veterinarians to use the word *chiropractic* to describe their work; however, some states are allowing veterinarians certified through the AVCA to use the term. State veterinary boards are mixed in their acceptance and regulation of nonveterinarian chiropractors, although a few states consider the AVCA course acceptable. An ideal situation would involve referral from the veterinarian to an AVCA-trained chiropractor, with a treatment form to be sent back to the veterinarian. All veterinarians should know state regulations because many veterinarians make referrals to chiropractors. If these chiropractors are practicing illegally, the veterinarian's own license may be jeopardized (see Chapter 42).

The AVMA guidelines state the following:

> Veterinary chiropractic is the examination, diagnosis, and treatment of nonhuman animals through manipulation and adjustments of specific joints and cranial structures. The term *veterinary chiropractic* should not be interpreted to include dispensing medication, performing surgery, injecting medications, recommending supplements, or replacing traditional veterinary care. While sufficient research exists documenting efficacy of chiropractic in humans, research in veterinary chiropractic is limited. Sufficient clinical and anecdotal evidence exists to indicate that veterinary chiropractic can be beneficial. It is recommended that further research be conducted in veterinary chiropractic to evaluate efficacy, indications, and limitations. The assurance of education in veterinary chiropractic is central to the ability of the veterinarians to provide this service. Veterinary chiropractic should be performed by licensed veterinarians; however, at this time, some areas of the country do not have an adequate supply of veterinarians educated in veterinary chiropractic. Therefore it is recommended that, where the state's practice acts permit, licensed chiropractors educated in veterinary chiropractic be allowed to practice this modality under the supervision of, or referral by, a licensed veterinarian who is providing concurrent care (*J Am Vet Med Assoc*, 1997).

Incorporating Homeopathy into Your Practice

Homeopathy is the least understood of the holistic modalities, especially by conventionally trained medical community. Homeopathy is also the most difficult to learn. Homeopathy is fairly straightforward in the treatment of simple cases, but the treatment of complex cases requires much study and practice. The Academy of Veterinary Homeopathy (AVH) was recently formed to teach veterinarians classical homeopathy. Although primarily targeted toward small animal practitioners at the time of this writing, the AVH course is an excellent place to learn the principles of homeopathy. Introductory weekend courses are held around the country for interested veterinarians. These weekends provide a foundation for further study, but the treatment of chronic cases cannot be learned in a weekend. Educa-

tion is the key to good results and credibility among clients and fellow colleagues, and it is the only way to approach a chronic case.

After learning homeopathy, veterinarians should find a mentor to consult for complex cases. Many clients already believe that homeopathy can treat chronic problems after conventional medicine has failed, but those are not the cases for new practitioners to attempt to manage. Many complex cases are still difficult to solve even with homeopathy, and the beginning practitioner may be easily frustrated. A mentor can alleviate this frustration. The most difficult part of learning homeopathy is learning to wait long enough between remedies for the first remedy to have finished working. In a chronic case, waiting 1 to 2 months or longer is not uncommon. If remedies are repeated too often, the case may become confused and difficult to interpret. The major mistakes most practitioners make are repeating a remedy too often and frequently changing remedies without correctly evaluating the responses.

For the practitioner just learning homeopathy, acute cases such as trauma, wounds, beestings, overeating colic, pregnancy, and acute infections should be selected. These cases usually have few remedies from which to select, and the differentiation is relatively easy. Acute cases often respond noticeably in a few hours or days. The practitioner is familiar with the natural course of a typical acute condition and can often see that the use of homeopathy speeds resolution time. This quick progress makes the practitioner and client more confident.

Many homeopaths state that homeopathy should not be used with drugs, but clinical experience from most homeopathic practitioners indicates that the remedies may still retain efficacy and are a useful adjunct in decreasing the number and duration of conventional treatments. The homeopathic remedies should be given at least half an hour before or after a drug is administered. Certain drugs affect the action of remedies, particularly steroids and vaccines. Homeopathy can work even with these drugs, although much less clearly. If a case is not responding properly, however, it may be necessary to stop drug treatment before a homeopathic cure occurs. A beginning practitioner may administer a remedy for a condition such as a bruise, along with some phenylbutazone. Generally the swelling and pain heal significantly faster than would similar injury treated with drugs alone.

Strong-smelling herbs may also interfere with the action of homeopathic remedies. Herbs such as peppermint, the strong oils used in liniments, and some fly sprays (e.g., citronella, camphor) should be avoided when homeopathic treatment is being used. In most cases, these strong herbs do not cause problems, but their use should be noted, especially in cases when the remedies are not working. Mild compounds such as poultices without liniments, leg sweats, and alcohol rubs can still be used. Magnetic blankets, Bio-Scan units, high-tension power lines, and magnetic boots may interfere with the action of homeopathic remedies. The remedies should be stored in a dark place (except the refrigerator) and kept away from microwave or electromagnetic radiation whenever possible. However, remedies are often stored in less-than-ideal settings, and they still work, in most cases.

Legal aspects

As of this writing, state boards have not adequately addressed homeopathy. Many poorly trained lay people are practicing homeopathy, which may lead to the impression that homeopathy does not work and that advanced training is unnecessary. The AVMA guidelines state the following:

> Veterinary homeopathy is a medical discipline in which conditions in nonhuman animals are treated by the administration of substances that are capable of producing clinical signs in healthy animals similar to those of the animal to be treated. These substances are used therapeutically in minute doses. Research in veterinary homeopathy is limited. Clinical and anecdotal evidence exists to indicate that veterinary homeopathy may be beneficial. It is recommended that further research be conducted in veterinary homeopathy to evaluate efficacy, indications, and limitations. Since some of these substances may be toxic when used at inappropriate doses, it is imperative that veterinary homeopathy be practiced only by licensed veterinarians who have been educated in veterinary homeopathy (*J Am Vet Med Assoc*, 1996).

The veterinarian should keep track of local policies and should consider using release forms as discussed earlier. A malpractice claim concerning the use of homeopathy could be a difficult one to win because expert witnesses would probably consider it ineffective and might call the practitioner negligent for refusing to use conventional treatment. However, because homeopathy involves such extensive case-taking and contact with the clients, a lawsuit is probably much less likely because most lawsuits arise from poor client communication (see Chapter 42).

For the best interests of the horse a few precautions should be taken when homeopathy is used. In general, homeopathic remedies do not produce positive drug tests at any level of competition because of their dilute nature, so competitors like to use them. However, during an endurance ride or 3-day event, homeopathic remedies may mask signs the control veterinarian uses to determine whether a horse is fit to continue. Serious harm to the horse, with such sequelae as a bowed tendon, may result if masking of pain causes early warning signs to be missed.

Because homeopathic remedies do not result in positive drug tests, competitors often use certain remedies to calm excited horses. Tense, anxious horses may be reacting to back and saddle pain, whereas others are reacting to insufficient turnout and improper exercise. Whatever the reason, a natural calming agent is often preferable to the common practice of lunging a horse for 1 to 2 hours. The American Horse Show Association (AHSA) considers any agent that alters a horse's mental state to be illegal and strives to prevent the use of any calming compounds. However, show competitors tend to find new illegal drugs if they are not using natural agents. Certainly, the use of natural remedies is preferable to using an untested drug of unknown origin.

Some practitioners believe that homeopathy is well-suited to telephone consultation, and many homeopathic veterinarians perform this service. Quite a few legal ramifications surround this practice, although only a few practitioners have had problems. Veterinarians are required to maintain a physician-client relationship with all patients, and this does not occur over the telephone. If a local veterinarian is the referring veterinarian, a telephone consultation may be legal, but frequently the client has no local veterinarian who supports the use of holistic medicine. Telephone consultations often involve the crossing of state lines, which presents another potential legal problem (see Chapter 42). The demand from clients, however, is clear, and only a few equine homeopaths exist to meet this demand. The telephone consultations will continue but whenever possible the practitioner should establish a relationship with the local veterinarian. As more practitioners become interested in homeopathy, referrals to local homeopaths will be less difficult.

Incorporating Herbs into the Equine Practice

Herbal therapy is relatively easy to incorporate into a practice because herbs are generally safe and readily available. Horses seem to be responsive to herbs, requiring only about 2 to 4 times the human dose. Most health food stores have herbal products, and several products are prepared especially for horses. Some literature is available at the time of this writing (de Bairacli-Levy, 1976; Heinermann, 1977; Morgan, 1993; Self, 1996; Xie, 1994); however, few training courses in veterinary herbal therapy are available. Some excellent courses in human herbal medicine are offered throughout the United States, but IVAS offers the only veterinary course, an advanced Chinese herb course for certified members. Weekend courses are held as an introduction to the use of herbs but are not complete courses.

Every culture has an herbal history, and those herbs can generally be applied to horses. Some herbs that are safe for human use may not be safe for horses or are suitable only in certain preparations. The veterinarian should learn as much as possible about the cultural medical system before prescribing.

Because Chinese herbology is based on the principles of Chinese medicine, the practitioner is advised to study Chinese medicine to learn about herbs. However, herbal formulas are available to treat specific conditions based on symptoms; these may be used easily (Fratkin, 1986; Xie, 1994). Chinese herbs work well when combined with conventional drugs and therefore allow practitioners to use holistic medicine while still practicing orthodox medicine. (Chapter 22 provides a more complete discussion of Chinese herbs and herbal formulas most commonly used in horses.)

American and European herbal formulas are also available. Most are quite safe and broad spectrum but may not be specific enough for more complex cases. This is especially true with respiratory cases in which herbs are put into general formulas for coughs. When herbs that dry out the lungs are mixed with herbs that moisten the lungs, the body becomes confused. The action of herbs is often slow, and many clients prefer not to wait for the results or administer formulas for the long period of time required. Most clients familiar with holistic methods are more patient and appreciate the lack of side effects. Some nonspecific formulas only palliate the symptoms, and every time the herb is removed the problem will return. A more complete holistic workup is needed if herbs do not seem to be fully effective, although some clients are happy with palliation.

Legal aspects

The AVMA guidelines state the following:

Veterinary botanical medicine is the use of plants and plant derivatives as therapeutic agents. It is recommended that continued research and education be conducted. Since some of these botanicals may be toxic when used at inappropriate doses, it is imperative that veterinary botanical medicine be practiced only by licensed veterinarians who have been educated in veterinary botanical medicine. Communication on the use of these compounds within the context of a valid veterinarian/client/patient relationship is important (*J Am Vet Med Assoc*, 1996).

From a legal standpoint, herbal formulas fall under Food and Drug Administration regulation. There is little control of the products on the market, although the sale of certain herbs, such as comfrey and chaparral, may be restricted. State boards have no regulations at this time concerning herbs.

Many herbal formulations designed to calm nervous horses are available. The AHSA policy states that no product may be used that alters the performance of the horse, and the association plans to test for these natural relaxants. Testing for herbs may be difficult because many horses eat them daily in their natural form. However, clients should be warned that herbal compounds can sometimes cause positive drug tests.

As with any other holistic modality the use of release forms may protect the practitioner from misunderstandings because herbal medicine is considered an alternative form of medicine (see Chapter 42). The practitioner is advised to find appropriate legal counsel.

Incorporating Holistic Nutrition

Managing a change in nutrition for horses can be a major challenge to the holistic practitioner (see Chapter 33).

Many horses are kept at boarding stables where owners have little control over what their horses are fed or given to drink or the quality and availability of turnout. Furthermore, horse owners are influenced by trends in their particular sport and advertising for feeds or supplements. Many clients listen to their veterinarian only until the next person gives them advice. The next source of information could be a feed dealer or another horse owner with only slightly more experience than the client.

Organically grown feeds for horses are cost-prohibitive because of the large volume required, high cost, and lack of local availability. Many roughages are treated with chemicals, and the purchaser often has no knowledge of their source or chemical content. Hays should be grown locally because of the high cost of shipping, but each region has only certain types of hay available, regardless of whether it is good for horses. Grains, on the other hand, are shipped throughout the country, and feed manufacturers may use the cheapest ingredients available. Again, the horse owner has no way of knowing the source of the feed. The practitioner is generally left in a defensive position, trying to help the horse become as healthy as possible so it can withstand the onslaught of poor nutrition and toxins.

Little holistic nutrition information is published; most of what is on the market is too general to be of value. The horses of different sizes may require the same amount of food but different amounts of trace nutrients, vitamins, and minerals; however, if nutrition comes prepackaged, those horses will receive exactly the same thing. Little money is spent on equine nutrition research because horses are not food-producing animals. Practitioners must become educated not only about nutrition in general but also about requirements specific to the area of the country in which they live.

Although equine nutrition is not highly regulated, the FDA may attempt to influence nutritional supplements. If regulations are enacted that list vitamins or minerals as drugs for livestock, the equine industry will also be affected. There has been some discussion of limiting the amount of selenium available, not just in feeds but also in supplements. Performance horses have well-known selenium-deficiency problems in certain parts of the country and would be directly affected by such regulation. The practitioner should try to stay abreast of changes in the feed industry because nutrition is the foundation of all health.

Incorporating New Vaccine Protocols

Practitioners and clients alike are beginning to question the need for yearly vaccination because of the perception that vaccinations are unnecessary and detrimental to the animal's health (see Chapter 40 and Smith, 1995). Vaccination protocols should be carefully evaluated for each patient.

Most equine practitioners have vaccinated horses against flu and have then seen an upper-respiratory tract infection go through the same barn. An upper-respiratory tract infection should be a mild, self-limiting disease requiring minimal treatment in a normal, healthy horse. Typically, however, most horses experience a month or more off work, a lingering cough, and increased susceptibility to allergic coughs (e.g., COPD) forever. Horses who do not produce a healthy immune response to a simple infection certainly cannot produce a healthy immune response to a vaccine. Horses who have become truly healthy on holistic programs tend to resist acute diseases and, when they do fall ill, mount a quick immune response and recover easily. The practitioner should look more carefully at horses that become sick in the 2-month period following vaccinations and determine whether some of those cases are less responsive to treatment than they should be.

A great deal of fear surrounds the subject of not using vaccines. Equine clients may be more afraid of not vaccinating than any other animal-owning population. Perhaps this is because horses are large and powerful and to see them ill is frightening to the owner; perhaps it is because an illness can be so expensive with a horse. Horses also travel more than animals of other species because most people like to ride with friends, and many people compete. Whatever the reason, few horse owners are open to the concept of not vaccinating or even that of vaccinating less frequently. Many horse owners keep their horses at boarding stables, where they must abide by the rules, which generally involve yearly vaccinations. Clients who wish to cut back or eliminate vaccines are often forced to move or conform to the rules.

Homeopathic nosodes are one possible option, and there are various protocols for using this form of protection (see Chapters 40 and 42). As more data become available concerning nosodes, these recommendations may change. The options presented in my practice are as follows:

1. Use of homeopathic nosodes. This option is for those who are comfortable with homeopathy, committed to following a schedule, and willing to treat any chronic disease already present, preferably before starting the nosodes.
2. Use of conventional vaccines for the initial series of foal shots, then either following up with nosodes or giving no more vaccines but treating the animals with constitutional homeopathy and good holistic nutrition.
3. Reduction in use of conventional vaccines, with use of homeopathic Ledum Pal. (immediately after vaccination) or Thuja Occ. (within the next several weeks after vaccination) to combat some of the negative effects of the vaccines.
4. Careful scheduling of vaccines so that only one or two are given at one time.
5. Cessation of all vaccines, with adherence to a complete holistic program of constitutional homeopathy and nutrition.

Most clients use option 2, 3, or 4; few opt for 1 or 5 at this time, although increasing numbers of clients are becoming interested in nosodes and reduction of vaccine use. Horses with little potential for disease exposure need fewer vaccinations. Horses who travel frequently or train under stressful conditions generally do better with supplemental vitamin C, high-quality fermented probiotics, constitutional treatment, and good nutrition than with multiple vaccines. One option that can be used is to spread vaccines out over a period of time to decrease antigen load and the possibility of interference. Clients may be encouraged to prepay or pay installments for a series of vaccines. The vaccinations can be given several weeks or a month apart. Call fees for each visit might make the cost prohibitive; if a practitioner is serious about wanting to implement a program such as this, it is best to waive the call fee and organize travel time carefully. The use of educational newsletters and lectures allows practitioners to reduce the number of vaccinations they perform, leaving them more time to diagnose and treat medical and surgical cases.

Legal aspects

From a legal standpoint, conventional vaccination protocols are standard. If a horse becomes ill and dies while receiving nosodes and the client believes the nosodes are at fault, the practitioner may have a difficult time in court. At the time of this writing, no studies have documented the efficacy of nosodes in the horse. FEI passports for all international transport of horses require flu vaccination according to a strict schedule, with a record of batch numbers and the make of the vaccine. Veterinarians must comply with these rules or the client will be barred from international travel. If flu vaccines are used for international travel, homeopathic Ledum Pal. 30C or X immediately after the vaccination may be used to ameliorate side effects, and vaccination should occur as early as possible before the shipping or competition.

Rabies is an important zoonosis, and if rabies is a local problem, vaccination is sensible. However, if a 3-year vaccine becomes available, it may be preferable to a 1-year vaccine. Any vaccine requirements for interstate shipment must be respected. For a boarding stable, practitioners may issue a certificate of protection for horses receiving nosodes or a veterinary letter stating that a certain horse is under constitutional homeopathic care and cannot have vaccines for a period of time. Some barns accept these forms, although many do not. Asking clients to sign a release form may be helpful (see Chapter 42).

Practice Management

Promoting Holistic Medicine and Client Education

As practitioners begin to incorporate holistic medicine into their practice, they must also educate clients and arouse interest in the new treatments. Lectures, articles, handouts, and advertising all play a part in promoting holistic medicine. The most successful strategy to give free lectures to the local horse organizations such as pony clubs, 4-H, breed organizations, and sport-specific organizations. There may be only 10 or 15 people in attendance, but a few of these will become clients. They may merely want to try this new approach, but if they like the results, they will tell other prospective clients. A happy customer tells an average of 10 people about his or her experiences, and the same is true for holistic medicine. Free lectures not only promote the business but also build good will and community support, both of which indirectly promote the business.

The next-best promotional tool, and the best for those with a fear of public speaking, is to write short articles for local equine newsletters. The local newsletters are usually short and contain information on members' friends. In the local newsletter the article will be read quickly, and because local news is of great interest, potential clients are likely to call. When people call for information about a new holistic technique, practitioners should either devote some time to answering their questions or request that staff members do so. Once clients become accustomed to the new therapies, they will tell friends, and new callers will already know they want the treatment.

Sending clients a newsletter explaining the new treatments is an excellent approach to incorporating the holistic modalities or converting the practice to holistic medicine. Clients will read a newsletter if it is short and interesting and contains information they can put to use themselves, such as a recipe for homemade herbal fly spray or a nutritional supplement they can buy from either the veterinarian or a local supplier. A newsletter also keeps clients informed about the continuing education the practitioner is pursuing and will help sell these new modalities. The newsletter should be visually appealing; with the amount of user-friendly computer software available, there is no excuse for a poorly done newsletter.

Advertising is another option; local newsletters and newspapers are good targets. Advertising probably does the least in direct promotion of holistic equine practice because horse owners tend to operate primarily by word-of-mouth. Name recognition does help if the ad appears regularly. Sometimes an area has a holistic practitioner, usually an acupuncturist or chiropractor who travels through irregularly and often leaves clients frustrated because they cannot get follow-up care. In this situation, advertising can be beneficial because clients discover they have a local practitioner.

Handouts are an excellent way to promote business and educate clients. The handouts may be just a brochure describing the basics of a therapy and ways clients can recognize symptoms in their own horses, or it may be an extensive first-aid booklet for clients or audiences at lectures. Some homeopathic companies have basic handouts that describe how homeopathy works. Most nutritional companies have a brochure about their products available at no charge. The IVAS and AVCA organizations offer brochures that can be purchased for a nominal fee and given to clients.

Clients like access to information, so making up a reading list or referring them to recent magazine articles can be helpful. The more education clients gain in the different modalities, the more helpful they will be in keeping track of symptoms and calling for maintenance treatments instead of waiting for disasters.

Charging for Holistic Services

Veterinarians have traditionally never charged enough for their services, a fact documented in the practice-management literature. Veterinarians are good at charging for things like drugs, but they seem less able to charge for knowledge and time.

Because of the emphasis on time-consuming histories and physical examinations, holistic practitioners must learn to charge for their time, or they will starve. In the end, not charging enough for services rendered takes the fun out of the practice. Holistic veterinarians also have additional education costs that exceed normal continuing education costs. A practitioner who completes all the holistic veterinary medical training has the equivalent of another year or two of veterinary college in costs, both directly in tuition and indirectly in lost time from work. Veterinarians must first be fair to themselves. Then they should consider the locality in which their practice is based and its cost of living. A practice in New York City obviously requires a great deal more profit than one in rural Missouri. The practitioner should establish an hourly rate to use as a goal like those of lawyers, riding instructors, and other professionals who have knowledge to share. Equine practices rarely recover travel time costs, so an hourly rate cannot always be achieved.

Fees for an acupuncture or chiropractic treatment should be based on the length of the time required to perform a treatment. In other words, if a treatment takes an hour and $100 per hour is the targeted figure to meet expenses, the base cost is $100, with additional charges added if the practitioner thinks this is justified.

For homeopathic, herbal, and nutritional consultations that may require extensive history-taking, the same per-hour fee may be targeted, but only the time used should be charged. Clients become efficient when they are charged this way. The physical examination can be done on the farm and telephone consultation used for the extensive history; some clients have a hard time paying for time spent talking while the practitioner is standing at the farm but seem to understand they need to pay if they are talking on the phone. The consultation can be done before the farm visit or after; each policy has advantages and disadvantages. In the beginning, clients might protest, but this decreases once they are educated about the system. Veterinarians must remember that clients are used to paying veterinarians for drugs, not knowledge.

General Office Organization

Several things can be done to make telephone work more efficient. A dedicated fax line in the home can be used for receiving telephone appointments. The fax tone effectively keeps clients from calling at any hour other than the appointed one, and because the line is in the home, phone appointments are made at the beginning of each day, before the first farm call. If the practitioner is likely to be out on an emergency, someone or an answering machine should convey the message to reschedule the appointment. The length of the consultation should be recorded, and the office should send the bill with the correct hourly rate. A total dollar cost should not be calculated at the time of the consultation because veterinarians tend to charge less than the actual predetermined fee.

The most important factor in scheduling consultations or appointments, setting fees, and collecting those fees is having someone other than the veterinarian in charge of those responsibilities. Veterinarians are seldom skilled in collecting money and setting appointments. They tend to charge too little and overwork themselves. If the practice is new and not yet busy, the practitioner can do it all, but set fees should be established. When the practitioner is busy every day of the week, a secretary should be hired so the practitioner is seeing clients instead of going to the bank and post office, running errands, and doing paperwork.

Veterinary staff can tell clients the fees and policies concerning telephone time and send out the bills. Basically the office should protect veterinarians from themselves. As the practice gets busier, the staff can reschedule appointments when the doctor is overworked. To give the best treatment, the practitioner must be rested.

The office staff can send out newsletters describing new prices, policies, and procedures. Obviously, significant increases in prices cannot occur all at once, but they be accomplished in a few increments.

The principles of *Feng Shui*, the Chinese art of placement, have been used to increase the positive energy and prosperity in the practice. *Feng Shui* involves arranging everyday articles in such a way that the energy flows in a positive direction. According to these principles, rearranging the position of a desk can change the productivity of the person sitting at that desk; moving the client files can increase income. Most, if not all, of the international banks in China or Hong Kong have a *Feng Shui* expert to organize the entire bank's interior. The stories of changing luck and prosperity by the use of *Feng Shui* make it worth trying (Rossbach, 1993).

Association with Nonveterinarian Holistic Practitioners

Once the word gets out that a veterinarian is beginning to practice holistic medicine, nonveterinarian practitioners may approach the practice in search of referrals. Some of them may be good practitioners and could be an asset to a practice, particularly a good massage therapist or a good chiropractor. However, most lay therapists in the equine world lack appropriate professional training. Many feel they have the right to treat horses without the involvement of a veterinarian.

The most common lay practitioners are massage therapists, many of whom have had only 5 days of school despite their high hourly rates. These people, unlike veterinarians, have no overhead in education, legal (liability), or financial investments. A skill such as massage cannot be learned in 5 days. Veterinarians should look for a massage therapist with at least 500 hours of education. Most of this training will probably be in human massage, but this usually translates well to horses. If referrals are made, some line of communication should be open so the client realizes everyone is working together. State laws should be followed in establishing a referral relationship because some states consider massage an act of veterinary medicine. If that is the case, repercussions could occur if an illegal referral was made.

Chiropractors who have completed the AVCA course are often great adjuncts to a practice. Like any professional, they should respect the established physician-client relationship and work closely with them.

After making referrals to lay practitioners, veterinarians should carefully evaluate the handling of clients. Lay practitioners sometimes begin with professional intentions and then start using other forms of holistic healing in which they are not qualified. If lay practitioners ask to observe veterinary practice, the veterinarian is advised to be careful. This often results in inappropriate claims that they studied with or are approved by a veterinarian. This happens with great regularity and can cause distress to both veterinarians and clients. Look for well-qualified nonveterinarians with a comprehensive education who are willing to discuss cases. These practitioners can become an asset if they fit into the practice and have complementary skills. The veterinarian should consult state board regulations concerning lay therapists and keep current on those rulings.

The AVMA guidelines for massage and physical therapy are as follows:

> Massage therapy is a technique in which the person uses only their hands and body to massage soft tissues. Massage therapy on nonhuman animals should be performed by a licensed veterinarian with education in massage therapy or, where in accordance with state veterinary practice acts, by a graduate of an accredited massage school who has been educated in nonhuman animal massage therapy. When performed by a nonveterinarian, massage therapy should be performed under the supervision of, or referral by, a licensed veterinarian who is providing concurrent care.
>
> Veterinary physical therapy is the use of noninvasive techniques, excluding veterinary chiropractic, for the rehabilitation of injuries in nonhuman animals. Veterinary physical therapy performed by nonveterinarians should be limited to the use of stretching;

massage therapy; stimulation by use of (a) low-level lasers, (b) electrical sources, (c) magnetic fields, and (d) ultrasound; rehabilitative exercises; hydrotherapy; and applications of heat and cold. Veterinary physical therapy should be performed by a licensed veterinarian or, where in accordance with state practice acts, by (1) a licensed, certified, or registered veterinary or animal health technician educated in veterinary physical therapy or (2) a licensed physical therapist educated in nonhuman animal anatomy and physiology. Veterinary physical therapy performed by a nonveterinarian should be performed under the supervision of, or referral by, a licensed veterinarian who is providing concurrent care (*J Am Vet Med Assoc,*1997).

Conclusion

Incorporating holistic medicine into an existing practice can be extremely rewarding. For many veterinarians, the incorporation of holistic medicine, whether full time or as an adjunct to conventional practice, is exactly what their practice needs. When conventional medicine has become routine and somewhat frustrating, holistic medicine may offer the practitioner new options to solve frustrating cases and improve animal health.

Acknowledgments

I am grateful for the proofreading and editorial help given by Ann Harman.

References

AVMA guidelines, *J Am Vet Med Assoc* 209(6):1026, 1996.

Beck MF: *Theory and practice of therapeutic massage,* Albany, NY, 1994, Delmar Publishing.

Day C: *Homeopathic treatment of small animals,* Saffron Walden, England, 1984, CW Daniel Co.

de Bairacli-Levy J: *Herbal handbook for farm and stable,* Emmaus, Penn, 1976, Rodale Press.

Dodds WJ: Vaccine safety and efficacy revisited: autoimmune and allergic diseases on the rise, *Vet Forum,* May:68-71, 1993.

Dvorak J, Orelli F: How dangerous is manipulation to the cervical spine? *Manual Med* 2:1-4, 1985.

Dvorak J and others: Musculoskeletal complications. In Haldeman S, ed: *Principles and practice of chiropractic,* ed 2, Norwalk, Conn, 1992, Appleton & Lange.

Fratkin JP: *Chinese herbal patent formulas: a practical guide,* Boulder, Colo, 1986, Shya Publications.

Gray H: *Gray's anatomy,* Philadelphia, Penn, 1974, Running Press.

Harman JC, Shaefer EC, Ward M: Chronic disease signs in horses, *J Am Hol Vet Med Assoc* 1994.

Heinermann J: *Healing animals with herbs,* Provo, Utah, 1977, Biworld Publishing.

Lauro A, Mouch B: Chiropractic effects on athletic ability, *Chiropractic, J of Chiro Res and Clin Investigation* 6(4):84-87, 1991.

Leach RA: *The chiropractic theories: principles and clinical applications,* Baltimore, Md, 1994, Williams & Wilkins.

MacLeod G: *The homeopathic treatment of horses,* Saffron Walden, England, 1977, CW Daniel Co.

Meagher J: *Sports massage,* Barrytown, NY, 1980, Station Hill Press.

Meagher J: *Beating muscle injuries for horses,* Hamilton, Mass, 1985, Hamilton Horse Associates.

Morgan J: *Herbs for horses,* Buckingham, England, 1993, Kenilworth Press.

Porter M: *Equine sports therapy,* Wildomar, Calif, 1990, Veterinary Data.

Rossbach S: *Interior design with feng shui,* New York, 1993, Penguin Books.

Sandoz R: Some physical mechanisms and effects of spinal adjustments, *Ann Swiss Chiro Assoc* 6:91, 1976.

Schoen A: *Veterinary acupuncture: from ancient art to modern medicine,* St. Louis, 1994, Mosby.

Self HP: *A modern horse herbal,* Buckingham, U.K., 1996, Kenilworth Press.

Smith CA, ed: Are we vaccinating too much? *J Am Vet Med Assoc* 207(4):421-425, 1995.

Willoughby SL: *Equine chiropractic care,* Port Byron, Ill, 1991, Options for Animals Foundation.

Xie H: *Traditional Chinese veterinary medicine,* Beijing, 1994, Beijing Agricultural University Press.

Youbang C and others, eds: *Chinese acupuncture and moxibustion,* Beijing, 1987, Foreign Languages Press.

Chapter 35

Holistic Medicine in Exotic Species Practice

DAVID M. McCLUGGAGE

The primary focus of this chapter is avian holistic medicine. Reptiles, small mammals, and other exotics are briefly included. Birds are highly emotional, easily stressed animals who may sustain more adverse effects from the stress associated with conventional medical care than they might benefit from the positive results produced by that therapy. Alternative medicine is often less stressful and may be more appropriate in certain situations. Reptiles and amphibians are not as emotional but still respond well to holistic medicine. Alternative therapeutic modalities, when judicially combined with conventional treatments, significantly improve the success rate while limiting the untoward consequences of conventional medical care. Chronic diseases are rarely successfully cured with the use of conventional methods. Alternative modalities—including acupuncture, herbal medicine, homeopathy, and nutrition—show promise for increasing the success rate in the treatment of these chronic conditions. This chapter is based on clinical experience in incorporating various alternative and complementary therapies into practice. Further research is needed to document the efficacy and safety of these procedures.

Introduction

Birds are sensitive, emotional, intelligent animals. Consequently, they are prone to stress and the detrimental effects of restraint, medications, and many of the more invasive diagnostic or therapeutic modalities employed in conventional practice. Patients can literally be stressed to death during restraint, physical examination, or blood collection. The stress associated with any procedure must always be evaluated against the potential benefits to the patients. They must always be treated gently during any procedure.

The patient should be treated with respect and viewed as a whole being, not as a collection of discrete body parts, systems, and emotions. Practitioners can make therapeutic decisions only after assessing the patient's mental and emotional condition, physical disorders, nutritional status, and environment.

Birds are often not well understood by their caretakers, who are often unable to differentiate abnormal behaviors from normal behaviors. Birds appear to hide their illnesses as a preservation response (McCluggage, 1989b); in fact, wild birds often drive sick birds out of the flock because they attract predators. Birds often carry illnesses for extended periods before the disease reaches a critical point. Many patients have been ill for years before the veterinarian sees them. Therefore the avian patient is often quite ill when first seen by the veterinarian. When developing diagnostic and therapeutic plans, the veterinarian should always remember that patients are often sicker than they first appear.

Reptiles and amphibians are not as intelligent and far less emotional than birds. They are not as likely to experience stress resulting from handling, restraint, and treatment. However, they are just as likely to carry illnesses for protracted periods and are often quite sick at presentation.

Because of their ability to hide illnesses, exotic animals must be evaluated with the use of laboratory diagnostic testing (McCluggage, 1989b) in addition to the physical examination and history of illness. The physical examination alone is not sufficient to determine the health status of the exotic patient; clients should be made aware of the availability of laboratory diagnostic tests.

Nutrition

General Avian Nutrition

Research on the correct diet for the various avian species has not been conducted. It is clear, however, that the outdated method of feeding birds seed diets and then trying to "balance" the diet by adding vitamins and a calcium supplement should be abandoned. Available research relates primarily to poultry, and guidelines provided in the literature are extrapolated from general nutritional information. Recent studies at the University of California provide some limited nutritional guidelines specific to the cockatiel; however, quite some time will elapse before guidelines can be formulated for all of the various groups of birds (Grau, 1983; Nearenberg, Roudybush, Grau, 1985; Roudybush, 1986).

Until more information is available, practitioners must follow the theory that a large variety of food items should be fed and that food high in fat, sugars, salts, or preservatives should be avoided. Diet recommendations are primarily for psittacines, with some reference to passerines and other aviary birds; nutrition of carnivorous birds is not covered.

In their natural habitat, psittacine birds consume a variety of food items, including seeds, nuts, grains, sprouts and leaves, insects, and fruits (Forshaw, 1973). Some have even been known to consume meat (mice, small birds, and carcasses) (Jackson, 1962). Typically, all birds subsist entirely on one type of food if it is plentiful. When that food source is no longer available, hunger triggers the natural foraging instinct, and birds seek out new food sources. When provided free access to seeds, birds lose this foraging instinct and subsist entirely on seeds. Offering new foods often fails to broaden the diet. The most effective method of altering the diet of the "seed addict" is to limit the total amount of all the different food items provided.

Feeding schedule

Birds should be fed on a twice-daily schedule (Lafeber, 1977). This technique approximates normal food-gathering in the wild and encourages birds to sample new food items. Access to food throughout the day inhibits the foraging instinct and may produce obesity. For many bird owners the best routine is to feed seeds or other dry food items (e.g., pellets) in the morning. The food cup should be removed after an hour, or small portions should be provided to ensure that the bird will consume all available food early in the day. The evening meal might include foods such as cheeses, meats, eggs, vegetables, and fruits.

Formulated diets

Formulated diets (pelleted diets) are now commonly available. These products provide a more balanced diet than seed diets and are preferable. Most bird caretakers should use formulated diets as the basic diet, supplementing extensively with fresh foods.

A fully organic formulated diet—one that is grown organically and processed without any preservatives or artificial ingredients—is preferred.*

Home cooking for psittacines

As with all animals, fresh foods and variety are the cornerstones of good nutrition for birds. The basic diet should comprise equal portions of beans, rice, formulated diets, and corn. Whole grains such as quinoa can be cooked and added to the basic diet. Other items, such as green leafy vegetables, sweet potatoes, fruits, and cheeses, should be added daily. The mix will spoil if left out for more than 3 or 4 hours. Preparation can be simplified by freezing large batches and thawing daily portions slowly in the refrigerator. As might be expected, high-fat, salty, and processed foods should be kept to a minimum.

Canaries and finches

Canaries and finches are primarily seed eaters, and seed should make up approximately 50% of their diet. The seed should be a mix of smaller seeds such as canary, rape, niger, poppy, and millet. Alternatively, many canaries and finches can be taught to eat a formulated diet. Although widely espoused by aviculturists, the belief that these birds can subsist on 95% or more seeds is unjustified.

Some species of softbills (e.g., some finches and sparrows) need live animals such as mealworms and crickets in the diet.*

Mynahs and toucans

A formulated bird diet should make up 75% of the diet of the mynah or toucan with the remainder including fruits such as apple, raisin, grape, and banana. Some meat (such as ground beef) should also be included. A food-source multiple vitamin and mineral supplement† can be added to the soft foods daily. Mynahs and toucans often have hemochromatosis, in which excess iron is stored in the liver, leading to liver disease. Diets low in iron are recommended to help prevent this disease, so most vitamin and mineral supplements containing iron are contraindicated. Mice or other meat should be added to toucan diets.

Lories and lorikeets

Diets for lories and lorikeets are poorly understood. The long-standing recommendations for lories include the basic diet of nectar formula: 1 teaspoon evaporated milk and 1 teaspoon honey, stirred into 1 cup of water. The various commercial lory nectar diets are preferred. Vegetables and fruits are fed ad libitum (Axelson, 1981).

The commercial nectar formulas may be augmented with two supplements and psyllium, a small pinch of each with every feeding. The additions to the commercial feeding formulas are as follows:

---

*Harrison Bird Diet, Inc., 7171 Mercy Road, Suite 135, Omaha, Neb 68106; 800-346-1269.

---

*Nature's Way, 800-318-2611.
†Cyrofood, Standard Process West, Inc., PO Box 270547, Fort Collins, Colo, 800-321-9807.

1. Green food supplements*: Lory formulas often lack green food products such as blue-green algae and wheat grass. A supplement high in these types of products provides needed nutrition.
2. Gastrointestinal Acidifier†: The lory intestinal tract needs a more acidic environment than that provided with the typical nectar formula; pH imbalance may lead to chronic intestinal problems. Lories are prone to *Candida* infections; therefore a product that works on diminishing the pathogenic yeasts is preferred.
3. Psyllium: Most nectar formulas contain too little fiber. A bulk fiber source such as psyllium improves digestion.

Nutrition for Other Exotic Animals

Iguanas

Approximately 80% of the iguana's diet should consist of plant-based foods, and 20% should consist of protein (Barton, 1984; Boyer, 1987, 1993). Of the plant materials, 90% should be vegetables and 10% should be fruits. Dark-green leafy vegetables—including collards, alfalfa, broccoli, and dandelions—should predominate because of their high calcium content. Good fruits include fig, papaya, apricot, and cantaloupe. The protein could be insects, fish, and worms or a formulated diet such as dog food and bird food.

Rabbits

Rabbits are strict herbivores. They should be fed a diet primarily consisting of grass hay (Bermuda or timothy) and alfalfa. A high-fiber rabbit pellet (18% to 24% protein) can make up 60% of the diet. Fruits and vegetables (such as those listed for iguanas) are beneficial but should be fed sparingly (Jenkins, 1993).

Ferrets

Ferrets are carnivorous and have a short intestinal tract compared with most other mammals. They must be fed frequent small meals. Unless obesity is a problem, ferrets can be fed free choice (Brown, 1993). The ferret's diet should contain 30% or more protein and 20% to 30% fat (Fox, 1988). A raw-meat diet, including muscle and organ meat, is preferred. Other foods that may be fed include small amounts of fruits (cantaloupe), eggs, dairy products (yogurt), and some whole-grain cereals (organic breakfast cereals).

Antimicrobial Therapy

Antimicrobial therapy is indicated in exotic animals with overwhelming bacterial infections. Specific guide-lines for effective therapy are briefly covered, especially points that are different in exotic animals compared with dogs and cats.

Birds often have bacterial infections caused by the Enterobacteriaceae group. These bacteria are often resistant to many of the more common antimicrobial agents used in veterinary medicine. Effective antimicrobial agents that may be used in birds include enrofloxacin (Baytril; Haver/Diamond), 15 mg/kg every 12 hours; piperacillin (Pipracil; Lederle), 200 mg/kg; doxycycline (Vibrimycin; Pfizer), 50 mg/kg, orally, each day for 45 days; trimethoprim/sulfamethoxazole (Bactrim; Roche), 20 mg/kg, orally, every 12 hours.

Administration of an incorrect antimicrobial agent can cause death in rabbits and rodents. Dysbiosis, superinfections, and clostridial enterotoxemia often develop in rabbits and rodents when many of the common antimicrobial agents are used. Antibiotics that should not be used include ampicillin, amoxicillin, erythromycin, lincomycin, or any of the other narrow-spectrum antimicrobials. Safe antimicrobial agents include enrofloxacin (10 mg/kg every 12 hours), piperacillin (100 mg/kg every 12 hours), chloramphenicol palmitate (35 mg/kg every 12 hours), and trimethoprim/sulfamethoxazole (30 mg/kg every 12 hours).

During and especially after the use of antimicrobial agents, supplementation of diet with a high-fiber formula containing lactobacillus and slippery elm* benefits most exotic animals, including birds, rabbits, small mammals, and ferrets.

Homeopathy

Homeopathy in Avian Practice

Homeopathy appears to be quite effective in avian species (McCluggage, 1995). Birds are particularly responsive to energetic therapeutics. Using classical homeopathy, the veterinarian must find the correct remedy by analyzing not only physical symptoms but mental and emotional symptoms. Such work can be a challenge with birds because most owners know little about the normal behaviors of their companions, let alone abnormal mental and emotional symptoms.

The holistic practitioner must be well acquainted with Western medical examination and diagnosis for avian patients. Because many birds come to the veterinarian quite ill, the physician may not have a second chance if the first remedy fails. Conventional medications may be indicated for critically ill birds to get them through a crisis. Bacterial infections are more common in birds than in dogs and cats, so antimicrobial therapy is often essential.

The veterinary homeopath must have an in-depth understanding of the various species' normal behaviors. Only

---

*Super Green Formula, Harmony Formulas, PO Box 41751, Santa Barbara, Calif 93140.
†Zymex, Standard Process West, Inc., PO Box 270547, Fort Collins, Colo; 800-321-9807.

---

*Fiber Formula, 4Health, Inc., 5485 Conestoga Court, Boulder, Colo 80301.

then can the practitioner hope to select an appropriate remedy from a repertory.

Birds are not vaccinated, so the vaccinosis rubric is not appropriate. Their behaviors are very different from those of mammals, making selection of rubrics in the mental section difficult.

Most species of birds have not been inbred and have recently been removed from their natural habitats. Therefore chronic deep miasms appear to be less common. Short-term prescribing is often rewarding, producing a rapid resolution of the pathologic process.

Perhaps the greatest obstacle to accurate prescribing in birds is the difficulty of assessing the mental condition of the patient. Food procurement, social interaction, reproduction, nest procurement, and many other behaviors that are normal in wild birds are absent or dramatically altered in captive ones. Being highly social and emotional animals, birds may have significant psychologic difficulties arising from caging, sexual frustration, lack of exercise, and a need to engage in meaningful activity. The homeopath must differentiate between normal behaviors that have produced situational stress and dysfunctional behaviors that arise from a diseased state manifested on the mental or emotional plane. Only mental symptoms that are truly pathologic should be used in diagnosing the case. This determination can be extremely difficult and practitioners should remember that behaviors arising from situational stress (e.g., biting the caretaker in an attempt to drive the caretaker away from a perceived rival) are normal when the patient's mental state is otherwise good (Sankaran, 1991). Pathologic symptoms on the mental or emotional plane (e.g., fearful and erratic behavior from a formerly affectionate, trusting bird) are manifested by unusual, uncharacteristic responses to ordinary occurrences.

The beginnings of an avian repertory are included here. This repertory is incomplete and certain to be revised in light of future findings. This repertory was developed from a human repertory (Künzli, 1987), a materia medica (Hering, 1993), and clinical experience (Box 35-1).

BOX 35-1

An Avian Homeopathic Repertory

BEAK
Dryness—silicea, thuja
Exfoliation—arsenicum album, graphites
Overgrowth, distortion—calcarea carbonica, graphites, silicea, sulfur, thuja

EYES
Conjunctivitis—*Euphrasia officinalis, Pulsatilla pratensis, Rhus toxicodendron*
   Acrid—*E. officinalis*
   Thick discharge, pus—*P. pratensis*
   Watery discharge—*R. toxicodendron*
Lacrimation—graphites
   Photophobia with lacrimation—graphites

EXTREMITIES
Feet, red and ulcerated—sulfur

FEATHERS
Poor quality—sulfur, nux vomica, arsenicum album, *P. pratensis*, sepia, silicea
Bronzing—nux vomica, sulfur, arsenicum album
Retarded growth—arsenicum album, nux vomica, selenium
Plucking/chewing—arnica, arsenicum album, calcarea carbonica, folliculinum, ignatia amara, natrum muraticum, nux vomica, phosphoricum acidum, sepia, silicea, sulfur, thallium, tuberculinum avis, veratrum album
   African Greys—arsenicum album, natrum muraticum
      With separation anxiety—natrum muraticum

Cockatoos—arnica montana, arsenicum album, natrum muraticum, nux vomica, sepia
   Males—nux vomica
   Females—*P. pratensis*, silicea
Macaws—nux vomica, tuberculinum avis
Aggression, general—nux vomica
   Sexual—nux vomica, sepia
   Males—nux vomica
Frantic—belladonna, stramonium, veratrum album

FEMALE
Egg binding—calcarea carbonica, kali carbonicum, *P. pratensis*
   Blood on eggs—*P. pratensis*
   Soft-shelled eggs—calcarea carbonica, kali carbonica
Egg laying—kali carbonica, *Lycopodium clavatum*, *P. pratensis*, sepia
   Stopping of eggs—sepia
Infertility—natrum muraticum, sepia, silicea
Oviduct—kali carbonica, *P. pratensis*, sepia

GENERALITIES
Abscesses, granulomatous—tuberculinum avis
Cancer—calcarea carbonica, carcinosinum, graphites, *Lycopodium clavatum*, nitricum acidum, phosphorus, silicea, sulfur, thuja
   Budgies—calcarea carbonicum, carcinosinum, graphites, *L. clavatum*

BOX 35-1

AN AVIAN HOMEOPATHIC REPERTORY—cont'd

Familial history—carcinosinum, *L. clavatum*
Candida albicans infections—calcarea carbonica, calcarea phosphorica, china officinalis, helonias dioica, *L. clavatum*, medorrhinum, *P. pratensis*, natrum phosphoricum, nitricum acidum, sepia, thuja
Emaciation—arsenicum album, calcaria carbonica, calcaria phosphorica, iodium, natrum muraticum, nux vomica, *L. clavatum, P. pratensis*, phosphorus, sepia, silicea, sulfur, tuberculinum bovinum
    Ravenous appetite—baryta carbonica, baryta iodata, calcaria carbonica, calcaria phosphorica, causticum hahnemanni, china officinalis, cina, iodium, *L. clavatum*, natrum muraticum, nux vomica, silicea, sulfur
Pyemia—arsenicum album, calcaria carbonica, hippozaenium, lachesis, pyrogenium
Sepsis—arsenicum album, arsenicum iodatum, baptisia tinctoria, china officinalis, crotalus horridus, echinacea angustifolia, *Lachesis*
Trauma—aconitum napellus, arnica montana, Hepar sulphuris calcareum, *R. toxocodendron*, ruta graveolens, symphytum officinale
    Head, with seizures—belladonna
Weakness, unable to rise because of severe illness—*Carbo vegetabilis*

HEART
Heart, general—crataegus oxyacantha et monogyna, *Digitalis purpurea, R. toxocodendron*
Cardiomyopathy—crataegus oxyacantha et monogyna, *Digitalis purpurea*
Cyanosis—*D. purpurea*

KIDNEY
Gout—urtica urens
Paralysis—hypericum perforatum
    Renal tumors—hypericum perforatum, *L. clavatum*

LIVER
Liver disease, general—nux vomica, *L. clavatum*, phosphorus
Fatty-liver disease—calcaria carbonica, carbo vegetabilis, chelidonium majus, kali bichromica, kali carbonica, lyssinum (hydrophobinum), *L. clavatum*, mercurius solubilis, nux vomica, phosphorus, picricum acidum, sulfur

MIND
Aggression—nux vomica
Anger—nitric acid, nux vomica
    Underlying—nux vomica
Cowardliness—*L. clavatum*

Dependence on others—baryta carbonica, *P. pratensis*
Fear (violently throwing self around cage)—aconitum napellus, belladonna, *L. clavatum*, nux vomica, stramonium, veratrum album
Grief—causticum hahnemanni, natrum muraticum
Irritability—natrum muraticum, nitricum acidum, nux vomica, phosphorus
Idleness—calcarea carbonica
Jealousy, biting of owner when others approach—calcarea sulphuricum, hyoscyamus niger, lachesis, *L. clavatum*, nux vomica, *P. pratensis*, stramonium

MOUTH
Pharynx
    Chronic inflammation—graphites, sulfur
    Elongated choanae—phosphorus
    Eroded choanal papillae—phosphorus

NERVES
General—*R. toxicodendron*, hypericum perforatum
Ataxia—arsenicum album, calcaria carbonica, nux vomica, phosphorus, plumbum metallicum, silicea, stramonium, zinc
Paralysis—hypericum perforatum, lachesis, phosphorus, plumbum metallicum, zinc
    Renal tumors—hypericum perforatum, *L. lavatum*
Seizures—calcaria carbonica, ignacia, *Lycopodium clavatum*, silicea
    Status epilepticus—aconitum napellus, belladonna
Weak—iodium, nux vomica, plumbum metallicum, silicea, zinc, zinc phosphoricum

NOSE
Pharyngitis—nux vomica, phosphorus, sulfur
Sinusitis—arsenicum album, bryonia alba, hepar sulphuris calcareum, kali bichromicum, *L. clavatum*, mercurius solubilis, natrum muraticum, nux vomica, phosphorus, *P. pratensis*, silicea
Coryza—graphites
    Dry, obstructed nose—phosphorus
Catarrh—graphites
    Contracts colds easily—graphites

PEDIATRICS
Stunted growth—baryta carbonica
Infantile behavior—baryta carbonica
Slow development—calcaria carbonica
Separation anxiety—nux vomica

RESPIRATORY
Chronic colds—graphites

Homeopathy in Other Exotic Animals

Homeopathy has been found effective in other animals, including rabbits, ferrets, and reptiles. For instance, it has been reported anecdotally that several rabbits with gastric obstruction (hairballs) responded positively to fluid therapy and nux vomica. One iguana that viciously and repeatedly attacked its owner became a much more tractable animal after treatment with nitrcum acidum. A rabbit with mucopurulent, greenish ocular discharge recovered after treatment with *Pulsatilla pratensis*. However, clinical efficacy and controlled trials must be conducted to verify the efficacy of homeopathic treatments.

English Flower Essence Therapy

In the early 1930s, Dr. Edward Bach categorized 38 flowers according to their ability to alter the emotions of his patients. Flower essences are similar to homeopathic medications in that they are prescribed in accordance with the law of similars. Various flower essences are used to help patients deal with fear, anger, insecurity, stress, and many other emotions. Often several different flower essences are combined to treat multiple emotional symptoms. After analyzing the patient's conditions, practitioners of this modality dispense a flower essence formula, usually as an adjunct to other therapies.

A particularly effective combination, the five-flower remedy, comprises star of Bethlehem, rock rose, impatiens, cherry plum, and clematis. This formula is beneficial for all birds who are stressed—for example, most birds brought into the veterinary clinic. The five-flower remedy can be sprayed on the bird, sprayed in the room, or administered by dropper into the bird's mouth to help relieve anxiety and fear.

Traditional Chinese Medicine

Chinese Herbs

Herbs such as those used in traditional Chinese medicine (TCM) can be administered to birds with caution. Birds are more sensitive than mammals to medications and their more rapid metabolic rate predisposes them to some types of poisonings (Dumonceaux, Harrison, 1994). The practitioner with little experience in the use of Chinese herbs should proceed with caution. A variety of Chinese herbal combinations may be used with excellent success and without side effects when dosages are correct. Common sequelae of moderately excessive dosages usually include vomiting, diarrhea, or anorexia. Decreasing the dose usually stops the side effects, and the herb can then be continued at a lower dose.

Doses for birds and other animals are not known. A starting dose may be calculated by first determining what percentage of a typical adult the patient weighs (the average adult being perhaps 65 kg), calculating down from the recommended adult dose, and then starting by giving one

third of that dose. If no side effects result, the dose may be slowly increased over a few days to the full amount.

Administration of herbs

Because of the bitter taste of many herbal products, they are often a challenge to administer to birds. Herbs come in several forms, including alcohol extracts, powders, pills, extract granules, and capsules. Alcohol extracts have an excessively high level of alcohol for administration to animals. The alcohol should be boiled off in a double boiler before the herbal preparation is given to the patient. Addition of an equal amount of boiling water to the alcohol extract also removes the alcohol.

Alcohol-extracted liquids may be given by eye dropper after the alcohol is removed. Powders and capsules can be mixed into favorite foods such as yogurt, ice cream, and sweet potatoes. For more precise dosing, the pills may be ground up, or the powders from capsules mixed into one of the pharmaceutical suspension vehicles intended for such uses.

For calculation of capsule or tablet dosing: 12 capsules (a typical adult daily dose) placed in 60 ml of suspension vehicle = 0.15 ml three times daily for a 450 gram bird (usually placed in food given by eye dropper). Extract granules often can be dissolved in water and then given by eye dropper. Most commonly, powders can be mixed with foods or liquid extracts are used.

One company* produces a line of alcohol-free liquid products that are also free of food coloring, preservative, and sugars. These liquids are particularly useful in birds, rabbits, reptiles, and small mammals. Birds are given 0.01 ml/30 gram bird twice or thrice daily.

Some specific herbal combinations

Hundreds of herbal combinations are available, each with specific indications for use. For effective herbal prescribing an accurate Chinese medical diagnosis is required. Only a few examples of herbal combinations are mentioned here as examples of how herbs can be used.

HUANG LIAN JIE DU TANG

This herbal combination, also known by the name "coptis" and "scute," contains the herb coptis (*Coptis chinensis, Huang lian*), which is antibacterial in nature. Coptis has antimicrobial, antiviral, antiprotozoal, and antiinflammatory effects and would be expected to aid in the treatment of bacterial infections (Bensky). Scutellariae is another ingredient in this formula. Scutellariae is antiviral, antibacterial, antiinflammatory, and antipyretic. It can relieve Fire Toxins (infective organisms) from the Upper Jao (Bensky). The combination makes it an excellent choice for viral and bacterial diseases. It can be found as a liquid or a powder. It is indicated in febrile diseases with inflammation, congestion, and bleeding (diseases of excess in

*Plum Flower Herbal Extracts, Mayway Corporation, 1338 Mandela Parkway, Oakland, CA 94607.

TCM). It is also known as Coptis and Scute Combination and can be found as a liquid or a powder.

Side effects of overdose include vomiting, dyspnea, and convulsions. Severe overdose can produce respiratory paralysis when the active ingredient berberine is given intravenously.

BU ZHONG YI QI WAN

Bu Zhong Yi Qi Wan (Central *Qi* Drink) is a classic formula to strengthen Spleen and Stomach *Qi* and invigorate *Qi* in the Liver. Chronic diarrhea may respond to this formula; many diarrheas are considered to be Spleen *Qi* Deficiencies. It is also helpful in improving digestion and relieving bloating and for relieving prolapses of rectum and uterus. It has been used successfully in the treatment of oviduct and cloacal prolapses.

XIAO CHAI HU TANG AND LIVER DISEASE

Xiao Chai Hu Tang, or Minor Bupleurum formula, is a good formula for viral hepatitis. Several herbs that are known as hepatoprotectants and have been clinically shown to decrease alanine aminotranferase (ALT, also known as SGPT) and aspartate aminotransferase (AST, also known as SGOT). Two of the most powerful herbs in this category are *Silybum marianum* (milk thistle) and *Han Lian Cao* (eclipta) (Goeddert). These two herbs, bupleurum, and other herbs for liver regeneration are included in an American patent medicine called Ecliptex* that the author has used for chronic liver disease in birds.

LIU WEI DI HUANG WAN

Also called *Rehmannia Six* and *six-flavor tea pills, Liu Wei Di Huang Wan* is a major formula to treat *Yin* deficiency, working through the Kidney, Spleen, Liver, and Heart. It clears Heat and cools Blood and especially nourishes Kidney *Yin*. Birds are more *Yang* in nature; Heat syndromes and *Yin* Deficiency develop easily when *Yang* becomes excessively dominant. Thus many birds become *Yin* deficient, and this formula works well in a wide range of *Yin* and Kidney deficiencies. Western diagnoses that might respond at least in part to this formula include chronic egg binding, kidney disease (especially with excess urates), infertility in hens, and respiratory disease (sinusitis, airsacculitis) in which the discharge is particularly dry.

JIN GUI SHEN QI WAN

Jin Gui Shen Qi Wan, or Rehmannia Eight Formula, is a classic formula used to treat Kidney *Yang* Deficiency (Ebling). A close relative to this formula is *Ba Wei Di Huang Wan*. Birds are often cold and have watery droppings (polyuria). A Western medical diagnosis would be kidney failure. *Jin Gui Shen Qi Wan* has been used to treat this disorder. Birds with undigested food in their stools might also respond to this formula.

MAI MEN DONG TANG

Ophiopogon combination is a Lung-moistening formula that may be effective in birds with chronic tail bobbing and shortness of breath, dry mouth, and dry rhinitis.

BIDENS 6

Birds often have bacterial gastrointestinal disorders, especially diarrhea with a foul smell. Bidens 6* has been used by the author to treat these disorders with some success. This formula has antiviral and antibacterial properties.

YUNNAN PAIYAO

Yunnan Paiyao is a Chinese herbal patent medicine that is excellent for stopping bleeding (Fratkin, 1986). It can be used topically to arrest bleeding and help granulate wounds or given internally in preparation for surgery. It significantly reduces bleeding during surgery. The dose one author uses is 1 capsule dissolved in water and given by gavage to a 400 to 1000 gram bird for 2 to 3 consecutive days before surgery and then again 3 hours before surgery. *Yunnan Paiyao* is routinely used to stop bleeding toenails during grooming and given systemically to birds who are prone to bleeding blood feathers during feather regrowth. It is also used in combination with aloe vera gel for topical treatment of self-induced granulomatous lesions.

Acupuncture Therapy

Traditional Chinese Medicine Basic Analysis

Birds have a high metabolic rate (heart rate often greater than 200) and a high body temperature (often greater than 103° F) and are light and relatively hollow because of the air sac system). These features make them more *yang* in nature. From an evolutionary view, birds have evolved from reptiles and are a younger class than the Class Mammalia. They appear to be more responsive or sensitive to acupuncture techniques (Partington, 1994a).

Tonification of points requires less manipulation and less time (Axelson, 1981). Because of birds' sensitive nature and relatively rapid and adverse response to restraint, acupuncture combined with vitamin B$_{12}$ (cyanocobalamin) is often used. Medium-sized parrots receive as much as 0.2 ml at each acupuncture point, and small birds usually as much as 0.05 ml. Dry needling is possible in birds and may be more effective in some conditions. Many birds leave the needles alone after being released from the restraint towel. Needles should be left in place for about 5 minutes for tonification and 10 minutes for sedation.

The example in Box 35-2 illustrates the way acupuncture produced significant therapeutic results when used in avian subjects.

Selected Problems and Points to Consider in Treatment

Crop binding

Crop binding can be considered primarily a disease of the Stomach (rebellious Stomach *Qi*) or Liver (failure of

---

BOX 35-2

CASE REPORT: A MACAW WITH POSSIBLE NEUROPATHIC GASTRIC DILATATION

A 5-month-old greenwing macaw *(Ara chloroptera)* had a history of an enlarged crop that was very slow to empty, marked weight loss, and a constant food-begging response. The bird's condition had worsened over the preceding 3 months. Before presentation the bird had received broad-spectrum antimicrobial therapy (courses of enrofloxacin at 15 mg/kg twice a day and piperacillin at 200 mg/kg twice a day, each for 10 days). The macaw had stopped maturing about 1 month before presentation.

PHYSICAL FINDINGS

On presentation the macaw was alert but moved slowly and behaved in an immature way. The bird was not sleeping excessively and was not fluffed. It begged constantly for food, as if starving. Once hand-feeding began, the bird ate little food. The bird's crop was full, and its contents had a normal, fluid feel. The bird's crop was still half full of food after 7 hours, suggesting a slow crop-emptying time. The bird had very watery droppings and was mildly dehydrated, although not thirsty. The skin was particularly dry. The abdomen was mildly distended.

The bird's feces were normal, as was the urinary portion of the droppings. The bird weighed 770 grams—subjectively, 25% less than normal. Feather development was mildly stunted. The bird's extremities felt cold, although its core temperature seemed normal. TCM pulse diagnosis is not possible in birds. The tongue had a moderately thick, whitish coating.

DIAGNOSTICS

Bacterial culture and sensitivity testing revealed no significant pathogens. Complete blood count showed a moderate leukocytosis (24,300 white blood cells). Blood-chemistry analysis revealed that aspartate aminotransferase (AST or SGOT) was increased at 495 and creatinine phosphokinase was increased at 1150 IU/L. Radiographs showed a dilated, thin-walled ventriculus; mild proventricular dilation; and a normal-sized liver.

WESTERN MEDICAL DIAGNOSIS

A presumptive diagnosis of neuropathic gastric dilatation (NGD; macaw wasting disease or psittacine proventricular dilation syndrome) was made. The cause of this disease has not been determined. According to one theory, it has an underlying viral origin (Gerlach, 1986; Lutz, Wilson, 1991) with a secondary autoim-

mune reaction that leads to lymphocytic and monocytic infiltration of intrinsic and extrinsic splanchnic nerves of the muscularis tunics of the alimentary tract (Graham, 1991; Lumeij, 1994). The loss of the splanchnic innervation produces decreased muscle tone and subsequent enlargement (flaccid paralysis) of the affected organs. The entire gastrointestinal tract may be involved; however, the proventriculus is most prominently affected, followed by the ventriculus and ingluvies.

EASTERN MEDICAL DIAGNOSIS

TCM diagnosis of Interior, Cold Deficiency affecting the Stomach and Spleen was made. An Interior diagnosis was made because the process was chronic and involved the internal organs. Deficiency was evident in the general lethargy, weakness, and retardation of development. Cold was manifested in the chilly limbs, watery stools, and lack of thirst.

The Stomach's functions of "rotting and ripening" food were impaired, with Rebellious Stomach *Qi* (the food was sitting in the crop instead of moving downward). Stomach *Qi* Deficiency was affecting the Middle Burner, producing symptoms of fatigue and weakness of the limbs (food essences were not being transported to the limbs) (Maciocia, 1989). Stomach *Qi* Deficiency also produces Spleen *Qi* Deficiency. Food was retained in the Stomach (an Excess pattern) and manifested as slow crop emptying, lack of appetite, crop distention, and poor digestion.

The spleen's function of Transformation and Transportation was adversely affected with deposition of Phlegm. A spleen *Qi* Deficiency was present because the Stomach *Qi* was not sending *Gu Qi* down to the Spleen. The Spleen is responsible for transporting *Gu Qi* to the muscles. Spleen Deficiency was exhibited as general dehydration, muscle weakness, abdominal distention, and fatigue.

Because the Spleen was not transporting the refined essence upward to the Lungs, the bird was dehydrated, most noticeably on the skin. The weak movement of the muscles and general fatigue were also due to the Spleen's failure to control the muscles (Maciocia, 1989).

Phlegm was seen as excess fluids throughout the abdomen and in the gastrointestinal system.

TREATMENT PRINCIPLES, TREATMENT, AND RESULTS

The points used included ST 36, SP 6, PC 6, LI 11, BL 13, and BL 14.

BOX 35-2

CASE REPORT: A MACAW WITH POSSIBLE NEUROPATHIC GASTRIC DILATATION—cont'd

ST-36 *Zu San Li* is located just lateral to the tibial crest, in the belly of the cranial tibial muscle (Vanden Berge, Zweers, 1993). It is the He-Sea point and the Earth point (and the Horary point) on the channel and the master point of the upper abdomen (Partington, 1994). In this case, ST-36 was used to benefit the Stomach and Spleen, tonify Stomach *Qi,* strengthen the body, regulate and harmonize Nutritive and Defensive *Qi,* and regulate the intestines.

SP-6 *San Yin Jiao* is located at the caudal border of the tibiotarsus, superior to the medial epicondyle (palpation reveals a small depression at the caudal border of the tibiotarsus) (Axelson, 1981; Boyer, 1987). It is the meeting point of the three *Yin* channels of the leg and the master point of the lower abdomen. Here, SP-6 was used mainly to tonify the Spleen to treat the Spleen Deficiency and resolve Damp.

PC-6 *Nei Guan* is found on the ventral surface of the wing, between the radius and the ulna, in a relatively large depression, three *cun* proximal to the ventral condyle of the ulna (Axelson, 1981; Boyer, 1987). It is the *Luo* point on the channel, the opening point of the *Yin* Linking *(Yin Wei)* channel, and the master point of the Chest and Heart (Taylor-Limehouse, 1994). Here, PC-6 was used to harmonize the Stomach and subdue rebellious Stomach *Qi.*

LI-11 *Qu Chi* is found on the dorsal surface of the wing, with the wing moderately extended, in the angle formed by the humerus and the radius, just dorsal to the brachialis muscle and caudal to the tensor propatagialis pars brevis tendon (Axelson, 1981; Boyer, 1987). Deep needle insertion must be avoided at LI-11 because the radial nerve lies just ventral to this point. It is the tonification point and the He-Sea point on the channel (Maciocia, 1989). LI-11 was used here as an immune modulator and immune booster to address the autoimmune sequelae of NGD.

BL-13 Avian *Wei Shu* is found immediately caudal to the transverse process and medial to the costa vertebralis: process uncinatus of the second thoracic vertebra (Axelson, 1981; Boyer, 1987). It is the Association point for the proventriculus and the ventriculus (Axelson, 1981). BL-13 was used in this case to benefit the proventriculus and ventriculus (the bird's Stomach), benefit Stomach *Qi,* and relieve the retention of Stomach food.

BL-14 Avian *Pi Shu* is found immediately caudal to the transverse process and medial to the costa verte-

bralis: process uncinatus of the third thoracic vertebra (Axelson, 1981; Boyer, 1987). It is the Association point for the spleen. It also affects the pancreas (Axelson, 1981). BL-14 was used here to tonify the Stomach and Spleen and benefit the Spleen's *Qi.* BL-14 is effective in benefiting the Spleen's functions of Transportation and Transformation.

DISCUSSION

Weekly acupuncture sessions produced marked improvements for the bird, which gained weight and feathered out. Before the weekly acupuncture sessions, the crop motility was poor and the bird was weak. After each session, the bird's digestion improved markedly and the bird became stronger. After 4 weeks the bird appeared normal and seemed to develop to normal maturity.

The point formula used addressed the Interior, Cold Deficiency that was affecting the Stomach and Spleen. After each acupuncture session, the Stomach's digestive function improved. The Spleen's function of Transformation and Transportation of the food essences improved, manifested as an improved state of hydration and strength. The refined essences were again being transported up to the Lungs, where they were then disbursed to the surface of the body.

Approximately 3 months after the sessions stopped, the bird again became very ill, lost weight, and eventually died. NGD is believed to have 100% mortality. Death is usually caused by starvation or secondary bacterial infection. A bird as severely affected as this macaw was when first presented would be likely to die within 30 days of a tentative diagnosis of NGD. Living for 6 months would be exceptionally rare with the use of conventional therapies (antimicrobials, gastrointestinal motility modifiers, and corticosteroids).

To shorten this case report, only one bird has been mentioned until this point. Actually, a total of four birds with the same disease process were being treated at the same time. Two of the birds eventually died, two are alive at this writing, 2 years later. The findings of gross necropsy in the two birds who died were consistent with NGD. A histopathologic study was not performed because of the cost.

Acupuncture using cyanocobalamine injected at the acupuncture points was shown to be a valuable treatment method in this case. The points used were effective for the birds in this report and should be considered in the future for other birds with similar disorders.

Liver to ensure the smooth flow of *Qi* to the Spleen and Stomach). Points to use might include the following:

- LI-11 Tonification point and the Earth point of the Meridian
- BL-13 Back-*Shu* Point for the proventriculus and ventriculus
- BL-16 Back-*Shu* Point for the Liver
- ST-36 Master Point for the upper abdomen, including Stomach and Spleen
- SP-6 Master Point for the lower abdomen; tonifies the Liver
- CV-6 Tonifies *Qi* and Blood; moves *Qi* and dispels stagnation

Egg binding

Egg binding constitutes a failure of the oviduct to pass the egg down into the cloaca. From a TCM perspective, egg binding represents a failure of the Kidney *Qi* to warm the Lower Burner, producing a weakness in the Fire of the Gate of Vitality and thus weakening the uterus. The Spleen fails to transport fluids as needed (the uterus is often too dry and the egg becomes stuck) and cannot produce the necessary *Qi* for egg laying (the Spleen is the Root of the Post-Heaven *Qi*). Egg binding is an interior Cold Deficiency with a buildup of phlegm. Egg binding can be treated by applying acupuncture techniques to the following points:

- SP-6 Strengthens the Spleen, tonifies the Kidneys, calms the Mind
- ST-36 Master Point of the abdomen, tonifies the Spleen, strengthens the body, tonifies *Qi*
- GV-20 Lifts the spirits, clears the Mind, tonifies *Yang*
- PC-6 Calms the Mind and opens the Penetrating Meridian, thereby tonifying the uterus

Bacterial infections

Infections are considered an invasion of the body by the Pathologic Factor. This is similar to Pathogenic Heat in nature, being rapid, causing dryness, damaging *Yin,* and causing lassitude and shortness of breath. As the disorder progresses, the *Wei Qi* is compromised. The Liver is often involved, inhibiting its main function of dispersing and ensuring the smooth flow of *Qi* to the other organs of the body. This leads to *Qi* Deficiency throughout the body. Of particular clinical significance is Spleen Deficiency, which leads to *Qi* Deficiency, Phlegm, and Stasis of Blood. Acupuncture points to consider include the following:

- LI-11 Clears Heat, resolves Dampness, regulates Nutritive *Qi* and Blood, benefits the sinews and is the Earth Point
- LI-4 Expels Wind Heat and releases the Exterior; tonifies *Qi;* Source Point; tonifies the Defensive Qi

- ST-36 Master Point of the Abdomen; treats any Deficiency; regulates *Wei Qi;* dispels Cold; tonifies *Qi* and Blood

Feather-plucking disorders

The causes of feather plucking are highly variable and include systemic diseases, organ failure, allergies, parasitism, and psychogenic causes. Most cases are psychogenic, but all feather pluckers should have a complete diagnostic workup to rule out other causes.

The cause of the feather plucking dictates the selection of acupuncture points (Figs. 35-1 to 35-3). Formulas for psychogenic plucking also vary among individual birds, but a common point selection might include the following:

- ST-36 Master Point of the Abdomen; treats any Deficiency; regulates *Wei Qi;* dispels Cold; tonifies *Qi* and blood
- LI-4 Expels Wind Heat and releases the Exterior; tonifies *Qi;* Source Point; tonifies the Defensive *Qi*
- LI-11 Clears Heat; resolves Dampness; regulates Nutritive *Qi* and Blood; benefits the sinews and Earth Point
- PC-6 Calms the Mind; regulates Heart *Qi;* relieves irritability caused by stagnation of Liver *Qi*
- HT-7 Calms the Mind; regulates other emotional problems; improves thinking

Other points that might be included are GV-20, LIV-3, SP-6, and BL-12. Each point formula must be individualized according to the patient's diagnosis and may change as the acupuncture sessions continue. Birds can often be divided into various TCM diagnostic categories, including those in Box 35-3. Some points listed above, combined with some points mentioned in each category, might be included in a bird's point formula.

Western Herbs, Glandulars, and Supplements

Western Herbs

Western herbs can be administered to exotic animals with reasonable success. The same cautions already mentioned for Chinese herbs apply. Dosing is determined as detailed for Chinese herbs. All herbs vary in potency, so exact dosing recommendations are difficult. Idiosyncratic reactions to specific herbs, both Eastern and Western, have not been researched in exotic species. Idiosyncratic reactions are possible, and professional discretion is advised. Beginning at a lower dose and slowly working up to a dose that produces the desired therapeutic result is recommended. Hundreds of possible herbs may be considered; only a few are described here. The pharmacologic effects of these herbs are discussed in Chapter 20. Some Western

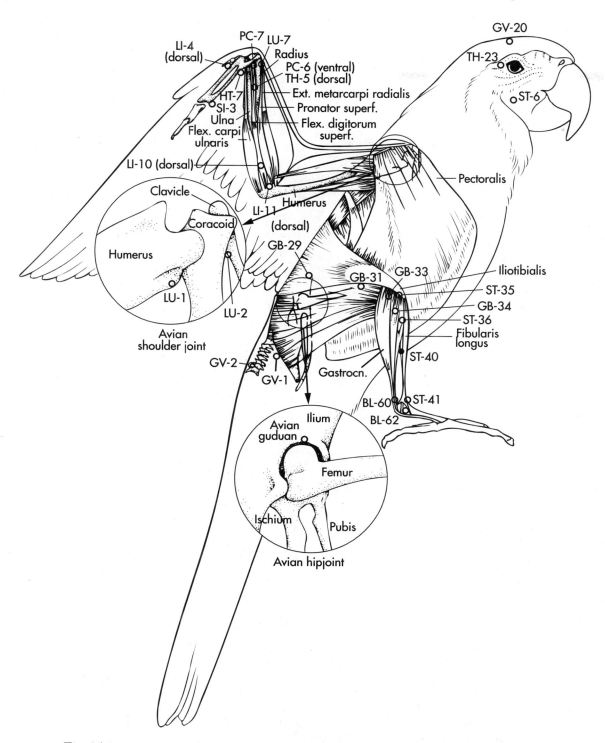

Fig. 35-1 Acupuncture points of birds, lateral view. (From Schoen AM: *Veterinary acupuncture: ancient art to modern medicine,* St Louis, 1994, Mosby.)

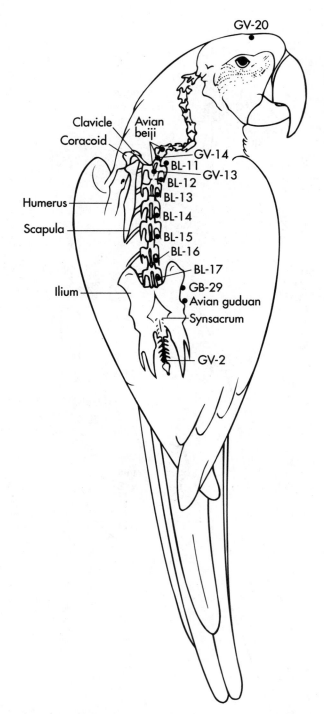

Fig. 35-2   Acupuncture points of birds, dorsal view. (From Schoen AM: *Veterinary acupuncture: ancient art to modern medicine,* St Louis, 1994, Mosby.)

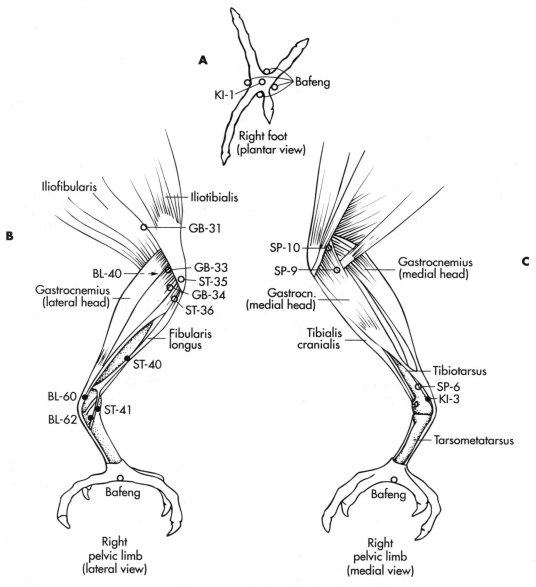

Fig. 35-3 Acupuncture points of the avian leg and foot. **A**, Right foot, plantar view. **B**, Right pelvic limb, lateral view. **C**, Right pelvic limb, medial view. (From Schoen AM: *Veterinary acupuncture: ancient art to modern medicine,* St Louis, 1994, Mosby.)

herbs used with birds and their possible beneficial effects (Kidd, 1995; Tierra, 1988) are as follows:

- Slippery elm bark—gastrointestinal antiinflammatory effects, parasites
- Echinacea—antibacterial and antiviral effects
- Garlic—antimicrobial effects
- Valerian—sedative and calming effects
- Milk thistle—hepatoprotective and hepatoregenerative effects
- Goldenseal—antiinflammatory, astringent, diuretic, and laxative effects
- Calendula—topical treatment of wound healing
- Aloe vera—topical treatment for burn wounds to feet, accelerated healing of skin; improves stamina
- Dandelion—liver and gallbladder problems; stimulates production of bile; excellent tonic

Glandulars

Glandulars are used extensively and appear to be efficacious in birds, rabbits, ferrets, and other small mammals. Birds often have liver-associated pathologic conditions, so liver glandulars are commonly prescribed. The scientific basis of glandular therapy is discussed in Chapter 6.

TCM Diagnostic Categories

STAGNATION OF LIVER *Qi*
Signs might include melancholy, frustration, depression, moodiness
Points used might include LIV 3, GB 34, PC 6, SP 6

LIVER *Yang* RISING
Signs might include irritability, anger
Points used might include SP 6, PC 6, LI 11, BL 40, ST 36

FEAR
Injures Kidneys and Adrenals
Points used might include HT 7, KI 3, SP 6, PC 6

ANXIETY AND WORRY
Points used might include HT 7, SP 6 (worry depletes Spleen *Qi*)

Correct use of glandulars requires a diagnosis of inflammation or damage to a specific body organ. The glandulars given correspond to the organs that are diseased. Diagnostic tests are indicated to determine the type of glandular needed. In birds the most common glandulars used are as follows:

- Liver disease—liver glandular
- Impaired feather development—thyroid glandular
- Renal disease—kidney glandular

Supplements

Supplements are nutritional products containing vitamins, minerals, coenzymes, and cofactors. They are administered to improve a body system function (e.g., immune system function). It is beyond the scope of the chapter to discuss the great number of supplements that can be used in birds and other exotic animals. Only a select few of the more common, particularly important supplements are discussed here. The pharmacologic basis of various nutritional supplements is discussed in Chapter 3.

- Beta-carotene—excellent for epithelial tissues, respiratory system, kidney system, alimentary tract; a good choice for general supplementation because many birds are vitamin A deficient
- Selenium—required for thyroid function; can help produce better skin, hair, and feathers, especially when combined with vitamin E and zinc; can be given only in trace amounts because toxicity is possible
- Vitamin E—a free radical scavenger; needed in conjunction with metalloenzymes (zinc, copper, iron,

selenium); cellular respiration; adenosine triphosphate metabolism; sulfur amino acid metabolism (Scott, Nesheim, Young, 1982)
- Vitamin C—an essential vitamin that cannot be produced by the guinea pig and must be provided in the diet
- Psyllium husks—provide fiber (rabbits are susceptible to enterotoxemia at least in part because of a lack of fiber in the diet) (Jenkins, 1993)

In addition to individual herbs and supplements, many products on the market are combinations of herbs, glandulars, and other supplements. These products are often very useful. To prescribe combination products effectively, the veterinarian must become acquainted with some of the various companies, their product lines, and the indications for use. The reader is referred to the Resources section for more information.

Integrating Holistic Therapies into the Avian and Exotic Species Practice

Holistic medicine is as difficult to learn as Western medicine. Acupuncturists and homeopaths study for years to become highly proficient in their practices. Exotic-animal veterinarians must choose a place to begin when they decide to incorporate holistic therapies into a traditional Western practice.

Herbal medicine and nutritional supplements are perhaps the easiest and safest areas to begin adding holistic therapies to general practice. Veterinarians may order catalogs from suppliers of herbs and nutritional supplements (see the reference section of this book) and can expect to see gratifying results immediately.

Acupuncture is more difficult and poses a real danger of producing untoward sequelae. Before using acupuncture, veterinarians should receive training. The best source for this training is the International Veterinary Acupuncture Society (IVAS).

Homeopathy is usually safe when used by a novice, but effective results are difficult to achieve. Training in veterinary homeopathy is available from the Academy of Veterinary Homeopathy.

Further research must be conducted to evaluate efficacy, appropriate dosage, and safety of the various therapies specifically for exotic species. Veterinarians should receive additional postgraduate training in these modalities and should be cautious when prescribing specific nutritional and botanical supplements, reviewing the appropriate literature for dosages and toxicity. Appropriate permission and release forms should be signed by pet owners before the veterinarian administers botanical and nutritional supplements that have not been approved for exotic species.

With training and effort, holistic therapies can be effectively added to Western veterinary medical practice. The results for the patient are increased health and recovery from disease. For veterinarians the ability to treat diseases that were previously considered untreatable is perhaps the most gratifying reward.

REFERENCES

Axelson RD: Caring for your pet bird, Toronto, 1981, Canaviax Publications.

Barton SL: Reptile nutrition: herbivorous species. In *Chicago Herpetological Society members handbook,* Chicago, 1984, CHS.

Bensky D: *Chinese herbal medicines: formulas and strategies,* Seattle, Eastland.

Boyer DM: An overview of captive reptile diets. Proceedings of the Student American Veterinary Medical Association Symposium, Fort Collins, Colo, 1987.

Boyer TH: *A practitioner's guide to reptilian husbandry and care,* The Professional Library Series, Lakewood, Colo, 1993, American Animal Hospital Association.

Brown SA: *A practitioner's guide to rabbits and ferrets,* The Professional Library Series, Lakewood, Colo, 1993, American Animal Hospital Association.

Dumonceaux G, Harrison G: Toxins. In Ritchie B, Harrison G, Harrison L, (eds): *Avian medicine: principles and applications,* Lake Worth, Fla, 1994, Wingers.

Ebling D: *The Chinese herbalist's handbook,* Santa Fe, NM, Inword Press.

Forshaw JM: *Parrots of the world,* Neptune, NJ, 1973, T.F.H. Publications.

Fox JG: *Biology and diseases of the ferret,* Philadelphia, 1988, Lea & Febiger.

Fratkin J: *Chinese herbal patient formulas: a practical guide,* Boulder, Colo, 1986, Shya Publications.

Gerlach H: Update on the macaw wasting syndrome, Miami, 1986, *Proc Assoc Avian Vets*

Goeddert A: *Chinese herbs in the Western clinic,* Dublin, Calif, 1994, Get Well Foundation.

Graham DL: Wasting/proventricular dilation disease: a pathologist's view, Chicago, 1991, *Proc Assoc Avian Vets,* Miami, Fla.

Grau CR: *Exotic bird report no. 1,* Davis, Calif, 1983, Department of Avian Sciences, University of California.

Hering C: *The guiding symptoms of our materia medica,* New Delhi, India, 1993, B. Jain.

Hsu H: *Commonly used Chinese herb formulas with illustrations,* Long Beach, Calif, 1990, Oriental Healing Arts Institute.

Huang KC: *The pharmacology of Chinese herbs,* Boca Raton, Fla, 1993, CRC Press.

Jackson FR: The life of the kea, *The Canterbury Mountaineer,* vol 31, 1962.

Jenkins JR: *A Practitioner's guide to rabbits and ferrets,* The Professional Library Series, Lakewood, Colo, 1993, American Animal Hospital Association.

Kidd R: Using herbs in pets. In *Proceedings of the Annual Conference of the Am Holistic Vet Med Assoc,* Snowmass, Colo, 1995.

Künzli J: *Kent's repertorium generale* (English edition), Berg, Germany, 1987, Barthel & Barthel.

Lafeber TJ: *Tender loving care for pet birds,* Park Ridge, Ill, 1977, Dorothy Products.

Lumeij JT: Gastroenterology. In Ritchie B, Harrison G, Harrison L, (eds): *Avian medicine: principles and application,* Lake Worth, Fla, 1994, Wingers.

Lutz ME, Wilson RB: Proventricular dilatation syndrome in an umbrella cockatoo, *J Am Vet Med Assoc* 198:1962, 1991.

Maciocia G: *The foundations of Chinese medicine: a comprehensive text for acupuncturists and herbalists,* New York, 1989, Churchill Livingstone.

McCluggage DM: Avian holistic veterinary medical care. In *Proceedings of the Annual Conference of the American Holistic Veterinary Medical Association,* Snowmass, Colo, 1995a.

McCluggage D: Presurgical Evaluation and Intraoperative Support Techniques. In *Proc Annu Conference Assoc Avian Vet,* Phoenix, 1989b.

McCluggage D: Efficacy of avian diagnostic tests. In Proceedings of the American Animal Hospital Association, 56th Annual Meeting, St. Louis, 1989c.

Mitscher LA: Plant-derived antibiotics. In Weinstein MJ, Wagman GH, editors: *Antibiotics,* vol 15, New York, 1978, Plenum Press.

Nearenberg DS, Roudybush TE, Grau CR: Hand-fed vs. parent-fed cockatiels: a comparison of chick growth. In Proceedings of the 34th Western Poultry Disease Conference, Davis, Calif, March 3-6, 1985.

Partington M: Avian acupuncture. In Schoen AM, editor: *Veterinary acupuncture: ancient art to modern medicine,* St Louis, 1994a, Mosby.

Partington M: The stomach meridian and its acupuncture points. In *Veterinary acupuncture course manual,* ed 3, Nederland, Colo, 1994b, IVAS.

Partington M: The spleen meridian and its acupuncture points. In *Veterinary acupuncture course manual,* ed 3, Nederland, Colo, 1994c, IVAS.

Roudybush T: Growth, signs of deficiency, and weaning in cockatiels fed deficient diets. In Proceedings of the 1986 Annual Meeting of the Association of Avian Veterinarians.

Sankaran R: *The spirit of homeopathy,* Bombay, 1991, Homeopathic Medical Publishers.

Scott ML, Nesheim MC, Young RJ: *Nutrition of the chicken,* Ithaca, NY, 1982, Scotts & Associates.

Taylor-Limehouse P: Pericardium meridian of hand-jueyin. In *Veterinary acupuncture course manual,* ed 3, Nederland, Colo, 1994, IVAS.

Tierra M: *Planetary herbology,* Twin Lakes, Wisc, 1988, Lotus Press.

Vanden Berge JC, Zweers GA: Myologia. In Baumel JJ (ed): *Handbook of avian anatomy: nomina anatomica avium,* Cambridge, Mass, 1993, Nuttall Ornithological Club.

Chapter 36

Integration into Surgical Practice

ELAINE R. CAPLAN

Surgical practice presents veterinarians with many challenges. Alternative therapies have been used perioperatively for pain control (musculoskeletal, spinal, and visceral), respiratory and cardiovascular stimulation, circulatory enhancement, bone healing, acceleration of wound healing, anorexia, nausea, and immune stimulation. Therapies include acupuncture, homeopathy, herbal medicine, chiropractic, and physical therapy.

Every case must be approached individually. A complete history and physical examination are imperative whether a surgery is as routine as a castration, as complicated as a total hip replacement, or as critical as a gastric dilatation volvulus. All surgical cases must be worked up appropriately to establish a definitive diagnosis and identify concurrent or preexisting conditions (e.g., coagulopathic disorders, anemia, immune-mediated diseases, cardiac disease, neoplasia) that may complicate surgery, anesthesia, or healing. Concurrently administered drugs such as corticosteroids may interfere with healing and drugs such as aspirin with hemostasis.

Alternative therapies may be used alone, in conjunction with conventional medical therapies, or in conjunction with other alternative therapies. For example, a dog with cervical pain may receive a corticosteroid trial (conventionally) and acupuncture (or other alternative therapy) to control neurogenic pain or muscle spasms. If the animal does not respond to this treatment trial, a myelogram, cerebrospinal fluid tap, and computed tomography scan may be necessary to rule out intervertebral disk disease, inflammatory or infectious etiology, tumor, and caudal cervical vertebral instability. If surgery is necessary, acupuncture, herbal, homeopathic therapy, and physical therapy may be incorporated into the immediate postoperative period and long-term rehabilitation process. This chapter discusses the use of alternative therapies in surgical practice. Theories, practical applications, and contraindications are discussed.

Acupuncture

Acupuncture can be used in many situations in surgical practice, such as pain management, rehabilitation after spinal surgery or orthopedic surgery, and postoperative convalescence problems such as anorexia and nausea. It can be included in the treatment of anesthetic complications such as respiratory and cardiac arrest or cerebral hypoxia. Moreover, experimental and clinical trials have found acupuncture-induced surgical anesthesia to be efficacious in many species.

Pain management is a common indication for acupuncture. Examples include perioperative pain management for thoracolumbar and cervical intervertebral disk disease, spinal fractures, and various orthopedic conditions. Nervous system dysfunction can result from disorders that cause pain or impaired function (Joseph, 1994). Pain results from pathologic processes that irritate meninges, ligaments, dorsal nerve roots, and periosteum of the vertebral canal with their innervation by nociceptive receptors. The most common neurologic disease treated for pain at the Animal Medical Center is intervertebral disk disease (Joseph, 1994).

The effectiveness of acupuncture for thoracolumbar disk disease varies according to the degree of the condition. In grade I disease (back pain only) a success rate of approximately 90% occurs within 1 to 2 weeks and with 1 to 3 treatments. In grade II disease (pain, paresis, ataxic gait, and conscious proprioceptive deficits) a success rate of 90% occurs in 3 weeks with 3 to 4 treatments. In grade III disease (paralysis, inability to stand or bear weight, and possible loss of conscious bladder control) a total recovery occurs in approximately 80% of patients within 6 weeks with 5 to 6 treatments. Only 10% of animals do not recover; the other 10% partially recover (e.g., no conscious bladder control). In grade IV disease (paralysis and no conscious pain perception in the rear toes) a recovery rate of less than 25% occurs within 3 to 6 months and with 10 or more treatments. Overall, 90% of animals with grades I to III disease recover over an average of 4 to 5 weeks with an average of 4 treatments (at 1 treatment a week). However, patients with grades III and IV disease should have a myelogram and surgery if seen within 24 to 36 hours after the onset of symptoms. For grade IV disease, treatments with acupuncture are only half as effective as rapidly performed surgery. Acupuncture should be used in grade IV cases if patients are seen at a later stage of grade IV disease. The effectiveness of acupuncture in grades I to II disease is comparable with that of surgery, drug therapy, or both (Janssens, 1994).

The effectiveness of acupuncture treatment for cervical disk disease also varies. In Grade I disease (neck pain only) a success rate of approximately 80% occurs within 1 to 2 weeks with 3 to 4 treatments. For grade II disease (neck pain and proprioceptive deficits) a success rate of 66.6% occurs within 3 to 4 weeks with 5 to 6 treatments. Too few cases of grade III disease (paralysis and neck pain) have been described to report adequate results. About one third of the successfully treated acupuncture patients with cervical disk disease relapse within 3 years (a higher percentage than for thoracolumbar disk disease and in agreement with results described for other conservative cervical disk disease treatments). Supplemental treatment (e.g., rest, bladder monitoring, padding, physical therapy) may be required. Surgical decompression for cervical disk disease is probably more effective than acupuncture. However, surgical treatment is expensive and sometimes risky, so acupuncture may be tried first. In a rapidly deteriorating situation a workup and surgery are recommended.

Acupuncture mechanisms may include local analgesia and antiinflammation, which decreases local spinal inflammation, edema, vasodilation or constriction, and histamine or kinin release. This lessens scar tissue formation, cord compression or hypoxemia, and pain. Acupuncture can abolish trigger points, thus abrogating muscle pain and shortening, stiffness, and referred pain. Axonal regrowth and thus regeneration of destroyed axons in the spinal cord can also be activated by acupuncture (Janssens, 1994).

Orthopedic conditions such as chronic degenerative joint disease are often seen in surgical practice. One study found that 70% of canine patients with chronic degenerative joint disease showed more than 50% improvement in mobility and ambulation after acupuncture. The 65 dogs in this study were no longer responding to conventional medications or surgery and were either recommended for euthanasia or consigned to chronic pain (Schoen, 1994).

Acupuncture is an option for patients with diseases usually treated with surgery but who are poor surgical candidates because of concurrent medical problems (e.g., a 10-year-old poodle with a chronic ruptured cranial cruciate ligament; patients with concurrent Cushing's disease, diabetes mellitus, congestive heart failure, renal disease). Some owners wish to pursue acupuncture for pain control before undertaking a more invasive procedure, such as in the case of a 7-year-old German shepherd with severe canine hip dysplasia and osteoarthritis in which a total hip replacement is the surgical option.

Rehabilitation is an important use of acupuncture, particularly in patients recovering from neurologic and orthopedic procedures. Animals who are paralyzed or paretic as a result of intervertebral disk disease (e.g., diffuse spinal cord swelling) or trauma (e.g., spinal fractures, radial nerve paralysis) benefit from tonification techniques. In contrast to sedation techniques (pain control), acupuncture stimulates nerves and nerve healing. The goal is to improve sensory and motor function, resulting in improved ambulation and resolution of other neurologic dysfunctions such as urinary and fecal incontinence. An important concept in orthopedic rehabilitation is the prevention of fracture disease. An immobilized limb may result in fracture disease, which manifests as atrophy of bone, soft tissue, nails, and skin (Herron, 1993). Stable fixation that allows the limb the most rapid return to normal weight bearing and function should be used. Patients undergoing fracture repair or joint surgery may need physical therapy postoperatively, and acupuncture can assist by increasing circulation and decreasing pain and muscle spasms, thereby promoting early return to function. Another perioperative application of acupuncture is wound healing. Delayed wound healing may result from infection, poor circulation, poor nutrition, and dehydration (Pavletic, 1993). Local cold laser on healthy tissue at the edge of the wound improves local vasodilation and phagocytosis, enhances cell metabolism (e.g., mitosis, local protein synthesis, local antibody formation, and activity of local tissue enzymes), and has an analgesic effect. Transcutaneous electrical nerve stimulation, acupuncture, and electroacupuncture across the wound have similar effects (Rogers, 1994).

During convalescence, animals may experience anorexia, nausea, vomiting, and regurgitation depending on the procedure performed or condition. For example, cats may become anorexic and develop hepatic lipidosis, and a dog with a gastric or an intestinal foreign body may experience ileus. Acupuncture stimulates the appetite and controls nausea and vomiting. A clinical study by Lao and others (1995) has shown that an effective antiemetic effect against morphine in the ferret results when electroacupuncture is used at the point *Neiguan* (P-6). In addition, acupuncture has a reported effect on postoperative nausea and vomiting (Dundee, Ghaly, 1989; Ho and others, 1989; Watcha, White, 1992). Common points used for anorexia include ST-36 and SP-6.

Some surgical patients may be immunocompromised as a result of neoplasia, concurrent infections (FeLV, feline immunodeficiency virus, Lyme disease, bacterial), or concurrent autoimmune disease. Acupuncture points exist for immune stimulation and immunosuppression and for enhancing production of white blood cells and phagocytosis. Acupuncture activates specific and nonspecific immune reactions (e.g., leukocytosis, phagocytosis, antibody production, complement, bactericidal factors) and controls many of the main symptoms in bacterial diseases in humans and animals. Acupuncture with conventional therapies also may be beneficial in patients with sepsis (e.g., septic abdomen resulting from ruptured pyometra, intestinal perforation, prostatic abscess) (Rogers, 1994).

Anesthetic complications can be addressed with acupuncture in conjunction with conventional drugs. Apnea or cardiac arrest can be treated with points that have sympathomimetic effects (e.g., GV-26, KID-1). The practitioner can use any small-gauge hypodermic needle if acupuncture needles are not available. GV-26 is located on the midline in the nasal philtrum at the level of the ventral borders of the nasal orifices. The practitioner inserts the needle and vigorously manipulates it by simultaneously twirling and inserting the needle in a delicate jabbing motion for up to 10 minutes. Acupuncture stimulation at GV-26 may be performed without interfering with conventional treatments. After cesarean section, respiration can be stimulated in newborn puppies with acupuncture (GV-26) (Schoen, 1992). A patient may experience cerebral anoxia as a result of deep, prolonged anesthesia. Clinically these patients may be cerebrally dull to comatose. In addition to conventional drugs, acupuncture points such as GV-20, GB-20, and LI-4 may be used to hasten recovery.

Acupuncture-induced surgical analgesia (AISA) has been reported in humans, horses, cattle, sheep, dogs, and cats. No apparent negative physiologic effects are associated with AISA, including respiratory depression and decreased blood pressure and cardiac output, which are produced by various injectable and inhalant anesthetics. Intraoperative bleeding seems to be less than normal with AISA. Acupuncture may be a suitable alternative for patients who have experienced drug reactions to a particular anesthetic or analgesic (Klide, 1994).

Treating postoperative pain with acupuncture may also be an alternative for high-risk respiratory compromised patients. For example, use of an opioid that produces respiratory depression may be a serious concern in brachycephalic dogs (e.g., bulldogs) and a geriatric patient with chronic pulmonary disease (Klide, 1994).

Acupuncture can reduce minimum alveolar concentration for halothane in dogs by 11% to 17%. This enables a patient to remain on a lighter level of anesthesia throughout a procedure, which is especially advantageous in high-risk patients physiologically compromised by disease. This same reduction has been shown in dogs for various agonist/antagonist analgesics such as pentazocine, butorphanol, and nalbuphine. However, an opiate pathway may not be involved in the mechanism by which acupuncture caused the decrease in halothane minimum alveolar concentration. Potential problems in using AISA include lack of restraint, inadequate or inconsistent analgesia, and lack of information on points to use for analgesia in a particular surgical site (Klide, 1994).

The International Veterinary Acupuncture Society certification course has certified several hundred veterinarians in acupuncture. The AVMA Guidelines for Alternative and Complementary Veterinary Medicine approved by the AVMA House of Delegates in 1996 state that "Veterinary acupuncture and acutherapy involve the examination and stimulation of specific points on the body of nonhuman animals by use of acupuncture needles, moxibustion, injections, low-level lasers, magnets, and a variety of other techniques for the diagnosis and treatment of numerous conditions in animals. Veterinary acupuncture and acutherapy are now considered an integral part of veterinary medicine. These techniques should be regarded as surgical and/or medical procedures under state veterinary practice acts. It is recommended that educational programs be undertaken by veterinarians before they are considered competent to practice veterinary acupuncture" (AVMA, 1997).

Herbal Medicine

Chinese herbs have been used in veterinary medicine in China for thousands of years. Chinese herbs can be used as the primary treatment of a disorder, in conjunction with acupuncture protocols, and with standard veterinary medicine. Herbs can be prescribed according to Western diagnosis; more preformulated mixtures are being produced with Western indications. Herbs are more versatile if the diagnosis is based on traditional Chinese medicine (TCM) (Schwartz, 1994).

The herbal system uses parts of plants, animals, or minerals and extracts their essences in alcohol or water. According to TCM, each herb has its own flavor and taste, energy or characteristic, meridians of influence, direction, categories, and actions. A particular active constituent is not sought, but rather the plant itself, along with environmental experience, is considered therapeutic. According to Western pharmacology, herbs contain constituents that are responsible for their therapeutic actions. Four categories of active constituents are polysaccharides, flavonoids, steroids, and alkaloids (Schwartz, 1994).

In TCM, herbal formulas are used more frequently than single herbs. In veterinary medicine, using prepared formulas available commercially is more practical. Formulas are provided as freeze-dried granules, powdered raw herbs, liquid tinctures, tablets, or capsules (Schwartz, 1994).

Applications of patented herbs in surgical practice include correction of hemostasis, swelling, pain, and circulation (blood activating). Geriatric patients or animals with chronic debilitating diseases undergoing surgery can benefit from tonification effects of herbs (e.g., ginseng, astragalus). These patients may experience generalized weakness, anorexia, anemia, or immune deficiency.

Huang (1993) describes the benefits of ginseng as follows:

> **Ginseng is reputed to be effective in treatment of shock, collapse of the cardiovascular system, hemorrhage, and heart failure. Ginsenocides have been**

used in the treatment of *Escherichia coli* endotoxin–induced septic shock in dogs, preventing the inhibitory effect of endotoxin on myocardial function and restoring falling blood pressure. Ginseng can reduce the effects of oxygen deprivation on brain tissue and improve mental and neurologic performance.

Yunnan Paiyao is a hemostatic preparation used for internal and external bleeding and traumatic swelling. It can be used as a first-aid treatment in animals with internal bleeding from tongue lacerations, aural hematomas, perianal surgery, or any procedure where profuse bleeding is expected. Postoperatively, *Yunnan Paiyao* can be given to enhance healing (Schwartz, 1994).

Kang Gu Zeng Shen Pian (combat bone hyperplasia pill) is used to treat ventral bridging spondylosis (including cervical, thoracolumbar, and lumbosacral). After surgery for intervertebral disk disease, *Kang Gu Zeng Sheng Pian* can be used for pain relief and to enhance healing. In TCM, it strengthens yang and *Qi*, fortifies the marrow, and decreases tendon and ligament dampness and pain (Schwartz, 1994).

San Qi 17 or *Chin Koo Tieh Shang Wan* (over-the-counter patented form) is used to activate blood circulation. These formulations are also useful in reducing swelling and pain and occasionally for soft tissue bruising (Schwartz, 1994).

Most herbal formulas used in the West on animals are based on human prescriptions and not approved in animals. AVMA policy states that "Veterinary botanical medicine is the use of plants and plant derivatives as therapeutic agents. It is recommended that continued research and education be conducted. Since some of these botanicals may be toxic when used at inappropriate doses, it is imperative that botanical medicine be practiced only by licensed veterinarians who have been educated in veterinary botanical medicine. Communication on the use of these compounds within the context of a valid veterinarian/client/patient relationship is important" (AVMA, 1997).

Homeopathy

Homeopathy uses remedies from plants, animals, and minerals and seeks to stimulate the innate healing power (vital force) or the immune system of the body. It is a philosophy of health and a formal system of drug therapeutics that traces its origins to Samuel Hahnemann (1755-1843). According to Hahnemann the proper remedy for an illness is the substance that produces the same symptoms in a healthy person as those exhibited by the sick patient (Weiner, 1996). Unlike orthodox medical practice the higher the potency of a homeopathic preparation, the smaller the amount of the medicinal substance present in solution. The process of potentiation (repeated subdivision and dilution with succession) releases the curative powers of the medication. Through administration of remedies carefully selected to match all the patient's symptoms, homeopathy treats disorders of the body, mind, and

emotions (Weiner, 1996). Only one remedy should be given at a time, although combination remedies are available. Several homeopathic remedies, including *Arnica Montana, Symphytum,* and *Hypericum,* are considered useful in the perioperative surgical period.

> *Arnica Montana* (leopard's bane) is a perennial herb of the family Compositae. *Arnica* promotes healing, controls hemorrhage, and reduces swelling. After trauma (especially injury to soft tissues with swelling and bruising) and shock, *Arnica* is the first remedy the practitioner should consider. It is useful in the immediate postoperative period to minimize bruising and swelling (Castro, 1991).
> *Symphytum* (comfrey) is of the plant family Boraginaceae. *Symphytum* is from the Greek word *sympho,* "to unite." The plant contains the substance allantoin, which stimulates cells to heal faster. *Symphytum* is administered to speed fracture healing in long bones and for pain relief. It is particularly useful in delayed healing or nonunion fractures (Castro, 1991).
> *Hypericum perfoliatum* (St. John's wort) is an herb from the family Hypericacaea. It is the first remedy practitioners should consider in patients with neurologic trauma. Thus perioperative administration is an application in patients undergoing neurologic surgery. Administration of Arnica first to prevent swelling and bruising and then Hypericum is often necessary (Castro, 1991).

AVMA policy states that "Veterinary homeopathy is a medical discipline in which conditions in nonhuman animals are treated by the administration of substances that are capable of producing clinical signs in healthy animals similar to those of the animal to be treated. These substances are used therapeutically in minute doses. Research in veterinary homeopathy is limited. Clinical and anecdotal evidence exists to indicate that veterinary homeopathy may be beneficial. It is recommended that further research be conducted in veterinary homeopathy to evaluate efficacy, indications, and limitations. Since some of these substances may be toxic when used at inappropriate doses, it is imperative that veterinary homeopathy be practiced only by licensed veterinarians who have been educated in veterinary homeopathy" (AVMA, 1997). A certification course in veterinary homeopathy is available through Richard Pitcairn, DVM.

Chiropractic

Chiropractic deals with the relationship between the nervous system and spinal cord and the role of this relationship in the restoration and maintenance of health. Hippocrates reportedly used spinal manipulation along with medication. In the late nineteenth century, B.J. Palmer maintained a veterinary hospital "to prove to ourselves that the chiropractic principles did apply." The scientific rationale for chiropractic is that homeostasis and an inherent recuperative ability exist within the body. The nervous system controls homeostasis. Faulty musculoskeletal relationships cause neurologic dysfunction (Willoughby, 1994).

The vertebral subluxation complex is the basis of chiropractic theories. *Subluxation* in chiropractic is defined as the disrelationship of a vertebral segment in association with contiguous vertebrae resulting in a disturbance of normal biomechanical and neurologic function. Clinically, subluxations can manifest as lack of joint play, palpable soft tissue changes, muscle contraction, and aberrant function of associated neural elements. The vertebral subluxation complex results in neuropathy and kinesiopathy. Neuropathy can result in facilitation (increased stimulation of end organs) such as muscle hypertonicity, increased glandular function, and paresthesia or pain. Kinesiopathy is a change in motor function. Hypomobility, or fixation, is the inability of the vertebra to move freely in the correct range of motion. Hypermobility is an increased range of motion in vertebral joints with increased stress on joint structures and supporting ligaments (Willoughby, 1994).

A chiropractic adjustment is a short-lever, specific, high-velocity, controlled, forceful thrust by a hand or an instrument directed at specific articulations to restore biomechanical and neurologic function (Willoughby, 1991). Only one motor unit is adjusted at a time. (A *motor unit* is defined as two adjacent vertebrae, ligaments, muscles, joints, nerves, blood vessels, and contents of the vertebral foramen.) The force of the adjustment relies on acceleration or speed to move a vertebral segment (Willoughby, 1994).

Clinical application of chiropractic has primarily been associated with control of back pain, radiculopathies (sciatic neuralgia), and autonomic nervous dysfunction (incontinence). Back pain may be caused by muscle spasms, facet syndrome, joint capsule pain, or subluxations. Iatrogenic subluxations are possible when an animal is under anesthesia and loss of muscle tone occurs. Subluxations may result because of improper patient positioning or failure to support the neck during transport to and from the operating room. Temporomandibular joint problems may result iatrogenically during intubation or from excessive manipulation during dental procedures. These animals may experience pain and have difficulty chewing after the dental procedure. Postoperatively, chiropractic is useful in rehabilitation, especially to counter the effects of compensation (such as an animal favoring one leg, thus putting more stress on other areas such as the back or other limbs). This is particularly important in athletic animals to correct movement aberrations. Chiropractic may be contraindicated in acute intervertebral disk disease, trauma, spinal compression, and neoplasia (in which it may cause pathologic fracture). Chiropractic can be performed in conjunction with acupuncture with synergistic and longer lasting results (Willoughby, 1994).

AVMA policy states that "Veterinary chiropractic is the examination, diagnosis, and treatment of nonhuman animals through manipulation and adjustments of specific joints and cranial sutures. The term *veterinary chiropractic* should not be interpreted to include dispensing medication, performing surgery, injecting medications, recommending supplements, or replacing traditional veterinary care. While sufficient research exists documenting the efficacy of chiropractic, research in veterinary chiropractic is limited. Sufficient clinical and anecdotal evidence exists to indicate that veterinary chiropractic can be beneficial. It is recommended that further research be conducted in veterinary chiropractic to evaluate efficacy, indications, and limitations. The assurance of education in veterinary chiropractic is central to the ability of the veterinary profession to provide this service. Veterinary chiropractic should be performed by licensed veterinarians; however, at this time, some areas of the country do not have an adequate supply of veterinarians educated in veterinary chiropractic. Therefore, it is recommended that, where the states' practice acts permit, a licensed chiropractor educated in veterinary chiropractic be allowed to practice this modality under the supervision of, or referred by, a licensed veterinarian who is providing concurrent care" (AVMA, 1997). Currently the American Veterinary Chiropractic Association administers the only certification course in veterinary chiropractic for veterinarians and chiropractors.

Physical Therapy

A 1995 article by Nicoll reviews the benefits of physiotherapeutic techniques. Physical therapy uses cold or heat, massage, and therapeutic exercises to treat disease or trauma. The goal is early return to function or ambulation after various orthopedic procedures and neurologic conditions. Rehabilitation is important after joint surgery, fracture repair, neurologic conditions such as traumatic injury (radial nerve paralysis, spinal fractures), and other spinal cord disease (intervertebral disk disease, caudal cervical vertebral instability, spinal tumors). Recumbent patients are especially responsive to physical therapy. Physiologic benefits include increased blood and lymph flow in the area undergoing treatment, early resolution of inflammation, increased collagen production, prevention of periarticular contraction, promotion of normal joint mechanics, and prevention or reduction of muscle atrophy. Passive range of motion exercises, massage, swimming or hydrotherapy, local hypothermia and hyperthermia, ultrasonography, and neuromuscular stimulation are physical therapeutic techniques used in veterinary medicine.

The movement of joints through a complete range of motion can reduce tissue adhesions, promote normal joint mechanics, enhance venous and lymphatic drainage, and prevent muscle and joint capsule contracture. These exercises should not be performed on unstable fractures, luxations, hypermotile joints, osteopenic bones, and areas with recent skin grafts (Nicoll, 1995).

Massage is extremely beneficial in postoperative rehabilitation and recumbency. Physiologic benefits include increased circulation and decreased edema. In addition, massage loosens and stretches tendons and minimizes scar tissue. The sensation of touch may also lessen anxiety in patients (Nicoll, 1995).

Swimming provides a relatively non–weight-bearing environment. Swimming enhances joint mobility and muscle action. Special therapy pools equipped with an electric pump create a current against which the animal swims (Nicoll, 1995).

Both cold and heat therapy provide physiologic advantages to the patient. Pain perception is decreased by presynaptic inhibition of pain stimuli and reduction of nerve conduction velocity as a result of local hypothermia. Cold therapy also decreases tissue enzyme activity and resultant enzymatic destruction. Local hyperthermia (heat therapy) provides analgesia, local vasodilation, and relaxation of muscle spasm. Caution should be exercised to prevent iatrogenic thermal injury, especially in patients with sensory nerve impairment (Nicoll, 1995).

Ultrasonography provides the most penetrating form of physiologic heat. When ultrasound waves contact living tissue, the energy is converted to heat. This modality is indicated for a variety of musculoskeletal problems, including muscle spasms, adhesions, and tendon or ligament injuries. In dogs, muscle spasms and fibrosis associated with femur fractures can be prevented by ultrasound (Nicoll, 1995).

Neuromuscular stimulation recruits more contracting muscle fibers and can increase the maximal contractile force of each muscle, thus improving muscle strength. The reduction of disuse muscular atrophy resulting from neurologic injury and prolonged immobilization is an important application of neuromuscular stimulation (Nicoll, 1995).

AVMA policy states that "Veterinary physical therapy is the use of noninvasive techniques, excluding veterinary chiropractic, for the rehabilitation of injuries in nonhuman animals. Veterinary physical therapy performed by nonveterinarians should be limited to the use of stretching; massage therapy; stimulation by the use of a) low-level lasers, b) electrical sources, c) magnetic fields, and d) ultrasound; rehabilitation exercises; hydrotherapy; and applications of heat and cold. Veterinary physical therapy should be performed by a licensed veterinarian or, where in accordance with state practice acts, by 1) a licensed, certified, registered veterinary or animal health technician educated in veterinary physical therapy or 2) a licensed physical therapist educated in nonhuman animal anatomy and physiology. Veterinary physical therapy performed by a nonveterinarian should be performed under the supervision of, or referral by, a licensed veterinarian who is providing concurrent care.

"Massage therapy is a technique in which the person uses only their hands and body to massage soft tissues. Massage therapy on nonhuman animals should be performed by a licensed veterinarian with education in massage therapy or, where in accordance with state veterinary practice acts, by a graduate of an accredited massage school who has been educated in nonhuman animal massage therapy. When performed by a nonveterinarian, massage therapy should be performed under the supervision of or referral by a licensed veterinarian who is providing concurrent care" (AVMA, 1997).

Conclusion

A variety of alternative therapies are available to aid in the management of surgical diseases in veterinary medicine. The primary goal of the clinician must always be to make an accurate diagnosis so that all options, conventional as well as alternative, be successfully used in treating the individual patient. Complementary and alternative therapies can greatly aid in the favorable outcome of many curable diseases and contribute to the comfort and function of those patients with chronic diseases. The veterinarian must know the limitations of each modality and communicate these to the client. As more veterinarians are certified in various alternative therapeutic modalities, they will incorporate these therapies into perioperative protocols and patients will reap the benefits of an expanded armamentarium to facilitate recovery and healing.

Bibliography

AVMA: *AVMA directory and resource manual: guidelines for alternative and complementary veterinary medicine,* Schaumburg, Ill, 1997, AVMA.

Castro M: Interna materia medica. In *The complete homeopathy handbook,* New York, 1991, St. Martin's.

Dundee JW, Ghaly RG: Does the timing of P6 acupuncture influence its efficacy as a postoperative antiemetic? *Br J Anaes* 63:630, 1989.

Herron AJ: Fracture disease. In Bojrab MJ, ed: *Disease mechanisms in small animal surgery,* ed 2, Philadelphia, 1993, Lea & Febiger.

Ho RT and others: Electroacupuncture and postoperative emesis, *Anaesthesia* 45:327-329, 1989.

Huang LC: *The pharmacology of Chinese herbs,* Boca Raton, Fla, 1993, CRC.

Janssens LAA: Acupuncture for thoracolumbar and cervical disk disease. In Schoen AM, ed: *Veterinary acupuncture,* St Louis, 1994, Mosby.

Joseph R: Acupuncture for neurologic disorders. In Schoen AM, ed: *Veterinary acupuncture,* St Louis, 1994, Mosby.

Klide AM: Acupuncture for surgical analgesia. In Schoen AM, ed: *Veterinary acupuncture,* St Louis, 1994, Mosby.

Lao L and others: Electroacupuncture reduces morphine-induced emesis in ferrets: a pilot study, *J Altern Compl Med* 1(3):257-261, 1995.

Nicoll SA, Remedius AM: Recumbency in small animals: pathophysiology and management, *Compendium* 17:1367, 1995.

Pavletic M: Common complications in wound healing. In Pavletic M, ed: *Atlas of small animal reconstructive surgery,* Philadelphia, 1993, JB Lippincott.

Rogers PM: Immunologic effects of acupuncture. In Schoen AM, ed: *Veterinary acupuncture,* St Louis, 1994, Mosby.

Schoen AM: Acupuncture for musculoskeletal disorders. In Schoen AM, ed: *Veterinary acupuncture,* St Louis, 1994, Mosby.

Schoen AM: *Acupuncture for cardiac and respiratory arrest,* Proceedings of The North American Veterinary Conference, Orlando, Fla, Jan 1992.

Schwartz C: Chinese herbology in veterinary medicine. In Schoen AM, ed: *Veterinary acupuncture,* St Louis, 1994, Mosby.

Watcha MF, White PF: Postoperative nausea and vomiting, *Anesthesiology* 77:162-184, 1992.

Weiner M: The complete book of homeopathy, Garden City Park, NY, 1996, Avery.

Willoughby SL: Veterinary chiropractic care. In Schoen AM, ed: *Veterinary acupuncture,* St Louis, 1994, Mosby.

Alternative and Complementary Perspectives

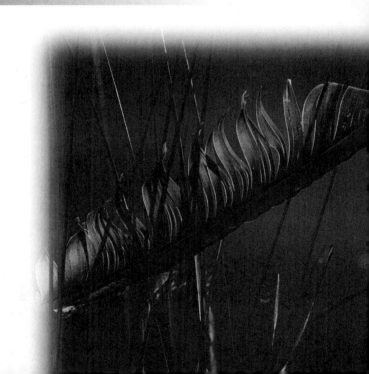

Chapter 37

Veterinary Bioethics

MICHAEL W. FOX

We live in a world of such biologic and ecologic complexity that the element of uncertainty is as omnipresent as intelligent organization in nature's systems, processes, and life-forms. Human society is similarly complex but not always as intelligently self-organizing as natural ecosystems. Human society relies on laws and moral codes to maintain functional integrity and well-being of its members. Advances in the natural (i.e., biologic and physical) sciences have enabled us to overcome to some degree the uncertainty principle and exercise a measure of control over the natural world. However, such knowledge is always incomplete, and the more we learn, the more we realize that we can never gain absolute control. Advances in the scientific domain of understanding are considerable, from the advent of pyrotechnology and petrochemistry to nuclear fission and genetic engineering biotechnology.

We have not advanced to the same degree in the science of human awareness and behavior, or ethics. The discipline of ethics comprises various schools and traditions of questioning, reasoning, and discourse, the most relevant of which is *bioethics*. The science of bioethics considers our roles and responsibilities and the consequences of our activities, products, processes, policies, lifestyles, attitudes, and values in a much wider scope than do other ethical systems. The scope is not limited to a consideration of human rights and interests. Equal and fair consideration* is given to all sentient life-forms, especially in terms of human demands on them and the environment.

---

*Equality of consideration is an animal's basic right. This does not mean that animals are the same as humans, which is the fallacy of anthropomorphic and anthropopsychic thinking. All animals have the right to humane treatment, but animal rights are not always the same as human rights because animals have different needs and interests.

The basic principles of bioethics can be summarized as seven Golden Rules (Box 37-1). These rules are generic in that they apply to public policies, personal lifestyles, and professional and corporate activities. They are therefore relevant to the practice and principles of veterinary medicine. It should be noted that bioethics is a synthesis of scientific and empathic knowledge, especially from the fields of ecology, ethology, cultural anthropology, and social economics.

Veterinary Responsibilities

Veterinarians belong to a unique professional guild that, compared with most other academic and business professions, has considerable empathic and scientific knowledge about animals. Veterinarians therefore have a significant yet largely unexplored role to play in both society and science.

Veterinarians have existed for thousands of years. As interlocutors between people, animals, and nature, their empathic, scientific, and instrumental knowledge was highly valued by society. Indeed, according to Professor Calvin Schwabe in his book *Cattle, Priests and Progress in Medicine* (1978), the earliest veterinarians were the priest-healer members of ancient Egypt's many dynasties. However, few of today's farm animals receive the same quality of veterinary care and husbandry that their ancestors enjoyed. Few veterinary experts have sufficient knowledge of good livestock husbandry, ethology, pasture and range management, and ecologic farming practices to advise society in these areas. Such veterinarians are no longer highly valued, and most were forced out of business along with family farms as Western agriculture became increasingly industrialized.

Seven Golden Rules of Bioethics

1. Compassion
2. Reverential respect
3. *Ahimsa* (avoidance of harm or injury)
4. Social justice and transspecies democracy (equal and fair consideration)
5. Ecojustice, or environmental ethics
6. Protection and enhancement of biocultural diversity
7. Sustainability

Livestock and Agriculture

Whereas extreme overcrowding and deprivation of natural behaviors in intensive systems of production threaten the welfare of farm animals in developed countries, animals in less industrialized countries face different problems. There, intensive systems of production are fortunately not yet prevalent, but poor nutrition, inadequate preventive and therapeutic veterinary medicine, climatic extremes, parasitic diseases, and a lack of adequate and uncontaminated water are all too common. Long, arduous journeys to slaughter, poor handling and slaughter facilities, and inhumane slaughtering methods also need to be rectified, and market infrastructures improved. The welfare of draft animals deserves equal attention for both ethical and economic reasons.

In most parts of the world the use of meat as a dietary staple is not cost-effective. Moreover, humane treatment of large numbers of animals raised for meat is not economically possible. In poorer countries the grain used to feed livestock raised for meat (a luxury few can afford) could be used more effectively to feed people. The veterinary profession must acknowledge the benefits of reduced meat consumption and vegetarianism to public health, environmental conditions, and the welfare of farm animals. This change in diet is increasingly important because the human population has reached 5.6 billion and will soon double.

Veterinarians have public health responsibilities and play a valuable role in helping control zoonotic diseases (Schwabe, 1984). However, those involved in the livestock industry should be aware of the link between excessive consumption of animal fat and protein (including seafoods) and a host of health-related problems common in all industrialized nations (Temple, Burkitt, 1994) (Box 37-2). These problems can be prevented and even reversed by a diet that includes more organic fresh fruits and vegetables, more high-fiber cereals, and less refined foods, sugar, salt, animal fat, and protein. With the industrialization of developing countries, the dangerous temptation to produce and consume more animal products increases.

Western Diseases of Known and Possible Dietary Origin

GASTROINTESTINAL
Constipation, hiatus hernia, appendicitis, diverticular disease, colorectal polyps, Crohn's disease (regional ileitis), celiac disease, peptic ulcer, hemorrhoids, ulcerative colitis

CARDIOVASCULAR
Coronary heart disease, cerebrovascular disease (stroke), essential hypertension, deep vein thrombosis, pulmonary embolism, pelvic phleboliths, varicose veins

METABOLIC
Obesity, diabetes (type II or non–insulin-dependent), cholesterol gallstones, renal stones, osteoporosis, gout

CANCER
Colorectal, breast, prostate, lung, endometrium, ovarian

AUTOIMMUNE DISEASES
Diabetes (type I or insulin-dependent), autoimmune thyroiditis

OTHER DISORDERS
Allergies, immunoinsufficiency, infantile hyperactivity, migraine, multiple sclerosis, pernicious anemia, rheumatoid arthritis, spina bifida, thyrotoxicosis

Modified from Burkitt DP: in Temple NJ, Burkitt DP, editors, *Western diseases: their dietary prevention and reversibility,* Totowa, NJ, 1994, Humana.

Other Veterinary Services

In more affluent countries the veterinary profession has benefited from the recent boom in the popularity of companion animals (primarily cats and dogs). Most veterinarians now practice in this field. Others inspect meat or work in livestock-disease surveillance and control. Some veterinarians specialize in exotic pets, racehorses, prize livestock, endangered and rare captive species in zoos and wildlife parks, and animals used in the biomedical technology industry. Many work for this industry researching and developing new products for veterinary and medical use.

Ethics of Drug Use

Most pharmaceutical products are not subjected to ethical evaluation, even though they are approved by the government and appreciated by clients. Many of these products have led to the annihilation of invaluable ethnoveterinary and ethnobotanical knowledge in colonially exploited developing countries. The iatrogenic, economic, and ecologic consequences have been calamitous, from the overuse and abuse of steroids, antibiotics, and growth stimulants to the environmental damage caused by insecticides such as DDT and other organochlorines, dioxins, chemical fertilizers, fungicides, fumigants, and other harmful agrochemical products. However, the veterinary profession is still divided over the ethics of using drugs for nonveterinary purposes (such as the genetically engineered bovine growth hormone) to increase animals' productivity at the expense of their health.

New Educational Initiatives, Roles, and Services

More textbooks and courses in ethnoveterinary medicine are clearly needed in the veterinary teaching curriculum, especially in developing countries (International Institute for Rural Reconstruction, 1995; McCorkle, Mathias, Schillhorn van Veen, 1996). More regional centers dealing with animal (including wildlife) health problems caused by environmental pollution would also be helpful. Marine and terrestrial life-forms, many of which people consume, are contaminated with chemical pollutants that affect their ability to reproduce and resist disease; similar effects are passed on to consumers. Farm animals contain high concentrations of agrochemicals and industrial pollutants that are as harmful to them as to consumers. All veterinary colleges worldwide should include introductory courses in veterinary ecology or eco-veterinary medicine, veterinary ethology, bioethics, animal welfare science, and the law. Postgraduate diploma courses for advanced study in these areas should also be developed.

Veterinarians in both urban and rural areas, especially those in developing countries, have a vital role in public health and humanitarian issues. Rabies, a potentially fatal disease, is a serious problem in many parts of the world. The dog, the closest companion of millions of people, is the main carrier in third-world countries. Every country should have a postgraduate center to train veterinarians for urban and rural work in animal welfare and population control. The delivery of vaccines and other essential materials necessitates closer cooperation (McCorkle, 1995) between the human and veterinary medical professions, especially in developing countries. No county or state public health authority should be without a full-time veterinarian who has expertise in epidemiology, zoonoses, and environmental medicine.

Veterinary Students

Many young people become veterinarians because they like the company of animals and want to help relieve and prevent their suffering. However, in the course of their education, students often find that their ideals are challenged and sometimes disparaged. They frequently drop out or conform to serve less idealistic and more conventional—if not pecuniary—ends.

These ends are seldom subjected to ethical appraisal. All students should have the opportunity to question ethical issues in an atmosphere of openness and trust, and all teaching staff should participate. A required course in veterinary bioethics would be an ideal vehicle for this student-faculty forum. Students often fear recrimination when their views conflict with those of their teachers and the establishment. Because of this fear, they may hesitate to suggest alternatives to invasive procedures routinely performed on healthy animals. However, without openness and mutual respect, students cannot learn and educators cannot learn from them.

Inviting a controversial speaker or two speakers with opposing views is a Socratic approach that can revitalize our higher educational system. Monolithic organizations, such as monocrop farming, and monocultures of mind and taste proliferate only in an ethical vacuum. Veterinary education has become as monolithic, pedantic, mechanistic, and reductionistic as the training of human doctors in conventional allopathic medicine. A revolution in the veterinary curriculum is both timely and ethically imperative.*

Veterinary Ethical Issues and Dilemmas

The veterinary profession is caught in an ethical dilemma, forced to serve the often conflicting interests of both clients and animals. Conflicts of interest and responsibility cannot be resolved without ethical deliberation. However, veterinary ethics boards deal only with professional codes of conduct such as malpractice, illegal use of drugs, and unfair competitive advertising.

Every veterinary specialty gives rise to unique ethical questions, and veterinarians must decide whether to prohibit or promote related practices and policies. The following examples are typical: ear-cropping and tail-docking of dogs; euthanizing healthy animals; breeding mutant animals with semilethal and lethal deformities; housing laying hens in battery cages and veal calves and pregnant sows in narrow crates and pens; keeping arboreal primates in hygienic but socially impoverished laboratory cage environments; and developing new vaccines and drugs to promote livestock production in spite of its hazards. An ethical approach to veterinary education and practice will

---

*The word *imperative* was chosen carefully; I do not believe that there are any absolutes, in terms of truth or understanding, except compassion and reverence for all life. I believe this is an imperative because, as a veterinarian for over 30 years, I am convinced that the profession and society in general would benefit immeasurably if the role of veterinarians were better defined, funded, and appreciated.

play a significant role in helping society become more humane, compassionate, economically viable, and ecologically sustainable.

The following examples show the importance of bioethics in the objective evaluation of the risks, benefits, and long-term consequences of various activities before their implementation. Colonial veterinary services, especially in Africa, have for decades focused on increasing the health and productivity of livestock. This emphasis, along with aid and development programs in agriculture has caused a decrease in the use of traditional ways of treating and preventing animal (and crop) diseases. Indigenous methods decline with the appearance of more costly and not always reliable vaccines and drugs and less sustainable agricultural practices. Poor management and overstocking have caused serious environmental degradation, even desertification. The demise of wildlife and biodiversity has been well documented. The combined loss of biologic and cultural diversity (i.e., biocultural diversity) is one of the unforeseen consequences of veterinary participation in increasing livestock populations around the world (Bayer, Waters-Bayer, 1989; Bostid/NRC, 1991; Fox, 1992a; McCorkle, 1992).

The veterinary teaching curriculum should include courses in ecology, as well as cultural anthropology and ethnoveterinary medicine. Veterinary schools in developing countries should pay special attention to these subjects and not unquestioningly adopt Western standards.

Veterinary ethology is another important area. Without a greater understanding of the behavior and social and environmental requirements of animals, veterinary education remains extremely deficient. A purely mechanistic and reductionistic approach to animal health, disease prevention, and treatment is inevitable if the profession fails to address animals' emotions, behavioral and socio-environmental needs, psychologic stress, and well-being. This deficiency in veterinary education is demonstrated by the fact that the profession has voiced little concern for or opposition to inhumane intensive methods of livestock production—factory farms, feedlots, and livestock handling, transportation, and slaughter methods—and until recently has done little to address the plight of primates and other animals kept in impoverished zoo and laboratory environments.

Humans, as well as the animals under our dominion, need veterinary experts who can speak impartially but as informed and qualified authorities about the treatment of animals. Every community and corporation that has any business with animals should employ veterinary experts who have had postgraduate education in veterinary bioethics, ethology, animal welfare science, and the law. Every community and corporation should aim to meet the highest standards of animal care and be open to consultation, public scrutiny, and accreditation by national animal welfare agencies.

International Bioethical Standards

With the advent of GATT and the World Trade Organization, international standards governing animal health and welfare are critically important. Protection of endangered species, the global environment, and biodiversity is essential for our survival. The contributions of veterinarians are necessary in this arena, and every country should be represented to prevent unfair trading practices in countries that refuse to adopt basic codes protecting animal welfare, endangered species, and the environment.

The importance of the veterinary profession is apparent in the *Codex Alimentarius,* the international standards currently being formulated to establish global food quality and safety. Humane and sanitary slaughter facilities and practices designed to reduce stress and pathogen proliferation are significant *Codex* considerations. International standards for organically certified foods should, with respect to meat, eggs, and dairy products, include reference to animals' living conditions (notably outdoor access) and the farming systems themselves, which should be ecologically sound. Practices involving livestock, crop production, and range management should be ecologically integrated.

International standards based on veterinary bioethics would also help resolve cultural differences in animal use and abuse. As we move toward a more integrated fair trade and world market system, cultural differences in attitudes toward animals and their treatment will become increasingly apparent. Although some countries have better laws and enforcement policies than others, no country is without some traditional or commercial form of animal exploitation that causes unjustifiable suffering.

Animal Health and Well-Being

Veterinary education includes the integration of many different disciplines. Because most veterinary diseases have multiple facets and causes, the best approach to animal health and welfare is interdisciplinary, or holistic. Health is not the absence of disease but a state of harmony or homeostasis between mind and body (psyche and soma) and between the animal and its social relationships. Applied animal ethology is relevant in understanding "ethostasis," wherein the animal's ethos, or intrinsic nature and behavioral needs, is in harmony.

The animal's ethos is linked with its telos, its final end or purpose. This telos (Fig. 37-1) is the animal's role in the ecosystem (the ecos) to which it is biologically preadapted. Applied veterinary ecology seeks to provide optimal environments that satisfy the animal's ethos in the context of a sustainable agricultural system. From a scientific and an ethical perspective, the use of intensive confinement systems that ignore the animal's ethos, telos, and ecos is unacceptable. The flawed theory that an animal can be changed to fit the system must be challenged, and environments should be created that better fit the animal's

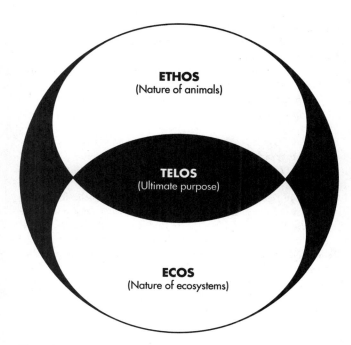

Fig. 37-1 Schematic representation of the codependent and coevolving components of animal or plant existence that determine the organism's health and well-being.

health and behavioral needs. The same criticism applies to the way animals are kept in most zoos and laboratory animal research facilities (Fox, 1986).

From the more holistic perspective of veterinary ecology, healthy soils mean healthy crops and forages, which in turn mean healthier animals and people. Nutrient deficiencies in soils, exacerbated by the misuse of agrochemicals and poor farming practices (especially monoculture/monocrop farming), increase the vulnerability of crops and livestock to disease, which leads to overuse and misuse of pesticides and veterinary medicines.

A nutrient deficiency of zinc, selenium, or vitamin E impairs an animal's immune system. Overcrowding, poor stockmanship, fear, contaminated water, and heat stress are among the many factors that increase an animal's susceptibility to disease. In immunocompromised animals, bacteria can mutate and become more virulent. The problem is often compounded by parasitic infestation and viral and mycoplasma infections.

The four pillars of holistic veterinary preventive medicine are therefore right environment, right nutrition, right attention and understanding (i.e., good stockmanship), and right breeding (because heredity plays an important role in stress and disease resistance). However, no matter how well the animals are fed, bred, and housed, the quality of their relationship with their caretakers is the ultimate determinant of their well-being (Kilgour, Dalton, 1984).

Attitude of Caretakers

Several studies have shown that a positive, affectionate human-animal bond helps enhance disease resistance in laboratory animals. This phenomenon is also apparent in the health and productivity of farm animals and the trainability of dogs and other species. When caretakers express a positive attitude toward farm animals and are not feared by them, sows have more piglets, hens lay more eggs, and cows produce more milk. Meat quality and growth rates in broilers, piglets, and beef calves also improve (Hemsworth and others, 1993).

Despite these advantages, agribusiness ignores the importance of the social bond and concentrates instead on short-term economic benefits. Large-scale, labor-saving livestock and poultry systems put one person in charge of hundreds, even thousands, of animals and rely on drugs to make animals productive and less prone to disease. A good stockperson with a positive attitude toward animals on a large factory farm may do a better job than one who is indifferent or frightening to the animals. However, working in large, intensive production systems can adversely affect the behavior and attitudes of stockpersons. One noticeable effect is increasingly aggressive behavior toward animals, which reduces their productivity and overall well-being (Seabrook, 1994) but not to such a degree that profits decline.

Animals have served us in many ways over millennia, and we owe them gratitude. We have yet to express this gratitude in a compassionate, egalitarian, and mutually enhancing relationship. The bond we share with animals today is primarily one of domination and exploitation rather than service and communion. Exploitation of animals has grown to include even genetic parasitism, wherein human genes are incorporated into the genomes of animals. Such transgenic creatures are being developed to serve as models for various genetic and developmental disorders in humans, to be blood and organ donors, and to produce "humanized" milk (i.e., milk produced by cows injected with human genes) and various pharmaceutical products (Fox, 1992b).

Scientific research confirms the many benefits humans can obtain from the company of animals. A variety of studies have documented that animals can help people overcome great emotional difficulties and physical and psychologic handicaps (Edney, 1992). Humans should therefore reciprocate by protecting endangered species and their habitats and alleviating or preventing the suffering of animals through the combined efforts of veterinary medical science and bioethics.

*R*EFERENCES

Bayer W, Waters-Bayer A: *Crop-livestock interactions for sustainable agriculture,* Gatekeeper Series Briefing Paper, Sustainable Agriculture Programme, London, 1989, International Institute for Environment and Development.

Bostid/NRC: *Microlivestock: little-known small animals with a promising economic future,* Washington, DC, 1991, National Academy Press for the Board on Science and Technology for International Development, The National Research Council.

Edney ATB: Companion animals and human health, *Vet Record,* p 285, April 4, 1992.

Fox MW: *Laboratory animal husbandry: ethology, welfare and experimental variables,* Albany, NY, 1986, State University of New York Press.

Fox MW: *The place of farm animals in humane sustainable agriculture,* Washington DC, 1992a, The Humane Society of the United States.

Fox MW: *Superpigs and wondercorn: the brave new world of biotechnology and where it all may lead,* New York, 1992b, Lyons & Burford.

Hemsworth PH and others: The human-animal relationship in agriculture and its consequences for the animal, *Animal Welfare (Universities' Federation for Animal Welfare)* 2:33-51, 1993.

International Institute for Rural Reconstruction: *Ethnoveterinary medicine in Asia,* Silang Philippines, 1995, YC James Yen Center.

Kilgour R, Dalton C: *Livestock behavior: a practical guide,* Boulder, Colo, 1984, Westview Press.

McCorkle CM, editor: *Plants, animals and people: agropastoral systems research,* Boulder, Colo, 1992, Westview Press.

McCorkle CM, Mathias E, Schillhorn van Veen TW, editors: *Ethnoveterinary research and development,* London, 1996, Intermediate Technology Publications.

McCorkle CM: Intersectoral health care delivery. In Chesworth J, editor: *Alternative perspectives on health: an ecological approach,* Thousand Oaks, Calif, 1995, Sage Publications.

Schwabe C: *Cattle, priests and progress in medicine,* Minneapolis, 1978, University of Minnesota Press.

Schwabe C: *Veterinary medicine and human health,* ed 3, Baltimore, 1984, Williams & Wilkins.

Seabrook JF: The effect of production systems on the behavior and attitudes of stockpersons. In *Biological basis of sustainable animal production,* Proceedings of the Fourth Zodiac symposium, 1994, EAAP Publication No. 67, Waneningen, The Netherlands.

Temple NJ, Burkitt DP: *Western diseases: their dietary prevention and reversibility,* Totowa, NJ, 1994, Humana.

Chapter 38

The Human–Companion Animal Bond

SUZANNE HETTS, DANIEL Q. ESTEP

The organization and content of this chapter are different from those of the other chapters in this book. This chapter does not deal with a specific treatment modality or protocol but rather with a theoretic conception of the way people and their companion animals relate to one another. A holistic approach to medical treatment for people or animals includes consideration of all factors that may influence an individual's well-being, including social relationships. In people, social isolation, bereavement, and relationships filled with conflict seem to affect many aspects of health negatively, ranging from the immune system to mortality. A significant body of literature has accumulated regarding the benefits people gain from positive social interactions with animals. Scientific studies have explored the way relationships between zoo animals and their keepers and farm animals and their owners affect the animals. For companion animals, interactions with their owners and other people may be significantly more frequent than interactions with members of their own species (Fig. 38-1). However, little is known about the way social interactions and relationships with humans affect the health and well-being of companion animals.

History of Human–Companion Animal Bond Studies

Scientific interest in the relationship between people and their pets was stimulated by the work of psychologists Samuel Corson and Boris Levinson in the 1960s and early 1970s (Corson, 1975; Levinson, 1961). Both observed that animals could be a beneficial addition to psychologic therapy for both children and adults. These observations motivated professionals in other fields, including social work, nursing, sociology, comparative psychology, veteri-

nary medicine, and ethology, to begin scientific investigations about the nature of the relationships between people and their pets. The Delta Society was formed in the United States in 1977. Its current mission statement is as follows: "To promote animals helping people improve their health, independence, and quality of life." In 1979 the Group for the Study of the Companion Animal Bond met in Scotland, and as a result of this meeting the first symposium on the Human–Companion Animal Bond was held in Britain in 1980. The study group developed five objectives for itself, one of which was to study the consequences of the emotional and psychologic bond between people and companion animals on *the emotional well-being and physical and mental health of pet owners* (Fogle, 1993; italics added). Interestingly, there was no corresponding objective to study such consequences on the health and well-being of companion animals. As its mission statement suggests, the Delta Society tends to focus on promoting animal-related services and activities that benefit people.

Scientific Basis for the Human–Companion Animal Bond

Since it was coined in the 1970s, the phrase "human–companion animal bond" has given rise to a number of sometimes unspoken assumptions. The bond is generally assumed to be a good thing, something that has positive consequences for both people and animals. The bond is assumed to be a type of mutual relationship, and its existence frequently seems to preclude acknowledgment of other types of relationships that may exist between people and their pets. A more balanced understanding is necessary to explore the possible effects of the

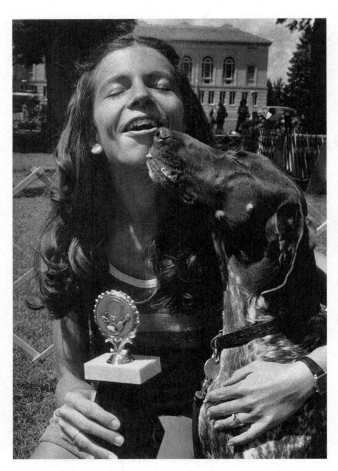

Fig. 38-1 A traditional view of the human–companion animal bond.

human–companion animal bond and other types of interspecies relationships on the health and well-being of companion animals. A good place to begin is with a review of the scientific literature on attachment.

Defining a Social Bond

In both human and animal behavior literature, the terms *bond* and *attachment* are often used interchangeably. Definitions for these terms are often lacking; when they are provided, they may differ substantially depending on the author and the context. *Attachment* can refer to an emotional feeling, process, or behavior (Estep, Hetts, 1992; Voith, 1985). The definition used here is drawn from animal behavior literature, which views attachment as an internal process motivating behaviors that keep an individual close to the object of attachment, as well as behaviors that reflect emotional distress triggered by involuntary separation (Cairns, 1972). This definition calls into question some of the implied assumptions about the human–companion animal bond mentioned earlier.

The term *human–companion animal bond* implies a mutual relationship. This mutuality may not in fact always be

the case. For example, animals may be bonded to their owners, but not vice versa, as evidenced by the millions of animals who are voluntarily surrendered to animal shelters every year. Conversely, people who feed feral cats may be attached to them, but the cats are relying on their caretakers only for food. Feral cats are not usually socialized to people and often will not even approach them.

Second, interactions on which a bond is based are not necessarily positive or friendly. A bond implies the existence of a relationship, and relationships are based on a series of interactions over time (Hinde, 1976). In a relationship, several kinds of interactions are possible. Some may be positive and affiliative; others may be negative, involving threats, fear, or aggression. Even in the closest and most positive of human relationships, occasional negative interactions sometimes occur (e.g., conflicts involving threats and punitive interactions between parents and children). Similarly, conflicts, threats, aggression, and fear occur in human-animal relationships. Dogs and cats who are very attached to their owners may purposely bite or scratch them. Owners who love their pets deeply may still strike them or use painful equipment to train them.

Third, a bond is not the only possible relationship that can exist between people and their pets. People perceive animals in almost limitless ways, or, as Hediger (1965) has put it, "from dead merchandise up to a deity." Animals in turn perceive humans in different ways as well—as predator, prey, insignificant part of the environment, symbiont, conspecific, or some combination of these (Hediger, 1965). Some pet owners clearly regard their animals as nothing more than living property, an attitude that often results in neglect or cruelty. Some owned pets behave as if they perceive their owners as enemies, reacting to them with extreme fear. Others behave as if their owners were just part of the inanimate environment and ignore them. Still others seem to treat their owners as symbionts, another organism that can supply them with vital necessities but nothing more. Practicing veterinarians and other animal specialists frequently see these other kinds of relationships between people and pets but may minimize them or even forget them when discussions center on human–companion animal bonds and the joys of pet ownership.

Factors Influencing Bond Formation

The factors that facilitate or inhibit the formation of attachments between people and animals have been the object of much theorizing. Some of these factors are common to both people and pets, whereas others are unique to one or the other.

Sensory contact

Among the factors that affect the human-animal bond, perhaps the most important is prolonged sensory contact (Cairns, 1966). In other words, the more time a person and an animal spend together, the more likely they are to form attachments to each other. Although objective data are not available, it would follow that strong attachments may not form between owners and companion animals when the animals spend most of their time outside and do not share time and activities with their owners.

Communication systems

Another factor that can influence attachment between individuals is the similarity in communication systems (Cairns, 1966). Animals of the same species have identical communication systems and signals, which can facilitate attachment. Animals of different species that are not closely related will have dissimilar communication systems and signals and therefore will be less likely to form attachments. People and earthworms rarely form strong attachments, partly because of the inability to engage in complex communication. Conversely, one of the reasons the dog has been treasured for so long as a companion animal is because its social structure and communication signals are more like those of humans than any other domestic animal.

Age

The age of the animal can influence how readily it forms attachments to other animals, both of its own species and others. In most social species, including humans, a sensitive period for socialization occurs early in life, during which individuals most easily form attachments to others. Species identity is also learned at this time, meaning that animals learn which individuals to treat as members of their own species (conspecifics) and which to treat differently, such as predators or prey (heterospecifics) (Scott, 1963). Attachments may be formed at later ages, but this is usually a much more difficult process if early experiences with the species were lacking or inadequate. For example, dogs who have many positive experiences with other dogs, people, and other species of animals such as cats between 4 to 12 weeks of age bond more readily with individuals of these species than dogs who have not had such experiences (Scott, Fuller, 1965). For cats, this sensitive period for socialization occurs between 2 and 7 weeks of age (Karsh, Turner, 1988). Dogs and cats who are not socialized to people often never form social attachments to people. Those who have had limited socialization experiences may strongly bond to a few individuals but act fearful and timid when exposed to unfamiliar people and environmental stimuli. In other words, they are unable to generalize their responses from the familiar to the unfamiliar. Many owners conclude—most likely erroneously—that such animals have been abused, when in fact it is more likely they have simply not been well socialized. From the human perspective a recent study suggests that one factor predicting the likelihood of pet ownership in adulthood is whether a pet was present in the home during childhood (Illmann, 1995).

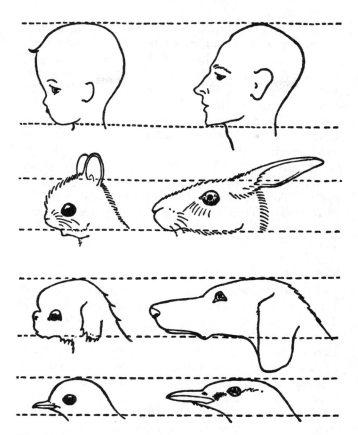

Fig. 38-2 Examples of neotenic and nonneotenic features in humans and nonhuman animals. (From Lorenz K: *Studies in animal and human behaviour,* vol. 2, Cambridge, Mass, 1971, Harvard University.)

Physical and behavior traits

Some experts have suggested that humans have selectively bred companion animals for those traits that make them better companions (Messent, Young, 1985; Serpell, 1981) and cause humans to form attachments more readily to them. For example, certain breeds of dogs and cats possess neotenic physical and behavioral characteristics (Fig. 38-2). *Neoteny* is the persistence of infantile or juvenile characteristics into adulthood. Examples of neotenic physical characteristics include large, round eyes; a rounded, sloping forehead; large ears; and a short muzzle or nose. Many toy breeds of dogs (e.g., the cavalier King Charles Spaniel) and long-haired breeds of cats (e.g., the Persian and Himalayan) possess these characteristics.

It has been stated that companion animals are neotenic versions of their wild ancestors. Neotenic behavioral traits include increased frequency of play behavior and vocalization. Adult domestic dogs and cats display increased frequencies of these behaviors compared with the wolf and the African wildcat from which each was domesticated. These neotenic features and behaviors tend to elicit caregiving responses from humans and thereby strengthen the attachment, possibly because they resemble the characteristics of human infants (McFarland, 1987).

Other behavioral traits that influence attachment have been described by James Serpell. By surveying dog owners, Serpell found that the characteristics owners believe would describe the "ideal dog" focus on the expression of attachment (Serpell, 1983, 1986). Owners rated affectionate behavior, intense greetings behaviors, highly expressive behavior, and attention to what the owner said or did as most desirable. Notably, owners rated signs of separation distress, which is often a consequence of the strong attachment behaviors that they rated as most desirable, as undesirable. This important paradox is discussed later in this chapter. Positive behavior characteristics in cats are also associated with attachment, although negative characteristics apparently do not affect attachment strength (Zasloff, Kidd, 1994).

Social support

Pet owners commonly rely on their companion animals for social support. The results of a survey conducted in 1985 revealed that most dog and cat owners talk to their pets at least once a day, talk to them about important subjects at least once a month, and believe their pets are aware of their mood changes (Voith, 1985). Pet owners also state that their animals have helped them make friends and become acquainted with more people (McNiell-Taylor, 1983). This is not surprising; several studies have documented that people with pets are perceived as happier and more approachable and indeed are more likely to be engaged in conversation by unfamiliar people than people without pets (Hunt, Hart, Gomulkiewicz, 1992; Lockwood, 1983; Messent, 1983; Rossbach, Wilson, 1992). Clinical experience in a grief-counseling program for pet owners at Colorado State University suggests that owners who believe their pets pulled them through difficult periods in the lives, rescued their pets from death or possible death, spent their childhoods with their pets, or relied on their pets for their most important means of social support and who anthropomorphize their animals to a significant degree may be more attached to their pets than owners whose relationships with their pets do not share any of these characteristics (Lagoni, Butler, Hetts, 1994).

Traditional Medical Theory

Until relatively recently, acknowledgment of the importance of the human–companion animal bond was not a part of formal veterinary medicine, although some veterinarians, such as Michael Fox, were studying and writing about human–companion animal interactions before this time (Fox, 1967). During the last 20 years the bond and its importance to veterinary practice have been recognized and are slowly becoming a part of traditional veterinary medi-cal practice. Evidence for this is the formation of the American Veterinary Medical Association Human–Animal Bond Committee and the Association of Human–Animal Bond Veteri-

narians and the many books and articles published in veterinary journals dealing with this subject.

Even with this recognition, veterinarians and other scientists have typically focused on just a few aspects of human-animal interactions and have neglected others. Most research and written materials on human–companion animal interactions have focused on the human–companion animal bond (just one kind of relationship)—specifically, the positive consequences of the bond for people and, to a lesser extent, on the negative consequences of the bond. The consequences of other kinds of human–companion animal interactions and relationships for people and the consequences of bond and nonbond interactions for animals have been largely neglected. As Andrew Rowan (1992) has pointed out, a thorough understanding of human-animal interactions will come only when all aspects of the phenomenon are understood, both positive and negative, and both sides of the interaction are considered.

Controversial Issues

This section reviews current knowledge about the positive and negative consequences of human-animal interactions for both people and companion animals. Most reviews and textbooks emphasize the positive consequences of the human–companion animal bond, and the subject of potentially negative consequences for both people and animals has been controversial.

Consequences of Human–Companion Animal Interactions

In the 20 years since interactions between people and their pets became a source of scientific inquiry, many studies have been conducted to determine the effects of the human–companion animal bond and other human-animal interactions on the physical and emotional health and well-being of people. These studies have focused more on dogs than on any other domestic or companion animal species. Human-animal interaction studies have not been restricted to pet owners and their animals but also have included interactions with domestic animals not owned as pets by the human participants. An in-depth review of this literature is beyond the scope of this chapter. Readers interested in a more complete sampling of the literature are referred to other sources (e.g., Anderson, 1975; Anderson, Hart, Hart, 1984; Davis, Balfour, 1992; Fogle, 1981, Katcher and Beck, 1983; Serpell, 1986; the journal of the Delta Society).

Positive Consequences for People

In a pioneering study Dr. Erika Friedmann found that among people hospitalized for heart attacks, pet owners had better 1-year survival rates than non–pet owners (Friedmann and others, 1980). This phenomenon has yet to be fully explained. Other investigators have focused on the beneficial effects of companion animals on the elderly. One study found that retirees with pet birds had better survival rates than those without birds (Mugford, M'Comsky, 1975), whereas another found decreased rates of depression among older people strongly attached to their pets (Garrity and others, 1989). Pets apparently also help lower blood pressure during stressful situations (Friedmann and others, 1983; Wilson, 1991) and can increase self-esteem in children and adolescents (Covert and others, 1985). One of the areas discovered most recently in which animals have beneficial effects involves children with attention deficit disorder (ADD) (Rowan, 1994). Dr. Aaron Katcher, a psychiatrist working with children with ADD in Pennsylvania, has found a significant improvement in behavior when the children were allowed to interact with animals.

In some studies, whether the presence of animals was beneficial depended partly on the degree of owners' attachments to their pets or participants' perceptions of animals. For example, in a sample of older women, those who were unattached to their pets were more likely to report being unhappy than those who were attached or those who did not own pets (Ory, Goldberg, 1983). During stressful situations, cardiovascular responses in college students who had positive perceptions of animals were significantly lower with an animal present than the responses of students with more negative perceptions (Friedmann, Locker, Lockwood, 1993). Such results suggest that the degree of attachment, the type of relationship, and people's perceptions of animals are important factors that influence the consequences of human–companion animal interactions. Human–companion animal relationships cannot be viewed as "magic bullets" for everyone.

Negative Consequences for People

When the interest in human–companion animal relationships was sparked 20 years ago, people were most interested in discovering the ways relationships with animals benefit people. Aside from the obvious zoonotic diseases, which are not discussed here, questions were not specifically posed about possible negative effects from these relationships. Negative effects have been found, but they are often neglected in literature about the human–companion animal bond.

For example, the authors of one study found that people between the ages of 21 and 34 who were strongly attached to their pets were at risk of having less social support from human relationships (Stallones and others, 1990). The same study reported that strong attachments to pets in people between 35 and 44 years of age were associated with emotional distress when no concurrent sup-

portive relationships with people existed. Negative effects of children's relationships with pets include inappropriate interactions with the animals for which the children were blamed and emotional reactions when their pets died or were given away (Bryant, 1990).

Emotional distress in reaction to the death of a pet is well documented (Carmack, 1985; Quackenbush, Glickman, 1983). Just as attachment and perception influence the occurrence of beneficial effects, these and other factors influence the intensity of grief. Pet owners referred to a counseling program at a veterinary teaching hospital after the death of their animals had more depressive symptoms than nonreferred owners. Referred owners were also more likely to have owned dogs, to have owned their pets longer, to have fewer household members, to have been more strongly attached to their pets, and to have experienced more negative life events than owners who were not referred (Stallones, 1994). However, in a national probability sample of adults 65 years of age and older, the death of a pet was not associated with depressive reactions as great as those displayed in reaction to the death of a significant person, especially a spouse (Rajaram and others, 1993).

Distress also occurs when an animal is lost for reasons other than death. Owners of guide dogs who were experiencing a transition between dogs were more distressed if the dog had died, had been involuntarily removed from the home, or had been placed in another home by the guide dog agency than owners whose dogs had retired but still lived with the owner or were placed in another home chosen by the owner (Nicholson, Kemp-Wheeler, and Griffiths, 1995). In addition, owners who were experiencing other life stressors at the time were more distressed, regardless of the reason the dog was leaving the home.

Clinical experience also suggests that normal animal behaviors regarded as problematic by owners are often a consequence of the human–companion animal bond (Voith, 1981). According to some researchers, behavior problems are so common in companion animals that it is hard to find an animal without one (Hart, Hart, 1985). Questions related to behavior are among those veterinarians are asked most frequently. Of dog owners, 43% have reported they are either "worried" about or "dissatisfied" with their dogs' behavior (Wilbur, 1976). At least 25% of the dogs and 10% of the cats surrendered to animal shelters are given up because of behavior problems (Hetts, unpublished data, 1993). Destruction of property, injuries from animal bites and scratches ranging from minor to severe to fatal, damage from house soiling, and fines and court summonses from violation of animal-control ordinances are all possible outcomes of living with a companion animal. Reports from professional behaviorists document the financial cost of such behaviors for owners (Serpell, 1986; Voith, 1981). Behavior problems are not restricted to animals owned by irresponsible, inexperienced owners. In fact, they can be the result of very strong human–companion animal bonds. A common example is separation anxiety.

Dogs with separation anxiety become anxious when apart from their owners and may soil the house, be destructive, or vocalize excessively. Dogs with separation anxiety tend to display frantic greeting behaviors and focus excessively on their owners, often following them from room to room (McCrave, 1991). According to Serpell (1986), owners find these attachment behaviors desirable. However, separation distress behaviors that owners find undesirable are also natural consequences of these attachments (Borchelt, Voith, 1985).

Positive Consequences for Animals

Most domestic animals and wild captive animals who are properly cared for probably live longer as a result of their close association with humans, although no carefully controlled study has documented this. This increase in longevity is most likely the result of the improved nutrition, disease prevention, medical care, and protection from predators that humans can provide. Research aimed at documenting this supposition, as well as other health benefits for domestic and companion animals, would be valuable.

Surprisingly few systematic studies have been conducted to investigate the positive consequences for domestic and companion animals resulting from human-animal interactions or, more specifically, the human–companion animal bond. This paucity is surprising, given the research focus on positive consequences of the bond for humans. Only one of the studies specifically measured attachment, so the nature of the human-animal relationships in these studies is unclear.

In noncompanion domestic animals, researchers have documented positive effects after gentle human handling. Gross and Siegel (1979) found that frequent human handling of chicks from 5 weeks of age on resulted in higher growth rates and better immune responses to disease challenges. In dairy cattle, Seabrook (1972) showed a correlation between the stockman's personality and milk production; introverted, confident stockmen had the best-producing cows. Presumably, these personality traits are expressed as human behaviors that produce more relaxed and compliant cows. In another study, rabbits were fed a high-cholesterol diet, which was expected to damage the cardiovascular system. Half the rabbits were handled, talked to, and played with by their human caretakers; the other group was not. The handled group had 60% less cardiovascular damage then the nonhandled group (Nerem, Levesque, Cornhill, 1980).

The most systematic work conducted with companion animals concerns changes in heart rate as a result of petting and gentle handling. In laboratory dogs, petting produced cardiac deceleration (Gantt, 1944). Petting has also been shown to ameliorate cardiac acceleration and blood pressure increases produced by aversive stimulation (An-

derson, Gantt, 1996; Lynch, Gantt, 1968). Kostarczyk (1992) has argued that ". . . heart rate deceleration is associated with a state of well-being . . ." Lynch and others (1974) found that petting produced a similar effect on heart rate in horses.

Positive effects may be inferred from the results of other studies. For example, a positive correlation was found between the intensity of attachment to a pet and the likelihood that the pet would be taken with a military family on transfer to a new location (Chumley and others, 1993). In this context, companion animals benefit from the human–companion animal bond by not being abandoned.

This relative lack of research on the animal side of human-animal interactions, especially regarding companion animals, is in part due to an unspoken assumption that if the bond is good for people, it must also be good for animals. This assumption should be tested. Among the questions that could be addressed are the following:

- Are animals who are more strongly bonded to their owners healthier, or do they live longer lives than animals who are not as bonded?
- Do strongly bonded animals have fewer behavior problems than less attached ones?

Similar questions might be asked about the consequences of the bond for the animal on the basis of the strength of the owner's attachment.

Negative Consequences for Animals

More research has been conducted on the possible negative consequences of human interactions with livestock and wildlife than with companion animals. Wildlife may be negatively affected by seemingly harmless interactions with people. Increased water-based tourism in Southern Florida, driven by interest in manatees, has been cited as an important cause of injury and death among these animals (Shackely, 1992). The use of short camera lenses, which require tourists to get closer, was more disruptive to mountain goats than the use of longer lenses (Lott, 1992).

In livestock, Hemsworth, Brand, and Willems (1981) showed that reproductive performance in sows was negatively correlated with the intensity of their fear of people. The authors also demonstrated that aversive handling could produce fear and a chronic physiologic stress response in pigs, leading to depressed growth and reproduction rates (Hemsworth, Barnett, Hausen, 1981, 1986). Surprisingly, studies have shown that seemingly harmless acts, such as approaching pigs in an erect posture while wearing gloves, could produce fear and reduce growth rates (Hemsworth, Barnett, Hausen, 1986). Inconsistent handling comprising 80% pleasant and 20% aversive interactions produced the same results (Gonyou, Hemsworth, Barnett, 1986).

Gantt (1944) found that when dogs were petted by a person who had previously punished them, cardiac acceleration occurred, presumably detracting from their well-being.

The implication of these studies is that a person's perception of an interaction and an animal's perception of the same situation may be quite different. Humans may assume an interaction has positive or neutral consequences for the animal, whereas in fact it may be quite detrimental. Sufficient research has not been conducted in companion animals to investigate the effects of typical human–companion animal interactions. However, the results of the limited research on companion animals, as well as findings from livestock and wildlife studies, certainly call into question the assumption that many of the routine interactions we have with companion animals are not having negative effects.

Many of the ways in which humans typically try to train and control animals are based on negative reinforcement or punishment, both of which use aversive stimuli. With punishment techniques an aversive stimulus is presented when an animal displays a particular behavior, resulting in a decrease in this response. With negative reinforcement, an animal can escape or avoid an aversive stimulus by performing a particular behavior. Both techniques use aversive stimuli; however, the former is used to decrease the frequency of a behavior, whereas the latter increases the likelihood a behavior will occur. "Traditional" training techniques for both dogs and horses are based mainly on negative reinforcement. Considering the fact that inconsistent aversive stimuli were found to produce stress, the following questions might be asked regarding the treatment of companion animals:

- What are the effects of hitting a dog for being destructive?
- Do obedience classes that use aversive teaching methods such as choke chains, pinch collars, and negative reinforcement produce physiologic stress responses? What is the impact on well-being?
- Are positive reinforcement training methods less stressful?
- What are the effects of aversive handling at the veterinary clinic?
- What are the effects of stress-producing relationships on health, immune function, and recovery from disease, illness, and surgery?

No research has been conducted to answer these questions.

Many human interactions with companion animals are based on anthropomorphic interpretations of animal behavior. For example, owners often justify punishing their pets after the misbehavior because they believe the animal "knows" it has done wrong because it "looks guilty" or avoids the owner when evidence of the misbehavior is apparent (Borchelt, Voith, 1985). An etiologic rather than anthropomorphic interpretation reveals that the animal is displaying fearful appeasement behavior in an attempt to prevent the punishment it has learned will follow on the basis of the owner's behavior and discriminatory cues.

Some animals learn an additional discriminatory cue that allows them to predict punishment based on the presence or absence of the evidence of earlier misbehavior. In other words, the animals makes the following discrimination: In the presence of evidence (e.g., urine, feces, chewed objects) and the owner, punishment will occur. In the presence of only one of these factors, punishment does not occur. This is the reason that some animals display the fearful appeasement behaviors even before the owner is aware of the evidence. It also accounts for the assumption that animals do not "look guilty" when they are home alone. It is the owner's arrival that triggers the submissive reaction, not the misbehavior itself.

From the animal's perspective, these interactions result in an unpredictable environment; the animal cannot prevent the negative interaction from occurring because it is not contingent on its own behavior. Many studies in laboratory animals have shown that lack of control over the environment is a stressor that negatively affects well-being (Levine, 1985).

Anthropomorphism can also result in people wanting their pets to behave as people, rather than animals. Most pet owners consider their animals family members (Voith, 1985); in many respects, this can be considered good for the animal because the animal will most likely be well cared for and integrated into the social structure of the family. However, this perception of pets as people may cause negative outcomes as well.

For example, Serpell (1986) relates an anecdote about a woman who induced an ulcerated colon in her dog by forcing it to sit at the dinner table and be spoon-fed instead of ingesting food as it normally would. An animal's ability to engage in normal, species-typical behavior has been considered one way to measure its well-being in captivity (Hetts, 1991). Although no evidence suggests that animals are compromised if they cannot display their entire behavioral repertoire (Novak, Suomi, 1988), evidence does show that preventing animals from displaying certain behaviors important to them may compromise their well-being (Dawkins, 1990). Thus, it may be asked whether the perception of pets as people can be too much of a good thing. Companion animals may need to display certain species-typical behavior patterns. Although animals should not be allowed to act aggressively, run unleashed, and breed indiscriminately, people may expect too much from their companion animals. The way service animals and those in animal-assisted therapy programs are affected by their work has been questioned (Ianuzzi, Rounn, 1991). Savishinsky (1983) commented, "One can perhaps feel some compassion for the poor neurotic pet who may have to be, for its owners, a mother, father, husband, wife, son, daughter, brother, sister, therapist, playmate, and lover—an all purpose person—all within a single household and a single lifetime."

Not only do specific human-animal interactions have the potential to create a negative effect on animals, but requiring animals to be exposed or adapt to environmental factors created by living in association with humans may also influence their health. For example, primary lung cancer in dogs is extremely rare, but it occurs significantly more in dogs whose owners smoke (Rife and others, 1992). Dogs and most birds, much more so than cats, are highly social. Yet many companion animals spend long time periods in social isolation, a condition considered one of the most potent stressors for social species (Fox, 1986). The effect of environmental changes such as moving or social disruptions such as divorce or tensions between human family members on the health and well-being of companion animals is not known.

Research has shown that strong attachments to animals do not always lead to positive outcomes. Strong attachments are also associated with animal-collecting, bestiality, and dog- and cock-fighting competitions (Rowan, 1992). Some people wrongly assume that only people who do not care about animals abuse, neglect, abandon, or kill them (Arkow, Dow, 1984). Rowan (1992) made the following remark: "We must be careful not to let ourselves become so caught up by the rosy side of human-animal attachments that we ignore the other side."

Conclusions and Practical Implications

This review may suggest to some that human–companion animal interactions have more negative than positive consequences. This is probably not the case. However, it is probably true that "the dark side of the force" (Rowan, 1992) has been largely ignored. Because the subject of this book is alternative and nontraditional veterinary medicine, this chapter describes alternatives in human-animal relationships that are frequently neglected in other reviews of research in this area. In addition, the ways human–companion animal relationships are created and the effects of those relationships are much more complex than some recent articles imply. Many factors on both the human and the animal sides influence the development of a bond or other type of human-animal relationship. The way the human perceives the relationship may be very different than the way the animal perceives this relationship. The strength of attachment is variable, not absolute (Fig. 38-3). Points representing the relative strength of attachments in a human–companion animal relationship can fall anywhere on the graph. No scientific evidence indicates that a linear relationship between attachment strengths is a necessity or even a probability. A person may be very attached to a pet and experience positive outcomes as a result of the relationship, whereas this may not be the case at all for the animal. How positive and negative outcomes correlate with relative attachment strengths is not fully understood. Awareness of all these possible outcomes from both the animal and the human perspectives and application of this awareness to a veterinary practice setting are an expanded version of the concept of a "bond-centered practice" proposed by Lagoni, Butler, and Hetts (1994). Box

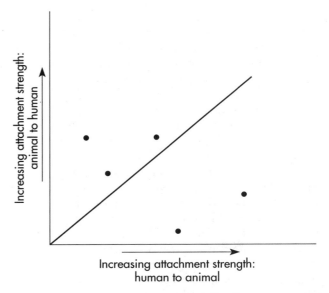

Fig. 38-3 Relative attachment strengths of human to animal and animal to human.

BOX 38-1

A BRIEF DESCRIPTION OF A BOND-CENTERED PRACTICE

In a bond-centered practice, veterinary care is focused where the medical needs of animals and the emotional needs of humans coincide. In a bond-centered practice the unique significance of each human-animal relationship is assessed and respectfully acknowledged.

Veterinarians understand that the levels of attachment between companion animals and their owners translate into various human behaviors, needs, and expectations, especially when the bonds are threatened by illness, injury, misbehavior, or death. This correlation often causes the medical needs of patients and the emotional needs of clients to arise concurrently. In a bond-centered practice the needs of animal patients and human clients are addressed simultaneously. This is accomplished by providing both medical and support-based services, thus extending veterinary care beyond the medical treatment of companion animals.

Modified from Lagoni L, Butler C, Hetts S: *The human-animal bond and grief,* Philadelphia, 1994, WB Saunders. Used with permission.

38-1 explains the basic premises of this concept. The primary tenets of the original concept of a bond-centered practice focus on acknowledgment and provision for the emotional needs of clients when relationships with pets are threatened as a result of disease, illness, or death. In a bond-centered practice, this kind of client support becomes an integral part of veterinary medical care. (For additional details and understanding of the skills and procedures involved, see Lagoni, Butler, Hetts, 1994.)

On the basis of the concepts presented and questions raised in this chapter, a broader term might be relationship-centered practice. In this view the relationship between the client and companion animal should be assessed and considered not only as it relates to the client but as an additional factor that may be affecting the health status of the animal. Veterinarians have long done this in a narrow sense by considering factors such as the amount of money a client will invest in veterinary care. However, a much broader view involves consideration of the way the entire set of interactions that make up a particular human–companion animal relationship may affect patient and client care and outcomes. This includes the interactions and relationships not only between clients and their pets but between the veterinary staff and the animals as well. (Human-human relationships between clients and staff are also important, but not the scope of this chapter.) A few examples of the many contexts in which human–companion animal relationship issues should be assessed to the degree possible follow:

Examine the way in which animals are handled at your veterinary clinic. Can animals be encouraged more often with positive reinforcers to perform certain behaviors or tolerate certain procedures? Can aversive handling and restraint methods be minimized? When such methods are necessary, can they be paired with something more pleasant for the animal? Which procedures do individual animals find most aversive? How can this be determined?

Carefully evaluate the resource people to whom clients are referred for obedience training and behavior counseling. Are you and your staff familiar with the training and behavior-modification techniques used by the professionals to whom you refer clients? Are trainers using primarily physically forceful methods relying on choke chains or pinch collars? How are aggressive animals handled? How will clients feel about your clinic if you are referring them (knowingly or not) to someone who recommends "stringing a dog up," the excessive use of crates or confinement, or throwing or pinning an animal to the ground?

Are you concerned about the effects these methods may have, especially when more effective, positive alternatives are available? What problems might you expect in handling an animal that has been subjected to these types of experiences?

Consider how animals that are strongly attached to their owners may be affected by hospitalization. What behaviors might you observe that would suggest an animal is being adversely affected? How might you ameliorate adverse affects? Can visits by owners be encouraged and planned for? In "gray areas," can animals be sent home for nursing care provided by a competent pet owner rather than being hospitalized? Are you willing to take the extra time to instruct these clients on the proper way to care for their pets?

Will owners who are strongly attached to their pets be more or less likely to make decisions for their animals' care with their animals' best interests in mind? Will strongly attached owners be able to say goodbye to their pets when euthanasia is necessary? How can you help them? How can you ensure that your practice will not take advantage of strongly attached owners who are willing to spend any amount of money to care for their pets? Alternatively, will owners who are strongly attached refuse a treatment such as amputation or other disfiguring surgery because of the potential effects on their relationship with the pet? What might you look for to determine if a relationship characterized by a strongly bonded owner is affecting the animal in a positive or negative way?

A seemingly infinite number of scenarios can be imagined in which an assessment of the human–companion animal relationship affects the way veterinarians interact with animals and clients. Systematic research on the positive and negative consequences of human–companion animal interactions and bonds is badly needed so that answers to the preceding questions can be based on scientific knowledge rather than unproven assumptions.

REFERENCES

Anderson RK, Hart BL, Hart LA, editors: *The pet connection*, Minneapolis, 1984, CENSHARE.

Anderson RS, editor: *Pet animals and society*, London, 1975, Baillière Tindall.

Anderson S, Gantt WH: The effect of person on cardiac and motor responsivity to shock in dogs, *Cond Reflex* 1:181, 1996.

Arkow PS, Dow LS: The ties that do not bind: a study of the human-animal bonds that fail. In Anderson RK, Hart BL, Hart LA, editors: *The pet connection*, Minneapolis, 1984, University of Minnesota, CENSHARE.

Borchelt PL, Voith VL: Diagnosis and treatment of separation-related behavior problems in dogs, *Vet Clin North Am Small Anim Pract* 12:625, 1985.

Cairns RB: Attachment behavior of mammals, *Psychol Rev* 73:409, 1966.

Cairns RB: Attachment and dependency: a psychobiological and social-learning synthesis. In Gewirtz JL, editor: *Attachment and dependency*, Washington, DC, 1972, Winston.

Carmack BJ: The effect of family members and functioning after the death of a pet, *Marriage Family Rev* 8:149, 1985.

Chumley PR and others: Companion animal attachment and military transfer, *Anthrozoos* 6:258, 1993.

Corson SA: Pet-facilitated psychotherapy in a hospital setting, *Current Psychiatric Ther* 15:227, 1975.

Covert AM and others: Pets, early adolescents and families, *Marriage Family Rev* 8:95, 1985.

Davis H, Balfour AD, editors: *The inevitable bond*, New York, 1992, Cambridge University Press.

Dawkins MS: From an animal's point of view: motivation, fitness and animal welfare, *Behave Brain Sci* 13:1, 1990.

Estep DQ, Hetts S: Interactions, relationships, and bonds. In Davis H, Balfour AD, editors: *The inevitable bond*, New York, 1992, Cambridge University Press.

Fogle B, editor: *Interrelations between people and pets,* Springfield, Ill, 1981, Charles C. Thomas.

Fox MW: The place and future of animal behavior studies in veterinary medicine, *J Am Vet Med Assoc* 151:609, 1967.

Fox MW: *Laboratory animal husbandry: ethology, welfare and experimental variables,* Albany, NY, 1986, State University of New York Press.

Friedmann E and others: Animal companions and one-year survival of patients after discharge from a coronary care unit, *Public Health Rep* 95:307, 1980.

Friedmann E and others: Social conditions and blood pressure: influence of animal companions, *J Nerv Ment Dis* 171:461, 1983.

Friedmann E, Locker BZ, Lockwood R: Perception of animals and cardiovascular responses during verbalization with an animal present, *Anthrozoos* 6:115, 1993.

Gantt WH: Experimental basis for neurotic behavior, *Psychosom Med Monogr,* vol 3, New York, 1944, Woeber.

Garrity TF and others: Pet ownership and attachment as supportive factors in the health of the elderly, *Anthrozoos* 3:35, 1989.

Gonyou HW, Hemsworth PH, Barnett UL: Effects of frequent interactions with humans on growing pigs, *Appl Animal Behav Sci* 16:269, 1986.

Gross WB, Siegel PB: Adaptation of chickens to their handlers and experimental results, *Avian Dis* 23:708, 1979.

Hart BL, Hart LA: *Canine and feline behavioral therapy,* Philadelphia, 1985, Lea & Febiger.

Hediger H: Man as a social partner of animals and vice versa. In Ellis PE, editor: *Symposia of the Zoological Society of London,* vol. 14, London, 1965, Social Organization of Animal Communities.

Hemsworth PH, Barnett JL, Hausen C: The influence of handling by humans on the behavior, growth and corticosteroids in the juvenile female pig, *Horm Behav* 15:396, 1981.

Hemsworth PH, Barnett JL, Hausen C: The influence of handling by humans on the behavior, reproduction and corticosteroids of the male and female pigs, *Appl Animal Behav Sci* 15:303, 1986.

Hemsworth PH, Brand A, Willems PJ: The behavioural response of sows to the presence of human beings and their productivity, *Livestock Prod Sci* 8:67, 1981.

Hetts S: Psychologic well-being: conceptual issues, behavioral measures, and implications for dogs, *Vet Clin North Am Small Anim Pract* 21:369, 1991.

Hinde RA: Interactions, relationships and social structure, *Man* 11:1, 1976.

Hunt S, Hart L, Gomulkiewicz R: Role of small animals in social interactions between strangers, *J Social Psychol* 132: 245, 1992.

Iannuzzi D, Rowan AN: Ethical issues in animal-assisted therapy programs, *Anthrozoos* 4:154, 1991.

Illmann J: Experts say it's dog's life without a pet, *The Rocky Mountain News,* Sept. 9, 1995.

Karsh EB, Turner DC: The human-cat relationship. In Turner DC, Bateson P, editors: *The domestic cat: the biology of its behaviour,* New York, 1988, Cambridge University Press.

Katcher AH, Beck AM, editors: *New perspectives on our lives with companion animals,* Philadelphia, 1983, University of Pennsylvania Press.

Kostarczyk E: The use of dog-human interactions as a reward in instrumental conditioning and its impact on dogs' cardiac regulation. In Davis H, Balfour AD, editors: *The inevitable bond,* New York, 1992, Cambridge University Press.

Lagoni L, Butler C, Hetts S: *The human-animal bond and grief,* Philadelphia, 1994, WB Saunders.

Levine S: A definition of stress. In Moberg GP, editor: *Animal stress,* Bethesda, Md, 1985, American Physiology Society.

Levinson BM: The dog as "co-therapist," *Mental Hygiene* 46:59, 1961.

Lockwood R: The influence of animals on social perception. In Katcher AH, Beck AM, editors: *New perspectives on our lives with companion animals,* Philadelphia, 1983, University of Pennsylvania Press.

Lott DF: Lens length predicts mountain goat disturbance, *Anthrozoos* 5:254, 1992.

Lynch JJ, Gantt WH: The heart rate component of the social reflex in dogs: the conditioned effects of petting and person, *Cond Reflex* 3:69, 1968.

Lynch JJ and others: Heart rate changes in the horse to human contact, *Psychophysiology* 11:472, 1974.

McCrave EA: Diagnositic criteria for separation anxiety in the dog, *Vet Clin North Am Small Anim Pract* 21:247, 1991.

McFarland D: Anthropomorphism. In McFarland D, editor: *The Oxford companion to animal behavior,* New York, 1987, Oxford University Press.

McNiell-Taylor L: *Living with loss,* London, 1983, Fontana.

Messent PR: Social facilitation of contact with other people by pet dogs. In Katcher AH, Beck AM, editors: *New perspectives on our lives with companion animals,* Philadelphia, 1983, University of Pennsylvania Press.

Messent PR, Serpell JA: An historical and biological view of the pet-owner bond. In Fogle B, editor: *Interrelations between people and pets,* Springfield, Ill, 1981, Charles C Thomas.

Mugford RA, M'Comsky JG: Some recent work on the psychotherapeutic value of caged birds with old people. In Anderson RS, editor: *Pet animals and society,* London, 1975, Baillière Tindall.

Nerem RM, Levesque MJ, Cornhill JF: Social environment as a factor in diet-induced atherosclerosis, *Science* 208:1475, 1980.

Nicholson J, Kemp-Wheeler S, Griffiths D: Distress arising from the end of a guide dog partnership, *Anthrozoos* 8:100, 1995.

Novak MA, Suomi SJ: Psychological well-being of primates in captivity, *Am Psychol* 43:765, 1988.

Ory MG, Goldberg EH: Pet possession and life satisfaction in elderly women. In Katcher AH, Beck AM, editors: *New perspectives on our lives with companion animals,* Philadelphia, 1983, University of Pennsylvania Press.

Quackenbusch JE, Glickman L: Social services for bereaved pet owners: a restrospective case study in a veterinary teaching hospital. In Katcher AH, Beck AM, editors: *New perspectives on our lives with companion animals,* Philadelphia, 1983, University of Pennsylvania Press.

Rajaram SS and others: Bereavement: loss of a pet and loss of a human, *Anthrozoos* 6:8, 1993.

Rife JS and others: Passive smoking and canine lung cancer risk, *Am J Epidemiol* 135:234, 1992.

Rossbach KA, Wilson JP: Does a dog's presence make a person appear more likeable?: two studies, *Anthrozoos* 5:40, 1992.

Rowan AN: The dark side of the "force," *Anthrozoos* 5:4, 1992.

Rowan AN: The psychiatric connection, *Anthrozoos* 7:222, 1994 [editorial].

Savishinsky JS: Pet ideas: the domestication of animals, human behavior, and human emotions. In Katcher AH, Beck AM, editors: *New perspectives on our lives with companion animals,* Philadelphia, 1983, University of Pennsylvania Press.

Scott JP: The process of primary socialization in canine and human infants, *Soc Res Child Dev Monogr* 28:1, 1963.

Scott JP, Fuller J: *Dog behavior: the genetic basis,* Chicago, 1965, University of Chicago Press.

Serpell JA: The personality of the dog and its influence on the pet-owner bond. In Katcher AH, Beck AM, editors: *New perspectives on our lives with companion animals,* Philadelphia, 1983, University of Pennsylvania Press.

Serpell JA: *In the company of animals,* Oxford, 1986, Basil Blackwell.

Shackely M: Manatees and tourism in southern Florida: opportunity or threat? *J Environ Management* 34:257, 1992.

Stallones L: Pet loss and mental health, *Anthrozoos* 7:43, 1994.

Stallones L and others: Pet ownership and attachment in relation to the health of U.S. adults 21-64 years of age, *Anthrozoos* 4:100, 1990.

Voith VL: Attachment between people and their pets: behavior problems of pets that arise from the relationship between pets and people. In Fogle B, editor: *Interrelations between people and pets,* Springfield, Ill, 1981, Charles C Thomas.

Voith VL: Attachment of people to companion animals, *Vet Clin North Am Small Anim Pract* 15:289, 1985.

Wilbur R: Pets, pet ownership and animal control: social and psychological attitudes. In *Proceedings of the National Conference on Dog and Cat Control,* 1976, Denver, Colo, National Association of Animal Control Officers.

Wilson C: The influence of a pet as an anxiolytic intervention, *J Nerv Ment Dis* 179:482, 1991.

Young MS: The evolution of domestic pets and companion animals, *Vet Clin North Am Small Anim Pract* 15:297, 1985.

Zasloff R, Kidd AH: Attachment to feline companions, *Psychol Reports* 74:747, 1994.

SELECTED READING

Arkow PS, Dow S: The ties that do not bind: a study of the human-animal bonds that fail. In Anderson RK, Hart BL, Hart LA, editors: *The pet connection,* Minneapolis, 1984, CENSHARE.

Borchelt PL, Voith VL: Punishment, *Compend Cont Vet Ed* 7:780, 1985.

Bryant BK: The richness of the child-pet relationship: a consideration of both benefits and costs of pets to children, *Anthrozoos* 3:253, 1990.

Fogle B: How did we find our way here? In Katcher AH, Beck AM, editors: *New perspectives on our lives with companion animals,* Philadelphia, 1993, University of Pennsylvania Press.

Seabrook MF: A study to determine the influence of the herdsman's personality on milk yield, *J Agric Lab Sci* 1:45, 1972.

Chapter 39

Small Animal Euthanasia: Behavioral Perspective

LAUREL LAGONI, CAROLYN L. BUTLER

The term *euthanasia* is derived from two Greek words: *eu,* meaning "good," and *thanatos,* meaning "death." Together, these words qualify euthanasia as a "good death" (Fogle, 1981). Words such as humane, painless, and loving are also associated with a good death by euthanasia. However, putting these positive attributes aside, euthanasia is nonetheless the purposeful act of terminating a life. Because of this reality, the euthanasia of a companion animal affects the individuals involved in intensely emotional ways.

No other medical procedure performed by veterinarians has as great an impact on them, their staffs, and the quality of the veterinarian-client relationship as the procedure of euthanasia. When euthanasia is performed well, it can help reassure all involved that the decision to end an animal's life was the right one. However, euthanasia done poorly—thoughtlessly, or without compassion and sensitivity—can deepen, complicate, and prolong grief for everyone.

During the last decade progressive veterinarians, animal health technicians, and grief counselors have worked together to create and perfect euthanasia protocols that address the comfort and well-being of patients, clients, and veterinarians. These teams of professionals have taken many variables into consideration, including the attitudes of those involved in the euthanasia process, the physical surroundings and emotional ambience of the euthanasia site, and the combination of drugs and methods used to induce peaceful and painless death. Effective ways to prepare clients for the death of their companion animals and help them plan the circumstances surrounding the euthanasia procedure have also been studied.

This chapter covers practical methods veterinarians can use to help clients before and during small-animal euthanasia. Many of these methods involve helping clients prepare and plan ahead for their pets' deaths, once it is clear that death is inevitable. This preparation may occur over a period of days, weeks, or even months in cases of long-term, chronic illness. On the other hand, preparation might be collapsed into a matter of hours or even minutes in cases of acute illness, injury, or trauma. Whatever the time frame, euthanasia can be conducted so that the needs of patients, clients, and staff members (including the veterinarian) are given sensitive consideration.

Grief

Just as it is almost impossible for pet owners to escape the experience of loss, it is also impossible for them to escape the experience of grief once a pet has died. As veterinarians begin to play more active roles in their clients' experiences with pet loss, they often find that most people know very little about coping with grief. In addition, they often find that what they do know—believe they know—is generally inaccurate.

Research and clinical experience show that what people say and do during bereavement is based on myths and misinformation about grief that are passed along in families from generation to generation (*Psychology Today,* 1992). One of the most prominent of these myths is that the best way to handle loss is to be strong and composed during grief. Another is the belief that staying busy and distracting oneself is the best way to feel better and recover more quickly.

These methods of grieving, however, can actually prolong the process of grief and cause grief to become complicated and even pathologic. To avoid reinforcing myths and misinformation, veterinarians must become knowledgeable about the normal, healthy grieving process.

Companion Animal Death

The death of a companion animal may be among the most significant losses of a person's life. The findings of recent studies illustrate this impact. In one study, for example, it was shown that the grief pet owners feel when companion animals die is often overwhelming and resembles their responses to the loss of human companions. In this study, 75% of pet owners reported experiencing difficulties or disruptions in their lives after their pets died. One third of the owners experienced difficulties in their relationships with others or needed to take time off from work because of their feelings of grief (Gage, Holcomb, 1991).

In a study conducted by the University of Minnesota Center for the Study of Human-Animal Relations and Environment, researchers examined the responses of 242 middle-aged couples who reported the death of a pet in the preceding 3 years. Couples were asked to rate the stress level associated with 48 events they had endured, including death of a spouse, divorce, marriage, loss of children, an arrest, loss of a job, and the death of a pet. Researchers found that the death of a pet was the most frequently reported trauma experienced by the couples participating in the study. Survey participants said the deaths of their pets were less stressful than the deaths of human members of their immediate families but more stressful than the deaths of other relatives. Forty percent of wives and 28% of husbands reported that the loss of a pet was "quite" or "extremely" disturbing (Frey, Lanseth, 1985).

Normal Grief

Although everyone experiences loss and grief repeatedly over a lifetime, loss and grief may be the two normal life processes about which the least is known. Historically, conversations about loss, death, and grief have been viewed as morbid, morose, and socially unacceptable.

However, grief is a natural and spontaneous response to loss. It is the normal way to adjust to endings and change. Grief is necessary to heal the emotional wounds caused by loss. Grief is a process, not an event, and because grief often begins with the anticipation of loss, its origin may not always be clear.

The end of the grief process is as unclear as its beginning. The progression of normal grief has no specific time frame. In fact, normal grief may last for days, weeks, months, or even years, depending on the significance of the loss.

The grief response is unique to each individual. There is no right or wrong way to grieve. Grief is also unique to different groups, societies, and cultures. In most cases the variables of age, sex, and developmental status greatly affect expressions of grief. For instance it has been conclusively confirmed that women shed more tears and cry more often during grief than men (Frey, Lanseth, 1985), probably because men are socially conditioned to maintain their composure during emotional times, whereas women are conditioned to express their feelings more openly. Research also confirms that children grieve just as deeply as adults. Because of their shorter attention spans, however, they do so more sporadically. Children most often express their grief through behavior rather than through words. They act out their grief through artwork, play, and expressions of anger and irritability. This is primarily because children do not possess the cognitive development and language capabilities necessary to express grief verbally until the age of 8 or 9 (Cook, Dworkin, 1992).

Clinical experience shows that the healing time for recovery is prolonged when the expression of grief is restricted in some way. Likewise, when grief is freely expressed, the healing time for recovery from loss is generally greatly reduced (Lagoni, Butler, Hetts, 1994). Veterinarians can best help clients by encouraging them to openly express their grief-related thoughts and feelings. They can also give their clients permission to grieve by encouraging them to cry, ask questions, be present during euthanasia, view their companion animals' bodies after death, and reminisce about the animals' lives. Permission from an authority figure such as the veterinarian reassures pet owners that grief over the death of a pet is not immature, overly sentimental, or crazy.

Noted grief expert Murray Colin Parkes makes the following statement: "It is important for those who attempt to help the bereaved to know what is normal" (1972). Box 39-1 provides an overview of the normal manifestations of grief.

Euthanasia: A New Paradigm

In traditional veterinary medicine the participation and presence of owners during euthanasia have often been discouraged. Euthanasia has been conducted as a routine, albeit uncomfortable, medical procedure with no one except the members of the veterinary staff present. However, contemporary veterinary medicine is beginning to see euthanasia in a new light. Because of a new perspective on euthanasia the procedure is evolving into more than a dreaded clinical task. More and more often, euthanasia is viewed—by veterinary professionals and clients alike—as a privilege and a gift, one that can be lovingly bestowed on dying animals. Modern veterinarians recognize "client-present" euthanasia as a potent grief-intervention tool. Thus many euthanasias performed by today's compassionate practitioners are conducted as ceremonies, with the process treated with the respect and reverence it deserves.

In the old model of euthanasia the standard practice was to talk about the process as little as possible, involve clients as little as possible, and complete the procedure as quickly as possible. Euthanasia was often referred to only indirectly or euphemistically, and clients were encouraged simply to leave pets at the veterinary clinic and thereby

BOX 39-1

The Manifestations of Grief

PHYSICAL

Crying, sobbing, wailing, shock and numbness, dry mouth, a lump in the throat, shortness of breath, stomachache or nausea, tightness in the chest, restlessness, fatigue, exhaustion, sleep disturbance, appetite disturbance, body aches, stiffness of joints or muscles, dizziness or fainting

INTELLECTUAL

Denial, sense of unreality, confusion, inability to concentrate, preoccupation with the loss, hallucinations concerning the loss (visual, auditory, and olfactory), a need to reminisce about the loved one and discuss the circumstances of the loss, a sense that time is passing very slowly, a desire to rationalize or intellectualize feelings abut the loss, thoughts or fantasies about suicide (not accompanied by concrete plans or behaviors)

EMOTIONAL

Sadness, anger, depression, guilt, anxiety, relief, loneliness, irritability, a desire to blame others for the loss, resentment, embarrassment, self-doubt, lowered self-esteem, feelings of being overwhelmed or out of control, feelings of hopelessness and helplessness, feelings of victimization, giddiness, affect that is inappropriate for the situation (nervous smiles and laughter)

SOCIAL

Feelings of withdrawal, isolation and alienation, a greater dependence on others, a rejection of others, rejection by others, a reluctance to ask others for help, change in friends or living arrangements, a desire to relocate, a need to find distractions from the intensity of grief (to stay busy or overcommit to activities)

SPIRITUAL

Bargaining with God in an attempt to prevent loss, feeling angry at God when loss occurs, renewed or shaken religious beliefs, feelings of being either blessed or punished, searching for a meaningful interpretation of a loved one's death, paranormal visions or dreams concerning a dead loved one, questioning whether or not souls exist and wondering what happens to loved ones after death, the need to "finish business" with a purposeful ending or closure to the relationship (a funeral, memorial service, last rites ceremony, goodbye ritual)

Although grief responses generally differ among individuals, many predictable manifestations of grief exist. These manifestations occur on physical, intellectual, emotional, social, and spiritual levels. Before, during, and after loss, grief may appear in several of the above forms.

avoid the upsetting details. This impersonal, clinical approach to euthanasia was believed to protect both clients and veterinarians from dealing with their emotions, thus making the process as painless as possible for all involved.

This paradigm probably worked for some, but for others it created different kinds of emotional pain. For many clients and veterinarians, it created feelings of guilt, shame, depression, and unresolved grief. The old model of euthanasia was particularly difficult for veterinarians because it placed the bulk of the emotional burden on their shoulders. Usually, with owners' permission, veterinarians were the ones to decide when, why, how, and where animals should die. In addition, veterinarians usually refrained from formally acknowledging their patients' deaths and contacting their clients afterward. Thus the old model forced everyone to grieve in isolation and generally prevented both veterinarians and clients from experiencing closure. Clinical experience reveals that many veterinarians resent this overwhelming responsibility and many clients resent their lack of control over the process (Lagoni, Butler, Hetts, 1994).

In the new model of euthanasia the standard operating procedure is just the opposite. With the new model, veterinarians and clients discuss euthanasia together, directly and at length. Veterinarians take the necessary time to complete the procedure and involve clients in the process as much as possible. The new paradigm is much more congruent with research regarding healthy grief resolution and effective practice management (Boss, 1988; Rando, 1984). Therefore the new model is both sensitive and pragmatic.

The key word when conducting euthanasia in the new paradigm is *choice.* As much as clients love their companion animals, they are probably undereducated consumers of veterinary services. Consequently, they may not always realize that they have choices. For clients to make wise and timely decisions when faced with a pet's death, they must be provided with information and choices by their veterinarians. In the new paradigm, clients are given choices about as many details as possible. The emotional burdens are shared and veterinarians and clients decide as a team when, why, how, and where companion animals should die.

When people make conscious choices, they feel empowered (Gershon, Straub, 1989); they are more likely to believe they are making decisions that are right for them. Even in loss-related crises, clients believe they have an element of control when they are presented with options and choices to consider. However, veterinarians should remember that not all clients want or require this kind of time or attention when having a companion animal euthanized. Clinical experience shows that different clients make different choices. Some choose total involvement and orchestrate a fairly complex euthanasia process. Others choose minimal involvement, opting for only a good-bye hug as they leave the examination room. However, all clients appreciate the option to be as actively involved as they choose in the euthanasia-planning process and the procedure itself.

Planning Client-Present Euthanasia

Once clients decide to proceed with euthanasia, veterinarians must take time to prepare them for what lies ahead. Research shows that longer preparation time diminishes the intensity of grief reactions (Ball, 1977) and that anticipatory grief acts as a mitigating influence on postdeath grief (Ball, 1977; Parkes, 1975). Client-present euthanasia, then, begins with thorough preparation. Preparation minimizes the regrets, the "what-ifs," and the "if-onlys" that inevitably follow the death of a companion animal.

Making the Decision

Both clients and veterinarians struggle with the timing of euthanasia. Yet, as veterinary professionals wait and watch the deterioration of companion animals, they are obligated to discuss with owners the signals for approaching death. In doing so, veterinarians dispel clients' anxiety and also prepare them for the consequences. Veterinarians can facilitate the decision-making process in many ways. For example, when clients ask, "What would you do if this were your pet?," veterinarians can let them know that they will be supportive, regardless of the decision. This message can be conveyed by a statement such as the following:

> Max isn't my pet, and what I might do if he were and what you should do now are probably two different things. You are the expert on Max. I know how hard you've tried to save him, and I know that this is one of the most difficult decisions you will ever face. However, I can't make this decision for you. I can only support you through it.

During decision making, clients may also ask how they will know when the time comes for euthanizing their pet. At this time, they are usually asking the veterinarian for guidance and structure. Anticipating death and knowing it is near can be intimidating, overwhelming, and stressful. Having solid information about signs to observe and actions to take may make the process seem more manageable.

For this reason, veterinarians must answer their clients' questions concretely and specifically. If clients can watch for specific medical signs such as seizures, disorientation, or particular responses in the animals, veterinarians should provide this information. Veterinarians may find it helpful to make a list of these symptoms as a reminder for clients. Beyond reviewing the medical aspects of the case, veteri-

narians might suggest that clients determine guidelines to assess the pet's level of deterioration and quality of life. For some, criteria might include a pet's lack of interest in drinking, eating, or going for walks. Others may identify the agony of watching a pet struggle to breathe or get comfortable in bed. For many clients, the bottom line is incontinence, the inability to walk or get up from the floor, or the failure to respond to their caretakers in the usual way.

One technique for aiding clients during the decision-making process is to call on the power of the human-animal bond—for example, by reminding clients that their relationship with the pet remains an available source of support. For instance, veterinarians might explain this to clients as follows:

> I believe you will know when it is time because Max will tell you. You and Max have always been able to communicate. That hasn't changed. Even now, if you get down on the floor, lie beside him, and look into his eyes, he will tell you when he is ready to go. Together you can make the decision about when it is time to help him die.

Client Presence

During medical treatment, veterinarians, staff members, and clients often function as a team and develop relationships based on mutual respect and trust. When treatment efforts fail and it is time to consider euthanasia, the desire for all involved to say goodbye to the animal is normal. Saying goodbye allows everyone to achieve closure in the relationship. Client-present euthanasia provides opportunities for pet owners to say goodbye to the companion animal, not only before or after death but at the moment that death occurs.

A common myth about grief is that people can be spared pain if they are protected from a painful experience. Without question, the experience of watching a beloved pet die is emotionally painful. However, clinical experience shows that owners undergo increased pain and distress when they are not present when companion animals die. Being present can facilitate resolution of the loss and the grieving process.

Although client presence has value, encouraging clients to witness the euthanasia must be done with care. Veterinarians should never aggressively persuade clients to be present at a euthanasia. Some clients clearly decide to leave their animals in their veterinarian's hands to be euthanized. In many cases this option is still acceptable, and clients should not be deterred from this decision when they have made an informed choice.

On the other hand, some owners want to be or feel they should be present at euthanasia but doubt their ability to do so. They have been told by friends or family that they should spare themselves the distress. They may also fear that death is too frightening to witness. Such misconceptions about euthanasia are damaging to the field of veterinary medicine. They imply that the methods used are less than humane. Pet owners should know that their animals' deaths are facilitated with sensitivity and compassion. In such cases, it is the veterinarian's responsibility to describe the euthanasia experience so the owner can make an educated and informed choice.

Explaining the Procedure

In deciding whether to be present, clients usually need specific information about the actual euthanasia procedure. The veterinarian's role during this time is to provide detailed information about the process and demonstrate nonjudgmental support during the decision-making process. This information should not be delivered in a dry, continuous monolog because owners sometimes cry or interrupt with questions during the veterinarian's explanation. The following is an example of an effective explanation of the euthanasia procedure:

> Betty, we know that Max is very important to you and your family. We are committed to making this experience as meaningful and as positive for you as possible. To decide whether you want to be with Max when he dies, you need accurate information about euthanasia. Would you like me to explain the procedure to you now? [With the owner's permission, the veterinarian continues.] The first thing we may do in preparation for Max's euthanasia is to take him back to our treatment area, shave a small area of fur, and place an intravenous catheter in a vein, most likely in one of his rear legs. The use of a catheter simply means that we can administer the euthanasia solution more smoothly. It also means that we can accomplish what we need to accomplish without interfering with your desire to pet or to hold Max's head and front paws.
>
> After this, Max will be brought back to you, and you will be given time to spend with him if you would like. Then, when all of us agree that it is time to proceed, we will begin the euthanasia process. The method we prefer to use involves three injections (Fig. 39-1). The first is merely a saline solution flush to ensure that the catheter is working. The second is a barbiturate, usually thiopental, which places Max in a soothing state of relaxation. The third injection is the euthanasia solution, usually pentobarbital sodium. This injection will actually stop Max's heart, brain activity, and other body functions and ultimately cause his death. Many people are surprised by how quickly death takes place because it occurs within seconds.
>
> You should also know that, although humane death by euthanasia is painless and peaceful, Max may urinate, defecate, twitch, or even sigh a bit. He will not be aware of any of this, though, and he will not feel any pain. In addition, Max's eyes may not close. Do you have any questions about any of this? [If the owner expresses understanding, the veterinarian concludes] Betty, after Max has died, you can stay with his body for as long as possible.

This conversation is greatly enhanced when it is conducted in a private, quiet setting with both the owner and

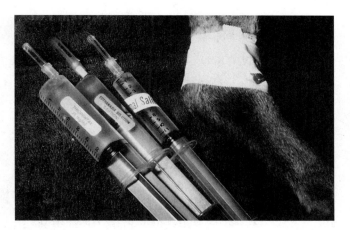

Fig. 39-1. Three injections (saline, thiopental, and pentobarbital) are given during the euthanasia procedure. A catheter is placed in the animal's rear leg to facilitate the smooth injection of drugs and allow the owner to stay near the animal's head.

veterinarian sitting or standing at eye level. It is also enhanced when the veterinarian demonstrates compassion by offering tissues or a gentle touch to an owner who cries or openly expresses emotion.

The American Animal Hospital Association offers a videotape portraying a version of client-present euthanasia similar to the one described in this example. It is called "The Loss of Your Pet." In addition to hearing the veterinarian's explanation, the client might view this tape at the clinic or check it out for viewing at home.

Euthanasia Logistics

The final set of choices clients face when preparing for euthanasia is planning and agreeing on the logistic details of the procedure. For example, the appropriate time and setting for the procedure must be determined. Owners must also decide whether anyone else will accompany them to the euthanasia, and if so, who. With proper preparation, children often choose to be present when their companion animals die.

As more clients choose to be present when their pets are euthanized, veterinarians and staff members must plan carefully. A euthanasia that occurs smoothly and with compassion and sensitivity is no accident; it requires members of the clinic staff to work together as a team.

Appointment timing

Although it may be difficult, scheduling a definite time for euthanasia is actually beneficial to the client and pet. An appointment ensures that a client's beloved companion animal will die in the way the client has chosen, with all who wish to be there in attendance.

Ideally, euthanasia appointments are scheduled for the least busy times of the day—early morning, over the lunch hour, the last appointment in the afternoon, or even after

BOX 39-2

An Examination Room Designed for Client Comfort

A standard examination room can be modified to provide pet owners with a private, comfortable area when visiting their companion animals or during euthanasia. The following is a list of items used in a modified examination room at the Colorado State University Veterinary Teaching Hospital. These costs are estimates. Many items may be donated by student and community organizations and clients who wish to memorialize their pets.

ITEM	ESTIMATED COST
Warm color of paint (or wallpaper border)	$20
Adjustable miniblinds for the door windows	$75
"Please Do Not Disturb" signs for the doors	$10
Small pad for exam table, large pad or mat for floor	$120
Washable pad covers (three small, two large)	$70
Comfortable seating (loveseat, wooden corner bench with cushions)	$675
System for lowered lighting	$100
Television monitor, VCR, and educational videos	$500
Display rack stocked with materials (brochures, pet cemeteries, counselor referrals, etc.)	$50
Pictures	$90
Bulletin board or scrapbook for pictures and cards	$50
Miscellaneous (clock, mirror, used blankets, towels)	$50
Sample urns, caskets, etc. (demonstration models)	no charge
Total	**$1810**

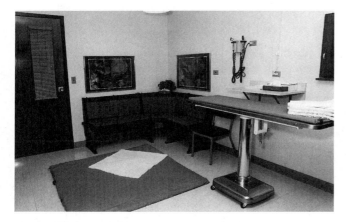

Fig. 39-2 An examination room set up for client-present euthanasias.

hours. Veterinarians should consider themselves as well as their clients when scheduling appointments, however. Client-present euthanasia requires a certain amount of energy and should be scheduled with this in mind.

Clients who bring their animals to the clinic for a euthanasia appointment should be given priority over everything except medical emergencies.

Location

Clients should never be left to sit in a busy waiting area but should be escorted to the euthanasia site. This site might be an examination room, especially one equipped with some or all of the features described in Fig. 39-2 and Box 39-2. If the veterinarian already knows the client's preferences, the site can be prepared in advance. For example, if the veterinarian knows that the client prefers an outdoor setting, tissues, handout materials, and some type of covering for the ground can be brought to the site ahead of time (Fig. 39-3).

Some veterinarians find that many clients prefer euthanasia to be conducted at the client's home. Home euthanasia is sometimes offered as a special service. It should be conducted by a team of at least two veterinary professionals. This allows one member to attend to medical needs and the other to attend to emotional needs.

Procedural details

Regardless of the euthanasia site, procedural matters should be dealt with before the day of euthanasia, if possible. Consent forms should be signed and arrangements for payment made. If the veterinarian knows and trusts the client, a bill may be sent after the event. However, a

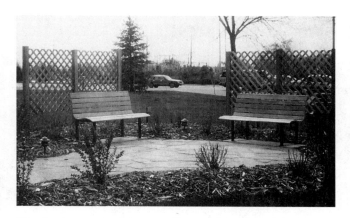

Fig. 39-3. Many clients are comforted when they can help their animals die in nonclinical, natural settings.

condolence card or letter should never accompany request for payment. Before the appointment, the veterinarian should also suggest that a friend or a less-involved family member accompany the owner for support and assistance during the drive home.

Saying goodbye and memorializing

Clients should be encouraged to consider the way they want to say goodbye to their pets. Many owners want to spend special time with their pets, engage in favorite activities, or take pictures or make videotapes of their companion animals. When an owner is prepared for a pet's death, the last days can be very special and can become a treasured memory.

Some pet owners also want to make plans to memorialize their pets. Memorializing helps bring meaning to loss and closure to relationships (Rando, 1988). Companion animals can be memorialized in countless ways. Several of these are explained in Box 39-3.

Body disposition

Whenever possible, decisions dealing with the pet's body should be made before euthanasia. Owners should be offered all available options, and each should be explained with honesty and sensitivity. Veterinarians should also disclose the cost of each option. Visual aids are often helpful during this explanation. For example, the veterinarians may show samples of caskets or urns, if these are available for purchase.

Facilitating Client-Present Euthanasia

Client-present euthanasia should always be conducted by a team of at least two veterinary professionals. This practice allows the person assisting the veterinarian to focus on owner needs and allows the veterinarian to concentrate on the medical aspects of the euthanasia procedure.

If an owner has elected to be present, the drug combination discussed earlier in this chapter and the use of a catheter must be carefully evaluated. Catheters are not always necessary, and they do not always improve the medical procedures involved with euthanasia. However, a catheter often enhances the emotional side of euthanasia because it provides extra insurance that an animal will die peacefully, without adverse side effects and the appearance of a struggle. As previously explained, if the veterinarian decides to use a catheter, it should be placed in the rear leg of a small animal. If the veterinarian is concerned about the added cost of using a catheter for euthanasia, he or she may opt to place a nonsterile, previously used one.

After the intravenous catheter has been placed and the animal has been returned to the euthanasia site, the owner should be given the opportunity to spend a short time alone with the animal. If the owner is left alone to say goodbye, the veterinarian should state specifically when he or she will return. For instance, the veterinarian may say, "I will be back in about 10 minutes." If the client wants more time and the veterinarian can afford to give it, he or she should do so.

Alternatively, the veterinarian might ask the owner to signal a member of the staff when he or she is ready to proceed. If the owner is asked to signal, the task must be made as simple as possible. During this time of intense grief, the owner will probably be able to do no more than crack open a door or wave a hand in a staff member's direction. Therefore at least one member of the veterinary team must remain close by to watch for the client's summons.

If, after about 10 minutes, the owner is still saying goodbye, the veterinarian may approach and gently say, "It is time for us to proceed. May we begin?" Most owners will indicate their answer by either nodding or shaking their heads. If the answer is no, the veterinarian may allow 5 or 10 minutes more. Such permission, however, must be made in an calm, quiet voice with no overtone of impatience. Owners often report feeling rushed through the euthanasia process by their veterinarians and feel this negated the positive aspects of their experiences.

When the owner is ready to proceed, veterinary team members often feel somewhat awkward as they enter the environment in which the euthanasia is to be performed. Many wonder what they should say or do to comfort the grieving client. Sometimes, no words are necessary. A touch on an owner's arm or a hug around the shoulders communicates support and understanding quite well.

When the veterinarian is about to begin the lethal injections, he or she should tell the owner so. Whenever possible, syringes should be kept out of sight (e.g., in the pocket of a laboratory coat or a smock) and handled very discreetly; some owners become alarmed at the sight of syringes and needles. Anxiety is usually high at this point, and sometimes owners have momentary episodes of panic. If this happens, the veterinarian should halt the procedure

BOX 39-3

Memorialization

Dedicated to and in loving memory of Barney

Below are a variety of ideas for memorializing a pet. The ideas were contributed by volunteers of the Pet Loss Support Hotline at the University of California at Davis, School of Veterinary Medicine. I was inspired to create this when I learned of the impending death of my beloved cat Barney. Barney died on June 30, 1990. This is intended to be a living document such that ideas are continually being added to it.

Leah M. Hertzel, Class of 1991
UC Davis School of Veterinary Medicine

Take many photographs, and when you think you have taken enough, take some more. Use the photos to fill an album, place them in your pet's favorite spots in the house, make a collage with them, fill a multipicture frame with them, or carry pictures in your wallet.

Write a poem, story, or song based on or dedicated to your pet.

Write down your special memories of your pet. Add to these stories or anecdotes from friends and family. Alternatively, you could make a tape recording of these memories.

Chronicle your pet's life with photos or a journal of its life.

Write a letter to your pet expressing feelings with which you may be struggling.

Videotape your pet doing anything and everything—eating, sleeping, playing, and just sitting there.

Make something that reminds you of your pet (e.g., a drawing, a clay sculpture, a needlework project).

Have a professional portrait, sketch, or sculpture done of your pet. This can be done after the pet's death from a photograph. You can also have a photo of your pet transferred to a t-shirt, clock, button, or mug (check advertisements in magazines like *Dog Fancy* and *Cat Fancy*).

Keep baby teeth, whiskers, or fur (from shaved areas) and place in a locket.

For horses, you can save shoes and tail and mane hairs.

Have fur spun to make yarn, and then knit or crochet something in memory of your pet. (Pet needs to have medium-to-long hair.)

Keep pet tags. You can attach these to your key ring so that you will always be carrying the memory of your special friend with you.

Have a plaque made to honor your pet. Place it in a special place—next to your pet's ashes, on a tree near your pet's grave, in the hospital where your pet was cared for, and so on.

Make a donation to a special cause in memory of your pet.

Volunteer your time at a humane organization, and help find homes for strays and unwanted pets.

Start a pet loss support group in your area.

Plant a bush, shrub, tree, or flowers over or near the location where the body or ashes are buried.

Place a bench with an engraved nameplate or an inscription beside your pet's grave.

Place ashes in a potted houseplant.

Scatter ashes in an area that was special to you and your pet.

Place ashes in a locket with your pet's name engraved on it. Ashes need to be sealed in an airtight bag and then placed in the locket, which must also be airtight.)

Collect pet's collars, tags, bowls, blankets, and other effects, and place them in a special area in honor of your pet. Ashes, sympathy cards, and other items may also be included.

Send out cards with a photograph of your pet informing those close to you and your pet of your loss.

If your pet is not buried near you, take pictures of the grave and place these in a special spot, which you can "visit."

and attend to the client before continuing. The veterinarian may say something such as, "This is always the most anxious and difficult moment, Betty, but we have all decided this is best for Max. Let's all take a deep breath and say goodbye one more time." Alternatively, the veterinarian may take advantage of this moment to share a personal experience with euthanasia. A statement such as, "I was with my own dog when she was euthanized last year, and I had a moment of doubt, too. But, looking back on it now, I know I did the right thing for her. This is the hard-

est part, Betty, and, for Max's sake, I'm going to continue now." However, it goes without saying that if the client becomes adamant about stopping the procedure, it should be stopped if it is still medically possible to do so.

Once the procedure has begun, the drugs should be injected quickly, with little or no lapse of time between them. As they are injected, each should be named so the owner knows how the procedure is progressing. For example, the veterinarian might say, "Betty, I am injecting the first solution, the saline flush, to make sure the catheter we have inserted is working properly." The veterinarian might next announce, "Now I am giving Max a barbiturate that will make him sleepy and help him drift off and relax." When it is time for the last injection, the veterinarian might say, "Now I am injecting the final drug." Aside from these statements, the veterinarian should remain silent. Most owners want to focus on saying goodbye to their animals and find comments, questions, and chatter distracting.

While the veterinarian is performing the euthanasia, the assistant should stand or sit quietly near the owner. The owner should be allowed to focus on the pet and to say goodbye, but the assistant should stay close by and lend emotional and physical support should the client need it.

This method of facilitating euthanasia usually goes so quickly and smoothly that most owners do not realize when their pets have actually died. It is very important, then, for the veterinarian to use a stethoscope to listen for a final heartbeat. When the veterinarian can do so with certainty, the animal should also be pronounced dead. The veterinarian should do this with a clear, simple statement such as "Betty, Max is dead." At this time, the owner may gasp, cry, sob, or sigh with relief. He or she may remark about how quickly death came and about how peaceful the experience was. This is a good time for the veterinarian to reassure the owner about the decision to euthanize the pet. It is also a good time for the veterinarian to express feelings of affection and respect for the animal. For example, the veterinarian might say, "I'm going to miss Max, too. His tail always wagged when he saw me come into the waiting room." Such a statement may prompt the owner to reminisce about the pet, sharing special or funny stories. Many owners appreciate the opportunity to talk a bit about their pets and reminisce about the life that has just come to an end.

Many veterinarians strive to create a "wake" atmosphere in the room after a euthanasia has occurred. At Irish wakes, it is acceptable to say not only positive but gently negative things about the deceased. This balance helps prevent the bereaved from overidealizing the one who has died. A more balanced perspective is desirable because idealization of the deceased is closely related to chronic grief (Stroebe, Stroebe, 1987).

After an animal has died, at some point during the conversation the veterinarian may say something like, "I'll bet this guy got into his share of trouble," or "I can only imagine the tricks this old girl used to play on you." Most pet owners pick up the conversation at this point and relate wonderful stories about the good and "bad" sides of life with their companion animals. For instance, one pet owner said, "I know I really loved this dog because he chewed up my $3000 leather couch, and I didn't kill him on the spot!" Another said, "This cat brought home little presents, like snakes and mice, and left them all over the house. Sometimes I wouldn't find them for days."

Most of these stories make everyone laugh. However, as owners realize they will never again witness their pets' hi-jinks, in the midst of their laughter their tears begin again. Animal wakes often go through several of these crying-laughing-crying cycles before everyone feels ready to bring them to an end. Under these circumstances, humor should not be used as a way to break the tension in the room or cheer people up after loss. Rather, it can be used to make the euthanasia experience real and human by helping pet owners recall all dimensions of their pets' personalities.

After-Death Follow-Up

After a pet's euthanasia, some owners want to leave the veterinary facility or site quickly, whereas others need more time alone with their pets. Because many owners have invested so much in the physical care of their companion animals, even after death, their pets' bodies remain important to them. Sometimes, family members who were not present at the euthanasia may want to view an animal's body before it is buried or cremated. As stated earlier, grief experts agree that seeing the body helps people accept the fact that death has occurred (Glick, Weiss, Parkes, 1974; Rando, 1988). If a pet's body is to be viewed, the client must be prepared for the scene. For example, depending on the situation, the client may need to be told whether the body will feel warm or cold, whether the eyes will be open or closed, and whether stroking or even holding the pet's body is appropriate. The client may also need to be told about wounds or surgical incisions on the pet's body.

Clients may also want the veterinarian to accompany them during the viewing. If so, the veterinarian should lead the way and make the first move to touch, pet, and talk to the animal. After the veterinarian has spent some time talking with and listening to the client, he or she may ask again whether the client would like some time alone. If the answer is yes, the veterinarian should leave the room and tell the client how soon he or she plans to return.

When a client wishes to view a pet's body, the body should be positioned so it will be pleasing to see. One way is to curl the body slightly, with the head and limbs tucked into a sleeplike position. Positioning the body is especially important if the animal is to be placed in a casket or other container for burial or transport at a later time. This is vitally important if the veterinarian has agreed to keep an animal's body in a cooler until other family members can view it or pick it up.

If the owner is not taking the pet's body away, a staff member should stay with the animal's body at the euthanasia site. Clinical experience has shown that almost every owner takes one last look back at the pet before leaving the euthanasia site (Lagoni, Butler, Hetts, 1994). When the owners see a friendly, familiar face next to the pet, they feel reassured that the pet will not be forgotten or treated with disrespect once they leave.

If an owner attended the euthanasia alone, the veterinarian should be certain the client is able to drive home. Some owners appreciate time to drink a glass of water or make a telephone call to a friend or family member as a way to calm themselves before leaving. When owners are ready to leave, they should be escorted out a side or back door, if possible, instead of through the busy waiting area. It may be embarrassing and awkward for a client who has been crying to walk through a crowded waiting area filled with unfamiliar people. It may also be emotionally difficult to see other pet owners with healthy companion animals.

Conclusion

Obviously the client-present euthanasia procedures discussed in this chapter represent the ideal. With practice, forethought, and organization, however, they can be implemented. For instance, when the members of a veterinary staff are well trained, technicians, receptionists, and even kennel help can be responsible for making sure that many preparatory and after-death tasks are accomplished.

Some circumstances call for modifications of these procedures. For example, sometimes the veins of very old or ill cats cannot be catheterized. In these cases the veterinarian should explain to clients the reason that a catheter cannot be used and several attempts may be necessary before an acceptable vein is found. In some cases, clients have special needs of their own or have nontraditional pets. Large animals such as horses and llamas also require some special preparation and techniques, but clients should still be given the option of being present at euthanasia (Lagoni, Butler, Hetts, 1994).

Client-present euthanasia can take more time. However, when client-present euthanasia is well planned and sensitively conducted, no other part of veterinary medical care engenders more loyalty to a veterinary practice. When clients are given choices, have their emotional needs anticipated and met, and witness their pets dying while surrounded by people who love and care about them, they are forever grateful.

Acknowledgment

We gratefully acknowledge the WB Saunders Company for granting permission to publish excerpts from their textbook *The Human-Animal Bond and Grief,* 1994.

References

Ball JF: Widow's grief: the impact of age and mode of death, *Omega* 7:307, 1977.

Boss P: *Family stress management,* Beverly Hills, Calif, 1988, Sage Publications.

Cook AS, Dworkin DS: Helping the bereaved: therapeutic interventions for children, adolescents, and adults, New York, 1992, Basic Books (Harper Collins).

Fogle B: Attachment—euthanasia—grieving, In Fogle B, editor: *Interrelations between people and pets,* Springfield, Ill, 1981, Charles C. Thomas.

Frey WH, Lanseth M: *Crying: the mystery of tears,* Minneapolis, Minn, 1985, Winston Press.

Gage G, Holcomb R: Couples' perceptions of the stressfulness of the death of the family pet, *Family Relations* 40(1):103, 1991.

Gershon D, Straub G: *Empowerment: the art of creating your life as you want it,* New York, 1989, Dell Publishing.

Glick IO, Weiss RS, Parkes CM: *The first year of bereavement,* New York, 1974, Wiley.

Lagoni L, Butler C, Hetts S: *The human-animal bond and grief,* Philadelphia, 1994, WB Saunders.

Loss: an interview with University of Chicago's Froma Walsh, *Psychology Today* 25(4):64, 1992.

Parkes MC: *Bereavement: studies of grief in adult life,* New York, 1972, International University Press.

Parkes MC: Unexpected and untimely bereavement: a statistical study of young Boston widows and widowers. In Schoenberg B and others, editors: *Bereavement and its psychological aspects,* New York, 1975, Columbia University Press.

Rando TA: *Grieving: how to go on living when someone you love dies,* Lexington, Mass, 1988, Lexington Books.

Rando TA: *Grief, dying and death: clinical interventions for caregivers,* Champaign, Ill, 1984, Research Press.

Stroebe W, Stroebe MS: *Bereavement and health: the psychological and physical consequences of partner loss,* Cambridge, Mass, 1987, Cambridge University Press.

Chapter 40

Vaccine-Related Issues

W. JEAN DODDS

Definition of Therapeutic Modality

Traditional methods of controlling the clinically important infectious diseases of humans and animals have involved epidemiologic and public health approaches aimed at improving general hygiene, sanitation, and nutrition and minimizing the risk of exposure to affected or asymptomatic carrier individuals (Stratton, Howe, Johnson, 1994). These techniques for managing infectious disease outbreaks began centuries ago and are still used today. Since the 1800s, however, another approach based on the principle of vaccination has been used. The exposure of individuals at risk for a particular infection to a very small "immunizing" dose of the offending organism or to an inactivated preparation made from it causes the person or animal to mount an antibody response that protects against future exposure (Halliwell, Gorman, 1989; Tizard, 1992).

Today, vaccines are the main conventional modality used to protect humans and animals against the more prevalent infectious diseases. Nevertheless, concerns about vaccine efficacy and safety have arisen recently, suggesting increasingly difficult international challenges. Top vaccine researchers attribute this problem to lack of world leadership and funding, and they face difficult scientific hurdles in developing future vaccines (Bloom, 1994; Cohen, 1994). Despite the urgent need to develop an effective vaccine for AIDS, the goal remains elusive. These issues have culminated in a moratorium on the use of oral polio vaccine and a questioning of the overall safety of childhood vaccines such as those for pertussis and measles (Gibbons, 1994; Gorman, 1995; Stratton, Howe, Johnston, 1994).

In veterinary medicine, evidence implicating vaccines in the triggering of immune-mediated and other chronic disorders (vaccinosis) is growing (Dodds, 1983, 1990,

1993, 1995a,b; Duval, Giger, 1996; Phillips, Schultz, 1992; Schultz, 1995a, 1995b). Although some problems have been traced to contaminated or poorly attenuated batches of vaccine that revert to virulence, others apparently reflect the host's genetic predisposition to adverse vaccinal events following use of the monovalent or polyvalent products given routinely to animals (Dodds, 1993; Gloyd, 1995; Smith, 1995; Wilbur and others, 1994).

History

The concept of vaccination to protect against common infectious diseases began many years ago with the landmark studies of Edward Jenner and Louis Pasteur. Since then, vaccines have been developed that significantly reduced the scourge of infectious diseases in humans and animals around the world (Bloom, 1994; Cohen, 1994; Stratton, Howe, Johnston, 1994). Today, however, there is heightened awareness of the potential for adverse effects from vaccination. In human and veterinary medicine an increasing frequency of immunologic disorders, acute and chronic, has been recognized in association with a recent viral infection or vaccination (Dodds, 1983, 1992; May and others, 1994; Sinha, Lopez, McDevitt, 1990; Stratton and others, 1994; Tomer, Davies, 1993).

These adverse reactions to vaccines can appear 24 to 72 hours afterward, in contrast to an acute hypersensitivity or anaphylactic reaction, which occurs immediately; 10 to 30 days later in a more delayed immunologic response (Dodds, 1983, 1990; Phillips, Schultz, 1992; Tizard, 1990); or even later, as evidenced by mortality resulting from high-titer measles vaccination in infants (Garenne and others, 1991), canine distemper antibodies in joint disease of dogs (May and others, 1994), and feline injection-site fibrosarcoma (Kahler, 1993; Kass and others, 1993). In delayed hypersensitivity from modified-live virus (MLV) vaccines the increasing antigen load during the period of viremia is presumed to be responsible for this immunologic challenge to the host animal (Phillips, Schultz, 1992; Tizard, 1990). The extent to which adverse events can be causally associated with vaccines has been discussed in depth (Stratton, Howe, Johnston, 1994) (Box 40-1).

Scientific Basis and Literature Review

In veterinary medicine, increasing concern about adverse reactions to vaccines has posed a dilemma in the selection of the appropriate approach to protect susceptible individuals or family members from the common infectious diseases.* Because of the recognized genetic predisposition to immunologic diseases and the role of environmental factors in triggering these disorders in susceptible individuals (Dodds, 1983; Sinha, Lopez, McDevitt, 1990; Tomer, Davies, 1993), it is not surprising that the frequency of adverse reactions to conventional vaccines is increasing.† A particular immunologic burden is presented to susceptible individuals when they are exposed to combination MLV products that also may contain killed bacterins administered at the same time in the diluent (Brenner and others, 1988; DVM Vaccine Roundtable, 1988; Halliwell and Gorman, 1989; Phillips and others, 1989; Schultz, 1995b). Although vaccines of killed viral or bacterial origin have been said to be more safe than MLV vaccines, this issue remains controversial.‡ (Gor-

man, 1995; Schultz, 1995b; Smith, 1995; Tizard, 1990). Most products available for vaccination of animals today are of MLV origin because they are easier and less expensive to produce, and they elicit a more sustained and complete antibody response (Greene, 1990; Hoskins, 1996; Schultz, 1995a, 1995b).

Additional points should be considered, however, before the adverse effects of vaccines can be said to outweigh their benefits in protecting animals from disease.

- First, innumerable animals have been vaccinated routinely and repeatedly without obvious untoward effects. In that regard, however, the veterinarian must determine what constitutes "acceptable" harm (Smith, 1995). Typical adverse reaction rates has been stated to be as high as 1:50,000 to 100,000 (animals) or as infrequent as 1:1 to 3.5 million (humans) (Schultz, 1995b; Stratton, Howe, Johnston, 1994). Thus the relatively few cases of documented or apparent reactions may have involved only those with susceptible genetic or physiologic makeups. This theory makes sense because current concepts of autoimmune disease invoke four interrelated causes: genetics, viral infection or exposure, hormonal balance (especially of sex and thyroid hormones), and stress (Dodds, 1993; Sinha and others, 1990). Unfortunately, predicting susceptibility or identifying susceptible individuals is not easy. Reducing the frequency of booster MLV and killed vaccines or the number of vaccine antigens given to close relatives of known adverse immune reactors may be one way to reduce the risk of immune-mediated problems. Increasing the periodicity between booster immunizations directed against only the clinically significant infectious disease agents or using alternative approaches such as monitoring of serum antibody can be implemented as a means of protecting against disease.

---

*Alderink and others (1995); Dodds (1993); DVM Vaccine Roundtable (1988); Duval, Giger (1996); Ellis and others (1995a,b); Greene (1992); Greene (1990); McDonald (1992); Olson, Klingeborn, Hedhammar (1988); Phillips, Schultz (1992); Rosenthal, Dworkis (1990); Schultz (1995a, 1995b); Smith (1995); Tizard (1990); Wallace, McMillen (1985); Wilbur and others (1994).
†Dodds (1993); Phillips, Schultz (1992); Smith (1995); Tizard (1990).
‡DVM Vaccine Gorman (1995); Greene (1990); Roundtable (1988); Schultz (1995a, 1995b); Tizard (1990).

BOX 40-1

ADVERSE EFFECTS OF VACCINES: CAUSALITY QUESTIONS

CAN IT? (POTENTIAL CAUSALITY)
- Strength of association
- Analytic bias
- Biologic gradient (dose-response effects)
- Statistical significance
- Consistency
- Biologic plausibility and coherence

DID IT? (RETRODICTIVE CAUSALITY)
- General experience with the vaccine
- Alternative causative candidates

- Susceptibility of vaccine recipient
- Timing of events
- Characteristics of adverse events
- Dechallenge
- Rechallenge

WILL IT? (PREDICTIVE CAUSALITY)
- Magnitude of risk difference
- Attributable risk
- Dependent on Can it?
- Difficult to quantitate

Modified from Stratton KR, Howe CJ, Johnston RB, Jr, editors: *Adverse events associated with childhood vaccines: evidence bearing on causality,* Washington, DC, 1994, National Academy Press.

- Second, the fact that the observed reactions often included a recent history of vaccination may be coincidental and not causal. Although the reactions clearly were associated with the use of vaccines in some of these cases, causality cannot be proved without studying a matched control group.
- Third, some of the adverse reactions may have resulted from frequent revaccinations given to induce protective titers in so-called nonresponsive animals. If so, the veterinarian should determine the "safe" number of repeated doses and the optimal interval between vaccinations for such cases. It would be interesting to conduct a survey of veterinarians to determine the number who vaccinate their own pets as often as they do client-owned animals, especially geriatric ones. Certainly the advantages and possible risks of repeated vaccination should be carefully weighed before the type and frequency of vaccines to be used are selected (Smith, 1995).

Typical signs of adverse vaccine reactions include fever, stiffness, sore joints, abdominal tenderness, susceptibility to infections, neurologic disorders, encephalitis, uveitis, collapse with autoagglutinated red blood cells and icterus (autoimmune hemolytic anemia [AIHA]), and generalized petechial and ecchymotic hemorrhages (idiopathic thrombocytopenic purpura [ITP]) (Dodds, 1993; Duval, Giger, 1996; Gloyd, 1995; May and others, 1994; Phillips, Schultz, 1992). Liver enzyme concentrations may be markedly increased, and liver or kidney failure may occur independently or accompany bone marrow suppression. Furthermore, MLV vaccination has been associated with the development of transient seizures in puppies and adult dogs of breeds or crossbreeds susceptible to immune-mediated diseases, especially those of hematologic or endocrine tissues (e.g., AIHA, ITP, autoimmune thyroiditis) (Dodds, 1983, 1993). Postvaccination polyneuropathy is a recognized entity occasionally associated with the use of distemper, parvovirus, rabies, and poliovirus, and presumably, other vaccines.* This neuropathy can result in various clinical signs, including muscle atrophy; inhibition or interruption of neuronal control of tissue and organ function; muscle excitation, incoordination, and weakness; and seizures (Collins, 1994; Gorman, 1995; Stratton, Howe, Johnston, 1994). Adverse reactions to vaccination are increasingly reported in cats (Kahler, 1993; Kass and others, 1993). Breeders should be advised of such occurrences because the genetic susceptibility to adverse vaccine reactions may place littermates and other relatives at greater risk (Dodds, 1983, 1990, 1993; Schultz, 1995b).

Perhaps the most alarming adverse events resulting from vaccinations are the tragic deaths from other infections following high-titer measles vaccinations of human infants (Garenne and others, 1991), development of sub-

acute sclerosing panencephalitis in Canadian infants given measles vaccine at less than 12 months of age (Stratton, Howe, Johnston, 1994), and experiences with refractory injection-site fibrosarcoma in cats (Kahler, 1993; Kass and others, 1993). Contamination of commercial vaccines with other adventitious viral agents has also been a long-standing problem, presumably as a result of inadequate quality control during vaccine production (Tizard, 1990). Such contamination has been of particular concern in cattle, in which contamination of bovine respiratory disease and rotacoronavirus vaccines with bovine viral diarrhea virus has occurred with unacceptable frequency (DVM Vaccine Roundtable, 1988; Ellis and others, 1995; Tizard, 1993). Another serious problem arose from a commercial canine parvovirus vaccine contaminated with blue-tongue virus (Wilbur and others, 1994). When given to pregnant dogs, the contaminated vaccine caused abortion and death. An important causality here related to the ill-advised but common practice of vaccinating pregnant animals (Wilbur and others, 1994). A question remains about the frequency of other chronic disease states induced in nonpregnant dogs given this lot of vaccine and about whether the blue-tongue virus could have been shed into the environment and induced disease in susceptible target species. More recently a commercial manufacturer of distemper vaccines was required to recall all biologic products containing distemper antigens that had been marketed through two different companies. This action was taken because "the vaccines have been associated with a higher than normally observed rate of CNS [central nervous system] postvaccination reactions," which were observed 1 to 2 weeks after vaccine administration (Gloyd, 1995). Clearly, veterinarians should be cautious in vaccinating patients.

For those killed vaccines available for veterinary use, potent adjuvants are usually added to produce a more sustained humoral immune response and compete favorably with the longer protection typically afforded by MLV products (Ellis, Hassard, Morley, 1995; Hoskins, 1996; McDonald, 1992). These adjuvants may also induce adverse effects (Halliwell, Gorman, 1989; Phillips, Schultz, 1992; Schultz, 1995b; Smith, 1995). Although killed or inactivated products make up about 15% of the veterinary biologicals used, they have been associated with 85% of the postvaccination reactions, mainly because of the acute adverse responses induced by the leptospira bacterin in dogs (DVM Vaccine Roundtable, 1988). Several years ago, an "all-killed" combination vaccine for dogs was marketed, but some users encountered minor problems with discoloration of the adjuvant and local reactions at the injection site. The product has since been withdrawn. At this writing, no other source of killed combination vaccine is available for dogs, although such a product is now offered for cats. Ringworm and chlamydia vaccines recently introduced for use in cats are advertised as having the safety advantage of a killed product (Wasmoen and others, 1992). This debate about the relative merits and safety of

*Collins (1994); Dodds (1993); Gloyd (1995); Gorman (1995); Phillips, Schultz (1992); Stratton and others (1994); Tizard (1990).

killed versus MLV vaccines has been ongoing in the veterinary literature* and recently was hotly debated in a comparison of the risks, costs, and convenience of killed versus modified live human polio vaccines (Gorman, 1995).

Overvaccination

A landmark editorial review on the subject of overvaccination was recently published (Smith, 1995). This editorial prompted several letters taking supporting and dissenting views, which were answered by Ronald D. Schultz, one of the experts interviewed for the editorial (Alderink and others, 1995). The increased cost of overvaccination, in time and dollars, must be considered in spite of the well-intentioned solicitation of clients to encourage annual booster vaccinations so that pets can also receive a wellness physical examination (Smith, 1995).

Giving already immunized animals repeated booster vaccinations when they are not necessary results in the client paying for a service that will do little if anything to improve the pet's level of protection. Moreover, the animals run the risk of adverse reactions as increasing amounts of foreign substances are injected into them (Alderink and others, 1995; Smith, 1995). Vaccination yields false-positive test results in viral or bacterial screening assays (e.g., feline leukemia [FeLV], canine borreliosis, feline coronavirus) (Smith, 1995). The experts also agree that the use of certain vaccines such as canine coronavirus, Lyme disease, and leptospira bacterin has little justification, and others so rarely cause disease today (e.g., infectious canine hepatitis) that the need for them is questionable (Alderink and others, 1995). Furthermore, only cats at high risk of exposure require vaccination for feline infectious peritonitis (FIP) or FeLV. A new canine rotavirus vaccine is about to be introduced, although no recognized canine rotavirus disease exists except perhaps in newborns. The important point, as stated by Dennis W. Macy, is to avoid the fallacy that recommending annual vaccination will cause a greater percentage of the pet population to be vaccinated (Smith, 1995). In fact, this results in conscientious clients coming in regularly and their pets being overvaccinated, with the attendant higher risk of adverse reaction (Smith, 1995).

Adverse Immunologic Effects of Vaccines

The combination of viral antigens—especially those of the MLV type, which multiply in the host—elicits a stronger antigenic challenge to the animal (Greene, 1990;

Hoskins, 1996; Phillips, Schultz, 1992; Schultz, 1995a, 1995b; Tizard, 1990). This stronger response is often viewed as desirable because a more potent immunogen should mount a more effective and sustained immune response. However, it can also overwhelm the immunocompromised host or even a healthy host that is regularly exposed to environmental stimuli and has a genetic predisposition to adverse response to viral challenge (Brenner and others, 1988; Dodds, 1993; Garenne and others, 1991; Phillips, Schultz, 1992). This scenario may have a significant effect on the recently weaned puppy or kitten being placed in a new environment. Furthermore, although the frequency of vaccinations is usually 2 to 3 weeks apart, some veterinarians have even advocated vaccination once a week in stressful situations (McDonald, 1992; Smith, 1995; Wilford, 1994). This practice makes little sense from a scientific or medical perspective. Although young animals exposed this frequently to vaccine antigens may not demonstrate overt adverse effects, their relatively immature immune systems may be temporarily or more permanently harmed (Schultz, 1995a, 1995b). Consequences in later life may include increased susceptibility to chronic debilitating diseases.

The immune response of dogs with preexisting inhalant allergies (atopy) to pollens has been shown to be augmented by vaccination, as a natural example of the "allergic breakthrough phenomenon" (Frick, Brooks, 1981). Furthermore, some veterinarians trace the increasing problems with allergic and immunologic diseases to the introduction of MLV vaccines some 20 years ago (Tizard, 1990). Although other environmental factors no doubt have a contributing role, the introduction of these vaccine antigens and their environmental shedding (Tizard, 1990) may provide the final insult that exceeds the immunologic tolerance threshold of some individuals in the pet population (Fig. 40-1).

Hormonal State During Vaccination

Relatively little attention has been paid to the hormonal status of the patient at the time of vaccination. Although veterinarians and vaccine manufacturers are aware of the general rule not to vaccinate animals during any period of illness, the same principle should apply in times of physiologic hormonal change (Greene, 1990; McDonald, 1992; Phillips, Schultz, 1992). This is particularly important because of the recognized role of hormonal influences along with infectious agents in triggering autoimmune disease (Dodds, 1992; Sinha, Gupta, 1990). Vaccination at the beginning, during, or immediately after an estrous cycle is as unwise as vaccination during pregnancy or lactation (Box 40-2). The abortions and deaths of dogs vaccinated during pregnancy with a blue-tongue virus–contaminated parvovirus vaccine are but one example (Wilbur and others, 1994). With respect to lactating bitches, adverse effects can accrue not only to the dam but also to the puppies, because a newborn litter is exposed to shed vaccine virus. Even the

---

*Brenner and others (1988); Dodds (1990, 1993); DVM Vaccine Roundtable (1988); Ellis and others (1995); Hoskins (1996); Olson, Klingeborn, Hedhammar (1988); Phillips, Schultz (1992); Rosenthal, Dworkis (1990); Schultz (1995a, 1995b); Smith (1995); Wallace, McMillen (1985); Wasmoen and others (1992); Wilford (1994).

CANINE IMMUNE SYSTEM IN NORMAL EQUILIBRIUM

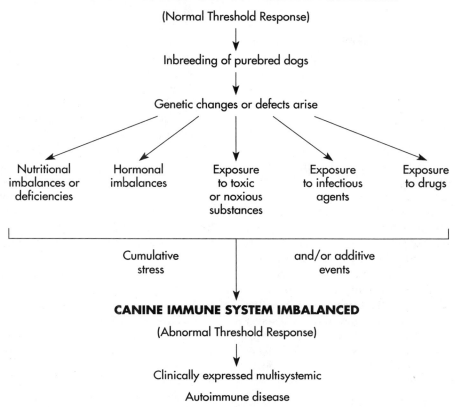

Fig. 40-1   The threshold model for inducing autoimmune disease.

*A*VOID *V*ACCINATING *P*ET *A*NIMALS

- Period (30 days) before estrus
- During or immediately after estrus
- During pregnancy
- Postpartum (lactation)

wisdom of using MLV vaccines on adult animals in the same household is questionable because of exposure of the mother and her litter to shed virus. Recent studies with MLV herpesvirus vaccines in cattle have shown that the vaccines induce necrotic changes in the ovaries of heifers vaccinated during estrus (Smith and others, 1990). The vaccine strain of this virus was also isolated from control heifers that apparently became infected by sharing pasture with the vaccinates. Furthermore, vaccine strains of these viral agents are known to cause abortion and infertility in the wake of herd vaccination programs. When these findings are extrapolated from cattle to dogs, the implications are obvious, although no evidence exists on this point.

Route of Vaccination

Although most vaccines used routinely in veterinary medicine are administered subcutaneously, other routes are preferred for some vaccines (e.g., measles and rabies vaccines), and intranasal (e.g., bordetella; "kennel cough" complex), inhalant or nebulized (e.g., respiratory disease), and oral and water delivered (e.g., porcine salmonella) vaccines are available or under development (Baer, Brooks, Froggin, 1989; Inhaled vaccine therapy for animal respiratory problems, 1995; McCracken, 1996; Roof, 1995; Smith and others, 1993). Previously, vaccination of wildlife against rabies virus involved the oral route, although this practice was controversial until recently, when a recombinant oral rabies vaccine for wildlife was approved for use in this country. The oral route is also being advocated for the vaccination of children in developing countries. However, other than the Sabin oral polio vaccine, which is now in disfavor (Gorman, 1995), such vaccines are not yet available and are unlikely to be produced without a worldwide cooperative effort (Gibbons, 1994). The cost benefits of these alternative routes of vaccination derive from ease of use and reduced handling of the animals—particularly livestock—which greatly reduces the labor involved (Roof, 1995).

Controversial Issues

Killed Versus MLVs

Most single and combination canine vaccines available today are of MLV origin, mainly because they are more economical and they produce more sustained protection.* A long-standing question remains, however, about the comparative safety and efficacy of MLV versus killed (inactivated) virus vaccines.† The author of an examination of the risks posed by MLV vaccines concluded that they are intrinsically more hazardous than inactivated products (Tizard, 1990). The residual virulence and environmental contamination resulting from the shedding of vaccine virus is a legitimate concern especially with regard to canine parvovirus (DVM Roundtable, 1988; Hoskins, 1996; Schultz, 1995b), but it should be weighed against the even more significant shedding of virulent virus by animals with clinically inapparent infection. More important, the ability of new infective agents to develop and spread poses a threat to both wild and domestic animal populations.

Viral infections and exposure have been recognized for many years to induce changes in hematologic cells and hematopoiesis (Axthelm, Krakowka, 1987; Sinha, Lopez, McDevitt, 1990; Young, Mortimer, 1984). Similar effects occur during the viremic period following MLV vaccination (Dodds, 1983; Jones, 1984; Phillips and others, 1989). A strain of parvovirus was recently shown to induce type I diabetes in rats (Guberski and others, 1991). The potential immunosuppressive effects of vaccination in humans and animals carrying latent infections, especially those with retroviral or parvoviral agents, has prompted discussion and specific recommendations.‡

Today, protection against the fatal public health hazard of rabies virus infection is afforded exclusively by killed vaccine products. Other inactivated vaccine products include those for canine parvovirus, coronavirus, and borreliosis; feline parvovirus; and leukemia virus. Although the duration and level of immunity produced by most of these vaccines has been questioned (Greene, 1992; Hoskins, 1996; Rosenthal, Dworkis, 1990; Schultz, 1995b), newer products on the market include the "all-killed" combination vaccines for cats, which are touted as having a safety advantage, and inactivated feline ringworm and chlamydia vaccines (Wasmoen and others, 1992).

Vaccine manufacturers seek to achieve minimal virulence (infectivity) while retaining maximal immunogenicity (protection) (Schultz, 1995a). This desired balance may be relatively easy to achieve in clinically normal, healthy animals but may be problematic for those with even minor immunologic deficit. The stress associated with weaning, transportation, surgery, subclinical illness, or a new home can also compromise immune function (Mockett, Stahl, 1995; Smith, 1995). Furthermore, the common viral infections, such as distemper in dogs and feline leukemia and immunodeficiency viruses in cats, cause significant immunosuppression. Dogs and cats harboring latent viral infections may not be able to withstand the additional immunologic challenge induced by MLV vaccines. The increase in vaccine-associated distemper and the enhanced susceptibility to latent parvovirus disease after parvovirus vaccination are but two examples of this potential (Gloyd, 1995; Greene, 1990; Halliwell, Gorman, 1989; Tizard, 1990). The same scenario applies to animals with subclinical disease or chronic disease states in temporary remission. The question of whether successful vaccination can occur in this situation and its safety has become significant for HIV-infected human populations, especially children (Onorato, Jones, Orenstein, 1988; Stratton, Howe, Johnston, 1994).

Veterinarians, scientists, breeders, and owners must voice their concern and discontent with the present industrial vaccine practices. They need to urge manufacturers to seek alternatives. All killed vaccines on the market today have passed current efficacy and safety standards to be licensed for use by the U.S. Department of Agriculture. The issue concerns the extent to which certain MLV vaccines, with their greater efficacy, convey an unacceptable risk along with the benefit of more sustained antibody level.

The future will see the evolution of new approaches to vaccination, including subunit vaccines, recombinant vaccines involving DNA technology, and killed products with new adjuvants to boost and prolong protection. These are not simple solutions to a problem, however; early data from recombinant vaccines against some human and mouse viruses have shown potentially dangerous side effects (e.g., damage to T-lymphocytes) (Oehen, Hengartner, Zinkernagel, 1991). The genetic background of the host, the time or dose of infection, and the makeup of the vaccine have been shown to be contributing factors.

Genetic factors have also been shown to contribute to the humoral and cell-mediated immune responses of swine and calves following immunization against salmonellosis (Lumsden and others, 1993; Smith and others, 1993). A significant challenge remains, in both human and veterinary medicine, to produce a new generation of improved and safe vaccines,* although the viral vector-subunit vaccines may generally be safer (Schultz, 1995a, 1995b).

Vaccine Dosage with Respect to Body Mass and Age

Manufacturers of polyvalent and monovalent vaccines recommend using the same dose for animals of all ages and sizes. However, the question remains as to whether it

---

*Halliwell, Gorman (1989); Hoskins (1995, 1996); Mockett, Stahl (1995); Phillips, Schultz (1992); Schultz (1995b); Tizard (1990).

†Dodds (1993); DMV Vaccine Roundtable (1988); Gloyd (1995); Gorman (1995); Rosenthal, Dworkis (1990); Schultz (1995b); Tizard (1990).

‡Frick, Brooks (1981); Garenne and others (1991); Onorato, Jones, Orenstein (1988); Rosenthal, Dworkis (1990); Stratton, Howe, Johnston (1994); Tizard (1990).

---

*Bloom (1994); Cohen (1994); Dodds (1993); DVM Vaccine Roundtable (1988); Katz, Gellin (1994); Littledike (1993); Schultz (1995b), Stratton, Howe, Johnston, (1994); Tizard (1990).

makes sense to vaccinate toy and giant-breed puppies (two extremes) with the same dose of vaccine. These products are stated to provide a sufficient excess of antigen for the average-sized animal, so they are likely to be either too much for the toy breeds or too little for the giant breeds. Although the minimum immunizing doses have been established, the optimum dosages required for protection have yet to be determined. Researchers are still uncertain as to whether these dosages should be based on body mass. It apparently depends on whether the vaccine is of MLV or killed viral origin because of the differing immunogenic principles involved (Schultz, 1995a, 1995b). Nevertheless, substantiating field evidence on this important issue is necessary.

Similarly, the administration of identical vaccine dosages for animals in all age groups is questionable. The combination of certain specific viral antigens such as distemper with adenovirus-2 (hepatitis) or parvovirus has been shown to influence the immune system by reducing lymphocyte numbers and responsiveness (Phillips and others, 1989) and causing thymic depletion (Brenner and others, 1988). What is the potential effect of those findings on vaccine dosage or age of vaccination, given the wide divergence of size among dog breeds? In humans, questions of the vaccine dosage necessary to elicit full protection in infants rather than adults have been addressed for hepatitis B vaccine (Moyes, Milne, 1988). The investigation was made for economic reasons to determine whether the standard vaccine dosage could be split and still afford protection for more than one infant (to reduce costs of vaccinating children in socioeconomically deprived countries). One fifth of the adult dose of hepatitis B vaccine was found to protect infants vaccinated during the first 6 months of life. Similarly, optimum vaccine dosage in infants was addressed by the well-intentioned but misguided attempt to overcome maternally conferred immunity to measles by giving a vaccine containing 10 to 50 times the usual titer of measles virus (Garenne and others, 1991; Katz and Gellin, 1994). Tragically, this approach was associated with increased infant mortality, especially in girls, caused not by measles but by other infections (Garenne and others, 1991).

The immune system is relatively immature at birth. At what age do young animals respond optimally to vaccine challenge? What is the earliest age at which vaccination is generally safe and effective, given the blocking effect of maternal passive immunity? How should this timing be adjusted if the newborn failed to receive adequate colostral antibodies? Do young animals of widely varying size or breed type mature at the same rate? If not, is there an optimal age at which to begin vaccinations for different breeds of dogs, especially in light of the primary concern about the levels of maternal immunity? At 22 weeks of age, most puppies and kittens have fully mature immune systems (Schultz, 1995a) and so are less likely to experience serious disease on exposure to infectious agents. Manufacturers recommend that rabies vaccination be given first between 3 and 6 months of age, although the National Association of State Public Health Veterinarians recommends its use at 3 months of age. At this age, most puppies and kittens are also receiving other vaccines, may be undergoing deworming, and are adjusting to a new environment. Is this a wise practice for urban centers where the risk for rabies exposure may be quite low compared with that of rural feral animals? The answer is yes for urban areas with a high risk for raccoon rabies. Box 40-3 lists points regarding age and vaccination.

Periodicity of Booster Vaccinations

Few published studies have addressed the necessary interval between initial and booster vaccinations, although 3 to 4 weeks has been suggested as ideal, despite the common practice of giving boosters every 2 weeks (Box 40-4).* In fact, little information has been published about the duration of protection after vaccination (Alderdink and others, 1995; Olson, Klingeborn, Hedhammer, 1988; Schultz, 1995; Smith, 1995; Sprent, Tough, 1994). Most veterinarians recommend that annual booster vaccinations be given after completion of the initial vaccine series and continued through old age. However, most experts currently advocate lengthening the interval between boosters, espe-

---

*Alderink and others (1995); Dodds (1990, 1993); DVM Vaccine Roundtable (1988); Ellis and others (1995); Halliwell, Gorman (1989); McDonald (1992); Olson, Klingeborn, Hedhammer (1988); Phillips and others (1989); Phillips, Schultz (1992); Schultz (1995a, 1995b); Smith (1995); Tizard (1990); Wallace, McMillen (1985); Wilford (1994).

BOX 40-3

VACCINE DOSAGE

BODY MASS
- Same dose intended for toy and giant breeds
- Why?
- MLV vaccines—immunogenic principle not based on body mass
- Killed vaccines—should be adjusted for body mass
- Minimum/optimum doses for protection
- Excess antigen present

AGE
- Optimal age for response
  12 weeks+ for puppies
  10 weeks+ for kittens
  Same for all breeds and sizes?
- Earliest age to promote safety
  6 weeks for puppies and kittens
- Effective age varies
- Blocking effects of maternal immunity

BOX 40-4

PERIODICITY OF BOOSTER VACCINATIONS

- No evidence supports the need for annual boosters
- The interval between boosters must be lengthened (e.g., every 3 years for healthy adults)
- Geriatric animals should be vaccinated with caution, especially if chronically diseased
- Veterinarians should consider monitoring serum antibody titers instead

cially for geriatric animals.* Others reason that the waning immune function of older animals should be boosted by vaccination more frequently. It seems obvious that the latter suggestion is unwise and unnecessary, especially in light of the long-term immunologic memory elicited by earlier vaccination or exposure (Alderink and others, 1995; Etlinger and others, 1990; Sprent, Tough, 1994).

A detailed study from Sweden (Olson, Klingeborn, Hedhammar, 1988) examined the duration of serum antibody response to canine parvovirus, adenovirus-1, and distemper virus immunizations. Only killed canine parvovirus vaccine was used, whereas the canine distemper virus vaccines were MLV and the adenovirus-1 was either killed or MLV. The study involved three groups of dogs: nonvaccinates less than 12 months old, vaccinates less than 12 months old, and adults over 12 months old. The groups varied in size from 110 to 296 animals. A fourth group of 110 pregnant bitches was studied during the immediate postpartum period. Several interesting conclusions arose from this work. For adult dogs vaccinated with killed parvovirus vaccine, no significant difference in antibody titer was detected between vaccinated and nonvaccinated animals. Although protective levels of immunity induced by the killed vaccine were of relatively short duration, two optimally spaced vaccinations (21 to 35 days apart) should adequately protect against parvovirus disease (Olson, Klingeborn, Hedhammar, 1988; Wallace, McMillen, 1985). By contrast, the MLV distemper and adenovirus-1 vaccines induced more long-lasting protective immunity. However, equating the effectiveness of vaccination with humoral antibody concentration alone is fraught with problems because cell-mediated immunity can fully protect against disease in the absence of circulating antibody titers (Halliwell, Gorman, 1989; Hoskins, 1996; Schultz, 1995a, 1995b; Tizard, 1992). Furthermore, antibody titers have a certain defined level that correlates with protection against infection and disease (Alderink and others, 1995; Hoskins, 1996) but also prevents anamnestic booster re-

sponses to many vaccines so that few animals actually benefit from annual boosters (Alderink and others, 1995; Smith, 1995). Regardless of the type of vaccine used, persistence of maternal immunity that interferes with active immunization remains the main cause of vaccine failures.*

In North America, annual revaccination of animals with a combination (polyvalent) product is typically practiced, although less frequent (every 2 years) or more frequent (every 6 months) vaccination is also given. The latter may be advised in high-risk exposure situations or with use of inactivated products such as killed canine parvovirus vaccine. In other countries the routine practice is to give booster vaccinations annually or biannually (Olson, Klingeborn, Hedhammar, 1988), although MLV vaccines are recognized to give long-lasting immunity and revaccination may be needed only every 3 to 5 years, if at all (Etlinger and others, 1990; Phillips, Schultz, 1992; Smith, 1995; Sprent, Tough, 1994; Tizard, 1992). The protection afforded by most MLV vaccines and by the MLV vaccines used in the Swedish study lasted at least 3 years (Olson, Klingeborn, Hedhammar, 1994). In humans, once the series of vaccinations in preschool- and school-aged children is completed and college students are revaccinated during disease outbreaks (e.g., measles), protection against these diseases is generally assumed to be lifelong (Stratton, Howe, Johnston, 1994). Furthermore, a recent study (Etlinger and others, 1990) showed that long after an individual is vaccinated, immunologic memory will be recalled on renewed exposure to the constituents of the vaccine. Prior immunization can be successfully exploited to elicit memory responses, as well as to help immunize individuals against new vaccines (Etlinger and others, 1994; Sprent, Tough, 1994).

Alternatives to Conventional Vaccination

This background on the adverse reactions associated with conventional vaccination justifies the need to seek alternative approaches to protection against the common infectious diseases of animals. Approaches to be considered include periodic measurement of serum antibody titers, avoidance of vaccination or overvaccination of animals at increased risk for adverse effects, and alternative methodologies (Box 40-5).

Monitoring serum antibody titers

For animals who previously experienced an adverse reaction to vaccination or are at genetic or physiologic risk for such reactions, one alternative to revaccination is annual monitoring of serum antibody titers.† Such testing

---

*Alderink and others (1995); Dodds (1993); Frick, Brooks (1981); Halliwell, Gorman (1989); Schultz (1995a); Smith (1995); Tizard (1990).

*DVM Vaccine Roundtable (1988); Garenne and others (1991); Greene (1990); Halliwell, Gorman (1989); Hoskins (1996); McDonald (1992); Schultz (1995a, 1995b); Smith (1995); Tizard (1992).
†Alderink and others (1995); Greene (1990); Hoskins (1996); Olson, Klingeborn, Zinkernagel (1988); Schultz (1995a); Smith (1995); Wallace, McMillen (1985).

Alternatives to Conventional Vaccination

MEASURE SERUM ANTIBODY TITERS
- Annual titers against common infectious agents
- Offered as alternative to routine boosters
- Used for chronically ill, allergic, geriatric, and immunocompromised animals

AVOID VACCINATION AND OVERVACCINATION
- Sick, very old, debilitated animals
- Immunocompromised animals
- Febrile animals
- Certain breeds/families (e.g., Akita, Weimaraner, harlequin Great Dane)

ALTERNATIVE METHODOLOGIES
- Require informed consent and doctor-client-patient relationship
- Clients informed that homeopathic alternatives (nosodes), although safe, require controlled trials for efficacy to be established

is generally available only for dogs. Titers can be determined for distemper virus IgG and IgM and parvovirus vaccine–induced IgG. If protective titers are found, the animal should not need revaccination until some future date. Rechecking of antibody titers can be performed at 6-month or yearly intervals thereafter. This alternative to vaccination can also be offered to owners who object to conventional vaccination.

Avoid vaccination and overvaccination

Common sense dictates that sick, very old, and debilitated animals should not be vaccinated. Similarly, immunocompromised and febrile animals should not be immunologically challenged with vaccines until their physiologic state returns to normal. Animals of certain susceptible breeds or families (e.g., Akitas and Weimaraners) and including those with coat color dilutions (e.g., double-dilute Shetland sheepdogs, harlequin Great Danes, albinos) appear to be at increased risk for severe and lingering adverse reaction to vaccines (Dodds, 1995; Wynn, Dodds, 1995).

Alternative methodologies

Appropriate rationale and justification appear to exist in certain situations for use of alternative methodologies to protect against the common infectious diseases of animals (Dodds, 1995; Pitcairn, 1993). These alternative techniques must be performed under the supervision of a licensed veterinarian with an established doctor-client-

patient relationship and requested by pet owners after appropriate informed consent. Obtaining a signed disclaimer and release form from the client is also advisable.

HOMEOPATHIC NOSODES

Nosodes are homeopathic remedies that offer a reasonable alternative to conventional (allopathic) vaccines, other than those that are required by law (e.g., rabies). Nosodes are typically prepared from an isolate of the particular disease agent selected (e.g., distemper, parvovirus, heartworm). A small amount of the infectious isolate is prepared as a tincture and then "potentized" by a series of serial dilutions and "succussions" (a specified type of shaking that adds kinetic energy to the dilutions) (Priest, 1996). The potentized nosode retains only the energy memory of the starting isolate and affords the medicinal properties of the remedy without the infective consequences of the original material (Pitcairn, 1993). Nosodes have been used in Europe since the 19th century and more recently have been introduced to North America.

The acknowledged leader in this field is the English researcher Christopher Day, who has long-standing experience with the use of homeopathic nosodes as alternatives to conventional vaccines (Day, 1984). His studies include the use of homeopathic nosodes in dogs and cattle for protection against kennel cough and bovine mastitis (Day, 1986, 1987). Another expert from England, John Saxton, has used the canine distemper nosode for disease control (Saxton, 1988, 1991). Work from India by Singh and Gupta (1985) showed potent antiviral effect of homeopathic drugs when tested in vitro against two animal viruses and a variable degree of viral inhibition in vivo. The person in North American most experienced with homeopathic approaches to vaccination is Richard Pitcairn (1993), who provided an in-depth review of the subject.

Properly designed controlled trials have yet to be performed to establish the efficacy of homeopathic nosodes as an alternative to conventional vaccination. Emphasis of this fact is particularly important with clients who specifically request alternative approaches for their pets. The literature provides the medical and scientific justification for selecting an alternative approach for those individual animals or closely related family members in whom a documented clinical illness has closely followed the use of conventional vaccination.* Another situation justifying an alternative approach applies to the patient who has a chronic immunologic disease, a previously experienced immune dysfunction, or an autoimmune disease now in remission. Use of conventional vaccines could trigger or exacerbate the existing medical condition (Dodds, 1983, 1993; Halliwell, Gorman, 1989; Stratton, Howe, Johnston, 1994; Tizard, 1992). Similarly, closely affected family members may be at genetic risk for adverse reactions associated with vaccination, particularly if they have an

---

*Day (1984, 1986, 1987); Pitcairn (1993); Priest (1996); Saxton (1988, 1991); Singh, Gupta (1985).

underlying subclinical metabolic imbalance such as that which would occur with autoimmune thyroid disease or deficiency of IgA or IgM (Halliwell, Gorman, 1989; Tizard, 1992; Tomer, Davies, 1993). It is prudent in such situations to delay the use of conventional vaccines or consider alternatives such as monitoring of serum antibody titers and the use of homeopathic nosodes for protection against infectious diseases. However, a word of caution is necessary: In a recently conducted, preliminary controlled trial, a parvovirus nosode failed to protect against street virus challenge (Schultz, Wynn, 1996). Clearly, additional trials are needed fairly to assess the efficacy of the nosodes in current use.

The guidelines of the American Veterinary Medical Association on the use of complementary and alternative therapies indicate that homeopathy is a medical discipline used by some veterinarians and that, although clinical and anecdotal evidence exists to indicate that veterinary homeopathy may be beneficial, research in this area is limited. The recommendation is that further research be conducted to evaluate efficacy, indications, and limitations and that veterinary homeopathy should be practiced only by a licensed veterinarian because inappropriate use may result in mismanagement of the case. As more veterinary teaching institutions have begun to include courses in complementary and alternative veterinary medicine in their curriculum, increased awareness and an open mind about other considerations for the practice of medicine and prevention of disease will be forthcoming.

Incorporation into Conventional Veterinary Practice

In certain situations, use of alternative methodologies to protect against the common infectious diseases of animals appears to be justified. Reducing the exposure risk of susceptible animals to known infectious agents is a basic epidemiologic principle that should be emphasized (Greene, 1990; Tizard, 1990, 1992). Other alternative techniques should be performed under the supervision of a licensed veterinarian with an established doctor-client-patient relationship and requested by the owner of the pet after receiving appropriate informed consent. Obtaining a signed disclaimer and release form from the client is also advisable, until such time that these alternatives are generally accepted as suitable options by the profession.

Finally, the issues raised in this chapter are timely and germane to parallel concerns about childhood vaccination.* In humans, this topic is equally important and controversial (Bloom, 1994; Cohen, 1994; Stratton, Howe, Johnston, 1994). The recent two-volume publication from an expert advisory panel of the National Academy of Sci-

ences offers fascinating and troubling reading (Stratton, Howe, Johnston, 1994).

Conclusions

Veterinary practitioners are confronting increasing numbers of patients exhibiting signs of immunologic dysfunction and disease. In an increasing number of cases the onset occurs within 30 days of vaccination. The evidence implicating vaccines as potential triggering agents is accumulating. A multifaceted approach to furthering the recognition of this situation, along with alternative strategies for containing infectious disease and reducing the environmental impact of conventional vaccines, is clearly needed. As a beginning, the periodicity between adult booster vaccinations can be increased to 3 years and monitoring of serum antibody levels (as an indirect assessment of protection against the clinically important infectious agents) can be implemented.

*R*EFERENCES

Alderink FJ and others: Letter to the editor, *J Am Vet Med Assoc* 207:1016, 1995.

Axthelm MK, Krakowka S: Canine distemper virus induced thrombocytopenia, *Am J Vet Res* 48:1269, 1987.

Baer GM, Brooks RC, Froggin CM: Oral vaccination of dogs fed canine adenovirus in baits, *Am J Vet Res* 50:836, 1989.

Bloom BR: The United States needs a national vaccine authority, *Science* 265:1378, 1994.

Brenner J and others: A thymic depletion syndrome associated with a combined attenuated distemper-parvovirus vaccine in dogs, *Israel J Vet Med* 44:151, 1988.

Cohen J: Bumps on the vaccine road, *Science* 265:1371, 1994.

Collins JR: Seizures and other neurologic manifestations of allergy, *Vet Clin North Am: Sm Anim Pract* 24:735, 1994.

Day CEI: *The homeopathic treatment of small animals,* London, 1984, Wigmere Publishers.

Day CEI: Clinical trials in bovine mastitis using nosodes for prevention, *J Int Assoc Vet Homeopathy* 1:15, 1986.

Day CEI: Isopathic prevention of kennel cough. Is vaccination justified? *J Int Assoc Vet Homeopathy* 2:1, 1987.

Dodds WJ: Immune-mediated diseases of the blood, *Adv Vet Sci Comp Med* 27:163, 1983.

Dodds WJ: Vaccine, drug and chemical-mediated immune reactions in purebreds challenging researchers, *DVM Newsmagazine* 21:41, 1990.

Dodds WJ: Genetically based immune disorders: autoimmune diseases (parts 1-3) and immune deficiency diseases (part 4), *Vet Pract STAFF* 4(1):8; 4(2):1; 4(3):35; 4(5):19, 1992.

Dodds WJ: Vaccine safety and efficacy revisited: autoimmune and allergic diseases on the rise, *Vet Forum* 10:68, 1993.

Dodds WJ: More bumps on the vaccine road, *Proc Am Holistic Vet Med Assoc* 74, 1995.

Dodds WJ: Vaccine-associated disease in young Weimaraners, *Proc Am Holistic Vet Med Assoc* 85-86, 1995.

Duval D, Giger U: Vaccine-associated immune-mediated hemolytic anemia in the dog, *J Vet Int Med* 10:290, 1996.

DVM Vaccine Roundtable: Safety, efficacy heart of vaccine use: experts discuss pros, cons, *DVM Newsmagazine* 19:16, 1988.

---

*Bloom (1994); Cohen (1994); Garenne and others (1991); Gibbons (1994); Stratton, Howe, Johnston (1994).

DVM Vaccine Roundtable: Measles vaccination: a different perspective, *DVM Newsmagazine* 20(1):33, 1989.

Ellis JA and others: Cellular and antibody responses to equine herpesvirus 1 and 4 following vaccination of horses with modified-live and inactivated viruses, *J Am Vet Med Assoc* 206:823, 1995.

Ellis JA, Hassard LE, Morley PS: Bovine respiratory syncytial virus-specific immune responses in calves after inoculation with commercially available vaccines, *J Am Vet Med Assoc* 206:354, 1995.

Etlinger HM and others: Use of prior vaccinations for the development of new vaccines, *Science* 249:423, 1990.

Frick OL, Brooks DL: Immunoglobulin E antibodies to pollens augmented in dogs by virus vaccines, *Am J Vet Res* 44:440, 1981.

Garenne M and others: Child mortality after high-titre measles vaccines: prospective study in Senegal, *Lancet* 338:903, 1991.

Gibbons A: Children's vaccine initiative stumbles, *Science* 265:1376, 1994.

Gloyd J: Distemper vaccines recalled, *J Am Vet Med Assoc* 207:1397, 1995.

Gorman C: Medicine: when the vaccine causes the polio, *Time* 146:83, 1995.

Greene CE: Immunoprophylaxis and immunotherapy. In Greene CE, ed: *Infectious diseases of the dog and cat*, Philadelphia, 1990, WB Saunders.

Greene RT: Questions "push" for vaccination against *Borrelia burgdorferi* infection, *J Am Vet Med Assoc* 201:1491, 1992.

Guberski DL and others: Induction of type I diabetes by Kilham's rat virus in diabetes-resistant BB/Wor rats, *Science* 254:1010, 1991.

Halliwell REW, Gorman NT: *Veterinary clinical immunology*, Philadelphia, 1989, WB Saunders.

Hoskins JD: Canine parvovirus: the evolving syndrome, *Pedigree Breeder Forum* 4(2):3, 1995.

Hoskins JD: Vaccination protocol for canine parvovirus, *Vet Forum* 13(1):60, 1996.

Inhaled vaccine therapy for animal respiratory problems, *Emerg Sci Technol* 1:10, 1995.

Jones BEV: Platelet aggregation in dogs after live-virus vaccination, *Acta Vet Scand* 25:504, 1984.

Kahler S: Collective effort needed to unlock factors related to feline injection-site sarcomas, *J Am Vet Med Assoc* 202:1551, 1993.

Kass PH and others: Epidemiologic evidence for a causal relation between vaccination and fibrosarcoma tumorigenesis in cats, *J Am Vet Med Assoc* 203:396, 1993.

Katz SL, Gellin BG: Measles vaccine: do we need new vaccines or new programs? *Science* 265:1391, 1994.

Larson LJ, Wynn SG, Schultz RD: *A canine parvovirus nosode study*, Milwaukee, Nov. 2-3, 1996, Proceedings of the Midwest Holistic Veterinary Conference.

Legendre AM, Mitchener KL, Potgieter LND: Efficacy of a feline leukemia virus vaccine in a natural exposure challenge, *J Vet Intern Med* 4:92, 1990.

Levy SA, Dreesen DW: Lyme borreliosis in dogs, *Canine Pract* 17(22):5, 1992.

Littledike ET: Variation of abscess formation in cattle after vaccination with a modified-live *Pasteurella haemolytica* vaccine, *Am J Vet Res* 54:1244, 1993.

Lorenz K: *Studies in animal and human behaviour*, vol. 2, Cambridge, Mass, 1971, Harvard University Press.

Lumsden JS and others: The influence of the swine major histocompatibility genes on antibody and cell-mediated immune responses to immunization with an aromatic-dependent mutant of *Salmonella typhimurium*, *Can J Vet Res* 57:14, 1993.

May C and others: Immune responses to canine distemper virus in joint diseases of dogs, *Br J Rheumatol* 33:27, 1994.

McCracken D: Development of an oral vaccine delivery system, *Emerg Sci Technol* 2(1):34, 1996.

McDonald LJ: Factors that can undermine the success of routine vaccination protocols, *Vet Med* 87:223, 1992.

Mockett APA, Stahl MS: Comparing how puppies with passive immunity respond to three canine parvovirus vaccines, *Vet Med* 90:430, 1995.

Moyes CD, Milne A: Should the dose of hepatitis B vaccine be reduced in newborn babies? *Lancet* 20:415, Feb 1988.

Oehen S, Hengartner H, Zinkernagel RM: Vaccination for disease, *Science* 251:195, 1991.

Olson P, Klingeborn B, Hedhammar A: Serum antibody response to canine parvovirus, canine adenovirus-1, and canine distemper virus in dogs with known states of immunization: study of dogs in Sweden, *Am J Vet Res* 49:1460, 1988.

Onorato IM, Jones TS, Orenstein WA: Immunizing children infected with HIV, *Lancet* 1:354, 1988.

Phillips TR and others: Effects on vaccines on the canine immune system, *Can J Vet Res* 53:154, 1989.

Phillips TR, Schultz RD: Canine and feline vaccines. In Kirk RW, Bonagura JD, editors: *Current veterinary therapy XI*, Philadelphia, 1992, WB Saunders.

Pitcairn RH: Homeopathic alternatives to vaccines, *Proc Am Holistic Vet Med Assoc* 39-49, 1993.

Pollock RVH, Scarlett JM: Randomized blind trial of a commercial FeLV vaccine, *J Am Vet Med Assoc* 196:611, 1990.

Priest SA: Holistic remedies are getting a shot in the arm, *Dog World* 81(1):24, 1996.

Roof M: Species specific vaccines: swine, *Emerg Sci Technol* 1(3):22, 1995.

Rosenthal RC, Dworkis AS: Incidence of and some factors affecting adverse reactions to subcutaneously administered Leukocell, *J Am Anim Hosp Assoc* 26:283, 1990.

Saxton J: Vaccination: the hidden enemy? *J Int Assoc Vet Homeopathy* 3(1):1, 1988.

Saxton J: The use of canine distemper nosodes in disease control, *J Int Assoc Vet Homeopathy* 5(1):8, 1991.

Schultz RD: Theory and practice of immunization. In *Small animal immunology: new faces of immune-mediated diseases and current concepts in vaccine immunology*, Proc San Diego Spring Vet Conf, pp 82-99, May 6-7, 1995a.

Schultz RD: Canine vaccines and immunity: important considerations in the success of vaccination programs. In Small Animal Immunology: New Faces of Immune-Mediated Diseases and Current Concepts in Vaccine Immunology, Proc San Diego Spring Vet Conf, pp 100-113, May 6-7, 1995b.

Singh LM, Gupta G: Antiviral efficacy of homeopathic drugs against animal viruses, *Br Homeopathic J* 74:168-174, 1985.

Sinha AA, Lopez MT, McDevitt HO: Autoimmune diseases: the failure of self-tolerance, *Science* 248:1380, 1990.

Smith CA, editor: Are we vaccinating too much? *J Am Vet Med Assoc* 207:421, 1995.

Smith PB and others: Vaccination of calves with orally administered aromatic-dependent salmonella dublin, *Am J Vet Res* 54:1249, 1993.

Smith PC and others: Necrotic oophoritis in heifers vaccinated intravenously with infectious bovine rhinotracheitis virus vaccine during estrus, *Am J Vet Res* 51:969, 1990.

Sprent J, Tough DF: Lymphocyte life-span and memory, *Science* 265:1395, 1994.

Stratton KR, Howe CJ, Johnston RB, Jr, editors: *Adverse events associated with childhood vaccines: evidence bearing on causality,* Washington, DC, 1994, National Academy Press.

Tizard I: Risks associated with use of live vaccines, *J Am Vet Med Assoc* 196:1851, 1990.

Tizard I: *Veterinary immunology: an introduction,* ed 4, Philadelphia, 1992, WB Saunders.

Tomer Y, Davies TF: Infection, thyroid disease, and autoimmunity, *Endocrine Rev* 14:107, 1993.

Wallace BL, McMillen JK: An inactivated canine parvovirus vaccine: duration of immunity and effectiveness in presence of maternal antibody, *Canine Pract* 12(1):14, 1985.

Wasmoen T and others: Demonstration of one-year duration of immunity for an inactivated feline *Chlamydia psittaci* vaccine, *Feline Pract* 20(3):13, 1992.

Wilbur LA and others: Abortion and death in pregnant bitches associated with a canine vaccine contaminated with blue tongue virus, *J Am Vet Med Assoc* 204:1762, 1994.

Wilford C: Vaccines revisited, *AKC Gazette* 111(1):62, 1994.

Wynn SG, Dodds WJ: Vaccine-associated disease in a family of young Akita dogs, *Proc Am Holistic Vet Med Assoc* 81, 1995.

Young N, Mortimer P: Viruses and bone marrow failure, *Blood* 63:729, 1984.

Chapter 41

*E*thnoveterinary Medicine*

CONSTANCE M. McCORKLE

Ethnoveterinary Research, Development, and Extension

Ethnoveterinary research, development, and extension[1] (ERD&E) has emerged as a fertile field for the generation (or regeneration) and transfer of appropriate and sustainable animal health technologies to rural and even peri-urban[2] stockraisers everywhere but especially in the Third World. After a brief introduction of this branch of study, this chapter outlines some of the fundamental lessons learned from ERD&E, along with their implications for understanding and then applying local knowledge (McCorkle, 1989a; Warren, 1991) to solving contemporary problems among primary producers.

What is ERD&E? In broad terms, it can be defined as follows:

> The holistic, interdisciplinary study of local knowledge and its associated skills, practices, beliefs, practitioners, and social structures pertaining to the healthcare and healthful husbandry of food-, work-, and other income-producing animals[3], always with an eye to practical development applications within livestock production and livelihood systems and with the ultimate goal of increasing human well-being via increased benefits from stockraising.

Although these benefits appear to be little understood or appreciated in today's First World (McCorkle, 1994d), they are legion. Unlike most livestock production in industrialized countries, animal agriculture in the developing world uses the full range of livestock outputs (e.g., meat, milk, hides), many of which are returned as essential inputs (e.g., manure, muscle power) into the overall farm-ing system. These outputs and inputs are vital to the economic, social, and cultural—as well as the physical-nutritional—survival of the vast majority of the globe's primary producers, virtually all of whom keep some species of livestock. Benefits embrace the pursuit of plant agriculture, plus the environmentally sound and sustainable management and use of the natural-resource base. Box 41-1 summarizes some of the multiplex returns to stockraising around the world.[4] Although there is not space here to discuss each of these categories, several merit some comment in relation to rural Third World livelihoods.

The importance of energy from livestock, for example, cannot be emphasized enough. Produced on the farm with little or no external inputs, it provides the power needed to work 52% of cultivated land in all developing countries, excluding China (Sansoucy, 1994). Given the rarity of roads in many Third World countries, pack and riding animals may be the only alternative to travel by foot in large parts of the world. For people living in extremely arid areas or above the timberline, energy from livestock, in the form of dung, may be the only fuel.

Also scarce in remote rural areas is remunerative employment. However, stockraising generates a wide variety of employment possibilities for both men and women: weaving, cobbling, smithing, tanning, saddlery, veterinary care, breaking and training, contracting for animal services (e.g., plowing, hauling, milling), and of course, direct or middleman marketing of food, work, breeding, and sporting animals; raw or processed animal products; and livestock inputs such as feed, hay, and natural minerals. Income can be earned in still other ways (e.g., from stud fees and winnings at sporting or show events).

Besides employment, income, and savings in household expenditures from home production and consumption of livestock goods and services that would otherwise have to be purchased in the marketplace, one of the most impor-

*This chapter was originally published by McCorkle CM: Back to the future: lessons from ethnoveterinary RD&E for studying and applying local knowledge, *Agriculture and Human Values* 12(2):52, 1995.

BOX 41-1

Benefits of Stockraising in the Developing World

Food: Animals provide dairy products, eggs, meat and related products, blood, fats, oils, gelatins, and, in some cultures, skins.

Clothing, shoes: Skins, leather, pelts, and wool or other fibers from animals are frequently used in apparel.

Shelter: Skins, hides, leather, and woven and felted goods serve as tenting and flooring; thong and rope are used for binding; dung is used in adobe-style construction and in plasters.

Energy: Animals provide traction (e.g., for plowing, threshing, milling, oil-pressing, water-lifting) and transport of people, water, farm products, and supplies. Their dung is used as fuel for home heating, lighting, and cooking. Tallow candles and biogas are also made from animal products.

Household and farm goods: Animal products such as leather, skin, organs, horn, bone, teeth, hair, hooves, and feathers are used for household and other items such as bedding, furnishings, containers, ropes, yokes, saddles, other tack, cups, needles, jewelry, brushes, musical instruments, and pillows. Products such as chyme and urine are employed in food processing; fish and livestock feed supplements are made from poultry and swine manure.

Employment: Often recompensed in kind as well as in cash, stockraising generates part- or full-time work, fully specialized or semispecialized professions based on livestock products, services, and health care and husbandry needs. Stockraising also contributes to full employment on the farm of family labor.

Money: Sale of foods, goods, and services provides money. In some cultures, animals or their products are themselves used as a sort of special-purpose money.

Savings, investment, and credit: For much of the developing world, livestock represent one of the few available savings and investment instruments. They are also a well-accepted form of collateral.

Social security: In many societies, animals are required as dowry, brideprice, or wedding gifts for young adults to marry and start a family on a secure economic footing. The gifting, lending, or shareherding of livestock or their products is vital for cementing kin and community mutual-aid relationships that can later be called on in time of need.

Cropping: Besides plowing and water-lifting, through their grazing, livestock clear croplands and irrigation canals, control weeds and insects that attack crops, and directly manure fields. Through consumption of crop residues, thinnings, and wastes, livestock increase returns to investments in crop inputs generally. Grazing can also recapture some of the value of such investments in failed fields; in times of crop surplus or market disturbances, livestock can serve as "living granaries."

Environment: Energy from livestock is fully renewable and reduces use of forest resources. Through manuring, livestock promote nutrient recycling and enhance soil structure. Fallow-land cover crops planted in forage for livestock reduce wind and water erosion; leguminous crops also enhance soil fertility. Herd animals can be deployed to control wildfires or restore natural vegetative cover, and many wild plants depend on livestock to disperse and germinate their seed.

Physical health: Foodstuffs from livestock make for a more diverse, high-energy diet, providing protein, fats, and essential amino acids lacking in local plant foods. These nutrients are especially critical for maternal health, child development, and physiologic stresses (e.g., prolonged heavy labor, freezing weather). Livestock also provide local materia medica and ethnomedical models. Their grazing or foraging can help control agents of human disease that breed in brushy or fouled grounds and waterways.

Mental health: Animal foods may be helpful for some types of psychologic stress, such as that produced by grieving or warfare. In some cultures, an individual's health, fate, wisdom, or skills are linked to a livestock familiar. Typically, a person's ability to raise large and healthy herds or flocks leads to pride, prestige, and a sense of security. People everywhere take pleasure from favorite, named animals, and interactions with animals can produce positive psychosomatic effects in humans.

This list is by no means exhaustive, and the classification of benefits is somewhat arbitrary.

BENEFITS OF STOCKRAISING IN THE DEVELOPING WORLD—cont'd

Safety: Livestock may do double duty as "burglar alarms" (e.g., guineafowl, geese), disaster warning devices (e.g., storms, floods, earthquakes), and guards (e.g., work dogs and llama placed in flocks of sheep to warn against and fend off predators).

Recreation: Especially in rural areas, livestock provide entertainment in the form of races, rides, fights, and exhibitions.

Religion and culture: In virtually all societies, livestock sacrifices and feast meats are imperative for the fulfillment of social and religious obligations, rites of passage, and secular holidays. Livestock also figure as icons, metaphors, totems, and other symbols in the language (oral or written), song, and art of all cultures.

tant functions of livestock is as savings, investment, and credit instruments in the Third World, where banking systems are often absent, disorganized, or intimidating; where currencies are unstable; and where land is not a commodity. In these fiduciary roles, livestock offer some unique advantages. Animals are readily fungible—there is almost always a market for them, and they come in different "denominations" that can be liquidated according to the size of a given cash need. Microlivestock (e.g., poultry, rabbits, guinea pigs) may function as spending money or checking accounts, small stock (e.g., swine, sheep, goats) function somewhat like savings accounts and money markets, and large stock (e.g., cattle, water buffaloes, camels) constitute trust funds and blue-chip stocks, to be cashed in for major expenditures such as farm equipment or education. Microlivestock also make it easy for small investors to enter the "stock market" and, over time, trade up to higher denominations. In some cultures, investing in livestock is recognized as a good way to shelter savings that would, if held in cash, be subject to a "kin tax" (i.e., demands for funds from relatives). As investments, livestock generally hold their value and yield substantial interest (10%, on average) in the form of weight gains and new births.

For a great many rural dwellers, such "stockholdings" constitute the main source of social security from cradle to grave, functioning as medical and disability insurance, retirement and pension plans, and death benefits.

Stockraising also typically provides the only form of crop insurance available to Third World farmers. When fields fail, feeding animals on whatever biomass was produced can help farmers recover at least some of the value of the cropping inputs expended (see Box 41-1). Herd animals can be moved to escape the localized agroecologic disturbances that led to crop failure. All the while, livestock continue to provide food directly and through exchange for plant foods; later, they also furnish the cash, credit, or barter items with which the farmer can obtain supplies to begin crop farming again.

Conversely, in years of surplus crop production, impossibly low crop prices, or interruption of farm-to-market transport systems, livestock serve as living granaries to store a portion of the harvest in a more rot-, rodent-, and insect-resistant and interest-yielding form that, if necessary, can walk itself to market. In good and bad crop years, livestock can exploit fallowing fields, nonarable lands, and unique patches of natural resources (e.g., lake algae, reeds) that would otherwise be of less use for humans.

Background and Rationale of ERD&E

The variety of goods and services listed in Box 41-1 demonstrates that livestock production is critical to rural peoples worldwide. Indeed, livestock constitute "a driving force for food security and sustainable development" (Sansoucy, 1994). However, as agricultural scientists, developers, and, above all, stockraisers know well, gains in livestock production and productivity are difficult to realize without corresponding improvements in animal health.

Background

Beginning in the mid-1970s, ERD&E emerged as an internationally[5] recognized branch of research, largely in response to growing concern for animal health in the context of practical, field-level projects in animal agriculture. As investigators experimented with different approaches and the projects matured, evidence suggested that conventional formal-sector resources alone would be inadequate to meet the basic veterinary needs of many Third World stockraisers in a sustainable fashion.

Significantly, this finding paralleled similar conclusions by the World Health Organization (WHO) in 1978 with regard to the universal delivery of basic human health care (Bannerman, Burton, Wen-Chieh, 1983; WHO, 1991a,b). As much as 90% of the world's population today still relies mainly on local ethnomedicine for most of their health needs (Duke, 1992; Plotkin, 1988). Similar figures appear to hold for the livestock sector. In both sectors, given the burgeoning human and livestock population and the soaring costs of high-tech, Western medicine, scientists and developers have increasingly acknowledged the utility of building on and working with existing local health care resources—both technologic and sociologic.[6]

The origin and evolution of ethnoveterinary medicine as a recognized branch of research have been detailed elsewhere, along with the many disciplines and research topics it embodies (McCorkle, 1986). An illustrative but criticoanalytic annotated bibliography of 261 items on the subject is available (Mathias-Mundy, McCorkle, 1989), as well as a descriptive database of 300 items dealing mainly with ethnoveterinary botanicals (Zeutzius, 1990) and an analytic overview of ERD&E for the African continent (McCorkle, Mathias-Mundy, 1992).

Although the information amassed in these and other overview efforts is too great to detail here, some of the more systematic or sustained efforts in ERD&E are noted for further reference. These include the cumulative work of Calvin Schwabe and his students (see the Schwabe publications cited in the references list and in the 1989 bibliography); the studies in seven Asian nations supported by the Food and Agriculture Organization (FAO) of the United Nations (FAO, 1980-1992); the Tufts University interdisciplinary teamwork (Sollod, Wolfgang, Knight, 1984; Sollod and Knight, 1983; Stem, 1996); the growing corpus of ERD&E by the Intermediate Technology Development Group (Grandin, Young, 1996); and the Small Ruminant Collaborative Research Support Program (Mathias-Mundy, Murdiati, 1991; McCorkle, 1982; and various Mathias and McCorkle references). A sampling of other recent publications includes Bizimana, 1994; deMaar, 1992; IIRR, 1994; Matzigkeit, 1990; McCorkle and others, 1996; and Revue Scientifique et Technique de l'Office International des Épizooties, 1994. Several English-language journals on veterinary acupuncture and acupressure have also been launched during the last decade, in addition to the vast amount of related literature in Chinese.[7]

Rationale

The wealth of publications available on ERD&E signals a clear and growing consensus that this modality promises to assist stockraisers who have no, little, or declining access to conventional, Western-style veterinary care and supplies. Relying solely on Western-style medicine and delivery systems, governments in most of the developing world have proved incapable of meeting most of their population's needs for veterinary services (Cheneau, 1985; Daniels and others, 1993; de Haan, Nissen, 1985; Leonard, 1987, 1993; Schillhorn van Veen, de Haan, 1995). This situation exists for many reasons that are summarized as follows:

- Heavy external debt burdens and, more recently, structural-adjustment programs make for scarce foreign exchange with which to import veterinary supplies that cannot be produced locally.
- Management of public exchequers is often inept,

corrupt, or skewed, with little of the taxes from the livestock sector going to production-related services for rural stockraisers.
- Veterinary research and extension agencies are often bloated, top-heavy bureaucracies, with as much as 90% of the total budget for livestock services going mainly to staff salaries (CTA/GTZ/IEMVT, 1985).
- Corruption or inept management leaves little for basic operational costs such as veterinary drugs; surgical supplies; field equipment; infrastructure items such as public dipping tanks and cold-chains; clinics, diagnostic laboratories and laboratory equipment; computers, offices, and office supplies; and vehicles, spare parts, and fuel with which to reach clients or supervise field agents.
- An even smaller share of these already slim services reaches rural areas, which have scant political and economic power and limited infrastructure.
- Government professionals (veterinary and otherwise) resist postings to rural areas with minimal infrastructural and social amenities.
- Civil or political strife (widespread banditry, strikes, terrorism, intertribal warfare, coups d'état) may disrupt already fragile government delivery systems.
- If civil disruption cuts off supplies of imported drugs with which livestock have been treated for several generations, the animals may have lost much of their innate or acquired immunity, and the targeted diseases can then return with even greater virulence.
- In addition to zoonoses (i.e., diseases transmissible between humans and animals), many government livestock services have concentrated on infectious epidemic diseases—especially those that imperil foreign-exchange earnings from exports of animals or animal products by powerful citizens.
- This narrow focus has often been adopted even in "the conspicuous lack of economic data" (FAO, 1991c) indicating that the epidemic diseases in question are those most common or deleterious to most of the nation's stockraisers in terms of goods, services, and income from animals—thus further skewing the targeting of scarce veterinary resources.

Indeed, most governments have paid relatively little attention to other, less dramatic noninfectious and production diseases (e.g., metabolic disorders, nutritional deficiencies, plant and chemical toxicoses, reproductive ills, dairy-related problems such as mastitis). Yet, along with parasitism, in the aggregate these problems may cause larger economic losses. For most stockraisers, the effect of these problems is of equal or even greater concern than that of epidemic diseases (Schillhorn van Veen, 1993).

Of course, many valid questions have been raised concerning the extent to which governments should subsidize veterinary assistance that redounds to private rather than public good (Leonard, 1993; Umali, Feder, de Haan,

1992), as is the case for many production and parasitic diseases. Yet for some of the same reasons detailed earlier, conventional privatized veterinary services have also proved inadequate to meet the needs of poor, remote, or small-scale stockraisers. Moreover, private veterinarians in the Third World often do little clinical work, concentrating instead on the sale of drugs and other livestock supplies (Schillhorn van Veen, 1994).

Even when formal-sector, privatized, or government veterinary services and supplies are available, they are usually too expensive for the average producer. As stockraisers often wisely calculate, these services and supplies may not be worth the price or trouble, for a variety of reasons:

- Field-level veterinary workers in remote, rural parts of the developing world are typically inadequately trained, equipped, motivated, and supervised.
- Private veterinarians and drug vendors (including government employees with easy access to the livestock agency's supposedly free drug supplies) who hold local monopolies on livestock services and supplies may greatly inflate prices.
- Unscrupulous vendors may foist adulterated, expired, and even contraindicated drugs and agrochemicals on unsuspecting clients, particularly clients who are formally uneducated or politically oppressed.
- Formal-sector veterinary workers and suppliers may treat poor, rural, or illiterate clients in a condescending, supercilious manner.
- Depending on the species and class of animal involved, its place in the production system, its market value, and other variables (Mathias, McCorkle, 1997), the cost of professional veterinary attention or Western commercial pharmaceuticals may well outstrip the animal's value to the producer.

Taken together, these factors make for limited delivery of high-quality formal-sector health services in developing countries. Often services do not target the most pressing veterinary concerns of the small-scale stockraisers or indigenous stockraisers who make up the majority of producers. Indeed, in some situations, producers lose more than they would if they had not sought conventional veterinary services at all.

Together, these considerations suggest an urgent need for "practical, low-tech, and cost-effective methods" of veterinary care and extension attuned to stockraisers' own concerns (FAO, 1991c). Ideally, such methods should be amenable to application by stockraisers or other local residents themselves. Herein lies the value of ethnoveterinary medicine.

Subject Matter and Principles of ERD&E

The goal of ERD&E is to offset some of the previously discussed problems by building on local veterinary and husbandry knowlege and practice, the associated materia medica, and local human and socioorganizational resources. This approach can increase the number of reliable veterinary alternatives available to producers in a cost-effective and sustainable way.

Target groups for ERD&E are small-scale stockraisers—including many periurban and women stockraisers—and poor or remote peoples who cannot afford or gain access to conventional services that are available. However, medical alternatives are important to all people whenever a situation arises requiring prompt action to ameliorate a problem, slow disease progression, or at least ease the patient's pain until specialized help is available.

Box 41-2 lists the topics and themes addressed by ERD&E in the process of developing and delivering workable, locally based veterinary alternatives. Although a systematic review of each of these topics is beyond the scope of this chapter, many are touched on later, in the discussion of lessons learned.

Box 41-2 also serves to highlight one of the paramount principles of ERD&E: its interdisciplinary nature. Many factors impinge on animal health, including endogenous and exogenous variables, defined respectively as internal and external to causative agents and their hosts. The interplay of such variables lies beyond the ken of any one social, biologic, or technical science. Many of the themes and issues noted in the box are grounded in anthropology, sociology, economics, and political science, as well as veterinary medicine both inside and outside the laboratory. Others call for additional expertise in disciplines such as agricultural extension and education; linguistics; animal husbandry, genetics, and reproduction; range management and forage agronomy; and virtually all aspects of agroecology (e.g., botany, entomology, hydrology, soil science, geology).

Another fundamental principle of ERD&E is holism. To achieve significant and sustainable net improvements in the well-being of humans, veterinary needs must be defined and dealt with in the context of the biophysical, economic, social, cultural (including religious), and political systems in which animals and their owners are embedded. Otherwise, development efforts may end up merely "robbing Peter to pay Paul." Such efforts may succeed in increasing livestock productivity, but they may do so only by compromising environmental health or taking resources from other sectors, such as cropping, human health, and children's education (McCorkle, 1992, 1994a).

Closely related to these principles is the commitment of ERD&E to in-depth, firsthand fieldwork with stockraisers themselves, under the real-world conditions to which they and their animals are subject. Hence ERD&E tends to feature the use of time-tested methods of anthropologic fieldwork and the extension knowledge of rural sociology. These are synergistically combined with the clinical and laboratory expertise of veterinarians and animal scientists, as well as all these disciplines' skills in on-farm research and development.

BOX 41-2

TOPICS AND THEMES IN *ERD&E*

THE ETHNOVETERINARY SCIENCE SYSTEM
- Ethnoveterinary semantics and taxonomies: How people name and classify diseases, treatments and other health matters.
- Ethnopathophysiology: How people understand the interrelationship, functions, and malfunctions of different organs and systems (e.g., circulatory, nervous), often drawing on information garnered from practical necropsy at slaughter or ritual sacrifice.
- Ethnoetiologic and ethnoepidemiologic theories: The causes (supernatural as well as natural) that people assign to different diseases and their understandings about disease transmission (including zoonoses).
- Ethnodiagnostic knowledge and technique: Based on all the above factors, plus clinical observation of signs and syndromes, how people decide what the given health care problem is and thus how to treat or control it.

ETHNOTHERAPEUTIC AND PROPHYLACTIC KNOWLEDGE AND PRACTICE
- Ethnopharmacology and ethnotoxicology: What local drugs people prepare from given ingredients to produce certain medical effects and the administration, posology, storage, and known side effects of these drugs.
- Traditional immunizations: Including both direct (vaccination) and indirect (e.g., purposive exposure) methods.
- Local surgical techniques: For example, debridement, suture, cauterization, rumen trocarization, obstetric operations, bonesetting, and excision of tumors.
- Manipulative and mechanical techniques: For example, massage, exercise, conditioning, acupuncture or acupressure, and quarantine.
- Pest, parasite, and predator control and avoidance: Many different practices.

LOCAL HUSBANDRY AND MANAGEMENT PRACTICES WITH HEALTH IMPLICATIONS
- Forages, dietary supplements, feeding and watering regimens, herding strategies or movements, species mix, and quarantine.
- Management of animal reproduction and breeding: For example, selection for disease resistance or assurance of optimal health conditions for mating, birthing, and lactation by culling or castration (both open surgery and bloodless techniques) and controlled breeding (e.g., by subdividing herds by sex, placing aprons on male animals, deviating the penis).
- Carcass use and disposal and product handling: What people do with the carcasses or products of diseased animals and how they slaughter and butcher to ward against further spread of disease among livestock or humans.
- Other management tasks with health implications: For example, horn-training, nose-ringing, docking, and shearing; care and feeding of herd or farm dogs that can transmit livestock diseases; special handling of dairy animals.

MEDICORELIGIOUS OPERATIONS AND CULTURAL VALUES*
- Greater veterinary attention for "sacred" or culturally valued species or individuals.
- Codification of useful veterinary knowledge in religious idiom and ritual.
- Ideologic proscriptions and prescriptions on the breeding, handling, culling, slaughter, consumption, or curing of different species or diseased animals.

DELIVERY OF HEALTH CARE SERVICES
- Many standard extension issues.
- Inclusion in formal medical systems of paraprofessionals, traditional/informal practitioners, and stockraisers themselves as caregivers.
- Issues in intersectoral delivery of care.

SOCIAL STRUCTURES AND ORGANIZATION
- Distribution of ethnoveterinary knowledge and skills by social status.
- Social structures useful for health care delivery, cooperative husbandry and health care action, epidemiologic surveillance, transmission of health care knowledge, and collaborative RD&E.

---

*Insofar as these surround or influence health care and decision making.

BOX 41-2

Topics and Themes in ERD&E—cont'd

ECONOMIC, POLICY, AND INSTITUTIONAL ISSUES†
- Appraisal of economic and social costs and benefits at micro and macro levels of different delivery, disease treatment and control options, epidemiologic information systems, government imports, price controls, and subsidies to the health care sector(s).
- Reanalysis and adjustment of corresponding government policies.
- Organization of livestock agencies and veterinary training institutes to take greater account of producers' expressed health needs and ethnoveterinary resources.

EDUCATIONAL ISSUES†
- Inclusion of modules or demonstrations on the relevant ethnoveterinary science systems, their associated vocabularies, and beneficial local veterinary and husbandry knowledge and practice in primary or secondary educational curricula, literacy programs, and university, vocational, and in-service training for veterinary professionals, extensionists, and paraprofessionals.

ENVIRONMENTAL ISSUES
- Too numerous to list (see text) but spanning human and environmental health as well as animal health.

ETHNOVETERINARY RESEARCH AND DEVELOPMENT METHODS AND APPROACHES
- See text.

†In light of findings from ERDE.

This hybrid methodology is one of the major means of applying a fourth principle of ERD&E: its equal attention to and respect for both *emic* and *etic* (respectively, insiders', or ethnoscientific, and outsiders', or Western-scientific) perspectives and information in the definition, holistic description, and analysis of animal health and husbandry problems. Without such a balance, ERD&E may not meet its ultimate goal of ensuring that results are useful to and readily usable by stockraisers.

Ensuring thorough *emic* input into the ERD&E process and complementing the hybrid methodology outlined above, a fifth and final principle has come to characterize ERD&E: participation and empowerment, embodied in a collaborative approach in which native stockraisers work alongside outsider colleagues as coresearchers, codevelopers, and coextensionists. In this approach, producers have major input into the definition of RD&E problems; they assist in the design of on-farm research to address the problems identified and then participate in the experiments.

Participation may include identifying promising ethnoveterinary treatments, preparing different strengths and mixtures of local prescriptions to be tested on farm, and conducting pretest and posttest sampling of local pest or parasite populations.[8] Of course, participating producers also evaluate all results from their vantage point as the final authority on user satisfaction. In the dissemination of useful technologies or information thus validated or generated, interested stockraisers, traditional healers, and community storekeepers may also assume extension roles.

Thus an RD&E team is created that embraces not only scientists and the usual government or NGO (nongovernmental and non–business organization) extensionists but producers-*cum*-"ethnoscientists," local volunteers, health care practitioners, and businesspeople. Each of these groups contributes knowledge, skills, and collegial or community networks.[9]

As with the topics and themes of Box 41-2, these principles cannot be fully examined here. In any event, they are little more than the tenets of good, applied RD&E in agriculture or industry. However, the practical application of most of these principles is exemplified in the next section, which focuses on lessons learned from ERD&E. Both for ease and continuity of exposition and because of stockraisers' own concerns, the illustrations in the following sections are drawn mainly (but not exclusively) from the world's most economically devastating veterinary problem—parasitic disease. As summarized in Box 41-3, however, the lessons outlined hold for all ERD&E and the study and application of local knowledge in general.

Lessons Learned from ERD&E[10]

Fundamental Lessons

The first lesson learned from examining local knowledge—veterinary and otherwise—has already been enunciated: *the value of identifying and applying effective, inexpensive, and readily accessible local solutions to problems.* Such

BOX 41-3

LESSONS FROM *ERD&E* FOR THE *S*TUDY AND *A*PPLICATION OF *L*OCAL *K*NOWLEDGE

1. Many technologies and practices based in local knowledge are effective. They are generally cheaper and more accessible, comprehensible, socioculturally acceptable, and ultimately sustainable than their conventional equivalents.
2. Such technologies and practices can often be enhanced through technoblending.
3. The validation and application of effective local or blended technologies and practices that rely on native floral and fauna resources can lend impetus to the maintenance of both biologic and cultural (biocultural) diversity.
4. Likewise, local-knowledge RDE can help reinvigorate old professions and statuses (e.g., ethnomedical practitioners) or create new ones, stimulating local economies and industries (e.g., sustainable harvest or cultivation of ethnobotanicals, production of and trade in ethnopharmaceuticals, establishment of ethnoveterinary clinics).
5. Local knowledge and its associated technologies and practices may suggest environmentally (and possibly also biomedically) friendly solutions to some development problems, increasing health and safety among both humans and livestock.
6. Many such solutions are to be found in management/husbandry strategies—singly or in integrated disease management (IDM) packages—rather than in technologic hardware (i.e., materials, tools, infrastructure).
7. Attention must be given to the software (i.e., social organization, taxonomic and semantic systems, information networks) as well as the hardware with which local knowledge is operationalized.
8. For maximal understanding and impact in studying and applying local knowledge from one domain (e.g., animal health care), this domain must usually be examined in relation to other, associated ethnoscientific disciplines (e.g., ethnoecology) as well.
9. Emic definitions of local-knowledge domains and of intersectoral linkages (e.g., those between health care for livestock and humans) can point the way to innovative development approaches.
10. Synergisms can be realized between education and agricultural extension research surveillance systems by folding findings from local-knowledge research and development into training curricula and outreach programs.
11. A bonus of the foregoing is enhanced maintenance of cultural diversity and empowerment of people.
12. Local knowledge should not be dismissed out of hand just because it is sometimes couched in a seemingly nonscientific or supernatural idiom; it should always be investigated further.
13. As its bearers themselves often point out, local knowledge is not perfect or omniscient, no more than is conventional science.
14. Scientific validation of ethnoscientific (and perhaps especially ethnomedical) knowledge is important for both ethical and pragmatic reasons.
15. Validation need not imply denigration of local knowledge and culture.
16. More care should be taken in conventional methodologic approaches to validation. Creative, new research designs are needed.
17. Such methodologies and designs must be cost-effective and feasible for national research and development entities if an appreciable number of technologies and practices are to be validated and disseminated.

solutions are workable precisely because they are locally grounded. For example, ERD&E has repeatedly demonstrated that many treatments made from local plants and other materials to combat parasitic diseases of livestock are just as effective as their conventional counterparts, particularly in extensive stockraising operations. Yet unlike costly commercial drugs and agrochemicals that are usually imported, these local remedies can be had for little more than the labor (and, of course, the knowledge) involved in collecting and preparing the necessary ingredients.

Box 41-4 exemplifies this point, using participatory research by a sustainable animal agriculture project spanning 10 years (see endnote 1).

The findings presented in Box 41-4 are by no means

BOX 41-4

ERD&E in Action

In the mid-1980s, farmers of Peru's central Andes found that with inflation running at more than 2000% annually and with terrorists bombing key infrastructure such as roads and bridges, they could no longer afford or obtain the commercial sheep dips they had been using for the past decade at the urging of the agricultural extension service. As a result, ectoparasites had returned in force to plague their flocks. Farmers identified this as one of their top animal production problems. A village meeting was held for farmers to discuss possible solutions to this problem with Peruvian and U.S. veterinary, social, and economic researchers of the SR-CRSP. During the meeting, one young man mentioned an almost-forgotten home remedy with which his grandmother successfully cured bovine and equine ectoparasitism. It involved a strong black soap and a plant that grew wild in the communal lands. He suggested that perhaps this could work on sheep, too.

The plant in question turned out to be a native tobacco (*Nicotiana paniculata* L.). The ectoparasiticidal properties of the powerful alkaloids in tobacco have long been known and used around the world, even in twentieth-century Europe. Unsurprisingly, when farmers and researchers conducted tests of the treatment on-farm, it worked.

The next question was, could this therapy somehow be used as an effective and convenient substitute for the prophylactic commercial dips? Traditionally the tobacco remedy was applied topically. However, even for a small flock this is a time-consuming process, and it is more difficult to use on fleece-bearing animals than on species like cattle, horses, and burros. Indeed, dips were invented as a faster and more thorough alternative to topical applications. Community members naturally hoped the traditional therapy could be made into a modern-style dip because they were already familiar with this technique and had dipping facilities in the community.

Working together, farmers and researchers started a series of on-farm trials. First, they modified the traditional prescription for cattle to fit the smaller size of sheep and the plan to make an aqueous solution of the materia medica. For the trials, families agreed on methods to divide their flocks into experimental and control groups while holding husbandry variables constant; men, women, and children all helped gather the plant materials; the women ground them to a powder and prepared the different concentrations of dipping solutions; and the men performed the actual dipping of the sheep. A variety of dipping regimens were tested, with detailed records kept of parasite mortality rates and close checking for harmful side effects.

One formula tested proved to be as effective as the store-bought agrochemicals the farmers had previously used. Indeed, many people believed the homemade dip was even more effective. Certainly it was cheaper and no more time-consuming than making the long trek down and back up the mountainside to the agrosupply shops in the valley market town. Moreover, farmers knew they could rely on the quality of their homemade dip, in contrast to the often adulterated or outright fraudulent products in the shops.

Exhilarated by this success, the community went on to test other local remedies, tackling more recalcitrant problems of endoparasitism. Farmers had identified liver fluke disease (fasciolosis or distomatosis) as their major endoparasitic worry. A zoonosis endemic in the Andes, fasciolosis is prevalent among rural populations there and sheep do not develop resistance to this parasitic infection. One of the community's still-popular traditional remedies for this destructive trematode consisted of drenching (force-feeding liquid medicines to livestock) with a decoction of fresh artichoke (*Cynara scolymus*) leaves combined with salt and mineral or cooking oil.

In this case, people prepared the artichoke drench according to their traditional prescription, and both veterinary and social scientists assisted in selecting a random sample of mixed-sex sheep matched for age and management regime, dividing them into experimental and control groups from among the flocks of cooperating families. As before, dosing records were kept, along with corresponding fecal egg counts. Owners permitted several sheep from each test group to be killed so that counts of adult flukes (which are visible to the naked eye) could also be made.

For more information on these cases and related methods, consult Bazalar, McCorkle, 1989; McCorkle, 1989b; and McCorkle, 1990. *Continued*

BOX 41-4

ERD&E IN ACTION—cont'd

As with the wild tobacco treatment, the artichoke drench proved effective. Within a week, fecal counts of fluke eggs diminished by 71% and liver necropsies indicated an 89% reduction in adult flukes. In fact, these findings came as little surprise to the veterinarians on the team, given their pharmacologic knowledge of the high cyanide content in artichoke leaves. No negative side effects were evident, however. Community members were so enthusiastic about the validation of this local treatment that they decided to extend it to their communal flock as well, but with one improvement. From the Western-scientific inputs into the experiment, people learned that it would be helpful to increase the strength, frequency, and regularity of their drenching.

isolated or unusual. Throughout the Andes, traditional preparations containing sylvan or domesticated plants to combat parasites of livestock have been scientifically validated. Some may have been used for centuries. One well-studied example is the traditional use as an ectoparasiticide for camelids (llama and alpaca) of the alkaloid-laden water that remains after tarwi (*Lupinas mutabilis,* an ancient and highly nutritious Andean foodcrop) is steeped to detoxify it for human consumption. Technoblended to yield more powerful extracts, dosages, or modes of administration, tarwi has proved an excellent alternative to commercial products. The extract of another Andean plant *(Aspidium Filix-mas)* has had great success in treating Bolivian sheep for flukes. Traditional remedies made from the leaves of certain *Senecio* species and the seeds of the giant South American pumpkin *Cucurbita maxima Duch* have proved effective against gastrointestinal parasites of sheep.

However, the larger significance of experiments such as those discussed in Box 41-4 lies in their exemplification of the ERD&E enterprise at its best (or near best—see Box 41-15). These cases illustrate another vital lesson that has emerged from ERD&E worldwide: the value of *techno-blending,* or the combining of knowledge from different sources (here, Western and ethnoscientific) to achieve more powerful but still readily accessible solutions to development problems.

Such blended approaches often provide the best of both worlds. New uses for old remedies may be discovered (e.g., for sheep as well as for cattle and horses; for prophylaxis as well as therapy); a more efficient route of administration may be found (e.g., dipping versus topical application); or a more effective treatment regimen may be devised.

Several lessons relevant to environment and development problems have emerged from work in ERD&E worldwide. One is that validating the efficacy of traditional materia medica from local flora and fauna can provide an impetus to protect and maintain biodiversity (and also cultural diversity). As with the wild Andean tobacco, valuable traditional uses of such species may have been all but forgotten. Worse still, other-culture outsiders, such as agronomists or missionaries, may have branded such

species as weeds, pests, or even "sinful" and set about to eradicate them. When their usefulness is experimentally validated, however, their controlled harvest, semidomestication, and even varietal selection become of interest to governments and local residents (Box 41-5).

A closely related lesson is that initiatives like those described in Boxes 41-4 and 41-5 can ultimately lead to the creation or reinforcement of local trade and industry in products based on sylvan resources. This new emphasis brings more jobs, income, and status to rural inhabitants. This is particularly true of ethnopharmaceuticals (Box 41-6).

Such initiatives build on the fact that botanicals selected from the 10% (approximately 25,000) of higher plants used in traditional medicine worldwide (Farnsworth, 1983; Greaves, 1994) are 2 to 5 times more likely to be pharmacologically active than any random sample of plants (Daly, 1983). Because of the cost of random screening, perhaps only 1% of the higher plant species that have been used in ethnomedicine have been subjected to systematic scientific study for their therapeutic value in extract form (Farnsworth, 1983). Nevertheless, from this tiny portion have come at least one fourth of all prescription medicines in use in the West today (Goleman, 1991).[11]

Another lesson from ERD&E is that maintenance of biologic diversity implies maintenance of cultural diversity as embodied in the local peoples who garner and husband ethnopharmacologic knowledge and manage the associated, biodiverse habitats (Hyndman, 1994). Sadly, Western educational and cultural imperialism has led young people to abandon traditional knowledge and practices. In many societies today the young show little interest in taking up traditional medicine as a full- or even part-time profession (Hyndman, 1994; Salih, 1992). Ironically, this loss of interest in the Third World coincides with growing interest in the First World to alternative medicine, both for humans (see endnote 3) and animals.

Fortunately, some farsighted organizations have taken steps to stem this frightening loss of cultural diversity through scholarship programs such as those described in Box 41-7.[12] The goal is to preserve some of the precious

BOX 41-5

Maintaining Biocultural Resources

One outcome of the ethnoveterinary work described in Box 41-4 was Peruvian farmers' interest in organizing, with help from SR-CRSP social scientists, ways to ensure fair, community-wide, sustainable use of their wild tobacco and other sylvan materia medica. Such steps have already been initiated in other parts of the world. Working with Fulani stockraisers in Cameroon, for instance, Heifer Project International (HPI) has assisted traditional veterinary doctors there in documenting and classifying their medicinal plants and establishing zonal nurseries to secure supplies of these invaluable but fast-disappearing materials. HPI also helped these Fulani practitioners organize into a formal association and to win government certification of their services (Nuwanyakpa and others, 1989). Similar efforts are under way among traditional livestock healers in Kenyan farming communities, with assistance from London's Intermediate Technology Development Group (ITDG, 1989, 1992). These healers, too, have planted medicinal gardens—many on their own initiative. They are now looking to obtain government recognition and promotion of their professional status, on a par with that already extended to practitioners of human ethnomedicine in their country.

BOX 41-6

Creating Employment and Income

In Indonesia a thriving industry in jamu (traditional medicines for humans) has long existed. Now the industry is adding more veterinary botanicals to its product lines. For both human and veterinary medicine, nations such as China and India have long promoted the large-scale commercial production of traditional herbal preparations, hundreds of which have been scientifically proved effective. In India today, examples of such drugs for livestock include antifungals, tonics, fortifiers, digestives, and antiparasitics (Anjaria, 1996; Mazars, 1994).

Whether in India, Belize, Brazil, or Samoa, organizations of local people or traditional healers have formed for the protection, sustainable harvest, and direct sale of traditionally gathered botanicals used in both human and animal ethnomedicine. By cutting out exploitative middlemen, local residents are earning greater profits from these natural resources while safeguarding their continued supply (Cox, Balick, 1994; Greaves, 1994).

With various environment development organizations, rural people are exploring other ethnomedically related income-earning opportunities. Some examples are local or regional industries in chemical prospecting; jobs for women and men as forest rangers or as ethnobiologists and parataxonomists trained to collect, identify, and inventory local plant resources; reinforcement or expansion of traditional healers' practices) (see Boxes 41-5 and 41-7); and establishment of local paraveterinary practices, clinics, and drugstores offering a blend of traditional and modern services at affordable prices that are run by trained local healers or producers, stock associations, or businesspeople (Grandin, Thampy, Young, 1991; Greaves, 1994; Iles, Young, 1991).

ethnomedical knowledge amassed through centuries of empirical experience.

Programs such as those described in Box 41-7 can renew interest in the ethnomedical knowledge of local practitioners, along with a firmer resolve to protect and maintain the habitats from which they draw their materia medica. Although these programs have so far focused only on human ethnomedicine, they would be equally appropriate for ethnoveterinary medicine, alone or in combination with initiatives such as that described in Box 41-5.

Another environment-related lesson has emerged from ERD&E paralleling local-knowledge research and development in other agricultural arenas, such as integrated pest management for crops. Taken as a whole or perhaps judiciously combined with modern interventions, ethnoscientific practices may offer more environmentally

BOX 41-7

PRESERVING ETHNOMEDICAL KNOWLEDGE

The venture-capital firm Shaman Pharmaceuticals works directly with rural communities to identify and develop new therapeutic agents, compensating the people for any useful materia medica found in their ethnopharmacopoeia or local ecology. To help protect the vital link between biologic and cultural diversity on which this venture depends, in 1992 Shaman pioneered an innovative plan in one Amazonian community of Ecuador. The firm provided a stipend for the sole apprentice to the community's one traditional healer to continue his studies full-time, instead of constantly interrupting them to do migrant wage labor (Greaves, 1994). Similarly, in 1993 the environmental NGO Conservation International mounted its Sorcerer's Apprentice Program, which awards scholarships to young people to apprentice themselves to elderly medicine men and women of their communities (Goodstern, 1993; Krajick, 1993).

friendly solutions to pest problems of livestock, with fewer negative effects on animal and human health than those propounded by conventional science. A case in point is traditional biologic and other nondrug controls on ectoparasites and disease-bearing pests, compared with some of the dangerous and often economically impractical pesticides urged on much of the Third World by development agencies and governments following Western models now known to be ecologically unsound (Box 41-8).

Another environmentally benign form of disease control found in some stockraising traditions is breeding for genetic tolerance or resistance to disease (Box 41-9). By maintaining valuable animal germplasm, this strategy can greatly reduce or obviate the need for mass applications of Western-style agrotoxins and their attendant threats to human health and wildlife biodiversity (see Box 41-8). Overuse or irregular use of such agrotoxins can ultimately compromise the unique livestock germplasm created by traditional breeding practices. In the absence of disease pressure across multiple generations, indigenous or nativized breeds that enjoy some genetic protection against the diseases being addressed with commercial pesticides or drugs could lose this valuable safeguard. Assuming the presence of a carrier pool of untreated host animals (livestock or wildlife), stockraisers could be locked into long-term dependence on economically unsustainable and only irregularly available drugs and agrochemicals (especially if they are imported). The result can be chemoresistance and the evolution of new strains of pathogens or pests—

as has occurred with the use of such chemicals in plant agriculture.

When it comes to ethnomedicines, however, treatments based on natural local materials and prepared and administered according to time-tested prescriptions and regimens tend to be less toxic, biostable, or biocumulative (Bodeker, 1994b; Etkin, 1990; Ibrahim, 1996; WHO, 1991a,b). Nor do they involve any substances (e.g., fixatives, preservatives, steroids, hormones, broad-spectrum antibiotics) that have triggered First World fears about drug residues in human food or the vitiation of Western miracle drugs. Traditional herbal medicines are also said to produce fewer side effects than synthetics (Lin, Panzer, 1994).

WHO and pharmacologic and toxicologic experts on traditional pharmacopoeia generally agree on one thing: Because such pharmacopoeia have essentially undergone decades or even centuries of empirical clinical trials, they include few or no acutely toxic plants (aside from those purposely used as poisons) and produce no serious unanticipated side effects. Local practitioners and stockraisers know which of the plant materials they use as foods or medicines are mildly toxic or produce unwanted side effects, either singly or in certain compounds. They subject such materials to various mitigating procedures: extraction, as described for tarwi; detoxification—for instance, by making pH adjustments with ash or potash and botanical acids; and other techniques, such as combination in a polyprescription that includes the antidote or deactivator or administration in safe, low dosages. Moreover, local medicines mainly consist of crude botanicals, meaning that, except in very large amounts or especially purified concentrations, they are generally less potent than their Western commercial equivalents [13] (Box 41-10).

Without the preservatives and fixatives of commercial pharmaceuticals, crude botanicals are generally less biostable. This is especially true in hot or humid conditions such as those in much of the Third World. Compared with synthetics, crude botanicals are usually more easily transformed in vivo. These features probably also make for less bioaccumulation in the patient's body and the environment.

Ethnopharmaceuticals are often given only to effect a particular response: Once symptoms disappear, administration is ceased. Such a treatment regimen has potential disadvantages, but Third World stockraisers and healers have few ways to test for the continued presence in the body of many endoparasites or hemoparasites and other subtle or invisible agents of disease. Still, depending on the ailment, such regimens have potential advantages, too. With less medication, bioaccumulation is decreased. Incomplete treatment of certain diseases can also be beneficial insofar as it encourages tolerance or premunity to the infectious agents. It may also mean less opportunity for chemoresistance, depending on the agent. Moreover, for some kinds of parasitism a local treatment that is, for ex-

BOX 41-8

Biologic Controls

In parts of Africa, livestock are periodically treated against ectoparasites without use of drugs. The animals are merely herded into water (preferably salty or sulfurous) long enough for the parasites to drown or loosen their hold and be washed away. For the same reason, owners of water buffaloes in Asia make sure their animals wallow regularly.

Companion species that feed on livestock parasites and pests are a traditional biologic control used worldwide. For example, in Africa and Asia, chickens and ducks may be herded through an area to help clear it of snails and flies. In Malaysia and other parts of Asia, stockraisers keep cats in and around livestock quarters to hold down populations of potentially disease-bearing rodents and annoying insects—just like the barn cats of the Western world. Also in Asia, poultry are often kept in buffaloes' nighttime quarters, where the fowl gobble up any ectoparasites that survive wallowing; in fact, the buffaloes lie down and obligingly lift their legs so the birds can reach the parasites still clinging to difficult sites such as the britch and axillae (Anonymous, 1994). Bedouins in Sinai also keep poultry to eat ticks and other insects that transmit diseases to both livestock and humans (Hadani, Shimshony, 1994).

These nondrug controls stand in sharp contrast to conventional Western veterinary practice, which advocates dipping, spraying, or dusting livestock with potent commercial agrochemicals. These practices have been enthusiastically adopted in many parts of Africa for controlling cattle ticks. Indeed, African villagers have been known to dust themselves for lice with some of these "white man's medicines"—including highly toxic and biocumulative insecticides such as DDT (McCorkle, fieldwork in Niger, 1988; Ibrahim, 1996). On occasion, dip runoff has poisoned community drinking-water supplies for livestock and people; DDT has been found in the meat and fish sold in African markets (McCorkle, fieldwork in Niger, 1988; Ibrahim, 1996).

In parts of southern Africa, the extreme toxicity and long-term residual effects of such chemicals have led to a distressing environmental irony. There, ox-peckers (also known as *cowbirds*) provide a natural biologic control by feeding on the same ectoparasites the dips are intended to combat. However, because of dip residues, some species of these birds have been poisoned nearly to extinction (Glen-Leary, 1990). As if all this were not enough, cost-benefit studies of cattle-dipping programs in Africa have shown that dipping expenses can surpass annual revenues per head, with little gain in livestock productivity (de Haan, Bekure, 1991).

BOX 41-9

Genetic Strategies

When they move into a new area, Fulani cattle raisers of Nigeria usually purchase local studs to enhance their herds' adaptation to endemic diseases and other environmental conditions. Their genetic strategies have resulted in exceptionally hardy and disease-resistant breeds. An example is the Keteku, which the Fulani "genetically engineered" by crossing Bunaji (a savanna milch breed) with N'Dama (a trypanotolerant rainforest breed) to produce cattle who can thrive under a wider range of drought and disease challenge (Salih, 1994; Schillhorn van Veen, 1995). African stockraisers have also bred trypanotolerant (the Djallonké of West Africa) and hemonchosis-resistant (among East Africa's Maasai) sheep. African stockraisers appreciated and wisely husbanded the unique germplasm involved in these and other breeds long before it was recognized by Western researchers.

BOX 41-10

Traditional versus Modern Pharmacology

In 1994 a set of on-station trials was mounted in Indonesia to validate a local Javanese treatment for ovine endoparasitism, with the goal of making a commercial version for the market. The traditional treatment consists merely of periodically feeding the sheep whole, immature papaya fruits. On the basis of prior experiments and review of the pharmacologic literature, scientists knew the key parasiticidal constituent resided mainly in the fruit sap. Therefore they collected and administered only the sap, instead of following farmers' practice of feeding the whole fruit. In a matter of hours, 80% of the sheep in the high-dosage experimental group and 20% in the medium-dosage group died of acute poisoning (Anonymous, 1994).

ample, only 60% effective must be weighed against the additional costs and benefits of using a 90%- or 100%-effective commercial drug, given that a low-grade infestation may not seriously affect the stockraiser's production goals (de Haan, Bekure, 1991; deMaar, 1992).

Finally, because people are usually more familiar with indigenous medicines, they may be less likely to misuse or abuse these preparations than with alien Western drugs. As documented in many studies, comprehension of the proper indications, administration, posology, and actions of powerful Western commercial pharmaceuticals is often sketchy among Third World stockraisers (Box 41-11). At best, the mistaken application of such alien materia medica can mean wasting poor families' scarce time and money on drugs that produce little net benefit. At worst, it can foster chemoresistance and cause disease and death among livestock and sometimes humans.

Effective ethnopharmaceuticals may pose fewer dangers than do the more highly residual, poisonous, concentrated, and unfamiliar drugs and agrochemicals of the First World. Humans, livestock, local fauna, and the environment stand to benefit from ethnomedical alternatives.

Strategic Management Lessons

Many diseases can be prevented or adequately controlled with little or no recourse to traditional or modern chemotherapy (Donald, 1994). This brings us to another lesson from ERD&E: the potential environmental, economic, and other advantages of drawing more heavily on local knowledge as embodied in stockraisers' many astute management practices to promote livestock health and productivity. Traditional management and husbandry techniques often offer additional alternatives for combating such problems as parasitism.

Some of these practices have already been described (e.g., wallows and baths, companion species). Selective breeding is also valuable (see Box 41-9). In a related vein, many people attempt to control the timing of breeding (see Box 41-2) so that parturition occurs during seasons when parasites are less of a threat to dams and their young. Conversely, young animals may be purposely exposed to parasitic infection to build up tolerance. More common are herding strategies that entail pasturing, watering, and moving animals to avoid times, places, and conditions in which disease-bearing pests and parasites are most active, infectious, or numerous. Box 41-12 describes a number of such practices used in contemporary Africa, Latin America, and the Middle East.

Indeed, stockraisers generally endeavor to keep their herds away from moist, low-lying, and heavily wooded areas that provide prime habitat for parasites and their hosts and vectors. For example, livestock may not be allowed to graze in swamps or floodplains in which the aquatic snail host of liver flukes is common. African pastoralists do not permit their animals to rest in the shade of trees observed to harbor large numbers of wood ticks. Many herders know to avoid such sites precisely during the season or year when parasitic life cycles amplify the risk of infection (see Box 41-12).

When avoidance is not an option, stockraisers may take other measures appropriate to the ecozone to control pests and parasites. For example, pastures may be deliberately overstocked to check the growth of woody vegetation. Following the example of natural phenomena, herders may set

---

BOX 41-11

*P*ROBLEMS WITH *N*ONTRADITIONAL *M*EDICINES

Accustomed to the crude botanicals of their traditional medicine, Nigerian agropastoralists may administer Western drugs in dangerously large quantities (Ibrahim, 1996). Samburu pastoralists of Kenya, on the other hand, often calculate the dosages and dipping concentrations of potent modern drugs by trial and error; as a result, some animals have been literally dosed or dipped to death (Grandin, Young, 1996). Also, Samburu consider aqueous Western drugs less powerful than viscous ones. Thus they overdose with the former, again risking toxicoses, and underdose with the latter, possibly encouraging chemoresistance.

Unfamiliar with Western drugs' specificity, Kenya's Pokot and Maasai pastoralists often give livestock potentially dangerous "cocktails" of drugs in the hope that one or another or the combination will work (Grandin, Young, 1996). The Pokot administer Novidium tablets (a trypanocide) by inserting them in an incision in the skin, rather than dissolving them in water and injecting the fluid subcutaneously as they are designed to be used. This method of administration persists despite the fact that Kenyan pastoralists usually favor injections in the administration of Western drugs. However, they do not always know the appropriate site (e.g., subcutaneous, intramuscular, intravenous) for different injections (Heffernan, Heffernan, Stem, 1996). Sometimes, African herders even inject veterinary drugs into humans (Stem, 1996).

controlled fires, which destroy parasites and their habitats and encourage the growth of nutritious grasses while diminishing the risk of wildfires. They may also chop down brush known to harbor disease-bearing pests. Such strategies help break the life cycle and reduce the populations of ticks, flies, mosquitoes, and other insects that transmit diseases to humans and wild and domestic animals.

Another ethologically and ecologically astute husbandry strategy is mixed grazing, or temporarily or permanently herding different livestock species together. Because every species has different feeding or flocking habits and disease susceptibilities, this practice increases herd health as a whole. For instance, sheep can harmlessly ingest some parasites that would otherwise sicken cattle, and vice versa. Thus one species can dilute disease agents that would otherwise infect another species.[14]

BOX 41-12

Husbandry Methods

Along with African pastoralists, Quechua (Inca) Indian agropastoralists delay turning their animals out to pasture in the early morning until the dew has dried. By that time, the larvae or hosts of many kinds of parasites that emerge with the damp of the dew have retreated to the soil, where they are less likely to be ingested by the grazing herd. Tzotzil Maya shepherdesses of highland Mexico ward off such parasites in different and sometimes unique ways. Especially during the rainy season, before the early-morning trailing of their flocks to the day's grazing grounds, they place a hand-woven grass muzzle on each sheep. The muzzles prevent the hungry animals from nibbling on damp, infested vegetation (and on ripening crops) along the way. Another Tzotzil strategy is to water sheep from buckets rather than directly from streams or springs. This prevents ingestion of the aquaphilic vegetation that shelters infectious larvae or the snail hosts and metacercariae of liver flukes. Furthermore, this practice has multiple environmental benefits. It protects streams, their banks, and riparian habitats (plus their often unique floral and faunal species) from degradation or disturbance by livestock, and it keeps livestock from fouling water supplies also used by humans.

Tzotzil also take care to keep animal quarters clean. Shepherdesses who use temporary corrals move them every 6 weeks; women with permanent structures muck them out every 8 to 10 weeks. In a similar vein, nomadic or transhumant herders of Africa regularly change their campsites and vary their itineraries slightly from year to year. All such practices help prevent the damp, dirty, and crowded conditions under which many disease agents proliferate and spread.

In much of Africa, flies are a particular concern, especially during the rainy season and in humid locales. Besides causing productivity losses from fly worry and myiasis (the maggot-ridden lesions that result from flies' laying their eggs in the skin), flies bear parasitic and other diseases. A well-known example is the tsetse fly, which transmits the trypanosomosis hemoparasites. To diminish the risk of infection during the height of the fly season, stock may be watered at night, when the insects are less active. For the same reason, stockraisers drive their herds through known tsetse flybelts at night.

The hills of Israel are home to a tick that transmits a paralyzing caprine disease. The ticks breed mainly in the dense brush found on the northern slopes of canyons, where they reach infective maturity across a 3-year life cycle. Consequently, local shepherds avoid the northern slopes every third year, leading their goats instead to the much poorer grazing on the bare southern slopes. Knowing that the ticks prefer the head and neck area, shepherds also may tie rags soaked in kerosene around their goats' necks—just like the flea collars worn by pets in the First World (Hadani, Shimshony, 1994).

A cognate strategy is to raise a diverse mix of animals. Quechua Indian families, for example, keep as many as seven species of herd animals (sheep, llama, alpaca, cattle, burros, goats, and horses) in addition to their barnyard species (guinea pigs, swine, chickens, and sometimes, ducks). This diversity lessens the health risks to one species because many diseases are species-specific.

The art of herding represents a substitution of valuable local-knowledge "software" for the "hardware" (e.g., materials, medicines, tools, infrastructure) of veterinary medicine. In this context, *software* refers to the social structures necessary to translate knowledge into organized human behaviors for effectively applying this knowledge in the form of technologies and practices. In this computer metaphor, the knowledge base stands as the operating system. Local software "programs" may be as small as a single household or as large as an entire ethnic group.

For example, vast labyrinths of wood, wire, adobe, stone, and even live fencing constitute one means of controlling livestock movement in healthful ways, keeping animals clear of infested or otherwise unhealthy sites and locating them wherever the best forage, clean water, and key dietary minerals are available. These efforts promote optimal nutrition and therefore decrease animals' susceptibility to disease. However, this strategy has its drawbacks. Wood is not durable in most of the tropics; using it for extensive fencing may mean forest degradation and less wood for other purposes, such as fuel and construction. Like electric fencing, wire is too expensive for most stock-raisers in the Third World. Adobe, although strong and durable, is not cheap either because of the heavy labor expenditures its production and maintenance entail. Stone fencing is also labor intensive. Like adobe and stone, live fencing is a long-term proposition in which people rarely invest without secure land tenure.

An alternative is "human fencing" in the form of cooperative social structures. Indeed, in many production systems, such human structures are preferable because they are more flexible, thoroughly mobile, and less expensive. Unlike veterinary cordon fences, human fences are also more friendly to migratory wildlife. Human fences or other "software programs" may be constructed from kin or nonkin interhousehold, community, multicommunity, or tribal and ethnic relations; they may be erected along other lines, such as sex, age groups, and specialized caste or profession. Box 41-13 offers several examples of such software from one stockraising culture.

At the risk of overextending the computer analogy, functional equivalents of network databases, electronic

BOX 41-13

SOCIOORGANIZATIONAL STRATEGIES

Quechua Indian families combine as many as seven species of animals together in a herd. This mix makes for sharp interspecies differences in feed requirements and palatabilities, watering needs, altitude and temperature tolerances, and other vital differences in susceptibility to disease and predation. Quechua are able to rear such a variety of stock mainly because of the great ecologic diversity of their tropical mountain habitat. However, this ecology extends vertically across considerable distances—anywhere from 20 to 100 km or more. Cattle and camelids thrive best in the lowest (3000 m and below) and highest (between approximately 4000 and 5000 m) zones, respectively; the other species are most efficiently managed in the middle zone.

Constructing conventional fencing to paddock each species in the zone best suited to it is socioeconomically out of the question for Quechua. Neither does any one household have the labor power daily to deploy a family herder in each zone. Quechua therefore turn to socioorganizational solutions. They adopt a variety of reciprocal and contractual interhousehold herding arrangements to better meet each species' needs. These arrangements can be triggered or suspended according to shifts in the species composition of household herds or changes in the availability of household labor across a week, a month, a year, or even the entire domestic life cycle.

For example, especially among very young or very old households (who tend to be labor poor), one family may handle the daily herding of its own and several other households' cattle while another oversees their pooled flocks of small ruminants during the day; a third family may take charge of all three's camelids. A more expensive alternative for labor-poor families is to hire or take wardship of one or more child herders from other households. A different software solution is often used in the highest, most remote and dangerous rangelands, which are plagued by rustlers and large predators. There, several households may instead cooperate in establishing, staffing, and provisioning a shared herding outpost for their camelids. These and still other social structures overcome the fencing problem and make for healthier and safer stockraising (Mc-Corkle, 1987).

bulletin boards, and user groups also exist. These larger social units are particularly noteworthy among African pastoralists. Within territories that may span one or more nations, nomadic or transhumant members of the same ethnic group exchange information about places where disease is rife or good water, forage, and dietary minerals are to be found. Members of these larger units may also post markers warning others away from pestilential areas.

Another socioorganizational response to the threat of disease is herd dispersal. In this "networking program," one household places segments of its same-species herd with those of other, distant households. The host households have free use of the manure, milk, or stud services of these shared-out animals, and they typically receive a portion of the live births as well. This strategy greatly reduces the likelihood of any household's losing its entire herd to a devastating disease. At the same time, it saves labor. Even more important, it builds up invaluable social capital for use after a drought or an epidemic, when the lender household may need to get its animals back—and perhaps borrow a few themselves—to rebuild their herd.

Lessons for Interdisciplinary and Intersectoral Coordination

Taken together, all the lessons suggest the following: Local knowledge pertaining to a given problem spans a wide array of interrelated ethnoscientific disciplines. Although *emic* definitions of such disciplines typically differ from *etic* ones, disciplines relevant to animal health care include all the conventional ones associated with ERD&E,[15] plus others, such as cosmology and theology.

This lesson suggests a corollary: Local knowledge must be considered in all its forms (e.g., management practices, social structures, information networks, tools, infrastructure) within a single discipline and in terms of multiple disciplines. The same theorem holds true for the application of conventional science to solving real-world agricultural problems—ERD&E is emically and etically interdisciplinary.

In this regard, the investigations reported in Box 41-4 are again instructive, albeit this time by default (Box 41-14). Unfortunately, the investigators neglected to link their ethnopharmacologic findings to other relevant ethnosciences. Doing so might have greatly enhanced or prolonged treatment benefits by tying them into a more powerful integrated disease-management (IDM) paradigm.[16] With one or more packages of IDM options, different stockraising units (e.g., households, interhousehold groups, corporate communities) can adopt or adapt different combinations of package components depending on particular circumstances.

An adjunct lesson involves the value of investigating and applying *emic* definitions of disciplines and their associated sectoral and professional or practitioner distinctions. Rightly or wrongly, many Western cultures draw a fairly sharp line between human and animal health care practitioners, dividing them into medical doctors versus veterinarians.[17] This dichotomy does not exist in most ethnomedical systems. Instead, major medical disciplines and their practitioners are categorized by professional specialization (herbalists, bonesetters, surgeons, midwives, acupuncturists, masseuses, and so forth), and the same traditional health workers treat both humans and livestock.

Application of the software of local knowledge, now in the form of various types of traditional practitioners and

BOX 41-14

NEED FOR ETHNOSCIENTIFIC INTERDISCIPLINARITY

In working with Peruvian farmers (see Box 41-4), researchers investigated local pharmacology in detail but neglected other ethnoscientific disciplines. For example, what were farmers' understandings of entomology—especially in relation to the prevention and control of parasitism? It was discovered that people were largely unaware of the complex life cycle of the liver fluke. In consequence, they failed to take some simple but effective husbandry measures to complement their veterinary ones. Yet with increased understanding of parasite habitats and life cycles and perhaps added software in the form of larger-scale social structures for cooperation in range management and daily herding, these stockraisers might be able to institute an even more effective package of practices to combat their livestock's diseases.

Such practices might consist of something as simple as improved corral hygiene or as sophisticated as breeding for disease tolerance or resistance. The package might also incorporate husbandry and herding practices akin to those described for Tzotzil, Africans, and Israelis. Whether the failure of Peruvian farmers to institute such measures is primarily due to lacunae in ethnoveterinary knowledge or to other constraints (e.g., lack of natural bedding materials, land, suitable studs, labor) is not clear, however, because the associated ethnoscientific disciplines went largely unstudied.

social groups, requires attention to these *emic* definitions of disciplines. According to WHO, all appropriate human resources must be tapped if basic health services are to reach most of the world's humans; clearly, the same can be recommended for the livestock sector.[18] As many experts have observed, the Western model for delivery of animal health services has rarely worked well in developing countries. A consensus is now emerging that what is needed instead are " … new tools and innovative ways to integrate human and animal health care delivery," plus a "rethinking of Western models and anthropocentric biases" in this arena. This rethinking should incorporate "traditional healers … as part of the primary health care delivery team" (Ward and others, 1993).

Especially (but not exclusively) in places where practitioners treat both animal and human patients, training, medical infrastructure, service delivery, and national epidemiologic intelligence systems should be coordinated across health sectors as much as possible (Schwabe, 1981, 1984; Ward and others, 1993).

For instance, because many concepts and treatments of both conventional medicine and ethnomedicine are substantially similar for humans and animals, training in one sector can be easily extended to another. For example, if training is being offered on bonesetting midwifery, injections, or oral rehydration therapy in humans, such training could also include the appropriate application of these techniques to livestock, and vice versa. The indication and posology of drugs can be noted for all pertinent species of patients, given that many traditional-herbal and modern-commercial treatments are administered for similar problems in humans and (at least mammalian) livestock.

When it comes to establishing health clinics, diagnostic laboratories, cold chains, and drug procurement and supply systems, the cost savings that could result from intersectoral coordination are even more obvious (CTA, 1984; GTZ, 1983). Synergistic benefits to both sectors in the identification, treatment, and control of zoonoses will also ensue; the same is true for the integration of epidemiologic surveillance systems for disease threats to humans, livestock, or both. Investigations by the International Laboratory for Research on Animal Diseases suggest that ethnomedical methodologies can be useful in rapidly estimating variable disease risk in lieu of more accurate but expensive laboratory diagnostic surveys (Delehanty, 1996). A large and growing body of research indicates that when local practitioners are trained and motivated to participate in such systems and methods, epidemiologic intelligence is obtained more quickly, accurately, and cheaply than in conventional schemes relying on a distant, uncaring, and often poorly trained cadre of civil servants (Baumann, 1990; Schwabe, Kuojok, 1981; Sollod, Stem, 1991; Zessin, Carpenter, 1985).

A less obvious benefit of intersectoral collaboration, in terms of cost savings and increased delivery or use of hu-

man health services, is also suggested in the literature. Sometimes, poor people who are unwilling to pay for medical care of family members *will* pay for veterinary care. Also, some stockraising peoples are more likely to gain access to human medical services when these are extended alongside veterinary services. In a combined delivery system a portion of the revenues from veterinary services could be diverted to defray the expenses of human services. Moreover, joint delivery is more efficient when the cost of delivering services to animals or people alone surpasses the cost of the treatments rendered (Ward and others, 1993).

Intersectoral approaches that also incorporate local traditional healers can increase public recognition, remuneration, and status for these practitioners. These advantages may encourage existing healers to continue—and more young people to enter—technoblended but still localized health care professions. People are more likely to seek treatment when providers are familiar and respected local practitioners whom communities have empowered to serve as paraprofessionals.[19]

ERD&E also promotes intersectoral coordination between agriculture and education via the value of incorporating research and development findings into educational curricula at all levels (Ibrahim, Abdu, 1996). Throughout the developing world, primary schools and functional literacy programs suffer from a paucity of practical subject matters and reading materials that are relevant to the everyday lives and cultures of rural students. The result is low interest in literacy. However, literacy is a major prerequisite for teaching and extending information about agricultural technologies and practices, whether traditional or modern, veterinary or medical. Grounding education in findings from research and development involving local knowledge can facilitate learning (Box 41-15).

For related reasons, ethnoscientific information and vocabulary can be usefully incorporated into secondary curricula—and, specifically for livestock health and husbandry, into paraveterinary, vocational, and higher education programs in veterinary medicine and zootechnology. With a "knowledge of local knowledge" (McCorkle, 1989a), both extensionists and researchers gain a greater respect for their clients' existing veterinary practices and beliefs and a clearer understanding of the kind of outsider or scientific knowledge most and least useful to clients. Training, extension, and research may then be focused accordingly. Also, a shared vocabulary of local-language terms enhances communication and collaboration among all parties. Benefits to national disease-surveillance systems may result as well. Box 41-15 illustrates some potential synergisms that result from collaboration between education and agriculture when local knowledge, language, and culture are considered.

Another lesson that has repeatedly emerged from ERDE is the importance of not dismissing out-of-hand

BOX 41-15

Intersectoral Coordination: Veterinary Medicine and Literacy

Among the Fulbe pastoralists of Senegal, ERDE resulted in the production of two booklets in the local language (Pulaar) on Fulbe ethnoveterinary vocabulary and knowledge. The booklets were used by a national nongovernmental organization (NGO) in its functional literacy classes. Besides meeting the need for native-language reading materials, the booklets implicitly acknowledged the value of local culture and technical knowledge. This approach to literacy training also provided Fulbe students with a way to individually expand, collectively share, and reaffirm—but also think critically about—their fund of local knowledge in this domain (Bonfiglioli, Diallo, Fagerberg-Diallo, 1996).

The information in the booklets was also used to design postliteracy classes in which participants learned to keep records on the livestock diseases in their area. This practical application greatly increased herders' interest in maintaining their functional literacy skills. It also empowered them to do more systematic epidemiologic surveillance on their own, enabling them to apply or coordinate their traditional (and also modern) strategies of disease avoidance and control in more timely or effective ways. The resulting skills and records facilitated the work of national epidemiologic intelligence systems too.

Used by an international NGO (Oxfam) to train Pulaar-speaking veterinary auxiliaries, the same booklets established a shared vocabulary and knowledge base between trainers and trainees that significantly accelerated training and focused it on areas where all agreed that inputs of more "outsider" information would be most useful.

Numerous projects in Kenya have found similar advantages to working with and from local lexicons and practices in their paraveterinary training courses and other extension and surveillance efforts. For example, disease nomenclatures, indigenous immunization techniques, and ethnodiagnostic models have all proved invaluable as readily comprehensible references, analogies, and verbal aids for communicating about veterinary problems and alternatives with stockraisers (Delehanty, 1996; Grandin, Young, 1996; Stem, 1996).

---

local knowledge that is enunciated in a nonscientific or supernatural idiom.[20] Scientists are prone to shrug off such data as merely part of local cosmology or theology. However, this information often has sound etic underpinnings that stockraisers can verbalize when pressed. Just as often, the associated ethnoveterinary practices have solid practical effect, sometimes mirroring procedures recommended by Western veterinary and animal science.

For example, many stockraising peoples attribute some diseases to supernatural beings or forces such as evil spirits and winds that haunt certain locales or appear at certain times of the day or night. Frequently, these explanations correlate to situations in which parasites and their hosts or vectors abound; microclimatic conditions create stress for animals or foster bacterial proliferation, poisonous plants, or fungal mycotoxins; or infectious spores lie dormant in the soil, awaiting their next victims (e.g., anthrax, blackquarter).

In the case of such putatively supernatural ills, people tend to explain the workings of their associated ethnotherapies or ethnoprophylaxes and their control or avoidance strategies in the same idiom. Sometimes, they also surround these practical health measures with magi-

cal and religious ones, much as people in the First World offer up prayers or light votive candles for a hospitalized friend or relative. This does not mean that the ethnomedical response is any less appropriate to the etically identified health problem (Box 41-16).

In short, considerable epidemiologic knowledge and practical veterinary acumen may be encoded in local cosmology and theology. Thus these disciplines must also be investigated. Of course, many supernatural practices (e.g., praying over animals, decorating them with amulets or fetish bundles to ward off evil spirits, holding special curative rites) may produce no readily discernible health effects.[21] This brings us to a third set of lessons from ERD&E.

Cautionary Lessons

As with any medical modality, not all ethnoveterinary practices make good sense, work all the time, produce sufficient effect, or are readily transferable. A remedy or practice used in one local context may not be suitable for other times, places, or production and livelihood systems. For some problems or among some peoples, local knowledge

BOX 41-16

Medicoreligious Beliefs and Practices

Quechua Indians' ethnoetiology of contagious keratoconjunctivitis in sheep is expressed partly in sixteenth-century Iberian notions of hot and cold diseases and partly in Incaic concepts of evil winds. Their ethnodiagnosis of the condition is nevertheless 100% accurate. Moreover, their ethnoetiology directs them to treat the ailment using the cleanest, coolest water to be found within the village, along with certain medicinal plant juices. Quechua report that this cure is 100% effective when consistently applied.

Quechua also argue that some sheep habitually eat poisonous locoweed (*Astragalus* spp.) because the plants are "magnetic" and magically attract the animals to them. In effect, this is another way of saying that locoweed is addictive. Despite the difference in semantics, the management message is the same: try to keep your flock away from this substance.

Similarly, with regard to the common strategy of keeping cats in and around animal quarters, some Asian stockraisers say the cats serve to ward off pestilential spirits. Of course, this choice of terminology in no way impairs cats' patrolling for disease-bearing pests.

may be inadequate, misguided, or completely absent. In other words, local knowledge is not perfect. For example, not all medicinal plants flourish in all locales or in all seasons. Plants that must be used fresh pose further problems that cannot always be resolved through horticultural technology (e.g., potting, greenhousing).

The utility of ethnoveterinary treaments and practices also varies according to production and livelihood systems. Consider some of the Tzotzil techniques described in Box 41-12. These can be quite useful for small-scale stockraisers with low labor costs, but daily muzzling of each animal, even for one season, would prove infeasible or inefficient for larger-scale producers or stockraisers with more diverse production or employment possibilities. Ethnomedicines (or, for that matter, Western medicines) that entail prohibitively high labor expenditures (see the discussion of topical applications in Box 41-4) pose similar problems.

The utility of ethnoveterinary methods is also affected by shifts in production systems. The great pastoral peoples of the world are an example. As their migration routes are blocked, their movements increasingly circumscribed, and their traditional grazing grounds or water and mineral sources appropriated by governments, encroaching cultivators, and even international development projects (e.g., hydroelectric, irrigation, or cultivation schemes), they may find they can no longer fully implement many of their long-distance movement strategies for avoiding disease and ensuring good herd nutrition.[22]

Ethnoveterinary practices might be helpful for some, but not all, of the ailments to which they are applied. For instance, the globally popular use of cauterization and branding has therapeutic value for various kinds of wounds, sprains, some hoof problems, and postsurgical treatment. However, these techniques are inappropriate for many other conditions (including endoparasitic, hemoparasitic, and viral diseases) for which they are often applied. (Of

course, contraindicated treatments are not exactly unknown in Western medicine, either.)

Furthermore, a treatment that is effective for the problem to which it is applied occasionally leads to complications. (Again, however, the same is true of Western medicine.) An example is the popularity of ectoparasiticidal topicals containing substances such as kerosene and creosote (used in the United States until the 1950s and used today in the former Soviet Union), spent engine oil, and battery acid. To varying degrees, such substances do work, but they can cause chemical dermatosis, toxicity, and negative environmental effects. So-called dirty pharmacy also has drawbacks. All around the globe, whether for human or livestock ailments, urine is commonly used as a disinfectant for cuts and abrasions, and mud or animal feces serve as a dressing for wounds and bruises. All these materials can (and usually do) work as intended, but they also pose risks of secondary infection.

Sometimes, however, ethnomedical beliefs and practices are actually harmful; for example, some African and South American stockraisers withhold drinking water from stock suffering from diarrhea and concomitant dehydration. Another example is indiscriminate bloodletting. Various folk procedures to stimulate estrus or increase fertility in female animals can cause infection of the reproductive tract and tissue damage. Of course, mistakes have been made in Western medicine, both with livestock (e.g., commercial dips) and humans (e.g., the thalidomide tragedy). In fact, safety is one reason alternative medicine is receiving considerable attention from both veterinarians and human physicians.

Ethnoveterinary medicine may not be the best alternative for some diseases. This is the case in at least five circumstances.

First, some diseases strike so rapidly that, for animals unprotected by vaccination or other effective prophylaxes, lo-

BOX 41-17

*E*THNOVETERINARY *M*EDICINE VERSUS *N*EW *D*ISEASES

A classic example of the way local knowledge can be stymied when a new disease strikes is the response of Maasai pastoralists to rinderpest when it first appeared in their area. Rinderpest is a viral disease usually transmitted by close and immediate contact. Traditionally, all families of a given Maasai camp grazed and corralled their cattle together. However, this practice promoted the rapid spread of rinderpest. Some time elapsed before Maasai recognized this epidemiologic pattern, took steps to disperse their animals more widely, and instituted quarantine measures whenever rinderpest threatened (Waller, 1988).

In a similar vein, when Samburu pastoralists first encountered East Coast fever (ECF or theileriosis) in 1977, they did not know that it was a tick-borne disease. Thus they did not take extra care to prevent tick infestation. Samburu could only hypothesize that the new plague was a punishment visited on them by God in retribution for their break with traditional norms of in-traethnic herder cooperation during the previous drought period (Heffernan, Heffernan, Stem, 1996).

Mijikenda farmers of coastal Kenya exemplify a somewhat different kind of shortcoming in local knowledge. Many Mijikenda embarked on cattle-rearing only in the 1980s. Thus nearly all cattle diseases are new to them. For example, Mijikenda are uncertain about the cause and clinical signs of ECF. They speculate that in calves (for whom the disease is often fatal if untreated), ECF is caused by overconsumption of milk or overly vigorous suckling. Most Mijikenda cannot even recognize the disease in adult cattle. In any case, their standard folk treatment—cauterization with a hot iron or botanical acids—is inappropriate (Delehanty, 1996).

cating and preparing the ingredients for otherwise effective home remedies or reaching a local veterinary specialist by the time patent clinical signs appear may be impossible. However, especially for range stock, the same problems arise in gaining access to Western-style drugs and specialists. In such circumstances, both local and Western-style veterinary treatments are largely powerless. An example is acute plant poisoning (see Box 41-10). The solution lies instead in prevention, for which local knowledge in the aggregate offers a variety of useful husbandry and herding strategies: training animals not to eat such plants or purposely building up tolerance by feeding small amounts of the plant over time, burning off or grubbing out infested grazing grounds, and simply herding stock away from such areas.

Second, ethnomedicine is often stymied by ailments for which cause-and-effect relations are not readily discernible. Particularly among farmers and agropastoralists, this is often the case for viral and bacterial diseases that spread by no readily identifiable vectors, are not clearly and consistently correlated with any particular environmental (e.g., brushy or moist areas) or epidemiologic parameters (e.g., heavy fly or tick attacks), or leave behind no visible signs even on practical necropsy (e.g., botulism).

Third, even pastoralists and Western-trained veterinarians have difficulty dealing with multifactorial diseases. These complex syndromes arise from multiple immediate and proximate causes. Diagnosis is difficult, and treatment is often merely palliative (Ward and others, 1993).

Fourth, even profound ethnomedical traditions can be useless when the practitioner is confronted with a new disease. Of course, the same is true for Western-scientific medicine, as the furor over acquired immunodeficiency syndrome (AIDS) demonstrates. Box 41-17 gives two examples of this situation from among some of the world's most knowledgeable traditional stockraisers. Predictably, however, lacunae in ethnoveterinary knowledge are most common among groups who have only recently taken up animal husbandry or adopted a new species.

A fifth circumstance in which ethnoveterinary medicine may fall short is when, despite all efforts at prevention, an epidemic strikes. Even apparently effective local remedies may not be adequate to treat sufficient numbers of animals quickly enough to stop an epidemic. This may occur when all the ingredients for local prescriptions are not readily available or are available only in small quantities or when large numbers of stock must be treated very rapidly. However, the same problems can arise in Western veterinary medicine (for an example concerning modern vaccination, see Brisebarre, 1996).

One final lesson pertains to ethnoveterinary interventions that have positive qualitative effects but may still fall short of quantitative ideals. For example, research on indigenous Andean anthelmintics has shown that although these remedies do lessen parasite burdens significantly, the kill rate of juvenile and adult parasites may be considerably less than 100% (recall Box 41-1). When the only other option is to do nothing, a risky or only partially effective solution may be preferable to inaction. The relative benefits and costs of less potent local treatments, compared with more potent Western-commercial ones, must be considered (recall Box 41-8). For sustainable agriculture, another consideration is chemoresistance: the more powerful the drug, the more rapidly disease agents may adapt to it.

Similarly, traditional nondrug interventions (e.g., companion species, habitat modification, mixed grazing) by themselves are probably not completely effective at keeping health challenges below economic damage thresholds (Meltzer, 1995). Producers may take such measures mainly because they have nothing better. It may be that "economic damage," if defined solely as monetary profit, is not stockraisers' major concern for the species or production system in question; they may be unwilling to invest in more capital-intensive interventions (McCorkle, 1992). Another possibility is that such interventions have significant strategic or additive effects when holisticaly evaluated as part of the totality of local IDM techniques keyed to seasonal shifts, parasite life cycles, animal nutrition needs, or other variables.

Of course, as noted at the beginning of this chapter, solid production-economic data supporting the efficacy of many Western-style commercial treatments are also lacking, but this has not stopped people or governments from using these treatments. The problem in accurately evaluating packages of ethnoveterinary (or conventional) IDM practices is one of Western-scientific reductionism.

Ethical and Methodologic Lessons

The flaws of conventional science make the next issue, which concerns the need to scientifically validate local knowledge and practice, controversial. For a variety of reasons, little research has been conducted in ethnoveterinary medicine compared with human ethnomedicine. The literature is rife with unassessed and incomplete descriptions of ethnoveterinary technologies and practices, and although anecdotal reports of ethnoveterinary successes abound, reporters have not always been qualified to comment on the biomedical basis of their findings. For local knowledge to be broadly and responsibly put to use, some means of discriminating between effective and ineffective methods is required.

An important reason to study local knowledge is to be able to recommend and more widely extend less expensive, readily available, easily understood development options, especially to people who live at or below the poverty line. Ethical and humane considerations must also be considered. Researchers and developers have a clear responsibility to ascertain the cost-effectiveness and safety (or, at a minimum, the relative risks of administering the treatment compared with doing nothing at all) of local or techno-blended options before widely promoting them.[23]

This view differs from that of some students and na-tive proponents of local knowledge, who believe the application of etic standards to emic phenomena is invalid (Thrupp, 1989). They feel that translating local knowledge into Western-scientific referents devalues ethnoscientific concepts and damages cultural and religious integrity. (Ironically, a few stalwart Western veterinary academicians have made much the same complaint about subjecting their professional canons and dogma to scrutiny from an ethnoveterinary perspective.)

A thorough discussion of this controversy is beyond the scope of this chapter.[24] In brief, properly designed and conducted local-knowledge ERDE integrates social-scientific and biologic-technical understandings, with as much input from insiders (emic) as outsiders (etic). This approach need not invalidate either alternative or conventional medical realities (see Box 41-1).

Of course, if the usefulness of local knowledge were limited to narrowly defined geographical and sociocultural settings, its study would be merely of academic interest. Instead, people everywhere have spontaneously and successfully adopted technologies, practices, and socioorganizational ideas from distant and nearby sources, adapting them to suit their own agroecologic, economic, and sociocultural circumstances.

Ethnomedicine itself provides an excellent example of such processes. It gave the world invaluable drugs such as aspirin, codeine, curare, and quinine and hundreds of other medicines (e.g., antifungals, antivirals) and molecular models (Cox, Balick, 1994). Moreover, it continues to do so, with new discoveries that fight cancer, AIDS, and recalcitrant neurologic disorders, among many others. In fact, of all modern drugs in use today, at least 50% contain substances of natural origin and many more are modeled on the molecular patterns provided by such substances. Most of these substances were first identified and used by local peoples (Conservation International, not dated). To take an example other than botanicals, in Western veterinary (and also human) medicine, farmer-stockraisers were the first to discover and successfully apply the principles of vaccination (deMaar, 1992; Schillhorn van Veen, 1996).

Whether in the First or the Third World, the potential for wider application of local knowledge underscores the importance of further research for both ethical and practical reasons. Validation is necessary to prevent the "dual knowledge" syndrome, in which local knowledge is labeled second rate (Lalonde, Morin-Labatut, not dated), with the implication that its inventors and users are second-rate as well.

However, scientific validation of local knowledge and practice has sometimes been problematic. In practice, methodologic difficulties have been especially common in the study of botanicals, even though research protocols for their formal pharmacologic and clinical study have been codified since the turn of the century, if not earlier. Studies have sometimes failed to recognize important variables such as the precise forms and quantities in which botanicals are used, locale (e.g., soil quality, microclimate) and developmental stage at which botanicals are collected, the way in which botanicals are compounded (e.g., additive, synergistic, antagonistic, and bioavailability effects in polyprescriptions), and the processing tools used locally. All these factors—even whether the materia medica are chopped or pounded with metal instruments or traditional wooden or bamboo tools—can influence phytochemical balances and processes and, hence, pharmacologic effect.[25] Such considerations suggest some final methodologic lessons for ERD&E. One is the importance of duplicating local drugs and practices as closely as possible, which may prove challenging to Western scientists when local procedures are highly unorthodox (Box 41-18).

At another level, experiences in human ethnomedicine suggest that researchers using conventional scientific methodologies may overlook some mechanisms by which natural medicines produce their effect. This neglect probably results from a narrow conception of therapeutic action. (For a striking example from cancer research, see Bodeker, 1994b.) The larger lesson here is the need to devise new, innovative research designs rather than mindlessly cleaving to conventional methodologic dogma.

A further lesson is that research methods must be inexpensive and easily used by national agencies if any progress is to be made in bringing validated technologies and practices to significant numbers of people (McCorkle, 1994b). Among other things, this focus on economy and ease of use implies that isolation of active ingredients should not be an automatic precondition for the validation of ethnopharmaceuticals. Such research is not only costly but also reductionistic because traditional prescriptions are often intended to produce simultaneous or synergistic actions such as a site-specific attack on the disease, enhanced immune response, increased cellular uptake, and repression of side effects. Such research may also raise ethical issues concerning intellectual property rights (McCorkle, 1994b; endnote 11). In any case, if systematic clinical observation of a treatment reveals positive benefits

with inconsequential or no side effects and its evaluation by collaborating stockraisers and ethnoscientists is satisfactory, this information should be sufficient for all but the most esoteric academic purposes.

The criterion of inexpensiveness also recommends a systematic search of the literature—oral as well as written—to identify the best treatments before investing scarce financial and human resources in validating a particular technology or practice. This criterion further argues for on-farm trials with stockraisers' or traditional healers' own animals whenever feasible. This approach has several virtues besides its inexpensiveness compared with on-station trials. As in FSR&E (farming systems research and extension), it provides a truer test of a treatment's robustness in the context of stockraisers' often harsh environments and management regimes. It also permits greater participation and evaluation by stockraisers, which can in turn prevent costly or embarrassing errors such as that detailed in Box 41-10.

Of course, a participatory on-farm approach has some drawbacks. Small-scale stockraisers may not have enough animals for detailed statistical evaluation. It often entails reimbursing unanticipated losses to stockraiser coresearchers because poor smallholders who already live on the edge of economic survival cannot absorb much risk. However, with more involvement by social groups (e.g., traditional practitioners, community organizations, coops) that have an immediate interest in experimental outcomes, both the risks and the costs of on-farm trials can be spread.[26]

Back to the Future

The ultimate lesson ERD&E provides is that it is both socioeconomically and scientifically imperative to take advantage of the rich storehouse of local knowledge embodied in ethnoveterinary medicine and its human bearers and practitioners. These resources demonstrate a potential for wide-ranging benefits to humankind—a potential that now must be followed with concerted study and validation.

By validating and then reinforcing or simply transferring or extending useful local knowledge, more choices of technologies and practices (including socioorganizational strategies) may be made available to more people everywhere. If nothing else, where or when there are no other options, people can do something helpful to address an immediate problem. Often, however, many local or technoblended alternatives serve just as well as their conventional counterparts. Particularly for remote, rural, or poor inhabitants of the developing world, these alternatives may even be preferable when considerations other than purely technical ones are taken into account (e.g., ready comprehensibility and applicability, sociocultural acceptability, consistent availability, low price, and sustainability in the face of economic and political vagaries).

BOX 41-18

Unorthodox Administration

For example, Kenyan pastoralists prepare a reportedly effective eyewash by masticating medicinal plant materials and then spitting them into the afflicted animals' eyes (McCorkle, fieldwork in Kenya, 1994). Designing a controlled scientific experiment to test such nonconventional modes of preparation and administration necessitates some creativity on researchers' parts.

Whether in animal agriculture or other life and livelihood activities, access to a range of problem-solving options implies increased potentials for production, profitability, and peace of mind (i.e., social security and psychologic well-being). Specifically for animal health care, local knowledge and its associated hardware and software offer much-needed alternatives to the veterinary and husbandry technologies and practices typically transferred from developed countries despite the fact that such imports " ... have almost always failed to overcome the constraints imposed on local farming systems or to meet the socioeconomic requirements of the farmers" (Sansoucy, 1994). Such alternatives translate into increases in any or all of the many benefits enumerated in Box 41-1. Further benefits are to be had from ERDE in various arenas noted in Box 41-3. To recap, these include the following:

- Savings in public exchequers and growth in national revenues
- New or greater rural income-earning opportunities
- Biomedically benign alternatives that lower health risks to humans as well as animals[27]
- Environmental bonuses in the form of maintenance of biodiversity and decreased pollution
- From intersectoral linkages, increased or more relevant and economically sustainable delivery of a greater variety of services to more individuals and groups
- To the extent that respected local specialists and existing social orgnizations participate in health care delivery, greater public knowledge about, credence in, and use of such services
- Improved public perceptions of government

Finally, investments in the study and application of useful local knowledge, practice, and social organization can produce another important benefit: renewed respect for local cultures and technologic knowledge. As a corollary, formal-sector health care workers, extensionists, educators, scientists, and policymakers may also gain increased appreciation of the knowledge and experience that their clients, students, users, and citizens already possess. All these benefits can add up to a fresh sense of local confidence and control, stronger social structures, and empowerment of people to work together at the local level—whether independently or with nonhegemonic formal-sector support—to solve more of their own development problems.

None of this is to say that ethnoscience is perfect or that conventional science must be abandoned. Rather, each has much to learn from the other. As Last (1990) observes for medical systems cross-culturally, "In theory ... all systems may 'work'; in practice, all have successes and failures, with some systems scoring much higher in particular areas of medicine," depending on the social, cultural, and economic context in which they are applied, as well as on their biomedical bases.

Indeed, the assumption that either ethnoscience or Western science alone is likely to provide a sufficient prescription for all development ills in today's rapidly changing world is naive. The aim is not to impose one cultural tradition on another but rather to create contact points between them (Salih, 1992). In contemporary problem solving, all potentially helpful knowledge bases should be considered carefully because drawing on insider and outsider, site-specific and universalistic, and old and new understandings can take us back to a brighter future.

*E*NDNOTES

1. This article represents a combined and greatly expanded version of several earlier papers presented to the EC exhibit on the Medical Rainforest in Leiden, The Netherlands, as the keynote address opening the exhibit in December 1993; the March 1994 National Symposium on Indigenous Knowledge and Contemporary Social Issues, held in Tampa, Fla; the International Workshop on Traditional Health Systems and Public Policy of Canada's International Development Research Centre, March 1994, in Ottawa; and the Animal Production and Health Division (AGA) of the United Nation's Food and Agriculture Organization in Rome in October, 1994. I am grateful to participants at all these events for their comments and reactions.

   Thanks are also due the Sociology Project and the Veterinary Medicine Project of the Small Ruminant Collaborative Research Support Program (SR-CRSP) at the University of Missouri–Columbia (UMC) and Colorado State University, respectively, for their long-standing support to the study of ethnoveterinary medicine. Along with a Fulbright CIES Faculty Scholar Grant in 1987-88, the SR-CRSP supported my ethnoveterinary investigations in highland Peru between 1980 and 1990 under USAID grants AID/DSAN/XII-G-0049 and AID/DAN/1328-G-SS-4093-00, with substantial additional support from UMC.

   Much of the thinking behind this article derives from the cumulative collaboration between 1986 and the present with my veterinary colleagues, Evelyn Mathias of the International Institute of Rural Reconstruction in the Philippines and Tjaart W. Schillhorn van Veen of the World Bank. Special thanks are also due David Ward of FAO for his coaching on technical details. Also appreciated were the insightful comments and queries of the editors and reviewers of *Agriculture and Human Values*. However, any errors of fact or judgment are solely mine.
2. At least one study (Mathias-Mundy and others, 1992) has shown that periurban stockraisers have regular recourse to local veterinary treatment because they find the time, transport, and cost constraints associated with conventional veterinary services prohibitive.
3. In principle, pets could also be included, but in practice ERDE has so far focused on food and work animals.
4. For more information, consult McCorkle (1992), McDowell (1980, 1991), Sansoucy (1994), and Waters-Bayer and Bayer (1992).
5. Before the 1970s, veterinary medicine concentrated on high-tech approaches, shifting away from the concern with social and natural aspects of the art that had characterized it until the turn of the century. This shift was related in part to the intensification of livestock production, leading not only to less humane treatment of animals but to different suites of health and husbandry problems that resulted from practices associated with intensification (e.g., inbreeding, confinement, less varied diets). Also, diseases of intensification tended to be less responsive to traditional methods of treatment and

control, which had evolved largely under extensive (e.g., range stock) conditions. The shift to high-tech medicine was particularly pronounced in the Anglo-Saxon cultures. On the European mainland and throughout much of Asia and the former Soviet Union, however, traditional methods have remained in use and are still taught in veterinary schools.

6. For human medicine, this has led, among other things, to the establishment of a worldwide network of WHO Collaborating Centers for Traditional Medicine. Also, many international meetings and conferences pertaining to traditional human health care systems and their potential for the universal delivery of health care have been held in recent years, involving such entities as arboreta and botanical gardens, environmental and development nongovernmental organizations (NGOs), cultural and other research institutes, both established and venture-capital pharmaceutical firms, the U.S. government's National Institutes of Health (NIH), Canada's International Development Research Centre (IDRC), representatives of the U.S. Department of Agriculture, the Pan-American Health Organization (PAHO), WHO, the World Bank, advocacy groups such as the World Council of Indigenous Peoples, and many universities. Indeed, the International Congress on Traditional and Folk Medicine is now in its ninth year, with attendance greater than 1000. Several such events have featured the active participation of traditional healers and spokespersons. In 1993 the NIH established a new Office of Alternative Medicine to evaluate promising ethnomedical therapies. Curiously, however, no corresponding events or offices have emerged for traditional veterinary medicine. So far, few forums have explored the fact that ethnomedical traditions generally incorporate both human and animal health care (McCorkle, 1994b; Ward and others, 1993).

7. These techniques are not discussed in this chapter because they are well covered in other chapters of this book.

8. During on-farm research, stockraisers can assist in fecal egg counts using simple reflecting microscopes. On the basis of anthropologists' experiences in other arenas of local knowledge, promising opportunities appear to exist for villagers' hands-on collaboration at the computer, using programs based on icons, pictograms, and visual sorting- and ranking-techniques and equipment powered from car batteries. Participatory rural appraisal and research methods may soon move far beyond their original media of twigs, pebbles, earth, pencil, and paper.

9. For further discussion, details, and case examples of people's participation in ERD&E, see Bazalar, McCorkle (1989); Grandin, Thampy, Young (1991); ITDG (1989, 1992); Kirsopp-Reed, Hinchcliffe (1994); McCorkle (1989b, 1990); Nuwanyakpa and others (1990); and Stem (1996).

10. Except where indicated, all references for the ethnoveterinary examples in the remainder of the text can be found in the various publications by myself and my veterinary colleagues Mathias and Schillhorn van Veen. If not already referenced earlier in the text, these publications are cited only once, where first relevant. These sources provide many additional illustrations of the lessons discussed here.

11. Even less research has been devoted to ethnobotanicals for livestock. However, many of the same plants figure in human ethnomedicine and have been investigated in this context. As might be expected, such studies indicate that a significant number of ethnoveterinary plant materials display pharmacologic activity against viruses, bacteria, fungal infections, and parasites. More specifically, research on samples of African ethnoveterinary botanicals suggests

that at least 30% are effective against the diseases they are used to treat. A similar figure seems reasonable for the Andes, on the basis of my observations and investigations in 20 years of fieldwork there. Such estimates roughly parallel the 20% figure commonly cited for human ethnopharmacognascy, although in specific ethnopharmacopoeia as many as 80% to 86% of the plants have been reported to show pharmacologic activity (Cox, Balick, 1994; Greaves, 1994; Trotter, 1988).

12. These and other such agreements have been formulated within the debate on intellectual property rights (IPR). A thorny issue with no definitive solutions, the IPR debate lies beyond the scope of this chapter. Interested readers are referred to Art and others (1993), Greaves (1994), and the Crucible Group (1994).

13. However, this is not to say that people never make mistakes (Mathias, McCorkle, 1997) or that all people are equally knowledgeable. In desperate circumstances, people sometimes try anything to save an ailing animal (McCorkle, 1982). Also, less is known about chronic toxicity in traditional medicines after protracted use (Etkin, 1990).

14. Mixed grazing seems to be especially helpful in controlling gastrointestinal nematodes; all but one (*Trichostrongylus* spp.) of this class of parasites appear to be species-specific (Michel, 1969, 1976; Schillhorn van Veen, 1995).

15. Space is not available to illustrate the breadth and depth of such knowledge among the world's stockraisers. However, knowledge does vary in some predictable ways. One is by type of production system: as a rule of thumb, pastoralists know more than agropastoralists, who know more than farmers. Another is length of experience in stockraising. Another variable is biosocial status (e.g., sex, age, caste, professional specialization), according to the often changing husbandry roles assigned to people of different status in a given society. (See Mathias, McCorkle, 1997; Thompson, Scoones, 1994.)

16. The analogy here is that of integrated pest management, another field of environmentally friendly agricultural research and development that has arisen in large part because of scientific attention to local knowledge.

17. For an insightful discussion of similarities and differences in both theory and practice between the two, see Ward and others (1993).

18. Per capita ratios of modern versus traditional practitioners to patients underscore this point. For example, China has only one modern medical doctor for every 10,000 patients, but the ratio for traditional practitioners is 1:100 (Bodeker, 1994a); for Ghana and Swaziland, these figures are, respectively, 1:20,000 versus 1:200 and 1:10,000 versus 1:100 (Zhang, 1994). Similar magnitudes can be assumed to hold for the livestock sector in most of the Third World. Kenyan farming communities, for example, typically boast two or three traditional healers for livestock but no formally-trained veterinary workers.

19. The pros and cons of intersectoral health care delivery, its private versus public health focus, and issues of cost recovery merit several lengthy articles. This chapter permits only an introduction to this tantalizing idea. Although much of it is unpublished, literature on paraveterinarians is also vast. For an overview of this subject, see McCorkle and Mathias (in progress). For a discussion of different models of the professionalization of traditional healers, consult Last (1990). In general, these and many other topics in ERDE would benefit greatly from lessons learned in mainstream medical anthropology. Contextualization in that body of theory and research is a logical next step for ERD&E.

20. Although this lesson has long been appreciated in medical anthropology for humans, it has received much less attention in veterinary contexts. (See again endnote 19.)

21. Certainly, however, they comfort the worried stockowner, just as Western peoples' prayers and masses for ailing friends and family members comfort them. Moreover, all the evidence is not yet in on the ways extramedical or extranutritional care and attention to (especially highly social) animals may affect their physical well-being. Quite possibly, acts such as stroking, talking to, or even just staying nearby a suffering creature may have positive somatic effects. Ethologic studies are suggestive in this regard. Many social animal species lick, groom, and stand watch over their sick or wounded young or herdmates. Benign effects on animal physiology (e.g., slowing and regularizing of heart rate) have been demonstrated as a result of stroking and petting. Reportedly, animals suffer psychosomatic disorders (deMaar, 1992). Finally, supernaturally related ethnomedical acts must be thoroughly investigated (e.g., a fetish bundle might contain a pest-repelling substance).

22. This is not to say, however, that the principles undergirding such movement strategies are invalid. Depending on the circumstances, they may continue to be applied on a more geographically limited basis. For more on the problems faced by today's pastoral peoples, interested readers are referred to Fratkin, Galvin, Roth (1994); Galaty, Aronson, Salzman, (1981); Scoones (1995); and the references cited therein.

23. Ask yourself whether you would be willing to gamble with your own or your children's health or with your family's long-term economic security in the form of its hard-won "stock portfolio" in the absence of any such evidence. How, then, can we morally ask others to do so?

24. Some aspects of this debate appear overblown. The Western-scientific etic is really just another emic. Cognitive anthropology has repeatedly demonstrated a basic structural similarity in the two types of knowledge. At least since the domestication of plants and animals some 12,000 to 15,000 years ago, farmers and stockraisers have been conducting empirical agricultural experiments and exchanging their findings (McCorkle, Brandstetter, McClure, 1988). Interestingly, the historiography of agricultural inventions and recommendations at international agricultural research centers reveals that many of these derive directly from producer knowledge and practice. This is not the place for an exegesis on the sociology of knowledge or the universality of the scientific method, however. In short, stockraisers are mainly interested in whether a given intervention makes sense to them and works to their satisfaction (and then, of course, whether it is available, affordable, convenient, and so forth)—no matter what its source.

25. Etkin (1990) discusses these and other points in ethnomedical pharmacognosy and pharmacology. For some dramatic examples of the way inattention to such factors can lead to lost drugs and medical tragedy, see Plotkin (1988) and CUSRI/CESO (1988).

26. Appropriate on-farm methodologies for ERDE are the subject of several books. Fortunately, a growing number of publications now provide models, guides, and informative case studies for the design and conduct of participatory on-farm research and development generally and in animal agriculture specifically (Kirsopp-Reed, Hinchcliffe, 1994; McCorkle, 1990), or exclusively in ERDE (Bazalar, McCorkle, 1989; Grandin, Young, 1996; McCorkle, 1994b; McCorkle, Mathias, Schillhorn van Veen, 1996).

27. Again, however, further research is needed on the relative biostability, bioaccumulation, and toxicity of ethnomedicines.

*R*EFERENCES

Anciennes méthodes de prophylaxie des maladies animales—early methods of animal disease control—los antiguos métodos de profilaxis de las enfermedades animales, *Revue Scientifique et Technique de l'Office International des Épizooties* 13, 1994.

Anjaria J: Ethnoveterinary pharmacology in India: past, present, and future. In McCorkle CM, Mathias E, Schillhorn van Veen TW, editors: *Ethnoveterinary research and development,* London, 1996, Intermediate Technology Publications.

Anonymous: Various personal communications to McCorkle during The Workshop to Produce an Ethnoveterinary Information Kit, held at the International Institute of Rural Reconstruction, Silang, Cavite, the Philippines, July 11-25, 1994.

Art JR and others: *Biotechnology, indigenous peoples, and intellectual property rights: CRS report for Congress,* Washington, DC, 1993, Library of Congress Congressional Research Service.

Bannerman RH, Burton J, Wen-Chieh C, editors: *Traditional medicine and health care coverage,* Geneva, 1983, World Health Organization.

Baumann MPO: The nomadic animal health system (NAHA-System) in pastoral areas of central Somalia and its usefulness in epidemiological surveillance, master's thesis, Davis, Calif, 1990, University of California–Davis School of Veterinary Medicine.

Bazalar H, McCorkle CM, editors: *Estudios etnoveterinarios en comunidades altoandinas del Perú,* Lima, Perú, 1989, Lluvia Editores.

Bizimana N: *Traditional veterinary practice in Africa,* Robdorf, Germany, 1994, Deutsche Gesellschaft für Technische Zusammenarbeit (GTZ).

Bodeker GC (chair): Summary of Symposium on Traditional Health Systems and Public Policy, Ottawa, March 1-4, 1994, Washington, DC, National Museum of Health and Medicine, 1994a.

Bodeker G: Traditional health knowledge and public policy, *Nature and Resources* 30(2):5, 1994b.

Bonfiglioli A-M, Diallo YD, Fagerberg-Diallo S: Veterinary science and savvy among Ferlo Fulbe. In McCorkle CM, Mathias E, Schillhorn van Veen TW, editors: *Ethnoveterinary research and development,* London, 1996, Intermediate Technology Publications.

Brisebarre A-M: Tradition and modernity: French shepherd's use of medicinal bouquets. In McCorkle CM, Mathias E, Schillhorn van Veen TW, editors: *Ethnoveterinary research and development,* London, 1996, Intermediate Technology Publications.

Cheneau Y: The organization of veterinary services in Africa, *Revue Scientifique et Technique de l'Office International des Épizooties* 5(1):107, 1985.

Conservation International: Fact sheet, Washington, DC, Conservation International.

Cox PA, Balick MJ: The ethnobotanical approach to drug discovery, *Sci Am* 271:82, June 1994.

The Crucible Group: *People, plants, and patents: the impact of intellectual property on biodiversity, conservation, trade, and rural society,* Ottawa, 1994, IDRC.

CTA: *Le role des auxiliaires d'élevage en Afrique: rapport de séminaire,* Bujumbura, Burundi, 1984, Centre Technique de Coopération Agricole et Rural.

CTA/GTZ/IEMVT: A new policy for the development of livestock production in African [sic] south of the Sahara primary animal health care structure: summary report of a seminar on a primary animal health care structure, Bujumbura (Republic of Burundi), October 24-26, 1984, Bujumbura, 1985, Technical Centre for Agricultural and Rural Cooperation, The Netherlands; Deutsche Gesellschaft fr Technische Zusammenarbeit, Germany; and Institut d'Elevage et de Médecine Vétérinarie des Pays Tropicaux, France.

CUSRI/CESO: Reports on group discussions. In *Indigenous knowledge and learning: papers presented in the workshop on indigenous knowledge and skills and the ways they are acquired, Cha'am, Thailand, March 2-5, 1988,* Bangkok, The Hague, 1988, Chulalongkorn University Social Research Institute, Centre for the Study of Education in Developing Countries.

Daly DC: The National Cancer Institute's Plant Collections Program: update and implications for tropical forests. In Plotkin M, Famolare L, editors: *Sustainable harvest and marketing of rain forest products,* Covelo, Calif, and Washington, DC, 1983, Island Press for Conservation International.

Daniels PW and others: *Livestock services for smallholders: a critical evaluation of the delivery of animal health and production services to the small-scale farmer in the developing world.* Proceedings of an International Seminar held in Yogyakarta, Indonesia, November 15-21, 1992. Bogor, Indonesia, 1993, Indonesia International Animal Science Research and Development Foundation.

de Haan C, Bekure S: *Animal health services in sub-Saharan Africa: initial experiences with alternative approaches,* Washington, DC, 1991, World Bank.

de Haan C, Nissen N: *Animal health services in sub-Saharan Africa,* Technical Paper No. 44, Washington, DC, 1985, World Bank.

Delehanty J: Methods and results from a study of local knowledge of cattle diseases in coastal Kenya. In McCorkle CM, Mathias E, Schillhorn van Veen TW, editors: *Ethnoveterinary research and development,* London, 1996, Intermediate Technology Publications.

deMaar TW: Ask what's in those bottles, *Ceres: The FAO Review* 24(4):40, 1992.

Donald AD: Parasites, animal production and sustainable development, *Vet Parasitol* 54:27, 1994.

Duke JA: Tropical botanical extractives. In Plotkin M, Famolare L, editors: *Sustainable harvest and marketing of rain forest products,* Covelo, Calif, and Washington, DC, 1992, Island Press for Conservation International.

Etkin NL: Ethnopharmacology: biological and behavioral perspectives in the study of indigenous medicines. In Johnson TM, Sargent CF, editors: *Medical anthropology: contemporary theory and method,* New York, 1990, Praeger.

Farnsworth NR: The NAPRALERT data base as an information source for application to traditional medicine. In Bannerman RH, Burton J, Wen-Chieh C, editors: *Traditional medicine and health care coverage,* Geneva, 1983, World Health Organization.

Food and Agriculture Organization (based on the work of CG Sivadas): *Preliminary study of traditional systems of veterinary medicine,* Bangkok, 1980, Food and Agriculture Organization Regional Office for Asia and the Pacific.

Food and Agriculture Organization (based on the work of JV Anjaria): *Traditional (indigenous) systems of veterinary medicine for small farmers in India,* Bangkok, 1984a, Food and Agriculture Organization Regional Office for Asia and the Pacific.

Food and Agriculture Organization (based on the work of P Buranamanus): *Traditional (indigenous) systems of veterinary medicine for small farmers in Thailand,* Bangkok, 1984b, Food and Agriculture Organization Regional Office for Asia and the Pacific.

Food and Agriculture Organization (based on the work of DD Joshi): *Traditional (indigenous) systems of veterinary medicine for small farmers in Nepal,* Bangkok, 1984c, Food and Agriculture Organization Regional Office for Asia and the Pacific (reprinted in 1991).

Food and Agriculture Organization (based on the work of M Maqsood): *Traditional (indigenous) systems of veterinary medicine for small farmers in Pakistan,* Bangkok, 1986, Food and Agriculture Organization Regional Office for Asia and the Pacific.

Food and Agriculture Organization (based on the work of SB Dhanapala): *Traditional veterinary medicine in Sri Lanka,* Bangkok, 1991a, Food and Agriculture Organization Regional Office for Asia and the Pacific.

Food and Agriculture Organization (based on the work of S Poedjomartono): *Traditional veterinary medicine in Indonesia,* Bangkok, 1991b, Food and Agriculture Organization Regional Office for Asia and the Pacific.

Food and Agriculture Organization: *Report: expert consultation on food losses due to non-infectious and production diseases in developing countries,* Rome, 1991c, Food and Agriculture Organization of the United Nations.

Food and Agriculture Organization: *Traditional veterinary medicine in the Philippines,* Bangkok, 1992, Food and Agriculture Organization Regional Office for Asia and the Pacific.

Fratkin E, Galvin KA, Roth EA, editors: *African pastoralist systems: an integrated approach,* Boulder, Colo, and London, 1994, Lynne Rienner.

Galaty JG, Aronson D, Salzman PC, editors: *The future of pastoral peoples: proceedings of a conference held in Nairobi, Kenya, August 4-8, 1980,* Ottawa, 1981, International Development Research Centre.

Glen-Leary J: Oxpecker revival, *Farmer's Weekly* 11:30, May 1990.

Goleman D: Shamans and their lore may vanish with forests, *The New York Times Science Times* 11 June: C1, 1991.

Goodstern C: Sorcerers' apprentices, *Currents* March/April: 14-16, 1993.

Grandin B, Young J: Collection and use of ethnoveterinary data in community-based animal health programs. In McCorkle CM, Mathias E, Schillhorn van Veen TW, editors: *Ethnoveterinary research and development,* London, 1996, Intermediate Technology Publications.

Grandin B, Thampy R, Young J: *Case study: village animal healthcare: a community-based approach to livestock development in Kenya,* London, 1991, Intermediate Technology Publications.

Greaves T, ed: *Intellectual property rights for indigenous peoples: a source book,* Oklahoma City, 1994, Society for Applied Anthropology.

GTZ: *Key programme: primary veterinary care and liberalisation of veterinary services,* Internal document No. 142-Dr. b/Gr, August 26, 1983, Deutsche Gesellschaft für Technische Zusammenarbeit.

Hadani A, Shimshony A: Traditional veterinary medicine in the Near East: Jews, Arab Bedouins and Fellahs, *Revue Scientifique et Technique de l'Office International des Epizooties* 13(2):581, 1994.

Heffernan C, Heffernan E, Stem C: Aspects of animal healthcare among Samburu pastoralists. In McCorkle CM, Mathias E, Schillhorn van Veen TW, editors: *Ethnoveterinary research and development,* London, 1996, Intermediate Technology Publications.

Hyndman D: Conservation through self-determination: promoting the interdependence of cultural and biological diversity, *Human Organization* 53(3):296, 1994.

Ibrahim MA: Ethnotoxicology among Nigerian agropastoralists. In McCorkle CM, Mathias E, Schillhorn van Veen TW, editors: *Ethnoveterinary research and development,* London, 1996, Intermediate Technology Publications.

Ibrahim MA, Abdu PA: Ethnoagroveterinary perspectives on poultry production in rural Nigeria. In McCorkle CM, Mathias E, Schillhorn van Veen TW, editors: *Ethnoveterinary research and development,* London, 1996, Intermediate Technology Publications.

IIRR: *Ethnoveterinary medicine in Asia: on traditional health care practices,* Silang, Philippines, 1994, International Institute for Rural Reconstruction.

Iles K, Young J: Decentralized animal health care in pastoral areas, *Appropriate Technology* 18(1):20, 1991.

ITDG: *Traditional healers' workshop: Intermediate Technology Development Group Utooni Development Project,* Nairobi, March 30-31, 1989, Unpublished manuscript, 1989.

ITDG: *Report on discussions with traditional healers: Mtito Andei, Nairobi, October 1992,* Unpublished manuscript, 1992.

Kirsopp-Reed K, Hinchcliffe F: *RRA notes: special issue on livestock,* London, 1994, International Institute for Environment and Development with ITDG, Oxfam, and VetAid.

Krajick K: Sorcerer's apprentices, *Newsweek Focus* Jan 2-4, 1993.

Lalonde A, Morin-Labatut G: *Indigenous knowledge, innovation and sustainable development: an information sciences perspective,* Unpublished manuscript.

Last M: Professionalization of indigenous healers. In Johnson TM, Sargent CF, editors: *Medical anthropology: contemporary theory and method,* New York, 1990, Praeger.

Leonard DK: The supply of veterinary services: Kenyan lessons, *Agricultural administration and extension* 26:219, 1987.

Leonard D: Structural reform of the veterinary profession in Africa and the new institutional economics, *Development and Change* 24:227, 1993.

Lin JH, Panzer R: Use of Chinese herbal medicine in veterinary science: history and perspectives, *Revue Scientifique et Technique de l'Office International des Épizooties* 13(2):425, 1994.

Mathias E, McCorkle CM: Animal health. In Bunders J, Haverkort B, Hiemstra W, editors: *Biotechnology: building on farmers' knowledge,* Basingstoke, UK, 1997, MacMillan Education Publishing.

Mathias-Mundy E, McCorkle CM: *Ethnoveterinary medicine: an annotated bibliography,* Bibliographies in Technology and Social Change No. 6, Center for Indigenous Knowledge and Agricultural and Rural Development (CIKARD), Ames, Iowa, 1989, Iowa State University Research Foundation.

Mathias-Mundy E, Murdiati TB, editors: *Traditional veterinary medicine for small ruminants in Java,* Bogor, Indonesia, 1991, Indonesian Small Ruminant Network.

Mathias-Mundy E and others: *Traditional animal health care for goats and sheep in West Java: a comparison of three villages,* Working Paper No. 139 of the Small Ruminant Collaborative Research Program/Indonesia, Bogor, Indonesia, 1992, SR-CRSP and Balai Penelitian Ternak.

Matzigkeit U: *Natural veterinary medicine: ectoparasites in the tropics,* Weikersheim, Germany, 1990, Verlag Josef Margraf Scientific Books for AGRECOL.

Mazars G: Traditional veterinary medicine in India, *Revue Scientifique et Technique de l'Office International des Épizooties* 13(2):443, 1994.

McCorkle CM: *Management of animal health and disease in an indigenous Andean community,* SR-CRSP Publication No. 4. Columbia, Mo, Department of Rural Sociology, University of Missouri, 1982.

McCorkle CM: An introduction to ethnoveterinary research and development, *J Ethnobiology* 6:129, 1986.

McCorkle CM: Punas, pastures, and fields: grazing strategies and the agropastoral dialectic in an indigenous Andean commnity. In Browman D, editor: *Arid land use strategies and risk management in the Andes: a regional anthropological perspective,* Boulder, Colo, 1987, Westview Press.

McCorkle CM: Toward a knowledge of local knowledge and its importance for agricultural R&D, *Agriculture and Human Values* 6(3):4, 1989a.

McCorkle CM: Veterinary anthropology, *Human Organization* 48(2): 156, 1989b.

McCorkle CM, editor: *Improving Andean sheep and alpaca production: recommendations from a decade of research in Peru,* Columbia, Mo, 1990, University of Missouri Printing Services for the SR-CRSP.

McCorkle CM: The roles of animals in cultural, social, and agroeconomic systems. In James VU, editor: *Sustainable development in Third World countries: applied and theoretical perspectives,* Westport, Conn, 1997, Greenwood Publishing.

McCorkle CM: Agropastoral systems research in the SR-CRSP Sociology Project. In McCorkle CM, editor: *Plants, animals and people: agropastoral systems research,* Boulder, Colo, 1992, Westview Press.

McCorkle CM: *A framework for analysis of gender and other socioeconomic variables in Ag&NRM,* Working Papers on Women and International Development No. 241, East Lansing, Mich, 1994a, Women in Development Program, Center for International Programs, Michigan State University.

McCorkle CM: Ethnoveterinary R&D and gender in the ITDG/Kenya RAPP (Rural Agricultural and Pastoral Development Programme), Unpublished consultancy report, Nairobi, 1994b, Intermediate Technology Development Group.

McCorkle CM: *Intersectoral action and policy directions in traditional health systems for humans and animals.* Paper presented to the International Workshop on Traditional Health Systems and Public Policy, Ottawa, 1994c, International Development Research Centre.

McCorkle CM: The "cattle battle" in cross-cultural context, *Culture Agriculture* 50:2-4, 1994d.

McCorkle CM, Brandstetter RH, McClure GD: *A case study on farmer innovations and communication in Niger,* Washington, DC, 1988, Academy for Educational Development for AID/S&T and USAID/Niger (partially reprinted in 1994 under the title *Farmer innovation in Niger: studies in technology and social change no. 12,* Ames, Iowa, Iowa State University Research Foundation in collaboration with the Center for Indigenous Knowledge for Agriculture and Rural Development [CIKARD] and the Leiden Ethnosystems and Development Programme [LEAD] of the Institute of Cultural and Social Studies, University of Leiden, The Netherlands.)

McCorkle CM, Mathias E: *Paraveterinary healthcare,* London, Intermediate Technology Publications (in progress).

McCorkle CM, Mathias-Mundy E: Ethnoveterinary medicine in Africa, *Africa: Journal of the International African Institute (London)* 62:59-93, 1992.

McCorkle CM, Mathias E, Schillhorn van Veen TW, editors: *Ethnoveterinary research and development,* London, 1996, Intermediate Technology Publications.

McDowell RE: The role of animals in developing countries. In Baldim RL, editor: *Animals, feed, food and people,* Boulder, Colo, 1980, Westview Press.

McDowell RE: *A partnership for humans and animals,* Raleigh, NC, 1991, Kinnic Press.

Meltzer M: Personal communication by letter to C McCorkle, January 5, 1995.

Mesfin T, Obsa T: Ethiopian traditional veterinary practices and their possible contribution to animal production and management, *Revue Scientifique et Technique de l'Office International des Épizooties* 13(2):417, 1994.

Michel JF: The epidemiology and control of some nematode infections of grazing animals, *Advances in Parasitology* 7:211, 1969.

Michel JF: The epidemiology and control of some nematode infections of grazing animals, *Advances in Parasitology* 14:355, 1976.

Nuwanyakpa M and others: Traditional veterinary medicine in Cameroon: a renaissance in an ancient indigenous technology, unpublished manuscript, Cameroon, 1990, HPI.

Perezgrovas R: Sheep husbandry and healthcare among Tzotzil Maya shepherdesses. In McCorkle CM, Mathias E, Schillhorn van Veen TW, editors: *Ethnoveterinary research and development*, London, 1996, Intermediate Technology Publications.

Plotkin MJ: Conservation, ethnobotany, and the search for new jungle medicines: pharmacognosy comes of age … again, *Pharmacotherapy* 8:257, 1988.

Roepke DA: Traditional and re-applied veterinary medicine in East Africa. In McCorkle CM, Mathias E, Schillhorn van Veen TW, editors: *Ethnoveterinary research and development*. London, 1996, Intermediate Technology Publications.

Salih MAM: Pastoralists and planners: local knowledge and resource management in Gidan Magajia Grazing Reserve, northern Nigeria, Dryland Networks Programme Paper No. 32, London, 1992, International Institute for Environment and Development.

Sansoucy R: Livestock: a driving force for food security and sustainable development, Unpublished working paper, Rome, 1994, Animal Production and Health Division (AGA) of the Food and Agriculture Organization of the United Nations.

Schillhorn van Veen TW: The present and future veterinary practitioners in the tropics, *The Veterinary Quarterly* 15(2):43, 1993.

Schillhorn van Veen TW: Changing paradigms in the delivery of livestock services. Paper presented to the Pan-American Health Organization's Animal Health Workshop on Alternative Models for Delivery of Official Livestock Services, Acapulco, Oct 8-10, 1994.

Schillhorn van Veen TW: Personal communications, Jan-Feb 1995.

Schillhorn van Veen TW: Sense or nonsense? Traditional methods of disease prevention and control in the African savanna. In McCorkle CM, Mathias E, Schillhorn van Veen TW, editors: *Ethnoveterinary research and development*, London, 1996, Intermediate Technology Publications.

Schillhorn van Veen TW, de Haan C: Trends in the organization and financing of livestock and animal health services, *Preventive Vet Med* 25:225-240, 1995.

Schwabe CW: Animal diseases and primary health care: intersectoral challanges, *WHO Chronicle* 35:227, 1981.

Schwabe CW: *Veterinary medicine and human health,* ed 3, Baltimore, 1984, Williams & Wilkins.

Schwabe CW, Kuojok IM: Practices and beliefs of the traditional Dinka health healer in relation to provision of modern medical and veterinary services for the southern Sudan, *Human Organization* 40:231, 1981.

Scoones I, editor: *Living with uncertainty: new directions in pastoral development in Africa,* London, 1995, Intermediate Technology Publications.

Sollod AE, Knight AJ: Veterinary anthropology: a herd health study in central Niger, Proceedings of the Third International Symposium on Veterinary Epidemiology and Economics, Edwardsville, Kan, 1983, Veterinary Medicine Publishing.

Sollod AE, Stem C: Appropriate animal health information systems for nomadic and transhumant livestock populations in Africa, *Revue Scientifique et Technique de l'Office International des Épizooties* 10(1):89, 1991.

Sollod AE, Wolfgang K, Knight JA: Veterinary anthropology: interdisciplinary methods in pastoral systems research. In Simpson JR, Evangelou P, editors: *Livestock development in subsaharan Africa: constraints, prospects, policy,* Boulder, Colo, 1984, Westview Press.

Stem C: Ethnoveterinary R&D in production-systems context. In McCorkle CM, Mathias E, Schillhorn van Veen TW, editors: *Ethnoveterinary research and development,* London, 1996, Intermediate Technology Publications.

Thrupp L: Legitimizing local knowledge: from displacement to empowerment for Third World people, *Agriculture and Human Values* 6(3):13, 1989.

Trotter RT: Seminar on Mexican ethnomedicine, Ames, Iowa, October 1988, Iowa State University.

Umali DL, Feder G, de Haan C: The balance between public and private sector activities in the delivery of livestock services, Discussion Paper No. 162, Washington, DC, 1992, World Bank.

Waller R: Emutai: crisis and response in Maasailand 1883-1902. In Johnson DH, Anderson DM, editors: *The ecology of survival: case studies from northeast African history,* London and Boulder, Colo, 1988, L Crook Academic Publishers and Westview Press.

Ward DE and others: One medicine: practical application for nonsedentary pastoral populations, *Nomadic Peoples* 32:55, 1993.

Warren DM, editor: Indigenous agricultural knowledge systems and development, *Agriculture and Human Values* 8(1/2):1991.

Waters-Bayer A, Bayer W: The role of livestock in the rural economy, *Nomadic Peoples* 31:3, 1992.

WHO: *Guidelines for the assessment of herbal medicines,* Geneva, 1991a, World Health Organization.

WHO: *Report of the consultation to review the draft guidelines for the assessment of herbal medicines,* Munich, 1991b, World Health Organization.

Zhang X: WHO's policy and activities on traditional medicine. In Islam A, Wiltshire R, editors: *Traditional health systems and public policy: proceedings of an international workshop,* Ottawa, Mar 2-4, 1994, IDRC.

Zessin K-H, Carpenter TE: Benefit-cost analysis of an epidemiologic approach to provision of veterinary service in the Sudan, *Preventive Vet Med* 3:323, 1985.

Zeutzius I: Ethnobotanische Veterinrmedizin: Literaturrecherchen-konventionell und online-zur ethnobotanischen Veterinrmedizin: Aufbau einer strukturierten Bibliographie: Diplomarbeit im Studiengang Biowissenschaftliche Dokumentation an der Fachhochschule, Hannover, Germany, 1990.

Chapter 42

Legal Issues in Holistic Veterinary Practice

GREGG A. SCOGGINS

As the use of complementary and alternative therapies has become more common in human medicine, so too has this trend appeared in veterinary medicine. Alternative modalities such as acupuncture, chiropractic, homeopathy, herbalism, and others have gradually increased the diagnostic and treatment options available to veterinarians and their clients. However, although alternative therapies have become more popular, they have yet to gain widespread acceptance by the public and, more important, the mainstream medical establishment. In the context of veterinary medicine, for example, the American Veterinary Medical Association (AVMA) until recently referred to the practice of holistic veterinary medicine and homeopathy as "unconventional" (AVMA, 1996a).

Many veterinarians find the use of complementary or alternative veterinary medicine (CAVM) personally and professionally rewarding, but the widespread belief that many of these alternative therapies are unconventional poses a legal conundrum. Because many theories of liability are based on an analysis of customary practices within the profession, veterinarians who use CAVM in their practices may be at an increased risk for liability exposure. Of course, the degree of risk depends largely on the extent to which a given procedure or treatment is considered to be unconventional. For example, chiropractic and acupuncture have gained a higher level of recognition as viable modalities than applied kinesiology and iridology.

The purpose of this chapter is to explore some of these legal issues and discuss the way practitioners can address and help minimize the risks posed by the use of CAVM. Because of the great variability among jurisdictions, the body of law on this subject cannot be treated comprehensively. Rather, the purpose of this chapter is to discuss some general legal concepts that may apply to the practice of CAVM and various issues that may arise. Before

following any suggestion offered in this chapter, veterinarians should first consult a lawyer familiar with the laws in the jurisdiction in which they practice.

The Concepts of Malpractice and the Standard of Care

When clients are dissatisfied with veterinary care and treatment, they can file a lawsuit or submit a complaint to the state veterinary licensing or disciplinary board. Historically the judicial system has judged the acts or omissions of most professionals such as veterinarians primarily according to a fault-based concept of liability known as *negligence* (King, 1990). In a broad sense, negligence simply is the failure to act as a reasonably prudent person (American Law Institute, 1965). Negligence by a professional is often referred to as *malpractice*.

The Standard of Care Defined

To determine whether a veterinarian has committed malpractice, the court compares the veterinarian's conduct with a legal standard that describes the way a reasonably prudent veterinarian with similar training and expertise would have behaved under the same or similar circumstances. This is known as *the standard of care*. When a veterinarian's conduct falls below the standard of care and damages follow as a result, the veterinarian may be held liable for paying those damages.

The standard of care incorporates several important considerations that may affect whether a given act or omission was negligent. First, the standard of care does not demand excellence or perfection; rather, it defines the minimal degree of skill and care required for an individual to avoid liability (Keeton, 1984). Because the standard of care represents a minimal threshold, it often does not distinguish between people who have different levels of experience. Therefore many courts judge students and new graduates according to the same standard of care as that applied to practitioners who have been in practice for 20 years.

Second, the standard of care distinguishes between veterinarians who possess different levels of expertise. In other words, someone who claims to be an expert in a particular area will be held to a higher standard of care (Keeton, 1984). Even if veterinarians are not board-certified in a particular area, they can be held to a higher standard of care if they profess expertise (Hannah, 1986).

Third, the applicable standard of care depends on the circumstances surrounding the particular incident in question (Keeton, 1984). In other words, a veterinarian faced with an emergency is not judged according to a standard of care that assumes no emergency. In this way the law attempts to account for the variations that exist in real life.

Finally, and perhaps most important for veterinarians who employ CAVM in their practice, the law in some states takes into account the fact that different schools of thought may exist within the profession with regard to the applicable standard of care. Where this difference of opinion is recognized, some state courts have judged practitioners according to the standard of care practiced by the particular school in which the defendant professes to be a member. However, Keeton (1984) makes the following observation:

> . . . [T]his does not mean, however, that any quack, charlatan or crackpot can set himself up as a "school," and so apply his individual ideas without liability. A "school" must be a recognized one within definite principles, and it must be the line of thought of a respectable minority of the profession.

This last consideration has obvious implications for the way the standard of care is defined in the context of CAVM. Because liability depends in large part on whether the veterinarian met the applicable standard of care, accurate definition of the standard of care in a case involving the use of alternative therapies is one of the most important objectives.

The fact that many forms of CAVM have not yet been recognized as conventional by a majority of the veterinary profession may mean greater risk for practitioners of CAVM. This is true particularly for veterinarians who choose to employ more controversial alternative therapies. In those states that recognize the potential for varying views within a profession and thereby apply different standards of care, the veterinarian's risk may be less.

The Standard of Care and the "School of Thought" Doctrine

Several courts have been asked to define the standard of care as applied to the practice of alternative medicine. Unfortunately, however, no reported case law exists that addresses the use of alternative therapies in veterinary med-

icine. Whereas several cases have addressed this issue in the context of human medicine and can be used as a model for discussing the issue in veterinary medicine, differences between the clinical and regulatory aspects of veterinary and human medicine prevent a uniform application of these principles.

Rationales used in support of the "school of thought" doctrine

In many cases involving practitioners of alternative medicine such as chiropractors, homeopaths, osteopaths, and other drugless healers, courts have held these practitioners to a standard of care that requires them to use "the same degree of care, diligence, and skill in the treatment of his patient as is possessed and used by prudent, skillful, and careful practitioners of the same school" (Liability of chiropractors and other drugless practitioners for medical malpractice, 1990). Thus a chiropractor's conduct will be judged according to that of a reasonably prudent chiropractor, and a homeopath's conduct will be judged according to that of a reasonably prudent homeopath. Courts adopting this approach generally point to one or more of the following rationales.

First, some courts have recognized the potential for philosophic differences between schools of medicine as to "the origin of discomfort and the means of relief ... " (*Sandford v. Howard*, 1982). The mere existence of a philosophic difference between two branches of medicine, however, may not justify holding a practitioner to a different standard. Generally, the philosophy must be held by a recognized school of medicine. Where none exists, the person employing those therapies may be held to the same standard as a medical doctor.

Alternatively, as the Supreme Court of New Jersey has held, even if a school of medicine is recognized as a branch of the healing arts, practitioners will be held to a broader standard of care and practitioners from other branches of the profession may be permitted to offer expert opinion testimony to establish the applicable standard of care if the therapy in question is considered to be a subset of the larger practice of medicine (*Rosenberg v. Cahill*, 1985).

A second rationale recognizes that practitioners of a particular school of medicine are licensed by the state to provide that specific type of medical care. Courts adopting this rationale reason that by providing for separate licensing statutes and regulation, the state has recognized the inherent differences among various schools of medicine that should be reflected in the standard of care applicable to each school (Rian, 1983). In fact, the Supreme Court of Illinois has held that in order for a proposed witness to be eligible to offer expert testimony on the standard of care of a given school of medicine, the proposed expert must be licensed in that school (*Dolan v. Galluzzo*, 1979).

Unfortunately, this second rationale may not apply in the context of veterinary medicine because in most states the practice of veterinary medicine is broadly defined and limited solely to licensed veterinarians. If a state requires the existence of parallel licensure before it will judge a defendant veterinarian according to a standard of care that differs from the standard followed by the entire profession, veterinarians who practice CAVM could face an uphill struggle.

An example from human medicine reflecting the current status of state veterinary licensing laws can be seen in the case of *Rosenberg v. Cahill*. In *Rosenberg* the plaintiffs attempted to use the testimony of a medical doctor regarding the interpretation of radiographs in support of their claim against a chiropractor. In ruling that a medical doctor was qualified to testify on the standard of care applicable to a chiropractor in the interpretation of radiographs, the court found persuasive New Jersey's lack of a specific statutory scheme for licensing chiropractors separate from the other healing arts. Specifically the court made the following judgment:

> Although chiropractic is philosophically different from and more limited than medical healing, chiropractors have been held to be one type of medical practitioner governed generally under Title 45, which codifies the legislative scheme for all persons involved in the healing fields (*Rosenberg v. Cahill*, 1985).

According to the *Rosenberg* analysis, theoretically any veterinarian licensed to practice veterinary medicine may be qualified to testify as an expert on the standard of care in a case involving CAVM even if the purported expert has no training in the use of CAVM. Therefore in states that apply a rule similar to the one applied in *Rosenberg*, a veterinarian who practices CAVM risks facing experts who will attempt to define the standard of care according to more accepted forms of therapy, which may not include the use of alternative therapies.

A third rationale cited by some courts in support of using a standard of care geared toward the specific school of medicine practiced by the defendant recognizes the existence of associations or medical schools designed to provide practitioners of a particular healing art with education and training. Courts also have considered the existence of organizations that strive to develop standards of practice within a particular branch of the healing arts.

Again, as with the existence of state licensing acts, this rationale may not apply with equal force to all alternative veterinary therapies. Although some forms of CAVM have specific educational programs, such as that offered by the International Veterinary Acupuncture Society, few schools provide specific training to persons interested in the application and use of a particular alternative modality in veterinary medicine. Furthermore, few recognized associations exist that promote standards and guidelines for practitioners of a particular form of alternative veterinary medicine. Thus until more groups are available to educate practitioners in the application and use of a given alternative therapy, the use of these therapies may be evaluated from the perspective of a more conventional type of veterinary medicine.

Finally, some courts have held that by choosing to seek medical care from a practitioner of alternative medicine, the patient or client is presumed to know the differences between the alternative form of medicine and more conventional types. Furthermore, the patient is presumed to have accepted the tenets followed by the school and to expect that the practitioner will perform according to the standard of care of the practitioner's particular school of medicine. This view is often characterized as a variation on the doctrine of assumption of risk. In other words, the patient assumes the risks of undergoing any treatment that is not considered mainstream.

Each state recognizing the "school of thought," or "school of medicine," doctrine has used one or more of the preceding rationales to justify its decision to apply a different standard of care to a case involving alternative therapies. For example, an appellate court in North Carolina, in precluding a board-certified orthopedic specialist from testifying as an expert on the standard of care for a podiatrist, cited the fact that podiatrists are regulated by state statutes, must graduate from podiatric medical schools, and have their own associations such as the American Podiatry Association (*Whitehurst v. Boehm*, 1979). Because not all the preceding rationales apply with equal force to veterinary medicine, the more rationales that a court finds persuasive, the more likely it is to apply the "school of thought" doctrine to the case.

Exceptions to the school of thought doctrine

Many courts have recognized an exception to the school of thought, or "school of medicine," doctrine for cases in which the procedures or principles of two schools of medicine concur. In those cases, many courts have held that a practitioner in one school of medicine can testify as an expert witness on the standard of care of a practitioner of a different school of medicine (Physicians and surgeons, 1981). The Supreme Court of Alabama has stated the exception as follows:

> [E]ven if the defendant and the [expert] witness are of different schools of practice, the witness may nevertheless be competent to testify on those standards as to which the principles of the schools do or should concur, such as matters of diagnosis or the existence of a condition that should be recognized by any physician (*Wozny v. Godsil*, 1985).

Under this exception, therefore, if a party presenting an expert witness who adheres to a school of medicine different from that of the defendant can prove the two schools of medicine share similar principles regarding the treatment in question, the court may permit the proffered expert to testify as to the defendant's standard of care.

Applying the Standard of Care Principles to the Practice of CAVM

The standard of care applies in a variety of settings, from diagnosis to treatment and everything in between. This section addresses the application of standard of care principles to the areas of veterinary practice in which the use of alternative therapies is relevant. These areas include obtaining informed consent, referring clients, and serving as a consultant.

The Standard of Care and Informed Consent

The law in most states provides that clients who seek veterinary medical care for their animals are entitled to know (to the extent known or knowable) the nature of the animal's condition, the diagnostic tests and treatment options available, and a reasonable prognosis. Generally, any explanation of the diagnostic or treatment alternatives available should include a discussion of the associated risks and the results that can be reasonably expected with each alternative. This concept is commonly known as *informed consent.*

In many jurisdictions the veterinarian's duty to obtain a client's informed consent is considered to be a part of the applicable standard of care (Keeton, 1984). The doctrine is based on the assumption that clients have the right to choose the health care their animals receive. To make this choice, a client must have sufficient information regarding the various diagnostic or treatment alternatives available, including the cost of those alternatives. The law, therefore, requires health care providers, including veterinarians, to furnish clients with sufficient information to enable them to make these informed choices (Wilson, 1989). The precise amount of information required, however, depends on the facts of the case and laws applicable in that particular jurisdiction.

The use of less conventional therapies in veterinary medicine often involves the doctrine of informed consent. As discussed previously, some courts have justified defining the standard of care according to the standard followed by the defendant's particular school of thought, or school of medicine, on the basis that clients who seek out practitioners of alternative medicine accept the tenets of the school. Presumably, this rationale is based on an underlying assumption that the client is fully aware of the benefits and limitations associated with a particular branch of medicine. If clients lack this knowledge and their animals suffer injury, however, a court may choose not to accept this justification and hold the practitioner liable for not discussing these matters beforehand.

In a case involving the use of alternative therapies, if the veterinarian can show that the client received information regarding the application and limitations of the therapy and the client still elected to proceed, defending a malpractice case may be less difficult. In general, the best way to present this evidence to a court or disciplinary board is through the use of a consent form.

Although the use of a consent form does not guarantee that a veterinarian will escape a lawsuit or even liability, failing to use one increases the risks substantially (Wilson, 1989).

For optimal effectiveness, consent forms should provide the client with a description of the specific procedure, a list of alternatives available (both conventional and nonconventional), a list of the risks associated with the procedure, a reasonable prognosis, and, where applicable, a statement that the procedure is not widely recognized by most veterinarians as a conventional form of therapy. In short, the veterinarian should take every step to ensure that if a jury or disciplinary board reviews the consent form, it will conclude that the client's decision to pursue the treatment was made after the veterinarian's full and fair disclosure. Vague or general consent forms afford little protection to the veterinarian if clients complain they were not advised of a specific risk. Likewise, a form that is too exculpatory may not find favor with the court either (Hannah, 1986).

In any practice the need to give clients full and complete disclosure must be balanced against the practical constraints of doing so. Most veterinarians cannot afford to spend 30 minutes or more with each client discussing proposed diagnostic or treatment alternatives. Furthermore, some veterinarians may find it difficult to communicate with clients. Although one-on-one discussions are preferable, veterinarians may consider alternatives, such as providing written educational materials on the procedure.

The Standard of Care and the Duty to Refer

In human medicine, many courts have held that the standard of care imposes a duty on the physician to refer a patient to a specialist if the physician has insufficient training or experience in an area. As the number of veterinarians with advanced training and board certification in particular specialties increases, the same duty will likely be imposed on veterinarians.

As with any issue involving the standard of care, whether the standard of care requires a veterinarian to seek a referral depends on the facts and circumstances surrounding the case. Factors to consider include the defendant veterinarian's own level of skill and competence, the availability of a specialist who possesses the needed expertise, whether the animal's condition permits it to travel, and the client's willingness to seek a referral.

As particular alternative therapies gain wider acceptance in the veterinary profession, the standard of care may impose on veterinarians a duty to refer clients to other veterinarians who offer these types of therapies. On the other hand, when a practitioner of alternative veterinary therapies encounters a case that cannot be treated adequately with alternative therapies, the standard of care may require the veterinarian to refer the client to a practitioner who uses more conventional therapies.

A Washington court recognized this duty in its ruling on a case in human medicine, in which the patient consulted a naturopath for abdominal pain and nausea. After several days of unsuccessful treatment the patient's wife called a medical doctor, who diagnosed the patient with appendicitis. The patient eventually died from complications of appendicitis. The plaintiff alleged that she had asked the defendant several times to refer her husband to a physician, but the defendant refused.

In ruling for the patient's family, the Washington Supreme Court stated the following:

> A drugless healer is in a position of trust and confidence as regards his patient, and if he knows or should know that any treatment he is permitted to use will be of no benefit to the patient, it is his duty to so advise. If there is another mode of treatment that is more likely to be successful, which treatment he does not have the right to give, it is his duty to send the patient to a doctor (*Kelly v. Carroll*, 1950).

Thus veterinarians who practice CAVM must determine carefully whether a given therapy is indicated for the patient's condition. If it is not, the veterinarian should consider whether a more conventional therapy would be more appropriate. If the veterinarian does not have sufficient skill or training in the recommended conventional therapy, he or she should consider referring the client elsewhere.

The Standard of Care and the Role of the Consultant

The increased presence of specialists in veterinary medicine has given more veterinarians the opportunity to consult on cases for which they do not have the added training or expertise. In many respects, practitioners of alternative therapies serve as specialists in the application and use of specific alternative modalities. Although few recognized specialty colleges for the practice of CAVM currently exist, veterinarians who claim expertise in these areas may be held to a higher standard of care.

Many specialists provide their services as consultants, relying on information provided by the referring veterinarian or the client and having no opportunity to examine the animal themselves. Coupled with the need to meet a higher standard of care, specialists who consult over long distances have additional liability issues to consider over those normally encountered in general practice. Many practitioners of CAVM also serve as consultants and must consider the risks involved.

The first test to determine liability depends on whether the consulting veterinarian owed a legal duty to the plaintiff-client. The formation of a veterinarian-client-patient relationship is usually a prerequisite to the recognition of a duty. Therefore the injury hinges on whether the defendant formed a veterinarian-client-patient relationship with the plaintiff.

The American Veterinary Medical Association defines the veterinarian-client-patient relationship as follows:

> A) The veterinarian has assumed the responsibility for making medical judgments regarding the health of the animal(s) and the need for medical treatment, and the client (owner or other caretaker) has agreed to follow the instruction of the veterinarian.

> B) There is sufficient knowledge of the animal(s) by the veterinarian to initiate at least a general or preliminary diagnosis of the medical condition of the animal(s). This means that the veterinarian has recently seen and is personally acquainted with the keeping and care of the animal(s) by virtue of an examination of the animal(s) and/or by medically appropriate and timely visits to the premises where the animal(s) is (are) kept.

> C) The practicing veterinarian is readily available for follow-up in case of adverse reactions or failure of the regimen of therapy (AVMA Membership Director, Model Practice Act, 1996b).

Many states have adopted this definition of the veterinarian-client-patient relationship in their veterinary practice acts.

This definition, however, does not appear to apply when veterinarians are asked to consult on a case without the opportunity to examine the animal or visit the premises where the animal is kept. Although the AVMA's definition of the veterinarian-client-patient relationship implies that consultants have no legal duty, reported cases in human medicine suggest otherwise.

In human medicine the courts asked to determine whether a physician-patient relationship exists have considered the following: (1) whether the consultant knew the patient or the patient's name; (2) whether the doctor ever saw the patient's records; (3) whether the patient and the consulting physician actually saw or talked to each other; (4) whether the physician actually examined the patient; and (5) whether he was paid a fee (*Hill v. Kokosky*, 1990). In *Hill* the court ruled that a consultant who communicated only by telephone with the referring physician and never examined the patient or the patient's chart owed no duty to the patient because no physician-patient relationship had been established. Several cases from states such as Alabama, California, Michigan, Nebraska, New York, and Texas have led to similar conclusions on this issue.

Other courts asked to analyze this issue, however, have held that a physician-patient relationship existed even when the doctor never saw the patient (*Davis v. Weiskopf*, 1982). The same conclusion was reached recently by a federal court in New York (*Gilinsky v. Delicato*, 1995). In the *Gilinsky* case the court found persuasive the fact that the consultant neurologist "exercised his professional judgment in a matter bearing directly upon the plaintiff" and that it was foreseeable to the consulting physician "that his exercise of judgment ultimately would determine the precise nature of the medical services to be rendered to the plaintiff."

Similar circumstances can easily be imagined in cases involving CAVM consultations. Often practitioners of CAVM are brought in strictly because the referring veterinarian is unfamiliar with the modality. If this is the case, practitioners of CAVM would be expected to exercise their own judgment, which, according to the *Gilinsky* court, would determine the nature of the medical services rendered to the client.

The liability risks associated with consultation underscore the need for a clear and open line of communication between the referring veterinarian and the client, if possible. Establishment of a valid veterinarian-client-patient relationship is also important so the veterinarian has the opportunity to examine the animal and its surroundings as necessary. Additionally, consultants should remember to document their conversations and their opinions, including any limitations, especially when such limitations result from the lack of client or patient contact.

The Impact of State Veterinary Practice Acts on the Practice of CAVM

Like most professions, the veterinary profession is regulated by state government. To protect the public health and welfare of its citizens, each state has developed a statutory and regulatory scheme to ensure that practitioners of veterinary medicine are properly trained and qualified. To assist in regulation of the profession, most states have created licensing or disciplinary boards, at least partly composed of practicing veterinarians. These state boards are responsible for promulgating regulations, or rules, to foster the goals of the enabling legislation. The state board also may hear complaints seeking to discipline licensed members of the profession when the member's conduct violates the state's practice act or the regulations promulgated by the state board.

If clients, colleagues, or members of the general public feel that a veterinarian has committed malpractice or violated the state's practice act, they may file a complaint with the state licensing board. In most states the board is dutybound to investigate the complaint to determine its validity. Depending on the nature of the complaint, the ultimate outcome for the veterinarian ranges from the dismissal of the complaint with no action to censorship, fine, license suspension, or revocation.

At this time, very few states even address the use of CAVM in their practice acts or the regulations promulgated by the state board, short of including it in the definition of the practice of veterinary medicine. Furthermore, some states define the term *malpractice* differently from the common law definition discussed above. For example, in Arizona, one of the applicable definitions of malpractice provided by the state's practice act defines *malpractice* as "treatment in a manner contrary to accepted practices and with injurious results" (Ariz. Rev. Stat. § 32-2201). Requiring veterinarians to use "accepted practices" could be interpreted as a subtle yet significant deviation from the traditional common law definition of the standard of care. Whether the Arizona practice act in fact differs from the traditional common law definition depends on the interpretation of "accepted practices."

The Treatment of CAVM by State Practice Acts

Most states define the practice of veterinary medicine very broadly. A good example appears in the AVMA's Model Veterinary Practice Act, which has been adopted by a number of states (AVMA, 1996b). According to the Model Veterinary Practice Act, the practice of veterinary medicine is defined, in part, as follows:

> [T]o diagnose, treat, correct, change, relieve, or prevent animal disease, deformity, defect, injury, or other physical or mental conditions; including the prescription or administration of any drug, medicine, biologic apparatus, application, anesthetic, or other therapeutic or diagnostic substance or technique, and the use of any manual or mechanical procedure for artificial insemination, for testing for pregnancy, or for correcting sterility or infertility or to render advice or recommendation with regard to any of the above (AVMA, 1996b).

Noticeably absent from this definition is any specific reference to alternative forms of veterinary medicine. The definition, however, captures the essence of most medical procedures and treatments and therefore would presumably include alternative therapies.

A few states have practice acts that acknowledge the use of certain forms of alternative veterinary medicine. An example can be found in Alabama's practice act, which defines the practice of veterinary medicine as follows:

> To diagnose, treat, correct, change, relieve, or prevent animal disease, deformity, defect, injury, or other physical or mental condition; including the prescription or administration of any drug, medicine, biologic, apparatus, application, anesthesia, or other therapeutic or diagnostic substance or technique on any animal *including but not limited to acupuncture, dentistry, animal psychology, animal chiropractic, theriogenology,* surgery (including cosmetic surgery), any manual, mechanical, biological or chemical procedure for testing for pregnancy or for correcting sterility or infertility or to render service or recommendations with regard to any of the above (Alab. Code § 34-29-61(14)(a)(emphasis mine)).

A similar definition can be found in the practice acts of Arkansas, Kansas, and Missouri. To date, no state practice act has acknowledged other forms of alternative medicine, such as homeopathy or naturopathy. To the extent other forms have been acknowledged, they are addressed in the regulations promulgated by the state board.

As an example, the Texas veterinary practice act is silent on the subject of alternative therapies; however, regulations promulgated by the Texas State Board of Veterinary Medical Examiners address four specific alternative therapies: acupuncture, chiropractic medicine, holistic medicine, and homeopathy. With the exception of chiropractic medicine, the regulations restrict the use of these modalities to licensed veterinarians. As for chiropractic medicine, a veterinarian's employee or independent contractor may perform musculoskeletal manipulations if performed "under the direct or general supervision of" a licensed veterinarian (Texas Bd. of Vet. Med. Examiners Reg. 573.12(b)(2)).

The Texas regulations also require client education before any of the four modalities may be employed. Before the alternative therapies can be used, the veterinarian must first advise the client of conventional therapies available. The client must then read and sign a statement acknowledging that the proposed treatment is an alternate therapy and approve its use (Tex. Regs. 573.14(c), 573.15(c) 573.16(c)).

In apparent recognition of the benefit of evaluation by like-minded practitioners, the regulations also provide that in cases involving the use of acupuncture, holistic medicine, and homeopathy, the "investigation of the complaint may include opinions from other licensees who use [that modality] in their treatment of animals" (Tex. Regs. 573.14(d), 573.15(d) 573.16(d)). Notice, however, that the regulation only states that the board <u>may</u> consult a practitioner of that alternative modality. An example of a state <u>requiring</u> the Board to consult with practitioners of alternative therapies can be found in the context of human medicine in New York, where the New York Board of Medicine is required to include on its list of consultants at least two physicians "who dedicate a significant portion of their practice to the use of non-conventional medical treatments. . . ." (N.Y. Public Health § 230.1 (1995)).

Finally, the Texas regulations fail truly to embrace the concept of judging practitioners solely by their peers because the standard of care requires practitioners of alternative therapies to "exercise the same degree of humane care, skill, and diligence in treating patients as are ordinarily used in the same or similar circumstances by average members of the veterinary medical profession in good standing in the locality or community, or in similar locations or communities, in which they practice" (Tex Regs. 573.14(d), 573.15(d), 573.16(d)). By its own terms, this definition appears to invoke a standard of care that looks beyond the practitioner's own school of medicine.

Similar to the Texas Board's approach, the California Board of Veterinary Medicine has sought to address the concerns created by the ever-increasing number of nonlicensed persons offering alternative therapies to clients' animals by defining circumstances under which a nonlicensed person renders such treatment. Their attempt to address the situation, however, is limited to licensed chiropractors (Calif. Regulatory Law Reporter, 1995). The number of fields to which this approach will be applied may expand in the future.

The Practice of Veterinary Medicine by Nonveterinarians

The increased popularity of CAVM has resulted in a number of nonveterinarians who provide these services to animal owners. Most state practice acts, however, do not address specifically the use of alternative therapies, which has created some uncertainty as to whether the use of these therapies by nonveterinarians is prohibited.

As discussed above, the definition of the practice of veterinary medicine is often so broad that it would be hard to argue that such modalities are not included. While many practice acts provide for criminal sanctions to issue against a nonlicensed person practicing veterinary medicine, the practical reality is that most states only rarely pursue nonlicensed persons. Instead, the board usually pursues the veterinarian who associates or consults with an unlicensed person under a provision found in most practice acts or regulations that prohibits a veterinarian from aiding or abetting the unlicensed or unlawful practice of veterinary medicine.

Thus before veterinarians consider bringing in a third party to offer chiropractic, acupuncture, or other alternative therapies, they should analyze their state's practice act to ensure that doing so will not place them in jeopardy of losing their license.

As discussed previously, many veterinarians who employ alternative therapies in their practice provide consultation to veterinarians or directly to clients. Whether such conduct constitutes the unlawful practice of veterinary medicine when the consultant is not licensed to practice veterinary medicine in the state where the client resides is questionable. In most state practice acts, consulting veterinarians are exempted from the license requirement if they are licensed to practice in another state. Some restrictions apply, however, and practitioners must understand the given state's practice act, including exceptions, before agreeing to consult on a case in another state.

For example, most states require the consultant to provide services at the request of a veterinarian licensed to practice in the state. In Missouri, consultants are required to work "under the immediate supervision of a veterinarian" licensed in Missouri (Mo. Stat. § 340.216). Thus most practice acts do not address the possibility of a nonlicensed consulting veterinarians entering the state without first having been asked to consult by a licensed veterinarian in the state. This rule may have broad ramifications for veterinarians who are asked for advice by the prospective client.

The Impact of CAVM on Liability

Because of the differences in the way various states define *malpractice* and regulate the practice of veterinary medicine, it is difficult, if not impossible, to draw any broad, overarching conclusions regarding the risk of liability associated with CAVM. The lack of reported case law in the context of veterinary medicine and anecdotal evidence suggests, however, that the use of CAVM is not currently a common target for malpractice claims. Several suggestions can be offered to explain this phenomenon.

First, the widespread use of alternative therapies has only recently begun. Although this explanation does not seem relevant to modalities such as acupuncture that have existed for centuries, the use of these therapies in veterinary medicine is relatively new—so new, in fact, that no legal decisions on their use have been reported.

Second, as alternative therapies grow more popular, practitioners will face increased scrutiny from various licensing and regulatory boards. Like Texas, more states may, and probably should, adopt regulations or modify practice acts to address this trend. The proliferation of nonveterinarians practicing CAVM is of particular concern. In the future, the veterinary profession and state licensing boards will be challenged to restrict the use of CAVM to veterinarians.

Because of the concern for protecting consumers and preventing the practice of veterinary medicine by nonveterinarians, the most likely source of scrutiny and legal pressure will come from state licensing boards. This pressure will take two forms. First, regulatory efforts will attempt to define more clearly the practice of veterinary medicine. Second, armed with these stricter definitions, state licensing boards will look more carefully at alternative therapies. To minimize the increased risk they may face in the future, veterinarians should implement sensible risk-management principles in their practices.

The first and most important risk-management tool is to practice good medicine. Practicing good medicine ensures that the veterinarian is meeting the standard of care. This requires veterinarians to be knowledgeable about the latest developments in veterinary medicine through periodicals, texts, and continuing education seminars.

The second most important risk-prevention strategy is to maintain effective client communication. Most malpractice claims and complaints filed with state disciplinary boards are rooted in the veterinarian's failure to communicate effectively with the client (Dinsmore, 1993). Veterinarians should strive to communicate during all phases of the veterinary-client relationship. As stated previously, face-to-face communication is most effective, but when circumstances do not permit this level of attention, other vehicles for client education may be considered.

While communicating with clients, the veterinarian should elicit feedback to ensure that clients understand the nature of the procedure and its risks and alternatives that may be available. Often, when clients face a crisis, they are distressed or distracted and do not always give their undivided attention to the person talking to them. By seeking feedback and questioning the client about treatment recommendations, the veterinarian can determine whether the client is paying attention. Also, the veterinarian's questions may help focus the client on the problem and its possible solutions. By engaging clients in these types of discussions, the veterinarian may be able to prevent misunderstandings and potential legal problems.

A third risk-management tool is the clear and accurate documentation of all findings regarding the animal's treatment, including all communications with the client. At a minimum, this documentation should be included in the patient's chart or in the form of a written consent. Effective communication may be of little benefit if the client denies that this occurred. In these types of cases, the result often hinges on the veterinarian's word against the client's. If the medical record supports the veterinarian's testimony,

the jury or disciplinary board may be more willing to accept the veterinarian's representation of the incident.

A fourth important risk-management principle is knowledge of laws and regulations that apply to the practice of veterinary medicine. As discussed previously, great variation exists in the way states define and regulate the practice of veterinary medicine. An awareness of the laws and regulations that apply where they practice can help veterinarians who are developing policies and procedures for the use of CAVM.

In the context of malpractice, some jurisdictions follow the rule that when a person's conduct violates a statute, the person is negligent *per se.* Under this rule, plaintiffs are relieved of the burden to present expert testimony showing that the defendant met the standard of care. Instead, the burden shifts to defendants, who must prove that their actions were not negligent. Familiarity with and adherence to the state's practice act and regulations are therefore important in preserving a veterinarian's license to practice.

Finally, practitioners should be aware of the limitations inherent in a given alternative therapy. Like most treatments, no one therapy can be all things to all animals. When the therapy has little or no application to an animal's condition, the practitioner should suggest an alternative or recommend a referral.

Conclusion

The practice of veterinary medicine offers practitioners a great deal of flexibility and independence. Certain social and professional norms exist, however, that restrict the amount of independence the veterinarian can exercise without encountering some risk. Because CAVM is not yet widely accepted by the veterinary profession, its practitioners may face additional legal risks. Practitioners can minimize these risks by recognizing their existence and incorporating basic, common-sense risk-management strategies into their practices.

*R*EFERENCES

Alabama Code § 34-29-61(14)(Supp.) 1995.

American Veterinary Medical Association: *Guidelines on alternative therapies,* 1996a, AVMA.

American Veterinary Medical Association: Model practice act, AVMA, 1996b.

Arizona Revised Statute § 32-2201, 1996.

California Regulatory Law Reporter: *Regulatory agency action,* 1995, Board of Examiners in Veterinary Medicine.

Davis v Weiskopf, 439 N.E.2d 60 (Ill. Ct. App.), 1982.

Dinsmore JR: Veterinary lawsuits: trends and defense strategies, *Vet Clin North Am* 23(5):1019, 1993.

Dolan v Galluzzo, 396 N.E.2d 13 (Ill.), 1979.

Gilinsky v Delicato, 894 F. Supp. 86 (E.D.N.Y.), 1995.

Hannah HW: *Legal briefs,* 1986, AVMA.

Hill v Kokosky, 463 N.W.2d 265 (Mich Ct. App.), 1990.

Keeton WP: *Prosser and Keeton on torts,* ed 5, 1984, West Publishing.

Kelly v Carroll, 219 P.2d 79 (Wash.), 1950.

King JH: The standard of care for veterinarians in medical malpractice, *Tenn Law J* 58:1, 1990.

Liability of chiropractors and other drugless practitioners for medical malpractice, *American Law Reports* 4(77):273, 1990.

Physicians and surgeons, *American Jurisprudence,* ed 2, vol 61, § 353, 1981.

New York Public Health Laws § 230.1, 1995.

Restatement 2d of the Law of Torts, American Law Institute, §§ 282, 1965.

Rian HM: An alternative contractual approach to holistic health care, *Ohio St Law J* 44:185, 1983.

Rosenberg v Cahill, 492 A.2d 371 (N.J.), 1985.

Sandford v Howard, 288 S.E.2d 739 (Ga.), 1982.

Texas Board of Veterinary Medical Examiners' Regulations 573.12-573.16, 1996.

Whitehurst v Boehm, 255 S.E.2d 761 (N.C. App.), 1979.

Wilson JF: *The law and ethics of veterinary medicine,* 1989, Priority Press.

Wozny v Godsil, 474 So.2d 1078 (Ala.), 1985.

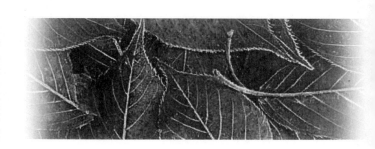

Appendixes:
Resources for Information

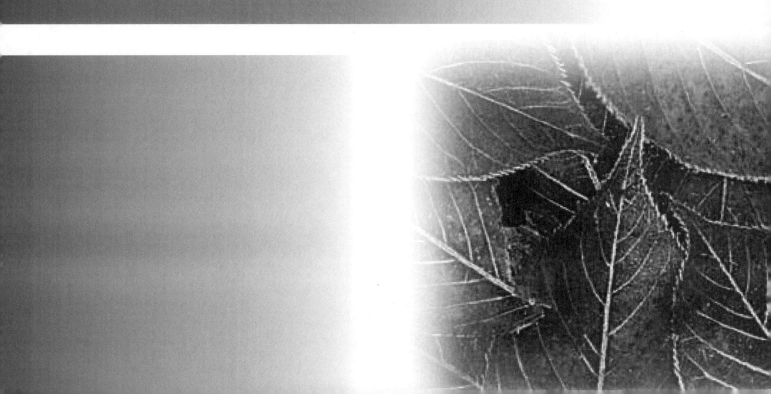

Suppliers

Books, Information

Homeopathic Educational Services
2124 Kittredge St.
Berkeley, CA 94704
800-359-9051

The Minimum Price
P.O. Box 2187
Blaine, WA 98231
1-800-663-8272

Redwing Book Company
44 Linden Street
Brookline, MA 02146
617-738-4664
Large and varied selection with concentration on TCM

Menaco Publishing Co.
P.O. Box 11280
Albuquerque, NM 87192-0280
800-963-6226
Mostly homeopathic books

Homeopathic Information Resources, Ltd.
Oneida River Park Drive
Clay, NY 13041

Ambrican Enterprises
P.O. Box 1492
Sumas, WA 98295
604-856-2050
Various veterinary titles

Eastland Press
1260 Activity Dr., Ste. A
Vista, CA 92083
800-453-3278
TCM and some physical manipulation texts

Lotus Light Publications
P.O. Box 325
Twin Lakes, WI 53181
414-889-8561
Mostly Ayurvedic

Homeopathic Resources and Services
P.O. Box 131
Old Chatham, NY 12136
(718) 784-3239
(518) 794-8653
Old, rare, and out-of-print homeopathic books

Primarily Veterinary

Vetri-Science Laboratories
20 New England Drive-C 1504
Essex Junction, VT 05453-1504
800-882-9993
Nutritional supplements (nutraceuticals)

Natural Animal Nutrition
2109 Emmorton Park
Edgewood, MD 21040
800-548-2899
Nutritional supplements (nutraceuticals)

Natural Animal, Inc.
P.O. Box 1177
St. Augustine, FL 32085
800-274-7387
Natural flea control products, Ester-C

Fleabusters/R$_x$ for Fleas
6555 NW 9th Avenue, Suite 412
Fort Lauderdale, FL 33309
800-666-3532
305-351-9244
Sodium polyborate powder

Halo
3438 East Lake Rd. #14
Palm Harbor, FL 34685
800-426-4256
813-854-2214
Herbal dip, ear wash, nutritional supplies for birds

Springtime Feed Company
10942-J Beaver Dam Rd.
P.O. Box 1227
Cockeysville, MD 21030
800-521-3212
Nutritional/herbal mixed supplements

Wysong
1880 North Eastman Road
Midland, MI 48640
800-748-0188
Foods, some herbal therapeutics

Dr. Goodpet
P.O. Box 4489
Inglewood, CA 90309
800-222-0032
Combination homeopathics, nutritional supplements

Ambrican Enterprises
P.O. Box 1492
Sumas, WA 98295
604-856-2050
Juliette Levy's Western herbal combinations for animals

Orthomolecular Specialties
P.O. Box 32232
San Jose, CA 95152-2232
408-227-9334
Nutritional supplements

Hilton Herbs, Ltd
Downclose Farm
North Perott, Crewkerne
Somerset TA18 7SH
England
(American distributor: Echo Publishing, 505-989-7280)
Western herbal combinations for dogs and horses

Advanced Biological Concepts
301 Main Street
P.O. Box 27
Osco, IL 61274
800-373-5971
Fax: 309-522-5570
Canada: 800-779-3959
Nutritional and herbal products for horses

Harmany Veterinary Products
P.O. Box 1376
Boulder, CO 80306-1376
303-541-9055
Fax: 303-541-9416
Herbs and nutraceuticals for horses and small animals

Nutramax
8304 Harford Rd
Baltimore, MD 21234
800-925-5187
Nutraceuticals

Green Foods Corporation
320 N. Graves Ave.
Oxnard, CA 93030
800-777-4430

PetSage, Inc.
4313 Wheeler Ave.
Alexandria, VA 22304
800-PET-HLTH

Animals' Apawthecary
P.O. Box 212
Conner, MT 59827
406-821-4090
Herbal glycerite formulas

Natural Products—Miscellaneous

Biotec/Biovet International
1215 Center Street
Honolulu, HI 96816
800-468-7578
Nutritional supplements

Nubiologics, Inc.
2470 Wisconsin Ave.
Downers Grove, IL 60515
800-332-3130
Nutritional/glandular supplements

Douglas Laboratories
600 Boyce Road
Pittsburgh, PA 15205
800-245-4440
Fax: 412-494-0155
Large selection of nutritional supplements, some herbs

Standard Process Laboratories
P.O. Box 22
St Joseph, MI 49085-0022
800-253-0864
Nutritional supplements, glandulars

P & D Nutritional Enterprises N.E. and S.E., Inc.
P.O. Box 270
Warrendale, PA 15086
800-245-1939
Nutritional and glandular supplements

Nutri-Dyn Products, Inc.
3300 Hyland Ave.
Costa Mesa, CA 92626
800-533-1033
Nutritional and glandular supplements

Immuno-Dynamics
P.O. Box 544
Perry, IA 50220
800-634-5229
Nutritional supplements

DMSC (Doctors Mutual Service Co.)
18722 Santee Lane
Valley Center, CA 92082
619-749-8609
Glandulars

Lotus Light
P.O. Box 1008
1100 Lotus Drive
Silver Lake, WI 53170
800-548-3824
Natural health care products

Torrance Co.
800 Lenox Ave.
Partage, MI 49002
800-327-0722
Injectable vitamins

For Your Health, Inc.
13215 S.E. 240th St.
Kent, WA 98042
800-456-4325
Nutritional supplements, herbs, glandulars, and books

Natural Health Resources
12729 S.E. 190th Pl.
Renton, WA 98058
Nutritional products

Professional Complementary Health Formulas
5112 SW Garden Home Rd.
P.O. Box 80085
Portland, OR 97280-1085

Advanced Medical Nutrition, Inc.
2247 National Ave.
P.O. Box 5012
Hayward, CA 94540-5012
800-437-8888

M.E.D. Servi-systems
8 Sweetnam Dr.
Stittsville, Ontario
Canada K2S 1G2
613-836-3004

En Garde Health Products, Inc.
7716 Balboa Ave., Ste. F
Van Nuys, CA 91406
800-955-4MED
Nutritional/herbal products

Second Opinion
P.O. Box 69046
Portland, OR 97021
800-999-6922
Nutritional/herbal products

Probiologics, Inc.
West Willows Technology Center
14714 N.E. 87th St.
Redmond, WA
800-678-8218
Nutritional/glandular products

Biotherapeutics, Inc.
P.O. Box 1745
Green Bay, WI 54305
800-553-2370
Nutritional/glandular/herbal products

PCI Press Containers
P.O. Box 204
College Point, NY
800-777-7241
Amber bottles for homeopathics

Lhasa Medical, Inc.
539 Accord Station
Accord, MA 02018-0539
617-335-6484
800-722-8775
Moxa and acupuncture needles

Norfields Magnets
632314 N. Doheny Dr.
Los Angeles, CA 90669
800-344-8400
Magnets

Herbs

East Coast Herbs Distributor
2525 South Mount Juliet Road
Mt. Juliet, TN 37122
800-283-5191
Brion herbs (Chinese)

Ayush Herbs, Inc.
2115 112th NE
Bellevue, WA 98006
206-637-1400
Ayurvedic herbs

ITM (Institute for Traditional Medicine)
2017 S.E. Hawthorne
Portland, OR 97214
800-544-7504
Chinese herbs

Ahmed Botanical International
14150-N.E. 20th St., Ste. 254
Bellevue, WA 98007
206-869-9243
206-869-9238
Herbal formulations

Nuherbs Co.
3820 Penniman Ave.
Oakland, CA 94519
800-233-4307
Chinese herb combos

Eclectic Institute, Inc.
14385 S.E. Lusted Rd.
Sandy, OR 97055
800-332-4372
Western herbs in the eclectic tradition

Health Concerns
8001 Capewell Drive
Oakland, CA 94621
800-233-9355

Physiologics
6565 Odell Place
Boulder, CO 80301-3330
800-765-6775

Crane Enterprises/Jade Pharmacy
45 Samoset Ave.
Plymouth, MA 02360
800-227-4118

McZand Herbals
P.O. Box 5312
Santa Monica, CA 90409
800-800-0405
310-822-0500

Herb Pharm
P.O. Box 116
20260 Williams Hwy.
Williams, OR 97544
541-846-6262
Western herb tinctures

Phytopharmacia
825 Challenger Dr.
Green Bay, WI 54311
800-553-2370

Flower Remedies

Ellon Bach, USA, Inc.
644 Merrick Rd.
Lynbrook, NY 11563
800-433-7523

The Source
2501 71st St.
North Bergen, NJ 07047
800-488-5177

Homeopathics

Standard Homeopathic Company
P.O. Box 61067
Los Angeles, CA 90061
800-624-9659

Hahnemann Pharmacy
828 San Pablo Ave.
Albany, CA 94706
510-527-3003

Biological Homeopathic Industries (BHI)
11600 Cochiti SE
Albuquerque, NM 87123
800-621-7644

Boiron
P.O. Box 449
6 Campus Blvd., Bldg. A
New Town Square, PA 19073
800-258-8823 (or 800-BLU-TUBE)
610-325-7464

Dolisos
3014 Rigel Ave.
Las Vegas, NV 89102
800-365-4767

ARNICA, Inc.
144 E. Garry Ave.
Santa Ana, CA 92707
714-545-8203
Wide variety of nosodes

Ainsworth Pharmacy
38 New Cavendish Street
London, WIM 7LH
United Kingdom
011-44-71-935-5330

Worldwide Web Sites

Acupuncture

http://www.Acupuncture.com
http://www.demon.co.uk/acupuncture/index.html
http://www.ida.com.au/amas/
http://www.med.auth.gr/~karanik/english/main.htm

Alternative Medicine

http://altmed.od.nih.gov
http://shell.idt.net/~drv/bookmark.htm
http://www.altmedicine.com/
http://www.pitt.edu/~cbw/altm.html
http://www.teleport.com/~amrta

Alternative Veterinary Medicine

http://home.earthlink.net/~fourwinds/
http://www.altvetmed.com
http://www.healthworld.com/pan/pa/vet/avca/index.html
http://www.med.auth.gr/~karanik/english/veter.htm
http://www.naturalholistic.com

Cancer

http://catalog.com/bri/bri.htm
http://www.ralphmoss.com/index.html
http://www.sph.uth.tmc.edu/www/utsph/utcam/index.htm

Chiropractic

http://www.amerchiro.org

Electrical Hypersensitivity

http://www.feb.se/

Herbs

http://biotech.chem.indiana.edu.botany/
http://chili.rt66.com/hrbmoore/HOMEPAGE/Home-Page.html
http://www.ars-grin.gov/~ngrlsb/
http://www.herbalgram.org/abcmission.html
http://www.herbs.org/index.html

Homeopathy

http://antenna.nl/homeoweb
http://community.net/~neils/faqhom.html
http://www.dungeon.com/~cam/homeo.html
http://www.lyghtforce.com/HomeopathyOnline/

Nutrition

http://arborcom.com/
http://www.ahsc.arizona.edu/nutrition/
http://www.mic.ki.se/Diseases/alphalist.html
http://www.thorne.com

Oriental Medicine

ftp://ftp.cts.com/pub/nkraft/ormed.html
http://www.pavilion.co.uk/jcm/welcome.html

Psychoneuroimmunology

http://pilot.msu.edu/user/chenhao/pniweb.htm
http://www.psy.aau.dk/bobby/

Subtle Energy Studies

http://vitalenergy.com/issseem

Traditional/Ethnobotanical Medicine

http://www.europa.com/~itm/index.html

Vaccination Issues

http://www.ihot.com/~via/

Recommended Texts

Complementary Medicine: General Reference

Alternative medicine: expanding medical horizons, Washington, DC, 1992, U.S. Government Printing Office.

Fugh-Berman A: *Alternative medicine: what works,* Tucson, 1996, Odonian Press.

Lewith G, Kenyon J, Lewis P: *Complementary medicine: an integrated approach,* New York, 1996, Oxford University Press.

Micozzi M: *Fundamentals of complementary and alternative medicine,* New York, 1996, Churchill-Livingstone.

Environmental Medicine

Chivian E and others: *Critical condition: human health and the environment,* Cambridge, Mass, 1993, The MIT Press.

Rea WJ: *Chemical sensitivity,* vols I-IV, Boca Raton, Fla, 1992, Lewis.

Vaccination Controversy

Stratton KR, Howe CJ, Johnston RB, editors: *Adverse events associated with childhood vaccines: evidence bearing on causality,* Washington, DC, 1994, National Academy Press.

Homeopathy

Bellavite P: *Homeopathy: a frontier in medical science: experimental studies and theoretical foundations,* Berkeley, Calif, 1995, North Atlantic Books.

Herbal Medicine

Bissett N: *Herbal drugs and phytopharmaceuticals: a handbook for practice on a scientific basis,* Boca Raton, Fla, 1994, CRC Press.

Tyler V: *Herbs of choice: the therapeutic use of phytomedicinals,* New York, 1994, Haworth Press.

Weiss R: *Herbal medicine,* Beaconsfield, England, 1994, Beaconsfield Publishers.

Werbach M, Murray M: *Botanical influences on illness: a sourcebook on clinical research,* Tarzana, Calif, 1994, Third Line Press.

Naturopathy

Murray M, Pizzorno J: *Encyclopedia of natural medicine,* Rocklin, Calif, 1991, Prima Publishing.

Nutrition

Werbach M: *Foundations of nutritional medicine,* Tarzana, Calif, 1997, Third Line Press.

Werbach M: *Nutritional influences on illness: a sourcebook of clinical research,* New Canaan, Conn, 1987, Keats Publishing.

Traditional Chinese Medicine

Huang KC: *The pharmacology of Chinese herbs,* Boca Raton, Fla, 1993, CRC Press.

Cancer Therapy

Boik J: *Cancer and natural medicine: a textbook of basic science and clinical research,* Princeton, Minn, 1995, Oregon Medical Press.

Complementary Veterinary Medicine

Schoen A: *Veterinary acupuncture: ancient art to modern medicine,* St Louis, 1994, Mosby.

appendix D

Periodicals

Journal of the American Holistic Veterinary Medical Association
2214 Old Emmorton Road
Bel Air, MD 21015
410-569-0795
Fax: 410-569-2346

Veterinary Acupuncture Newsletter
International Veterinary Acupuncture Society
268 West Third Street, Ste. 4
P.O. Box 2074
Nederland, CO 80466-2074
303-449-7936
Fax: 303-449-8312

Alternative Therapies in Health and Medicine
101 Columbia
Aliso Viejo, CA 92656
800-899-1712

Journal of Alternative and Complementary Medicine
Mary Ann Liebert, Inc., Publishers
1651 Third Avenue
New York, NY 10128
914-834-3100
Fax: 914-834-3688

Alternative and Complementary Therapies
Mary Ann Liebert, Inc., Publishers
1651 Third Avenue
New York, NY 10128
914-834-3100
Fax: 914-834-3688

Alternative Medicine Journal
Prime National Publishing Corp.
470 Boston Post Road
Weston, MA 02193

Alternative Medicine Review
Thorne Research, Inc.
P.O. Box 3200
Sandpoint, ID 83864
208-263-1337
Fax: 208-265-2488

The American Journal of Natural Medicine
Impakt Communications, Inc.
P.O. Box 12496
Green Bay, WI 54307-2496
414-499-2995
Fax: 414-499-3441

Clinical Pearls News
IT Services
3301 Alta Arden #3
Sacramento, CA 95825
800-422-9887

Nutrition Research Newsletter
Lyda Associates
P.O. Box 700
Palisades, NY 10964
914-359-8282
Fax: 914-359-1229

International Journal of Alternative and Complementary Medicine
Green Library
Homewood House
Guildford Road, Chertsey
Surrey KT 16 0QA
England

Herbalgram
American Botanical Council
P.O. Box 201660
Austin, TX 78720
512-331-8868

Medical Herbalism—A Clinical Newsletter for the Herbal
    Practitioner
Bergner Communications
P.O. Box 33080
Portland, OR 97233
800-231-9290

Protocol Journal of Botanical Medicine
P.O. Box 721
Ayer, MA 01432-0721
800-466-5422

American Herbalists Guild (newsletter)
P.O. Box 1683
Soquel, CA 95073

The Australian Journal of Medical Herbalism
The National Herbalists Association of Australia
Ste. 305, 3 Smail St.
Broadway NSW 2007
Australia

Canadian Herbal Practitioners Newsletter
302-1220 Kensington Road, NW
Calgary, Alberta
Canada T2N 3P5

The European Journal of Herbal Medicine
The National Institute of Medical Herbalists
9 Palace Gate
Exeter, EX1 1JA
UK

Fosters Botanical and Herb Reviews
P.O. Box 1343
Fayetteville, AR 72702

Herb, Spice, and Medicinal Plant Digest
University of Mass Cooperative Extension
Dr. LE Craker
Stockbridge Hall
University of Massachusetts
Amherst, MA 01003

Phytomedicine: International Journal of Phytotherapy and
    Phytopharmacology
VCH Publishers
NW 12th Avenue
Deerfield Beach, FL 33442-1788

International Journal of Pharmacognosy
University of Illinois at Chicago
M/C 781
833 S. Wood St.
Chicago, IL 60612-7231

Natural Products Letters
Dr. Ernest Wenkert
Dept. of Chemistry
University of California at San Diego
La Jolla, CA 92093

Phytotherapy Research
Heydon and Son Ltd.
Spectrum House
Hillview Gardens,
London, England NW 12 JQ
or
Dr. Fred J. Evans
The School of Pharmacy
University of London
29/39 Brunswick Square
London, WC1N 1AX
UK

Journal of Ethnopharmacology
Elsevier Science, Inc.
P.O. Box 882
Madison Square Station
New York, NY 10159
212-989-5800

Ethnopharmacologia
Bulletin of the Societé Française
d'Ethnopharmacologie
1, Rue des Recollets
57000 Metz
France 87-75-81-83
Fax: 87-36-41-98
E-mail: iee@pub.mairie-metz.fr

Health: State of the Art
Health Research
6 Alfred Road
Windmill Hill
Bristol
England BS3 4LE
0272-635109
Fax: 0272-538069

Quarterly Review of Natural Medicine
NPRC
600 First Avenue
Suite 205
Seattle, WA 98104
206-623-2520

Journal of Naturopathic Medicine
Journal Management Group
10 Morgan Ave.
Norwalk, CT 06851
203-866-7664
or
54 Lafayette Pl.
Greenwich CT 06830

Newsletter for the International Association for Veterinary Homeopathy
Dr. Andreas Schmidt
Sonnhaldenstr. 18
CH-8370 Sirnach
Switzerland
41 (73) 26 14 24
Fax: 41 (73) 26 58 14

Simillimun
11231 S.E. Market St.
Portland, OR 97216
503-829-7326

Resonance
2366 Eastlake Ave. East, Suite 325
Seattle, WA 98102
206-324-8230

Homeopathy Today
801 N. Fairfax #306
Alexandria, VA 22314
E-mail: nch@igc.apc.org

Homeopathic Research Reports
5916 Chabot Crest
Oakland, CA 94618

British Homoeopathic Journal
2 Powis Place
Great Ormond St.
London WC1N 3HT
England

New England Journal of Homeopathy
356 Middle Street
Amherst, MA 01002

European Journal of Classical Homeopathy
Athenian Centre of Homeopathic Medicine
Pericleous 1, Maroussi
Athens 15122
Greece
0030-1-80 52 6715

Homeopathic Links
Jean Pierre Jansen, Editor
De Ree 11
9753 BX Haren
The Netherlands
31-50-5347107, 10-12 CET
Fax: 31-50-5341252
E-mail: homeolinks@antenna.nl

Homeopath: The Journal of the Society of Homeopaths
Robin Logan, Editor
The Society of Homeopaths
2 Artizan Road
Northampton nni 4HU
United Kingdom
44-604-21400
Fax: 44-604-22622
E-mail: robinlogan@gn.apc.org

Journal of the American Institute of Homeopathy
George Guess, MD, Editor
1585 Glencoe
Denver, CO 80220
E-mail: gguess@igc.apc.org

The Prover: The Journal of the Chiropractic Academy of Homeopathy
6536 Stadium Drive
Zephyrhills, FL 33540
813-782-2690

The Journal of Chinese Medicine
Eastland Press
1260 Activity Dr., #A
Vista, CA 92083
800-453-3278

Oriental Medicine Journal
3723 N. Southport
Chicago, IL 60613
312-477-1000
E-mail: silkroad@ix.netcom.com

Journal of Chinese Medicine
22 Cromwell Road
Hove, Sussex BN3 3EB
England

Advances: The Journal of Mind-Body Health
John E. Fetzer Institute, Inc.
9292 West KL Ave.
Kalamazoo, MI 49009-9398
616-375-2000

Holistic Medicine: Magazine of the American Holistic Medical Association
4101 Lake Boone Trail, Ste. 201
Raleigh, NC 27607
919-787-5146

Frontier Perspectives
The Center for Frontier Sciences
Temple University, Ritter Hall 003-00
Philadelphia, PA 19122
215-204-8487
Fax: 215-204-5553
E-mail: <V2058A@vm.temple.edu>

Health Inform: Essential Information on Alternative Health Care
InfoLink
P.O. Box 306
31 Albany Post Road
Montrose, New York, 10548
914-736-1565
Fax: 914-736-3806

Massage Therapy Journal
American Massage Therapy Association
820 Davis St., Ste. 100
Evanston, IL 60201

Mind-Body Connection
Center for Mind-Body Medicine
5225 Connecticut Ave. NW, Ste. 414
Washington, DC 20015

FACT: Focus on Alternative and Complementary Therapies
Verlag PERFUSION Gmbh
Regensburger Str 44-46
90478 Nuremberg
Germany

Nutrition and Healing
c/o Publishers Mgt. Corp.
P.O. Box 84909
Phoenix, AZ 85071
800-528-0559
Fax: 602-943-2363

Alternatives
Mountain Home Publishing
P.O. Box 829
Ingram, TX 78025
210-367-4492

The Townsend Letter for Doctors
911 Tyler St.
Port Washington, WA 98368
206-385-6021

Complementary Therapies in Medicine
Churchill Livingstone
650 Avenue of the Americas
New York, NY 10011

Veterinary Complementary and Alternative Medicine (CAM) Organizations

American Holistic Veterinary Medical Association
2214 Old Emmorton Road
Bel Air, MD 21014
410-569-0795
Fax: (410) 569-2346
E-mail: 74253.2560@compuserve.com

International Veterinary Acupuncture Society
P.O. Box 1478
Longmont, CO 80502-1478
303-682-1167
Fax: 303-682-1168

Academy for Veterinary Homeopathy
1283 Lincoln Street
Eugene, OR 97401
503-342-7665

American Veterinary Chiropractic Association
623 Main
Hillsdale, IL 61257
309-658-2920
Fax: 309-658-2622

Florida Holistic Veterinary Medical Association
751 Northeast 168th Street
North Miami Beach, FL 33162-2427
305-652-5372
Fax: 305-653-7244

Georgia Holistic Veterinary Medical Association
334 Knollwood Lane
Woodstock, GA 30188
770-516-5954

Greater Washington Area Holistic Veterinary Association
6136 Brandon Avenue
Springfield, VA 22150
703-569-0300
Fax: 703-866-4962

International Association for Veterinary Homeopathy
Dr. Andreas Schmidt, General Secretary
Sonnhaldenstr. 18
CH-8370 Sirnach
Switzerland
41 (73) 26 14 24
Fax: 41(73) 26 58 14
or
Susan G. Wynn, DVM, U.S. National Secretary
334 Knollwood Lane
Woodstock, GA 30188
770-516-5954
E-mail: swynn@emory.edu

Rocky Mountain Holistic Veterinary Medical Association
311 S. Pennsylvania St.
Denver, CO 80209
303-733-2728
Fax: 303-733-2858

Veterinary Institute for Therapeutic Alternatives
(V.I.T.A)
15 Sunset Terrace
Sherman, CT 06784

Complementary Medicine Databases

AMED (Allied and Alternative Medicine)
Through the Health Care Information Service of the
    British Library
Boston Spa, Wetherby, West Yorkshire,
LS23 7BQ, U.K.
44-01937 546039
Fax: 44-01937458

CISCOM
Administered by the Research Council for Complemen-
    tary Medicine
60 Great Ormond Street, London, WC1N
3JF, U.K.
44-(0)171-833-8897
Fax: 44(0)171-278-7412
E-mail: <rccm@gn.apc.org>

Database of Biologically Active Phytochemicals and
    Their Activities
James A. Duke
Ethnobotanical Database
http://www.ars-grin.gov/~ngrlsb/

Hominform (Glasgow Homeopathic Hospital Library)
Mrs. Mary Gooch, Librarian
Faculty of Homoeopathy
Glasgow Homoeopathic Hospital
1000 Great Western Road, Glasgow G12 #0NR
2786/339 0382
E-mail: <ghl@gn.apc.org>

INRAT (International Network for Researach on Alter-
    native Therapies)
Helle Johannessen.
Institute of Anthropology
Frederiksholms Kanal 4
DK-1220 Copenhagen, Denmark
45 35 32 34 80
Fax: 45 35 32 34 65
http://inet.uni-c.dk/~inrathj
E-mail: inrat.network@anthro.ku.dk

Natural Therapies Database
37 Ashby Avenue, Chessington, Surrey KT9
2BT, UK
Fax: 44-(0)181-391-0150

World Research Foundation
15300 Ventura Blvd. Suite 405
Sherman Oaks, CA 91403

*D*iagnostic Software

Homeopathic Medicine

CARA
Chiron
P.O. Box 424
Port Townsend, WA 98368
360-385-1917
Fax: 360-385-1926
E-mail: chiron@olympus.net

Homeo21
Age of Reason
415-826-5078

Homeopathy @ Work
Biodesic
10444 Wiseacre Ln., NE
Aurora, OR 97002
800-678-5185

HomPath WIN
Dr. Jawahar Shah
10 Harish Kunj
46 Tagore Rd.
Santacruz (w), Bombay -400 054, India

MacRepertory
ReferenceWorks
Zizia
Kent Homeopathic Associates
P.O. Box 39, Fairfax, CA 94978
415-457-0688

Radar
Homeovia
P.O. Box 56603
8601 Warden Ave.
Markham, Ontario, L3R-ON6, Canada
905-513-0619 or 1-800-668-7543
Fax: 905-513-0626
E-mail: homeovia@homeovia.com

Similia
Chiron
P.O. Box 424
Port Townsend, WA 98368
360-385-1917
Fax: 360-385-1926
E-mail: chiron@olympus.net

Eclectic (Complementary Medicine)

IBIS (Interactive BodyMind Information System)
AMR'TA
GAIA Multimedia, Inc.
P.O. Box 14641
Portland, OR 97214
503-291-6155
E-mail: ibis@teleport.com
http://ftp.teleport.com/vendors/ibis

Herbal Medicine

The Formulary for Chinese Medicine
Chiron
P.O. Box 424
Port Townsend, WA 98368
360-385-1917
Fax: 360-385-1926
E-mail: chiron@olympus.net

Genusys: The Electronic Pharmacopeia
(for Mac or Windows)
Datalogics
215-794-7486

GlobalHerb
Steve Blake, ND
5831 S. HiWay 9, Box 9 EW
Felton, CA 95018
408-335-9011

The Interactive Herbal
(CD-ROM)
Terry Willard, PhD
Mosby
11830 Westline Industrial Dr.
St. Louis, MO 63146
800-325-4177
http://www.mosby.com

The Herbalist
(CD-ROM)
David Hoffmann
Hopkins Technology, LLC
421 Hazel Lane
Hopkins, MN 55343-7116
612-931-9376
Fax: 612-931-9377

The Herbal Prescriber
Botanica Press
10226 Empire Grade
Santa Cruz, CA 95060
408-457-9095

Index